Paramedic Field Care:

A Complaint-Based Approach

THE AMERICAN COLLEGE OF EMERGENCY PHYSICIANS

The American College of Emergency Physicians (ACEP) is the oldest and largest national medical specialty organization representing physicians who practice emergency medicine. With more than 19,000 members, the College is the leading source of continuing education for emergency physicians and the primary information resource for developments in the specialty.

ACEP exists to support quality emergency medical care and believes that emergency medical services (EMS) and prehospital medical care are integral components of emergency medical care. Through its development and promulgation of policies to improve the quality of prehospital patient care, by promoting effective EMS organizational development, and by maintaining active outreach/liaison programs with various organizations and federal agencies, the College strives to provide meaningful support and leadership to the EMS industry.

A highly visible manifestation of the College's committment to EMS is its annual sponsorship of EMS Week—a national campaign to educate the public about the EMS system and injury prevention, how to recognize and respond to a medical emergency, and to show appreciation for the contributions of every member of the EMS team.

About the Chief Editors

Peter T. Pons, MD, FACEP is an emergency physician at Denver Health Medical Center in Denver, Colorado. He has been active in EMS throughout his entire career and served as the Medical Director for the Denver Paramedic Division for over eight years. Before that, he was the physician director for the Glendale, Colorado, Fire-Rescue system and the Jacksonville, Florida, Fire-Rescue system. In addition, he has been a member of and chaired ACEP's EMS Committee.

Debra Cason, RN, MS, EMT-P began her professional career as an emergency department nurse at Parkland Memorial Hospital in Dallas, Texas, eventually serving as Head Nurse, after which she entered EMS, in which she has been involved for more than 19 years. She currently serves as the program director, Division of Emergency Medicine Education, and associate professor, Health Care Sciences Department, at the University of Texas Southwestern Medical Center, Dallas, Texas.

ACEP Paramedic Field Care Editorial Board

Phil Fontanarosa, MD, FACEP
Carol Goodykoontz, RN, MS, EMT-P
S. Scott Polsky, MD, FACEP
Jedd Roe, MD, FACEP
William R. Roush, MD
Michael P. Wainscott, MD, FACEP

Paramedic Field Care:

A Complaint-Based Approach

American College of
Emergency Physicians

Chief Editors:

Peter T. Pons, MD, FACEP

Debra Cason, RN, MS, EMT-P

Editor-in-Chief: Claire Merrick
Director EMS/Fire/Rescue Publishing: William Metcalf
Managing Editor: Nancy Peterson
Senior Assistant Editor: Carla Goldberg
Production Editor: Mark Flanagan
Design: OX and Company, Incorporated
Production Director: Douglas Bruce

Printed in the United States of America

Composition by GTS Graphics

Printing/binding by Von Hoffmann Press, Inc.

Mosby-Year Book, Inc.
11830 Westline Industrial Drive
St. Louis, Missouri 63146

Library of Congress Cataloging-in-Publication Data

Paramedic field care : a complaint-based approach / chief editors.
    Peter T. Pons, Debra Cason.
        p.   cm.
    Includes index.
    "American College of Emergency Physicians."
    ISBN 0-8016-6361-X (hardcover)
    1. Medical emergencies.   2. Emergency medical personnel.
I. Pons, Peter T: II. Cason, Debra.   III. American College of
Emergency Physicians.
    (DNLM: 1. Emergencies.   2. First Aid.   3. Emergency Medical
Services.   4. Emergency Medical Technicians.   WA 292 P2218 1997)
RC86.7.P363   1997
818.02'5—dc21
DNLM/DLC
for Library of Congress
                                                                97-21620
                                                                CIP

This book is dedicated to all who labor long and hard to bring knowledge to students and emergency medical care to patients, but above all, to DC and SM whose vision, perseverance, and humor brought this project to completion.

PP

To my husband and best friend, Kenny, who is my lifeline of love, encouragement, and renewal. To my son, Christopher, who inspires me by his enthusiasm for life and his excitement for learning. To my daughter, Kate, who makes me laugh and reminds me why I love being a mother. To my father and the memory of my mother, who lived and taught the values of God, family, and perseverance. I love you all.

DC

NOTE TO THE READER

The author and publisher have made every attempt to ensure that the drug dosages and patient care procedures presented in this text are accurate and represent accepted practices in the United States. They are not provided as a standard of care. Paramedics perform advanced life support procedures under the authority of a licensed physician. It is the reader's responsibility to follow patient care protocols established by a medical direction physician and to remain current in the delivery of emergency care, including the most recent guidelines set forth by the American Heart Association and printed in their textbooks.

The scene photographs in this text were taken during past emergency responses. Therefore they may depict some patient care activities that do not accurately represent the current practice in prehospital emergency care.

The American College of Emergency Physicians makes every effort to ensure that contributors to College-sponsored publications are knowledgeable authorities in their fields. Readers are nevertheless advised that the statements and opinions expressed in this publication are provided as guidelines and should not be construed as College policy unless specifically referred to as such. The College disclaims any liability or responsibility for the consequences of any actions taken in reliance to those statements or opinions.

Contributors

The Author and Publisher gratefully acknowledge the following individuals for their written contributions to this text:

Barbara Aehlert, RN
Phoenix, Arizona

James M. Atkins, MD
Professor of Internal Medicine
Internal Medicine, Division of Cardiology
University of Texas Southwestern Medical School
Dallas, Texas
and
Professor and Director of Emergency Medicine Education
Health Care Sciences, Division of Emergency Medicine
    Education
University of Texas Southwestern Allied Health School
Dallas, Texas

William K. Atkinson, MPH, MPA, EMT-P
President and Chief Executive Officer
Aurora Regional Medical Center
Columbia/HCA
Aurora, Colorado

David Barillo, MD
Clinical Assistant Professor of Surgery;
University of Texas Health Sciences Center at San Antonio
San Antonio, Texas

John George Barron, BA, NREMT-P
Paramedic Instructor and Guest Lecturer
Sherrill, New York

Nicholas H. Benson, MD, FACEP
Professor & Chair
Department of Emergency Medicine
East Carolina University School of Medicine
Greenville, North Carolina

Thomas H. Blackwell, MD, FACEP
Medical Director
The Center for Prehospital Medicine
Carolinas Medical Center
Charlotte, North Carolina
and
Medical Director
Mecklenburg County EMS

Michelle Blanda, MD, FACEP
Attending Physician
Department of Emergency Medicine
SUMMA Health System (Akron City Hospital)
Akron, Ohio
and
Assistant Professor of Emergency Medicine
Department of Emergency Medicine
Northeastern Ohio Universities College of Medicine
Akron, Ohio

Marilyn Bourn, RN, MSN, CEN, NREMT-P
Senior Instructor, Department of Surgery
EMS Educator, Division of Emergency Medicine
Rocky Mountain Regional Burn Education Coordinator,
    Department of Rehabilitation Medicine
University of Colorado Health Sciences Center
Denver, Colorado

Rocky Mountain Regional Burn
Education Coordinator
Department of Rehabilitation Medicine
University of Colorado Health Sciences Center
Denver, Colorado

Barbara N. Camp, MD
Resident Physician
Department of Emergency Medicine
Albany Medical Center
Albany, NY

Robert J. Carter, NREMT-P
Clinical Associate, Pediatric Intensive Care Unit
John Hopkins Children's Center
Paramedic, Baltimore City Fire Department
Baltimore, Maryland

Norman C. Christopher, MD
Director, Division of Emergency/Trauma Services
Department of Pediatrics
Children's Hospital Medical Center of Akron
Akron, Ohio

Paul J. Clancy, MD
Attending Physician
Department of Emergency Medicine
Charleston Area Medical Center
Charleston, West Virginia
and
Clinical Instructor for the Department of Emergency Medicine
West Virginia University School of Medicine
Charleston, West Virginia

Keith Conover, MD, FACEP
Department of Emergency Medicine, Mercy Hospital
Pittsburgh, Pennsylvania
and
Clinical Assistant Professor
Department of Emergency Medicine
University of Pittsburgh
and
Medical Director, Wilderness EMS Institute

Ellen C. Corey, MD

Elizabeth Criss, RN, MEd
Base Hospital Coordinator, Emergency Services
University Medica Center
Tuscon, Arizona
and
Senior Research Associate, Section of Emergency Medicine
Arizona Health Sciences Center
University of Arizona

Alice (Twink) Dalton, BSN, NRPM
Trauma Nurse Coordinator
Department of Surgery
St. Joseph's Hospital
Creighton University Medical Center
Omaha, Nebraska

Captain Forrest D. Dalton, Sr.
Captain – Duty Shift Infectious Disease Control Officer
Omaha Fire Department
Omaha, Nebraska

Kathleen A. Delaney, MD, FACEP
Associate Professor and Assistant Medical Director,
    Parkland Hospital
Department of Surgery, Division of Emergency Medicine
University of Texas Southwestern Medical School
Dallas, Texas

Kate Dernocoeur, BS, EMT-P
Partner
Team Dernocoeur
Grand Rapids, Michigan

Edward T. Dickinson, III, MD, NREMT-P
Director of EMS
Colonie, NY

Jennifer L. Erich, MD
Department of Emergency Medicine
Medical Center of Delaware
Wilmington, DE

Donna Fehrenbach, DO
Resident Physician
Albany Medical Center
Albany, New York

Phil Fontanarosa, MD, FACEP
Associate Professor of Medicine
Division of Emergency Medicine
Northwestern University Medical School
Chicago, Illinois

Marion Angell Garza, BA
Editorial/News Coordinator
Editorial, Jems Communications
Carlsbad, California

Carol Goodykoontz, RN, MS, EMT-P
Associate Professor
Assistant Program Director
Emergency Medicine Education
University of Texas Southwestern Medical Center
Dallas, Texas

Mark Hauswald, MD, FACEP
Associate Professor
Aeromedical Director
Department of Emergency Medicine
The University of New Mexico, School of Medicine
Albuquerque, New Mexico

James E. Hayes, MD, FACEP
Chairman, Division of Emergency Medicine
Associate Professor, Surgery
University of Texas Southwestern Medical Center at Dallas
Dallas, Texas

Richard C. Hunt, MD, FACEP
Associate Professor and Vice Chair
Department of Emergency Medicine
East Carolina University School of Medicine
Greenville, North Carolina

John C. Johnson, MD, FACEP
Clinical Associate Professor
Division of Emergency Medicine
University of Chicago Hospitals and Clinics
Chicago, Illinois
and
Clinical Assistant Professor of Medicine
Department of Medicine
Associate Professor, School of Public and
    Environmental Affairs
Indiana University
Bloomington, Indiana

Robert C. Jorden, MD, FACEP
Chairman, Emergency Department
Maricopa Medical Center
Phoenix, AZ

Eugene E. Kercher, MD, FACEP
Assistant Clinical Professor, Department of Emergency
    Medicine
University of California, Los Angeles
and
Chairman, Department of Emergency Medicine
Kern Medical Center
Bakersfield, California

Mark A. Kirk, MD
Director, Medical Toxicology Fellowship
Indiana Poison Center
Methodist Hospital of Indiana
Indianapolis, Indiana

Debra Lejeune, BS, NREMT-P
Publishing Coordinator
Center for Emergency Medicine
Pittsburgh, Pennsylvania

Ralph B. "Monty" Leonard, MD, PhD, FACEP
Associate Professor
Department of Emergency Medicine
Bowman Gray School of Medicine
Winston-Salem, North Carolina

Dwight Lodge, MS, EMT-P
Richmond, Virginia

Michael Mackan, MD, FACEP
Associate Professor of Clinical Emergency Medicine,
    Northeastern Ohio Univertsity College of Medicine
Emergency Medicine Core Faculty
SUMMA Health Systems
Akron, Ohio

Peter A. Maningas, MD, FACEP
Medical Director
Emergency Medical Services
Oklahoma City and Tulsa, Oklahoma

Gregg Margolis, MS, NREMT-P
Associate Director of Education
Center for Emergency Medicine
Pittsburgh, Pennsylvania
and
Clinical Instructor, Emergency Medicine
University of Pittsburgh School of Medicine
Pittsburgh, Pennsylvania

Vince Markovchick, MD, FACEP
Director, Emergency Medical Services
Denver Health Medical Center
Professor of Surgery, Division of Emergency Medicine
University of Colorado Health Science Center
Denver, Colorado

Craig Marsden, MD, MA, FACEP
EMS Director, Emergency Preparedness Committee Chair
Department of Emergency Medicine
Maricopa Medical Center
Phoenix, Arizona

Loren Marshall, MA, EMT-P
Treeline Writers Group
Anchorage, Alaska

Greg D. Mears, MD, FACEP
Assistant Professor
Head, Division of EMS
Department of Emergency Medicine
University of North Carolina–Chapel Hill
Chapel Hill, North Carolina

Larry Mellick, MD, FAAP, FACEP
Chair and Professor
Department of Emergency Medicine
Director of Pediatric Emergency Medicine
Medical College of Georgia
Augusta, Georgia

Francis R. Mencl, MD, FACEP
Associate Director of EMS Activities
Department of Emergency Medicine
SUMMA Health System (Akron City Hospital)
Akron, Ohio

Jeffrey T. Mitchell, PhD
Clinical Associate Professor
Emergency Health Services
University of Maryland
Baltimore County
Baltimore, Maryland
and
President,
International Critical Incident Stress Foundation
Ellicott City, Maryland

Richard N. Nelson, MD, FACEP
Associate Professor and Medical Director
Department of Emergency Medicine
The Ohio State University College of Medicine
Columbus, Ohio

Lawrence D. Newell, Ed.D., NREMT-P
President, Newell Associates, Inc.
Educational Consultants
Ashburn, Virginia
and
Faculty, Paramedic Education
Department of Health Technologies
Northern Virginia Community College
Annandale, Virginia

David J. Orban, MD, FACEP
Associate Professor and Chief
Division of Emergency Medicine
Department of Surgery
University of Florida College of Medicine
Gainesville, Florida
and
Director of Emergency Services
Shands Hospital and Shands Care Flight Program
Gainesville, Florida

Robert E. O'Connor, MD, FACEP
Medical Director
Office of Paramedic Administration
Dover, DE
and
Clinical Associate Professor
Department of Emergency Medicine
Medical Center of Delaware
Wilmington, DE

James L. Paturas, EMT-P
Director
Bridgeport Hospital
Bridgeport, CT
and
Executive Director
Prehospital Trauma Life Support
National Association of Emergency Medical Technicians
Bridgeport, CT

Chris Perrin, BA, EMT-P
Program Director, School of EMS
Mercy College of Health Sciences
Des Moines, Iowa

Thomas Platt, BA, NREMT-P
Assistant Director of Education
Center for Emergency Medicine
Pittsburgh, Pennsylvania
and
Lecturer, Emergency Medicine
University of Pittsburgh, School of Medicine
Pittsburgh, Pennsylvania

S. Scott Polsky, MD, FACEP
Regional Director, E.C.I.
Traverse City, Michigan
and
Consulting Educational Faculty
Emergency Medicine
SUMMA Health Systems (Akron City Hospital)
Akron, Ohio

Sandra M. Race, RN, BSN, CEN
EMS/Trauma Coordinator
SUMMA Health System (Akron City Hospital)
Akron, Ohio

William Raynovich, MPH, BS, NREMT-P
Senior Program Director
EMS Academy
University of New Mexico
Albuquerque, New Mexico

Janet Reich, RN, MSHSA
President
Reich Consulting
Flagstaff, Arizona

Jedd Roe, MD, FACEP
Attending Faculty, Emergency Medical Services
Denver Health Medical Center
Denver, Colorado
and
Assistant Professor, Division of Emergency Medicine,
    Department of Surgery
University of Colorado School of Medicine
Denver, Colorado

S. Rutherfoord Rose, PharmD
Director, Carolinas Poison Center
Carolinas Medical Center
Charlotte, North Carolina

William R. Roush, MD
Currently Medically Retired

Previous Positions:
Director EMS/Consulting Teaching Staff
Department of Emergency Medicine
Akron City Hospital
Akron, Ohio
and
Program Director/Medical Director Paramedic Training
Institute of Summit and Portage Counties, Ohio

Carol J. Shanaberger, JD, EMT-P
(deceased)

Robert Sherard, BA, EMT-P
Director of Emergency Medical Services Training
Collin County Community College
McKinney, Texas

Mahesh Shrestha, MD, FACEP
Adjunct Professor of Surgery and Medicine
Division of Emergency Medicine
University of Texas Southwestern Medical Center
Dallas, Texas

Currently practicing at:
Crozer-Chester Medical Center
Upland, Pennsylvania

Daniel R. Smiley, MPA, EMT-P
Chief Deputy Director
Emergency Medical Services Authority
State of California
Sacramento, California

Mike Smith, REMT-P
Vice President, Emergency Medical Training Associates
Olympia, Washington

Andrew W. Stern, NREMT-P, MPA, MA
Senior Paramedic/Flight Paramedic
Town of Colonie Emergency Medical Services
Albany, New York

Charles E. Stewart, MD, FACEP
Associate Professor of Emergency Medicine
University of Rochester Medical Center
Rochester, New York

George M. Stohr, BS
New York College of Osteopathic Medicine
Old Westbury, New York
and
Empress Ambulance Service
Yonkers, New York

Daniel Louis Storer, MD, FACEP
Professor, Clinical Emergency Medicine
Emergency Medicine
University of Cincinnati, College of Medicine
Cincinnati, Ohio
and
Medical Director, Clinical Operations
Center for Emergency Care, University Hospital
Cincinnati, Ohio

Walt Alan Stoy, PhD, EMT-P
Director of Educational Programs
Center for Emergency Medicine
Pittsburgh, PA
and
Research Assistant Professor of Medicine
Department of Emergency Medicine
University of Pittsburgh, School of Medicine
Pittsburgh, Pennsylvania

Robert E. Suter, DO, MHA, FACEP
Chief, Emergency Services
Providence Hospital and Medical Centers
Southfield, Michigan

Medical Director, Southfield Fire Department
Sothfield, Michigan

Medical Director, East Central Georgia (Region VI)
Augusta, Georgia

Robert Swor, DO, FACEP
Director, EMS Programs
Department of Emergency Medicine
William Beaumont Hospital
Royal Oak, Michigan

Mark Terry, BA, NREMT-P

Patricia L. Tritt, RN, MA
System Director EMS & Trauma
Healthone
Englewood, Colorado

Bruce S. Ushkow, MD
Assistant EMS Director
Assistant Residency Director
Department of Emergency Medicine
Albany Medical Center
Albany, NY

Vincent P. Verdile, MD, FACEP
Associate Professor and Vice Chairman
Department of Emergency Medicine
Albany Medical College
Medical Director
City of Albany Fire and Emergency Services
Albany, NY

Frederick H. Veser, III, MD
Associate Professor of Emergency Medicine
Medical University of South Carolina
Charlston, South Carolina
and
Attending Physician
Charlston Memorial Hospital
Charlston, South Carolina

Michael P. Wainscott, MD, FACEP
Associate Professor and Associate Residency Director
Division of Emergency Medicine
University of Texas Southwestern Medical Center
Dallas, Texas

Daniel J. Weeks, MD
Department of Emergency Medicine
Medical Center of Delaware
Wilmington, DE

Howard A. Werman, MD, FACEP
Associate Professor of Clinical Emergency Medicine
Department of Emergency Medicine
The Ohio State University, College of Medicine
Columbus, Ohio
and
Co-Medical Director
MedFlight
Columbus, Ohio

Lena C. Williams, RN, BS
Director, North Texas Poison Center at Parkland Memorial
    Hospital
Dallas, Texas

Richard Wolfe, MD, FACEP
Attending Physician
Brigham & Womens Hospital and Massachusetts General
    Hospital
Boston, MA
and
Program Director
Harvard Affiliation Emergency Medicine Residency
Boston, MA

N.R. Zenarosa, MD
Division of Emergency Medicine
Parkland Memorial Hospital
University of Texas Southwestern Medical Center
Dallas, TX
and
Department of Emergency Medicine
Carolinas Medical Center
Charlotte, North Carolina

Foreword

Ronald D. Stewart, OC, MD, FACEP, FRCPC, Dsc(hon)

It is a great pleasure to welcome this text to the growing literature of emergency health services. To the experienced eye, this text marks a milestone along the path leading to improvements in delivering emergency care, in teaching caregivers, and in promoting research in the field management of emergencies.

Even a quick perusal of the contributor list provides assurance that this text is the work of respected experts in emergency medical services (EMS). These are not "dreamers" only—they are "doers" and "dreamers." Their great practical experience is reflected not only in the approach taken in the text, but in the content of the chapters. They have nicely balanced theory with practice, and knowledge with street sense. They consistently work *forward* in the solution to a clinical problem, not backward from diagnostic labeling. In this alone, this text could be considered landmark.

Woven through the text is a repeated emphasis on assessment and evaluation. Assessment of the scene, the situation confronting the team, the immediate needs of patients, and the presenting complaints all form the base of the text's approach. The foundation laid out early in the work is fundamental to safe and effective prehospital care—knowledge of the human condition and the disease processes that often afflict us. In every way, this text works by lifting and supporting the reader from this foundation, rather than oppressively dictating dogma from above. The basic sciences are not neglected, but presented in a way relevant to the practice of the street paramedic. This text is in every way patient-focused. The special needs of many people cared for in EMS are dealt with in a spirit of understanding and realistic expectation.

Supported by colorful photographs and technically accurate illustrations, this text is a treasure of practical good sense coupled with a realistic view of the work of field teams. Combine this refreshing approach with the solid advice and sound teaching in every section, and there is good reason to cheer its introduction to this important and growing discipline.

Foreword

Alice "Twink" Dalton, BSN, NRPM
Mike Smith, REMT-P

For years after the publication of the 15 module DOT National Standard Paramedic curriculum, a single textbook dominated the market, and was the primary educational resource for paramedic instructors across the country. Following the 1985 revision of the curriculum, four publishers threw their hats in the ring with textbooks focused on presenting information to the paramedic student in a form that was useable and relevant to the reader, the field paramedic. Most were written by paramedics, (or former paramedics), usually in cooperation with a physician or two. To a certain degree, instructors gravitated toward the text that seemed to be best suited for their needs. However, there remained a group of students and educators that needed something more, something that was missing from the previous textbooks.

With the introduction of this text, the American College of Emergency Physicians (ACEP) has moved in to fill the gap, the "something" that was missing. The educational resources assembled to produce this text were extensive. Over 75 contributors, represented by paramedics, educators, emergency physicians, and program directors from across the country, shared their knowledge and expertise. The galvanizing of such a huge pool of talent provided the opportunity for this text to move in a direction of *contextual learning* that is quite unique: teaching patient care and treatment by use of chief complaint, just as patients actually present. Additional areas such as fever, syncope, headache, and back pain are new sections to any paramedic text, but are common complaints encountered in the field. Other chapters on geriatric care, rural EMS, interpersonal communication skills and issues of personal violence offer unique perspectives on previously unavailable or glossed over topics, and provide essential material for the paramedic.

A previously untouchable area, *diagnosis,* is pointedly included. The fact that paramedics must make a determination of what is actually wrong, a working diagnosis, if you will, is not ignored, but is openly addressed by its own section, "Conditions by Diagnosis." This approach is a milestone in paramedic education. Paramedics do in fact diagnose, certainly not to the same extent as a physician, but to the extent necessary to their profession, paramedicine.

It is hoped that using this approach will encourage linkage of information from book learning to actual field practice. Of course no text can ever replace street smart, field wise instructors, or bookwise in-field preceptors as they work in harmony to help students make the transition from theory to actual practice. However, this text may very well pave the way and ease the book-to-street transition that makes the goal of field competent paramedics a more accessible and achievable reality.

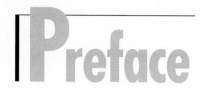
Preface

by Peter Pons, MD, FACEP, and Debra Cason, RN, MS, EMT-P

Reality. The word conjures up many different images and thoughts to many different people. Let's concentrate on educational reality. If you think back over your educational history, how much of what you were taught bore any semblance to reality? We suspect that you'll probably say "not much." Even as you reflect upon your early educational experiences in EMS, how much reality was there? Did your preparation to become an EMT-Basic provide a sense of the reality of the prehospital medical practice that you would participate in?

Traditional EMS education requires the student to learn disease-specific content, pathophysiology, signs and symptoms and then management. The student thus works "backward" to learn how the signs and symptoms fit the patient presentation. The Editorial Board of *Paramedic Field Care: A Complaint-based Approach* feels that reality is more appropriate to teach, and that is exactly what we have attempted to provide in this text. We feel that a more logical and thus learnable approach is to start with how the patient presents to the paramedic—through the patient's chief complaint. If the patient is unable to describe a chief complaint, the patient is assessed by a certain set of steps that either rules out or manages critical life threats.

Having said this, let's again talk about reality. Evaluating the chief complaint, performing an assessment based on that complaint, and treating that complaint only takes you so far. Traditional teaching in EMS is that EMTs, in general, and paramedics, in particular, don't diagnose patients. How about reality? Paramedics do need to make more definitive assessments or even diagnose in order to treat with advanced life support therapies. A good understanding of the pathophysiology of disease, the signs and symptoms that manifest from that disease or condition, as well as drug actions and interactions are all part of what paramedics need to know in order to make educated decisions about using their arsenal of patient care modalities. This text was written with those things in mind.

The patient's presenting signs and symptoms, as well as other findings at the scene, must be thoroughly assessed and evaluated in order to determine appropriate management. The Patient Presentation section of this text (broken down into medical and traumatic presentations) focuses the reader on these chief complaints and their appropriate assessment and management.

"Key Conditions and Findings" sections in most of these chapters outline the most likely and most concerning conditions and findings that may be present given the patient's chief complaint.

Since different conditions can present in a variety of ways, the indepth information about each condition is not repeated in each chapter in which it is mentioned. Rather, the reader is referred to the Conditions by Diagnosis section of the book for this additional information. As such, the CBD section (presented by body systems) can be a valuable reference for students and professional providers.

For example, a patient who is having a stroke can present with an altered mental status, dizziness, or a headache (these are all Patient Presentation chapters). In order to reduce repetition in the text and to prevent disruption of the chapter flow, the assessment and management of the patient complaint continues in each chapter. The reader may at another time refer to the CBD section for reference or review on the topic of stroke.

Reality. The reality of paramedic care is that in addition to providing emergency medical and trauma care, there are many special situations that you will confront. Some of these include issues of personal violence; patients with disabilities and those with specialized treatment adjuncts; multiple casualty incidents; and rescuers experiencing critical incident stress. The reality of paramedic care is that much of what you do will be routine — or at least routine for you. But there will also be the satisfaction of knowing that you comforted a frightened elderly woman with a broken hip who speaks no English, or eased the wrist pain of a 7 year-old roller blader. And then there are the incredible but infrequent moments of actually saving a life, as well as the emotional impact of realizing that some of your patients will die in spite of your best efforts. The reality of paramedic care is that in order to effectively take care of your patients, you must take care of yourself. We have attempted to provide you, the paramedic student, with information on these various topics to give you a sense of the realities that you will deal with in your profession.

Unfortunately, many students pursue paramedic education with expectations of their future as a paramedic that are not based in reality. If we, by virtue of this text, can help even one paramedic better handle just one situation because he or she was prepared for the reality, we will have accomplished our task.

EDITOR ACKNOWLEDGMENTS

We would like to express our gratitude to many individuals for their contributions to this team approach textbook.

First and foremost is ACEP's managing editor, Susan Magee. Susan was our coach and cheerleader. Her wit and wisdom helped to keep the project moving, despite constant setbacks. Susan's educational expertise provided insight and clarity during the process.

Nancy Peterson, Mosby Lifeline's developmental editor, was the team's coach and manager. She had the ability to gently crack the whip, problem solve, and assist when securing additional resources was necessary.

Claire Merrick, Mosby Lifeline's editor-in-chief, was our owner and "ruled" with a calm, helpful approach. We appreciate her insight and support.

Denise Fechner, Carla Goldberg, Cynthia Ramirez, and Karen Murdock were important players who kept track of volumes of chapter drafts, word processed and re-word processed manuscripts, letters, tracked team players and other details too numerous to list.

Patti Hicks Ryder, our team artwork coordinator, and the talented illustrators and photographer who made changes and more changes in order to provide the quality artwork in this textbook.

Loren Marshall, our "lines" man, for his excellent editing of the entire textbook.

The many authors and section editors who were all brave team players and willing to try a new approach to paramedic education. Their patience throughout this process was remarkable.

The reviewers who offered many helpful suggestions, including Larry Newell; Rob Carter who was our able and willing Pediatric Perspective team member; and Jedd Roe who deserves a special thank you as designated hitter with his editing of the Patient Presentation section.

We gratefully acknowledge the pinch hitting of Dr. E. Jackson Allison, Jr., Dwight Polk, Mary Gardner, Dr. Richard C. Hunt, and Dr. N. Heramba Prasad for allowing us to use many of the skill procedures from their excellent skills text, *Advanced Life Support Skills*. We couldn't have done it better ourselves!

The American College of Emergency Physicians who made this project possible. ACEP's support and vision are appreciated.

Parkland Memorial Hospital BioTel nurses and paramedics, and EMS instructors from the University of Texas Southwestern Medical Center who willingly helped us secure ECG strips and other helpful educational information .

And, last but certainly not least, we gratefully acknowledge our families and colleagues, for they contributed the largest part by their encouragement, patience, and acceptance of our absence during the development of this innovative publication.

PUBLISHER ACKNOWLEDGMENTS

The development of a textbook of this magnitude with such a unique presentation took the creativity, scrutiny, diligence and hard work of many special people. We extend our thanks and deep appreciation to the following individuals who gave so much of themselves to make a difference in paramedic education:

- To the American College of Emergency Physicians (ACEP) for making this tremendous joint publishing venture possible and giving us the opportunity to work with Chief Editors Debra Cason, RN, MS, EMT-P and Peter Pons, MD, FACEP. We are fortunate to have worked with such talented editors so driven to excellence. Their expertise, superb judgment, and patience with a sometimes arduous process made this textbook possible.
- To Susan Magee, ACEP's Manager of EMS Education, whose focus, drive and talents as a developmental editor were out shined only by the sheer pleasure of working with her.
- And to the ACEP Editorial Board members, for their support and insight from the very beginning of this project to pull together the contributions of so many talented individuals in the emergency medical services field.
- To Loren Marshall, for his superb editorial skills and gentle diplomacy.
- To Patti Hicks Ryder, MS, NREMT-P, Art Coordinator, for her creativity, for sharing her talents as an educator, and for sticking with us for so long. Thanks also to Angel Clark Burba, BS, EMT-P, for her timely help with this art program.
- To our extremely talented medical illustrators, Mark Wieber and Caitlin and Rob Duckwall, and photographer Rick Brady, whose beautiful work added to the attractiveness and functionality of this book.
- Special thanks to Jedd Roe, M.D., Lawrence Newell, Ed.D., and Barbara Aehlert, R.N., for reviewing and revising some key content for us, often in a pinch. We are immensely grateful.
- To Rob Carter, EMT-P, for his invaluable insight as an experienced paramedic and pediatric specialist.
- To Benita Boyer, RN, MS, CIC, for her technical assistance regarding body substance isolation and proper representation of personal protection in our art program.

In addition, the following individuals served as reviewers for part or all of the manuscript process. Their comments, questions, and suggestions were a great help in shaping this textbook and ensuring its accuracy, consistency, practicality and applicability. Their candor, time, and dedication are greatly appreciated.

Barbara Aehlert, RN, BS
Phoenix, Arizona

John G. Barron, BA, NREMT-P
Paramedic Instructor and Guest Lecturer
Sherrill, New York

Phillip L. Currance, EMT-P, RHSP
Prehospital Supervisor/Hazmat Operations Officer
United States Public Health Service
Denver, Colorado
and
Emergency Response Training Coordinator
Department of Environmental Science
Front Range Community College
Westminster, Colorado

Bob Elling, MPA, EMT-P
Synergism Associates, Ltd.
Niskayuna, New York

Jonathan Epstein, MEMS, NREMT-P
Assistant Director, North East Emergency Medical
    Services (MA Region III)
Reading, Massachusetts
Paramedic, Cataldo Ambulance Service, Inc.
Somerville, Massachusetts

Robert A. Felter, MD, FAAP
Chairman, Department of Pediatrics and Adolescent
    Medicine
Tod Childrens Hospital
Youngstown, Ohio
Professor of Pediatrics
Northeast Ohio Universities College of Medicine

Jeffery L. Hayes, BS, NREMT-P
Department Head, Emergency Medical Services
    Technology
Austin Community College
Austin, Texas

Benjamin Honigman, MD
Interim Head, Division of Emergency Medicine
Associate Professor of Surgery
University of Colorado Health Sciences Center
Denver, Colorado

Lawrence D. Newell, Ed.D., NREMT-P
President, Newell Associates, Inc.
Educational Consultants
Ashburn, Virginia
and
Faculty, Paramedic Education
Department of Health Technologies
Northern Virginia Community College
Annandale, Virginia

James E. Pointer, MD
Staff Physician, Emergency Department
North Broward Medical Center
Pompano Beach, Florida
Associate Editor, *Prehospital and Disaster Medicine*

William Raynovich, MPH, BS, NREMT-P
Senior Program Director
University of New Mexico
Albuquerque, New Mexico

David M. Reeves, BS, AAS
Instructor, Emergency Medical Science
Guilford Technical Community College
Jamestown, North Carolina
and
Chairman, Rescue Subcommittee, Certification Board
North Carolina Department of Insurance, Fire and
　　Rescue Division
Raleigh, North Carolina

Patricia H. Ryder, MS, NREMT-P
Continuing Education Coordinator
Department of Emergency Health Services
University of Maryland Baltimore County
Baltimore, Maryland

David S. Smith, Ph.D.
President, Smith Aquatic Safety Service
Charlevoix, Michigan

Katherine H. West, BSN, MSEd, CIC
Infection Control/Emerging Concepts, Inc.
Springfield, Virginia

Douglas M. Wolfberg, BS, J.D.
Attorney at Law, Duane, Morris & Heckscher
Harrisburg, Pennsylvania
Former Prehospital Systems Consultant
Division of Trauma and Emergency Medical Systems
United States Public Health Service
Rockville, Maryland

Barack Wolff, MPH
Chief, EMS Bureau
New Mexico Depatment of Health
Santa Fe, New Mexico

The following individuals representing the emergency
medical services, fire, law enforcement, and specialty
rescue arenas assisted in the photography for this
textbook:

MARYLAND

Anne Arundel County Fire Department
Emergency Medical Services
Michelle DeLalla

Captain Frank Stamm, NREMT-P
Lieutenant Michele DeLalla, RN, NREMT-P
Lieutenant David W. Berry, CET
Carol Rabinowitz, NREMT-P
Battalion Chief Michael F.X. O'Connell
Lieutenant Conrad Listman

Anne Arundel County Hazardous Materials Response
　　Team

Orchard Beach Volunteer Fire Department

Anne Arundel County Police
Corporal Ron Hines

City of Annapolis Emergency Services
Captain Dale A. Crutchley, NREMT-P
Lieutenant David O. Colburn, Jr., NREMT-P

Howard County Fire and Rescue Department
Battalion Chief Don Howell

Montgomery County Fire Department

Baltimore County Fire Department
Captain Dennis Krebs

Kent Island Volunteer Fire Department and Rescue
　　Squad Dive Team

Branchville Volunteer Fire Company

Prince Georges County Fire Department
James R. Miller, EMS Training Coordinator
Captain J.P. Medani, NREMT-P
Mark E. Brady, Public Information Officer

Anne Arundel Medical Center
Annapolis, Maryland

Bowie Health Center
Pat Brady, RN, CEN

Maryland State Police Aviation Division
Sergeant Mark Gabriele, NREMT-P

HazMat Training, Inc.
Columbia, Maryland

University of Maryland Baltimore County
Department of Emergency Health Services
Baltimore, Maryland

VIRGINIA

Sterling Park Volunteer Rescue Squad
Jose V. Salazar, EMT-P
Larry Newell, EdD, NREMT-P

City of Fairfax Fire and Rescue Services

Battalion Chief Don R. Barklage, Jr.

WASHINGTON DC

Providence Hospital
Suzanne Felder, MSN
Kathleen Yano, RN, Certified IV Therapist

Huntemann Ambulance Service, Inc.

United States Park Police Aviation Section

NEVADA

Mercy Medical Services
Barbara Murphy, EMS Nurse Specialist, Director
*　　Clinical Services*
Ralph Gilliam, Jr., NREMT-P

Preface to the Student

When the American College of Emergency Physicians (ACEP) set out to develop a new paramedic textbook, its Editorial Board members decided on a challenging goal — to prepare paramedic students for the realities of the prehospital setting. After much discussion and feedback from experts in education and emergency medical services, the complaint-based approach of this textbook was formulated. We are pleased to present you with this innovative textbook to facilitate your understanding of the subject matter and to serve as a helpful reference during your career as a paramedic.

Sections I and II of the text set the stage for your paramedic education, including information on the paramedic's level of involvement in emergency care systems, as well as build a foundation of knowledge on topics such as "Infection Control" and "Basic Body Systems." This section also includes a comprehensive **Prehospital Medications Appendix** to the "General Pharmacology" chapter, which presents drug profiles of more than 40 commonly administered emergency drugs.

In Section III, you will learn how to ensure your safety at the prehospital scene and to evaluate the mechanism of injury or nature of the patient's illness. By taking clearly outlined steps, you will learn how to assess patients, beginning with the immediate identification and appropriate management of life threats, such as the "Patient Without a Pulse." Assessment of the critical patient is thoroughly explained, followed by the focused examination and continued assessment of stable patients. This section also includes separate chapters on **special patient groups,** such as "Geriatric Assessment" and "Pediatric Assessment."

You are now ready to "learn at the patient's side." In Section IV, the complaint-based approach is laid out by **Patient Presentations,** both medical and trauma (for example, "Syncope" and "Orthopedic Injuries"). How does the patient present when you arrive on the scene? Depending on this presentation, you will learn the most pertinent aspects of the patient's history to elicit, as well as what physical examination findings are most significant. Key conditions and findings related to that presentation are outlined, followed by appropriate management strategies.

Critical Issues boxes within many of these patient presentation chapters highlight critical assessment and management issues posed by potential life threats and how to best manage them during the assessment, management and transport phases of emergency care. In addition, **Pediatric Perspective** boxes integrate pertinent information about that presentation that is unique to the pediatric population.

Section V presents **Specialized Chapters,** such as "Issues of Personal Violence," "Specialized Adjuncts to Therapy," and "Rural EMS." Throughout this textbook, we have taken care to include information based on the most current research, such as 12-lead ECGs and Paramedic Well Being. We have paid careful attention to the illustration of key concepts so you can gain a clearer understanding of them. We have also included **sidebars** on items that may be of special interest to you, such as "The Paramedic's Role in Research" and "Bicycling and In-line Skating Injuries."

The **Conditions by Diagnosis** (CBD) section in Section VI is particularly exciting. This section is similar to an encyclopedia, containing entries for more than 200 specific diagnosed conditions, such as chronic obstructive pulmonary disease. Entries are organized alphabetically by body system. While you are reading the text chapters, you will encounter terms that are printed in the same yellow color as the CBD section. This will alert you to a corresponding entry in the CBD section. At your leisure, rather than disrupting the flow of the chapter and distracting you with lengthy medical explanations, you can look up additional information about these specific conditions. This section will also serve as an excellent reference after you complete your paramedic education.

The **Skills Section** in Section VII provides you with ready access to 37 detailed and fully illustrated, step-by-step skill procedures from "Needle Cricothyrotomy" to "Thoracic Decompression." This is followed by the **Patient Medications Appendix,** where you can quickly locate commonly prescribed medications by generic name, as well as the trade name and the medication categories. The text **Glossary** and **Index** will be of great help as you use this book in the classroom and later as a reference.

Finally, a challenging **Student Workbook** is available that tests your knowledge through case studies and expands on your learning with comprehensive answer rationale.

We are confident that the bold new direction we have taken in this textbook will be an enjoyable learning tool and will prepare you for a successful, rewarding career as a paramedic.

Contents

SECTION 3

Scene and Patient Assessment

SECTION 3A

Scene Assessment

SECTION 4B

Patient Presentations—Trauma

SECTION 5

Special Situations

Section

The Paramedic and EMS

1

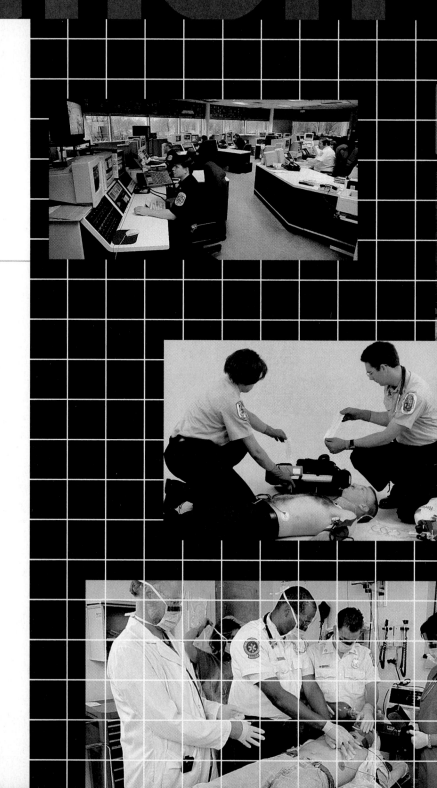

Included In This Section:

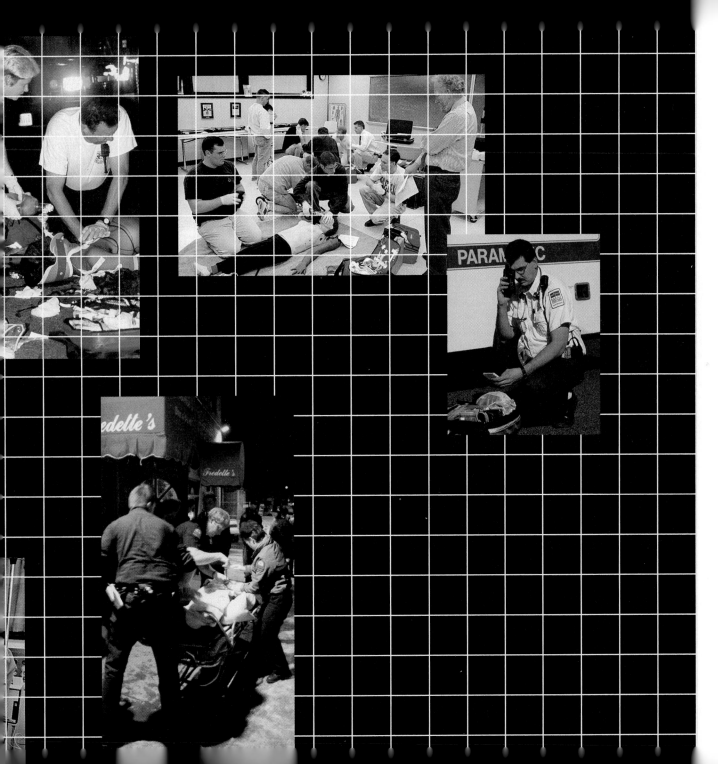

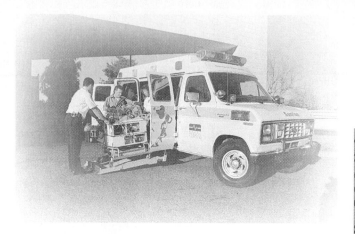

OBJECTIVES

A paramedic should be able to:

1. Explain the development of EMS in the United States including important legislative and other developments.
2. Identify the five stages of the EMS system from a patient's perspective.
3. List the 15 components of an EMS system.
4. Explain the relationship between medical direction and the quality of prehospital health care provided within an EMS system.
5. List the different funding mechanisms in EMS.
6. Outline the role of regulatory agencies in EMS systems.
7. Describe the use of standards in EMS, including the various mechanisms for certification and licensure.
8. Define the terms "mutual aid" and "reciprocity."
9. Explain the need for system planning and identify five system goals.
10. Identify various EMS system participants and standards.
11. Describe the four components of EMS Communications.
12. Describe the role of research in EMS.

KEY TERMS

1. **Advanced Life Support (ALS)**—provision of care rendered by medical personnel that includes advanced airway maneuvers, defibrillation, intravenous therapy, and medication administration.
2. **Basic Life Support (BLS)**—care provided by prehospital providers that includes first aid, cardiopulmonary resuscitation, and other noninvasive therapies.
3. **Emergency Medical Services (EMS) Systems**—a system that provides for the arrangement of personnel, facilities, and equipment for the effective and coordinated delivery in an appropriate geographic area of health care services under emergency conditions (occurring either as a result of the patient's condition, natural disasters, or similar conditions) and which is administered by a public or nonprofit private entity that has the authority and the resources to provide effective administration of the system.
4. **Mutual Aid**—concept of using neighboring EMS resources to assist when local resources are overwhelmed.
5. **Reciprocity**—free movement of EMS personnel from one jurisdiction to another without further testing.

Two major changes have occurred in the delivery of emergency health care since 1966. The first was the development of new allied health personnel, called emergency medical technicians (EMTs). These dedicated and talented individuals represented a trend toward increased training for all levels of providers, as well as the development and application of new technology designed to decrease morbidity and mortality for persons suffering from emergent illness or injury.

The second change, which involved the delivery of emergency health services, was development of the emergency medical services (EMS) system. Federal, state, and local governments increased their efforts to plan for the delivery of emergency health services and to coordinate the various provider organizations into functional systems. EMS councils and "system lead agencies" were developed and charged with determining system needs, assigning roles and responsibilities to system participants, and coordinating their system-related activities. With these changes, the role of the paramedic was established—to provide patient care as part of an organized EMS system.

Development of EMS in the United States

The provision of emergency medical services can be traced back to early military medicine, particularly the use of horse-drawn carts, which were first used to remove battlefield casualties during the Napoleonic wars. The first ambulance services in the United States were hospital based, in Cincinnati prior to 1860 and New York City in 1869. These services were limited to transportation of patients to a medical facility.[15]

Modern EMS is generally viewed as beginning with the 1966 publication of the "White Paper" by the National Academy of Sciences' National Research Council, formally titled *Accidental Death and Disability: The Neglected Disease of Modern Society*. The White Paper served as a needs statement for the national effort to improve emergency care. In preparing the White Paper, the council found that the techniques and equipment used in emergency health care were lacking. Specifically, the council found:

- The available information (regarding ambulance services) showed a diversity of standards, which were often low, frequent use of unnecessarily expensive and usually ill-designed equipment, and generally inadequate supplies.
- There was no generally accepted standard for the competence or training of ambulance attendants.
- Although it is possible to converse with the astronauts in outer space, communication was seldom possible between an ambulance and the emergency department that it was approaching.
- For decades, the "emergency" facilities of most hospitals consisted only of "accident rooms"—poorly equipped, inadequately manned, and ordinarily used for limited numbers of seriously ill persons or for charity victims of disease or injury.[12]

The White Paper called for an organized response similar to the intense efforts to conquer cancer, heart disease, and mental disease. Two federal programs were enacted to overcome the perceived problems in EMS. The first established the National Highway Traffic Safety Administration (NHTSA) in the Department of Transportation (DOT). NHTSA has been responsible for setting standards by developing training curricula for prehospital providers (EMS Dispatchers, First Responders, EMTs, EMT-Intermediates, and EMT-Paramedics). Through grant monies to each state, NHTSA has funded ALS program development, ambulances, communications equipment, and other EMS system improvements.

The primary push at the federal level to develop EMS systems came from the EMS Systems Act of 1973 (Public Law 93-154). The US Department of Health, Education, and Welfare (now known as the Department of Health and Human Services or DHHS) provided the funding to develop regional EMS organizations. These organizations were intended to plan, implement, and coordinate EMS systems. The regional boundaries ignored city and county borders in order to include sufficient EMS resources to treat the majority of patients. Three hundred and four EMS regions were identified, which, if fully developed, would have provided "wall-to-wall" emergency health care. Unfortunately, many were never fully funded or organized because of political considerations.

The federal EMS program provided three types of grants: 1) feasibility studies and system planning; 2) implementation and initial operation; and 3) system expansion and improvement. In 1981, the Consolidated Omnibus Reconciliation Act was passed, which changed the funding process. Instead of funding the regional organizations directly, the federal EMS grant monies were now included in the DHHS Preventive Health and Health Services block grant program and the funds were distributed by the states.[5] Many states continue to fund EMS system-related activities using these DHHS funds or other state monies.

Systems Approach to EMS

The Federal EMS Systems Act defined an EMS system as "a system which provides for the arrangement of personnel, facilities, and equipment for the effective and coordinated delivery in an appropriate geographic area of health care services under emergency conditions (occurring either as a result of the patient's condition or of natural disasters or similar conditions) and which is administered by a public or nonprofit private entity which has the authority and the resources to provide effective administration of the system."

The delivery of emergency health care requires the participation of numerous independent organizations, including public safety agencies, ambulance services, and hospitals. Despite their autonomy, these organizations enjoy high degrees of functional interdependence as they work to provide care, sometimes simultaneously, to individual patients. However, managing such interdependence requires planning, standardization, and mutual adjustment.[10]

Each community can employ five possible approaches to manage the interdependence of its EMS providers. The first—ignoring it—results in conflicts, inefficiencies, and in the end, a lower level of patient care. The second approach involves the creation of voluntary networks (e.g., EMS councils) to coordinate system participants. This approach depends heavily on the willingness of the participants to cooperate. A third approach, started under the federal EMS initiative, creates an independent agency to develop a system plan and encourage providers to participate in the plan. Under the fourth approach, this same planning agency is granted regulatory powers, such as the franchising of ambulance services and formal designation of specialty hospitals, to assign roles and responsibilities to system participants in order to enforce implementation. The fifth approach places the entire EMS system under a single agency. This method is not fully used, even in systems such as New York and San Francisco, where government owns or manages most of the system's resources.[9]

Under the third and fourth approaches, the job of the lead agency (regardless of its specific regulatory powers) is to plan for the entire EMS system to provide the optimal response to the emergency patient. In doing so, it must consider all potential patient needs and all resources required to meet those needs. In many ways, the lead agency must act in the same capacity as the upper management of a large corporation, coordinating the activities of its various divisions.[9]

System Response Stages

The EMS system can be generally broken down into five stages from a patient's perspective (Fig. 1-1): 1) preresponse (initial access to the system, with first aid and cardiopulmonary resuscitation performed by members of the public prior to the arrival of first responders); 2) prehospital (fire, law enforcement and other public safety "first responder" agencies, dispatch, and basic and advanced life support ambulances); 3) hospital (emergency department and secondary-level inpatient hospital care); 4) critical care (intensive and cardiac care); and 5) rehabilitation (services necessary to return the patient to a productive place in society).

Not all of the participants in these stages are involved with patients during the emergent phase of their illnesses, nor may they be under the regulatory control of EMS organizations. Yet the relationships among providers, and the policies and procedures needed to ensure proper patient care, make them all links in the chain to ensure patient survival.

Service Areas

The National Academy of Sciences defined regionalization in EMS as "the process of identifying and developing resources on an area-wide basis to meet the needs of all the acutely ill and injured for prompt, efficient, and effective medical care," which is "achieved by areawide organization, coordination, and integration" of system components.[12] The American Society for Testing and Materials (ASTM) committee on EMS defined a region as "the geographic or demographic area that is a natural catchment area for EMS provision for most, if not all, patients in the designated area."[1]

Using these definitions, a regional EMS system is a natural system, based on day-to-day response patterns and hospital catchment areas. A catchment area is the natural area from which patients normally travel to receive services. Wherever possible, the boundaries of the responsible EMS council or lead agency should match the natural system. Within that area, providers should be coordinated to ensure that, regardless of geopolitical boundaries, the closest appropriate providers are sent to a medical emergency, and that patients are taken to the closest facility appropriate for their condition. These natural boundaries do not necessarily share any relationship with county or state lines. Rather, the system should include metropolitan areas along with suburban and rural areas to ensure availability of specialty care services. In remote areas, transfer agreements will need to be used to ensure access to specialized tertiary care services.

System Components

Most EMS system models focus on functional components. The Federal EMS Act identified 15 components that needed to be addressed[16] (Box 1-1).

As with the system stages previously noted, establishing the components does not identify the individuals or the organizations involved. Although a system design can address the components generically, an effective plan requires that the roles and responsibilities of specific participating organizations be addressed. Some states have created EMS system standards and guidelines to assist EMS planners.

Medical Direction and Oversight

The concept of medical direction extends medical accountability, clinical leadership, and quality improvement over the entire EMS system.[6] The medical direction of the EMS system is the responsibility of the EMS Medical Director who authorizes the medical practice of the EMS providers and takes responsi-

BOX 1-1	Fifteen Components of the EMS System

1. Manpower
2. Training
3. Communications
4. Transportation
5. Facilities
6. Critical care units
7. Public safety agencies
8. Consumer participation
9. Access to care
10. Patient transfer
11. Coordinated patient record keeping
12. Public information and education
13. Review and evaluation
14. Disaster linkage
15. Mutual aid

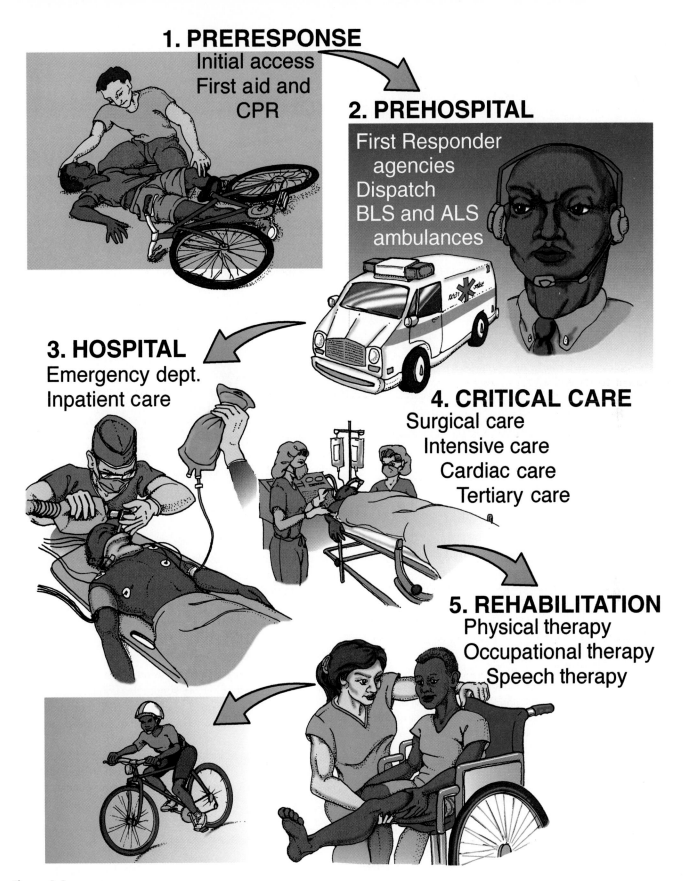

1. PRERESPONSE
Initial access
First aid and
CPR

2. PREHOSPITAL
First Responder
agencies
Dispatch
BLS and ALS
ambulances

3. HOSPITAL
Emergency dept.
Inpatient care

4. CRITICAL CARE
Surgical care
Intensive care
Cardiac care
Tertiary care

5. REHABILITATION
Physical therapy
Occupational therapy
Speech therapy

Figure 1-1

System response stages as seen from a patient's perspective.

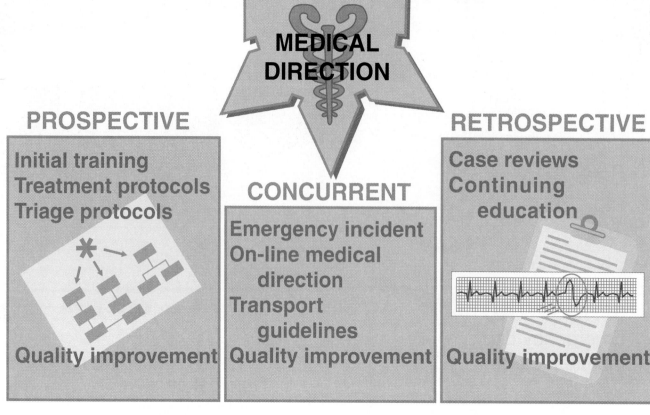

Figure 1-2

Types of medical direction and oversight.

bility for the quality of health care provided. Medical direction can be provided prospectively, concurrently, and retrospectively.[3,6] (Fig. 1-2)

Medical accountability is the process by which the medical community ensures that prehospital procedures and the actions of the providers are in accordance with acceptable medical practice.

Treatment Protocols

Treatment protocols provide standards of practice for the entire EMS system and are the yardstick by which all actions are measured. These standards apply to all segments of the system, including online physicians and prehospital personnel. Medical treatment can often be provided without direct, online medical direction. Standing orders are used in many areas to authorize medical procedures to be performed prior to attempting base hospital contact.

Triage Protocols

Also known as patient destination policies or "point of entry" plans, triage protocols specify the hospital to which patients should be transported. Some triage policies identify patients who are to be preferentially transported to a specialty center, such as a trauma center or a pediatric critical care center. In other cases, triage policies provide guidelines to ensure that a medical direction facility does not use its status to influence patient destination decisions.

Transfer Guidelines

Transfer guidelines provide direction to physicians in identifying patients who should be transferred to a tertiary facility or for whom consultation with a specialist is appropriate. Transfer guidelines must be specific to each hospital, based on its own capabilities and the distance to specialty centers.

Recordkeeping and Evaluation

Records should cover the patient's entire treatment sequence—from initial access to the EMS system through final disposition. Records should be designed to allow for such individual tracking and to allow for data to be extracted, compiled, and analyzed.[17]

Evaluation must include both system-wide reviews of the overall appropriateness, adequacy, efficiency, and effectiveness of the system's response to medical emergencies and reviews of the quality of care offered to individual patients.

System Coordination and EMS Organization

State EMS Office

One of the goals of the federal EMS program was to establish an EMS "lead agency" in each state. Each state now has such an agency, with most located in the state's health department or an equivalent organization. Most states also have an EMS advisory committee, often appointed by the governor, which provides both professional and consumer input to the administrative agency.

ASTM's standard on "Structures and Responsibilities of EMS System Organizations" identifies the setting of EMS standards as the primary responsibility of the state EMS agency. In addition, many state EMS agencies are responsible for enforcing EMS-related laws and regulations, such as licensure or certification of prehospital care personnel, licensure of ambulance services, approval of training programs, and designation of specialty care centers.

BOX 1-2   **Funding Sources for EMS**

- General tax revenues
- Special district revenue
- Subscription services
- Health insurance
    Medicaid (State)
    Medicare (Federal)
    Health insurance
    Other private insurance
- Direct payment by the patient
- Donations/fundraising

Regional and Local EMS Organizations

In 1969, the American Medical Association's Commission on Emergency Medical Services recommended that a community council on EMS bring together the leaders providing such care for the purposes of planning, education, and funding. Council members were to represent providers, payers, patients, public agencies (including first responders, health departments, health planning agencies, and local governments), and community leaders. This concept evolved into what is now recognized as the Regional EMS Organization (REMSO), which is responsible for the coordination of all system participants.

Due to the number of independent organizations involved with the care of emergent patients and the strong interdependencies that exist within the system, an external coordinating body is needed to create an overall system plan, to identify roles and responsibilities of participants, to standardize policies and procedures in areas in which independent organizations interact, and to evaluate the overall system. REMSOs are usually developed as units of local government, nonprofit organizations, or divisions of the state EMS agency, and may be responsible for single- or multiple-county areas.

In some states, direct authority for establishing medical direction standards, approving advanced providers, certifying personnel, and overseeing other regulatory functions is delegated to the REMSO. Although the concept of the REMSO under the federal EMS initiative was that these organizations should have full authority over the system participants, many REMSOs are currently limited to strictly planning functions.

Numerous sources are used for the funding of regional EMS organizations, including the federal Preventive Health and Health Services Block Grant, state and local taxes, and fees. The Federal EMS Act required grantees to develop a plan for ongoing funding at the end of their federal grants, but such plans had limited success in ensuring financial stability. Some states have developed special sources for funding EMS programs, such as a surcharge on traffic violations, driver's licenses, or vehicle registrations. In several states, the regional agency is operated by the state EMS office and its staff are state employees.

Funding of EMS

In general, financing of emergency services is similar to health care financing, but is complicated by several factors. Multiple funding sources, both public and private, may be used to pay for ambulance services (see Box 1-2). Some communities use a competitive bid process to award an exclusive franchise for ambulance service, which can include the setting of rates by a government body, a subsidy from local taxes, or other payment systems. Other communities provide EMS as a government service, public utility, private ambulance service, or some combination.

EMS Regulatory Authority

Authority for EMS

Authority for EMS activities, such as certification or licensure of personnel, vehicle licensure, facility designation, and approval of advanced life support providers, is governed by various state laws. EMS rules and regulations may be found in an EMS act, medical and nursing practice acts, hospital licensure laws, or other sources.

Although most state EMS offices are created by a statute, some were created by regulation or executive orders. Regional agencies are authorized through several sources, including statutes, regulations, and formal recognition by the same office.

The amount of direct control exercised by state and regional EMS organizations over system participants varies. Several states have delegated specific regulatory powers to their regional organizations, whereas others maintain this at the state level. Regulatory powers such as ambulance franchising are local options in some states and are not allowed in others. Some EMS organizations have authority to designate trauma centers, whereas other states use a less formal approval process.

Licensure or Certification, and Revocation of License

EMS personnel are licensed or certified in all states. The state EMS office or state health department is usually responsible for this process, although in some states, advanced life support personnel are licensed or certified through the state's medical board. Suspension, revocation, or denial of licenses or certifications is based on regulations governing those actions to ensure that "due process" of law is applied.[14]

A paramedic licensed or certified in one state may be able to practice in another. Some states readily accept another's licensure as proof of competency to practice without further testing. The concept that no further testing is necessary in order to become licensed or certified is called *reciprocity*. The National Registry of EMTs is a nongovernmental, nonprofit entity established to certify EMTs and paramedics according to a national standard. Some states use the National Registry testing as the state certification examination. Some states accept National Registry Paramedic Certification to gain reciprocity, whereas others require further written and skills testing.

Delegated Practice

Most states require a local medical director for each EMS system or for advanced life support service providers. Several states require that this person "recommend" certification or provide an additional "authorization to practice." This process is analogous to the granting of hospital privileges to a physician who is already licensed to practice by the state. To participate, the individual must be oriented to the system (including local treatment protocols and operating policies), be introduced to the system's medical direction, and be part of the quality improvement process.

Facility Designation and Categorization

One of the goals of the EMS system is to transport the patient to a facility that can provide appropriate treatment, even if it is not the closest one. One of the recommendations in the 1966 White Paper was to categorize emergency departments according to the level of care available. Toward this end, several professional organizations, such as the American College of Surgeons, have developed criteria for rating hospital services for specific clinical target groups, including burns, spinal cord injuries, pediatrics, and trauma.

Through categorization has sprung the notion of designating specific facilities to treat particular patients. Patients meeting predetermined clinical criteria are triaged directly from the prehospital setting to these centers or, in rural areas, are transferred after assessment and stabilization at a nearby hospital. In some areas, all hospitals that meet the criteria are approved; in other systems, a competitive process is used to select one or more hospitals to serve the system.

EMS Boards and Committees

As the community EMS council evolved into the REMSO, various mechanisms developed to ensure appropriate input into system development. EMS advisory councils may include consumer representatives, as well as various professional groups representing physicians, hospital administrators, ambulance providers, fire chiefs, and other essential system participants. Council members are generally appointed by their respective groups to represent their point of view. Unfortunately, this can sometimes create a problem if the decisions to be made substantially affect a council member's agency or company.

When the REMSO is a unit of government, these groups may nominate members who are then appointed by the appropriate elected officials. When the REMSO is not a unit of government, the group council may also serve as a board of directors and oversee the agency's staff.

System Planning, Goals, and Objectives

One of the primary tasks of both state and regional EMS organizations is to develop a system plan. This plan should set overall system goals and consider financial, technical, and political constraints. Based on these goals and constraints, attainable objectives can be established. The plan should identify the resources that are available and needed to develop the system. It should also establish short- and long-range work plans to achieve the objectives and to determine the roles and responsibilities of the system participants.

Goals are broad statements of purpose, whereas objectives are more specific and measurable. A goal statement might be "to provide short ambulance response times to the entire system," whereas its related objective might be "to provide an 8-minute response time for 90% of all responses in the urban area."

Realistic and attainable objectives will result in a higher level of care than holding out for an unobtainable optimum. Although having a trauma surgeon in-house might be optimal, one who is available on call within a short period of time is better than employing a nonmandatory call list. An EMT-Intermediate (EMT-I) may not provide the same level of care as a paramedic but is still preferable to a basic life support provider. The reasonableness of minimum standards and the availability of alternative levels should be considered when developing laws, regulations, and professional guidelines as well as the EMS system design.

Tiered Response

Nearby responders can begin patient stabilization while awaiting the arrival of higher trained but more distant providers (Fig. 1-3). For example, firefighters can begin cardiopulmonary resuscitation when awaiting ambulance arrival. In some areas, basic life support ambulances respond along with advanced units and transport less serious patients, keeping advanced life support available for more serious emergencies. Air ambulances may respond along with ground ambulances.

A tiered response requires that all providers be designated according to their capability and that dispatch policies specify the appropriate responders for each type of call. When multiple transporting units are available, the decision among them and the choice of the patient's destination must be based on the patient's needs and should be the responsibility of the medical direction facility.

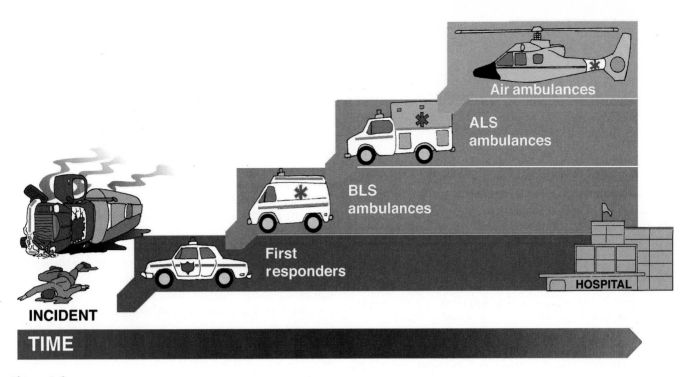

Figure 1-3

A tiered response system allows for rapid patient intervention and efficient use of varying levels of resources.

Response Times

In addition to providing an immediate first response using any available responder, many systems work to decrease ambulance response times. This can be accomplished through strategic placement of ambulance stations, the establishment of ambulance "standby positions" to serve areas left uncovered by another emergency response, mutual aid agreements with providers in other jurisdictions, or the merging and coordinating of small providers to improve efficiency. System Status Management is a technique designed to match resources to the projected demand; historical call data is used to calculate the estimated number of units and specific locations for placement based on time of day and day of the week.[16]

Advanced Life Support

Advanced life support (ALS) care extends the emergency department into the prehospital setting. ALS providers are able to provide early invasive care under the direct or indirect direction of physicians. Scopes of practice vary widely, but include capabilities for defibrillation, invasive airway techniques, and administration of intravenous fluids and medications. Many states recognize several levels of EMS providers to extend the benefits of ALS service to rural areas that cannot afford full EMT-Paramedic training or staffing.

Early ALS programs focused on cardiac patients and were able to improve the outcome of cardiac arrest and prearrest patients through the use of early defibrillation and pharmacologic intervention. ALS treatment of trauma patients is more controversial, with many experts recommending that transport of the patient to definitive treatment should not be delayed by prehospital invasive procedures.

Early Defibrillation

Defibrillation has become a skill expected of any EMS provider who responds to a cardiac arrest patient. EMTs, first responders, and even the lay public are using lightweight, portable automatic external defibrillators (AEDs). Clear scientific evidence now exists that early defibrillation is the single most critical intervention for the patient in ventricular fibrillation. Some airlines and highrise buildings have AEDs available for use by minimally trained individuals.

Mutual Aid and Disaster Medical Response

Mutual aid and disaster medical response are forged through agreements among individual providers and linkages with neighboring EMS systems. Mutual aid is the concept that neighboring EMS providers will assist when the resources of an area are overwhelmed. On a day-to-day basis, a mutual aid agreement might provide for emergency response by a closer ambulance from another jurisdiction, or for back-up for multiple calls. During significant medical incidents or disasters, mutual aid agreements may provide for provision of additional units to the affected area, as well as coverage of areas left uncovered by initial response to the incident.

System Participants and Standards

First Responders

Public safety agencies such as fire departments, police agencies, and parks and recreation departments, which serve as nontransporting first responders, are often able to respond more quickly than an ambulance and begin stabilization before arrival of the ambulance. In some systems, first responders are trained to the ALS level and either accompany the ambulance to the hospital or turn the patient over to an ambulance crew with an equal or higher level of training.

Sending multiple responders to each call has been criticized as unnecessary duplication, but in cardiac arrests and other true emergencies, the few minutes saved can mean the difference between a viable patient and one who suffers hypoxic brain death. First responders are particularly important in rural areas with long ambulance response times.

Ambulance and Ambulance Crews

Ambulances have transformed from "horizontal taxis" to an extension of the emergency department. In many communities, both urban and rural, they are staffed and equipped to provide initial and invasive treatment for a variety of emergencies. Air ambulances and water rescue craft may also be available in some areas.

In 1993, 35% of the ambulance services in the 200 most populous US cities were operated by fire departments and 24% by private ambulance services. Another 16.5% used a combination of fire and private services, 16% were municipal "third party services," and 7% were hospital based.[3]

Although EMS systems run the gamut from public to private to volunteer, they all do essentially the same job, and no single type of provider has been shown to be more effective than any other. Rather, appropriate coordination of all providers and their integration into the EMS system are the key components to ensuring that the service is appropriate for the patient's needs.

In many states, ambulances must conform to the Federal DOT standards for ambulance construction known as the KKK 1822C standards. These standards reflect the minimum standard for ambulance operation and include lighting and patient compartment specifications. These standards identify three types of vehicles as acceptable ambulances, depending on the type of chassis (van or truck) and patient compartment (van conversion or modular) (Fig. 1-4).

Ambulance services can also be nationally accredited by the Commission on the Accreditation of Ambulance Services (CAAS). This process includes a review of the service to ensure that standards for the operation and quality of services are met.

Critical Care Transport Units and Interfacility Transfers

The interfacility transfer of patients is a component of many EMS systems. Some public services only respond to emergencies, leaving nonemergency calls to the private sector. There is

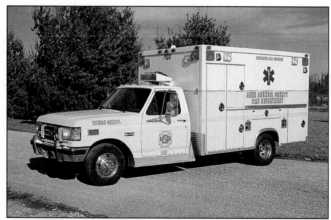

A

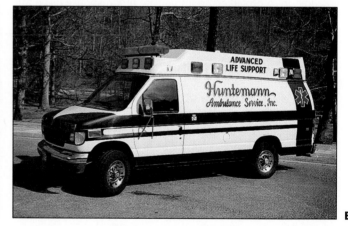

B

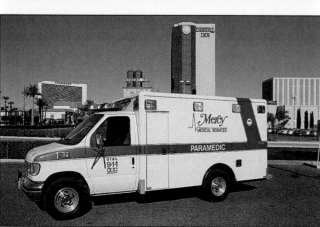

C

Figure 1-4

Three types of ambulances as specified by the Federal DOT KKK 1822C standards. A, Type I. B, Type II. C, Type III.

some question as to who is responsible for the actions of a provider transferring a patient after evaluation by a physician. If the patient is unstable or requires treatment not specifically approved for EMS by the state, a physician or other representative of the hospital should accompany the patient during transfer.

Hospitals and emergency physicians are required to assess all emergency patients and women in active labor when they arrive at the emergency department. This federal requirement, Consolidated Omnibus Budget Reconciliation, (COBRA 1987 and COBRA 1989) was enacted to ensure that patients are stabilized prior to transfer to another hospital and that the sending and receiving physician are in agreement concerning the transfer of the patient. COBRA mandates that the transferring physician do the following:

- Certify that the patient is stable or that the risks of remaining at the first facility outweigh the risks of transfer.
- Certify that the patient is not in active labor.
- Contact the receiving facility to ensure that it is willing and able to accept the patient.
- Send appropriate records.
- Certify that the personnel transporting the patient are appropriate for the care needed during transport.

If these conditions are not met, both the transferring physician and hospital may be assessed large fines.

In some areas of the country, Critical Care Transport units staffed with nurses or physicians transport patients between facilities (Fig. 1-5). Some specialty systems, such as neonatal critical care groups, have developed specialized vehicles and specially trained personnel for interfacility transfers. Fixed or rotary wing aircraft may also be used under certain circumstances for the transfer of critical patients.

Hospitals

When considering the link between the emergency department and the community emergency response system, it is clear that the continuum of care begins in the prehospital setting.

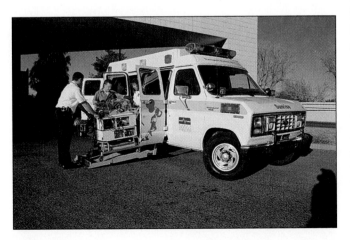

Figure 1-5

Critical care transport units have special equipment and are staffed by specially trained EMS providers and nurses or doctors. Both air and ground transport units serve as critical care transport units.

In addition to the recognition of emergency medicine as a specialty and other improvements in hospital emergency department services, the role of in-patient and critical care services has changed. Military experience in Korea and Vietnam has been translated into civilian trauma systems in which patients are preferentially triaged to a hospital that is specially staffed and equipped to provide rapid surgery. Tertiary-level centers for burns, neonatal and pediatric intensive care, spinal cord injuries, and other specialties have been identified in some communities. Patients are transported directly to these centers from community hospitals.

In rural areas, even where nearby specialty centers have been designated, patients are generally transported to a closer hospital and then transferred as appropriate. Hospitals should develop agreements with specialty centers for the transfer of patients who require care beyond that available at the transferring facility.

Trauma Centers and Systems

Trauma centers are specialized hospitals with the capability to treat victims of traumatic injury quickly. These facilities are categorized as Level I, II, III, and IV, following standards developed by the American College of Surgeons (ACS). Trauma systems should be planned so that the system includes the proper number of trauma centers to ensure efficiency and effectiveness.[11]

The DHHS Trauma and EMS Division provided financial grants from 1991 to 1994 to states to develop comprehensive statewide trauma systems consistent with the model trauma care plan developed as part of the 1990 Trauma Systems Planning and Development Act (PL 101-590).

Medical Direction Facilities

The remote practice of medicine by prehospital personnel requires access to a facility with a physician who provides medical direction for the care of patients. Known as *base hospitals* or *resource hospitals,* these facilities also participate in training and continuing education of prehospital personnel and in the medical audit process. Some states allow specially trained nurses to provide medical direction to prehospital providers.

Educational Programs

With increasing standardization of titles, scopes of practice, and training standards, education of prehospital personnel is nearing that of other allied health professionals. Some areas provide on-the-job training for employees, but most people pursuing an EMS career now seek education prior to employment. The cost of education may be borne by the employer, subsidized through an EMS organization, or paid for by the student.

In many states, education is still considered to be the major function of regional EMS organizations. Standards for educational programs are drawn from the DOT curriculum. Curriculum revisions occur periodically to ensure that the latest information and method of presentation are integrated into prehospital training programs. Additionally, the Joint Review Committee for EMT-Paramedic Educational Programs sets standards for paramedic programs and reviews the programs for national accreditation. The Review Committee functions in conjunction with the Commission on Accreditation of Allied Health Educational Programs (CAAHEP).

Several universities have developed bachelor's and master's programs in EMS to prepare the EMS professional for advancement to leadership positions. These programs generally incorporate training in prehospital medical care with general education topics and business management, administration, and research courses.

EMS Communications

The communications component of an EMS system is the most crucial link to an effective system. An organized response to an urgent medical situation requires a number of people working together for a common purpose from remote locations. Without a communications system, these individuals cannot bring their collective expertise together.

The basic concept underlying all communication is that there are three parts to any transaction: a sender, a message, and a receiver. In EMS, the goal is to accurately and quickly transmit the message that will provide information crucial to a medical incident. To achieve this goal in EMS a communications system should be comprised of five components:

System Access

Any individual who perceives that an urgent medical need exists should have a simple and reliable method to access the EMS system. In many states, 9-1-1 has become the universally recognized number to obtain law enforcement, fire department, or EMS assistance in an emergency. Areas that have not yet developed 9-1-1 should still have a well-publicized number for citizen access to EMS.

The basic emergency number, 9-1-1, became available in 1967 from American Telephone and Telegraph. It is a toll-free telephone service that enables the caller to access a public safety answering point (PSAP). Because the basic system allows the caller to reach the PSAP only, an enhanced system (E 9-1-1) provides the dispatcher with automatic location and phone number of the caller. It also instantly routes the call to the appropriate emergency service after the type of emergency is identified.

Dispatch Centers

A single dispatch or communications center that can communicate with and direct all emergency medical services units within the system is ideal. It should link personnel, facilities, and vehicles through a common communications system. The EMS dispatcher should be in charge of all emergency vehicle movements in the area to ensure system readiness, and should dispatch the closest, most appropriate unit to the scene. Most high-performance dispatch control centers are equipped with computer aided dispatch (CAD) and automatic vehicle locator (AVL) systems, and staffed by trained EMS dispatchers (Fig. 1-6).

Trained Dispatchers

The term *dispatch* means to assign units and direct appropriate medical resources to the victim of an illness or injury. Trained and certified emergency medical dispatchers, or system status managers, should be a part of any EMS system. The dispatcher often functions in two distinct roles: as call taker and radio dispatcher. The EMS dispatcher has the responsibility for maintaining the status of all units in the system, positioning vehicles for optimal coverage of the service area, receiving calls, giving prearrival instructions to callers, prioritizing calls, and dispatching and tracking the response of a unit until it clears the hospital and is available for the next call. Dispatchers also provide operational data for quality improvement and system evaluation.[4]

EMS dispatchers should be trained in both telecommunication and medical techniques. Emergency Medical Dispatch (EMD) training should include telecommunications, caller interrogation, prearrival instructions, and call prioritization. Dispatch personnel are also trained to determine whether an ALS ambulance is required and whether a first responder should be dispatched along with the ambulance. "Priority medical dispatch" requires that communications personnel be able to elicit adequate information from the reporting part and, based on medically acceptable policies, determine the appropriate response and give prearrival instructions. Several standardized courses are available nationwide.[4]

Dispatch and Medical Communications System

Every EMS system should have communications equipment that links the dispatch center to each EMS field unit, field units to hospitals, and units and hospitals to their counterparts.[2] To

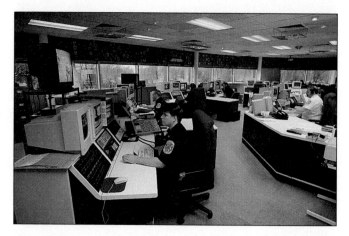

Figure 1-6

Specially trained dispatchers are required to coordinate the delicate operations taking place within the modern dispatch center.

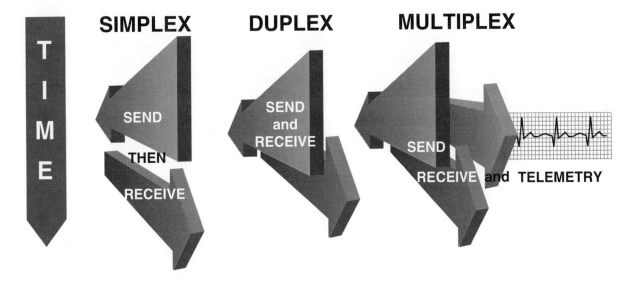

Figure 1-7

Communication systems can be simplex, duplex, or multiplex, allowing for varying types of transmission.

achieve this, certain radio frequencies have been designated by the Federal Communications Commission (FCC) for medical emergency communications. EMS transmissions are assigned to either a very high frequency (VHF) or ultra high frequency (UHF) band for dispatch and medical communications, including telemetry. In addition to these designated channels, other channels may be used locally to achieve the same purpose.

Most systems are set up as duplex rather than simplex systems. In a simplex system, a single channel is used that allows communication between two points (Fig. 1-7). Unfortunately, communication can only go in one direction at a time. A duplex system uses two "paired" channels, one to send and one to receive, similar to a telephone. It allows for the simultaneous reception and transmission between two points. If the duplex system is engineered to simultaneously send and receive telemetry, it is called a *multiplex system.*

Some systems use commercial cellular phone systems to achieve reliable backup communications, including ECG telemetry. However, the EMS system will not necessarily have priority access in the event the cell site or system becomes congested.

Research

The use of research to validate existing treatment techniques and to choose new methods in prehospital care is important for the EMS system. The implementation of closely supervised clinical trials and the published results should be part of the EMS system to identify better ways to provide patient care and improve survival. These clinical trials must be completed and analyzed prior to adding a device or medication to the paramedic scope of practice. Research can also yield new system configurations and new responsibilities for providers.

SUMMARY

With cutbacks in both health care and government funds, the need for rational planning of the EMS system is more important than ever. Through the planning process, cooperation among services is essential to provide the best response with the available resources. By increasing overall system efficiency, higher levels of care can be maintained for more areas.

REFERENCES

1. American Society for Testing and Materials: Standard Guide for Structures and Responsibilities of Emergency Medical Services System Organizations, Philadelphia, 1988, ASTM.

2. Braun O, Callahan ML: Direct Medical Control. In Kuehl A (ed), EMS Medical Directors' Handbook, St. Louis, 1989, Mosby–Year Book.

3. Cady G: EMS in the United States 1994 Survey of Providers in the 200 Most Populous Cities. JEMS, 19:1, 1994.

4. Clawson JJ, Dernocoeur KB: Principles of Emergency Medical Dispatch, Englewood Cliffs, 1988, Brady.

5. Consolidated Omnibus Reconciliation Act (COBRA) of 1981, Public Law 97-35.

6. Holroyd BR, Knopp R, Kallsen G: Medical Control: Quality Assurance in Prehospital Care. JAMA, 256:1027–1031, 1986.

7. Guidelines for Cardiopulmonary Resuscitation and Emergency Cardiac Care. JAMA, 1992, 268, No. 16.

8. McSwain NE: Indirect Medical Control. In Kuehl A (ed), EMS Medical Directors' Handbook, St. Louis, 1989, Mosby–Year Book.

9. Narad RA: Emergency Medical Services System Design. Emerg Med Clin North Am, 8:1–14, 1990.

10. Narad RA: Managing Functional Interdependence between Multiple Autonomous Organizations, Dissertation, University of Southern California, 1991.

11. Narad RA, Smiley DR: Trauma Care: System in Crisis? California Policy Choices, 7:125–151, 1991.

12. National Academy of Sciences/National Research Council: Accidental Death and Disability: The Neglected Disease of Modern Society, Washington ED, National Academy of Sciences, 1966.

13. Polsky S (ed), Continuous Quality Improvement in EMS, American College of Emergency Physicians, Dallas, 1992.

14. Smiley DR: Remediation. In Polsky S (ed), Continuous Quality Improvement in EMS, American College of Emergency Physicians, Dallas, 1992, Mosby–Year Book.

15. Stewart RD: The History of Emergency Medical Services. In Kuehl A (ed), EMS Medical Directors' Handbook, St. Louis, 1989.

16. Stout J: System Status Management. *JEMS,* 14:65–67, 1989.

17. United States Public Health Service Act, Title XII (EMS System), Section 1201(1).

18. Valenzuela TD, Criss EA: Data Collection and Ambulance Report Design. In Kuehl A (ed), EMS Medical Directors' Handbook, St. Louis, 1989, Mosby–Year Book.

Mike Smith, REMT-P

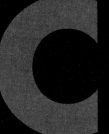

Chapter 2

Roles and Responsibilities

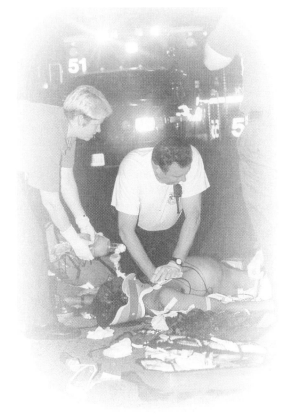

KEY TERMS

1. **Certification**—A process in which an individual, an institution, or an educational program is evaluated and recognized as meeting certain predetermined standards. Certification is usually made by a nongovernmental agency. The purpose of certification is to assure that the standards met are those necessary for safe and ethical practice of the profession or service.

2. **Ethics**—A system of moral principles or standards governing conduct.

3. **Licensure**—The process by which permission is granted by a competent authority (usually a government agency) to an individual to engage in a specific profession or occupation that would otherwise be illegal.

4. **The White Paper**—A landmark study, "Accidental Death and Disability: The Neglected Disease in Modern Society" by the National Academy of Sciences and National Research Council. This document identified key issues and problems facing the US in providing emergency care, and proposed recommendations for comprehensive and organized EMS development.

A paramedic should be able to:

OBJECTIVES

1. Apply the principles of the EMT Code of Ethics to specific patient care situations.

2. Discuss the impact of the "White Paper" on EMS.

3. Describe the differences among the education and training of an EMT-Basic, EMT-Intermediate and EMT-Paramedic.

4. List eight major functions of the paramedic and the tasks associated with each function.

5. Describe the benefits of continuing education.

6. Identify three national EMS organizations that promote the advancement of prehospital emergency care.

7. Define the terms *certification, licensure* and *reciprocity.*

8. State the major purpose of a national registry agency in EMS.

ntering paramedic training solely out of a desire to save lives would be a mistake. On the other hand, a genuine desire to help people and to meet the challenge of providing prehospital emergency care, under often unique and adverse conditions, can lead to a rewarding career as a paramedic.

A paramedic is a health care professional, and as such has an obligation to adhere to the standards of the profession of EMS. This is not a legal obligation, because no law can require that a paramedic behave as a professional. It is a voluntary choice that once made will increase one's credibility not only as a member of an EMS team, but also as part of the total health care team (Fig. 2-1). It also helps to further the continued growth and development of the EMS profession.

A competent paramedic knows how to perform skills, knows why to perform the skills and when they need to be performed. A common misconception holds that being a professional requires some form of compensation, which is simply not true. Full-time versus volunteer status is not what defines professionalism. Adherence to the standards of the profession marks the true professional.

Medical Ethics

Ethics is the study of moral principles and values. A professional code of ethics is a set of standards designed to guide or

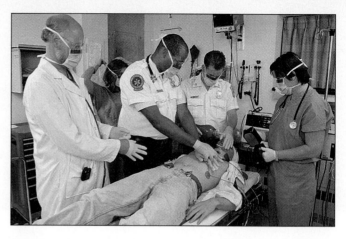

Figure 2-1

The EMT-Paramedic is an integral part of the professional patient care team.

govern the behavior of that profession's members. Over the years, there have been a number of published codes of ethics for health care professionals. In 1978, the National Association of Emergency Medical Technicians issued the code of Ethics for EMTs (Box 2-1).

Although these principles outline ideal conduct, paramedics often find themselves faced with ethical dilemmas. For instance, a burglar is shot twice in the chest as he attacks a po-

---

BOX 2-1   **The EMT Code of Ethics**

Professional status as an Emergency Medical Technician and Emergency Medical Technician-Paramedic is maintained and enriched by the willingness of the individual practitioner to accept and fulfill obligations to society, other medical professionals and the profession of Emergency Medical Technician. As an Emergency Medical Technician at the basic level or an Emergency Medical Technician-Paramedic, I solemnly pledge myself to the following code of professional ethics:

A fundamental responsibility of the Emergency Medical Technician is to conserve life, to alleviate suffering, to promote health, to do no harm, and to encourage the quality and equal availability of emergency medical care.

The Emergency Medical Technician provides services based on human need, with respect for human dignity, unrestricted by consideration of nationality, race, creed, color, or status.

The Emergency Medical Technician does not use professional knowledge and skills in any enterprise detrimental to the public well-being.

The Emergency Medical Technician respects and holds in confidence all information of a confidential nature obtained in the course of professional work unless required by law to divulge such information.

The Emergency Medical Technician, as a citizen, understands and upholds the law and performs the duties of citizenship; as a professional, the Emergency Medical Technician has the never-ending responsibility to work with concerned citizens and other health care professionals in promoting a high standard of emergency medical care to all people.

The Emergency Medical Technician shall maintain professional competence and demonstrate concern for the competence of other members of the Emergency Medical Services health care team.

An Emergency Medical Technician assumes responsibility in defining and upholding standards of professional practice and education.

The Emergency Medical Technician assumes responsibility for individual professional actions and judgment, both in dependent and independent emergency functions, and knows and upholds the laws which affect the practice of the Emergency Medical Technician.

An Emergency Medical Technician has the responsibility to be aware of and participate in matters of legislation affecting the Emergency Medical Technician and the Emergency Medical Services System.

The Emergency Medical Technician adheres to standards of personal ethics which reflect credit upon the profession.

Emergency Medical Technicians, or groups of Emergency Medical Technicians, who advertise professional services, do so in conformity with the dignity of the profession.

The Emergency Medical Technician has an obligation to protect the public by not delegating to a person less qualified any service which requires the professional competence of an Emergency Medical Technician.

The Emergency Medical Technician will work harmoniously with, and sustain confidence in, Emergency Medical Technician associates, the nurse, the physician and other members of the emergency medical services health care team.

The Emergency Medical Technician refuses to participate in unethical procedures, and assumes the responsibility to expose incompetence or unethical conduct of others to the appropriate authority in a proper and professional manner.

Courtesy National Association of Emergency Medical Technicians. Kansas City, Missouri.

lice officer with a knife. The police officer sustains a minor stab wound. Should the responding paramedic treat the critically injured burglar first or begin with the police officer, as the officer's partner insists? The paramedic may never see the burglar again, but could have to work with the injured officer and his partner for years.

As another example, emergency care is often needed by someone who cannot pay for the services, such as a homeless person. Should the paramedic consider the drain on the ambulance service or the effects on paying patients, insurance companies and taxpayers? How should these patients be treated? Are they deserving of less care because of their financial status?

With the decision to become a paramedic comes a responsibility to provide the same quality care to every patient, regardless of financial status, race, creed, gender, age, and so on. This can be one of the more challenging parts of a paramedic's job.

The Myth of Saving Lives

Somewhere along the way, the myth of saving lives found its way into the EMS profession. There are indeed times when paramedics save lives, but even in large EMS systems, this is by no means a daily occurrence. The vast majority of the time, paramedics are called upon simply to take care of people in need. Sometimes those needs are met with a combination of advanced invasive procedures, sophisticated pharmacology, and technical expertise. Other times, what a patient may need is a caring attitude, a few kind words, or safe transportation to an extended care facility (Fig. 2-2).

Between these two extremes lie many shades of gray. One measure of an outstanding paramedic is the ability to perceive a patient's real needs and to meet them. Along with each technique performed or drug administered there are certain inherent risks. For example, with the initiation of an IV line comes an added risk of rescuer infection. It is important for the paramedic to keep in mind that it can be just as dangerous to overtreat patients as it is to undertreat them.

Turn a Page of History

Some experts say EMS first started in Biblical times when a Good samaritan stopped to provide aid to an injured person. Others say that EMS actually began when Napoleon's army began to transport injured soldiers from the battlefront lines

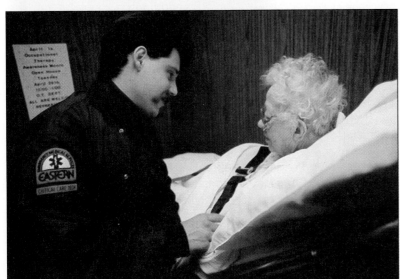

Figure 2-2

A, Life and death situations in EMS are infrequent when compared with the total call volume. B, Compassion and comfort for a sick or injured person is a skill that is used on nearly every EMS call. *Photographed by Craig Jackson.*

back to medical treatment areas. During the Korean and Vietnam conflicts, this concept had been refined with the development of mobile intensive care medicine. The trademark of this unique brand of medicine was rapid identification and correction of life-threatening emergencies, coupled with short on-scene times and the use of helicopters for rapid transport to mobile army surgical hospital units. With advanced life support (ALS) during transport, battlefield mortality of seriously injured soldiers in Vietnam was significantly reduced. In fact, the care was far better than that being provided in the civilian sector of America.

The organizational seeds of modern EMS were first planted in 1966 by a group convened by the National Academy of Sciences/National Research Council. The efforts of these participants culminated in publication of a landmark document titled *Accidental Death & Disability: The Neglected Disease of Modern Society,* now referred to as The White Paper.[1] This document put forth the conceptual model of an organized and coordinated system to deliver EMS. This setup was quite different from earlier ambulance services, which were often run by funeral homes and provided virtually no emergency care. The White Paper set the stage for an organized system that would reduce morbidity and mortality among trauma victims by ensuring continuity of emergency care. The system response began with recognition of the emergency and activation of the system. An EMS team responded and provided ALS care, both at the scene and enroute to the hospital. Treatment continued in the emergency department, operating room, critical care unit, or wherever the patient's specific needs could best be addressed. Last came the process of rehabilitation. One of the hallmarks of this coordinated system was the idea that the hospital could be delivered to the patient rather than delaying care until the patient was delivered to the hospital.

With this innovative approach, the term "ambulance driver" was finally laid to rest, and the EMT and paramedic were born. Currently, EMT-Basics are entry-level prehospital providers who provide both emergency care and transportation to ill or injured patients. Their education and training usually consist of a minimum of 110 hours of noninvasive medicine. EMT-Is, or Intermediates, are EMT-Basics with additional training and education that, depending on local policy, may prepare them to perform tasks such as placing intravenous lines, defibrillating a patient, providing invasive airway care, and administering a limited selection of medications. The training time spent in upgrading certification from EMT-Basic to EMT-Intermediate ranges from 40 to several hundred hours.

A paramedic is an EMT-Basic who has returned to school and completed a comprehensive education program that either meets or exceeds the knowledge and skill objectives in the Department of Transportation National Standard Curriculum for the EMT-Paramedic. Paramedics perform the same skills as EMT-Basics, as well as advanced and invasive skills such as endotracheal intubation, electrocardiogram (ECG) interpretation, cardioversion, and defibrillation. They can also initiate intravenous therapy and administer an extensive list of medications. The length of paramedic programs varies from 400 hours to over 2500 hours. Some paramedic programs offer associate or bachelor degrees.

Shortly after the White Paper was published, another major cultural event occurred in EMS. In the early 1970s, a television series called "Emergency" premiered, featuring two firefighter/paramedics named Johnny Gage and Roy DeSoto. Every week, these two health care professionals responded to a new set of emergencies. Their professional image and the quality of care they rendered remains a big part of the public's perception and expectations of EMS today.

Paramedic Functions

The practice of paramedicine is not simple. As a key member of the emergency medical services team, the paramedic extends the reach of a physician through the concept of delegated practice, which permits the performance of specific tasks while operating under the physician's license. The functions of a paramedic (Fig. 2-3) are:

1. Preparation
2. Activation
3. Evaluation
4. Stabilization
5. Communication
6. Transportation
7. Documentation
8. Education

The performance of these functions and other associated tasks requires that paramedics master the practical skills and develop a good foundation of medical knowledge in keeping with the current state-of-the-art prehospital practice. In some cases, paramedics may also be employed outside the prehospital setting in emergency departments, industrial clinics, or even performing physical examinations for insurance companies. The more conventional role of the paramedic is as a prehospital care provider. The remainder of this chapter covers prehospital functions in more detail.

Preparation

A lot of behind-the-scenes work goes into preparation for handling an emergency call (Fig. 2-4). Some of the preparatory tasks include:

- Assuring that the ambulance is cleaned and fully stocked with equipment and supplies. This is done before and after each call.
- Completing the vehicle maintenance check to assure the ambulance is in working order for a safe response.
- Studying the response area and noting any circumstances that might effect the emergency response, such as road construction and flooded underpasses.
- Learning the medical protocols and standard operating procedures of the EMS system.
- Exercising to maintain a level of physical fitness adequate for safe performance of the various physical tasks involved in prehospital care.

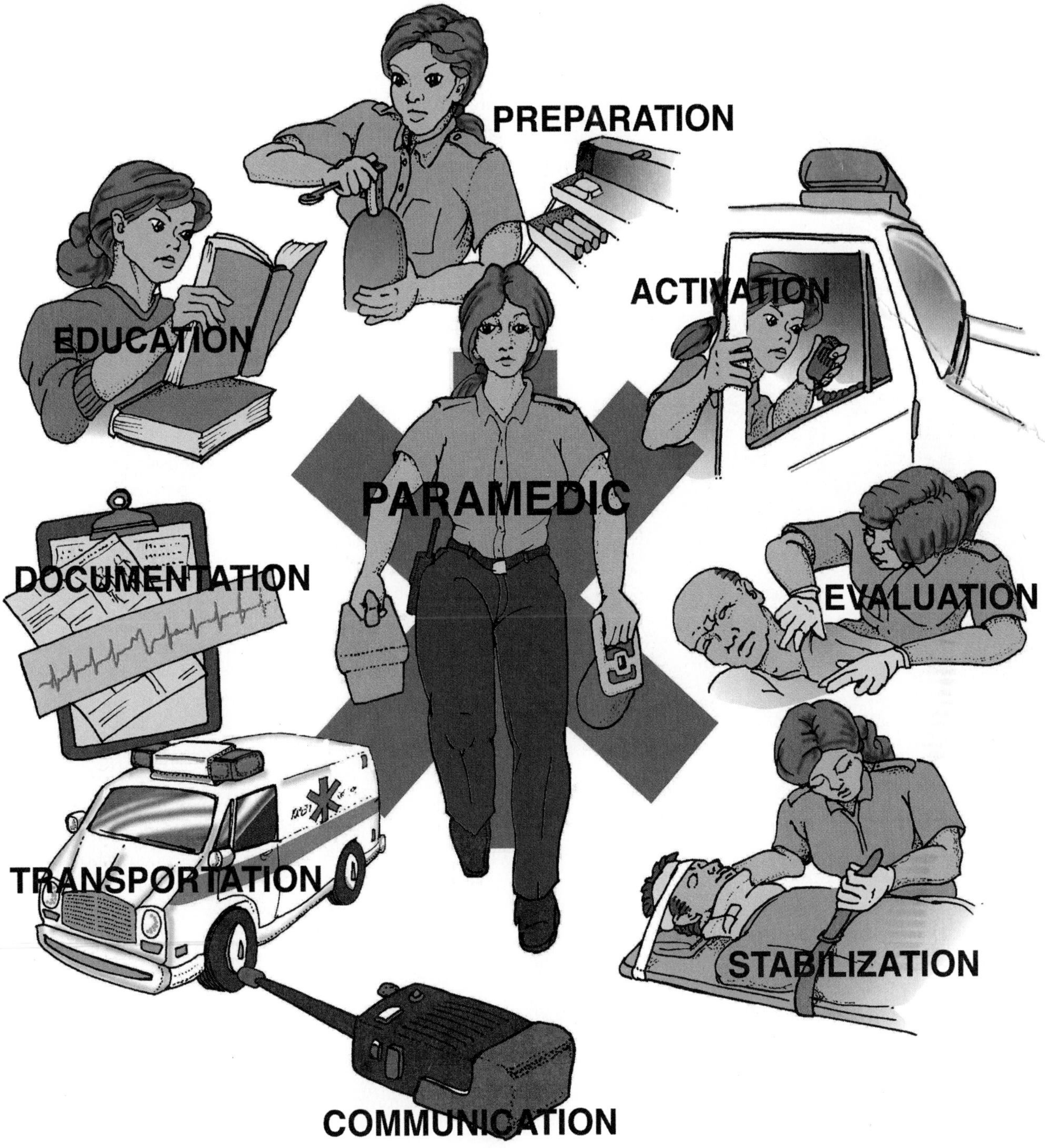

PREPARATION

ACTIVATION

EDUCATION

PARAMEDIC

DOCUMENTATION

EVALUATION

TRANSPORTATION

STABILIZATION

COMMUNICATION

Figure 2-3

The circle of function for a paramedic requires that the provider be skilled in many areas other than patient care. The image of an "ambulance driver" no longer exists and has been replaced by one of a highly trained and efficient health care professional.

- Maintaining mental well-being.
- Educating the public about how and when to activate the EMS system.

Activation

Within moments of receiving the call for assistance, the EMS team should be enroute. The first priority is a safe response to the scene. This is not guaranteed by simply turning on the red lights and sirens. A close look at "red light" laws shows that many are similar. In most places, an ambulance can exceed the posted speed limit, drive against the flow of traffic, and so on, as long as doing so does not endanger life or property. Red lights, sirens, and high-speed driving contribute very little to saving lives. When the call is within city limits, a high-speed response usually only saves a few seconds. Repeatedly

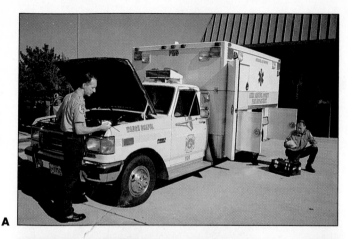

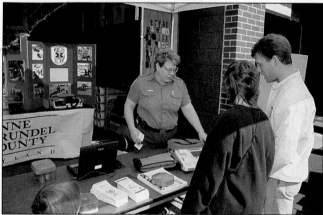

Figure 2-4

Preparation includes: A, ensuring that the vehicle and equipment are in proper condition and B, educating the community about the EMS system.

accelerating and slowing provides an uncomfortable ride, makes patient care more difficult, wears out the vehicle more quickly, and increases the risk of injury to the rescue team, the patient, and the public. The EMS system doesn't work if the ambulance doesn't arrive at the scene, and the patient should not have to survive the rescue delivery.

On the way to the scene, the paramedic should be considering the possible problems that may be encountered and what equipment will be needed to handle the situation.

Evaluation

This aspect of a paramedic's job consists of two main components: survey of the scene and patient assessment (these topics are covered in further detail in subsequent chapters). The survey, or assessment, of the scene includes:

1. *Scene safety.* Identification and control of anything that poses a threat or creates a hazard to the patient or the rescue team.
2. *Mechanism of injury or illness.* Observation of the mechanics of an incident to predict possible injuries.
3. *Hints at the scene.* Are there clues to the patient's problem, such as unvented heaters or empty pill bottles?

4. *Mutual aid needs.* What additional units, specialized equipment, or personnel will be needed?

Patient evaluation consists of initial assessment, focused history and physical exam, and continued assessment. The purpose of the initial assessment is identification and correction of life-threatening injuries. After life threats are addressed, the focused history and physical examination and continued assessment identify other problems.

Stabilization

In most cases, definitive care is not provided in the prehospital setting. It usually occurs in the hospital, where surgical intervention, blood replacement, and other advanced procedures can be provided. Even the patient in ventricular fibrillation, whose immediate need—defibrillation—is within the realm of prehospital intervention, requires intensive hospital treatment for myocardial infarction. Part of a paramedic's competency lies in understanding the appropriate time, place, and limitations for the application of prehospital care.

As a general rule, treatment of the trauma patient in the field should be kept to a minimum (e.g., spinal immobilization, airway management, control of bleeding) until the patient can be treated in the more controlled hospital environment. Scoop and run is not always appropriate, but unnecessary time in the field may place the patient at further risk by delaying definitive care.

The paramedic is the on-scene leader of patient care, but does not dictate how law enforcement or rescue personnel should do their jobs. EMS personnel must work closely with all involved parties to coordinate patient care with other aspects of the scene (Fig. 2-5). Disagreements about who is in charge will detract from patient care. Good rescuers understand that cooperative scene management best serves the patient.

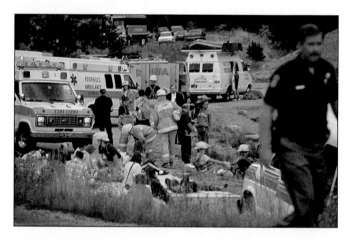

Figure 2-5

Intra-agency cooperation is essential to provide optimum levels of patient care and to ensure the safety of all the rescuers involved in the call. *Photographed by Howard Paul.*

Communication

The ability of the paramedic to communicate with the patient is fundamental to quality care. This can be difficult enough with a patient who is thinking clearly, but when hypoxia, illicit drugs, or head trauma alter cerebral function, the ability to communicate effectively becomes even more challenging (see Chapter 13).

The ability to communicate with family members and bystanders is equally important. These people may have little understanding of prehospital care but are often vocal at emergency scenes. Failing to spend a few moments communicating with the family can result in a very difficult scene as family members become uneasy.

Another key person in the communication loop is the paramedic's partner, who may be an EMT-Basic, Intermediate, or another paramedic. Other key professionals in the EMS system include first responders, fire, rescue, and law enforcement personnel. Each group has specific responsibilities, and effective communication among them is crucial to providing the best possible patient care.

Often described as the "eyes, ears, and hands of the physician," the paramedic must also be able to communicate efficiently with the receiving hospital. The best patient assessment means nothing if the information is not relayed effectively. Remember, the person receiving the report cannot see, hear, or feel what is being done in the field. The ability to paint the picture is important to the continuity of patient care in the emergency department (see Chapter 14).

Transportation

After making the decision to transport the patient, the paramedic also accepts the responsibilities of providing safe transportation and maintaining the continuity of care. Even the most routine transfer patient returning home or moving to an extended care facility should at least have their vital signs checked. The paramedic must never assume that a call will be problem free simply because a patient is going home. A basic life support (BLS) transfer can quickly deteriorate into a critical ALS situation.

Until the patient is turned over to someone of equal or higher certification or licensure, the patient's well being is the paramedic's responsibility. A good report at the receiving facility is essential to update the receiving staff on the patient's status, even if the status has not changed (see Chapter 14).

Documentation

As with many medical skills, the ability to write a clear, concise prehospital care report is an important part of a paramedic's job. Once completed, the prehospital care report becomes both a part of the patient's medical record and a legal document. It should be legible, grammatically correct, and whenever possible, paint a clear picture of everything that occurred from dispatch to delivery at the receiving facility.

The information contained in the report may also be a paramedic's best defense should legal action arise. Litigation usually occurs long after the actual call. Depending on the state's statute of limitations, several years may elapse before the complaint is filed and even more time before the case goes before a court. The report will probably be the only way to refresh one's memory about the details of the call (see Chapter 14).

Education

The paramedic course represents only one phase in the education and development of a paramedic. Depending on the call volume of the system in which the graduate works, it may be several months to a year before he or she becomes fully proficient in the field. Additional time, experience, and training will allow the proficient paramedic to take further steps toward becoming an expert in prehospital medicine.

After completing the paramedic course, the student takes written and practical examinations. Successful completion results either in certification or licensure, depending on state laws. This approval creates the expectation that the paramedic will remain competent throughout the certification period. Continued competency is accomplished through the process of continuing education.

A leading-edge drug therapy today may be considered "routine" in 6 months and "obsolete" next year. The field of medicine is always changing and the scope of paramedic practice changes with it. Some hospitals already employ paramedics in their emergency departments. Other areas are using them to provide public health services such as immunizations. As additional changes occur, more continuing education will be required. Professional journals and conferences, workshops, or seminars help to keep providers current. Participating in run reviews or audits is also an integral part of quality improvement for a paramedic. As the saying goes, "What gets you to the top doesn't keep you there . . . at least not for long."

Professional Organizations

Within the EMS profession, there are a number of professional organizations including:

1. American Ambulance Association (AAA)
2. American College of Emergency Physicians (ACEP)
3. National Association of EMS Educators (NAEMSE)
4. National Association of EMS Physicians (NAEMSP)
5. National Association of EMTs (NAEMT)
6. National Association of Search and Rescue (NASAR)
7. National Association of State EMS Directors (NASEMSD)
8. National Council of State EMS Training Coordinators (NCSEMSTC)
9. National Flight Paramedic Association (NFPA)

Each group works for the growth and advancement of prehospital emergency care.

by Marion Angell Garza

The push for health care reform, the rise of managed care organizations, and the consolidation of health care services, including ambulance services, have caused health care and EMS planners to reexamine the role of paramedics. How can their practice be expanded to help fill some of the gaps in the United States health care system?

While Congress debates how to provide "universal access" to health care, paramedics and other emergency personnel know that uninsured and underinsured patients have already found the key to universal access—A call for an ambulance provides transportation to a hospital emergency department, where primary and emergency care are given. There has been no incentive to halt this costly and inefficient system.

But managed care organizations, and the ambulance services that contract with them, have a huge incentive for reforming the system. Since managed care organizations are paid a lump sum in advance for all of the health care needs of a patient, they lose money every time they unnecessarily transport or treat a patient. Consequently, some ambulance services and managed care organizations have begun to develop plans in which paramedics can treat certain patients on the scene, referring them to an appropriate facility for follow-up care rather than transporting them to a hospital.

In rural areas, where hospitals may be hours away and where some are closing their doors, paramedics or EMTs are sometimes the only available health care providers. People living in such areas might even drop in at their local firehouse or rescue squad headquarters to ask emergency personnel for informal medical advice or care, rather than driving many miles to see a physician. Some EMS planners believe that, if this practice is legitimized and paramedics are given more assessment and treatment skills, they can help fill the gap in rural health care.

In a few rural areas, other local health care practitioners, such as physicians, nurses, and physician assistants, have formed consortiums to help support and craft new programs for paramedics. Overtaxed and underfunded public health organizations are realizing the advantage of teaching paramedics new skills and using them for immunization programs, TB screenings, and medication compliance programs. Paramedics have also learned new skills, such as how to maintain IV pumps and central lines, to care for critical patients during long transports.

Pilot projects aimed at expanding the scope of practice of paramedics are cropping up in rural and urban areas. Curricula are being developed, based in large part on the Community Health Aide/Practitioner Program that has been providing the bulk of health care in rural Alaska since the 1970s. A few paramedics at a time are learning to perform more in-depth patient assessments, use new tools, perform simple lab tests, suture wounds, and monitor chronically ill patients.

As paramedics accept new roles in the US health care system, even the language they use is changing. For example, the term "prehospital care" is being replaced with "out-of-hospital care" and "EMS" and "ambulance services" are becoming "mobile health services" or "mobile community health services" to reflect their expanding role. It is an exciting time to begin a career as a paramedic. In the future, paramedics will likely have the authority and training to help patients

Reciprocity

When paramedics move to another state, or in some cases to another county in the same state, they must transfer their license or certification. This process is called reciprocity. It usually involves written and practical testing and in some cases may require the applicant to obtain additional education. The National Registry of EMTs is an agency that prepares and administers standardized national testing materials for four levels of prehospital providers: First Responder, EMT-Basic, EMT-Intermediate, and EMT-Paramedic. Currently, this is the only agency that has established a national minimum standard of competency. Most states accept National Registry registration as an equivalent to their state certification/licensure. Thus, designation of a National Registry EMT (NREMT) can serve as a means of obtaining reciprocity between states or counties in the same state.

Career Opportunities

Many people believe that working as a paramedic in the field is a young person's job. Although many people enter the profession in their mid-twenties, there is no hard-and-fast rule that says it must be that way. As with any other job that requires a large amount of physical work, the paramedic must be in good physical condition and have the desire to do the work.

There are a number of possibilities for the paramedic who wishes to change job focus. One option is a move to a management position. Typically, the first step is to move to a field or shift supervisor position. Another possibility is to shift toward education, possibly starting as a field training officer or continuing education instructor. There are also teaching opportunities in paramedic education programs at colleges, universities, and hospitals. Continuing education and street experience are usually needed to pursue these goals.

Finally, there is the choice of moving into a different branch of medicine altogether. Nursing, physician assistant practice, other allied health professions, and medical school are all options, depending on the individual's interests. Almost all of these changes in career path require additional education.

SUMMARY

The paramedic's profession is a challenging one. The long-term commitment to maintaining the knowledge and skills is not easy to make. Leadership, teamwork, and decision-making skills come naturally to some paramedics; others have to work at them. The field of prehospital medicine is filled with caring people and the profession is maturing year by year. Few other jobs offer the rewards and diversity of being a paramedic.

REFERENCES

1. National Academy of Sciences, National Research Council: Accidental Death and Disability: The Neglected Disease of Modern Society, Washington, 1966, United States Department of Health, Education, and Welfare.

SUGGESTED READINGS

1. Brown E, Sindelar J: The Emergent Problem of Ambulance Misuse. *Ann Emerg Med,* 22:4, April 1993.

2. Cummins RO: Moving Toward Uniform Reporting and Terminology. *Ann Emerg Med,* 22:1, January 1993.

3. Dernocoeur K: Streetsense—Communications, Safety, and Control, ed 2, Brady-Prentice Hall.

4. Dick T, Federoff L: Why Do Paramedics Intimidate Their Leaders? *JEMS,* 17(2), 1993.

5. Federeriuk CS, *et al:* Job Satisfaction of Paramedics: The Effects of Gender and Type of Agency of Employment. *Ann Emerg Med,* 22:4, April 1993.

5. Haller J: The Beginnings of Urban Ambulance Service in the United States and England. *JEMS,* 1990.

6. MacLean C: The Future Role of Emergency Medical Services Systems in Prevention. *Ann Emerg Med,* 22:11, November 1993.

7. Page JO: The Paramedics, Morristown, 1979, Backdraft Publications.

8. Page JO: The Magic of 3 AM, Solana Beach, 1986, JEMS.

9. Page JO: Twenty Years Later, Solana Beach, May 1986, JEMS.

10. Rosemurgy AS, *et al:* Prehospital Traumatic Cardiac Arrest: The Cost of Futility. *J Trauma,* 35(3), 1993.

11. Rosen RA: Jewels—The Peanut Butter Kid and the Girl With the Rose. *Ann Emerg Med,* 22:11, November 1993.

12. In Roush W (ed): Principles of EMS Systems, Dallas, 1989, American College of Emergency Physicians.

13. Sampalis JS, *et al:* Impact of On-Site Care, Prehospital Time, and Level of In-Hospital Care on Survival in Severely Injured Patients. *J Trauma,* 34(2), 1993.

14. Shuster M, Shannon HS: Differential Prehospital Benefit of Paramedic Care. *Ann Emerg Med,* 23:5, May 1994.

15. Sosna DP, *et al:* Implementation Strategies for a Do Not Resuscitate Program in the Prehospital Setting. *Ann Emerg Med,* 23:5, May 1994.

16. Staten C: A Vision of Tomorrow. *JEMS,* July 1993.

17. Werdman MJ, Paturas J: Prehospital ALS, What Next? *Emergency,* November 1993.

Chapter 3

The EMS Call

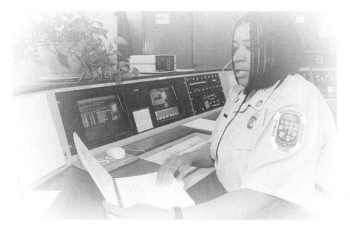

A paramedic should be able to:

OBJECTIVES

1. Describe the role of the public in the EMS system.
2. Describe the main functions of dispatch.
3. Identify vital information needed from dispatch in order to prepare for patient care.
4. Identify the key factors that should be assessed when evaluating the scene.
5. Given a set of patient situations, identify appropriate transport decisions.
6. Describe the appropriate transfer of responsibility for patient care in the receiving emergency department.
7. Describe prerun and postrun activities.

KEY TERMS

1. **Computer-aided dispatch**—an enhanced dispatch communication system in which electronic (computerized) data is used to assist dispatchers in selecting and directing EMS resources.
2. **Emergency medical dispatcher**—1) a program for educating dispatchers in the appropriate use of emergency medical dispatching, including prearrival instructions, radio terminology and triage; 2) a person trained in asking the caller standard questions, prioritizing the call and providing prearrival instructions.
3. **Prearrival instructions**—patient care instructions given to the caller prior to the arrival of EMS resources.
4. **Enhanced 911**—a fully integrated, computerized 9-1-1-access telephone system.
5. **Patient care report**—a prehospital patient chart that establishes pre-set criteria of patient demographics, vital signs, treatment modalities, etc.

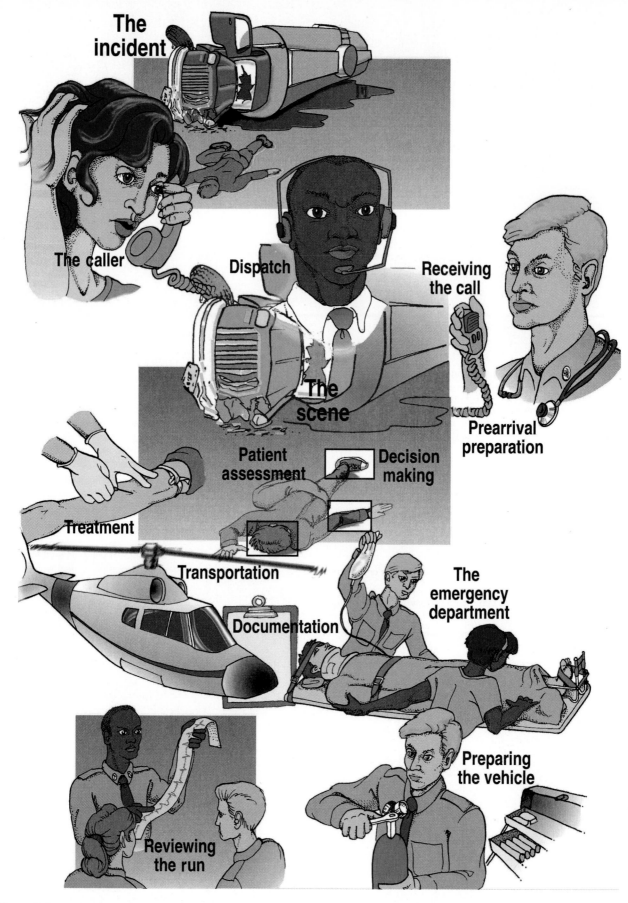

The incident

The caller

Dispatch

Receiving the call

The scene

Prearrival preparation

Patient assessment

Decision making

Treatment

Transportation

Documentation

The emergency department

Reviewing the run

Preparing the vehicle

Figure 3-1

Components of the EMS call.

EMS is unique in that, in any given day, no two calls will be exactly the same. However, there is a natural history to each EMS call. In this chapter, the call and its components will be discussed. By understanding the components of the call, the paramedic can manage time efficiently.

The EMS call can be broken down into the components shown in Figure 3-1.

The Incident or Illness

Each EMS call begins with a reported incident or illness (Fig. 3-2). Unfortunately, the person initiating the call does not always perceive the problem in the same fashion as a trained paramedic. Because the average caller has no medical training, the situation is typically considered an emergency, even though it may seem minor to the paramedic. The caller's perceptions are further colored by fear and helplessness. Many of the calls received by an EMS system clearly do not require an emergency response. However, paramedics must look at the situation from the perspective of the untrained patient or bystander. From this vantage point, many more runs appear appropriate.

No matter what situation is encountered, paramedics must be prepared to identify and manage patient problems with the ultimate goal of providing efficient, high-quality patient care. Patients come in all sizes and present with varying degrees of severity. Certain EMS systems have a higher percentage of specific types of incidents, such as violent trauma in the urban setting or cardiac emergencies in retirement communities. Paramedics must exercise flexibility to adjust to each patient and the needs of the specific environment.

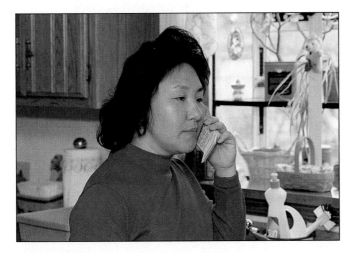

Figure 3-2

The caller reports an incident or illness.

The Caller

The person initiating the 9–1–1 call may be the patient, a family member, a friend, or even a stranger. Therefore, the quality of information available to the dispatcher can vary. The caller may be delayed in accessing the EMS system due to lack of familiarity with emergency phone numbers or knowledge of who provides EMS care in the area. Fear, despair, and other emotions can also interfere with the caller's ability to provide vital information. When the patient is the caller, the medical condition itself can interfere with the ability to express what is wrong. Although some of these variables cannot be controlled by the EMS system, two variables can: access and public education.

Access

All calls for emergency care begin with citizen access. The public is a vital member of the emergency health care team. Calling 9–1–1 or a seven-digit telephone number is the common method for accessing EMS. Because of the time that elapses from the point the call is placed to the arrival of the ambulance, it is imperative that EMS access begin as soon as possible.

Most states are partially covered by the standard or enhanced universal 9–1–1 telephone number.[5] As of December 1996, the National Emergency Number Association estimates that 85 percent of the US population, mostly urban areas, has 9–1–1 access. Advances in cellular technology have allowed citizens to access 9–1–1 by some cellular phones[3]. Many EMS services have also incorporated cellular technology into their communication systems.

Public Education

EMS can and should be involved in educating the public to maximize patient care in the field. The better the care prior to EMS arrival, the more likely a favorable outcome. The two areas that can have the greatest impact on the outcome are first aid and CPR training. Bystanders or family members trained in first aid can control bleeding, open an airway, immobilize a trauma patient, and activate the EMS system in a more efficient fashion. CPR can extend the window of opportunity for resuscitation by several minutes.

Dispatch

EMS systems strive to have a paramedic crew on scene within minutes from the time the call is received at the emergency communications center. Communities with a tiered response system can send both an EMT-Basic and paramedic crew to each emergency. Fire service personnel and police officers are also often dispatched either as first responders or as the primary EMS provider. Dispatch serves three main functions: information gathering, EMS contact, and prearrival instructions.

Dispatch must also coordinate other public safety services, mutual aid requests, and disaster response.

Information Gathering

Emergency medical dispatch (EMD) and citizen use of 9–1–1 have evolved as key components of an effective EMS system. Several EMD training programs have been developed to provide dispatchers with training, quality assurance or total quality management (QA/TQM), and medical direction. A good dispatch system functions by adhering to protocols designed to guide the dispatcher in gathering necessary information using standardized questions based on the patient's complaint (Fig. 3-3). This information can then be used to determine the appropriate level of response and the required prearrival instructions.

EMS Contact

When sufficient information has been gathered, the dispatcher must determine the proper level of response and contact the appropriate prehospital providers. The EMS unit dispatched must receive sufficient information to allow them to prepare for the call and arrive safely at the scene.

One of the key obstacles faced by dispatchers is the determination of the level of care required (e.g., basic or advanced) and the response configuration (response code and number of vehicles). This requires that the dispatcher recognize the patient's needs based upon established medical criteria. This is best accomplished by following a preestablished protocol. One form of protocol that is widely used is Criteria Based Dispatch. Computer Aided Dispatch (CAD) systems that include protocols in their programs are also now being integrated into EMS communication systems around the country.

Once dispatch determines the appropriate level of response, information must be exchanged with the responding

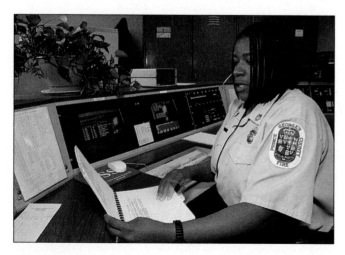

Figure 3-3

Emerging as a subspecialty of EMS, dispatchers have a variety of tools at their disposal and often are able to greatly impact the outcome of an emergency situation.

EMS unit. The goal is to present sufficient information and not waste time with unnecessary details.

Prearrival Instructions

Even in the best EMS systems, paramedics cannot arrive at the patient's side immediately. To improve the patient's chances of survival, dispatchers must be able to provide prearrival instructions to the caller. The EMD can give instructions on performing CPR, administering mouth-to-mouth resuscitation, controlling bleeding, and even delivering a baby.

Resources other than EMS may be needed on certain calls. Dispatch may need to access fire, police, helicopter mutual aid, or disaster services.

Receiving the Call

Given the limitations of the information available to the dispatcher, paramedics must be sure to receive enough information enroute to prepare for the patient's care. Vital information includes the nature of the complaint, the status of the patient (e.g., awake and breathing), the location of the incident, the safety and accessibility of the scene, and the type of resources available. Sometimes, specific information about the medical complaint will be available.

Prearrival Preparation

While enroute to the scene, the paramedic must fully prepare for the patient and the situation. All potential problems, impediments, and possible hazards should be anticipated. There are six principal elements to consider: the number of patients, patient access, scene safety, role assignments, patient condition, and required equipment and medications.

Multiple Patients

Early in the paramedic's communication with dispatch, the potential number of patients must be established. The paramedic must consider the resources available and how to divide patient care among prehospital personnel, make triage decisions, and go into disaster mode if the number of patients exceeds the resources available.

Patient Access

The paramedic must consider potential patient access problems and be prepared to address them. Access problems can occur both outdoors and indoors. Outdoor restrictions that may impede access include mountains, heavy woods, steep inclines, water rescue, wilderness, mud, and distance from the road. Indoor factors include tall buildings (especially if the elevators aren't operating), narrow stairs, obese patients, and working in cramped spaces. The paramedic must also be knowledgeable about street locations, traffic hazards, special events in progress, railroad crossings, drawbridges, and any other information that will impact quick, unobstructed access to the patient.

Scene Safety

Scene safety issues must also be considered before arrival. Any police, fire, heavy equipment, extrication, or electric company backup needed must be contacted before the paramedic arrives, to shorten access time to the patient.

Role Assignments

ALS system configurations vary from a first responder with one paramedic to two or more paramedics responding as a team. Regardless of the configuration, each prehospital provider must play a defined role in the patient's care. If the paramedic tries to do everything alone, care will be slow and inefficient. Patient care can be maximized by preassigning roles to each member of the team.

Patient Condition

Enroute to the scene, serious thought should also be given to the patient's potential condition and the steps required to handle it. For example, if the patient's complaint is chest pain, then airway problems, respiratory distress, cardiogenic shock, and hypovolemic shock should be considered and prepared for. Serious secondary conditions that could develop based on the patient's complaint should also be anticipated. For example, in the case of chest pain, the paramedic should be prepared to manage cardiac arrest. Procedures that may be needed should be reviewed prior to arrival on scene to foster smoother patient care.

Required Equipment, Supplies and Medications

Once the worst potential problems have been considered, the equipment, supplies, and medications required can be determined. The prehospital team should bring these supplies to the patient to expedite treatment. Significant time can be wasted if someone has to run back to the ambulance for needed equipment. Equipment and supplies can include (but are not limited to) extrication equipment, splints and other immobilization devices, backboards, a stair chair, stretchers, medication box, airway kit, oxygen, and IV equipment.

The Scene

Upon arrival at the scene, a comprehensive evaluation of the scene should occur. At this time, scene safety and access can be more precisely assessed, the scope of the incident determined, environmental factors considered, leadership estab-

lished, and communication and scene control initiated. Information previously provided by dispatch should not bias future decisions or result in tunnel vision.

Scene Safety

No scene should be approached until it has been determined safe for prehospital personnel. The last thing needed is for providers to join the number of patients, thereby decreasing the available resources at hand (For more on scene safety, *see* Chapter 15).

Patient Access

The fastest, safest method for getting to the patient must be coupled with the best method for removing the patient from the environment. For example, although it may be possible to reach and extricate a patient trapped in a car over a large embankment, it may still be difficult to transport the patient back to the ambulance. Instead, a helicopter may be able to land in a field nearby so that the patient will not be lifted up the embankment. The paramedic evaluates the access problems, designs the best possible solution, and determines the equipment and personnel needed. It is important that the paramedic constantly reassess the scene to ensure that he or she is continually aware of any changes in the scene situation.

Scope of the Incident

The paramedic must also determine the potential scope of the incident. Are there multiple victims? Are hazardous materials present? Are scene resources insufficient? Should additional resources such as police, first responders, and BLS personnel be considered? These questions must be answered before patient assessment begins.

Environmental Factors

Paramedics are often forced to work in less-than-desirable situations that challenge the ability to provide the most effective patient care. The most dramatic example of this would be a mass-casualty incident, where large numbers of patients are injured or killed in the aftermath of an earthquake, flood, or tornado. Attempting to treat patients in severe weather conditions, such as cold, snow, rain or severe heat, poses similar challenges for paramedics.

Upon arrival at each scene, paramedics must take note of the surroundings and the factors that will positively or negatively affect their work. Often, a few simple preliminary adjustments will greatly improve the working environment. For example, if the area is cluttered, clear away a space that permits a more comfortable and safe environment. If the patient is found on the street and can be moved safely, take a moment to move him or her into the ambulance. This will afford the patient some privacy as well as provide shelter for the patient and crew. Improving scene conditions may require calling for the assistance of specialized rescue or specialty units.

Leadership

A critical component of being a paramedic and responding to an EMS call is taking command of the situation. Leadership is the ability to influence others to perform assigned tasks according to job specifications. There is nothing as important as delegating authority in an emergency medical situation. For directives to be carried out, each team member must understand his or her individual assignment and believe in the ability to carry out those tasks.

Paramedics learn to lead by following the examples set forth by other leaders. Because prehospital care often requires working with limited support under somewhat adverse conditions, paramedics must accept leadership as a necessary fact of organizational life. Those with conflicting emotions about their leadership qualities will find it difficult to employ authority prudently and productively.

Communication

Effective communication is another form of influence and an equally important component of scene management. True communication hinges on creating a relationship in which all parties play distinct but complementary roles. The major purpose of effective communication is the transmission of information. For the paramedic, this will take the form of face-to-face conversations with patients, family, bystanders, and staff. It also requires written reports with history and treatment information properly documented, radio transmissions for medical direction, and additional patient care directives.

Scene Control

One of the biggest challenges in scene management is handling bystanders and the patient's family and friends. The paramedic must walk a fine line between accessing important information and getting bogged down with people other than the patient.

There are four straightforward rules to assist in these situations. The foremost rule is that the patient's welfare comes first. Second, the paramedic must determine exactly what information is needed and how much time should be spent gathering it. The third rule is to remember that family or friends of the victim are often under tremendous stress and must be dealt with gently. The fourth is to remain assertive but not aggressive (*see* Chapter 13).

Patient Assessment and Decision Making

Patient assessment and decision making are the core of prehospital care. The key factor is understanding what actions are available to the paramedics and then tailoring interventions to the assessment findings. To establish treatment priorities, the paramedic differentiates between conditions that can be treated in the field, and those that require hospital care.

One unique aspect of prehospital patient assessment is working in full view of the public (Fig. 3-4). This aspect affects

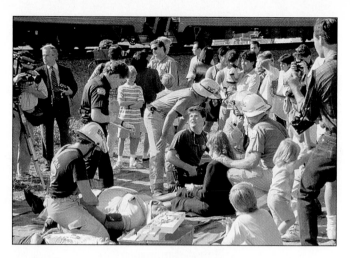

Figure 3-4

The presence of bystanders on emergency calls adds to the overall stress and safety concerns at the scene. *Photographed by Colin C. Williams.*

both the paramedic and the patient. From the paramedic's perspective, it is similar to working in a fish bowl, continuously scrutinized by others. The paramedic cannot afford to be self-conscious or arrogant. At the same time, the patient is faced with the humiliation of answering personal questions and being examined in public by a total stranger. To offset the patient's discomfort, the paramedic must be gentle and sensitive to the patient's need for privacy.

Reassessment and continued management of the patient are also essential during transport. Transport mode, hospital destination, and therapeutic interventions should be reconsidered if the patient's condition changes while enroute.

Treatment, Transport and Documentation

Often, treatment should begin during patient assessment. One of the most common errors made in the field is delaying vital life-saving treatment until the assessment is complete. Likewise, many paramedics wait until all treatments and procedures are complete before transporting the patient. Transport should be viewed as a form of treatment and as with all treatments, it must be prioritized.

Destination Decisions

Once a decision has been made to transport the patient, the paramedic must decide on the destination. The choice of one hospital over another may depend on patient request, proximity, specialized care, emergency department patient-diversion status, or local protocols. Although system protocols should include specific criteria to assist with this decision, preplanning and analysis of the available facilities are essential. Consideration must be given to the patient's needs, the capabilities of the potential receiving facilities, and the *effect* of the transport time on the patient. The decision must be made based on what is best for the patient, and not the wishes of a particular hospital health maintenance organization (HMO), insurance company, or paramedic.

Communication with Medical Direction

As the physician surrogate on the scene, the paramedic becomes the physician's eyes, ears, voice, and hands. The ability to quickly and accurately transmit patient assessment information allows a remote physician to form a mental picture of what is occurring at the scene.

Acuity and Transport Coding

To maximize use of system resources while protecting the patient, many EMS systems have developed levels of acuity for transport. Dispatch determines the unit level for response and the necessity for the use of lights and sirens. A second decision is made after patient assessment. In ALS systems, there are four possible choices regarding transport of the patient. The lowest acuity patients do not need transport by ambulance. The second level requires hospital transport but not paramedic care. The third level requires a paramedic on board but is stable and does not need emergent transport. The fourth level is unstable or may soon become so and requires both a paramedic and transport with lights and siren. These decisions can be made by the paramedic on the basis of protocols, or in conjunction with medical direction.

Air Medical Transport

When considering air medical transport, the risk/benefit ratio must be weighed. A helicopter is usually warranted if rapid access to a higher level of care is required. Another consideration is access to an adequate landing zone with no potential hazards. Unfortunately, it is not always possible to assess all conditions prior to contacting the helicopter. Generally, however, air medical transport should be considered if the following would be of benefit to the patient:

- Faster access or access to poorly accessible areas
- Faster transport to an appropriate facility
- Higher level of care

On occasion, a patient may be in a location that is more rapidly approachable by helicopter than by ambulance. If there is a need for rapid access, air medical transport may be warranted.

A helicopter can also provide rapid transport when a patient is a long distance from an appropriate facility. Keep in mind, though, that helicopter services are very expensive; the expense should be justified by the patient's condition.

Some helicopter services provide a physician on board. Others may have protocols for advanced airway procedures or other treatments not permitted by local protocols. If the patient requires such services, the helicopter should be called. (Air medical transport is further explored in Chapter 53.)

The Emergency Department

Paramedics may not leave the emergency department until the patient's care has been properly transferred. Proper transfer means that the nurse or physician has been given both the written and verbal reports on the patient's condition. The physician or nurse must also have the opportunity to further question the paramedic about the patient.

The primary concern should be that hospital personnel have all the information needed to properly care for the patient. To deliver a clear concise report, the following is suggested: If the hospital was contacted prior to arrival, ask the receiving personnel if they are aware of the report. If they are aware of the report, offer an update on what has transpired since that contact. The update should include significant changes in the patient's vital signs, complaints, and physical findings. If they are not aware of the report, repeat it.

If the paramedics are not needed immediately for new calls, they should remain at the hospital until the emergency physician has initially assessed the patient. This is an excellent opportunity to improve skills by comparing findings. Ask the physician if he or she agrees with the field assessment; this provides valuable feedback on field care. After the EMS unit leaves the hospital, the only means the ED staff has to determine what happened prior to arrival is the prehospital care report (PCR). Therefore, it is imperative that all findings be documented and any patient valuables or personal effects are turned over to the ED staff.

Preparing the Vehicle

Preparing the EMS vehicle for the next call involves restocking, cleaning, and performing maintenance. Restocking is replacing the materials used on the previous call which includes, but is not limited to, medications, IV supplies, airway materials, oxygen, disposable splints, dressings, linens, and gasoline. Both the vehicle and any nondisposable equipment used, such as back boards, PASGs, and traction splints, must also be cleaned and disinfected in accordance with federal guidelines. Contaminated needles and angiocaths equipment must be properly disposed of in appropriate containers. Biohazardous waste and linen must be placed in a designated biohazardous bag. All equipment, including defibrillators, splints, and the vehicle itself, require ongoing maintenance to ensure readiness for future calls.

Reviewing the Run

The time between the end of one call and the beginning of another should be used to review the call that was just completed. Run reviews should include discussion of both what was done well and what could be improved in the future to maximize patient care. The review should be accomplished in a nonthreatening, informal manner; no notes are necessary. Everyone's ideas should be heard and discussed, and the best suggestions should be incorporated into future action.

SUMMARY

Paramedics are confronted with a wide variety of calls, ranging in nature from minor to life threatening. To be effective, all aspects of the call must progress in a manner that expedites and contributes to proper patient care.

REFERENCES

1. American College of Surgeons Committee on Trauma: Advanced Trauma Life Support Course for Physicians, Chicago, 1993, American College of Surgeons.

2. American Heart Association: Emergency Cardiac Care Committee and Subcommittees, Guidelines for cardiopulmonary resuscitation and emergency cardiac care; I:Introduction. *JAMA,* 268:2172–2183, 1992.

3. Pies R, Weinberg A (ed): Quick Reference Guide to Geriatric Psychopharmacology, Branford, 1990, American Medical Publishing.

4. Commission on Accreditation of Ambulance Services: Ambulance Accreditation Standards, Dallas, 1992.

5. Emergency Medical Services, Sixteenth Annual EMS State and Province Survey. *JEMS,* 21(12): 196–199, 202–204, 207–218, 220–224, 226, 1992.

6. King County Emergency Medical Services Division: Criteria Based Dispatch, Washington, 1990, King County Medical Services.

7. National Institutes of Health: National Heart, Lung, and Blood Institute. 9−1−1; Rapid identification and treatment of acute myocardial infarction. US Department of Health and Human Services, 1994. (Pub. #94-3302).

Robert A. Swor DO, FACEP

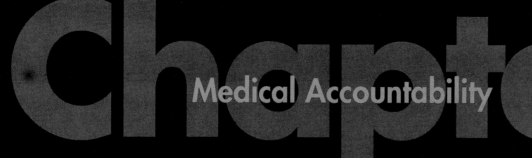

Chapter 4
Medical Accountability

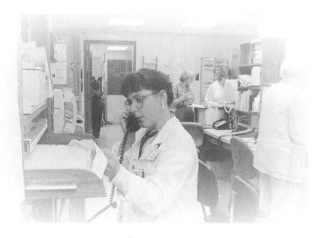

A paramedic should be able to:

OBJECTIVES

1. Describe the concept of delegated practice.
2. Describe the off-line and on-line responsibilities of a physician EMS medical director.
3. Compare and contrast prospective, concurrent and retrospective medical direction.
4. Discuss the role of medical direction in prehospital education, evaluation, policy and protocol development, and operational issues.
5. Define the term *protocol* and identify appropriate areas to consider in the development of medical protocols.
6. Explain why hospital categorization (designation) and destination policies are important to an EMS system.
7. Discuss the role of quality assurance and quality improvement processes in the EMS system.
8. Describe the role of field EMS providers in EMS research.

KEY TERMS

1. **Delegated practice**—Legal means by which a paraprofessional may provide patient care under the supervision of a physician.
2. **Medical accountability**—Refers to the fact that an individual practitioner, at whatever level that individual functions, must acknowledge and accept responsibility for the assessment and interventions performed on a patient by that individual.
3. **Medical direction**—A system of physician-directed quality assurance that provides professional and public accountability for medical care in the prehospital setting.
4. **Off-line medical direction**—Also called *indirect medical direction*. Refers to the medical oversight of EMS patient care, which occurs before and after the care of the individual patient.
5. **On-line medical direction**—Also called *direct medical direction*. Direct voice communications between a field unit and a physician or designee for the purpose of supervising the medical care of an emergency patient.
6. **Quality assurance**—A systematic evaluation method used to assure quality care and provide information to caregivers about how to improve it.
7. **Quality improvement**—A management method and philosophy which emphasizes quality as measured by customers, provision of resources to facilitate improvement, and improvement of processes as a means of improving patient care.

The provision of medical care in the field by paramedic personnel was a revolutionary concept when introduced in the late 1960s. Prior to that time, emergency care for patients outside of the hospital was limited to first aid measures rendered by bystanders and public safety personnel who were minimally trained and equipped. With the exception of care given on battlefields, the delivery of medical care by physician surrogates had no precedent.

Because EMTs and paramedics act as physician surrogates in delivering patient care and must practice sound medicine as determined by the medical community, medical accountability and physician involvement are essential. Emergency medical care has evolved dramatically in America. As the public has become more sophisticated regarding health care, the demand for accountability of actions by the medical profession has grown.

Prior to the mid-1960s, care was delivered only by someone known and trusted by the patient—the private physician. As emergency care systems have developed, more care of the critically ill and injured is delivered by providers unknown to the patient. The result is a demand for emergency care evaluation, both from within the medical community and from accreditation agencies such as the Joint Commission for Accreditation of Health Care Organizations (JCAHO). Emergency care in hospitals and in the prehospital setting is a highly scrutinized area of medicine.

This chapter examines the relationship of the field EMS provider to the broader scope of medicine.

Physician Involvement

The basis for the paramedic's action in the field is the practice of medicine, and sound medical practice is clearly the province of physicians. Because it is impossible within the confines of the paramedic curriculum to teach all aspects of emergency medicine as taught in medical school and residency training programs, there must be a solid relationship between the paramedic and the physician who provides medical accountability. Responsibility for oversight of medical care rendered in the field belongs to the medical director. A strong relationship between the paramedic, the EMS service, and the medical director is the basis of sound patient care in the field.

Authority to Provide Patient Care

Medical care of patients is tightly regulated by statute in the United States. Historically, this activity has been performed by individuals (physicians or nurses) or entities (hospitals and other health care facilities) licensed to do so by individual states. The authority to prescribe medications is restricted through state boards of pharmacy, and controlled substances are further regulated by the federal government through the Drug Enforcement Administration.

The authority to provide medical care is contained in laws called medical practice acts of the individual states. The specifics of these statutes vary significantly from state to state.

The role of prehospital care providers as defined by these medical practice acts depends on the level of provider and the state of licensure or certification. However, one aspect is consistent across the United States; the paramedic must function under the control, authority, or direction of a physician.

For most paramedics, the authority to care for patients is considered to be granted through the concept of delegated practice. This means that a paramedic renders care as a physician delegate, acting under the license of a physician who has agreed to supervise that care. EMS systems are now recognizing that all EMS care is medical in origin, and care rendered by first responders and EMT Basics should also be accountable to the medical community. The necessity of medical responsibility for care rendered outside of the hospital is the basis for the concept of medical direction.

Medical Direction/Medical Control

Medical control has been defined as "a system of physician-directed quality assurance that provides professional and public accountability for medical care in the prehospital setting."[7] Also called *medical command* or *medical direction,* the essence of medical control is ensuring that EMS activities provide medical benefit to patients. This broad mandate has resulted in a wide variety of EMS system configurations across the country.

The most common mechanism of medical direction in EMS throughout the country is a physician who oversees EMS. The Federal EMS Systems Act of 1973, which funded the development of modern EMS, defined medical control and left its implementation to regional EMS lead agencies. This allowed for development based on each region's unique needs and resources. This also represents a major weakness in medical direction in areas that do not allow the medical director the authority required to assure medical accountability. Initially, medical oversight of the new "EMS projects" was rendered by a single physician, the Project Medical Director, who was responsible for EMS care in the region. The term has since been replaced by the more appropriate term, *EMS Medical Director* (EMSMD), a reminder that EMS systems are no longer short-term projects.

The EMSMD position has evolved considerably. Early systems were directed by physicians from a variety of disciplines: surgeons, internists, cardiologists, orthopedic surgeons, emergency physicians, and others. Today, the EMS medical director is most commonly an emergency physician by training or active practice. In some areas (mostly rural), this role is filled by a family practitioner, surgeon, or other individual with interest or expertise in EMS. The American College of Emergency Physicians (ACEP) has published a position statement which asserts: "The primary role of the medical director is to ensure quality patient care. Responsibilities include involvement with the ongoing design, operation, evaluation, and revision of the EMS system from initial patient access to definitive patient care."[1]

Interest in EMS by the medical community has increased. With that interest, medical control boards, comprised of physi-

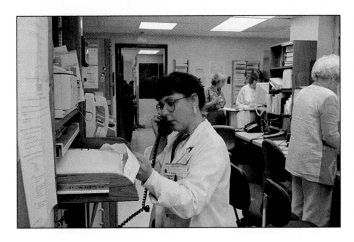

Figure 4-1

On-line medical direction from a physician at a hospital allows the physician to interact in the care of the patient on scene by using information supplied by the EMS provider.

cians who represent the medical community, have developed to supervise EMS activities. Depending on the local structure, these boards either select and oversee or merely advise the EMSMD and EMS lead agency.

Medical direction responsibilities can be characterized as either "on-line" or "off-line." On-line (or direct) medical direction refers to direct voice communications with a physician (or designee) at the time that care is being rendered to the patient (Fig. 4-1). Off-line (or indirect) medical direction refers to those activities that involve medical input into the EMS system and occur either before or after the care of that patient (Fig. 4-2).

On-line Medical Direction

The first EMS systems in the United States were developed with physicians actually staffing ambulances for emergency responses. Pilot programs in Miami, Columbus, Ohio, and

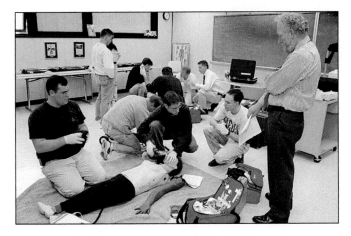

Figure 4-2

Off-line medical direction takes place at times other than during patient care and involves such activities as educating paramedics in new skills and case review.

Seattle first demonstrated that care delivered outside of the hospital was effective, and paramedics directly supervised by the physician could provide that care. The system then evolved to the stage in which the physician was not physically present but would be immediately available (on-line) for medical direction via two-way radio. This included interpretation of ECGs transmitted by radiotelemetry. In this way, the physician not only consulted on each case, but was medically accountable and responsible for patient care. Some states specifically identify that a physician-patient relationship exists when a paramedic is on-scene and calls for medical direction.

The practice of on-line medical direction varies significantly from region to region on issues such as what communication devices are used and if communications are established with a single facility, one of a number of regional receiving facilities, or a single individual. The provider of medical direction is also variable. Direction may be rendered by the system medical director or a designee such as an emergency department physician, a specially trained nurse (a Mobile Intensive Care Nurse, MICN), or a paramedic.

Even when a nonphysician provides on-line medical direction, the physician remains responsible for the direction given. The nonphysician is limited to a clarification of the protocols, whereas a physician may go beyond them. Systems require that the individual giving on-line medical direction be knowledgeable regarding emergency care, the local protocols, and the local EMS system.

One of the original purposes of radio communications was interpretation of ECG rhythm strips by radiotelemetry. While initially valuable, this specific application of radiotelemetry is becoming less common, and a number of large systems have stopped using telemetry entirely. Some states continue to require its capability for EMS communications.

The level of usage of on-line medical direction also varies. Some regions require radio communications for any paramedic-patient contact, and others only require it in cases involving advanced life support procedures. Some EMS researchers have argued that on-line medical direction consumes valuable personnel time and yields few benefits, and some systems do not use on-line medical direction at all, depending instead on protocols and retrospective physician oversight of paramedic care. A sampling of cases for which on-line medical direction may be of the greatest benefit is listed in Box 4-1.[5]

Off-line Medical Direction

The central role of medical direction is to assure timely, appropriate, and high-quality patient care. This requires medical input into virtually every facet of the EMS system. Direction during the emergency is useless unless general supervision ensures that the appropriate training, resources, and evaluation are in place. This occurs before and after each individual patient care contact and is "off-line" or indirect in its effect. This does not suggest that it is less important. It is, in fact, crucial to the development of a mature EMS system.

For off-line medical direction to be successful, there must be a commitment from the physician medical director, the

- Critical medical cases
- Patients with vague chief complaints or complaints with complicated differential diagnoses (e.g. Chest pain, abdominal pain, allergy)
- Field pronouncement
- Refusal of care
- Medical-legal issues
- Determination of destination

Adapted from Braun O, Direct Medical Control, in NAEMSP: Prehospital Systems and Medical Oversight, 2 ed, St. Louis, 1994, Mosby–Year Book.

EMS service, and the paramedic. The paramedic has an ongoing responsibility to maintain and heighten his or her knowledge and skills. This can only happen if the paramedic is willing to be critically evaluated and is willing to take training and assessment seriously. In dealing with human lives, "almost" is not good enough.

Prospective Medical Direction

The purpose of prospective medical direction is to assure that the system components are in place to provide quality medical care. Interpreted broadly, these structural components include everything from system access to patient delivery. Other components include initial training, testing, and certification of providers; continuing education; protocol development; operational policy and procedure development, and legislative activities (Fig. 4-3).[4]

Education

The bulk of initial education is medical; therefore, both its development and provision require direct input from physicians knowledgeable in emergency medicine and EMS. This must be done in cooperation with professional educators at all levels of EMS certification. Education must ensure that the provider is able to perform appropriate tasks and procedures and has adequate background to grow professionally in his or her field. The education must also be integrated with the evolving body of medical knowledge. This is often accomplished via special programs (e.g., Basic Trauma Life Support, Advanced Cardiac Life Support, and Pediatric Advanced Life Support) that may be required as part of initial training or subsequent to licensure. EMS educational requirements apply not only to EMT-Basics and paramedics, but also to calltakers and dispatchers, first responders and on-line medical directors.

Technical skills are usually practiced in the confines of a hospital. Often the medical director or designee must represent the prehospital community in its efforts to receive clinical training in the hospital. Specialty areas such as anesthesia, intubation training, and obstetrics are areas of critical need for initial training. These are often difficult for the EMS community to access without significant medical support.

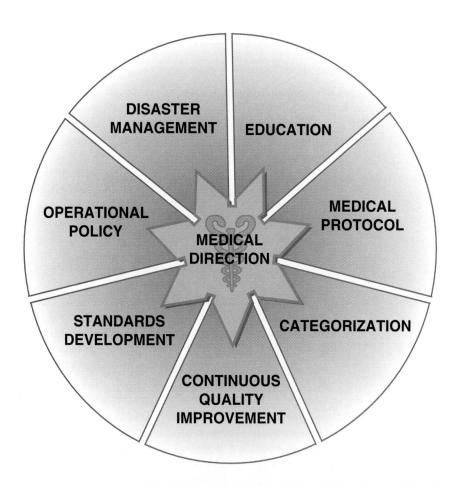

Figure 4-3

Prospective medical direction ensures that the components for quality medical care are in place.

Continuing education requirements must also be developed with direct medical input, based on the scope of EMS practice in the community. They should include education specific to the local environment and the field of EMS as a whole. Ideally, the educational program is tied directly to issues identified during review (quality assessment). Continuing medical education for providers whose days and shifts vary is extraordinarily difficult to deliver on a consistent basis. In one suburban Chicago EMS system, the EMS authority conducts approximately 60 conferences per month to reach providers.[14] There must be a clear administrative commitment on the part of the agency and a personal commitment by the individual paramedic to maintain a knowledge base and grow through professional education.

Education and conditions in the local medical community together define the "scope of practice" in an EMS system. This dictates the type of care rendered by providers individually and by the system as a whole.

Operational Policy

The involvement of the medical community in operational matters is viewed by some with suspicion and hostility. However, good medical care does not exist in a vacuum. Providers must be dispatched appropriately, arrive quickly, have adequate ancillary support on scene (e.g., extrication, scene safety, and first response), and have appropriate drugs and equipment available. When a medical voice articulates the need for this type of support, it is more likely to become a priority in the system. Ambulance service owners, fire chiefs and other providers must similarly have a voice in the development of medical protocols that are practical and medically appropriate (Fig. 4-4). The medical director must also have input into EMS personnel training and hiring practices.

Medical Protocols

Medical protocols form the backbone of the care rendered by the EMS field provider. They indicate which conditions to treat, procedures to perform, medications to give, and so on. Protocols provide a structured approach to important clinical issues faced in the field. Some authors further classify certain protocols as "standing orders," or orders that can and should be performed prior to any other therapy or intervention, such as an immediate quick look and possible defibrillation for a cardiac arrest victim and intubation for a patient with respiratory failure. Most systems will also have medical protocols for triage of the trauma patient, based on criteria that can be physiological (vital signs) or related to mechanism of injury (ejection from vehicle). These triage protocols go hand-in-hand with the designation of hospitals that will receive the seriously injured trauma patient.

In addition to clinical issues, protocols should address medical-legal and ethical issues (e.g., refusals of care, do not resuscitate orders, ambulance diversions, and abuse and neglect of children and adults). Protocols also must address when and how providers use radio communications and what mode of transportation they employ (e.g., ALS vs BLS, and lights and sirens vs nonemergency traffic). The distinction between medical and operational protocols is a subtle one and will vary in its interpretation among different EMS systems.

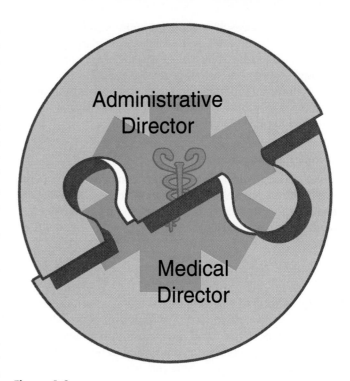

Figure 4-4
Administrative personnel and medical directors must work together and share the responsibility for the development of a quality EMS system.

System-Wide Standard Development

In addition to development of protocols, the EMS system must implement system performance standards. These must be developed through a consensus process that reviews national standards and decides which are applicable locally. Standards may apply to individual providers (e.g., training, continuing education and testing, and minimum procedural proficiency) or to the system itself (e.g., response times and staffing). This process is valuable in itself because it educates members about system function and what to expect.

Categorization/Designation

The procedure of designating which hospitals are appropriate to receive an individual patient is one of the more complex and politically charged issues facing medical directors and the medical control boards. This procedure by definition directs patients away from certain institutions and therefore may be perceived as "stealing" patients and revenue. For that reason, and because of the straightforward medical care issues involved, this process must be conducted as openly and objectively as possible. Some systems merely survey receiving facilities regarding the services they provide (e.g., surgery, obstetrics, and availability of specialized diagnostic equipment) and allow individual providers to make decisions based on that data. This is not inappropriate. The medical director must understand the capabilities of the hospitals served by the EMS agency and, based on this, must articulate clear policies.

A number of states have developed elaborate systems to care for trauma patients, based on research showing that trauma systems improve patient outcomes. The process of designation in states with trauma systems is complex and expensive. To become a Level I trauma center in accordance with criteria developed by the American College of Surgeons, a hospital must demonstrate extensive patient care capabilities, educational programs, and quality assurance procedures. This process assures a commitment by the hospital and its providers to provide high-quality trauma care.

Disaster Management

Disaster management is an important component of the EMS system. Procedures and protocols must be in place to respond and care for the victims of disasters and multi-casualty incidents (*see* Chapter 51).

Concurrent Medical Direction

Review of medical care at the time it is rendered can be referred to as concurrent medical direction. This provides education that is specific and direct to the individual circumstances. It also optimizes the quality of patient care. Many physicians see this as reviewing care when the patient arrives at the emergency department, but in fact this is retrospective. The patient who arrives in the emergency department with an endotracheal tube inserted can appear to be properly intubated, for instance, but that tube may have been placed with improper technique after long periods of apnea. To be effective, concurrent evaluation must truly take place at the time care is given.

In the best of all worlds, an EMSMD is physically available at each patient encounter, understands the limitation of the prehospital environment, and is experienced in the provision of medical care outside of the hospital. Policies and protocols are also designed with the appreciation of that environment in mind. This is rarely the case in practice. Efforts are needed to educate both providers on-scene and physician policymakers regarding the field environment. In large EMS services, scene response by the EMSMD should be a basic part of the responsibilities of the medical director or an assigned representative, such as a clinical supervisor. This person should be readily available to assist, assess, and teach at the time care is being rendered. In small services this may not be possible, although it remains desirable.

Direct communication between the paramedic and an on-line physician is another form of concurrent medical direction. It is therefore imperative that physicians providing on-line medical direction be properly trained and understand the EMS system and its protocols.

Retrospective Medical Direction

All of the topics above are important in designing a system that "should" provide quality field care. Equally important, but less fully developed in most systems, retrospective medical direction is a method of after-the-fact review to answer the questions, "Does the system actually provide quality medical care?" and "What can be done to provide better care?" This process is absolutely vital to the development of mature EMS systems.

The continued documentation of performance shows that the EMS system is accountable to the medical community and the community at large.

Quality assurance (QA) and quality improvement (QI) are important methods of achieving this accountability. The implementation of QA and QI methods appear to be very similar on the surface, and many use the terms interchangeably. However, they are, fundamentally different and have a very different impact on the individual provider and the system as a whole.

Quality Assurance

Quality assurance is a method of assuring that medical care is provided at a quality level consistent with standard medical practice. Its central concepts include routine review of care to assess its quality, clear documentation of problems identified, and an emphasis on feedback to the individual practitioner (Fig. 4-5). The basic assumption of the method is that most care providers try to do a good job, want to know if mistakes are made, and will work diligently to improve their performance if a problem exists. QA also assumes that medical practice is an art as well as a science, and the people best able to evaluate care are other professional practitioners. EMS literature has confirmed that review of care by EMS providers improves the practice of the provider and the system at large.[11] This concept of peer review is vital to the evaluation of care in any EMS system.

Traditionally, EMS QA activities have focused on paramedic care. This is because early EMS laws placed only paramedics under medical direction. As systems matured, it be-

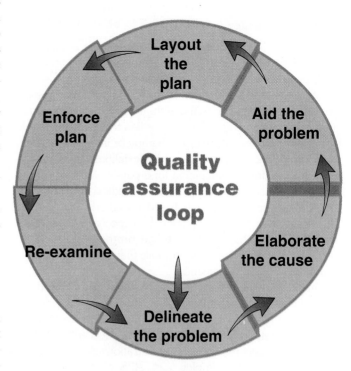

Figure 4-5

Quality assurance is a method of ensuring that superior medical care is provided.

came apparent that there are multiple components to quality EMS care and every portion of a system should be evaluated, including (at a minimum) dispatch, first response, paramedic care, and on-line medical direction.

However laudable the goals of QA programs, they suffer from a number of limitations. A review of care after the incident always has the potential of incorrectly second guessing the caregiver. Worse, retrospective reviews that look for individuals who consistently make mistakes take on the appearance of witch hunters, and in turn strain the entire system. QA also makes the rather dramatic assumption that the individual provider is able to improve care rendered and is solely responsible for the success or failure of that care. A failed intubation, for instance, is due to a "problem" with the paramedic who was unsuccessful. A second shortcoming is that QA programs often identify problems that cannot be solved. To assure public and professional accountability, QA programs will continue to be part of most EMS systems, but their shortcomings have led EMS leaders to search for other methods to improve care (Table 4-1).

Quality Improvement

Quality improvement is a method that Japanese industry embraced after World War II, and was introduced to American industry in the 1970s. This revolutionary approach to management emphasizes quality as measured by the "customer," improvement of systems of care, and the use of data (facts) to make management decisions. QI also stresses the role of management in creating the environment and the system that enable frontline personnel do their jobs effectively. The emphasis on faulty processes as a major impediment to quality (85% of problems in some studies) puts the focus on tools and environments rather than on individuals. In the example of the paramedic who was unable to intubate, there might have been problems with poor suction equipment, inadequate medical assistance on scene, or poor quality laryngoscopes.

The concept of the customer as the one who defines quality is foreign to many health care providers. QI philosophy identifies a customer as anyone who uses the goods and services of an individual. The patient, the nurse who receives that patient, and the first responder who depends on the paramedic for patient care might all be considered to be customers who evaluate the quality of the paramedic's function. The emphasis on facts for decisions requires semiscientific study to obtain "hard" data on specific items needing improvement.

The QI concept of problem solving is similar to the patient care process itself (see Box 4-2). The focus on the process places the frontline provider—the person who best understands patient care—in the central role. The ultimate QI goal is to empower field providers to continuously improve care by focusing on the needs of customers, and by focusing through improving the processes of care, the organizational culture will change so that all activities become channeled toward the goal of enhancing the quality of patient care.

For those reasons, it is absolutely vital that paramedics be committed to and actively involved in evaluating and improving the system. QA, QI, and other methods that assure accountability, improve patient care, and increase efficiency of the EMS system will all be integral parts of EMS systems of the future.

TABLE 4-1 Comparison of Traditional Management Ideas and Continuous Quality Improvement	
Traditional QA	**Continuous Quality Improvement**
Inspection is the key to quality.	Inspection is too late. Quality cannot be inspected into a process—it must be built in from the beginning.
Defects are caused by workers.	Most defects are caused by the system, specifically, by inputs into the process that are defective.
Fear and reward are proper ways to motivate.	Fear should be eliminated to encourage ideas for improvement.
Make purchases based on the lowest bid.	Buy from suppliers who offer the greatest value.
Quality is expensive.	Quality leads to lower costs.
Quality control experts and inspectors can ensure quality.	Quality is made by a commitment from management at the highest level.
People can be treated like commodities—add more when needed and lay off when fewer are needed.	People are on important resource.
Reward the best performers and punish the worst to motivate people for greater productivity.	Because most variation is caused by the system, judging people who perform as well as they are allowed to by the system destroys teamwork and is counterproductive.
Profit is the most important indicator of a company's health.	Running a company by profit alone is like driving a car by looking in the rearview mirror—it tells you where you've been but not where you're going.

From Polsky (ed): Continuous Quality Improvement in EMS, Dallas, 1992, American College of Emergency Physicians.

BOX 4-2 Comparison of the Function of a QI Team with the Process of Patient Care	
Quality Improvement Team	**Patient Care**
Problem	Chief complaint
Observable symptoms	History and physical examination
Theories of causes	Differential diagnosis
Tests of theories	Lab, x-ray
Identified causes	Final diagnosis
Recommended solutions	Treatment
Reexamination	Follow-up visit

From Wilson AG: Implementing Quality Improvement. In Swor RA, et al: Quality Management in Prehospital Care, St. Louis, 1993, Mosby–Year Book.

Sample Report #3, Generic Ambulance Service Report

Individual Personnel Summary

(Prehospital Report Date Range: 06/01/91 through 09/01/91)
(Total Number of Prehospital Reports: 70)

EMT Name: Wilton, George
EMT Level: EMT-Paramedic
EMT Certification Number: 0120361896
Current Squad Number: 0000000074

Certification Status

(* indicates certification expired or due to expire within 90 days)

EMT-Ambulance: 11/23/91 *   ACLS: 03/15/93

EMT-Advanced: 11/23/91 *   BTLS: 11/23/91 *

EMT-Paramedic: 04/15/91   PHTLS: 06/01/91 *

BCLS: 03/15/92

Field Procedures

Legend: {1} = Not Indicated but Done   {2} = Indicated but Not Done
              {3} = Indicated Unsuccessful   {4} = Indicated and Successful

Procedure	{1}	{2}	{3}	{4}
Oral/Nasal Airway	0	1	0	11
Assisted Ventilation	0	1	1	12
Tracheal Intubation	0	0	4	2
Esophageal Airway	1	0	1	1
Cricothyroidotomy	0	0	0	0
Needle Thoracostomy	0	0	0	0
Peripheral IV Catheter	0	1	2	21
Central IV Catheter	0	0	0	1
Defib/Cardioversion	0	0	0	4
PASG	1	0	0	7
Medication Administration	0	0	0	13
Oro/Tracheal Suctioning	0	1	1	10
Spinal Stabilization	0	0	0	13
Traction Splint Device	0	0	0	6
Total Field Procedures	2	4	8	101

Figure 4-6

Generic ambulance service report: Individual Personnel Summary. *In Polsky (ed): Continuous Quality Improvement in EMS, American College of Emergency Physicians, Dallas, 1992.*

Documentation

Any review of medical care must be based on clear, complete data. This data usually originates in the patient care record (PCR), which the provider completes as part of the care of that patient. The PCR communicates initial findings and pertinent data to providers in the hospital, serves as a legal record of the event, and provides data for review of individual and system performance (Figures 4-6 and 4-7) (*see* Chapter 14).

Commitment

The EMS system must be firmly committed to providing the time, personnel, and resources necessary to following through on issues raised by a QI program. This requires an organizational commitment from everyone—the medical director to the first responder. Giving lip service to quality is easy; the leaders of the system must be willing to support improvement both philosophically and financially and to integrate front-line personnel into programs to improve patient care.

Sample Report #1, Generic Ambulance Service Report

Prehospital Activity Summary

(Prehospital Report Date Range: 06/01/91 through 09/01/91)
(Vehicle Unit Number Range: 0000000045 through 5000000010)
(Total Number of Prehospital Reports: 113)

Patient Demographics

< 2 yrs:	4 (3.5%)	19-40:	37 (32.7%)	Avg. Patient Age:	48.5
2-10:	2 (1.8%)	41-65:	25 (22.1%)	Num/Pct Males:	76 (67.3%)
11-18:	0 (0.0%)	> 65 yrs:	45 (39.8%)	Num/Pct Females:	37 (32.7%)

Etiology (Num/Pct)

Respiratory:	16 (14.2%)	Gastrointestinal:	9 (7.9%)
Cardiovascular:	34 (30.1%)	Other Illness:	0 (0.0%)
Metabolic:	7 (6.2%)	Motor Vehicle Crash:	28 (24.8%)
Psychiatric:	4 (3.5%)	Gunshot/Stab Wound:	5 (4.4%)
Ob/Gyn:	4 (3.5%)	Other Blunt Trauma:	3 (2.7%)
Neurologic:	2 (1.8%)	Other Penet. Trauma:	1 (0.9%)

Occurrence Times

Time	Sun	Mon	Tue	Wed	Thu	Fri	Sat	Time: Total/Pct
0001-0400	5	2	1	0	1	3	4	16/(14.2%)
0401-0800	2	1	0	2	1	2	1	9/(7.9%)
0801-1200	1	4	3	2	2	5	2	19/(16.8%)
1201-1600	2	3	6	5	4	4	4	28/(24.8%)
1601-2000	5	4	2	1	1	4	5	22/(19.5%)
2001-2400	7	1	0	0	0	6	5	19/(16.8%)
Daily Total	22	15	12	10	9	24	21	113/(100.0%)

Figure 4-7

Generic ambulance service report: Prehospital Activity Summary. *In Polsky (ed): Continuous Quality Improvement in EMS, American College of Emergency Physicians, Dallas, 1992.*

Research

The ultimate responsibility of the EMS community is to provide its patients with the best possible care. This requires that the EMS system must continually evaluate and improve itself. QA and QI methods review care and compare it with established norms of care. These practices are researched to assess their relevance. As a field that has been in existence for less than 30 years, there are many areas of EMS care that must be critically evaluated. While not all medical directors and prehospital providers have the resources and expertise to do research, efforts to improve EMS in this capacity are the responsibility of all members of the system.

Future of Medical Direction

The EMSMD is a vital link in the provision of medical care on the street. The medical director must be able to assess medical care in the context of the EMS environment, educate providers, interact with the hospital community, make neces-

Prehospital Activity Summary

Transport Acuity Level

Level of Acuity		BLS	ALS
Level 1 (non-life-threatening):	78 (69.0%)	74 (94.9%)	4 (5.1%)
Level 2 (potential life-threatening):	29 (25.7%)	7 (24.1%)	22 (75.9%)
Level 3 (imminent life-threatening):	6 (5.3%)	1 (16.7%)	5 (83.3%)

Transport Disposition

Transported to Regional Facility:	88 (77.9%)	Treated at Scene, Not Transported:	8 (7.1%)
Transported to Nearest Facility:	5 (4.4%)	Dead at Scene, Not Transported:	2 (1.8%)
Transported to Specialized Care:	4 (3.5%)	Unknown Transport Disposition:	6 (5.3%)

Prehospital Time Intervals (in minutes)

Average Access Time:	9.8	Average Scene Time for Illness:	30.8
Average Response Time:	8.0	Average Scene Time for Injury:	24.2
Average Transport Time:	18.8	Average Vehicle Extrication Time:	23.7

Field Procedures Outcome

Procedure Indicated and Successful:	132 (83.5%)
Procedure Indicated but Unsuccessful:	14 (8.9%)
Procedure Indicated but Not Done:	3 (1.9%)
Procedure Not Indicated but Done:	2 (1.3%)
Unknown Procedure Outcome:	7 (4.4%)
Total Field Procedures:	158 (100.0%)

Patient Disposition

Discharged Directly to Home:	103 (91.2%)
Transferred to Acute Care Facility:	2 (1.8%)
Transferred to Skilled Nursing Facility:	3 (2.7%)
Transferred to Rehabilitation Facility:	3 (2.7%)
Left Hospital Against Medical Advice:	1 (0.9%)
Expired While in Hospital:	1 (0.9%)
Other Specified Disposition:	0 (0.0%)
Unknown Disposition:	0 (0.0%)

Figure 4-7

(Continued)

sary hospital training available to the system, be the local expert on EMS research, and act as the patient advocate in the system. In turn, the system must grant the medical director sufficient authority to carry out these responsibilities.

The 1980s produced a generation of medical directors in EMS. Many systems now employ full-time EMSMDs. Organizations such as the American College of Emergency Physicians (ACEP), the Society for Academic Emergency Medicine (SAEM), and the National Association of EMS Physicians (NAEMSP) have encouraged and supported physician interest and involvement in EMS. This interest has resulted in a wealth of EMS physician education and research and further led to the development of specialized training programs specifically designed to train physician leaders for EMS. These EMS subspecialists should become the leaders of the industry in the years ahead.

SUMMARY

Since the medical standard of care is determined by physicians, the EMS medical director should be an integral part of the system. The quality of care provided is the responsibility of the entire system; the provider shoulders a large part of this responsibility. Although there are many intermediaries to whom the provider answers (e.g., medical directors, supervisors, and courts), the patients and the communities in which they live are the ultimate authorities that will judge the care. The EMS provider should not be intimidated by that responsibility, but instead understand that the ability to render patient care is a privilege.

REFERENCES

1. American College of Emergency Physicians: Policy statement on Medical Direction of Prehospital Emergency Medical Services, Dallas, 1992.

2. In Polsky (ed): Continuous Quality Improvement in EMS, ACEP, Dallas, 1992.

3. Berwick DM, Godfrey AB, Roessner J: Curing Health Care: New Strategies for Quality Improvement, San Francisco, 1990, Jossey-Bass Publishers.

4. Boyd DR: The History of Emergency Medical Services Systems in the United States of America. In Boyd DR, Edlich RF, Micik S (ed): Systems Approach to Emergency Medical Care, Norwalk, 1983, Appleton-Century-Croft.

5. Braun O, Callahan ML: Direct Medical Control, In National Association of EMS Physicians, Prehospital Systems and Medical Oversight, ed 2, St. Louis, 1994, Mosby Lifeline.

6. Hoffman JR, Luo J, Schriger DL, et al: Does Paramedic-Base Hospital Contact Result in Beneficial Deviations From Standard Prehospital Protocols. West J Med, 153:283–287, 1990.

7. Holroyd B, Knopp R, Kallsen G: Medical Control: Quality Assurance in Prehospital Care. JAMA, 256:1027–31, 1986.

8. Committee on Trauma, American College of Surgeons: Resources for the Optimal Care of the Injured Patient, Chicago, 1993.

9. Stout JL: System Financing. In Roush WR (ed), Principles of EMS Systems: A Comprehensive Text for Physicians, Dallas, 1989, American College of Emergency Physicians.

10. Swor RA, Rottman SA, Pirrallo RG, Davis E: Quality Management in Prehospital Care, Philadelphia, 1993, Mosby Lifeline.

11. Swor RA, Bocka JJ, Maio RF: A Paramedic Peer-Review Quality Assurance Audit. Prehosp Dis Med, 6(3):321–326, 1991.

12. Wilson AG: Implementing Quality Improvement. In Swor RA, Rottman SA, Pirrallo RG, Davis E (ed): Quality Management in Prehospital Care, Philadelphia, 1993, Mosby Lifeline.

13. Zehnder WJ, Davidson SR, Kelly JJ, Cionni D: Non-Transports of Prehospital Patients: Is Stronger Medical Control Needed? Ann Emerg Med, 20(4):446 (abs), 1991.

14. Zydlo S, Personal Communication, 1991.

C.J. Shanaberger, EMT-P, JD

Chapter 5

Legal Accountability

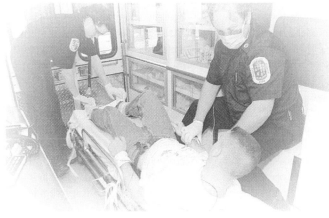

A paramedic should be able to:

OBJECTIVES

1. Describe the basic structure of the legal system in the United States.
2. Define negligence and recognize the four elements that must be proved in order to recover damages.
3. Explain standard of care as it pertains to prehospital care.
4. Identify statutory provisions pertinent to the paramedic.
5. Describe the paramedic's responsibilities in using and protecting a patient's medical information.
6. Differentiate among expressed consent, implied consent and involuntary consent.
7. Define abandonment as it relates to prehospital care.
8. Identify legal issues in the non-transport patient encounter.
9. Explain the principles of use of force and use of restraints.
10. Identify factors affecting resuscitation decisions in the prehospital setting.
11. Describe the paramedic's professional responsibilities related to preservation of evidence at a crime or accident scene.

KEY TERMS

1. **Abandonment**—Termination of the patient care without the patient's consent, at a time when there is a need for on-going care, and when the patient is harmed as a result.
2. **Implied consent**—The assumed consent of an unconscious patient or other person who is unable to participate in decision-making in an emergency medical condition.
3. **Informed consent**—Agreement to medical treatment that is based on sufficient information for a reasonable person to make a decision.
4. **Malpractice**—Professional misconduct, or violation of the standard of care, which is the cause of injury to another.
5. **Negligence**—A failure to act as a reasonably prudent person would, which directly causes harm to another.
6. **Scope of practice**—The specified medical practices that can be performed by a licensed or certified health care provider, usually established in statute or regulations.
7. **Standard of care**—The measure of competence of a professional in a malpractice practice action, based on the degree of knowledge, judgment, skill and care possessed by other professionals in the same field of practice.

A lthough it might be argued that the paramedic's role is confined by legal limitations, understanding the medical-legal aspects of the position actually enables the paramedic to lead a fulfilling career as a medical professional. Because some legal principles establish the foundation of the paramedic's everyday actions, a review of these concepts is important.

The Legal System

Sources of Law

There are four sources of law (Table 5-1). Constitutional law is based on the Constitution of the United States of America. Each state also has a Constitution, which is subject to the federal Constitution. A specific provision in the United States Constitution that is important to EMS includes the Fourteenth Amendment (*see* Box 5-1). The procedural steps that must be afforded to paramedics during disciplinary action, if employed by a public agency, are rooted directly in the "due-process" clause of the Fourteenth Amendment. In addition, the Constitution has been interpreted as assuring rights to citizens with which the government may not interfere, except under certain circumstances, such as the right to privacy, the right to refuse medical treatment, and the right to be free from racial discrimination. An important aspect of constitutional law is that no state may enact a law that nullifies the protections, rights, and privileges established by the US Constitution.

Statutes are another form of law. These are codifications established by Congress, the legislative branch of the federal government, and the state legislatures. Subcategory laws are ordinances, enacted by municipalities, and resolutions, enacted by counties. These are sometimes generically referred to as "local laws," which are subject to the "higher" law of state and federal statute and constitution. This means a county resolution may impose more restrictive conditions than a state or federal law, but may not conflict with it.

Governmental agencies, such as a state office for EMS, exist by the enactment of a statute establishing the agency and defining its powers, structure and responsibilities. Among the powers of an agency is the authority to enact regulations under which the agency operates. For example, a statute that empowers an EMS agency to certify persons as paramedics

may enact regulations regarding the specific procedural steps for doing so. Regulations or rules have the authority of law, but if a rule conflicts with the state statute, the statute overrides. Some state statutes are very detailed and lengthy, leaving little room for detailed regulations; other states have voluminous rules. Only the legislature can change a statute. Regulations or rules, in contrast, are created and changed by an agency after a public hearing.

Common law is also known as case law or "judge-made" law. This is law derived from the evolution of society's accepted customs and norms, as pronounced in the decisions of judges. The principle of stare decisis, which literally means "to stand by decided cases," establishes common law decisions as precedent for similar court cases in the future. Common law and its precedents change through time. In this way, law can change without the involvement of a legislature or regulatory body.

This evolution of law through case law is important as EMS evolves. There are very few federal statutes that directly pertain to prehospital emergency medical care, and state laws vary in scope and clarity. In addition, because EMS is a relatively young field, there are fewer precedents in prehospital care than in other areas of health care. As a result, there remains some uncertainty as to how a court will interpret EMS-related statutes and the actions of paramedics.

Court Systems

The American legal system is composed of criminal and civil law (Table 5-2). Criminal law refers to conduct or offenses that have been codified in statutes by the legislature (state and federal) as crimes or "public wrongs." A criminal case is prosecuted by an attorney for the government (the prosecutor) on behalf of the citizens. Violation of these laws can result in fines, imprisonment, or both.

Civil law involves private matters (e.g., contracts, domestic relations) between persons or legal entities such as corporations. An individual, called the plaintiff, may seek recovery of money or other forms of relief from another private person or entity, known as the defendant. "Tort" is a civil claim involving any wrongful act or injury done by a private person in a careless or reckless manner against another person or his property that causes injury or damage. A claim of medical negligence, or malpractice, is a tort action.

Another area of civil law is administrative, or regulatory law. This pertains to a governmental agency's authority to enforce the rules, regulations and statutes pertinent to its func-

TABLE 5-1	Sources of Law

Category	Source
Constitutional	Federal and State governments
Statute	Federal and State governments
Ordinance	Municipal government
Resolutions	County government
Regulations	Agency created by state
Common law	Societal norms decided by judges

TABLE 5-2	Types of Law		
Type	**Foundation**	**Action Initiated by**	**Penalty**
Criminal	Statute that codifies conduct or offenses as crimes or "public wrongs"	Government as prosecutor, on behalf of citizens	Fines, imprisonment
Civil	Private law between any two persons or entities	Individual plaintiff	Money, form of relief
-tort	civil law	Plaintiff claiming wrongful act or injury	Money, form of relief
-administrative (regulatory)	Governmental agency's regulations and statutes	Agency in front of administrative law judge	Revocation of privilege granted by agency

tion. The paramedic is granted certification by a state agency. Violation of the conditions and provisions of certification are typically reviewed in an administrative proceeding before an administrative law judge. If there is evidence of a violation of the provisions of certification, such as fraud in obtaining certification or substandard patient care, the certificate may be revoked or suspended.

Legal Accountability

There are a number of civil claims that can be brought against the paramedic based on his professional conduct. In any case, the plaintiff bears the burden of proof (must prove the claim). In most jurisdictions, the professional health care provider is presumed to act in an appropriate manner; the mere occurrence of an error or bad outcome does not constitute evidence of substandard care. Statutes and common law differ between states, but some common principles do exist. These are reviewed below.

Negligence is a civil claim in which the plaintiff may seek damages for injuries caused by someone who owed a duty of care. The plaintiff must prove four elements: 1) the defendant owed a duty to the plaintiff to act as a reasonably prudent person; 2) the defendant breached that duty; 3) an injury to the plaintiff occurred; and 4) the breach was the cause of the injury.

A closer look at each element is important. A paramedic usually becomes obligated to render care to a person because of the paramedic's position of employment or membership with an EMS agency. In turn, the EMS agency that promises to provide ambulance coverage for a municipality becomes obligated to perform. The paramedic should keep in mind that certification as a paramedic in and of itself usually does not create a duty to provide care. Consequently, a person who is a paramedic usually does not have a duty to render aid to a stranger when the paramedic is off-duty. There is no duty recognized by common law in this situation, although a duty could be established by enactment of a statute that required a person to render aid in such circumstances.

If the defendant owes a duty to the plaintiff, then the plaintiff must prove the second element—that the defendant failed to act as a reasonably prudent person would have acted under similar circumstances. The reasonably prudent paramedic is expected to anticipate whether or not his conduct or inaction would result in harm to a patient. For example, a

paramedic has a duty to apply a cervical collar in a careful manner and it is reasonably foreseeable that failure to do so could result in harm to the patient.

There must be a cause-and-effect relationship between the breach and the harm suffered by the plaintiff. Proximate cause is a legal term that refers to the legal cause of an injury; it is the link between the breach of duty and the other element of negligence: injury suffered by the plaintiff. Sometimes this is obvious, such as when a patient is dropped from a stretcher. On the other hand, separating the injury initially sustained by a patient injured in a motor vehicle collision from an injury caused by the paramedic's actions can be difficult to prove in a negligence claim.

The injury must be one that the law recognizes as compensable. The courts have been reluctant to recognize a claim for "wrongful life," when a person is kept alive against the patient's desires, because life is not considered an "injury." Where injury does occur, the law can provide compensation for loss of limb, pain and suffering, or reimbursement of medical expenses.

Thus, common law usually establishes negligence based on the principle of "due care." Sometimes, however, negligence is established by violation of a statute, which is called negligence per se. Either way, allegations of negligence are examined in light of the particular circumstances in which the paramedic was performing, such as the physical environment and degree of cooperation of the patient. However, the conduct is always judged by what a "reasonably prudent paramedic" would have done under the same or similar circumstances.

A very similar civil claim is malpractice. The elements of a malpractice claim are: 1) the defendant practitioner possessed and used the skill, knowledge, and experience of other practitioners engaged in the same practice, referred to as the standard of care; 2) the practitioner violated this standard of care; 3) this violation was a direct or (proximate) cause of 4) the plaintiff's injury. Malpractice is different from a negligence action. The duty in a negligence action is defined by what is prudent. In a malpractice action, the duty is defined by the standard of care. The difference can be slight, but it can change the proof the plaintiff is required to present at a trial (Table 5-3). In managing a patient with chest pain, for instance, expert testimony would be necessary to establish that the standard of care requires a paramedic to assess cardiac status, determine if medications are needed, and decide whether transport should be delayed while treatment is given.

TABLE 5-3	Comparison of Negligence and Malpractice	
Negligence	**Malpractice**	
1. EMS had duty to act.	1. EMS trained to standard of care.	
2. Breach of duty occurred.	2. Violation of standard of care occurred.	
3. Breach was proximate cause.	3. Violation was proximate cause.	
4. Injury to plaintiff.	4. Injury to plaintiff.	

The standard of care for paramedic prehospital care includes the knowledge and training provided through medical principles supported by the informed medical community and sound prehospital research. In addition, the paramedic is expected to act in accordance with state laws, rules, and regulations, and the medical direction of pertinent local protocols.

Because research and experience are constantly evolving in prehospital medical care, the standard of care is also subject to change. Consequently, the paramedic who is trained and certified today must be vigilant in maintaining knowledge and skills to continue to practice within the standard of care. The standard of care is consistent across state lines for many aspects of treatment, because of research that has either undermined previously untested patient care principles or proven other treatment modalities to be useful. The standard of care usually does not change according to geography, whether urban or rural, but environmental limitations do affect the options and efficacy of treatment involved in emergency medical care.

Negligence and malpractice claims against prehospital providers have often been related to emergency vehicle collisions. Claims that do involve patient care tend to involve failure to treat, rather than actions of negligent treatment. Claims are most frequent in cases of cervical spine injury, intoxicated patients, and cases of nontransport for patients with medical illnesses.

Pertinent Statutory Provisions

Scope of Practice

Every state has legislation that provides for establishment of an EMS regulatory body and the licensure or certification of EMS responders. These rules also address the specific medical procedures and functions that the paramedic is authorized to perform, called the scope of practice. The paramedic is allowed to engage in a limited medical practice, usually delegated by physicians who supervise prehospital care. In this "delegated practice," the paramedic is often referred to as a physician surrogate or physician extender, operating under a medical director who supervises the paramedic and oversees the prehospital EMS system (*see* Chapter 4).

The scope of practice for the paramedic varies somewhat from one state to another. However, it is generally understood that the paramedic may perform certain invasive medical procedures, as long as there are protocols indicating when to do so. It is the responsibility of the paramedic to have a clear un-

derstanding of regulations, statutes, and approved medical functions. Acting beyond or in violation of these statutory provisions may constitute the unauthorized practice of medicine, and could be a source of civil liability or administrative action by the state medical board or EMS authority.

Emergency Driving Statutes

Driving an ambulance or rescue vehicle in emergency mode (i.e., with flashing lights and siren on) is fraught with dangers even in the best of circumstances. The red lights and siren are intended to provide emergency vehicles with special use of the roadways, if other drivers yield to the emergency vehicle. The paramedic driving an emergency vehicle may be allowed to exceed the speed limit in limited situations, but this does not create a *right* to exceed the speed limit. State statutes usually allow an authorized emergency vehicle to be exempt from speed limits, parking restrictions, and traffic signals, but the operator is *never* exempt from the responsibility to exercise great caution (Fig. 5-1). In some states, the operator of an ambulance is held to a standard of extreme caution, not just reasonable care.

Liability may be established if emergency driving contributes to the injury of a patient or other persons. For example, the driver of the ambulance may fail to stop before proceeding through an intersection, or may drive too fast for weather conditions. In addition, if the red lights and siren are used when there is not a real emergency, any statutory immunity may be disallowed. Because there is no evidence that emergency status to or from an ambulance call improves patient outcome, emergency driving is increasingly subject to criticism. The operator of an emergency vehicle must still maintain control of the vehicle, drive in a safe manner, and know the state statutes pertaining to emergency driving.

Immunity Statutes

The concept of the Good Samaritan, derived from the Bible, has been codified in state statutes enacted to encourage

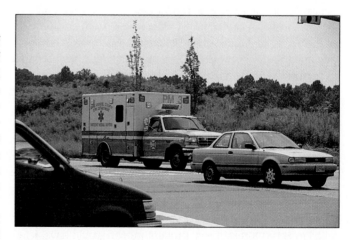

Figure 5-1

Emergency response is dangerous, and the paramedic should always use caution.

strangers to assist accident victims. To encourage the "Good Samaritan" to provide help, the victim is not allowed to seek damages for injuries caused by careless actions that worsened the victim's condition. Such laws also usually state that the Good Samaritan cannot seek payment for the assistance. Over the years, some immunity statutes have been broadened to include rescuers in some circumstances. There is often a distinction between the Good Samaritan who is under no obligation to offer assistance and the professional health care provider or rescuer who renders aid while employed by an EMS agency. Immunity statutes differ, and through case law can be interpreted in different ways. For example, a statute may allow rescuers who are on duty and compensated to be immune from liability as long as emergency care is rendered outside of a hospital or physician's office. Others specifically grant immunity as long as the paramedic is acting under the supervision of a medical director.

Governmental immunity, also known as sovereign immunity, is a form of statutory protection from liability granted to the publicly employed paramedic. Not every state provides this immunity, and the statutes that do exist are subject to limitations. The doctrine will not protect the paramedic who is off duty.

Almost every immunity statute, including Good Samaritan and governmental immunity laws, limits immunity to acts done in "good faith." Conversely, actions that the rescuer knows will cause harm, such as willful misconduct or reckless or intentional acts, will give rise to liability. The publicly employed paramedic whose conduct constitutes gross negligence or extreme departure from reasonable care, will also be subject to legal accountability.

Reporting Statutes

Most states have statutes that mandate reporting certain problems or conditions, such as situations of suspected child abuse, abuse of elderly persons, contagious diseases, sexual assault, animal bites, and gunshot wounds. Failure to report such situations may be grounds for both civil and criminal liability. The person who reports such matters is not required to believe that, for example, child abuse has in fact occurred. The paramedic need only have a reasonable suspicion or belief of the circumstances. As an example, Maine law requires EMS personnel to report cases of suspected child abuse, and grants immunity from civil liability for reporting done in good faith.[10]

Infectious Disease Statutes

Every paramedic should be aware of the risks of disease transmission, particularly involving infectious diseases. Because the awareness of acquired immune deficiency syndrome (AIDS) and human immunodeficiency virus (HIV) has increased, there have been numerous new laws that pertain to blood testing, sharing of information, and management of patients and rescuers when HIV infection is involved (see Chapter 10).

The common point in these statutes is an emphasis on confidentiality, whether it pertains to the report filed by a paramedic concerning possible exposure to infected blood or to a prehospital care report on a patient who is HIV positive.

The Paramedic-Patient Relationship

Confidentiality

As a member of the health care profession, the paramedic has responsibilities regarding the use and protection of a patient's medical information. It does not matter if this information is acquired from the patient's statements to the paramedic or from transfer documents. The paramedic has an ethical responsibility to keep any medical information about a patient confidential.

The principle of confidential communications applies to information shared with the assumption that the information will not be disclosed. The confidentiality of communications shared by a patient with his or her physician is based on society's recognition that the patient has a reasonable expectation and a valid need for medical privacy. Disclosure of this information can cause injury to the patient and discourage the candor and trust necessary for patient treatment. In general, the medical information acquired by the paramedic and documented in the prehospital care report should not be revealed to anyone not involved in the patient's care, unless the patient authorizes disclosure.

The protection from disclosures applies only to the personal medical information shared in a confidential environment. For example, if the patient makes a statement about something not relevant to the treatment or medical condition, that information is not privileged.

A claim of invasion of privacy or breach of confidentiality involves a disclosure about the patient where the patient has a reasonable expectation of privacy and the disclosure causes harm. An example would be release of a patient's diagnosis of infectious disease status to the news media, causing the patient to suffer embarrassment or loss of employment. Release of the prehospital care report to a patient's employer, without a subpoena or permission of the patient, could also lead to such a claim.

Consent

General Principles

In the United States, individuals have the constitutional right to accept or refuse medical treatment. This right is highly valued and protected by the courts as part of the right to freedom from unwanted intrusions. In a non-life-threatening situation, the patient is allowed to decide whether to accept or reject any treatment. In a true emergency, other principles of law define the nature and extent of treatment. Understanding the principles of consent are very important for the paramedic.

Forms of Consent

There are three forms of consent recognized by law: expressed, implied, and involuntary. The paramedic must be given one of these to proceed with treatment and transport. Although case law has not addressed in detail the issue of consent in the prehospital setting, it is accepted that the principles applied to the medical profession in general are valid. Of course, there are differences. For example, written consent forms are routinely used in the hospital setting but have not been considered necessary in the prehospital environment. The paramedic should be careful in situations in which a person's request for medical treatment is not clear.

Expressed consent is the clear voluntary expression by the patient of desire and willingness to be treated, made either verbally or in writing. The patient is seldom asked to sign a written consent form in prehospital care but verbally expresses consent for transport. The paramedic should not assume that permission to transport also means the patient consents to an intravenous line.[10] A request for assistance is not a blanket authorization for the paramedic to perform medical procedures.

A second form of consent, implied consent, is assumed when the patient is unable to give consent (e.g., is unconscious), but appears to have a life-threatening injury. In such circumstances, common law provides that treatment may be rendered despite the absence of the patient's expressed consent; it is assumed that the person would request treatment if able. This does not authorize treatment for non-life-threatening conditions.

The third form is involuntary consent. Under this principle, permission to treat is granted by the authority of law, such as a statute or a court order, regardless of the patient's desire. This occurs in situations of involuntary mental health "holds" for patients in need of emergency medical or psychiatric care, mentally or physically incompetent persons for whom a guardian has been appointed, alcohol treatment orders, and in some circumstances, prisoners in need of treatment.

Most states have laws that authorize the police, physicians, psychologists, or social workers to place persons under involuntary treatment holds for alcohol treatment or mental health evaluation. These laws are subject to important conditions and limitations. For example, there must be a factual basis—not speculation or unfounded fear—that the patient is dangerous to himself or others, and the patient must be evaluated by a physician within a specific number of hours or days. Beyond the specified time period, the need for the involuntary hold must be reviewed by a judge.

Statutes that authorize involuntary holds or treatment typically require probable cause to believe the patient is dangerous to himself or others, or gravely disabled because of a mental condition. Immunity is usually granted to persons who act in good faith when using these statutes to take a person into custody involuntarily, including the paramedic who complies with the police order.

Failure to obtain a patient's consent can result in a claim of battery, which is offensive contact with a patient without consent. This can create either civil or criminal liability. Physicians have faced claims of battery for performing surgery beyond that which was specifically consented to by the patient. The paramedic must not perform any invasive procedure, such as starting intravenous therapy, if the patient expresses unwillingness or expressly denies permission. A claim of battery may arise also if a paramedic improperly uses force or restraints on a patient.

Problems of consent and battery are generally avoidable if the paramedic clearly communicates his intentions to the patient and obtains the patient's cooperation before taking action. Compassionate interpersonal skills often save the patient and paramedic from misunderstandings and hostile encounters.

Consent for treatment should be based on an understanding of what treatment will be provided and the consequences of accepting or refusing it. The principle of informed consent requires that the patient be adequately informed of the planned treatment, of the risks and consequences of the treatment, and of alternative treatments, including no treatment. Unless the patient receives sufficient information to make an informed decision, the patient's agreement may be considered invalid.

The extent of information that must be given to the patient varies tremendously with the circumstance of the patient encounter, and may also depend on whether or not the proposed treatment is invasive.[20] In the prehospital environment, the extent of disclosure necessary for administering a medication or transporting would be substantially less than in the hospital. Time constraints and environmental factors are part of the emergency nature of the contact. Typically, brief but clear explanations are given and the patient's actions, such as walking to the ambulance, signify consent.

A closely related issue is the concept of informed refusal. Recognized in some case law, this principle states that the patient should be informed of both the consequences of the proposed treatment and of refusing treatment.[15]

Ability to Consent or Refuse

Our society assumes that an adult is able to make decisions regarding medical treatment. The term *competency* refers to the mental and emotional ability of a person to understand the process of decision-making. This involves understanding the consequences of treatment options, weighing the alternatives, and making a voluntary choice to accept or reject treatment.[12] Obviously, this decision-making capacity is necessary to give informed consent to, or refusal of, medical treatment.

In most situations, the paramedic will readily perceive the patient's ability to consent and can proceed to treatment and transport or refusal of treatment. However, in circumstances in which the patient's decision-making capacity is not obvious, a few guidelines may help. First, the paramedic should act in accordance with consent protocols, and mental status determinations should involve physician input whenever possible. Second, the paramedic must interact with the patient to gather sufficient information to establish the patient's decision-making capacity. This requires questioning a patient, rather than simply talking to him or her. The patient must be alert, oriented, and able to hear the paramedic.

Next, in the case of refusal, the paramedic must verify the patient's understanding of the information by asking the reasons for the decision. This enables the paramedic to evaluate the patient's ability to think logically. For example, if the patient states he can call a taxi to take him to the hospital, the reasoning may be sound. On the other hand, if the patient is not able to walk without assistance and there is no telephone in the apartment, such an option is not reasonable, and the patient's decision-making capacity is questionable.

If the patient is asked to respond with only "yes" or "no" answers to the paramedic's questioning, very little useful information is obtained. Therefore, the determination of the patient's decision-making capacity should be based on the content of the patient's explanations. Simply asking a patient why he or she is making a decision may reveal underlying causes of fear, money, religion, or confusion affecting the decision, as well as the patient's understanding of the situation. For meaningful communication to take place, the paramedic must also communicate with the patient in words that are specific and nontechnical. Alcohol, age, medications, anxiety, hypoxia, trauma, and intelligence must be considered by the paramedic in evaluating decision-making capacity.

The patient who lacks the ability to make medical treatment decisions but who does not have a life-threatening injury poses the greatest dilemma for the paramedic. There is no simple answer. To some extent options for management are guided by state law. Florida, for example, allows patients to be taken into custody by prehospital personnel for medical or psychiatric evaluation. However, most states do not have a statute that permits "protective custody," except for the patient who is a minor or a patient who is legally determined to be incompetent or mentally ill. Some states allow physicians to exercise control for limited circumstances if patient consent is not obtainable. There may simply be times when the patient insists on refusing treatment and is consequently left at the scene. The paramedic must warn and inform the patient, remembering that only in limited circumstances is it legal for the paramedic to make the patient's decisions.

Minors and Consent

Another consideration regarding who may give consent is the age of the patient. An adult, meaning a person of the "age of majority," may give consent to medical treatment. This age varies between states. In Alabama, for example, a person age 14 or older may consent to medical treatment but in most states, 18 is the age of majority.[1] Legally, a minor is deemed to lack the capacity to consent to or refuse treatment because a minor is thought to not appreciate the consequences of such a decision. Most states allow only the parent or legal guardian to give expressed consent on behalf of the child. Either parent can consent; if the parents are divorced, usually only the custodial parent may provide consent, unless otherwise provided by statute or a court order.

Some states also allow a person who is a minor, but who is married or in the armed services, to consent to treatment as an adult. The teenager who is an unmarried mother is generally allowed to consent to treatment for her child. She may be considered to be an adult for this limited purpose and for the purpose of consenting for her own medical treatment. In some states, college students are considered in a similar light, even if financially dependent upon their parents.

Another common exception is a minor who is emancipated (i.e., legally recognized as free of parental power). If the minor is living alone without financial dependence on the parents, then he or she is allowed to consent to treatment. The determination of emancipation can be difficult for the paramedic. There may be a court document acknowledging emancipation, but more likely there is not. This leaves the paramedic in the uncomfortable situation of questioning the individual and collecting as much information as possible to verify the minor's status. In most jurisdictions, if a minor misrepresents his age or emancipated status but consents to treatment, the courts will not permit the minor or the minor's parents to subsequently question the consent. On the other hand, the opposite has not generally been accepted: the paramedic who allows a minor to refuse treatment and leaves the patient without the support of police, social services, or another legally recognized substitute parent may later be held accountable to the parents.

Implied consent to treat a minor arises when the child is suffering from what reasonably presents as a life-threatening injury or illness. The child need not be unconscious, nor is the parents' permission needed in an emergency situation. The extent of the emergency in the case of a minor is not easily defined. However, if the minor patient is in pain and in need of medical care, the courts are not likely to punish those who provide care.[13]

The primary concern for the paramedic, as it will be in a court of law, is to respect the personal dignity of the young patient and act in his or her best interests. Common sense must prevail regarding the manner in which these encounters are managed. When treatment is not needed, the paramedic is likely relieved of responsibility by transferring the minor to the custody of police, social services or the hospital, who can contact the legal system for resolution if the parents are not readily located.

Involuntary consent for a minor, in which the consent of the parents is not required or not obtainable can occur in several circumstances. Under the doctrine of parens patriae, the state's child protective agency acts in place of the parents and has the authority to protect the welfare and health of a minor. Thus, if the parents cannot be located, the state may intervene to authorize treatment if requested by the physician, police, or social services. In addition, most states have legislation that prohibits a parent from denying a child emergency medical treatment.

Consent Problems in EMS

The Patient Refusal

A refusal to consent to treatment by the patient is a common occurrence in EMS that can be fraught with risk for both the patient and the paramedic. The risk to the patient arises because beneficial medical treatment is delayed. Risk to the paramedic arises because the patient, or patient's family, may blame the paramedic for conveying the impression that treatment was not necessary or for refusing to provide transport. Frequently, patients with injuries and illnesses fail to reach the hospital, and lawsuits can arise from these incidents. In such cases, it is often alleged that the paramedic failed to adequately assess the patient or failed to adequately warn the patient of the risks of nontransport. Consequently, the no-transport situation needs special attention (see Box 5-2).

There have been a number of studies about nontransports by prehospital agencies. In some systems, 50% to 90% of the patients contacted by prehospital personnel were not transported.[16] The outcome of patients not transported is often not good. In one study, of 93 patients not transported, 60 subsequently sought physician care.[3] Of these patients, 15 were hospitalized, two of whom died. Paramedics recommended or agreed to nontransport of 50 patients and these accounted for 11 of the 15 hospitalizations.

BOX 5-2 — Patient Refusal Guidelines

A. At minimum, the paramedic should do the following:

1. Be courteous with any patient who refuses an offer of transport or treatment.

2. Try to determine the reason(s) the patient does not accept transport by ambulance.

3. Evaluate the patient sufficiently to determine the urgency of the condition.

4. Assess the patient's ability to understand the medical condition and the information communicated.

5. Determine if the patient is capable of seeking assistance or taking actions for his own well-being.

6. Encourage appropriate medical follow-up or access to emergency medical services if the patient later wants medical assistance.

7. Be familiar with and follow agency protocol and local and state laws. Use medical direction when there is any question.

B. Essential documentation in patient refusal situations should include:

1. The patient's physical signs and symptoms, description of the scene.

2. Information from the caller (if not the patient) or reason EMS was contacted.

3. Summary of the options communicated as available to the patient (transport by ambulance, private car or other means).

4. The patient's stated reason for rejecting treatment or transport.

5. The paramedic's warning of risks and consequences of not receiving transport to the hospital.

6. The paramedic's observations or statements of the patient that indicate the patient is able and understands the risks and consequences.

7. Instructions from medical direction about the patient's refusal.

8. The patient's signature, if possible, acknowledging information communicated to the patient by the paramedic.

The paramedic should not do the following:

A. Insult or embarrass a patient for using emergency medical services or refusing to accept transport.

B. Ignore clues to potentially serious injuries or illnesses, such as abnormal vital signs, concern of family or witnesses, or inconsistencies in information obtained from different sources.

C. Assume a patient who is intoxicated has no other injuries or medical needs.

D. Ignore protocols and input from medical direction.

2. Conduct an assessment of the patient that enables him or her to adequately inform the patient of the possible risks of delaying treatment.

3. Solicit additional information from bystanders and family on scene or other witnesses, if possible. The paramedic can also use other crew members or persons to verify his or her own observation. For example, the paramedic may sense that the patient is slow to respond to questions and ask a partner or a first responder on scene to confirm the patient's responses.

4. If possible, document the observations and findings while still on the scene. This allows additional time at the scene, which may encourage a change of mind about transport. If the paramedic is eager to depart, the patient is less likely to believe the need for treatment.

Claims against paramedics in no-transport situations may be caused by poor communication. If the paramedic does not slight the patient who initially declines transport, and conveys professional concern and respect, misunderstanding may be avoided. As with any patient contact, there should be documentation of the encounter. The paramedic should document the physical and mental assessment, the need for medical care, and the patient's stated reason for refusing treatment and transport. Soliciting the patient's signature on the PCR is advised for the simple reason that it provides objective information about the patient. If the patient is able to follow commands, grasp a pen and sign, there is some indication of capabilities. Finally, the paramedic must inform the patient that EMS can be recalled at any time, should there be a change of mind.

Abandonment

Another claim that can arise from the patient relationship is that of abandonment. The patient generally has the right to terminate the services of a health care provider. However, if the paramedic stops rendering care without the patient's agreement, and the patient is injured as a result, then abandonment has occurred.

The paramedic has a duty to continue to provide care until relieved of the responsibility by the patient or another medically qualified person or until care is no longer needed. Although the patient must show the burden of proof to prove abandonment, inevitably in a claim of abandonment the paramedic will have to explain the reason(s) for ceasing to provide care to an injured or ill person. The method of discontinuing care is also important. A patient who is in the ambulance and abruptly decides he does not want to be taken to the hospital cannot simply be left in the roadway. The discharge of the patient relationship must be done in a reasonable manner with the patient's well-being in mind.

Abandonment can also occur if a paramedic begins caring for a patient who requires advanced life support therapies, but then turns the patient over to personnel who are not certified to provide that level of care. Finally, when transferring care to those who are properly qualified, the paramedic must ensure good care until the receiving caregivers are fully ready to take over. A time gap of inadequate care during the transfer could also lead to a charge of abandonment.

The termination of the patient encounter in the refusal situation should be preceded by several actions. The paramedic must:

1. Act consistently with local protocol, which often mandates contact with medical direction as a safeguard to assure that the paramedic's assessment and recommendations to the patient are appropriate.

False Imprisonment

Detaining a person without consent is a risky endeavor. False imprisonment is a claim based on an intentional and unjustifiable detention of a person against his or her will. Justification is difficult to define. Restraint of a person for medical purposes, even when the treatment would clearly be beneficial, may be inappropriate. However, circumstances in which the patient is unaware of the surroundings and unable to provide informed consent or refusal, may justify transporting a patient to a hospital for evaluation. False imprisonment can arise only if the patient knows he or she is being detained. The bottom line is that the competent adult has the right to make a refusal that results in his or her death.

Transport Issues

The delivery of patients to a hospital should be a medical decision, not complicated by financial considerations or the politics of physician or paramedic convenience. Although the paramedic is sometimes limited in the options of transport decisions, he or she must not surrender professional judgment when confronted with transport problems.

Consider the following example:

A paramedic is called to a physician's office for a routine transfer to the hospital. However, the patient's condition is unstable and the physician, rather than assisting the paramedic, insists that the paramedic depart quickly and that the patient be transported to a distant hospital instead of a closer appropriate facility.

What are the guiding principles in this situation? The paramedic is accountable to the EMS medical director, and may be negligent in accepting a patient who is not ready to transport. Bypassing the closest facility may also be negligent, and cannot be blamed on the private physician. The paramedic is expected to exercise independent judgment when deciding that a patient's condition is so unstable as to warrant transport to a closer appropriate facility, despite the inconvenience to the private physician.

A federal law, commonly referred to as antidumping legislation, was enacted to prevent hospitals from transferring patients without providing needed emergency care, especially based on the patient's ability to pay. The statute, whose sections are referred to as "COBRA" and "OBRA," also requires hospital emergency departments to provide appropriate evaluation for any patient who presents requesting care.[6] This law also prohibits a hospital from transferring a patient in an unstable condition unless certain treatment measures are taken first, and requires that "necessary and medically appropriate life support measures" accompany the patient during the transfer.

Antidumping statutes can benefit the paramedic as well as the patient. These precautionary measures may prevent an unstable patient from being transported carelessly and without appropriate precautionary treatment, stabilization, and monitoring equipment. The law provides that, if the unstable patient's condition warrants a higher level of care than the paramedic can provide during the transport, a physician, critical care nurse, or other qualified provider must accompany the patient, in addition to the paramedic. The imposition of heavy fines and other legal penalties are strong incentives to prevent dumping on the paramedic, as well as to prevent the patient from being denied necessary emergency care.

The COBRA/OBRA statute received considerable attention in a 1991 case involving Chicago paramedics who were instructed by a hospital base station to transport a child in cardiac arrest to a hospital that was not the closest.[9] The child died and the mother claimed the hospital was negligent in directing the paramedics to the more distant hospital. She also alleged violation of COBRA on the basis that the prehospital provider's communication with the base station was sufficient contact with the emergency department (ED) to constitute a violation of the law. The final court ruling in 1992 was that the base station was distinct from the ED and that base station contact did not equate to coming to the ED. Nonetheless, the case demonstrates how other aspects of health care, such as hospital and physician regulations, can entangle paramedics' patient contacts.

The issue of patient destination is a complex one. EMS systems should have protocols that guide paramedics in choosing the most appropriate patient destination. Patient preference further complicates destination decisions. In one court ruling, paramedics honored a patient's hospital choice even though they thought a trauma center would be better for the patient. The base station that acquiesced to the patient's choice was found not negligent.[17]

In general, when a patient is not in life-threatening condition and there are no system constraints, a patient's preference is accommodated. However, in a city EMS system with strained resources, patients with specialized needs or restrictions of health care plans, destination decision-making can be complex. In some states, statutes or regulations may dictate decision-making priorities for the paramedic. Otherwise, the paramedic should rely on protocols and medical direction for guidance.

Interveners in the Field

Among the more stressful encounters for the paramedic is the situation in which a well-meaning person at the scene, often called an intervener, insists on participating in patient care. An intervener who was attending the patient prior to paramedic arrival may feel an obligation to remain involved or even in control. Also, very few members of the public, including private physicians, understand the scope of paramedic practice and the link to a medical director and EMS system. It is this ignorance that tends to cause misunderstanding and even conflict.

ACEP has a position statement that addresses the issue of the physician intervener.[2] It is important that the paramedic maintain a professional attitude, without antagonism, when encountering someone who feels a need and willingness to assist.[15] At the same time, the paramedic cannot relinquish his own responsibilities to the patient, unless the patient makes a clear and competent refusal.

The potential liabilities in these situations must be kept in perspective. The intervener will be held accountable for his actions, but may be able to assert "Good Samaritan" status.

The paramedic, on the other hand, will be held accountable for his or her own actions, unless governmental or other immunity protections apply. In any event, discord that is allowed to compromise patient care will likely be seen unfavorably by a judge or jury. Cooperation and communication between the intervener and the paramedic will often resolve questions of authority and responsibility. The paramedic should invoke control measures (e.g., requesting the assistance of police or first responders) to remove the intervener only if the intervener becomes a danger to the patient's well-being.

Use of Restraints

Improper use of force may be a source of criminal or civil liability for the paramedic. The use of force is allowed only in circumstances that reasonably suggest an immediate risk of harm to the patient, responder, or another person (*see* Chapter 45). The paramedic should avoid the use of force, and the amount of force allowed is only that which is necessary to prevent harm or subdue the aggressor; any greater use of force is considered excessive.

Paramedics should consider the use of restraints as a means of patient protection in very limited circumstances. Our society considers liberty a right. Therefore, depriving a person of liberty without justification can give rise to claim of false imprisonment. Restraints should be applied only when the individual patient's behavior warrants the restriction of movement to protect the patient and the paramedic. The extent of restraints must be governed by what is reasonable under the circumstances, based as much as possible on objective observations. Consider the following questions when deciding what reasonable patient restraint should be:

- Are restraints necessary?
- What type of restraints are suitable?
- Are restraints necessary for the duration of the patient contact?
- Does the patient have any injuries or illnesses that must be considered before or during the use of restraints?

Conditions in which restraints might be appropriate include:

- A patient who is mentally retarded and easily angered when in the presence of strangers must be transported to the emergency department for treatment of a respiratory problem. An aide cannot accompany the paramedic during the transport.
- A patient is under police arrest or detention and has exhibited overt acts of violence toward people in a uniform. The police should accompany the patient in the ambulance.
- An elderly female patient, who has a tracheostomy and is disoriented, continues to pull the stoma out, causing compromise of the airway during transport.

In each situation, the paramedic may need to engage in both emotional or psychological management of the patient as well as the use of physical restraints. Antagonistic behavior by the paramedic when applying restraints is abusive and counterproductive. The paramedic should carefully consider the use of re-

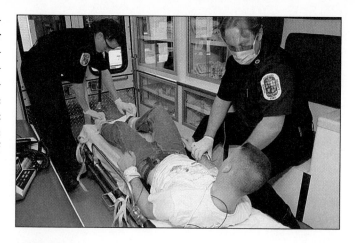

Figure 5-2

The paramedic must continuously monitor patient status when restraints are applied.

straints, never losing sight of the risk to the patient that can result from the use of such devices. It is imperative that the paramedic continuously monitor a restrained patient to ensure a patent airway and adequate circulation to extremities (Fig. 5-2). If the patient has scoliosis of the spine, caution must be used in any physical force that could result in fracture of brittle bones. Sometimes simple restraints with the use of pillows, to both minimize and protect the patient as well as limit movement, can be effective for the duration of a transport.

Paramedics can be subject to claims of battery if the application of restraints contributes to a patient's injuries. The use of restraints requires a careful balancing of risks. For example, a patient with a possible cervical spine injury should be immobilized with tape, cervical collar, or other devices. Failure to restrain this patient from movement may cause a stable cervical spine injury to develop into an unstable, debilitating, neurologic injury.

The guideline for the paramedic is always reasonableness. In addition, the paramedic must consider the relative size of the patient, the behavior known or reasonably anticipated, overt conduct, and the foreseeable consequences of both using restraints and not using them.[2] Finally, it is imperative that the paramedic receive training prior to application of any restraint device.

Issues in Resuscitation

General Principles

Considerable emphasis has been placed on saving lives in prehospital care. Cardiac resuscitation is considered the ultimate effort in the EMS response. Indeed, sometimes the desired goal-of-restoration of life occurs. Many times, however, the outcome is absence of cardiovascular response, and resuscitation efforts appropriately are stopped.

A principle of law that is acknowledged and revered in our country is that an adult of sound mind has the constitutional right to refuse treatment, even if it is life-saving. This includes the right to refuse resuscitation efforts by health care providers in a hospital as well as paramedics in the patient's home. This right has been upheld in numerous legal proceedings in which the patient, or the patient's guardian, petitions a court to authorize life-saving treatment to be withheld or withdrawn, thereby allowing the patient to die. In such rulings, the court weighs the rights of the individual against the interest of society to preserve life and prevent suicide.

A principle in medical care that has traditionally dictated treatment was the presumption that life is preferred over death; therefore, resuscitation was always deemed to be "in the best interests of the patient." However, medical technology now can prolong life artificially for months and even years. As a result, the courts have acknowledged the patient's right to refuse treatment, even if the result is death. A patient generally may refuse life-prolonging or life-saving treatment, such as CPR and defibrillation (see Chapter 57).

Case law regarding withholding or withdrawing life-saving or life-prolonging treatment has generally involved long-term situations and questions about ceasing treatment. There are no precedents related to nonresuscitation in the prehospital setting. Statutes pertaining to termination of treatment have also been silent regarding prehospital care, leaving prehospital providers concerned about liability. However, the 1990s have seen an increase in legislation expressly addressing out-of-hospital resuscitation dilemmas.

Finally, it is important to understand that the verbal statements of the patient's family regarding the patient's resuscitation preferences are not necessarily binding. If a patient is competent to make medical treatment decisions, the consent of spouse or family is not generally relevant or necessary.[11,13] When the patient is unconscious or incompetent, a court may grant authority to the family to make treatment decisions.[4] However, in emergency resuscitation situations, the desires of the family may not be a reason to cease or withhold treatment, although their information regarding the patient's specific treatment preferences may be useful.

Withholding and Stopping Resuscitation

Despite the sometimes low chance of success, paramedics are trained and expected to deliver a resuscitative effort unless there is a valid medical or legal reason not to. One such reason is that the resuscitative efforts have proven unsuccessful (e.g., cardiovascular unresponsiveness). To withhold treatment because it may be futile is simply unacceptable, unless other obvious signs of death are present (discussed further in Death on Scene). Termination of treatment can be done based on an attending physician's order, which is presumably based on the physician's decision that the patient did not want resuscitation or that cardiovascular unresponsiveness has been established. The paramedic's decision to stop resuscitation should be based on clear, physician-directed protocols or on-line medical direction. The paramedic must not make decisions about resuscitation based on personal religion, beliefs about brain damage that the patient may have suffered, or other subjective factors.

Another recognized justification for withholding resuscitative efforts is the physician's decision that the patient's condition is terminal, and death appears to be imminent.[7] If treatment is of no benefit to the patient's condition, then withholding resuscitative efforts is considered consistent with the standard of care in the medical profession. In such cases, the physician may order that cardiopulmonary resuscitation (CPR) not be initiated when the patient suffers cardiopulmonary arrest, or that CPR be stopped once started, by signing a "Do Not Resuscitate" (DNR) order.

Advance Medical Directives

Most paramedics have heard of "living wills." Although the term is commonly known, the document itself can be complex and may be interpreted differently from state to state, as well as region to region. Living wills are one form of advance medical directives, written patient statements of preference about medical treatments, to be administered or to be withheld. Usually these documents become effective when the patient suffers from a terminal condition and is comatose or unable to express treatment preferences. In addition, these documents sometimes appoint another person to make the necessary medical treatment decisions on behalf of the patient, called a proxy or surrogate decision-maker.

Some states have legally recognized these documents, but circumstances are usually limited and procedures can be restrictive. For example, the document may be operative only in the hospital setting after a patient is informed of diagnosis of a terminal condition. Consequently, the living will might not apply to a patient suffering from acute conditions such as a stroke or cardiac arrest caused by an airway obstruction.

An advance directive is only one method by which a patient expresses his treatment preferences, and there is no requirement that a person have such a directive. In the absence of a directive form which may be specifically recognized by state statute, the health care professional must be guided by the general principles of consent, and by the accepted standard of care, in determining what treatment is appropriate for the patient. The advantage of a patient who has expressed treatment preferences in an advance directive is that the physician, as well as the paramedic, can withhold specified treatments, so long as the document meets legal requirements.

The presence of these documents in the prehospital setting has had some disadvantages. Directives can appear in a variety of formats, such as preprinted forms, or be handwritten; family may present the document when it is not applicable to the patient's situation, such as when the patient has an acute, nonterminal condition. Experience has demonstrated that advance medical directives can be honored in the prehospital setting if certain conditions are established: advance arrangements in which the patient completes such a document, communicates desires to the local prehospital system, and involves family and caregivers in education efforts regarding the use of 9-1-1.

A Do Not Resuscitate order, also called a DNR, or No-CPR order, is a similar concept. A DNR order is commonly understood to mean that, when the patient suffers cardiopulmonary or respiratory arrest, CPR is not to be initiated.

The DNR order is usually written by the patient's physician in the patient's medical chart in the hospital or nursing home. If the patient is unable to communicate his or her desires because of illness, the physician may consult with close family members to determine the patient's probable treatment desires.

A DNR order does not mean that the patient does not want other forms of treatment before suffering an arrest. Because of the possible conflicts or confusion about a DNR order, the paramedic should depend on the medical director and the medical direction physician for guidance, both through protocol and on-line advice. Where possible, the paramedic should act consistent with the patient's preferences. However, when there is any reasonable question, it is appropriate to initiate full resuscitative efforts. Because the paramedic does not have the benefit of knowing the patient, or ensuring that the patient has made an informed decision and has not altered that decision, resuscitation should be withheld only when clear information reflects the patient's desires. Considerations for withholding or stopping CPR or any resuscitative efforts are included in Box 5-3. In summary, prehospital complexities regarding DNR status made it preferable that local protocol, on-line direction, and specific state law all be available to guide paramedics in decisions not to resuscitate.

Death in the Field Setting

The legal aspects of the out-of-hospital death can be complex. Most states have statutes that mandate certification of death by a licensed physician. The ability of a paramedic to make objective observations of death should not be confused with that legal certification. According to the American Heart Association, the three obvious signs of death, in which resuscitation efforts are not warranted, include only:[8]

1. Decapitation
2. Dependent lividity
3. Rigor mortis

When the paramedic encounters an apparent death in the field, the following are recommended as minimum appropriate steps:

- Verify death by ECG tracing, in at least two leads, unless otherwise directed by local protocol.

BOX 5-3 — Possible Considerations for Accepting a Prehospital DNR or Other Advance Medical Directive

- Is there a clearly valid prehospital DNR order in effect and present?
- Is the patient's personal, primary physician present to communicate the patient's resuscitation preferences?
- If the patient is incompetent or unable to communicate his treatment preferences, is there an advance directive that prohibits CPR which unquestionably applies to the current situation?
- Is the patient competent and informed as to the likely result of DNR status?

- Document the observations and findings of the scene, as well as ambulance dispatch and base station contact details.
- Notify appropriate authorities (e.g., police or coroner).
- Be courteous and respectful to family, witnesses, and bystanders, and remain sensitive to those who may be upset or confused by the absence or discontinuation of resuscitation efforts.
- Do not disturb the body or scene except as necessary to verify death.

Evidence and Accident Scene Responsibilities

The nature of the paramedic's work often involves crime scenes. It may be a call to an assault in an alleyway, a domestic dispute in a home or an attempted suicide in a garage. The paramedic's first and foremost concern, after personal safety, is to render care to the patient. Nonetheless, there is a professional responsibility at a possible crime scene to prevent unnecessary disturbance and destruction of evidence.

A common example of physical evidence is a shirt that has a tear in it above the patient's fatal stab wound. The location of the tear on the clothing and the condition of the fabric may be important in differentiating suicide from assault. However, the shirt will only be useful if it is left intact, as it was found at the scene, so that police specialists can examine it. Avoid the site of the tear when cutting away clothing to evaluate and treat the patient. Keep in mind that anything can be evidence, including testimony by the paramedic of his own personal observations of a scene. Placing paper bags on a patient's hands can be important in preserving evidence of gunpowder burns. The sooner such protective measures are implemented, the more reliable the information will be for use at trial. The position of a patient before cardiac resuscitation efforts are commenced may be critical evidence in examination of blood splatters on the walls or floor.

The paramedic is likely at some point to be requested to provide testimony in a legal proceeding, either criminal or civil. For example, the paramedic may note the simple fact that the ignition was on in a vehicle found at the bottom of an embankment. Or, the paramedic's testimony may be necessary if different versions of the causes of a child's injuries were given. The paramedic may be asked by law enforcement to draw a blood specimen from a person. Months or even years later, the paramedic may be asked to testify in court about observations and actions. Therefore, adherence to protocol and accepted standards, including accurate and detailed documentation can be critical.

A few simple guidelines are important:

- Disturb as little as possible in any potential crime scene.
- Inform appropriate law enforcement personnel if objects had to be moved or altered in the process of patient care. For example, a patient with a gunshot wound to the neck may require an emergency cricothyrotomy in which the exit wound to the anterior neck is obscured by the life-saving procedure. Both the police and the emergency room physician must be informed of this alteration.

- Adequately document pertinent information on the patient care record, including observations (through sight, sound, or smell) of the scene and how the patient appeared or was positioned when first encountered.

The paramedic's primary concerns are always personal safety and patient care. Then, preservation of evidence may be addressed.

SUMMARY

The rights of the individual patient, the broad range of laws that pertain to society, and the emerging professional image of EMS all mingle with the day-to-day medical responsibilities of the paramedic. A single ambulance call involves emergency driving statutes, consent issues, constitutional rights, and principles of evidence, legal documentation, and confidentiality. As is true of medical care, there is no substitute for practice and preparation, education and on-going training for the legal aspects of prehospital emergency care.

REFERENCES

1. Alabama Revised Statute, 22-8-4.

2. Bennett v. Wintrop Community Hospital, 489 NE 2d 1032, Massachusetts, 1986.

3. Bryan ED, Zachariah BS, Pepe PE: Follow-up and outcome of patients who decline or are denied transport by EMS. *Prehosp Dis Med* 7: 359–364, 1992.

4. Cruzan v. Director. Missouri, 110 S.Ct. 2841, Missouri, 1990.

5. Deel v. Syracuse Veterans Admin. Medical Center, 729 F. Supp. 231, New York, 1990.

6. Emergency Medical Treatment and Active Labor Act, 42 USCA, Section 1395dd, et seq., as amended by the Omnibus Budget Reconciliation Acts of 1987, 1989, and 1990.

7. Fox E, Seigler M: Redefining the emergency physician's role in Do-Not-Resuscitate decision-making. *Am J Med* 92:125, 1992.

8. Jaffe AS: Advanced Cardiac Life Support, ed 2, 1990, American Heart Association.

9. Johnson v. University of Chicago Hospitals, 982 F.2d 230, Illinois, 1992.

10. Maine Revised Statute Annotated, 22-4011.

11. Miller RD: Problems in hospital law, Rockville, 1990, Aspen Publishers.

12. O'Brien v. Cunard S. S. Co., 154 Mass. 272, 28 NE 2d 266, Massachusetts, 1981.

13. Rozovsky FA: Consent to treatment, a practical guide, Boston, 1990, Little, Brown, and Company.

14. Ryan White Comprehensive AIDS Resource Emergency Act of 1990, Public Law 101-381.

15. Scholendorff v. Society of New York Hospital, 211 NY 125, New York, 1914.

16. Selden, BY, Schnitzer PG, Nolan FX: Medico legal documentation of prehospital triage. *Ann Emerg Med*, 19:547–551, May 1990.

17. Smith v. East Medical Center, 585 So.2d 1325, Alabama, 1991.

18. Truman v. Thomas, 27 Cal 3d 285, 611 P 2d 901, California, 1980.

19. Vosk A: Physician intervention at the scene. *JEMS,* 14:60, 1989.

20. Wu v. Spence, 605 A.2d 395, Pennsylvania, 1992.

SUGGESTED READINGS

1. Ayres RJ: Issues of patient consent and liability for unauthorized treatment. *Prehosp Dis Med*, 5: 231–239, July/September 1990.

2. Goldstein RJ: EMS and the law, Maryland, 1983, Brady Company.

3. Hannah JH: Ambulance and EMS Driving, Reston, Virginia, 1983, Reston Publishing Company.

4. National Association of EMS Physicians, Prehospital Systems and Medical Oversight, ed 2, St. Louis, 1994, Mosby Lifeline.

5. President's Commission for the Study of Ethical Problems in Medicine and Biomedical and Behavioral Research: Deciding to Forego Life-Sustaining Treatment, Washington, 1983, United States Government Printing Office.

6. Shanaberger CJ: Why releases don't work. *JEMS*, 13:47–49, 1988.

7. Shanaberger CJ: Decision-making capacity. *JEMS*, 13:70–73, 1988.

Section 2

Foundations for Practice

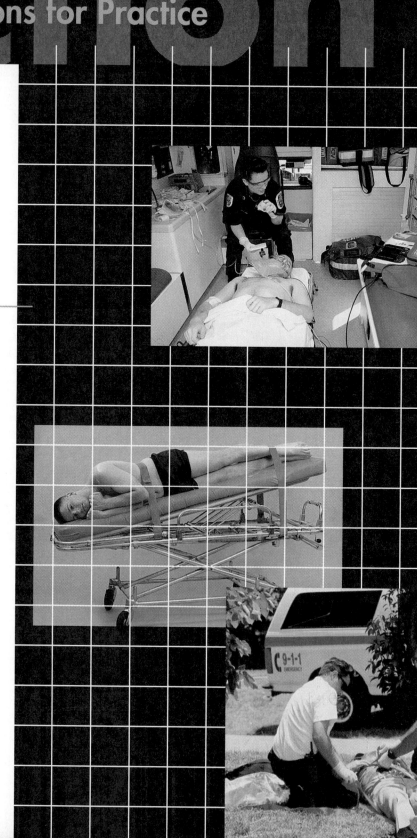

Included In This Section:

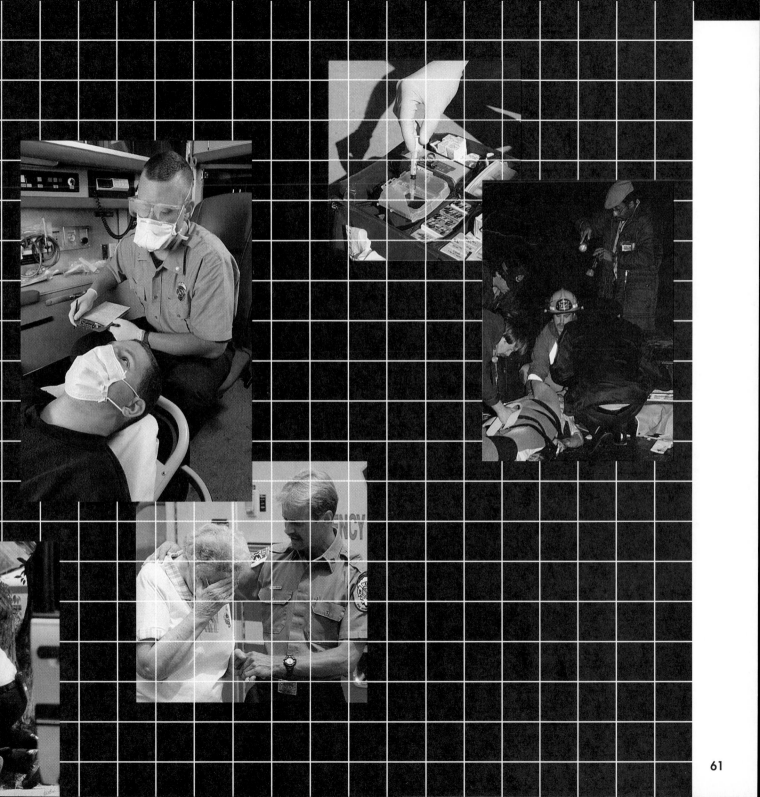

Chapter 6

Medical Terminology

Robert Sherard, BA, EMT-P
Dwight Lodge, MS, EMT-P

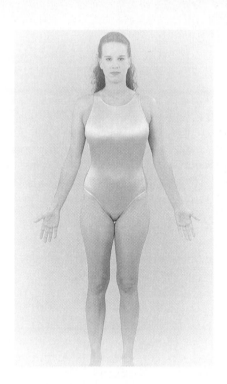

A paramedic should be able to:

OBJECTIVES

1. Identify and define commonly used prefixes, root words, suffixes and abbreviations.

2. Describe standard anatomical position.

3. Identify the imaginary planes and lines of the body and the relationships of body structures to these lines.

4. Describe anatomical relationships in the extremities.

5. Describe the various positions of the body at rest.

6. Describe movements of the body and extremities.

7. Recognize and use common terminology related to specific body systems and their diseases.

The paramedic, who serves as the eyes, ears, and hands of the medical direction physician, often enters urgent situations with little information and must rapidly conduct a physical assessment, gather pertinent history, and report these findings by radio so that appropriate therapy can be initiated. Neither the patient nor the medical direction staff has time for long descriptions of the patient's condition. In fact, time wasted in lengthy radio reports may be at the patient's expense. The use of proper terminology can help to shorten report time and add to accuracy. In addition, the use of proper terminology on a patient care report may add a degree of accuracy and professionalism that reduces liability.

The Origin of Words

Physicians in ancient times used Greek and Latin words to describe patients' conditions. Although the medicine of those times was primitive by today's standards, the language proved to be quite sophisticated. Even today, with high-tech medical equipment and a constant cascade of new information, much terminology has its roots in these ancient languages. Latin terms seem particularly well-suited for communication among health care professionals. Although most languages that evolved from Latin have changed through the centuries, the Latin language itself has remained unchanged. Words used hundreds of years ago to describe a medical condition or procedure still have the same meaning today.

Combining Words

Considering all of the information available today, it would be impractical to learn every medical term. Fortunately, ancient physicians devised a systematic approach to naming things. A term centers around a root word that describes the organ, system, process, or body part. These root words are combined with other words to give a specific meaning. Therefore, root words are more accurately referred to as combining words. Table 6-1 lists the most common combining words.

Combining words do not necessarily have to be added to other words to have meaning. They can be used alone to specify a body system or organ simply by adding an ending. Some examples are listed in Table 6-2.

Combining words can be added to one another when more than one body system or process is involved. The two words are often bridged by the letter "o." Table 6-3 illustrates the formation of a compound word using the letter "o" as a bridge.

Prefixes

Prefixes are words that are added to the beginning of a combining word to describe not only the system or process involved, but the extent of the involvement as well. Prefixes are used with combining words to indicate direction, quantity, degree or position. For example, the Greek word for slow is *brady*. When added to the beginning of the Greek word for heart, *cardia*, a new word, *bradycardia*, is formed that means

slow heart. Table 6-4 lists some of the most common prefixes, their meanings, and usage.

Suffixes, like prefixes, are added to combining words to expand their meaning. Suffixes are added to the end of the combining word to indicate the event, activity, origin, or pathology of the body part under discussion. For example, *-algia* means *pain.* When added to the end of the word for nerve, *neur-*, the new word, *neuralgia,* means pain originating from a nerve. Common suffixes are listed in Table 6-5.

Word combinations may use more than one prefix, root, or suffix to describe a condition. For example, paramedics may encounter a condition known as paroxysmal supraventricular tachycardia. When each word is broken down into its components, the meaning of the phrase becomes clear. *Paroxysmal* means sudden onset, *supra* means above, *ventricular* means the ventricles, *tachy* means fast, and *cardia* means heart. *Paroxysmal supraventricular tachycardia* is the sudden onset of a rapid heart beat originating somewhere above the ventricles.

By knowing the essential combining words, or roots, prefixes, and suffixes, medical professionals are able to use a vast library of words that clearly communicate their intended meaning to others. Although this textbook presents the foundation upon which to build a working vocabulary, it is beyond the scope of this text to list every word that the paramedic might encounter. A readily accessible pocket-sized medical dictionary will prove to be a valuable tool throughout a paramedic's career.

The Body at Rest

Without the availability of surgery or x-ray, the paramedic must make many decisions based on a knowledge of surface anatomy and its relation to structures that lie beneath. Descriptions of injuries or the location of pain are made in terms of known topographical landmarks. For example, in describing an injury to a patient's chest, it would be inadequate to state that the patient has a wound on the front of the chest on the left side. A more precise description would be: the patient has a wound on the anterior surface of the chest, two inches medial to the left nipple at the fourth intercostal space.

Standard Anatomical Position

As a standard reference, descriptions are based on the body alignment known as standard anatomical position. This is an erect posture, with the face, toes and palms of the hands facing forward (Fig. 6-1). These descriptions hold true regardless of the position in which the patient presents. Whether face-up, face-down, or slumped over a steering wheel, all descriptions should refer to the body in standard anatomical position. This minimizes confusion when reporting patient data.

Body Planes and Lines of Reference

To further clarify the location of surface structures, the body (still in anatomical position) is divided by several imaginary

TABLE 6-1   Common Combining (Root) Words

Combining (root) word	Meaning; pertaining to	Combining (root) word	Meaning; pertaining to	Combining (root) word	Meaning; pertaining to
Abdomin-	Abdomen	Gravid-	Pregnancy	Pneumo-	Lung
Acromi-	Acromion process of shoulder	Gynec-	Woman, female	Pulm-	Lung
Aden-	Gland			Pyr-	Fever
Adren-	Adrenal glands	Hallucin-	Mental wandering		
Angi-	Blood or lymph vessels	Hem, hemat-	Blood	Ren-	Kidney
Arteri-	Artery	Hepat-	Liver	Resuscit-	Revive
Arthr-	Joint	Hist-	Tissue	Retent-	Hold back
		Homeo-	Sameness, unchanging	Retin-	Retina
Bacteri-	Bacteria	Hyster-	Uterus	Rhin-	Nose
Brachi-	Arm				
Bronchi-	Primary airways	Ile-	Ileum of the small intestine	Sacchar-	Sugar
		Ili-	Ilium of the pelvis	Sacr-	Sacrum
Carcin-	Cancer	Immun-	The immune system	Saliv-	Saliva
Cardi-	Heart	Inguin-	Groin	Sanguin-	Blood
Cartilag-	Cartilage			Sarc-	Cancer
Cephal-	Head	Lact-	Milk	Scoli-	Curved, crooked
Cerebell-	Cerebellum	Lapar-	Abdomen	Sinus-	Cavity
Cerebr-	Cerebrum	Laryng-	Larynx, voice box	Skelet-	Skeleton
Cervic-	Neck, cervical spine	Ligament-	Ligament	Son-	Sound
Chole-	Bile	Lumb-	Lower back, lumbar spine	Spin-	Spine
Cholangi-	Bile duct	Lymph-	The lymphatic system	Spir-	Breathing
Cholecyst-	Gall bladder			Splen-	Spleen
Chondr-	Cartilage	Mamm-	Breast	Stern-	Sternum, the breastbone
Chrono-	Time	Mandibul-	Mandible, the lower jaw	Steth-	Chest
Clavicul-	Clavicle	Mast-	Breast, nipple		
Conjunctiv-	Conjunctiva	Maxill-	Maxilla, the upper jaw	Tars-	Ankle, instep
Constrict-	Draw tightly together, narrow	Meatus-	External opening	Tempor-	Temporal bone
Cost-	Rib	Mediastin-	Mediastinum, middle divider	Tendin-	Tendon
Crani-	Skull	Mening, meningi-	Meninges	Testicul-	Testicle
Cubit-	Elbow	Mictur-	Urination	Thalam-	Thalamus
Cyan-	Blue coloration	Myo-	Muscle	Therapeut-	Treatment
Cyst-	Bag, fluid sac, bladder	Myel-	Spinal cord, bone marrow	Therm-	Temperature
Cyt-	Cell			Thorac-	Chest
		Nat-	Birth	Thromb-	Clot
Dent-	Tooth	Necr-	Death	Trache-	Trachea
Derm-	Skin	Nephr-	Kidneys	Tract-	Bundle of nerve fibers
Duct-	Opening	Neur-	Nervous tissue	Trich-	Hair
		Noct-	Night	Tympan-	Tympanic membrane, eardrum
Edem-	Swelling	Occipit-	Back of the skull		
Embry-	Fertilized ovum, fetus	Occult-	Hidden	Ulcer-	Sore
Encephal-	Brain	Ocul-	Eye	Uln-	The ulna
Enter-	Intestinal tract	Odont-	Tooth	Umbilic-	Umbilicus
Erythr-	Red coloration	Oro/oral-	Mouth	Ureter-	Ureter
Esth-	Sensation	Orth-	Correct, straight	Urethr-	Urethra
		Os-	Mouth, bone	Urin-	Urine
Faci-	Face			Uter-	Uterus
		Palpat-	Touch		
Febr-	Fever	Pancreat-	Pancreas	Vagin-	Vagina
Femor-	Femur, thigh bone	Paroxysm-	Sudden onset	Valv-	Valve
Flex-	To bend	Part-	Labor	Varic-	Dilated, swollen
Foramin-	Opening	Patell-	Knee cap	Vas-	Vessel, duct
Foss-	Shallow depression	Path-	Disease, suffering	Vascul-	Vessel
Fract-	Break	Pector-	Chest	Ven-	Vein
Gangli-	Nerve bundle	Ped-	Foot	Ventricul-	Ventricle (brain or heart)
Gastr-	Stomach	Pedi-	Child	Vertibr-	Vertebra, spinal column
Genit-	Reproductive organs	Perme-	To pass through	Vesicul-	Small bladder-like structure
Geront-	Old age, elderly	Phag-	To swallow	Vestibul-	Entrance
Gingiv-	Gums	Pharmac-	Drug	Viscer-	Internal organ, viscera
Glott-	Opening of the larynx	Pharyng-	Throat, pharynx		
Glyc-	Glucose, sugar	Phleb-	Vein	Zygom-	Cheekbone

TABLE 6-2 Common Endings That Help Combining Words Stand Alone

Ending	Example	Meaning
-ac	Cardiac arrest	Cessation of heart activity
-al	Abdominal viscera	The organs contained in the abdomen
	Tibial tuberosity	The bony prominence of the tibia inferior to the knee
	Fermoral artery	The artery which lies close to the femur
-ar	Tonsillar abscess	A pus cavity or sore on the tonsil
	Valvular heart disease	A condition of weakening or stiffening of the heart valves
	Testicular torsion	Twisting of the testicle within the scrotum
-ic	Gastric ulcer	A lesion in the lining of the stomach
	Adrenergic nervous system	The sympathetic division of the nervous system, which secretes adrenalin and noradrenalin
	Cephalic presentation	Normal head-first delivery of a baby
	Chronic condition	A condition persisting over a long period of time

TABLE 6-3 Compound Words Formed by Bridging Two Combining Words

Word	Meaning
Cardiomyopathy	Disease of the heart muscle
Cardiopulmonary resuscitation	A procedure for reviving the functions of the heart and lungs
Cerebrovascular accident	A rupture or clot in the blood vessels of the brain, causing an interruption of blood flow to the brain; a stroke
Gastroesophageal reflux	A backflow of stomach contents into the esophagus
Laryngotracheobronchitis	Inflammation of the major respiratory passages
Musculoskeletal	Pertaining to muscle and bones, and their connections
Nasopharynx	That portion of the pharynx posterior to the nasal cavity

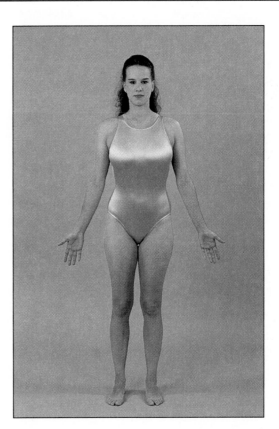

Figure 6-1

The anatomical position is the standard reference point used to describe body alignment. Note that the eyes, palms, and toes face forward and the patient is standing erect. When referencing "left" and "right," we refer to the patient's left and right sides.

planes (Fig. 6-2). The lines created by these planes are useful for descriptive reference. The median, or midsaggital, plane divides the body into right and left halves. The imaginary line that it creates, running down the middle of the body through the nose, umbilicus and the symphysis pubis, is called the midline. In describing anatomical relationships, structures close to the midline are described as medial, and structures away from the midline are lateral.

Another imaginary plane divides the body into front and back halves. This is frontal, or coronal, plane. The front surface of the body is the anterior surface, and the back is called the posterior surface. Each organ in the body can also be divided by a frontal plane, meaning organs have anterior and posterior surfaces as well. For example, the left anterior descending coronary artery feeds the anterior surface of the heart, and the right circumflex artery feeds its posterior surface.

A third plane, the transverse plane, divides the body into upper and lower sections. This plane may be imagined as transecting the body at any point. Structures above it are superior to those below, which are inferior. The diaphragm, for instance, makes up the inferior border of the thoracic cavity and the superior border of the abdominal cavity. The paramedic will seldom refer to these planes by name. It is much more important to know the terms medial, lateral, anterior, posterior, superior, and inferior.

TABLE 6-4 **Common Prefixes**

Prefix	Meaning	Example	Meaning
A-, an-	Without,	Asymptomatic	Without symptoms
Ab-	Away from	Abduction	Movement of a limb away from the body
Ad-	Toward	Adduction	Movement of a limb toward the body
Ante-	Before, forward	Antepartum	Before birth
Anti-	Against, opposed to	Anticholinergic	Opposes the action of acetylcholine
		Antiarrhythmic	A drug that prevents disturbances of the cardiac rhythm
Bi-	Two	Bisect	Divide into two parts
Brady-	Slow	Bradycardia	Slow heart beat
Circum-	Around	Circumoral cyanosis	Bluish discoloration around the mouth
Contra-	Against	Contraindication	Indication against (a drug or procedure)
Dys-	Difficult, painful	Dysuria	Difficult or painful urination
		Dyspnea	Difficult breathing
Epi-	Over, upon	Epidural hematoma	A swelling of blood over the dura mater of the brain
		Epigastric pain	Pain above the stomach
Hemi-	Half	Hemiplegia	Paralysis of one half of the body
Hyper-	Above, excessive	Hyperglycemia	Excessive glucose in the blood
Hypo-	Below,	Hypoglycemia	Inadequate glucose in the blood
Inter-	Between, among	Interstitial fluid	Fluid between cells
Intra-	Inside, within	Intraosseous infusion	Injecting fluids inside the bone
Multi-	Many	Multisystem failure	Failure of more than one body system
Post-	After	Postpartum	After birth
Pre-	Before	Prenatal	Before birth
Poly-	Many, too much	Polyuria	Excreting too much urine
Quad-	Four	Quadriplegia	Paralysis of all four extremities
Retro-	Behind	Retroperitoneal	Behind the peritoneum
Semi-	Half	Semiconscious	Half conscious
Sub-	Under, below, beneath	Substernal pain	Pain beneath the sternum
Super-	Above, in addition, in excess	Superinfection	A new infection added to one already present
Supra-	Above	Supraventricular tachycardia	A rapid heart rate originating above the ventricles
		Suprarenal glands	The glands found above the kidneys, the adrenal glands
Tachy-	Fast	Tachycardia	Fast heart rate
Trans-	Through	Transtracheal	Through the tracheal wall
Tri-	Three	Tricuspid valve	A heart valve with three flaps, or cusps
		Trigeminal PVCs	Premature ventricular contractions occurring every third beat
Uni-	One	Unifocal	Originating from one focus, or site (such as unifocal PVCs)

Surface Landmarks

There are many surface landmarks that improve the precise description of body location. On the anterior surface of the chest, for example, the clavicles and nipples are commonly used as landmarks. Midclavicular refers to an imaginary line that starts at the midpoint of the clavicle (about where the sharp bend is) and descends in a straight line down the anterior chest surface (Fig. 6-3). A needle thoracotomy, an emergency procedure for relieving a tension pneumothorax, is performed by inserting a 16-gauge IV catheter through the chest wall in the second intercostal space at the midclavicular line.

Another method for a needle thoracotomy is the midaxillary approach. Midaxillary refers to a line drawn straight down from the armpit (axilla) along the lateral surface of the chest wall (Fig. 6-4). In males, the nipples also serve as good landmarks. The nipple usually lies over the fifth rib.

The contents of the abdominal cavity are also frequently referred to in terms of topographical landmarks. By drawing a vertical and horizontal line through the navel, the abdomen can be divided into four quadrants, each containing specific organs (Fig. 6-5). Abdominal pain is most often referred to by the quadrant involved, since pain cannot be well localized to a specific organ in the abdomen.

TABLE 6-5   Common Suffixes

Suffix	Meaning	Example	Meaning
-algia	Pain	Neuralgia	Pain originating from a nerve
-ectomy	Surgical removal	Tonsillectomy	Surgical removal of the tonsils
-emia	Blood	Hyperglycemia	Excessive glucose in the blood
		Hypoxemia	Low oxygen levels in the blood
-genic	Causing, origin	Cardiogenic shock	Shock caused by failure of the heart muscle
-itis	Inflammation	Hepatitis	Inflammation of the liver
-osis	Process, state	Acidosis	A condition of excessive acid levels
-ostomy	Surgical creation of an opening	Tracheostomy	Surgical creation of an opening in the trachea
-plegia	Paralysis	Hemiplegia	Paralysis of one half of the body
-rrhage	Excessive flow	Hemorrhage	Excessive flow of blood
-rrhea	Excessive flow or discharge	Rhinorrhea	Excessive flow or discharge from the nose
-sis	State or condition	Ketosis	A condition of excessive ketone levels

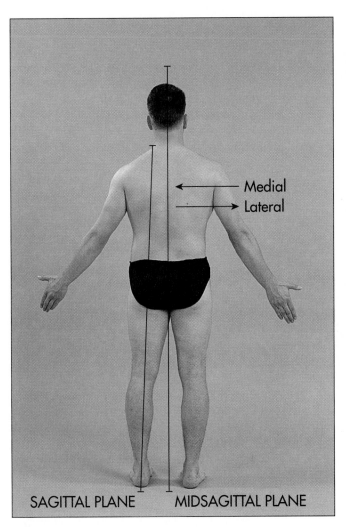

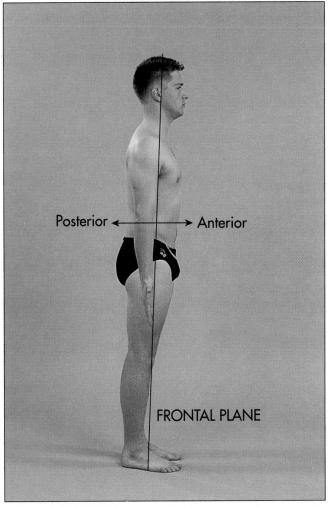

Figure 6-2

Imaginary lines drawn through the body structures provide descriptive references that serve to orient medical professional attention to the affected or described part of the body. Planes divide the body into left and right halves, front and back, and superior and inferior sections.

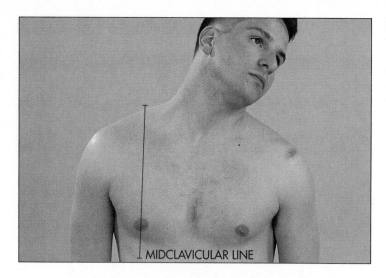

MIDCLAVICULAR LINE

Figure 6-3

The midclavicular line is found by identifying the distal and proximal points of the clavicle, the moving to the point midway between the ends. Identify the second intercostal space by palpation of the second rib, which lies directly below the clavicle. A needle thoracotomy is commonly performed at this site.

The Extremities

Two additional terms are used to describe anatomical relationships of the extremities (arms and legs). Proximal means nearer to the trunk. Distal means away from the trunk or nearer to the free end of the extremity. For example, the distal end of the humerus articulates (meets in a joint) with the proximal ends of the radius and ulna at the elbow (Fig. 6-6).

Positions of the Body at Rest

The paramedic seldom finds a patient in anatomical position. Several terms are used to describe the position of an individual who is not in anatomical position. An individual lying face up is said to be in a supine position. A person lying face down is in a prone position. A patient lying on either the right or left side is in a right or left lateral recumbent position. One who is lying supine with head elevated is in a semi-Fowler's position (Fig. 6-7).

Patients in shock are sometimes placed supine with the legs elevated 30 to 45 degrees. This is called Trendelenburg position (Fig. 6-8).

These resting positions may appear in various combinations. Patients suffering an air embolism are often placed in a head-down, feet-up position on their left side to prevent the air bubble from entering the pulmonary artery. This is accurately described as a "left-lateral recumbent with Trendelenburg" position (Fig. 6-9).

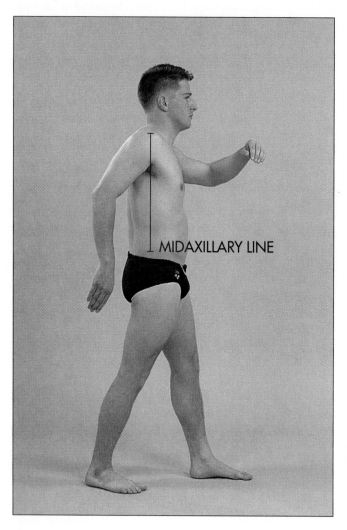

MIDAXILLARY LINE

Figure 6-4

The midaxillary line is found by drawing a line vertically from the armpit (axilla) along the lateral chest wall.

The Body in Motion

With more than 200 bones and 800 muscles, the human body is seldom totally at rest. Even simple movements such as pick-

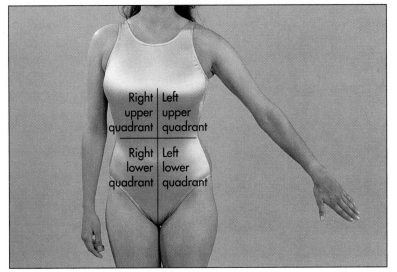

Figure 6-5

The umbilicus serves as the external landmark for the dividing point of the abdominal quadrants. The costal margin, formed by the bottom of the ribs, is the superior landmark of the upper abdominal quadrants. The bony symphysis pubis forms the inferior border of the lower abdominal quadrants.

ing up a glass of water involve the coordination of hundreds of nerve and muscle fibers. Describing the action of these groups of nerves and muscles would be a difficult task were it not for the adoption of certain single-word terms. For example, rotating the hand at the wrist so that the palm is facing upward is called supination. Rotating it downward is called pronation. Bending at a joint is called flexion, and straightening at a joint is extension. Pulling a limb in toward the midline of the body is called adduction, and moving the limb away from the midline of the body is called abduction (Fig. 6-10).

Injuries to muscles, bones, and nerves frequently cause pain with movement. Describing the specific movement that causes pain will aid the physician's diagnosis and also identify specific bandaging and splinting needs. Thus, instead of saying, "The patient has pain when he rotates the hand so that the palm is facing upward," we say, "The patient has pain upon supination."

Abbreviations and Acronyms

By necessity, patient care reports allow limited space for the paramedic to write a detailed narrative. Certain approved abbreviations and acronyms will aid in concisely describing perti-

nent findings and interventions. For example, the acronym for the heart condition paroxysmal supraventricular tachycardia is PSVT. A common treatment for PSVT is carotid sinus massage, or CSM. If written out, the condition and treatment would take 56 letters, but they have now been reduced to just seven—and the meaning remains clear.

The paramedic must be cautious, however, to use only abbreviations and acronyms that are approved by local medical direction. The use of terms known only by the paramedic writing the report makes the report more confusing and may create an unnecessary liability for the paramedic. Table 6-6 lists some commonly used medical abbreviations and acronyms.

Symbols

In addition to abbreviations and acronyms, certain symbols can take the place of words and phrases on a patient care report. Table 6-7 lists common symbols. Use of these terms should also conform to local standards.

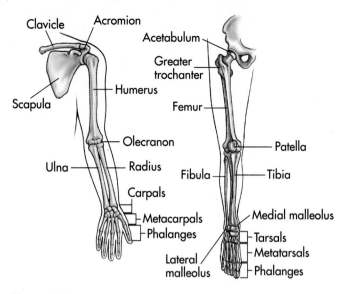

Figure 6-6

The upper and lower extremities have their proximal points of insertion into the body formed with joints. Note that one bone makes up the upper portion of each extremity and two make up the lower portion. Also note the similarity of the names for the bones of the hands and feet.

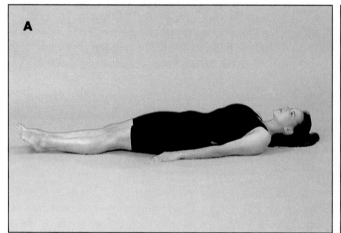

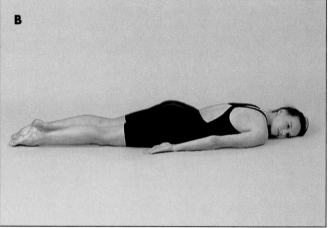

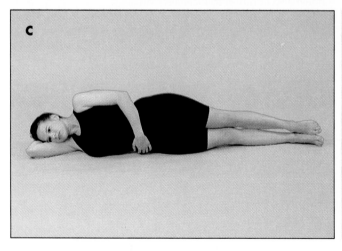

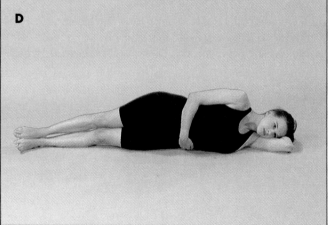

Figure 6-7

Positions of body at rest including A) supine B) prone C) right lateral recumbent D) left lateral recumbent E) Semi-Fowler's and F) High Fowler's.

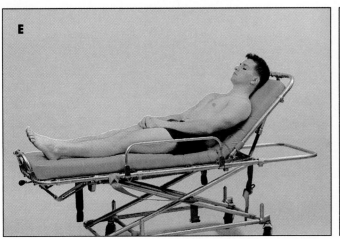

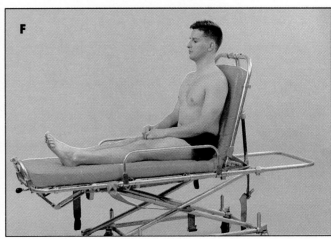

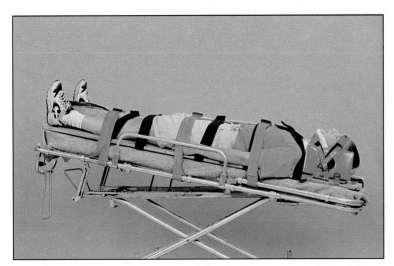

Figure 6-8

The Trendelenburg position is a common shock position and can be accomplished by elevating the end of the long board once the patient is securely immobilized.

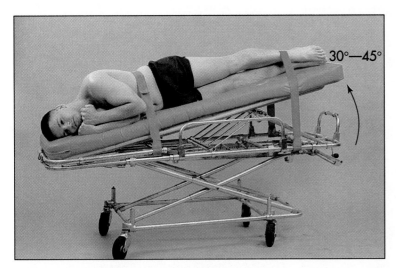

Figure 6-9

A combination of the left lateral recumbent and Trendelenburg positions prevents the introduction of an air embolism into the pulmonary artery, which could result in death. These positions are frequently used for diving emergencies.

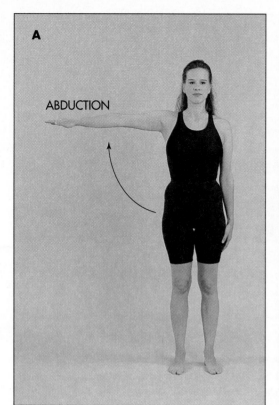

A

ABDUCTION

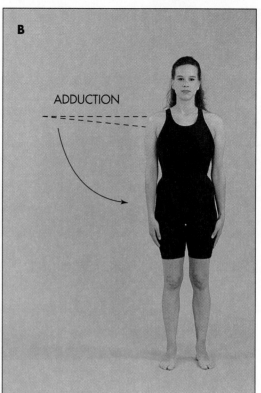

B

ADDUCTION

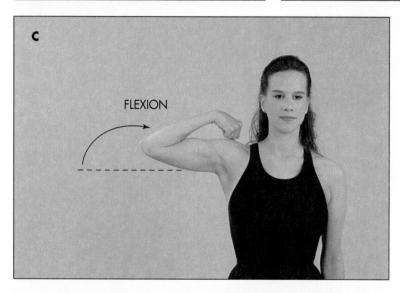

C

FLEXION

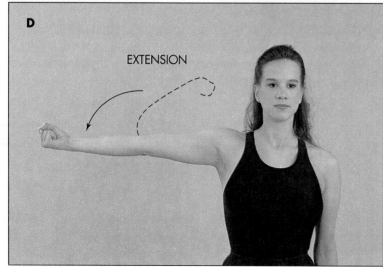

D

EXTENSION

Figure 6-10

Terms used to describe the motion of body parts and their relationship with the rest of the body include: A) abduction B) adduction C) flexion D) extension E) lateral rotation F) medial rotation G) supination H) pronation

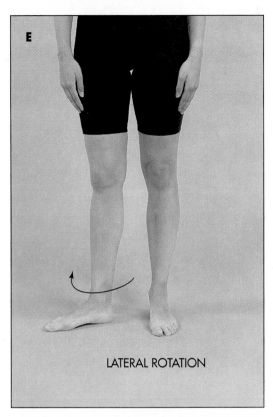

LATERAL ROTATION

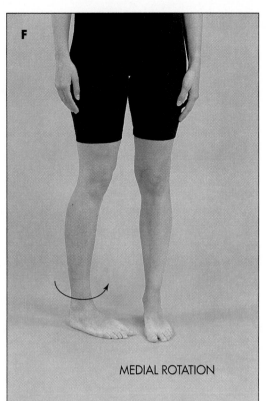

MEDIAL ROTATION

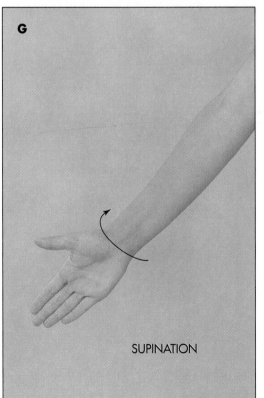

SUPINATION

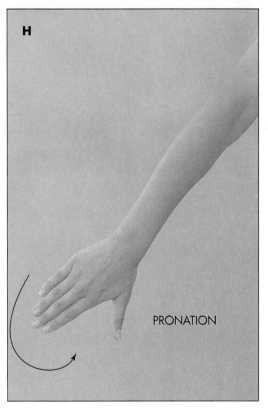

PRONATION

TABLE 6-6 Common Medical Abbreviations and Acronyms

Abbreviation/Acronym	Meaning	Abbreviation/Acronym	Meaning
a	Before	ED	Emergency department
ABCs	Airway, breathing and circulation	EEG	Electroencephalogram
ACLS	Advanced cardiac life support	e.g.	For example
AIDS	Acquired Immune Deficiency Syndrome	EGTA	Esophageal gastric tube airway
ALS	Advanced life support	EMD	Electromechanical dissociation
A.M.	Morning	ENT	Ears, nose and throat
AMA	Against medical advice	ER	Emergency room
AMI	Acute myocardial infarction	ET, ETT	Endotracheal, endotracheal tube
AO×3	Alert and oriented to person, place, and time	ETA	Estimated time of arrival
AP	Anterior/posterior	ETO	Estimated time out
ARDS	Adult respiratory distress syndrome	ETOH	Ethyl alcohol
ASAP	As soon as possible	EOA	Esophageal obturator airway
Ab	Abortion	F	Female
Abd.	Abdominal	F°	Degrees Fahrenheit
Adm.	Administration	FHT	Fetal heart tones
A-fib	Atrial fibrillation	fx	Fracture
A-flutter	Atrial flutter	G	Gravidity
A-tach	Atrial tachycardia	GB	Gall bladder
approx.	Approximate	GI	Gastrointestinal
BBB	Bundle branch block	Gm.	Gram
BM	Bowel movement	gr.	Grain
BOWI	Bag of waters (amniotic membrane) intact	GSW	Gun shot wound
BOWR	Bag of waters (amniotic membrane) ruptured	gtt/gtts	Drop/drops
BP	Blood pressure	GU	Genitourinary
BS	Breath sounds	GYN	Gynecological
BVM	Bag valve mask	h.	Hour
b.i.d.	Twice a day	H & H	Hemoglobin and hematocrit
bilat.	Bilateral	H & P	History and physical
C°	Degrees centigrade	H/A	Headache
c	With	Hb,Hgb	Hemoglobin
CA	Cancer	Hct.	Hematocrit
CAD	Coronary artery disease	HIV	Human immunodeficiency virus
C/C	Chief complaint	HR	Heart rate
CHF	Congestive heart failure	hr	Hour
CHI	Closed head injury	hs	At bedtime
CNS	Central nervous system	HTN	Hypertension
CO	Carbon monoxide	Hx	History
CO$_2$	Carbon dioxide	ICP	Intracranial pressure
COPD	Chronic obstructive pulmonary disease	ICU	Intensive care unit
CP	Chest pain	IM	Intramuscular
CPR	Cardiopulmonary resuscitation	inf.	Inferior
CSF	Cerebrospinal fluid	IPPB	Intermittent positive pressure breathing
CSM	Carotid sinus massage	IO	Intraosseous
C-spine	Cervical spine	IV	Intravenous
CVA	Cerebrovascular accident	IVP	Intravenous push
CXR	Chest x-ray	IVPB	Intravenous piggyback
D$_5$W	5% dextrose in water	JVD	Jugular venous distention
DC	Discontinue	Kg	Kilogram
DM	Diabetes mellitus	KVO	Keep vein open
DNR	Do not resuscitate	L	Liter
DOE	Dyspnea on exertion	Lt.	Left
DOS	Dead on the scene	lac.	Laceration
Dr.	Doctor	lb.	Pound
DTs	Delirium tremens	LBBB	Left bundle branch block
Dx	Diagnosis	L & D	Labor and delivery
ECG	Electrocardiogram	LLL	Left lower lobe of the lung

Abbreviation/Acronym	Meaning	Abbreviation/Acronym	Meaning
LLQ	Left lower quadrant of the abdomen	PSI	Pounds per square inch
LMP, LNMP	Last (normal) menstrual period	psych.	Psychiatric
LOC	Level of consciousness	pt.	Patient
LPM	Liters per minute	PVC	Premature ventricular contraction
L-spine	Lumbar spine	q	Every
LUL	Left upper lobe of the lungs	q.i.d.	Four times a day
LUQ	Left upper quadrant of the abdomen	R, RR	Respirations, respiratory rate
M	Male	RBBB	Right bundle branch block
M	Meter	RBC	Red blood cell
MAE	Moves all extremities	RL	Ringer's lactate solution
MAST	Medical (military) antishock trousers	RLL	Right lower lobe of the lungs
mcg.	Micrograms	RLQ	Right lower quadrant of the abdomen
MCL	Modified chest lead	RML	Right middle lobe of the lungs
MD	Medical doctor	R/O	Rule out
Meds	Medications	ROM	Range of motion
mEq.	Milliequivalent	Rt.	Right
MI	Myocardial infarction	RUL	Right upper lobe
MICU	Mobile intensive care unit	RUQ	Right upper quadrant of the abdomen
mL	Milliliter	Rx.	Prescription, treatment, therapy
mm	Millimeter	s	Without
MS	Morphine sulfate	SC, SQ	Subcutaneous
MVA	Motor vehicle accident	SIDS	Sudden infant death syndrome
MVC	Motor vehicle collision	SL	Sublingual
NaCl	Sodium chloride	SOB	Shortness of breath
NAD	No apparent distress	S/S	Signs and symptoms
NaHCO$_3$	Sodium bicarbonate	Stat	Immediately
NC	Nasal cannula	sub-Q	Subcutaneous
neg.	Negative	SVT	Supraventricular tachycardia
NGT	Nasogastric tube	tab.	Tablet
NKA	No known allergies	tach.	Tachycardia
NKDA	No known drug allergies	TB	Tuberculosis
NS(S)	Normal saline solution	tbsp.	Tablespoon
NSR	Normal sinus rhythm	Temp.	Temperature, temporary
NTG	Nitroglycerin	TIA	Transient ischemic attack
N/V	Nausea/vomiting	t.i.d.	Three times a day
O$_2$	Oxygen	TKO	To keep open
OB	Obstetrical	tsp.	Teaspoon
OBS	Organic brain syndrome	T-spine	Thoracic spine
OD	Overdose	Tx.	Treatment
oz.	Ounce	UA	Urinalysis
p	After	Unc.	Unconscious
P	Pulse	URI	Upper respiratory infection
PAC	Premature atrial contraction	USP	United States Pharmacopeia
PASG	Pneumatic anti-shock garment	UTI	Urinary tract infection
PAT	Paroxysmal atrial tachycardia	VD	Venereal disease
P.E.	Physical exam, pulmonary embolism	V-fib	Ventricular fibrillation
Pedi.	Pediatric	vol.	Volume
PERL(A)	Pupils equal and reactive to light (and accommodation)	V.S.	Vital signs
pH	Hydrogen ion concentration (measure of acid/base balance)	V-tach	Ventricular tachycardia
PID	Pelvic inflammatory disease	WBC	White blood cell
P.M.	After noon	WNL	Within normal limits
PND	Paroxysmal nocturnal dyspnea	W/S	Watt/seconds
p.o.	By mouth	wt.	Weight
POPTA	Passed out prior to arrival	y.o., y/o	Year old
PRN	As needed		

TABLE 6-7	Symbols to Shorten the Written Report While Maintaining Clarity

Symbol	Meaning
@	At
α	Alpha
β	Beta
μg	Microgram
↑	Increased, increasing
↓	Decreased, decreasing
→	Leading to, progressing to
∅	Lack of, none, no
≅	Approximately
(+)	Positive, plus
(−)	Negative, minus
=	Equals, equal to
≠	Not equal
>	Greater than
<	Less than
≥	Greater than or equal to
≤	Less than or equal to
♀	Female
♂	Male
△	Change
/	Per
∴	Therefore
#	Number

SUMMARY

Just as knowledge of anatomy and physiology is necessary in the care of the patient, correct terminology is necessary in communicating with other members of the health care team. By learning the meanings of combining words, prefixes, suffixes, acronyms, symbols, and common abbreviations, the paramedic makes better use of patient care time and can easily provide an accurate verbal or written picture of the patient's condition.

REFERENCES

1. Backhouse KM, Hutchings RT: Color atlas of surface anatomy, Baltimore, 1986, Williams & Wilkins.

2. Bledsoe BE, Porter RS, Shade BR: Paramedic emergency care, Englewood Cliffs, 1991, Prentice Hall.

3. Campbell JE: Basic trauma life support: advance prehospital life support, ed 2, Englewood Cliffs, 1988, Prentice Hall.

4. Caroline NL: Emergency care in the streets, ed 4, Boston, 1991, Little, Brown, and Company.

5. Ehrlich A: Medical terminology for health professions, ed 2, Albany, 1993, Delmar Publishers.

6. Hensyl WR: Webster's new world/stedman's concise medical dictionary, Baltimore, 1987, Williams & Wilkins.

7. Madigan KG: Prehospital emergency drugs pocket reference, St. Louis, 1990, C.V. Mosby.

8. Urdang L: Mosby's medical & nursing dictionary, St. Louis, 1983, C.V. Mosby.

Christopher Perrin, BA, EMT-P

Chapter 7

Basic Body Systems

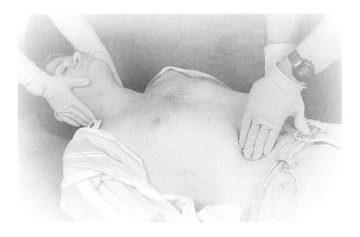

A paramedic should be able to:

OBJECTIVES

1. List the four major tissue types.
2. Describe the unique characteristics of each of the four major tissue types.
3. List the eleven major organ systems of the body.
4. Identify the key anatomic structures in each of the major organ systems of the body.
5. Describe the functions of the major anatomic structures of the eleven major organ systems of the body.
6. Describe how major anatomic structures of the eleven major organ systems of the body interact to perform the specified functions of the system.

KEY TERMS

1. **Anatomy**—the study, classification, and description of structures and organs of the body.
2. **Cell**—the fundamental unit of all living tissue.
3. **Central nervous system**—the brain and spinal cord, which are encased in and protected by bone.
4. **Circulatory system**—the dynamic cardiovascular network consisting of the heart, arteries, veins, capillaries, and blood.
5. **Connective tissue**—tissues that support and bind other body tissues and parts.
6. **Diffusion**—the random, passive distribution of particles in a mixture or solution; substances move in the direction of the concentration gradient. When all parts of the solution have equal concentrations, the solute is dissolved, and the solution is homogeneous.
7. **Digestive system**—the organ system of the body which prepares food and liquids for absorption; consists of the mouth and tongue, esophagus, stomach, small and large intestines, and the rectum.
8. **Endocrine system**—the network of ductless glands that secrete hormones directly into the bloodstream.

9. **Epithelial tissue**—the cellular covering of internal and external surfaces of the body, including the lining of vessels and other small cavities.
10. **Homeostasis**—a state of equilibrium in the body with respect to functions and composition of fluids and tissues.
11. **Hormone**—a complex chemical substance produced in one part or organ of the body that initiates or regulates the activity of an organ or a group of cells in another part of the body.
12. **Integumentary system**—skin, hair, and nails; the outer covering of the body.
13. **Lymphatic system**—the network of vessels, ducts, nodes, valves, and organs that are involved in protecting and maintaining the internal fluid environment of the body.
14. **Metabolism**—the aggregate of all chemical processes that take place in living organisms, resulting in growth generation of energy, elimination of wastes, and other bodily functions as they relate to the distribution of nutrients of the blood.
15. **Muscular system**—the complex, dynamic network of muscles, nerves, bones and tendons that function to maintain body posture and provide motion.
16. **Muscle tissue**—contractile tissue that provides kinetic energy for the body.
17. **Nervous system**—the network of conductive tissues which transmit impulses to and from the brain, and process thoughts, impulses and reflexes.
18. **Organ**—a structure made up of two or more kinds of tissues, organized to perform a more complex function than can any one tissue alone.
19. **Peripheral nervous system**—a major subdivision of the nervous system consisting of nerves and ganglia.
20. **Physiology**—the study of the processes and functions of the human body.
21. **Reproductive system**—the organ systems involved in conception (in males and females), and gestation, labor and delivery, and mammalian feeding (in females).
22. **Skeletal system**—the structure of bones which provide posture to the body.
23. **Tissue**—a collection of similar cells acting together to perform a particular function.
24. **Urinary system**—the organs of the body which filter, store, and then eliminate urine; includes the kidneys, ureters, bladder, and urethra.

his chapter describes the organization and major structures and functions of the human body. Other chapters will focus on the details of specific systems and their pathophysiology.

A fundamental understanding of the structure (anatomy) and function (physiology) of the human body can assist paramedics in conducting timely assessments and determining interventions. Such an understanding enables paramedics to predict how injury and illness can affect other structures and systems that are related structurally or functionally to the primary problem area.

Basic Building Blocks

The fundamental building block for the human body is the cell (Fig. 7-1). Trillions of these tiny factories of life unite to form the organism called the human body. Surrounded by a membrane and filled with protoplasm (proto: *original,* plasm: *substance*), each cell is independently alive—capable of growth, repair, or reproduction. Cells differ greatly in their life spans. Some intestinal cells may live an average of only 1 or 2 days while red blood cells average 120 days.

These cell building blocks are grouped together to form increasingly more complex structures. A group of cells with similar features or functions is called a tissue. Tissues, in turn, make up organs. Organs can be grouped together with those having similar functions and described collectively as systems (Fig. 7-2).

For example, cells that specialize in creating and secreting hydrochloric acid (grouped by function as tissue) combine with connective tissue and protective tissues (in this case, mucus-secreting cells) to form the lining of an enlarged pouch of smooth muscle tissue. Together these tissues mix their respective secretions with food and liquid. This collective function of tissues defines an organ, in this case, the stomach. By break-

ing down foodstuffs into useable products for cells, and eliminating the excess, the stomach shares a similar purpose with other organs and structures, such as the intestines. Their common function groups them together into the digestive system.

Cells, tissues, organs, and systems work collectively to balance the human organism, allow it to respond to internal and external changes, and return to the balanced state called homeostasis. Injury and illness often set predictable reactions into motion within the body as it attempts to restore itself to this state. These bodily reactions manifest themselves as signs and symptoms, which are discovered during patient assessment. Paramedics look, touch, listen, and smell for normal and abnormal tissue, organ and system functions, and consider how the abnormal findings may be affecting cells throughout the body. Understanding the unique and the common properties of these structures helps the paramedic to predict the impact of injury and illness.

Basic Tissues and Structures

The human body is composed of four basic tissue types: epithelial, muscle, connective, and nervous tissue (Fig. 7-3). This section describes each of these basic building blocks of tissue and how these tissues combine to form organs and systems (Fig. 7-4).

Epithelial Tissue

Epithelial tissue covers the body's surfaces and lines its cavities. Epithelium forms the skin, the lining of blood vessels and the respiratory, digestive, reproductive, and urinary systems, and is also the principal tissue that makes up glands, both endocrine and exocrine. A key characteristic of these cells is their ability to tightly join together to form surfaces; there is little intercellular material. Epithelial tissue is also noted for its ability to repair or replace itself rapidly.

Epithelial cells can have special functions beyond simply providing protective cover. Some of these cells purposely leak or secrete substances, such as mucus from respiratory or stomach epithelium. Other epithelial cells secrete and absorb substances, as with the digestive cells that form the lining of the small intestine. Other epithelial cells specialize in filtering and creating movement, such as the hair-like projections in the respiratory system known as cilia (Fig. 7-5). Still others are characterized by their ability to expand significantly, such as the urinary bladder and the uterus.

Epithelial tissues that specialize in secretion are considered either exocrine or endocrine glands. Exocrine glands produce secretions, such as saliva and digestive enzymes, that are delivered through ducts to their destinations. Endocrine glands secrete substances known as hormones directly into the bloodstream. Epinephrine, secreted by the adrenal gland, is an example. Hormones are chemical messengers that typically travel via the bloodstream to specific receptor sites to trigger a desired effect in the function or metabolism of the targeted tissue.

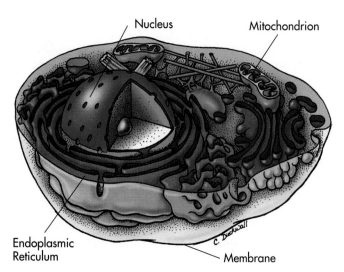

Nucleus

Mitochondrion

Endoplasmic Reticulum

Membrane

Figure 7-1

The cell: the fundamental building block for the human body.

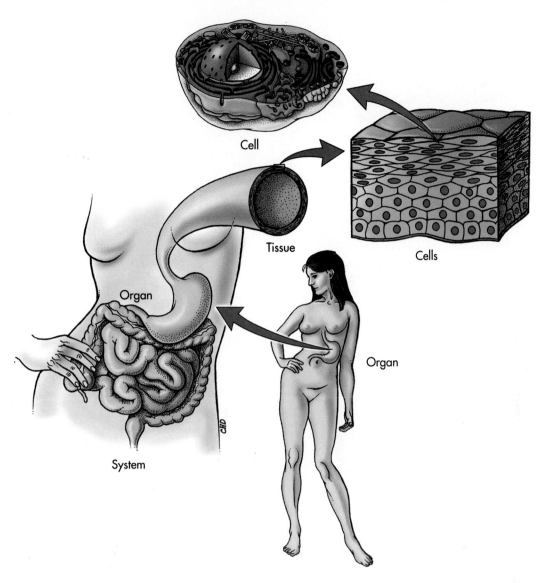

Cell

Tissue

Cells

Organ

Organ

System

Figure 7-2

Systems are made up of organs. Organs are made up of tissues. Tissues are made up of cells.
The combination of all body systems working together allows the individual to survive.

Connective Tissue

Connective tissue functions primarily to protect, connect, and support. It differs from epithelial tissue in that connective tissue contains significant amounts of intercellular material. The intercellular material may be fluid, gel, or solid and may be plastered to a network of fibers, as calcium is cemented to collagen fibers by bone-forming cells (Fig. 7-6). Included in this category are adipose (fatty) tissue, tendons, ligaments, fascia, cartilage, and bone. Special connective tissue includes the formed elements of blood: platelets and red and white blood cells.

Loose connective tissue, with soft intercellular material, is found throughout the body. Often the base of attachment for epithelial cells, it is highly vascular and frequently has varying layers of adipose, which is another form of connective tissue. The combining of sheets of epithelial and connective tissues creates a tissue membrane.

Dense connective tissue contains more fibers in its intercellular spaces than loose connective tissue. Tissues of this nature include tendons, ligaments, and membrane capsules that envelop organs such as the kidneys and liver. Cartilage is a special form of dense connective tissue; it has a firm gel-like base for the intercellular fibers with no blood supply of its own. Cartilage receives its nutrient supply through close contact with surrounding vascular tissue and through a process called diffusion, the flow of electrolytes from areas of higher concentration to areas of lower concentration.

Bones are composed of calcified dense connective tissue. Calcium and phosphorus salts are deposited around bone-forming cells (osteocytes) on collagen fibers. This process is continuous as cells are built up, torn down, and built up again. Collectively, the body replaces its skeleton the equivalent of once every 7 years. The mineral salts in bone give the tissue hardness, whereas the collagen framework is responsible for its flexible, shock-absorbing support. Insufficient amounts of

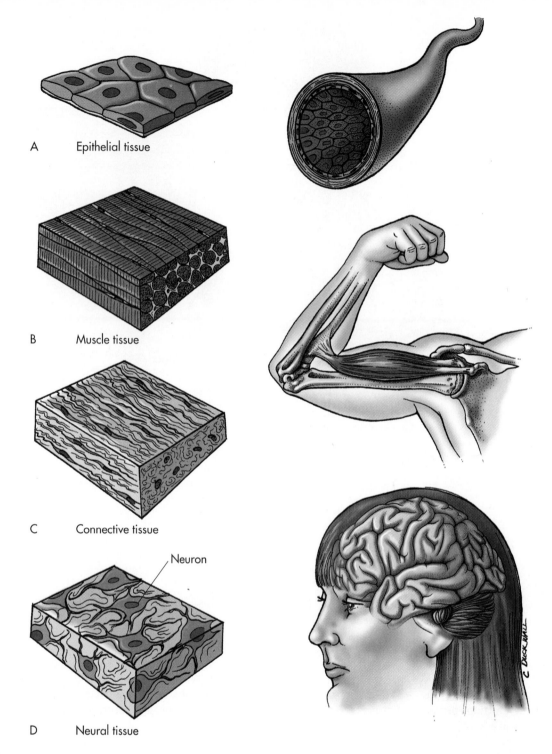

A   Epithelial tissue

B   Muscle tissue

C   Connective tissue

Neuron

D   Neural tissue

Figure 7-3

The four basic tissues types: A, Epithelial. B, Muscle. C, Connective. D, Neural.

calcium weaken bones and predispose them to breakage, as seen in the condition known as **osteoporosis.** (A paramedic may encounter this when treating a patient who has minimal trauma and yet shows evidence of fracture.) Generally, healthy bone has the same tensile (tearing) strength as reinforced concrete and a greater ability to withstand compression. Bones are coated with a thin fibrous tissue called the periosteum that serves as a place of attachment for ligaments, tendons, and muscles. The periosteum also has an extensive supply of nerve

fibers and nerve impulses known as innervation, including pain receptors. Individual bones are categorized by their overall appearance: short (carpals), flat (temporal bone in the skull), irregular (maxilla), long (humerus or femur), and sesamoid (patella).

Bone tissue is extremely vascular—the equivalent of 100 acres of surface area in the bones are in contact with the bloodstream. Inner canals (called bone marrow) of long bones and some flat bones are the production sites for red blood

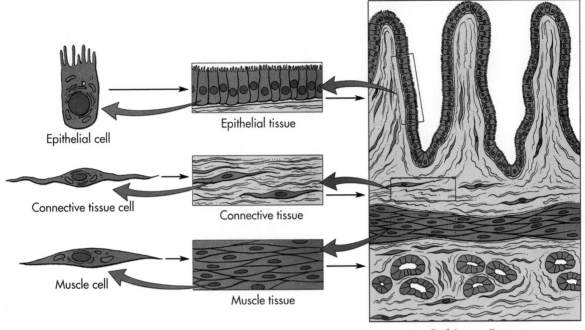

Epithelial cell

Epithelial tissue

Connective tissue cell

Connective tissue

Muscle cell

Muscle tissue

Wall of the small intestine

Figure 7-4

Combinations of two or more basic tissues types allows for the formation of organs. An example of this is shown by the wall of the small intestine.

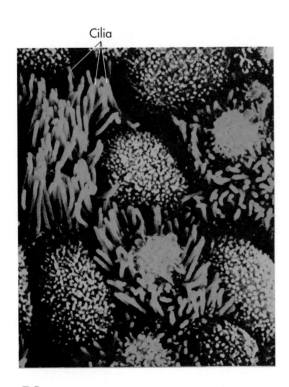

Cilia

Figure 7-5

Cilia are specialized epithelial cells found in the lining of the respiratory tract. Their hairlike projections are used to sweep away debris. *From Thibodeau: Anatomy and Physiology, ed 2, St. Louis, 1993, Mosby–Year Book.*

cells. Because of their vascularity, some bones are excellent sites for infusing fluids or administering medications. Described as the intraosseous route, this is a particularly effective alternative to intravenous routes in emergencies involving unconscious pediatric patients.

Muscle Tissue

There are three general types of muscle tissue: striated, smooth, and cardiac.

Striated, also known as voluntary or skeletal, muscle appears striped under microscopic examination. Its action can be voluntary (through conscious effort) or by reflex. Striated muscles are typically attached directly or indirectly to bone through cord-like attachments called tendons or flattened sheets of dense connective tissue. They may also attach to other muscles or skin, as do the facial muscles. Most muscles require opposing muscle groups; their counter-contraction modifies the primary group or returns the anchor points to their original position when the primary group relaxes.

The maximum contraction of a muscle fiber is 57% of its resting length; to create greater range of movement, longer parallel grouping of muscle fibers is necessary. Strength, the force or power of contraction, depends on mass; a more powerful contraction requires a greater diameter of muscle. Muscle contraction and relaxation in the extremities compresses veins within the compartments. This helps to propel blood through the vessels and their one-way valves back to the heart.

Smooth muscle is also known as involuntary, nonstriated, or visceral muscle. It is found in blood vessels and in the organs of the respiratory, digestive, and genitourinary systems.

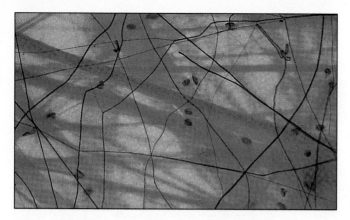

Figure 7-6

Loose, ordinary (areolar) connective tissue. Connective tissue has many different appearances. Adipose (fat), tendons, ligaments, fascia (the covering over muscles), cartilage, bone, and each type of blood cell are all examples of connective tissue. *From Thibodeau: Anatomy and Physiology, ed 2, St. Louis, 1993, Mosby–Year Book.*

Smooth muscle contractions are generally less powerful and slower, although more sustained, than striated muscle. The autonomic nervous system and the endocrine system typically control smooth muscle.

Faintly striated in appearance, cardiac muscle is found only in the heart. It is capable of spontaneous contraction. Although the cardiac muscle itself does not require outside innervation to initiate contraction, the rate can be modified by the autonomic system.

Nervous Tissue

Nervous tissue is constructed of two basic tissue types: neurons and neuroglial cells.

Neurons are the basic structural and functional units of the nervous system, responsible for message formation and transmission (Fig. 7-7). Individual neurons can be bundled together to form nerves (Fig. 7-8). Neurons receive incoming messages along fibers called dendrites that are sent to each cell's central switchboard (cell body), which then decides to pass the signal along its single outgoing fiber, or axon. Internally, cells conduct messages electrically: for the message to be able to jump the tiny gap or synapse, between cells requires the message to be ferried across by chemicals called neurotransmitters (Fig. 7-9). Through creation and transmission of chemical-electrical messages, neurons coordinate body activities. Sensory or afferent neurons take information in from outside the body or from other areas within the body. Efferent or motor neurons create and send responses to those stimuli. In addition, some neurons, called connector or interneurons, conduct impulses or messages between afferent and efferent neurons.

The body's neurons are all present at birth. They may grow in mass, connections, and support structures, but are not believed to be capable of multiplying except for peripheral neurons. They are capable of regeneration in limited circumstances.

Neuroglial cells are actually a type of connective tissue. They provide support functions, such as fiber insulation, which protects central nervous system tissue from contamination from exposure to toxins in the bloodstream. This creates a blood-brain barrier that selectively transports products to and from CNS tissue, including certain drugs.

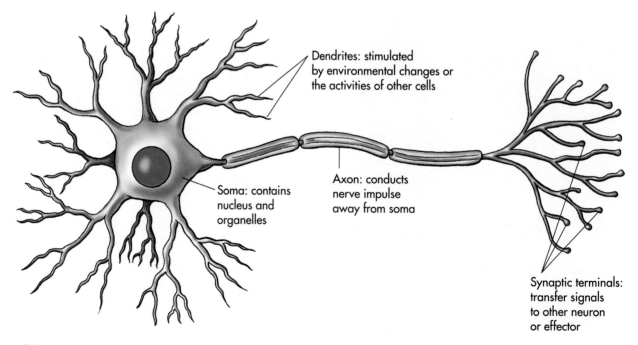

Figure 7-7

The neuron is the basic structural component of the nervous system. Some neurons reach several feet in length and are visible with the naked eye.

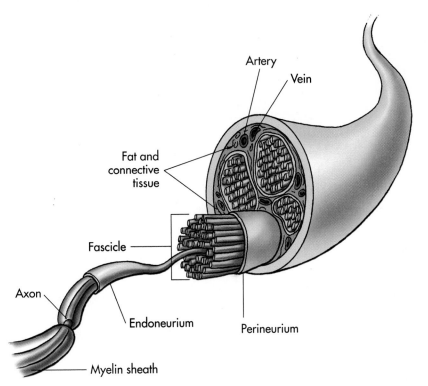

Artery
Vein
Fat and connective tissue
Fascicle
Axon
Endoneurium
Perineurium
Myelin sheath

Figure 7-8

Neurons bundled together form nerves.

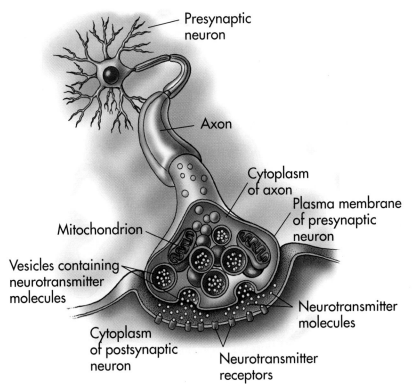

Presynaptic neuron
Axon
Cytoplasm of axon
Plasma membrane of presynaptic neuron
Mitochondrion
Vesicles containing neurotransmitter molecules
Neurotransmitter molecules
Cytoplasm of postsynaptic neuron
Neurotransmitter receptors

Figure 7-9

A synapse is formed in the space between two nerve cells, or a nerve cell with a gland cell, muscle cell, or sensory receptor. The function of the synapse is to transmit the action potential from one cell to the other.

Systems

As cells with similar structure or function group together to form tissues, tissues also combine their functions to create organs, which collectively function as body systems.

Nervous System

The nervous system is the communications network that provides the ongoing exchange of information to tie the other systems together. The nervous system is divided into two subsystems: the central nervous system and the outlying peripheral nervous system.

Central Nervous System

The CNS is composed of two of the most delicate and complex structures in the human body: the brain and the spinal cord (Fig. 7-10). Together they provide the primary processing units for coordination, interpretation, and regulation of body functions and interaction with the surrounding environment.

The cerebrum is the originator of all voluntary thought, memory, movement, perception, and emotion (Fig. 7-11). The cerebellum mediates balance, fine motor movement, and coordination. The midbrain and hypothalamus regulate such vital functions as temperature, appetite, and consciousness. The brainstem regulates overall control of breathing and heart rate. The brain is further divided into the right and left hemispheres. Hemispheres contain regions that specialize according to function (e.g., certain areas specialize in sensory interpretation, others in speech, movement, and vision) (Fig. 7-12). Each hemisphere receives and sends information to the opposite side of the body. Communication between hemispheres occurs through a bridge-like structure called the corpus collosum.

The human brain is a 3-pound jello-like mass composed of 85% water. The wrinkled outer ¼-to ⅛-inch thick shell, or cerebral cortex, consists of gray matter or cell bodies that are grayish in color. The inner core is supporting white matter,

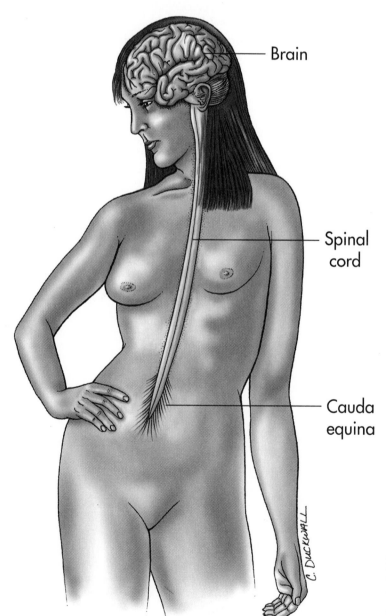

— Brain

— Spinal cord

— Cauda equina

Figure 7-10

The brain and spinal cord make up the central nervous system. The bulk, ropelike spinal cord ends approximately at the level of the first lumbar vertebra, and forms the cauda equina (horse's tail) from that point on.

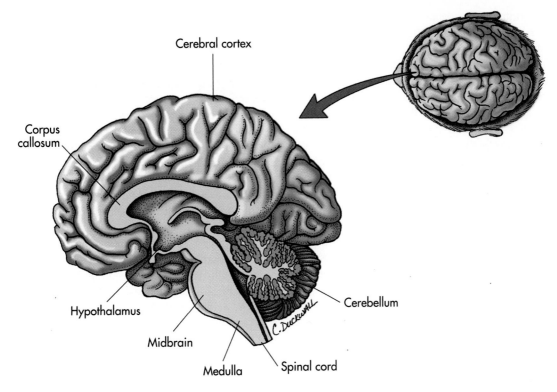

Figure 7-11

The structures of the brain.

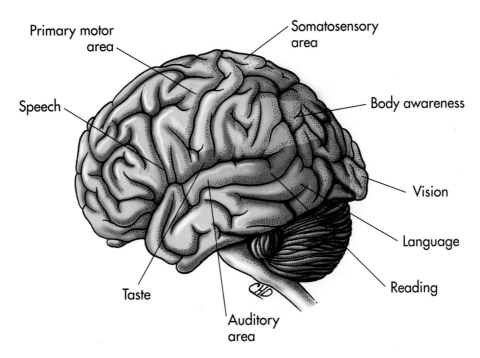

Figure 7-12

Specific areas of the brain responsible for bodily functions and sensations.

neuroglia. This white matter contains sheathed connections between the various cell bodies, with as many as 60,000 connections to a single cell body.

Extending from the base of the brain approximately 18 inches downward lies the spinal cord. Its primary function is to serve as a transmitter of information to and from the brain. Occasionally, it creates reflex pathways that do not require processing by the brain. Averaging ½ inch in diameter, the spinal cord consists of a butterfly-shaped inner core of gray matter encased in white matter. It extends down through its protective canal in the vertebral column almost to the second lumbar vertebrae. Below that level, the spinal canal is filled with nerve branches that cascade down from the end of the cord in a tail-like fashion, called cauda equina (Latin for "horsetail").

The brain and the spinal cord are the only body organs completely encased in bone (skull and vertebrae) for protection. Inside their bony fortresses are the meninges, three envelopes of membranes that also surround and protect (Fig. 7-13). In addition, approximately 120 cc of shock-absorbing, nutrient-filled cerebrospinal fluid (CSF) surrounds the brain and spinal cord. Without such protection, minor occurrences such as dropping a coin on the head from a few inches elevation could crush delicate brain and spinal tissue, resulting in permanent and significant damage to the CNS.

Peripheral Nervous System

Peripheral nerves branch out to and from the central nervous system. Twelve pairs of cranial nerves (Table 7-1) attach directly to the underside of the brain, and 31 pairs of spinal nerves branch off of the spinal cord. These major nerve bundles provide sensory input and motor output.

The peripheral nervous system is divided into two functional subsystems: the somatic (primarily under deliberate or voluntary control) and the autonomic (primarily under involuntary control). The autonomic system is further divided into two opposite or antagonistic divisions: the sympathetic system (the accelerator or stress response division) and the parasympathetic system (the brakes or vegetative response division) (Fig. 7-14).

The sympathetic system uses the hormones epinephrine and norepinephrine as neurotransmitters (synapse-jumpers) to create its adrenergic response. Adrenergic responses include fight-or-flight responses such as pupillary dilation, changes in blood vessel and bronchiole diameters, increases in heart rate, and strength of cardiac contractility. The parasympathetic system uses acetylcholine as the neurotransmitter to accomplish its cholinergic response. Cholingeric responses generally oppose adrenergic responses and include pupil constriction, decreases in the heart rate and strength of contractility, bronchiole constriction, and increased secretions.

The autonomic system directs activities that do not require conscious effort or awareness, such as overall regulation of heart rate in response to body needs, blood vessel diameter, breathing, digestion, and blood pressure maintenance. For example, paramedics may administer the drug epinephrine which affects both the diameter of blood vessels and air passages (bronchi).

Respiratory System

The respiratory system includes structures within the head and the trunk of the body. Its principal task is to facilitate the exchange of oxygen and carbon dioxide for the circulatory system, to deliver oxygen to and from the individual cells of the

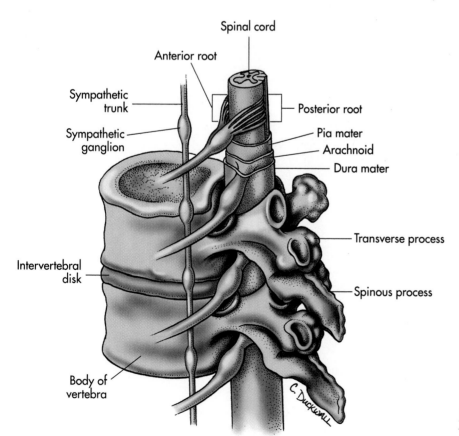

Figure 7-13

The meningeal layers cover the spinal cord.

body. Oxygen is needed by the body's cells, to convert nutrients to useable energy. The respiratory system is formed by a network of tubes with openings in the mouth and nose that end in tiny clusters of air sacs in the lungs (called alveoli) (Fig. 7-15). This network includes the nasal and oral passages, pharynx, larynx, trachea, lungs, bronchi, bronchioles, and alveoli.

The lungs are two large, sponge-like organs, each weighing only about 1 pound. Each lung has its own slippery visceral lining (visceral pleura) that is vacuum sealed with a small amount of fluid against a slippery cavity lining (parietal pleura). The right lung has three sections, or lobes, whereas the left lung has only two. This allows room for the left-tilted contents of the mediastinum (the heart and other structures in the center of the chest).

To facilitate movement of gases into and out of the system, the body uses the diaphragm, a dome-shaped muscle beneath the lungs. As the diaphragm contracts, the base of the lungs is drawn downward, which expands the respiratory container and creates an inflow of air into this reduced-pressure environment. This process is known as inspiration. Accessory muscles within the chest wall (intercostals) and the neck (sternocleidomastoids) can contract and further increase the size of the container and the resulting inflow of air. Expiration is typically a passive phase that requires only the relaxation of previously mentioned muscles; this then reduces the container's size and creates an outflow of air. Paramedics may encounter patients with abnormally narrow, damaged, or partially obstructed lower airways. Asthma and COPD are two conditions that often require the patient to actively work at exhaling the lung's contents.

Inspiration, expiration, and the resulting exchange of gases within the alveoli result in the processes known as respiration and ventilation. (Respiration also refers to the exchange of gases at the final destination between the capillaries and the cells of the body). The actual exchange of gases occurs within the alveoli, which are minute air sacs within the lungs. Alveoli are coated with a film of surfactant that creates surface tension and prevents collapse during exhalation. Thin-walled capillaries that drape over the alveoli allow red blood cells to pass over them single file. In a fraction of a second, the capillaries off-load carbon dioxide and take on oxygen to be sent back to the heart. The oxygen then travels to the area of the body in need of its cargo.

Circulatory System

The circulatory system of the average adult employs 60,000 to 72,000 miles of blood vessels, 5 to 7 quarts of blood, and a 10-ounce pump that is overseen by the central nervous system. The circulatory system circulates nutrients and collects wastes from the same tissue.

Blood is 78% water. It consists of plasma, and red blood cells (erythrocytes), white blood cells (leukocytes), and platelets. Plasma, a watery, colorless fluid, makes up approximately 50% of the total volume of blood. It carries the red and white blood cells and the platelets through the bloodstream, and is instrumental in maintaining the acid-base balance of the body. Red blood cells represent approximately 45% of the volume of blood, and are the most common cells in the body. Red blood cells transport hemoglobin, an iron compound that carries oxygen from the lungs to the cells, and carbon dioxide from the cells to the lungs for removal. White blood cells (including lymphocytes, neutrophils, and macrophages) number considerably less than the red blood cells and represent the main line of defense against invading organisms. Platelets are the blood's smallest cells. In wounds, they rush to replace surface cells and initiate the complex process of blood clot formation.

The heart has its own electrical system and uses approximately 5% of the body's oxygenated blood supply. Each contraction sends about 70 cc of deoxygenated, waste-laden blood

TABLE 7-1	Cranial Nerves and Their Functions		
Number	**Name**	**General Function**	**Specific Function**
I	Olfactory	S	Smell
II	Optic	S	Vision
III	Ocularmotor	M, P	Motor to four of six eye muscles and upper eyelid; parasympathetic: constricts pupil, thickens lens
IV	Trochlear	M	Motor to one eye muscle
V	Trigeminal	S, M	Sensory to face and teeth; motor to muscles of mastication (chewing)
VI	Abducens	M	Motor to one eye muscle
VII	Facial	S, M, P	Sensory: taste; motor to muscles of facial expression; parasympathetic to salivary and tear glands
VIII	Vestibulocochlear	S	Hearing and balance
IX	Glossopharyngeal	S, M, P	Sensory: taste and touch to back of tongue; motor to pharyngeal muscle; parasympathetic to salivary glands
X	Vagus	S, M, P	Sensory to pharynx, larynx, and viscera; motor to palate, pharynx, and larynx; parasympathetic to viscera of thorax and abdomen
XI	Accessory	M	Motor to two neck and upper back muscles
XII	Hypoglossal	M	Motor to tongue muscles

*S, sensory; M, motor; P, parasympathetic. From Seeley RR, et al: Essentials of anatomy and physiology, second edition, St. Louis, 1996, Mosby–Year Book, Inc.

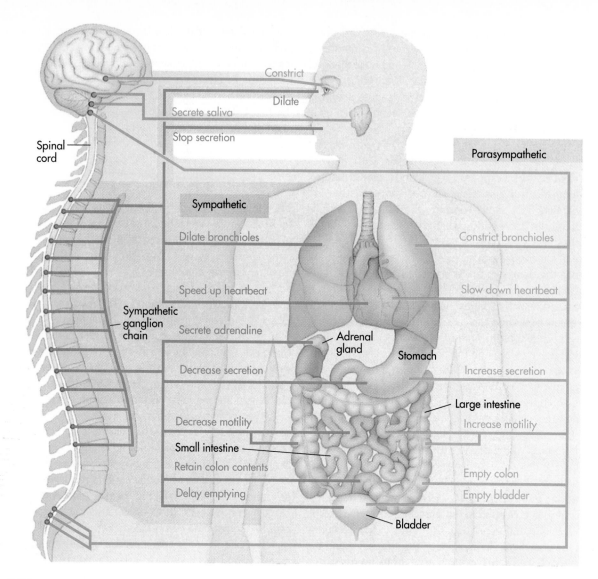

Constrict

Dilate

Secrete saliva

Stop secretion

Spinal cord

Parasympathetic

Sympathetic

Dilate bronchioles

Constrict bronchioles

Speed up heartbeat

Slow down heartbeat

Sympathetic ganglion chain

Secrete adrenaline

Adrenal gland

Stomach

Decrease secretion

Increase secretion

Large intestine

Decrease motility

Increase motility

Small intestine

Retain colon contents

Empty colon

Delay emptying

Empty bladder

Bladder

Figure 7-14

The two divisions of the autonomic nervous system, the sympathetic and parasympathetic, allow for involuntary control of body systems and function in maintaining homeostasis or balance. The parasympathetic fibers are highlighted with blue, and the sympathetic fibers are highlighted with red. *From Thibodeau: Structure and Function of the Body, ed 9, St. Louis, 1992, Mosby–Year Book.*

from the right side of the heart to the lungs; at the same time an equal amount of blood is collected from the lungs, cleansed, oxygenated, and returned to the body via the heart's more heavily muscled left side. The characteristic "lub-dub" sound heard with each contraction is the result of four sets of valves keeping the flow moving in one direction through the heart (Fig. 7-16).

The central nervous system helps regulate the heart rate and controls the diameter of the many miles of blood vessels through which the heart must pump blood. These vessels include arteries, capillaries, and veins (Fig. 7-17). At any given time, approximately two-thirds of the total blood volume is in the thin-walled, valved veins awaiting return to the heart.

Lymphatic System

The lymphatic system helps restore fluids and filter out waste from the body. Every 24 hours, the heart pumps thousands of liters of blood; it is estimated that almost 20 liters leak out of

the capillaries during the same time period. Capillaries reabsorb between 16 and 18 liters of this leakage, with the remaining 2 to 4 liters returned via the lymphatic system (Fig. 7-18). Interstitial fluid pressures rise when this leakage occurs. Excess water and escaped plasma proteins are absorbed by lymph capillaries. Lymph capillaries are thin walled and made of loosely connected endothelium that allows passage of the surrounding fluid inside. Once inside, this fluid becomes lymph. Lymph collects and travels through its own passive network of capillaries, vessels, and finally, ducts. Without its own pump, it must rely on one-way valves, movement of surrounding muscle groups, and position changes to create a slow lymphatic flow. During that flow, scattered clusters of lymphoid tissues (lymph nodes) filter out pathogens, remove dead blood cells, and manufacture antibodies and lymphocytes (about one fourth of the white blood cells). The filtered and revitalized lymph fluid and plasma proteins are then returned to veins entering the heart for redistribution.

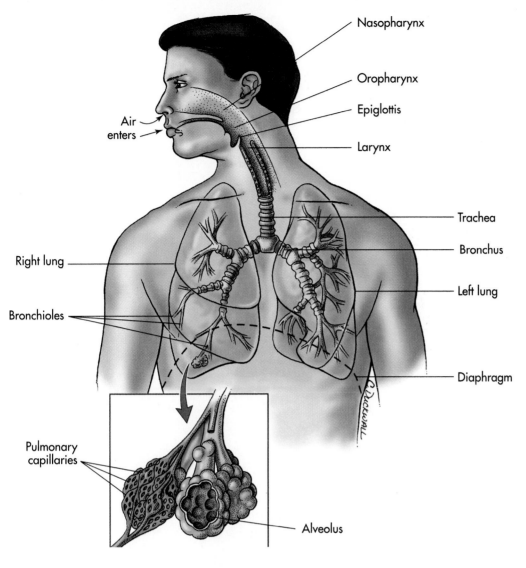

Nasopharynx

Oropharynx

Epiglottis

Larynx

Air enters

Trachea

Bronchus

Right lung

Left lung

Bronchioles

Diaphragm

Pulmonary capillaries

Alveolus

Figure 7-15

The respiratory system.

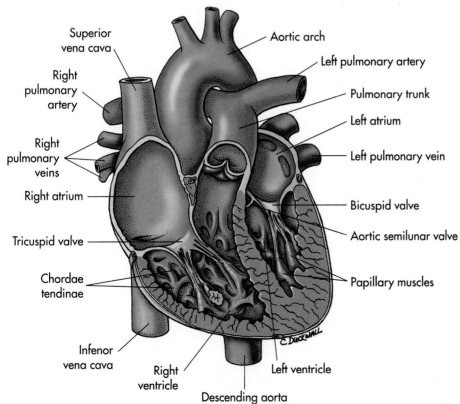

Superior vena cava

Aortic arch

Right pulmonary artery

Left pulmonary artery

Pulmonary trunk

Left atrium

Right pulmonary veins

Left pulmonary vein

Right atrium

Bicuspid valve

Tricuspid valve

Aortic semilunar valve

Chordae tendinae

Papillary muscles

Infenor vena cava

Right ventricle

Left ventricle

Descending aorta

Figure 7-16

The heart.

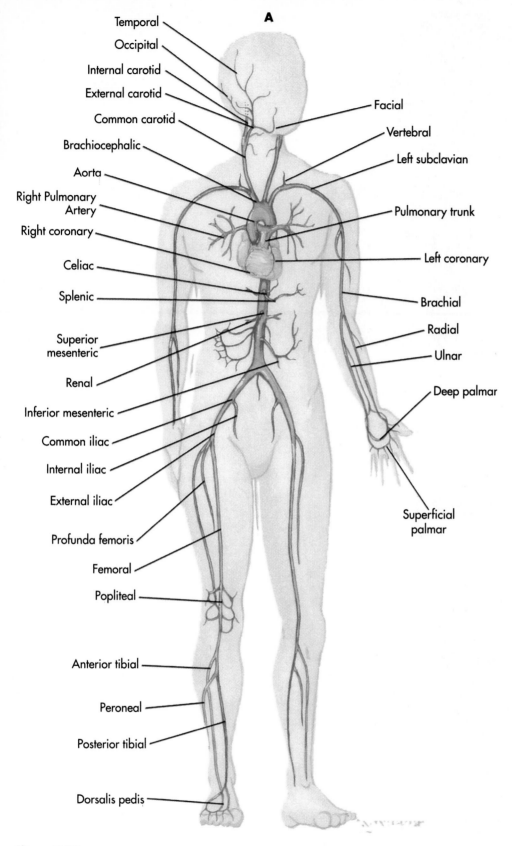

A

Temporal

Occipital

Internal carotid

External carotid

Common carotid

Brachiocephalic

Aorta

Right Pulmonary Artery

Right coronary

Celiac

Splenic

Superior mesenteric

Renal

Inferior mesenteric

Common iliac

Internal iliac

External iliac

Profunda femoris

Femoral

Popliteal

Anterior tibial

Peroneal

Posterior tibial

Dorsalis pedis

Facial

Vertebral

Left subclavian

Pulmonary trunk

Left coronary

Brachial

Radial

Ulnar

Deep palmar

Superficial palmar

Figure 7-17

The primary vessels of the circulatory system: A, Arteries. B, Veins. *From Sanders: Instructors Resource Kit to Accompany Mosby's Paramedic Textbook, St. Louis, 1995, Mosby–Year Book.*

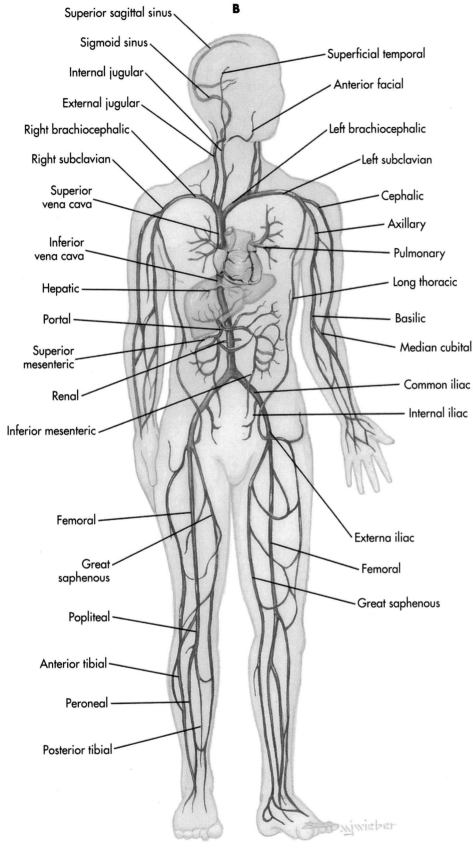

B

Superior sagittal sinus

Sigmoid sinus

Internal jugular

External jugular

Right brachiocephalic

Right subclavian

Superior vena cava

Inferior vena cava

Hepatic

Portal

Superior mesenteric

Renal

Inferior mesenteric

Femoral

Great saphenous

Popliteal

Anterior tibial

Peroneal

Posterior tibial

Superficial temporal

Anterior facial

Left brachiocephalic

Left subclavian

Cephalic

Axillary

Pulmonary

Long thoracic

Basilic

Median cubital

Common iliac

Internal iliac

Externa iliac

Femoral

Great saphenous

Figure 7-17

(Continued)

Lymph nodes are powerful elements in the body's defense system. With local infections, nodes in the area can become swollen (often externally palpable) and inflamed from the accumulation of bacteria and toxins swept into the nodes by local lymph.

Lymphoid tissue is also located in the tonsils, thymus (during early childhood), and the spleen. These structures filter body fluids directly rather than through channeled lymph.

Endocrine System

The endocrine system produces substances called hormones that regulate other glands, organs, and body processes. Endocrine cells are usually clustered together into special tissue called endocrine glands (Fig. 7-19). These glands are ductless, relying instead on the surrounding blood supply to pick up the hormones they produce and deliver them to their target sites.

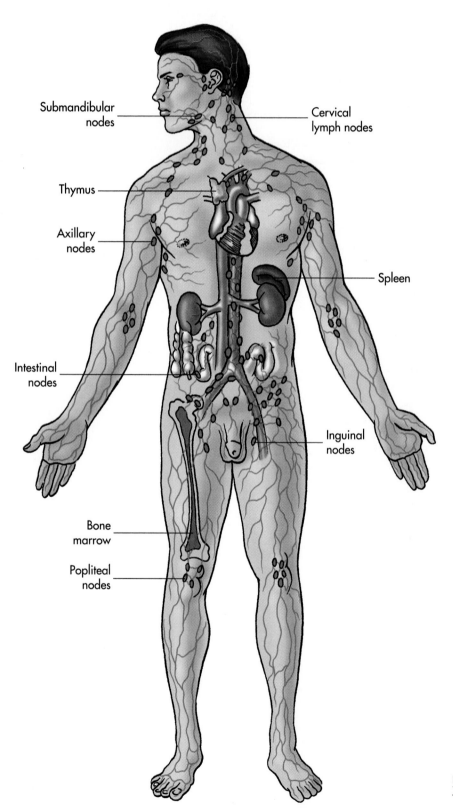

Submandibular nodes

Cervical lymph nodes

Thymus

Axillary nodes

Spleen

Intestinal nodes

Inguinal nodes

Bone marrow

Popliteal nodes

Figure 7-18

The lymphatic system.

Growth, development, reproduction, metabolism, water reabsorption, mineral distribution, and neurotransmitter production are some of the functions controlled by the endocrine system (Table 7-2). The primary endocrine glands include: pituitary (the anterior portion produces growth hormones and tropins, while the posterior pituitary produces antidiuretic hormone and oxytocin); the thyroid gland (produces the metabolism-regulating hormone thyroxine); the parathyroid (produces mineral-regulating parathormone); the adrenal cortex (produces the multifunctional corticosteroids); the adrenal medulla (produces the stress-response catecholamines such as epinephrine); the pancreatic islets (produce insulin and glucagon); the pineal gland (regulates pigmentation through melatonin); and the ovaries (producing female steroids); and testes (producing male steroids).

Endocrine cells are also found scattered throughout tissues with primarily nonendocrine functions. These include the thymus, hypothalamus, heart, stomach, kidneys, liver, and duodenum, each of which produces a unique hormone related to the functions of that organ.

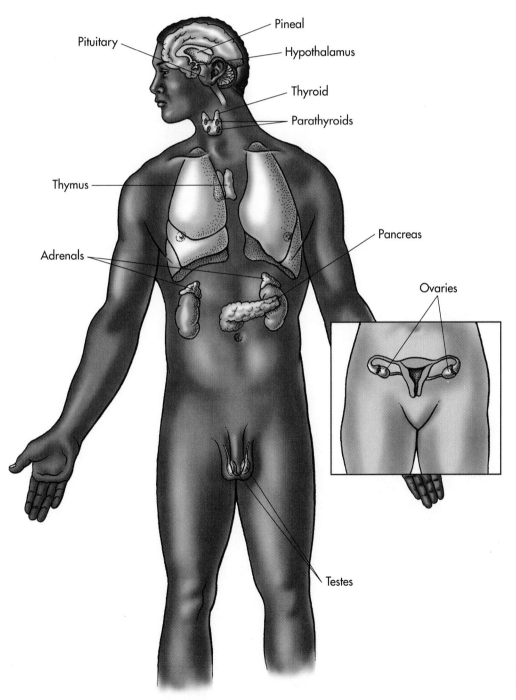

Figure 7-19

The endocrine system.

Reproductive System

Sexual reproduction is the mechanism that allows the human species to perpetuate itself. Both sexes are equipped with gonads, structures that produce reproductive cells; in the male, these are the testes, and in the female, they are the ovaries. Accessory organs and ducts assist in the growth, transport, and placement of the necessary ingredients for reproduction to take place (Figs. 7-20 and 7-21).

Muscular System

As a system, muscle and connective tissue combine to produce contraction following electrical stimulation. The energy necessary for this to occur comes from glucose (usually stored within the muscles as glycogen), which is obtained most efficiently through the presence of oxygen (aerobic metabolism). Without oxygen in the tissue, energy can only briefly and inefficiently be obtained through anaerobic metabolism. In either case, the spent energy results in movement (appoximately 25%) and the production of heat (75%). More than 400 skeletal muscles use the bones of the body as levers to accomplish movement (Fig. 7-22).

Urinary System

The urinary system consists of two kidneys, two ureters that connect each kidney to the urinary bladder, and the urethra (Fig. 7-23). The system helps filter and eliminate waste products, such as excess water, glucose, urea, and some salts from the blood. It also assists in regulating the acid-base balance of the body.

Each day, approximately 48 gallons of blood flow through 2 million tiny filtering units, or nephrons, within the kidneys (Fig. 7-24). The kidneys are located in the retroperitoneal space, with the right kidney located slightly lower than the left, to accommodate the liver. The kidneys launder the blood, with the proper amount of required nutrients being reabsorbed. Ninety-nine percent of the water is returned to the circulation. With normal hydration and circulation, 1.5 to 2 liters of waste fluid (urine) are produced in an average day (about 70 cc/hour). In the hospital setting, urine output is one of the key measurements for determining whether a patient is suffering from shock.

Urine flows from each kidney through a tube-like structure called the ureter to the urinary bladder in the pelvis. This hollow bladder stores the urine before releasing it from the body through the urethra. The characteristic odor of urine comes from the decomposition of ammonia, which is obtained from urea that is manufactured in the liver as a waste product of protein digestion. The typical yellow color comes from trace amounts of bile filtered from the blood.

Digestive System

The digestive system is responsible for the breakdown, conversion and absorption of foodstuffs into a form useable as fuel for cells (Fig. 7-25). It consists of one long (25 to 30 feet) canal and several organs that contribute ingredients to the process. The mouth breaks down substances mechanically and mixes them with saliva. The tongue propels the food into the esophagus. The smooth muscle of the esophagus continues the movement of the food downward through the cardiac sphincter and into the stomach. The food then mixes with hydrochloric acid and other enzymes in the stomach. These con-

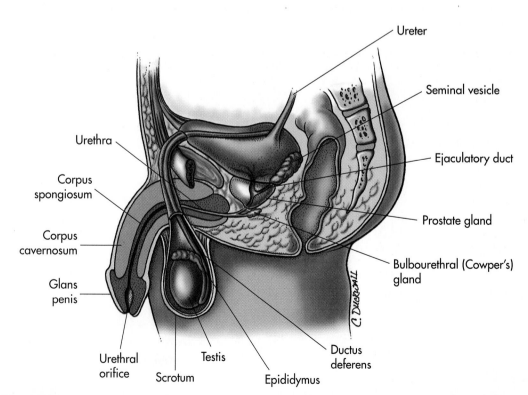

Figure 7-20

The male reproductive system.

TABLE 7-2 Endocrine Glands, Hormones, and Their Target Tissue

Gland	Hormone	Target Tissue	Response
Pituitary gland			
Anterior	Growth hormone	Most tissues	Increases protein synthesis, breakdown of lipids, and release of fatty acids from cells; increases blood glucose levels
	Thyroid-stimulating hormone (TSH)	Thyroid gland	Increases thyroid hormones secretion (thyroxine and triiodothyronine)
	Adrenocorticotropic hormone (ACTH)	Adrenal cortex	Increases secretion of glucocorticoid hormones such as cortisol; increases skin pigmentation at high concentrations
	Melanocyte-stimulating hormone (MSH)	Melanoctyes in skin	Increases melanin production in melanocytes to make the skin darker in color
	Luteinizing hormone (LH) or interstitial cell stimulating hormone (ICSH)	Ovaries in females, testes in males	Promotes ovulation and progesterone production in the ovaries, testosterone synthesis and support for the sperm cell production in testes
	Follicle-stimulating hormone (FSH)	Follicles in ovaries in females, seminiferous tubules in males	Promotes follicle maturation and estrogen secretion in ovaries; sperm cell production in testes
	Prolactin	Ovaries and mammary gland in females, testes in males	Stimulates milk production and prolongs progesterone secretion following ovulation and during pregnancy in women; increases sensitivity to LH in males
Posterior	Antidiuretic hormone	Kidney	Increases water reabsorption (less water is lost as urine)
	Oxytocin	Uterus	Increases uterine contractions
		Mammary gland	Increases milk "let-down" from mammary glands
Thyroid gland	Thyroid hormones (thyroxine and triiodothyronine)	Most cells of the body	Increases metabolic rates, essential for normal process of growth and maturation
	Calcitonin	Primarily bone	Decreases rate of bone breakdown; prevents large increase in blood calcium levels
Parathyroid glands	Parathyroid hormone	Bone, kidney	Increases rate of bone breakdown by osteoclasts; increases vitamin D synthesis, essential for maintenance of nromal blood calcium levels
Adrenal glands			
Adrenal medulla	Epinephrine mostly, some norepinephrine	Heart, blood vessels, liver, fat cells	Increases cardiac output; increases blood flow to skeletal muscles and heart; increases release of glucose and fatty acids into blood; in general, prepares the body for physical activity
Adrenal Cortex	Mineralocorticoids (aldosterone)	Kidneys; to lesser degree, intestine and sweat glands	Increases rate of sodium transport into body; increases rate of potassium excretion; secondarily favors water retention
	Glucocorticoids (cortisol)	Most tissues (e.g., liver, fat, skeletal muscle, immune tissues)	Increases fat and protein breakdown; increases glucose synthesis from amino acids; increases blood nutrient levels; inhibits inflammation and immune response
	Adrenal androgens	Most tissues	Insignificant in males; increases female sexual drive, pubic hair and axillary hair growth
Pancreas	Insulin	Especially liver, skeletal muscle, adipose tissue	Increases uptake and use of glucose and amino acids
	Glucagon	Primary liver	Increases breakdown of glycogen and release of glucose into the circulatory system
Reproductive organs			
Testes	Testosterone	Most tissues	Aids in sperm cell production, maintenance of functional reproductive organs, secondary sexual characteristics, and sexual behavior
Ovaries	Estrogens and progesterone	Most tissues	Aids in uterine and mammary gland development and function, external genitalia structure, secondary sexual characteristics, sexual behavior, and menstrual cycle
Uterus, ovaries, inflamed tissues	Prostaglandins	Most tissues	Mediates inflammatory responses; increases uterine contractions and ovulation
Thymus gland	Thymosin	Immune tissues	Promotes immune system development and function
Pineal body	Melatonin	At least the hypothalamus	Inhibits release of gonadotropin-releasing hormone, thereby inhibiting reproduction

*From Seely RR, et al: Essentials of Anatomy and Physiology, ed 2, St. Louis, 1996, Mosby–Year Book, Inc.

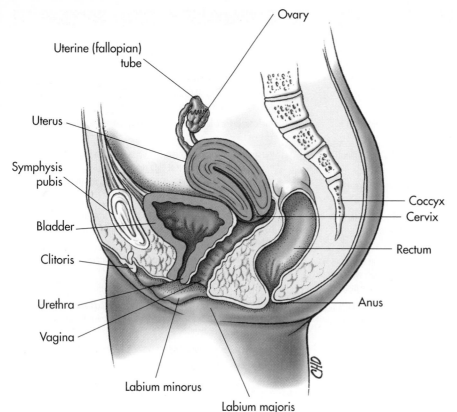

Ovary

Uterine (fallopian) tube

Uterus

Symphysis pubis

Bladder

Clitoris

Urethra

Vagina

Labium minorus

Labium majoris

Coccyx

Cervix

Rectum

Anus

Figure 7-21

The female reproductive system. *From McSwain, et al: Instructors Resource Kit to Accompany The Basic EMT: Comprehensive Prehospital Patient Care,* 1996, Mosby Lifeline.

tents are propelled through the pyloric sphincter into the first part of the small intestine, the duodenum, where products are added from the liver and pancreas. Although the liver and pancreas are not actually part of the GI tract, they act as accessory organs to digestion. Bile salts are produced by the liver and stored in the gall bladder, then mixed with the products of digestion as they pass into the duodenum. Bile salts help break down or emulsify large fat particles; they can then be digested more easily by the water-soluble enzyme, lipase, which is excreted by the pancreas.

Continuing through the small intestine (the jejunum and then the ileum), the food is broken down into basic nutrients (fats, carbohydrates, proteins, vitamins, minerals, and water). These are absorbed through special finger-like epithelial projections called villi that line the intestinal wall and help move the contents in a wave-like manner. After nutrients are absorbed, material remaining in the small intestine is propelled into the large intestine. Located just beyond the junction of the small and large intestine is the appendix, a small pouch of lymphoid tissue. When in the large-intestine, additional water is removed and bacteria remove nutrients. The remnants are then expelled through the rectum.

Skeletal System

Bones and their supporting connective tissues collectively create the skeleton. The adult skeleton is composed of 206 bones. It is divided into the axial skeleton, including the skull, spine, sternum, and ribs, and the appendicular skele-

ton, the pelvis and extremities (Fig. 7-26). Principal functions of the skeletal system include: 1) creating a framework for the body; 2) protecting fragile structures; 3) providing attachments for muscles and movement; 4) storing minerals, such as calcium and phosphorus; and 5) manufacturing red blood cells.

Integumentary System

Skin is the protective covering for most of the outer surface of the body (Fig. 7-27). The average adult has approximately 17 to 20 square feet of skin. The outer layer (epidermis), is an epithelium with a thin covering of dead cells. This layer is continually being shed and replaced from a deeper germinal layer. The underlayers of the epidermis have no direct blood supply; rather, they receive nourishment from diffusion from underlying dermis. Primary functions of the epidermis include protecting the body from trauma, water loss, ultraviolet light (skin pigmentation is found here), and direct bacterial contamination.

Under the epidermis lies the dermis, a layer of connective tissue that contains the hair follicles, blood vessels, sebaceous (oil) glands, lymph structures, and nerves. Underneath the dermis is the superficial fascia, a layer of loose connective tissue and of fat, as well as nerves, arteries, veins, and lymph structures. The final layer is the deep fascia, made up of dense connective tissue that helps compartmentalize and anchor muscles. It also provides attachments for muscles and keeps tendons in position as they cross over joints.

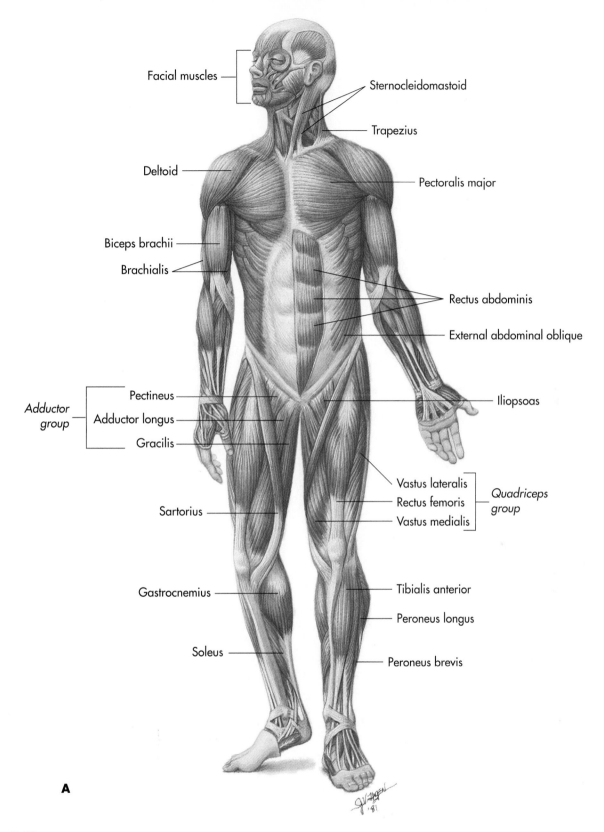

Facial muscles

Sternocleidomastoid

Trapezius

Deltoid

Pectoralis major

Biceps brachii

Brachialis

Rectus abdominis

External abdominal oblique

Adductor group

Pectineus

Adductor longus

Gracilis

Iliopsoas

Vastus lateralis

Rectus femoris

Quadriceps group

Vastus medialis

Sartorius

Gastrocnemius

Tibialis anterior

Peroneus longus

Soleus

Peroneus brevis

A

Figure 7-22

The muscular system. A, Anterior view. B, Posterior view. *From Thibodeau: Structure and Function of the Body, ed 9, St. Louis, 1992, Mosby–Year Book.*

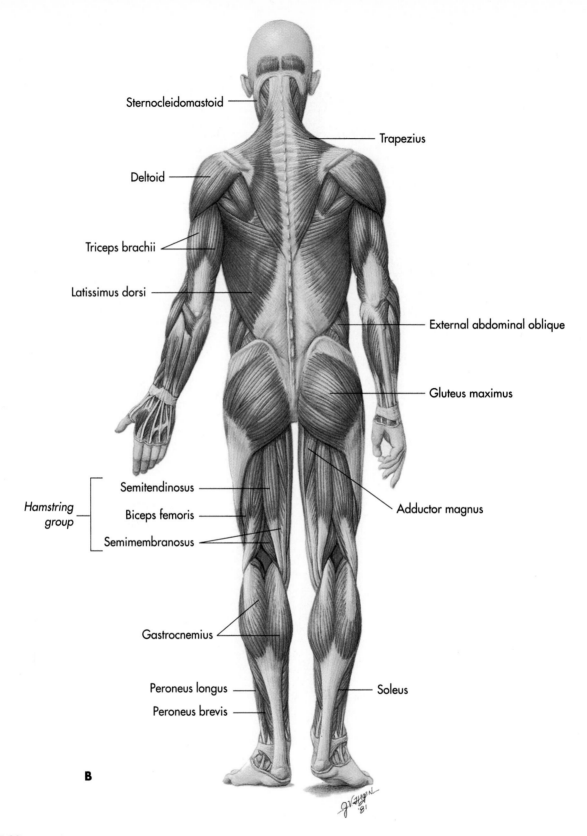

Sternocleidomastoid

Trapezius

Deltoid

Triceps brachii

Latissimus dorsi

External abdominal oblique

Gluteus maximus

Hamstring group

Semitendinosus

Biceps femoris

Semimembranosus

Adductor magnus

Gastrocnemius

Peroneus longus

Soleus

Peroneus brevis

B

Figure 7-22

(Continued)

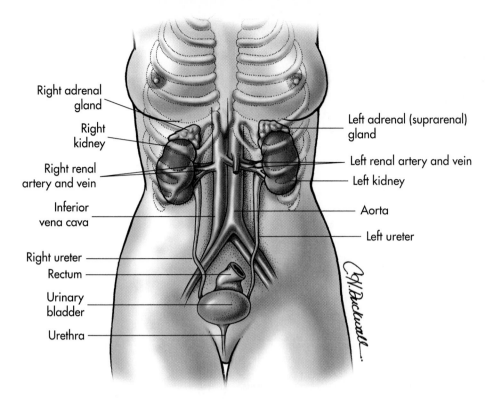

Right adrenal gland

Right kidney

Right renal artery and vein

Inferior vena cava

Right ureter

Rectum

Urinary bladder

Urethra

Left adrenal (suprarenal) gland

Left renal artery and vein

Left kidney

Aorta

Left ureter

Figure 7-23

The urinary system.

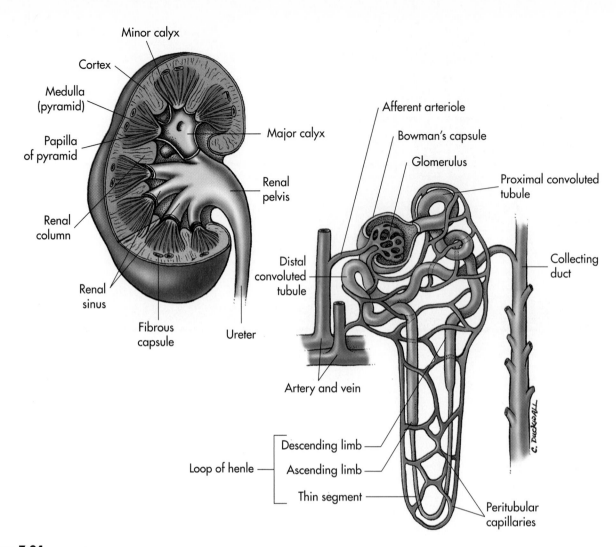

Figure 7-24

A cross-sectional view of the kidney with a close-up of a single filtering unit, called a nephron.

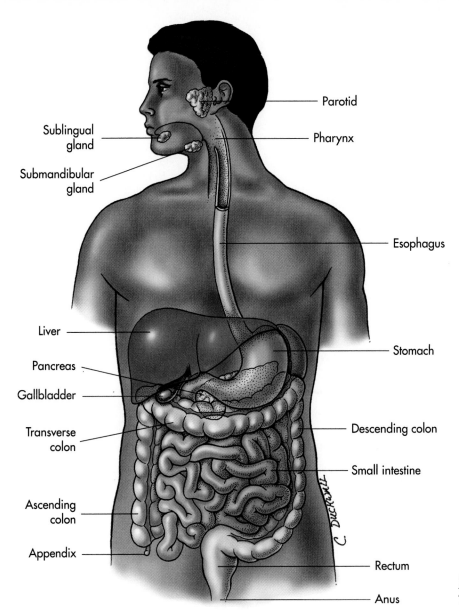

Parotid

Sublingual
gland

Pharynx

Submandibular
gland

Esophagus

Liver

Stomach

Pancreas

Gallbladder

Transverse
colon

Descending colon

Small intestine

Ascending
colon

Appendix

Rectum

Anus

Figure 7-25

The digestive system.

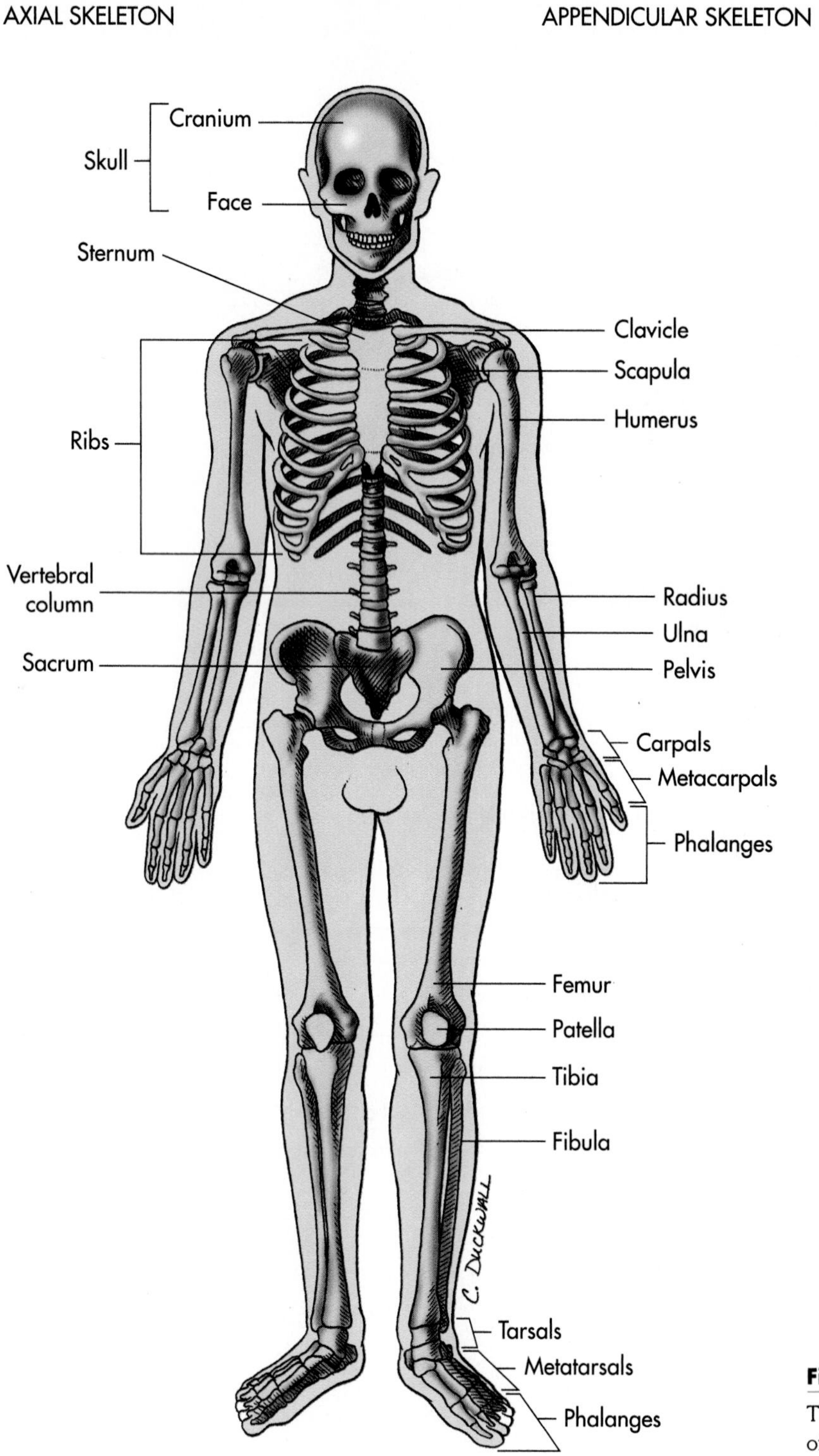
AXIAL SKELETON
APPENDICULAR SKELETON
Skull
Cranium
Face
Sternum
Ribs
Vertebral column
Sacrum
Clavicle
Scapula
Humerus
Radius
Ulna
Pelvis
Carpals
Metacarpals
Phalanges
Femur
Patella
Tibia
Fibula
Tarsals
Metatarsals
Phalanges
C. Duckwall

Figure 7-26

The axial and appendicular skeleton are the two divisions of the skeletal system.

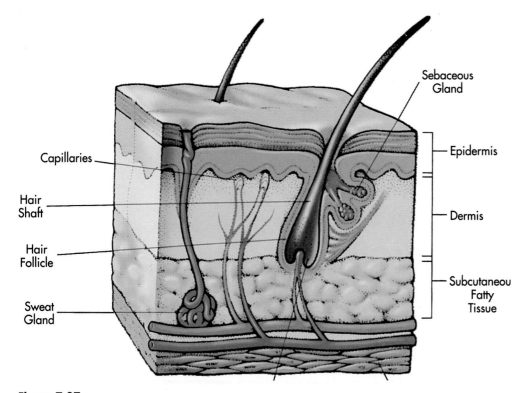

Figure 7-27

The skin is the largest organ of the body. *From McSwain, et al: Instructors Resource Kit to Accompany The Basic EMT: Comprehensive Prehospital Patient Care,* 1996, Mosby Lifeline.

SUMMARY

Starting with individual cells and four basic types of tissues, the human body is arranged into an amazing array of organs and systems. These structures work individually and collectively to carry out intricate and sometimes complex functions striving for balance and growth, as well as coordinated responses towards internal and external stimuli.

The actions and interactions of these systems in response to illness and injury create the signs and symptoms that are the object of patient assessment. Knowing the structures, functions, and relationships of tissues, organs, and systems assists the paramedic in connecting signs and symptoms with underlying pathophysiology and developing strategies for monitoring, intervention and treatment of patients.

SUGGESTED READINGS

1. Bisacre, Carlisle, Robertson, Ruck (ed.): The Illustrated Encyclopedia of the Human Body And How It Works, 1979, Exeter Books.
2. Bodanis D: *The Body Book—A Fantastic Voyage to the World Within,* 1984, Little, Brown, and Company.
3. Dienhart C: *Basic Anatomy and Physiology,* Philadelphia, 1979, WB Saunders.
4. Fox S: *Human Physiology,* ed 3, 1990, WC Brown Publishers.
5. Godling H, et al: *Atlas of the Human Body,* 1985, JB Lippincott.
6. Kahn F: *The Human Body,* 1965, Random House.
7. McAleer N: *The Body Almanac,* 1985, Doubleday.
8. Memmler, Wood D: *The Human Body in Health and Disease* ed 4, Philadelphia, 1977, JB Lippincott.
9. Smith A: *The Body,* 1986, Viking Penguin.

Alice "Twink" Dalton, BSN, NRPM

Chapter 8

Principles of Pathophysiology

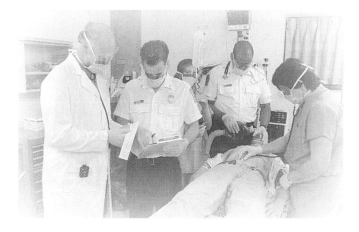

A paramedic should be able to:

1. Explain the primary function of the following:
   a. Plasma
   b. Plasma proteins
   c. Electrolytes
   d. Red blood cells
   e. White blood cells
   f. Platelets
   g. Spleen

2. Describe five key functions of blood.

3. Define hemoglobin and hematocrit, and describe their relationship to red blood cells.

4. State the normal blood volume for the average adult patient.

5. Explain the purpose and function of the lymph system.

6. Identify the universal donor and recipient.

7. Discuss the significance of the Rh factor in terms of blood typing and pregnancy.

8. Identify the average percentage of total body water for an adult.

9. Describe the following terms in relationship to total body water:
   a. intracellular
   b. extracellular
   c. interstitial
   d. intravascular

10. Correlate body fluid composition to the conditions of dehydration and overhydration.

11. List signs and symptoms for dehydration and overhydration.

12. Define the major function of the following electrolytes:
   a. sodium
   b. calcium
   c. potassium
   d. magnesium

13. Define the terms osmosis and diffusion, and explain the role of each process in human fluid dynamics.

Continued

KEY TERMS

1. **Acid**—a substance that has a sour taste, releases hydrogen ions when dissolved in water, and reacts with bases to form salts.

2. **Acidosis**—a concentration of acid substances in the blood; a pH less than 7.35.

3. **Active transport**—the movement of materials across the membrane of a cell through channels or "gates" by means of chemical activity that allows the cell to admit larger molecules than would otherwise be able to enter. This process requires energy.

4. **Alkalosis**—a concentration of alkali or bases in the blood; a pH greater than 7.45.

5. **Anions**—negatively charged ions.

6. **Base**—substance that has a bitter taste, releases hydroxyl ions (OH⁻) when dissolved in water, and reacts with acid to form salts.

7. **Catecholamines**—any one of a group of sympathomimetic compounds composed of a catechol molecule and the aliphatic portion of an amine.

8. **Cations**—positively charged ions.

9. **Colloid**—protein molecules or aggregates of protein molecules in a solution.

10. **Crystalloid**—electrolytes in a solution; this substance forms crystals.

11. **Electrolytes**—elements that, when dissolved in water, break up into positively or negatively charged ions.

12. **Extracellular fluid**—the portion of the body fluid comprising the interstitial fluid and blood plasma.

13. **Homeostasis**—a relative constancy in the internal environment of the body, naturally maintained by adaptive responses that promote healthy survival.

14. **Hypertonic**—having a greater concentration of solute (particles) than another solution, hence exerting more osmotic pressure than that solution, such as hypertonic saline solution, which contains more salt than is found in intracellular and extracellular fluid. Cells shrink in a hypertonic solution.

15. **Hypotonic**—having a smaller concentration of solute (particles) than another solution, hence exerting less osmotic pressure than that solution, as a hypotonic saline solution, which contains less salt than is found in intracellular and extracellular fluid. Cells expand in a hypotonic solution.

Continued

Cont.

14. Define the following and describe their relationship to body fluid balance:
    a. crystalloid
    b. colloid
    c. hypertonic
    d. hypotonic
    e. isotonic

15. Discuss the purpose of IV therapy in the prehospital setting.

16. Discuss the composition and rationale for use for the following IV fluids:
    a. 5% Dextrose in water
    b. Ringer's lactate
    c. Normal saline

17. Define the normal body pH range, metabolism, acidosis and alkalosis.

18. Explain the importance of acid-base balance in the body.

19. Briefly describe the mechanism of action for the following acid-base compensatory mechanisms:
    a. Bicarbonate-carbonic acid
    b. Respiratory
    c. Kidney

20. Identify the most important aspect of prehospital care that can positively affect acid-base imbalances.

21. Discuss the pathophysiology and the common causes of the following:
    a. Respiratory acidosis
    b. Respiratory alkalosis
    c. Metabolic acidosis
    d. Metabolic alkalosis

22. Describe the purpose and function of the autonomic nervous system.

23. Identify circumstances when the autonomic nervous system is activated.

24. Describe the two branches of the autonomic nervous system in terms of their specific effects and the target organs they mediate.

25. Describe the effects of the following receptor sites on the heart, veins, lungs, skin, and pupils:
    a. Alpha
    b. Beta 1
    c. Beta 2

Cont.

16. **Interstitial fluid**—an extracellular fluid that fills the spaces between most of the cells of the body and provides a substantial portion of the liquid environment of the body. Formed by filtration through the blood capillaries, it is drained away as lymph.

17. **Intracellular fluid**—a fluid within cell membranes throughout most of the body, containing dissolved solutes that are essential to electrolytic balance and healthy metabolism.

18. **Isotonic**—having the same concentration of solute or particles as another solution, hence exerting the same amount of osmotic pressure as that solution.

19. **Metabolism**—the aggregate of all chemical processes that take place in living organisms, resulting in growth, generation of energy, elimination of wastes, and other bodily functions as they relate to the distribution of nutrients in the blood after digestion.

20. **Osmolarity**—the osmotic pressure of a solution expressed in osmoles or milliosmoles per kilogram of the solution.

21. **Osmosis**—the movement of a pure solvent, such as water, through a semipermeable membrane from a solution that has a lower solute concentration to one that has a higher solute concentration. Movement across the membrane continues until the concentrations of particles in the solutions equalize.

22. **Plasma**—a watery, straw-colored, fluid portion of the lymph and the blood in which the leukocytes, erythrocytes, and platelets are suspended. Plasma is made up of water, electrolytes, proteins, glucose, fats, bilirubin, and gases.

23. **Tonicity**—the concentration, or size, of particles in solution compared to another. For example, a hypertonic saline solution has a tonicity greater than that of blood.

The regulation and maintenance of blood, body fluids, electrolytes, and acid-base balance are key to the basic cellular function and the health of the individual. To varying degrees, all injury and disease affect these elemental units of the body. Likewise, patient treatment and its success depends on a thorough understanding of these body units and their action and interaction.

Section 1: Blood and Its Components

Blood is the main element involved in the oxygenation of body cells, transport of nutrients, transport of control and maintenance factors (hormones), waste removal, and temperature regulation. Blood is also a major factor in the system designed to protect the body, the immunological system. The following is an overview of the components and functions of blood.

Components

Blood is a complex substance divided into two basic components—plasma and formed elements.

Plasma

Plasma is the complex fluid portion of blood. Plasma communicates continually through pores in the capillaries with the fluid circulating between the cells (interstitial fluid).[2] Plasma is approximately 92% water and contains a number of formed elements (Fig. 8-1). The concentration of these elements varies depending on diet, metabolic demand, hormones, and other factors.

Formed Elements

Formed elements consist of plasma proteins, plasma lipids, electrolytes, nutrients, and cellular elements such as red blood cells, white blood cells, and platelets. The formed elements make up approximately 45% to 50% of blood volume.[3] The continuous movement of blood keeps the formed elements dispersed throughout the plasma, where they are available to carry out five chief functions:

1. Respiratory—delivery of oxygen to the cells and exchange of carbon dioxide.
2. Nutritional—delivery of other substances needed for cellular metabolism (glucose and other carbohydrates, amino acids, fatty acids, vitamins, minerals, trace elements).
3. Regulatory—delivery of substances such as electrolytes and hormones.
4. Excretory—removal of cellular debris and waste products such as those of cellular metabolism (carbon dioxide, water, acids).
5. Protective—defense against injury and invading microorganisms.

Plasma Proteins

There are numerous plasma proteins in the blood. Three of the major groups include the albumins, globulins, and clotting factors. Albumin is a substance regulating the movement of water in the circulation. Globulins (immunoglobulins or gamma globulins) function as antibodies and are critical for defense against infectious diseases. Clotting factors, of which fibrogen is the most plentiful, are key components in the formation of blood clots that stop bleeding from damaged vessels.

Plasma Lipids

Plasma lipids include triglycerides, cholesterol, phospholipids, and fatty acids. They are carried through the blood as part of plasma protein complexes known as lipoproteins.

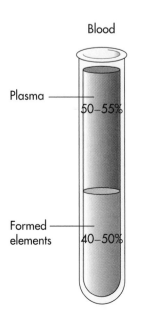

Blood

Plasma — 50–55%

Formed elements — 40–50%

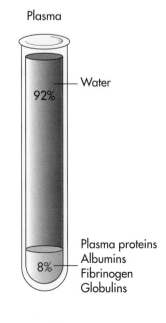

Plasma

Water — 92%

8%

Plasma proteins
Albumins
Fibrinogen
Globulins

Figure 8-1

Plasma, the liquid component of blood, is roughly 92% water. The remaining 8% is composed mainly of proteins, clotting factors, and electrolytes.

Electrolytes and Nutrients

Electrolytes (electrically charged particles, such as hydrogen, sodium, potassium, and calcium) in the plasma maintain the osmolarity and pH of blood within the physiologic range.[3] Nutrients include glucose and other carbohydrates, amino acids, vitamins, and individual trace elements.

Cellular Elements

Cellular elements are broadly classified as red blood cells (erythrocytes), white blood cells (leukocytes), and platelets (thrombocytes).

Red blood cells (RBCs) are the most abundant cells of the blood and are primarily responsible for tissue oxygenation. Hemoglobin, an iron-containing family of molecules contained in the RBCs, enables the blood to transport 100 times more oxygen than in plasma alone (Fig. 8-2).[3] Each hemoglobin molecule can carry four oxygen molecules when fully saturated.

RBCs also have the unique ability to alter their shapes when squeezing through capillaries.[3] This property is extremely important to the maintenance of perfusion. The mature RBC lacks a nucleus and other cell parts necessary to survive and multiply. At the end of its 12-day life span, the RBC dies and is replaced by a new one.

Laboratory tests can determine amounts of hemoglobin per deciliter of blood (measured in g/100 mL of blood). These methods are useful in identifying anemic problems. Measurements of hematocrit give the percentage of blood volume occupied by RBCs. This measurement helps to assess hemorrhage and other conditions that result in abnormal numbers of RBCs (see Table 8-1 for normal blood cell counts).

White blood cells (WBCs) are part of the immunological system that defends the body against infection and removes debris, including dead or injured cells. WBCs act primarily in the tissues, but they are also transported in the circulation.

Measurement of WBCs is useful when determining presence of disease or infection. By differentiating between the various types of WBCs, health care providers can often determine the inflammatory reaction or other disease process that is occurring (see Table 8-1).

TABLE 8-1	Normal Blood Cell Counts	
Red Blood Cells	**Men**	**Women**
Hemoglobin	16 ± g/100 mL	14 ± g/100 mL
Hematocrit	47% ± 5	42% ± 5
White Blood Cells	5000–10,000/μL	
Neutrophils	62.0%	
Eosinophils	2.3%	
Basophils	0.4%	
Monocytes	5.3%	
Lymphocytes	30.0%	

Note: These values vary slightly from reference to reference and institution to institution.

Platelets are not cells but disk-shaped fragments; they are essential for blood coagulation and control of bleeding. Like RBCs, platelets lack a nucleus and other cell parts necessary to multiply. A platelet lives approximately 10 days, and is removed by macrophages in the spleen.

Production and Regulation

Blood cell production, termed hematopoiesis, occurs in the liver and spleen of the fetus, but normally takes place only in red bone marrow after birth. In children, all bone marrow is red—the type that actively produces red and white blood cells. As the body matures, some red marrow is replaced by fat (yellow marrow) and becomes inactive. In adults, the majority of red bone marrow is found in the pelvis (34%).[3] The remainder of red bone marrow is found in the vertebrae, cranium, mandible, sternum, ribs, and proximal ends of the femur and humerus.

Blood cell production is stimulated by the hormone erythropoietin in response to anemia, hypoxia, high altitudes, or pulmonary disease. This mechanism explains why many pa-

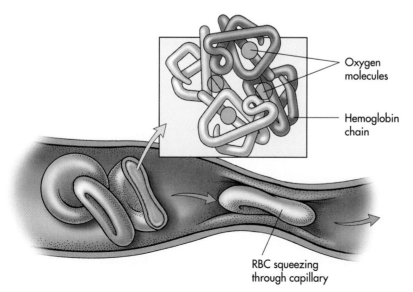

Oxygen molecules

Hemoglobin chain

RBC squeezing through capillary

Figure 8-2

Each hemoglobin molecule is capable of transporting four oxygen molecules. Each RBC has numerous hemoglobin molecules.

tients with chronic obstructive pulmonary disease (COPD) and congestive heart failure can compensate well for long periods of time. Hematopoiesis subsides when a sufficient number of mature RBCs enter the circulation. The process continues throughout life to replace blood cells that grow old and die, are killed by disease, or are lost through bleeding.

Blood is continually cleansed and filtered by the spleen. When RBCs grow old or their cell membranes become damaged, they are eliminated in the spleen along with other types of dead blood cells. The heme, or iron portion of the hemoglobin, is saved and recycled for use in the bone marrow. If the spleen is absent or dysfunctional, special cells in the liver take over the cleansing process.

Normal Blood Volume

Normal blood volume is determined by a number of factors. In general, adequate perfusion requires 80 mL of blood/kg of body weight. Thus the average blood volume of a 70 kg adult is approximately 5000 mL.[2]

Circulation

Plasma and formed elements move through two circulatory systems—the cardiovascular and lymphatic systems.

The cardiovascular system is composed of the heart, arteries, arterioles, capillary beds, venules, and veins. This system is discussed in greater detail in Chapter 7. The focus of this chapter is the lymphatic system. The lymphatic system is composed of the fluid, or lymph, and lymphoid organs such as the spleen, thymus, lymph nodes, and tonsils. The lymphoid organs serve as a link between the blood and the immune system. The lymphatic system is also explained and illustrated in Chapter 7.

As stated previously, plasma communicates continually with the interstitial fluid through pores in the capillaries. Once outside the vessels, this fluid is known as lymph and becomes part of the lymphatic system.

Most of the lymph fluid filtering from the arterial capillaries is reabsorbed back into the venous ends of the blood capillaries. Approximately one tenth of the fluid returns to the blood through the thoracic duct, or the right lymph duct, rather than the venous capillaries.

The lymphatic system performs two critical functions: 1) returns excess proteins and fluid volume to the circulation from the tissue spaces, and 2) immunologically defends the body.

The spleen is one of the most important lymphoid organs. It is a concave, encapsulated organ about the size of a fist, located in the upper abdominal cavity beneath the left ribs, and next to the stomach. The major function of the spleen is to filter and cleanse the blood, but it also serves as a reservoir, storing approximately 300 mL of blood that is available when needed.

Blood Types

An antigen is the protein identifier in most cells. The presence or absence of a particular antigen identifies that cell as either "self" or foreign. Once a cell is identified as foreign, specific antibodies to that cell are formed. Subsequently, all antigens (cells with that specific foreign identifier), are attacked and destroyed. This is termed an antigen-antibody reaction. When this occurs upon mixing two types of blood, it is called "transfusion reaction." At least 30 commonly occurring antigens, each of which can trigger antigen-antibody reactions, have been found in human blood cells, especially on the cell membrane surfaces.[3]

There are two groups of antigens in the blood that are more likely than the others to cause reactions; these are the ABO system of antigens and the Rh system.

ABO Type

The ABO group consists of two major antigens, labeled A and B, that are found on the surface of RBCs. These antigens can appear by themselves or together or be entirely absent. The result of their presence or absence is one of four blood types. Individuals with blood type A carry the A antigen on the RBCs; individuals with blood type B carry the B antigen; those people with blood type AB carry both antigens, and those with type O carry neither antigen. In the ABO system, the body spontaneously develops antibodies to the other blood types. This system determines which blood type or types each person can receive without triggering a transfusion reaction (Table 8-2).

Rh Factor

The second important system in blood transfusion is the Rh system. The Rh antigen, type D, is widely prevalent. People with this type of antigen are said to be Rh positive; those without the Type D antigen are Rh negative. Approximately 85% to 95% of Americans are Rh positive.[2]

Antibodies to the Rh factor do not occur naturally and must be acquired through exposure to Rh-positive blood. This process is most evident in Rh-positive babies born to Rh-negative mothers. The mother must be given a vaccine after each birth to prevent the formation of antibodies to any subsequent Rh-positive fetuses.

TABLE 8-2	ABO Blood Types		
Blood Types	**Antibody(ies)**	**Can Receive**	**Can Donate to**
Type A	B antibodies	Type A or O	Type A, AB
Type B	A antibodies	Type B or O	Type B, AB
Type AB	No antibodies	Type AB, A, B, O	Type A, B, AB
Type O	A and B antibodies	Type O	Type A, B, AB, O

In an adult Rh-negative patient, a similar but delayed reaction can occur if Rh-positive blood is received. Upon receiving the second Rh-positive transfusion, a severe and potentially life-threatening reaction may occur in the patient.

Section 2: Fluids and Electrolytes

This section describes the cellular environment and body fluid, including distribution, electrolytes, and methods of movement.

Distribution

Most of the body's weight is composed of fluid (body water). Approximately 56% to 60% of the adult human body is water.[2] Most of this fluid (two thirds) is inside the cells and is called intracellular fluid. Approximately one third of this fluid is found in the spaces outside the cells and is called extracellular fluid. Extracellular fluid is divided between the interstitial space (between the cells) and the intravascular space (inside the blood vessels).

The sum total of fluid in the intracellular and extracellular space (interstitial and intravascular) is termed total body water (TBW). In the 70-kg man, this amount is approximately 42 liters of fluid (60% TBW). The distribution and amount of TBW changes with the age of the patient. In newborns, TBW is approximately 75% to 80% of body weight. This amount falls to 67% during the first year of life. During adolescence, the percentage of TBW approaches adult proportions, and gender differences begin to appear. These differences center around the percentages of muscle mass and fat. Muscle mass requires more body water than fat. This explains why men, who generally have more muscle mass, have a greater percentage of body water than women. Along with gender and percent of body fat, aging also contributes to a decline in the percentage of TBW. Normal changes of aging result in an increased amount of fat and a decreased amount of muscle mass. With age, the kidneys also have a declining ability to regulate sodium and water balance.

Hydration and medication are the last major factors to influence TBW. Inadequate water intake and many medications (especially diuretics) used for blood pressure control may lead to chronic states of dehydration.

Water Balance

Body water is regulated by several mechanisms. Concentrations of particles within the extracellular and intracellular spaces regulate movement of body water. However, actual water volume is controlled by hormones, such as antidiuretic hormone from the pituitary and aldosterone from the kidney, by the kidney itself, and by the thirst mechanism.

Too much water volume is known as **hypervolemia**, or water intoxication, and has generalized edema as its primary symptom. Early symptoms include headache and seizures in infants. If untreated, heart failure with **pulmonary edema** may result. True overhydration is uncommon; it may be associated with a sodium imbalance, excessive water ingestion, or administration of too much IV fluid. Treatment is aimed at removing the extra water; diuretics are frequently prescribed for this treatment.

Too little water volume is known as **dehydration**, and its primary sign is poor skin turgor or "tenting" (Fig. 8-3). Dry mucous membranes, thirst, and in severe cases, tachycardia and decreased blood pressure may also occur. Dehydration is often associated with electrolyte losses. The condition is common and can occur gradually. Causes of dehydration include:

- GI losses, such as those that occur with vomiting or diarrhea, especially in infants. This condition also predisposes the patient to electrolyte losses.
- Rapid respiratory rates, especially in the presence of fever. This "insensible" water loss in the form of vapor contributes to dehydration.
- Sweating, especially if profuse and prolonged, as during heavy exercise in hot weather.
- Plasma losses, when draining from wounds or fistulas is prolonged, or when the phenomenon of "third spacing" occurs (most often with burns covering more than 10% of the body surface area, ascites, or **septic shock**).
- Polyuria from drug overdoses (especially of diuretics) or diseases such as **diabetes**.
- Insufficient water intake, which occurs in patients who have an impaired thirst mechanism, such as the elderly, or patients who cannot respond to thirst stimuli, such as the comatose, confused, or immobilized.

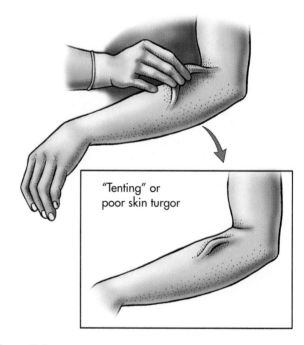

"Tenting" or poor skin turgor

Figure 8-3

Skin tenting, a sign of dehydration, is observed when pinched skin stays pulled up, or returns to normal slowly. Suspect that the patient has lost electrolytes as well as water.

Treatment is aimed at replacing body water and associated electrolyte losses.

Electrolytes

Electrolytes are among the principal components of body fluid. Electrolytes are substances that break up into electrically charged ions when dissolved in water. The charge can be positive or negative. Ions with a positive charge are known as cations, and negatively charged ions are anions. Opposite charges attract, and like charges repel. The action of repelling and attracting allows ions of similar charge to exist in the same area and yet not interfere with their individual function. The ability to carry a charge is important in both generating and transmitting nerve impulses, in muscle contraction and relaxation, and in maintaining fluid balance.

There are many electrolytes in body fluid. The amounts of various electrolytes such as sodium (Na^+), potassium (K^+), magnesium (Mg^{++}), calcium (Ca^{++}), chloride (Cl^-), and bicarbonate (HCO_3^-) vary between the fluid compartments. Extracellular fluid contains larger amounts of sodium, calcium, and bicarbonate ions. Intracellular fluid contains more potassium, magnesium, and phosphate (see Table 8-3). This difference is crucial to maintaining homeostasis in the body. Table 8-3 summarizes the concentrations and functions of electrolytes.

The major cations—sodium, calcium, potassium, and magnesium—are of special interest. Sodium (Na^+) and calcium (Ca^{++}) have their greatest concentration in the extracellular fluid, and potassium and magnesium are more concentrated in the intracellular space. Imbalances in any one of these electrolytes can result in major problems.

Extracellular Cations

Sodium

Sodium is the most abundant extracellular cation and is especially important in the regulation of body water. Sodium is also important in nerve impulse transmission and in the transfer of calcium into the cell. The most common source of sodium is sodium chloride or everyday table salt. Sodium is often found in conjunction with chloride (Cl^-) or bicarbonate (HCO_3^-).

Regulation of sodium occurs in the kidney, primarily through reabsorption in the tubules. Aldosterone is the hormonal regulator. Secreted by the kidney, aldosterone increases renal reabsorption of sodium. Because of sodium's high attraction for water, alterations in sodium and water balance are closely related. An imbalance in one leads to imbalance in the other.

Hypernatremia, too much sodium, may be due to either an acute gain in sodium, or a loss of water without corresponding loss of sodium.

Calcium

Calcium is necessary for the structure of bone and teeth. It also functions as an enzyme cofactor for blood clotting and is required for hormone secretion, membrane stability and permeability, and muscle contraction. One common source of calcium is dairy products.

Most calcium in the body is located in bone tissue, with the remainder found in the plasma and body cells. Inside the cells, calcium is necessary for energy used by muscle fibers to contract. The strength of contraction is directly related to the concentration of calcium. Calcium is often found in conjunction with phosphate (HPO_4).

TABLE 8-3	Distribution, Concentrations, and Functions of Major Cations and Anions in Body Fluid		
Electrolyte	Extracellular Fluid	Intracellular Fluid	Function
Cations			
Sodium (Na^+)	142 mEq/L	10 mEq/L	Principal extracellular cation; regulates water concentration and nerve impulse transmission
Calcium (Ca^{++})	5 mEq/L	< 1 mEq/L	Extracellular cation; structure of bone and teeth, enzyme cofactor for clot formation, and hormone secretion, essential for membrane stability
Potassium (K^+)	5 mEq/L	150 mEq/L	Principal intracellular cation; nerve impulse transmission, essential for muscle contraction, aids in glycogen storage
Magnesium (Mg^{++})	2 mEq/L	40 mEq/L	Intracellular cation; essential for cell membrane function, energy source for Na^+/K^+ pump
Anions			
Chloride (Cl^-)	103 mEq/L	4 mEq/L	Extracellular anion; formation of stomach acid and maintenance of acid-base balance
Bicarbonate (HCO_3^-)	24 mEq/L	10 mEq/L	Extracellular anion; major component of blood buffer system
Phosphate (HPO_4^-)	2 mEq/L	75 mEq/L	Intracellular anion; formation of energy, oxygen delivery (part of RBC) and acid-base balance

Blood levels of calcium are closely regulated by parathyroid hormone (PTH), vitamin D, and calcitonin (from the thyroid gland). Renal regulation of calcium requires PTH, which is secreted in response to low plasma levels.

Intracellular Cations

Potassium

Potassium is necessary in transmission and conduction of nerve impulses, maintenance of normal cardiac rhythms, and skeletal and smooth muscle contraction. It is also required for glycogen deposits in the liver and skeletal muscles. In this capacity, potassium works closely with sodium, momentarily trading places with sodium across the cellular membrane to maintain electrical neutrality. This action conducts nerve impulses from one end of the cell to the other. This becomes extremely important in the conduction of cardiac rhythms and the movement of calcium into the cell for muscle contraction.

Magnesium

Approximately 40% to 60% of magnesium is stored in muscle and bone. Most of the remainder is stored intracellulary and appears to be related to potassium and calcium. Magnesium activates the enzyme (ATP-ase) that is essential for normal cell membrane function and is the energy source for the sodium-potassium pump.[4] Physiologic effects include relaxing smooth muscle and increasing the stability of cardiac cells, thus reducing the potential for dysrhythmias.

Recent research suggests that hypomagnesemia is probably not as rare as previously thought.[4,5,6] As with potassium, serum levels of magnesium are often normal despite depletion of cellular magnesium. Hypomagnesemia has two distinct areas of effect—neuromuscular and cardiac.

Movement of Fluid

The fluid compartments—intracellular, interstitial, and intravascular—are separated by semipermeable membranes. These membranes are readily permeable to some substances, but not to others. In the body, water is one of only a few substances that moves freely across membranes. Other substances require the assistance of some mechanism to pass through a membrane. The body has several of these "assistants."

In some cases, cell membranes require activation of specialized "channels" or gates to enable a substance to pass through. Substances requiring channels usually also require energy use. This type of movement is termed active transport (Fig. 8-4). Energy is necessary for active transport because most of the substances that use it are moving from an area of lesser concentration to one of greater concentration.

In other cases, substances require special "carriers" before a substance can pass through a membrane, such as the insulin that carries glucose into muscle cells. This process, called facilitated diffusion (Fig. 8-5), may or may not require energy. Facilitated diffusion and active transport most often occur with substances entering the cells.

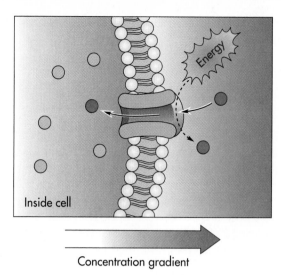

Figure 8-4

Active transport uses energy in the movement of molecules to allow movements against the normal concentration gradients.

Waste products and oxygen use another method of movement. They tend to flow from an area of greater concentration to one of lesser concentration. This method, called diffusion (Fig. 8-6), does not require energy or a semipermeable membrane.

Because extracellular fluid is in constant motion throughout the body, all cells essentially live in the same environment. Circulating blood is rapidly transported to all parts of the body; in the capillary beds, plasma mixes with the interstitial fluid by diffusion through the capillary walls.

The natural tendency of the body is to maintain a balance between the intracellular and extracellular fluid spaces, both in

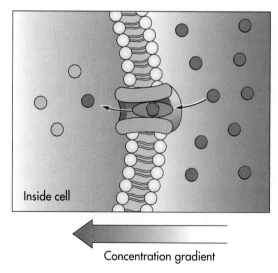

Figure 8-5

Facilitated diffusion occurs when "carrier" structures, such as membrane-bound proteins allow substances to move against a concentration gradient.

concentration of particles and electrical charge (Fig. 8-7). When the fluid concentration and charge are equal on both sides of a membrane, the fluids are called isotonic. When the concentration is unequal, the more concentrated side is hypertonic and the less concentrated is hypotonic. These terms are usually used in reference to the normal tonicity of the blood.

Tonicity refers to the concentration or the size of particles in a solution. In general, the more particles or the larger the particles in solution, the more pulling power the solution has for water. The solution with greater concentration of particles can literally attract or "pull" water from one fluid space to another. This movement of water is termed osmosis (Fig. 8-8). The natural tendency of osmosis is to maintain equal concentrations of particles by movement of water when the membrane is not permeable to the particles.

Proteins in the blood stream are large molecules that do not normally pass through the vessel walls. They aid in keeping a given amount of water volume inside the vessels. Thus, blood proteins, together with sodium, help to regulate the intravascular fluid volume. The protein structures inside the cells, together with potassium, similarly maintain the intracellular fluid volume.

Intravenous fluids fall into two categories—crystalloids and colloids, which vary in tonicity. Crystalloids contain non-protein particles. Colloids contain proteins or other large, osmotically powerful particles.

Colloids are used when intravascular volume must be maintained for an extended period. Whole blood is the ideal colloid. Although blood contains plasma, platelets, and red blood cells, these elements can also be administered separately for various patient needs. Plasma is often used in burn patients to treat the increased concentration of RBCs, WBCs, and other particles in the blood that occurs when fluid shifts out of the vascular spaces. Platelets are given to patients who need clotting factors. Red blood cells (known as packed cells when plasma is extracted) are the only substance that can carry oxygen. There is no substitute for red blood cells. Blood transfusion of either whole blood or packed cells requires blood typing prior to infusion.

There are other colloid products, including substances such as:

Intravenous Therapy

An isotonic solution must have concentrations of proteins and electrolytes similar to those in the blood. The ideal isotonic fluid is whole blood. There are, however, several other isotonic intravenous (IV) fluids.

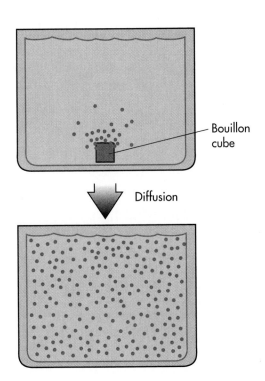

Figure 8-6

Diffusion naturally occurs when a substance is allowed to disperse its molecules through a solution without any barriers. Diffusion does not require energy.

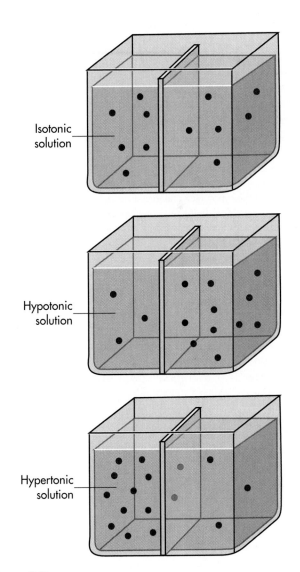

Figure 8-7

Tonicity. When the amount of particles (of a relative volume) is not equal between two solutions, there is a difference in tonicity.

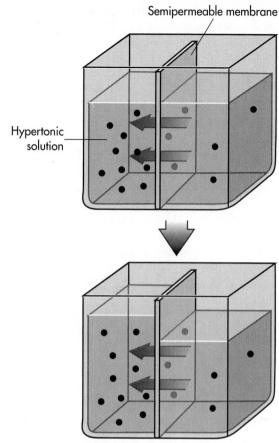

Semipermeable membrane

Hypertonic
solution

Figure 8-8

Osmosis. The movement of water, not particles, defines osmosis. A semipermeable membrane will allow water, a small particle molecule, to pass through, trapping larger molecules within its compartment. As the water moves, you will see a dilution of the hypertonic solution and a concentration of the hypotonic solution until an equilibrium of concentrations is achieved between the two compartments. The overall volumes of fluid on each side of the membrane will most likely change during this process as well.

The three primary crystalloids most commonly used in the field are 0.9% saline, or normal saline (NS), lactated Ringer's (LR) (sometimes known as Ringer's lactate), and Dextrose 5% and water (D_5W).

Consideration of tonicity is important in the selection of an IV fluid. A dehydrated patient given a hypertonic fluid will suffer additional intracellular dehydration, while a hemorrhaging patient given large amounts of a hypotonic solution may suffer further harm from RBC rupture. Dehydrated patients often have associated electrolyte losses, and acutely hemorrhaging patients have not had a chance for significant fluid shifts. Therefore, an isotonic fluid is generally the best choice for fluid replacement, although there are exceptions. Dehydration without sodium loss, such as that caused by fever, may require hypotonic solutions such as half-strength normal saline (0.45% NS).

Normal saline and LR are frequently used for fluid replacement and drug routes. NS contains sodium and chloride particles, and LR has lactate, sodium, calcium, potassium and chloride. Because of the natural movement of fluids and electrolytes in the body, NS and LR remain in the intravascular space for approximately 40 to 45 minutes. Although these solutions are useful for volume replacement, they cannot carry oxygen. The American College of Surgeons Committee on Trauma recommends an initial bolus of 1 to 2 L (in the adult) to a maximum of 2 to 3 L of crystalloid replacement for acute blood loss.[1]

Dextrose 5% and water (D_5W) is used as a drug route. Although D_5W has the same concentration of dextrose as plasma, the dextrose is rapidly absorbed by the cells, leaving water inside the vascular space. Thus, D_5W behaves as if it were hypotonic. For this reason, D_5W is not used for volume replacement.

The major shortcoming of crystalloids and colloids, with the exception of blood, is their inability to carry oxygen. Researchers are working to develop a cost-effective fluid that will bind to oxygen in the pulmonary capillaries and release it into the tissues.

• Plasma protein fraction (Plasmanate)—a saline solution whose principal protein is albumin.
• Dextran—an artificial sugar solution with osmotic properties similar to albumin.
• Hetastarch—an artificial starch solution, with osmotic properties similar to albumin but with fewer side effects.

Colloid products tend to be expensive, may interfere with blood typing, and have a short shelf life. For these reasons, they are not commonly used in the field.

Crystalloids are the fluids of choice for volume replacement in both the prehospital and hospital settings. They are also used as vehicles for drug administration. There are many crystalloid solutions available, classified according to their tonicity (Box 8-1). Tonicity is measured in milliosmoles (the concentration of solutes in water), abbreviated mOsm. Normal tonicity for body fluid is 290 mOsm/kg water. Therefore, any crystalloid that has approximately 280 to 310 mOsm/L of water is considered isotonic. Again, these values vary slightly from reference to reference.

BOX 8-1 **Tonicity of Crystalloids**

• Isotonic fluid has the same or similar concentration of particles as plasma, tends to remain within the vascular space longer than hypotonic fluid, and can be used effectively as a volume replacement for short periods of time.
• Hypotonic fluid has a lower concentration of particles than plasma and tends to migrate to the intracellular spaces, eventually causing particle migration. Too much IV hypotonic fluid may result in rupture of RBCs.
• Hypertonic fluid has a greater concentration of particles than plasma and tends to pull fluid from the intracellular and **interstitial spaces** into the vascular space, eventually causing particle migration.

Section 3: Acid-base Balance and Regulation of Waste Products

Blood, body fluids, and electrolytes form the environment for the body's chemical reactions. Nearly every process in the body related to growth, energy production, and repair is stimulated or regulated by some form of chemical reaction. The sum of all these reactions is termed metabolism. The by-products of metabolism include carbon dioxide, water, acids, and other waste products. The maintenance of a proper balance of these substances is essential to life.

Acids are formed constantly in the body as a result of cellular metabolism. Substances that form bases (sodium bicarbonate) are taken into the body in our food. A proper balance between acids and bases affects three main areas:

1. maintenance and support of an environment that enables cellular enzymes to work most efficiently;
2. maintenance of cell membrane potential and permeability;
3. oxygen uptake and release at the cellular level.

Because of the constant production and ingestion of acids and bases, the body has developed a system to "balance" these two substances within very narrow limits, called "acid-base balance."

Acids and Bases

An acid is a substance that releases hydrogen ions (H^+) when dissolved in water. Carbon dioxide, a common metabolic substance released during energy production, combines with water to form carbonic acid. Other common metabolic acids include lactic acid, released during aerobic and anaerobic metabolism, and ketones, which are formed when fats are metabolized for energy.

Bases, also known as alkalis, are H^+ acceptors. Like acids, the bases dissociate in water, but in this case, the hydroxyl ion (OH^-) is released. The hydroxyl ion is an avid hydrogen ion seeker. The most common metabolic base substance in the body is bicarbonate (HCO_3^-), which is formed by the combination of hydroxyl ions and CO_2: $OH^- + CO_2 = HCO_3^-$.

pH Scale

The relative concentration of hydrogen (H^+) and hydroxyl (OH^-) ions in solution in various body fluids is expressed on a scale called pH, which stands for potential of hydrogen. The pH scale runs from 1 to 14; each successive change of 1 pH unit represents a 10-fold change in hydrogen-ion concentration.

At a pH of 7, the midpoint of the scale, the number of hydrogen ions is the same as the number of hydroxyl ions and the solution is considered neutral, which is neither an acid nor a base. For example, water is a neutral solution, with an equal number of hydrogen and hydroxyl ions:

$$H^+ + OH^- = H_2O$$

Solutions with a pH lower than 7 (more H^+ ions) are considered acidic, and those above 7 (more OH^- ions) are basic, or alkaline.

Body cells are extremely sensitive to even slight changes in pH. Normal blood pH is slightly alkaline, varying within a narrow range from 7.35 to 7.45. A pH above 7.45 is considered alkalotic, and one below 7.35 is acidotic. The extreme limits considered compatible with life vary by only 0.4 pH units from the normal range. They are 6.9 on the acidic side and 7.8 on the alkaline side (see Fig. 8-9). This delicate balance is carefully regulated by three mechanisms—the lungs, the kidneys, and a system of blood chemicals called buffers.

Buffer System

The first and fastest means of controlling acid-base balance in the body is the blood buffer system. It responds within a fraction of a second to prevent large shifts in the hydrogen-ion concentration. A buffer may be considered a chemical "sponge" that accepts hydrogen ions when they are overabundant and releases them when they are scarce. Buffers do not prevent major pH changes, but can moderate such changes by replacing strong acids and bases with less harmful substances. These, in turn, can be eliminated more easily by the body. There are four sets of blood buffers, the most important of which is the bicarbonate-carbonic acid system.

Bicarbonate-Carbonic Acid System

Carbonic acid (H_2CO_3) is formed when water combines with carbon dioxide:

$$H_2O + CO_2 = H_2CO_3.$$

This reaction occurs primarily in the red blood cells. Carbonic acid can then dissociate into hydrogen (H^+) and bicarbonate (HCO_3^-). The majority of CO_2 is thus transported as bicarbonate in the plasma (Fig. 8-10). The bicarbonate is free to pick up another H^+ ion and either travel to the lungs, where the equation reverses and carbonic acid dissociates to be excreted as carbon dioxide (CO_2) and water vapor (H_2O), or travel to the kidneys where it dissociates into hydrogen ions (H^+) and bicarbonate (HCO_3^-). The kidneys can excrete the H^+ ion, and the bicarbonate ion is free to repeat the process in the blood.

Respiratory System

The respiratory system reacts within minutes to correct acid-base imbalances. This system is triggered by the action of chemoreceptors in the respiratory centers of the brain stem that detect pH in the cerebrospinal fluid. One of the most common examples of the respiratory system working to

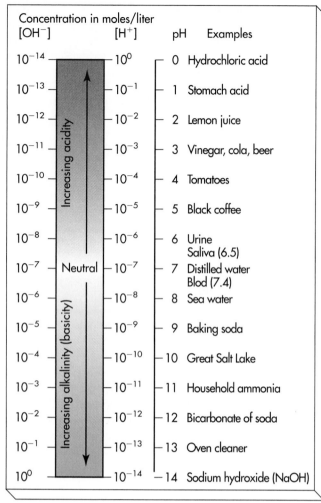

Figure 8-9

pH scale. The concentration of hydrogen (H$^+$) and hydroxyl (OH$^-$) ions determines the pH of solution. A solution with equal concentration of H$^+$ and OH$^-$ ions causes acidosis (pH lower than 7.0). More OH$^-$ ions causes alkalosis (pH higher than 7.0). Normal blood pH is slightly alkalotic (pH of 7.35–7.45). From Seeley, et al: Essentials of anatomy and physiology, ed. 2, St. Louis, 1996, Mosby-Year Book Inc.

Concentration in moles/liter [OH$^-$] [H$^+$] pH Examples:
10^{-14} 10^0 0 Hydrochloric acid; 10^{-13} 10^{-1} 1 Stomach acid; 10^{-12} 10^{-2} 2 Lemon juice; 10^{-11} 10^{-3} 3 Vinegar, cola, beer; 10^{-10} 10^{-4} 4 Tomatoes; 10^{-9} 10^{-5} 5 Black coffee; 10^{-8} 10^{-6} 6 Urine, Saliva (6.5); 10^{-7} 10^{-7} 7 Distilled water, Blod (7.4); 10^{-6} 10^{-8} 8 Sea water; 10^{-5} 10^{-9} 9 Baking soda; 10^{-4} 10^{-10} 10 Great Salt Lake; 10^{-3} 10^{-11} 11 Household ammonia; 10^{-2} 10^{-12} 12 Bicarbonate of soda; 10^{-1} 10^{-13} 13 Oven cleaner; 10^0 10^{-14} 14 Sodium hydroxide (NaOH). Increasing acidity / Neutral / Increasing alkalinity (basicity)

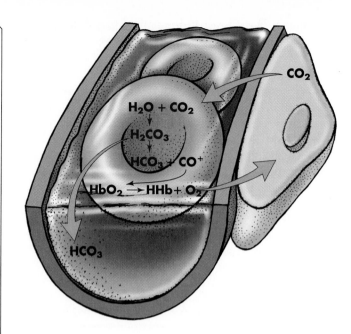

Figure 8-10

The breakdown of carbonic acid results in the presence of H$^+$ and HCO$_3^-$ ions, or H$_2$O and CO$_2$ ions in the blood stream. In the lungs, CO$_2$ is exhaled. In the kidneys, H$_2$O and H$^+$ is excreted. Bicarbonate continues to circulate and is used to make more carbonic acid.

Renal System

If the respiratory system cannot compensate for, or is the cause of, an acid-base imbalance, the kidneys begin to act. The renal system is comparatively slower, taking hours or days to become effective. The kidneys regulate pH by excreting excess hydrogen or bicarbonate ions. If the pH of the extracellular fluid falls, the kidneys eliminate more hydrogen ions. When pH rises, the kidneys eliminate more bicarbonate ions to re-

balance the acid-base concentration in the body is **diabetic ketoacidosis**. Chemoreceptors in the respiratory center of the brain stem detect pH changes and stimulate changes in respiratory rate and depth (Fig. 8-11). The characteristic rapid, deep respirations are evidence that the respiratory system is blowing off carbon dioxide and water to rid the body of excess acid by producing a respiratory alkalosis. Respiratory alkalosis is the body's method of compensating for metabolic acidosis. Even minor changes in pH will stimulate the chemoreceptors and trigger the process of hyperventilation. The respiratory system is most effective in compensating for sudden or acute pH changes due to disease or injury.

If the patient's lungs are damaged by disease or trauma, and respirations become ineffective or insufficient, carbon dioxide will build up, creating more carbonic acid. Although the pH changes stimulate the chemoreceptors, interference by disease or trauma may not allow the system to correct itself. The resulting acidosis is termed "respiratory acidosis," because it is directly related to ineffective or insufficient respirations.

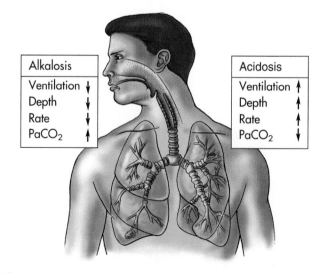

Figure 8-11

Chemoreceptors in the brain stem detect pH changes and alter respiratory patterns to treat acidosis or alkalosis.

store balance. The kidney tubules operate on an exchange system; when one ion is excreted, another is saved.

In acute disease or injury, the patient's renal system is too slow to be effective for quick correction of a pH imbalance. Such patients may deteriorate very quickly. However, renal regulation is the most important factor in long-term maintenance of acid-base balance. For example, the chronic **emphysema** patient who retains carbon dioxide as a normal part of the disease process depends entirely on the renal system for acid-base balance.

Blood Gases

Because carbon dioxide and oxygen are dissolved gases, their partial pressure in arterial and venous blood can be measured. The concentration of hydrogen ions can also be measured as pH. Bicarbonate on the other hand, is measured indirectly. Blood gas measurements are obtained from arterial blood. Calculations of concentration, especially of O_2, depend on barometric pressure. Normal values at lower altitudes are as follows:

$$PaO_2 = 90\% \text{ to } 100\%$$
$$PaCO_2 = 40 \pm 5$$
$$HCO_3^- = 24 \pm 2$$
$$pH = 7.35 - 7.45$$

Note: Because normal PaO_2 depends on altitude, the full range of normal for $PaO_2 = 70\%$ to 100%.

Acid-base derangements are common and often interfere with treatment. Although blood gas testing is not done in the field, there are methods to aid the prehospital provider in effective management of acid-base balance. The key component is management of the airway and ventilation.

An assessment tool known as pulse oximetry is very effective in measuring oxygen saturation (see Sidebar in Chapter 18). In patients with good peripheral circulation, pulse oximetry can guide the selection of oxygen delivery devices. In the absence of pulse oximetry, careful evaluation of the patient's ability to talk, respiratory rate and effort, lung sounds, skin color, temperature and moisture, level of consciousness, and pulse rate can instead guide the selection. It is equally important for the paramedic to know that any condition interfering with carbon dioxide elimination increases the acid level of the blood (decreases the pH). For instance, in the cardiac arrest patient, absence of spontaneous respirations greatly increases the carbon dioxide level in the blood and decreases the pH. To rid the body of this excess carbon dioxide, establish a patent airway and hyperventilate the patient. For the adult, at least an 800 mL tidal volume with a 1.5 to 2 second exhalation time seems to be effective. This equals a respiratory rate of 26/min to 30/min. Reducing the level of carbon dioxide is as important as increasing the oxygen level.

Acid-Base Derangements

Prehospital providers should have a working knowledge of the common causes of acid-base derangements. These causes can be divided into two groups—respiratory and metabolic—based on the general origin of the problem. Table 8-4 is a summary of acid-base derangements.

Respiratory Derangements

Respiratory derangements include respiratory acidosis and respiratory alkalosis. Of the two, respiratory acidosis is more common.

TABLE 8-4	Summary of Acid-Base Derangements	
Primary Cause of Problem	**Results in**	**Response to Adjust CO_2/HCO_3^- Concentrations**
Respiratory acidosis (retained carbon dioxide)	pCO_2 ↑ HCO_3^- normal pH falls	immediate ↓ CO_2 by hyperventilating 12 to 24 hours for HCO_3^- to ↑
Respiratory alkalosis (too much carbon dioxide blown off)	pCO_2 ↓ HCO_3^- normal pH rises	immediate ↑ CO_2 by hypoventilating usually no time for HCO_3^- to change prior to other corrective measures
Metabolic acidosis (retained metabolic acids)	pH falls pCO_2 and HCO_3^- normal to low	immediate CO_2↓ by hypoventilation 12 to 24 hours for HCO_3^- to ↑
Metabolic alkalosis (too many bases ingested or injected)	pH rises pCO_2 normal HCO_3^- high	immediate CO_2↑ by hyperventilation 12 to 24 hours for HCO_3^- to ↓

Normal Values of Arterial Blood Gases	
pH	7.35–7.45
PaO_2	90%–100%
$PaCO_2$	35–45
HCO_3	22–26

NOTE: Metabolic alkalosis is relatively rare, resulting hypoventilation usually at low end of normal.

Respiratory acidosis

In respiratory acidosis, carbon dioxide is retained for some reason (usually hypoventilation), because of respiratory depression, such as that which occurs with some drug overdoses or chronic pulmonary disease, such as emphysema. In the blood, retained carbon dioxide combines with water to form carbonic acid. The renal system will excrete the H^+ ion in urine and save the HCO_3^- ion. The carbonic acid-bicarbonate equation moves in the direction of hydrogen ion:

Retained CO_2: $\uparrow CO_2 + H_2O \rightarrow \uparrow H_2CO_3 \rightarrow \uparrow H^+ + HCO_3^-$

| Respiratory System | Blood Buffer | Renal System |

In the absence of adequate pulmonary function, the renal system takes over but not for several hours.

As long as the blood buffers and the renal system can maintain a relatively normal pH, the body will continue to function. However, when compensatory mechanisms fail or the onset of the problem is acute, rapid deterioration may occur. Causes of respiratory acidosis include pneumonia, emphysema, chronic bronchitis, flail chest, pneumothorax, lung contusions, pulmonary edema, pulmonary emboli, asthma, head injury, damage to the phrenic or intercostal nerves, central nervous system diseases (e.g., polio, myasthenia gravis), and drug overdose.

Respiratory alkalosis

In respiratory alkalosis, carbon dioxide is eliminated in excessive amounts, usually by increased respiratory rate. In the blood, decreased amounts of carbon dioxide decrease the hydrogen-ion concentration and leave an excess of bicarbonate. As long as there is enough circulating carbonic acid, the blood buffer system will compensate. When the blood buffer system cannot, the renal system will take hours to have an effect. This often results in a rapid onset of signs and symptoms of respiratory alkalosis. The carbonic acid-bicarbonate equation looks like this:

Decreased CO_2: $\downarrow CO_2 + H_2O \rightarrow \downarrow H_2CO_3 \rightarrow \downarrow H^+ + HCO_3^-$

| Respiratory System | Blood Buffer | Renal System |

If the episode lasts long enough, the renal system will secrete the HCO_3^- ion and save the H^+ ion.

Respiratory alkalosis is usually a compensatory response to metabolic acidosis. However, pure respiratory alkalosis is uncomplicated by any other disease condition or injury and is usually caused by anxiety (hyperventilation syndrome) or rapid ascent to a high altitude.

Metabolic Derangements

Metabolic derangements include metabolic acidosis and metabolic alkalosis. Of the two, metabolic acidosis is more common.

Metabolic acidosis

In metabolic acidosis, the body metabolism is producing more acid than normal. This condition can be caused by a severely increased metabolism, an abnormal metabolism resulting in excessive acid production, or the presence of a toxic substance that acts as an acid. The acid substance reacts with bicarbonate, forming carbonic acid which is then eliminated through the respiratory system.

As long as the buffers and the respiratory system can maintain a pH within relatively normal levels, the only symptoms will be increased respiratory rate and depth. If the respiratory system cannot keep up and the pH change increases, other signs and symptoms will occur. If renal mechanisms also cannot prevent a change in pH, signs and symptoms become pronounced. The symptoms include agitation and irritability, abdominal pain, muscle cramping, tachycardia, and dehydration. Other signs and symptoms vary according to specific causes. The most common general causes of metabolic acidosis are dieting and anaerobic exercise. Common medical conditions that lead to metabolic acidosis are diabetic ketoacidosis, seizures, and hypovolemia. Other causes include diarrhea and overdoses of aspirin and other medications.

Metabolic alkalosis

In metabolic alkalosis, there is too much bicarbonate in the body. This taxes the renal system and causes the buffer system to use up its stores of carbonic acid. To compensate, the respiratory system slows respirations to conserve carbon dioxide and create more carbonic acid.

Metabolic alkalosis is relatively rare. Because substances that form bases in our body are ingested, the most common cause of metabolic alkalosis is a drug overdose. Possible drugs include Milk of Magnesia, soda bicarbonate, and overzealous administration of sodium bicarbonate. Prolonged vomiting is another cause.

The key to field management of acid-base balance is management of airway and ventilation. Recognizing any visible change in a patient's respiratory status is an important assessment tool. Actual blood gas determinations are done at the hospital. Results can indicate the success of airway management to the prehospital provider and help guide future treatment of patients with similar conditions.

Section 4: Autonomic Nervous System

The nervous system is the master control and communications system of the body. It has direct control over the movement of blood and body fluids, short-term effect on metabolic rate, and an indirect effect on the body's acid-base balance.[3] It is a primary force in the compensation for disease and trauma. It communicates by electrical impulses that travel up or down the nerves to their target sites, either in the brain or in the various organs and glands. These impulses are rapid and specific, and they cause immediate responses.

The primary nervous system division responsible for mobilizing many of the body's compensatory mechanisms is the sympathetic division of the autonomic nervous system. This division is sometimes known as the "accelerator," or stress response, division. It is balanced by the other autonomic branch, the parasympathetic system. The parasympathetic system puts the "brakes" on the sympathetic division and is also called the "vegetative" side of the autonomic system. These two divisions work together to balance each other and provide for the varied needs of the body.

Both sympathetic and parasympathetic fibers serve the same organs. The only exceptions are the structures of the skin, some glands, and the adrenal medulla, all of which receive only sympathetic fibers. These two systems produce opposite effects in most organs; effects that are mediated by the chemicals, or neurotransmitters, they release. Parasympathetic fibers release acetylcholine at their endpoints, and sympathetic fibers primarily release norepinephrine.

The Parasympathetic System

The parasympathetic system keeps the visceral organs, such as the GI tract, working when the body is not threatened. This division promotes normal digestion and elimination and acts to decrease demands on the heart and circulatory system.

The parasympathetic system has its origin in the medulla of the brain. Its principal nerve is called the vagus nerve, which is one of the 12 cranial nerves. The vagus nerve supplies the atrium of the heart (SA and AV nodes), the stomach, and the intestine. The primary function of the vagus nerve is to slow the heart rate. Stimulation of the vagus nerve during a heart attack explains why some people complain of indigestion, nausea and vomiting, or develop a **bradycardia**. Bradycardia from vagal stimulation can also actually cause syncope or a **myocardial infarction**.

The Sympathetic System

The sympathetic system is also known as the "fight or flight" mechanism. When stimulated, it releases norepinephrine at the synapses of the sympathetic nerves and directly to the various organs it innervates.[2,3] The adrenal medulla, an extension of the sympathetic system, also releases norepinephrine but takes the reaction a step further. The majority of the norepinephrine in the medulla is transformed into epinephrine. These chemicals (norepinephrine, epinephrine, and dopamine), known as catecholamines, serve as the sympathetic neurotransmitters. The sympathetic system is responsible for activating sweat glands, increasing the heart rate, and causing bronchodilation.

Sympathetic nerve fibers originate in the spinal cord, exiting at the thoracic and lumbar levels. There are two types of adrenergic (sympathetic) receptors—alpha and beta. Beta is further subdivided into beta 1 (β_1) and beta 2 (β_2). Organs supplied by the sympathetic system have either one or both types of receptor sites. The various effects of the sympathetic system on the numerous organs and organ systems involved depend on which receptor site is stimulated and which cate-

cholamine (dopamine, norepinephrine, or epinephrine) does the stimulating. See Table 8-5 for a summary of the effects of neuroreceptors on the organs.[3]

Cardiovascular structures have predominantly more β_1 receptors, specifically in the conduction system. Coronary arteries have more β_2 receptors.[3] The effect of norepinephrine on β_1 receptors in the heart results in an increase in impulse generation (automaticity), the rate of conduction (conductivity), strength of myocardial contraction (contractility), and response to stimulus (irritability). As a consequence of increasing automaticity and contractility, oxygen demand of the myocardium also increases. To compensate, epinephrine's β_2 effect in the coronary arterioles causes vasodilation, thus providing more oxygen and nutrients to the working myocardium. Together these effects are designed to increase cardiac output, raise blood pressure, and maintain perfusion. Beta effects are easily summarized by the mnemonic CARDIO (see Box 8-2).

Stimulation of β_1 receptors causes the release of renin from the kidney. Renin stimulates another chain reaction that, together with alpha receptor stimulation, causes constriction of blood vessels supplying areas not critical for "fight or flight," such as those in the skin and gut. This constriction shunts blood to areas that require a higher oxygen supply, such as the heart and skeletal muscle, and helps maintain blood pressure. Beta-2 receptors dilate skeletal muscle and coronary arterioles, decrease the motility of the GI tract, and cause

TABLE 8-5	Sympathetic Nervous System	
Organ or Tissue	**Alpha Effect**	**Beta Effect**
Pupil of eye	Constriction	None
Heart		
SA node		Increase heart rate
Atria		Increase contractility
AV junction		Increase conduction
Purkinje system		Increase conduction
Ventricles		Increase conduction and contractility
Arterioles		
Coronary	Constriction	Dilation
Skeletal muscle	Constriction	Dilation
Renal	Constriction	None
Salivary glands	Constriction	None
Mesentery	Constriction	None
Mucosa	Constriction	None
Veins, systemic	Constriction	Dilation
Skin		
Arterioles	Constriction	Dilation
Sweat glands	Secretion	None
Lung		
Bronchial muscle	None	Relaxation
Stomach		
Motility	Decreases (usually)	Decrease (usually)
Sphincters	Contraction (usually)	None

BOX 8-2   Mnemonic for Beta Effects on the Heart

C — ↑ Contractility
A — ↑ Automaticity
R — ↑ Rate
D — Dilates coronary arteries
I — ↑ Irritability
O — ↑ Oxygen demand

---

bronchodilation in the lungs. Beta effects also release stored glucose in the form of glycogen. Alpha stimulation of sweat glands increases sweat production.

Together, alpha- and beta-receptor stimulation in the respiratory and cardiovascular systems supplies enough oxygen, glucose, and waste removal to ensure adequate energy production to maintain perfusion of the vital organs and thus compensate for injury or disease.

With age, the sympathetic nervous system gradually becomes less efficient, particularly in constricting blood vessels. Elderly people are more vulnerable to fainting when they stand, because the sympathetic system cannot react quickly enough to counteract the pull of gravity. The number of functioning beta receptors in the heart, vessels, and lungs also decreases with age.

The nervous system is the origin of many stimuli for compensatory mechanisms. If the paramedic learns to recognize compensatory mechanisms and understands the signs and symptoms found, problems can often be noted and treated when the body is still compensating, rather than after body systems begin to deteriorate.

SUMMARY

Together, these elemental parts of the body—the blood, body fluids, electrolytes, and acid-base balance—along with the controlling autonomic nervous system, enable us to function on a daily basis. When impacted by injury or disease, these components provide a highly sophisticated compensatory response in which the priority is survival of the organism. For most people, these actions take place entirely without conscious knowledge. For prehospital care providers, a functioning knowledge of the processes can enable the most efficient and effective approach to patient care.

REFERENCES

1. American College of Surgeons Committee on Trauma: Shock. In Advanced Trauma Life Support Course for Physicians Instructor Manual, ed 5, Chicago, 1993, p. 74–94.

2. Guyton AC: Human physiology and mechanisms of disease, ed 5, Philadelphia, 1992, WB Saunders.

3. McCance KL, Huether SE (ed): Pathophysiology: the biologic basis for disease in adults and children, St. Louis, 1990, CV Mosby.

4. Purvis JR, Movahed A: Magnesium disorders and cardiovascular diseases. *Clin Cardiol*, 15:556–568, 1992.

5. Reinhart RA: Magnesium deficiency: recognition and treatment in the emergency medicine setting. *Am J Emerg Med*, 10(1):78–81, 1992.

6. Tobey RC, Birnbaum GA, Allegra JR, Horowitz MS, Plosay JJ: Successful resuscitation and neurologic recovery from refractory ventricular fibrillation after magnesium sulfate administration. *Ann Emerg Med*, 21(1):120–123, 1992.

Alice "Twink" Dalton, BSN, NRPM

Chapter 9

Shock

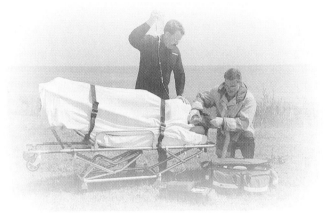

A paramedic should be able to:

OBJECTIVES

1. Describe the components necessary for normal tissue perfusion.
2. Describe the functions of the precapillary sphincters and the vascular system.
3. Define the following terms: afterload, aldosterone, baroreceptors, capacitance vessels, preload.
4. Discuss factors that affect peripheral vascular resistance.
5. Define and discuss the significance of the Frank Starling Law.
6. Define and describe the overall clinical picture of shock.
7. Discuss factors that affect compensation for shock in the a) elderly and b) pediatric age groups.
8. Identify patients and/or conditions that are at high risk for the development of shock.
9. Identify the most useful method to assess for the presence of shock in the prehospital setting.
10. Discuss the basic pathophysiology, signs and symptoms and complications of early shock and late shock (progressive, irreversible).
11. Discuss the compensatory mechanisms of shock exerted by the autonomic nervous system.
12. Discuss why blood pressure can be normal in early shock.
13. Describe assessment and management for shock in the prehospital setting.
14. Describe the types of shock (cardiogenic, hypovolemic, distributive) in terms of their pathophysiology, causes, specific signs and symptoms, complications, and general management.
15. Identify factors that can affect the body's ability to compensate for shock.

KEY TERMS

1. **Adrenergic**—pertaining to the sympathetic nerve fibers of the autonomic nervous system that use epinephrine or epinephrine-like substances as neurotransmitters.
2. **Afterload**—the load, or resistance, against which the left ventricle must eject its volume of blood during contraction.
3. **Anaphylactic shock**—shock caused by an exaggerated allergic reaction that results in widespread vasodilation and permeability.
4. **Baroreceptors**—one of the pressure-sensitive nerve endings in the walls of the atria, vena cava, aortic arch, and carotid sinus. Baroreceptors stimulate central reflex mechanisms that allow physiologic adaptation to changes in blood pressure caused by vasodilation or vasoconstriction. Essential for homeostasis.
5. **Cardiac output**—the volume of blood expelled by the ventricles of the heart, equal to the amount of blood ejected at each beat (the stroke output) multiplied by the heart rate per minute.
6. **Cardiogenic shock**—shock that occurs as a result of abnormal cardiac function (i.e., failing heart muscle, valvular insufficiency, or dysrhythmias).
7. **Compensatory mechanism**—mechanisms that cause or promote enhanced function to supplement decreased or inefficient function elsewhere.
8. **Distributive shock**—shock that occurs as a result of low resistance of blood vessels. Low resistance may occur from massive vasodilation or vasodilation with increased vessel permeability.
9. **Hypovolemic shock**—shock caused by a loss of fluid volume, either by frank blood loss or plasma loss.
10. **Neurogenic shock**—a type of distributive shock that results when sympathetic control of the vascular system is lost.
11. **Perfusion**—the circulation of blood to the tissues to provide for metabolic needs.
12. **Peripheral vascular resistance**—resistance created by the diameter of blood vessel walls in the periphery.
13. **Preload**—the stretch of myocardial fiber at end diastole. The ventricular end diastolic pressure and volume reflect this parameter.
14. **Septic shock**—shock caused by toxins released by infectious organisms. The effect is usually a combination of inhibition of compensatory mechanisms, vasodilation, and/or increased permeability of blood vessels.
15. **Shock**—inadequate tissue perfusion.

century ago, shock was described as "a rude interruption of the machinery of life."[3] This description remains meaningful today. Shock occurs because the "machinery of life"—perfusion—is inadequate to support life. Shock ultimately results in death unless compensatory mechanisms reverse the process or therapeutic interventions succeed. It is only with early recognition, treatment, and rapid transport that a positive effect on morbidity and mortality will occur. To recognize the signs and symptoms of shock and understand the process, the paramedic first must understand normal tissue perfusion.

Physiology of Normal Tissue Perfusion

Normal tissue perfusion implies that tissue cells have enough circulation to efficiently provide for their metabolic needs. Cellular metabolism requires that oxygen and sugar produce energy in amounts necessary to meet the demand, as well as remove waste adequately enough to maintain efficient cellular function.[5]

Oxygen, glucose, and waste removal are provided by the respiratory and cardiovascular systems. These systems can be further broken down into:

- Lungs—where oxygen and carbon dioxide exchange occurs at the alveolar level.
- Blood—the transport medium that carries oxygen and glucose to the cells, and carries carbon dioxide, lactic acid, and other wastes away from the cells.
- Vessels—the containers for the blood that regulate its distribution.
- Heart—the pump that keeps blood moving with enough pressure to reach all body tissues.

Respiratory System

The primary function of the lungs is to exchange oxygen for carbon dioxide in the alveoli. The rate and depth of ventilations control the amount of oxygen that reaches the alveoli.

Carbon dioxide is the primary waste product of cellular metabolism (Fig. 9-1). Once carbon dioxide has been produced, it diffuses into the blood stream and combines with water molecules to form carbonic acid. Carbonic acid and other acidic byproducts of metabolism are carried to the lungs or kidneys for excretion from the body. If the carbon dioxide concentration builds up, a threshold is reached at which cell damage begins.

The body alters the arterial concentration of carbon dioxide ($PaCO_2$) by altering the ventilation depth and rate,[5] which are under the control of the medulla's respiratory chemoreceptors. These are specialized cells sensitive to concentrations of oxygen, carbon dioxide, and hydrogen ions (pH).[5] The chemoreceptors stimulate regulators in the medulla to adjust the rate or depth of ventilation.

Normal hemoglobin saturation is influenced by pH, $PaCO_2$, and body temperature. During states of normal perfusion, these factors closely regulate the binding and release of oxygen. In anaerobic states, such as shock, decreased pH and

increased $PaCO_2$ interfere with the ability of hemoglobin to adequately deliver oxygen to the tissues and collect carbon dioxide for removal.[4]

Through effective management of the airway and ventilations, and appropriate use of assessment devices, such as pulse oximetry, pH, and the arterial concentration of carbon dioxide, this condition can be controlled. Use of these devices aids in the uptake and release of oxygen by hemoglobin and in removal of carbon dioxide from the tissues.

Cardiovascular System

The cardiovascular system is composed of three natural divisions—blood, vessels, and the heart. All three divisions must be functioning properly for adequate perfusion to occur.

Blood

Adequate perfusion requires roughly 80 mL of blood per kilogram of body weight.[1] To maintain that amount, blood volume as a part of total body water (TBW) is constantly regulated and maintained by normal fluid shifts and hormone systems. See Chapter 8, Section II on fluids and electrolytes for more information on fluid regulation.

Adequate perfusion also supplies clotting factors carried in the blood to the entire vascular system. In times of stress, clotting factors work at peak efficiency and clotting time actually decreases.

Vessels

The actual work of perfusion—the exchange of oxygen, nutrients, and waste products—occurs at the capillary level. Because the vascular system is so extensive and blood volume is relatively small in comparison, regulation of blood flow is an extremely important ongoing process.

The vascular system regulates flow by controlling two main factors—the size of the vessel and the amount of blood flow into the vessel. Both arteries and veins are involved in this

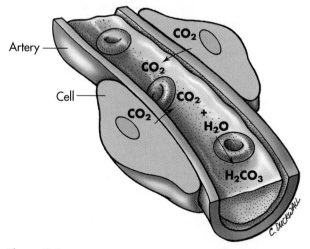

Figure 9-1

Carbonic acid is formed when the cellular waste product, CO_2, diffuses into the bloodstream and combines with water.

regulation, primarily through the sympathetic and parasympathetic systems.

Elastic arteries (i.e., the aorta, its major branches, and the pulmonary trunk) stretch and recoil, maintaining pressure within the vessels. Depending on the type of stimulation, muscular arteries—the remaining arteries and the arterioles—constrict (by stimulation of alpha receptors) or dilate (by stimulation of beta receptors or the parasympathetic system). Arteries thus regulate blood flow to the capillary beds (Fig. 9-2).[4]

Where the arterioles and capillaries meet, the precapillary sphincters contract and relax to control blood flow throughout the capillaries (Fig. 9-3). The sphincters are under the influence of cellular oxygen demand, accumulation of waste products, and nutrient needs. Precapillary sphincters perform three functions: 1) maintain arterial pressure; 2) oppose the effects of gravity on blood flow in the arteries; and 3) accomplish selective distribution of flow according to needs throughout the body.[4]

From the capillary beds, vessels branch into the venules and veins. Venules are the capacitance vessels that function together to regulate the capacity of the vascular system and serve as a blood reservoir. Venules and larger veins respond, primarily to alpha adrenergic stimulation, by constricting. In this manner, the body's blood "reserve" is mobilized when the system is stressed.

Peripheral Vascular Resistance. Resistance is the opposition to force. In the cardiovascular system, most opposition to the force of blood flow is provided by the diameter and length of the blood vessels themselves.[4] Changes in blood flow through an organ are therefore primarily affected by vascular resistance changes within the organ. The major mechanisms causing these changes are alterations in vessel diameter and the opening or closing of precapillary sphincters.[4] Another important factor in vascular resistance is the viscosity, or thickness, of the blood. The greater the viscosity, the lower the blood flow in a vessel, if all other factors are constant.[2]

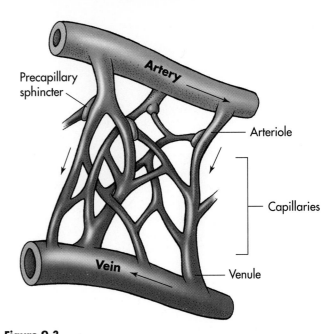

Figure 9-3

Precapillary sphincters, located on the arteriolar side of the capillary bed, dilate and constrict to control blood flow through the capillary beds.

Vascular resistance is most important when a special need arises to regulate blood flow to a given area or to maintain pressure throughout the system. Vasoconstriction occurs, initially in the periphery, when the body is trying to maintain an adequate blood return to the heart, so that it can produce perfusion pressure in the system. Sympathetic stimulation of blood vessels, primarily of the veins, can maintain enough pressure and reduce the dimensions of the circulatory system sufficiently, so that perfusion of vital organs continues almost normally even with loss of as much as 25% of the total blood volume.[2]

Heart

The heart functions as a pump that rhythmically generates pressure to circulate the blood through the vessels to the tissues. Properties such as preload, afterload, heart rate, cardiac output and contractility affect the heart's contribution to tissue perfusion (Fig. 9-4).

Preload. The amount of blood returning to the ventricles, or preload, is determined by the pressure in the venous system. Preload also determines the amount of stretch in the ventricle just before systole and is therefore a major factor in the Frank Starling Law.[4]

Afterload. The pressure against which the left ventricle—the main pumping chamber of the heart—has to pump is known as afterload. Afterload is determined by the volume of blood present and the amount of resistance created by the constriction level of arterial vessels.

Cardiac Output. Cardiac output is determined by the amount of blood ejected in each contraction of the left ventricle (stroke volume), and the rate at which the heart contracts. As an equation, cardiac output equals the stroke volume times the heart rate, or:

$$CO = SV \times HR.$$

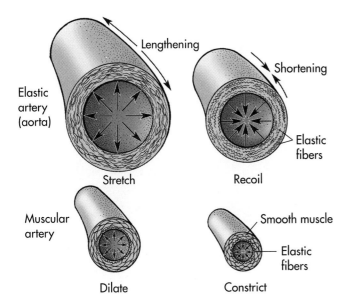

Figure 9-2

Elastic and muscular arteries respond to maintain blood flow.

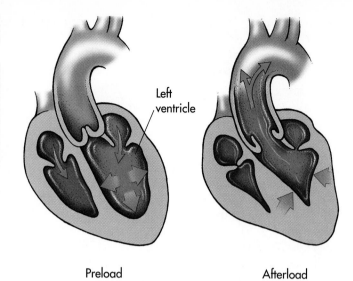

Left ventricle

Preload   Afterload

Figure 9-4

Preload is at maximum pressure at the end of ventricular filling. Afterload is measured as the amount of pressure the ejecting blood volume is working against as it leaves the ventricle and enters the aorta during systole.

Contractility. Two mechanisms influence the strength of cardiac contractions: 1) the Frank Starling Law; and 2) the sympathetic nervous system.

Briefly, the Frank Starling Law states that the more the ventricular wall is stretched, the stronger the contraction becomes (Fig. 9-5). When peripheral vascular resistance increases preload, the heart responds to the increase in blood return by contracting harder. Stroke volume also increases, as does myocardial oxygen demand.[4] However, there is a point at which preload will not result in further contractility gains.

Sympathetic stimulation of the heart muscle and coronary vessels enables the heart to keep up with tissue demands for oxygen and nutrients. The catecholamines, norepinephrine and epinephrine, increase cardiac contractility, automaticity, and rate, thus increasing cardiac output. To handle the increased workload, coronary arteries also dilate, primarily in response to epinephrine's beta effects. (For a more detailed discussion of the effects of alpha and beta stimulation, see Chapter 8.)

Together, the respiratory and cardiovascular systems supply enough oxygen, glucose, and waste removal to ensure efficient energy production and maintain tissue perfusion. These systems in turn are supported and maintained by a number of regulatory and compensatory mechanisms from the brain and the endocrine and nervous systems.

Shock

Shock is most simply defined as inadequate tissue perfusion.[1] Disease or injury interfering with normal function of any part of the respiratory or cardiovascular system can alter tissue perfusion. When that occurs, the body's regulatory and compensatory mechanisms work to help correct or maintain adequate cardiac output. However, if tissue perfusion remains inadequate, the cycle of shock begins.

Because tissue perfusion can be disrupted by any factor that alters heart function, blood volume, or vascular integrity, there are many causes of shock. Body tissues function and malfunction at different stages of metabolic impairment, so the signs and symptoms of shock are diverse and sometimes conflicting. Blood pressure is usually, but not always, decreased. The heart rate may be normal, and skin color can vary from pink and flushed to gray and mottled. Lung sounds can be clear or indicate the presence of fluid. Other variable signs of shock include changes in core temperature, skin temperature, and systemic vascular resistance. Signs such as dyspnea, diaphoresis, and altered level of consciousness may be more obvious.

Factors Affecting the Process of Shock

Just as there are differences between factors causing shock, there is diversity among individuals with a given type of shock. Differences include what signs and symptoms are seen, when they appear, and how rapidly the shock process advances. Determining factors include age, relative health, efficiency of compensatory mechanisms, and the organ system initially affected.

Age and relative health refer to the patient's general physical condition and the presence of pre-existing disease. Good physical condition improves the ability to compensate and can delay the onset of shock. If patient condition is poor or there is pre-existing disease, the onset of shock tends to be more sudden and can progress more quickly toward a bad outcome.

Compensatory mechanisms are less efficient in the elderly. Children tend to compensate longer, but they also deteriorate faster when compensatory mechanisms fail. Some drugs, such as beta blockers, may interfere with compensatory mechanisms and thus promote the advance of shock.

The organ system initially affected may determine rapidity of onset and the signs and symptoms first seen. For example, anaphylactic shock may occur within seconds as the patient literally suffocates; hypovolemic shock may take days to

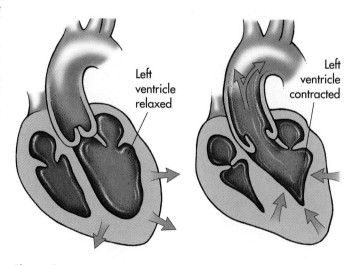

Left ventricle relaxed

Left ventricle contracted

Figure 9-5

The ventricles will have a more forceful contraction if they are stretched to their maximum during filling. If the ventricle is overfilled or underfilled, it loses contraction force, affecting cardiac output and blood pressure.

develop with a slow GI bleed and a chief complaint of dizziness; and cardiogenic shock may occur within hours of the first complaint of chest pain.

High-risk Groups

Those particularly susceptible include the very young and the elderly, because of altered or inefficient compensatory mechanisms or compromised immune systems. Other high-risk groups include victims of trauma with sufficient mechanism of injury (hemorrhagic or neurogenic shock); patients with a history of ulcers or GI bleeding (hemorrhagic shock); patients with acute MI (cardiogenic shock); allergic reaction, especially to bee sting or drugs (anaphylactic shock); patients with indwelling tubes or shunts, such as urinary catheters or venous access devices (septic shock); drug abusers, including alcoholics (septic or hemorrhagic shock); and diabetics and those with compromised immune systems (septic shock).

Pathophysiology

Of all the factors that can cause shock, decreased blood volume caused by hemorrhage is the most common. The process of hemorrhagic shock, and the stages the patient goes through, serve as baselines with which all other types of shock are compared. The process can be identified in two ways: 1) based on percent of blood lost, and 2) based on signs and symptoms seen in the different stages of shock.

The American College of Surgeons classifies hemorrhagic shock in terms of percent of blood loss.[1]

The field setting does not lend itself well to classifying shock in terms of percent of blood loss. For field care, the most useful method is to look at shock in terms of signs and symptoms.

Some have advocated grouping signs and symptoms into stages such as compensated, progressive, and irreversible. The stages and classes are compared in Table 9-1.

However, patients rarely fit neatly into categories, stages, or classes. It is more important to recognize the process of shock, manage the patient appropriately, and transport rapidly.

Early Shock (Compensated Phase)

In this phase, body systems are able to maintain perfusion to the vital organs and compensate for the bodily insult. A fall in cardiac output triggers two reactions. First, a drop in capillary pressure causes interstitial fluid to move into the vascular space.[4] Second, the baroreceptors, located in the arch of the

aorta and the carotid sinus, detect the pressure change almost immediately and initiate a signal to the adrenal glands to secrete epinephrine and norepinephrine. These hormones stimulate alpha and beta receptors in the heart, lungs, blood vessels, and sweat glands.

Alpha-receptor stimulation causes vasoconstriction in the least necessary parts of the body first, such as the skin, GI tract, and extremities. This effectively shunts blood to the core, increasing preload. Beta-receptor stimulation increases cardiac function. Together, alpha and beta stimulation work to increase cardiac output by increasing stroke volume, contractility, and heart rate, and to promote maximum oxygen/carbon dioxide exchange through bronchodilation. Combined effects also help increase the body's energy supply by converting glycogen to glucose, and increase the body's ability to take in oxygen and discard wastes. The goal is to preserve the vital organs—the brain, heart, lungs, and kidneys. Early clinical signs and symptoms include pale facial color, especially around the mouth and nose, increased heart rate, increased respiratory depth and rate, and sweating, usually starting on the upper lip and around the hair line.

If the compensatory efforts are successful, the body maintains perfusion and blood pressure remains within normal limits. This explains why this stage of shock is sometimes referred to as "compensated" shock; it corresponds to Class I and early Class II shock.

Late Shock (Progressive and Irreversible Phases)

If compensatory mechanisms are unsuccessful or the cycle continues, the progressive and irreversible phases (Class II and III) follow. Late shock begins when the body no longer can maintain adequate tissue perfusion, and the kidneys detect a drop in filtration pressure. The liver and spleen release stored supplies of red blood cells and plasma.[4] Stimuli are also sent to increase the release of epinephrine, norepinephrine, and antidiuretic hormone (e.g., ADH or vasopressin), and the synthesis of renin, angiotensinogen, and aldosterone.

The effects of epinephrine and norepinephrine become more pronounced at this stage. The blood vessels respond by maximal constriction to further reduce the circulating area for blood. Ischemia intensifies, and decreased oxygen availability results in anaerobic metabolism. As carbon dioxide and other toxic chemicals build up, respirations become increasingly rapid and shallow. ADH is released from the pituitary to help conserve water in the kidney. At the same time, renin and angiotensinogen produce angiotensin, a powerful vasoconstrictor. This process also stimulates aldosterone production. Aldosterone conserves sodium in the kidney and further helps to conserve body fluid. At this point, urine production is minimal.

As hypoxia, hypoxemia, and ischemia increase, high acid concentrations in the blood cause relaxation of precapillary sphincters. Ongoing contraction of the postcapillary sphincters causes blood to pool in the capillary beds. This eventually results in mottling of the tissues. The high levels of acid in the blood reduce its oxygen-carrying capacity. Deoxygenated red blood cells cluster together forming microemboli. Cyanosis begins, usually around the nose, mouth, earlobes, and the distal extremities.

It is during this stage of shock that the "classic" signs and symptoms are evident—a change in the level of

TABLE 9-1	Comparison of Classifications of Hemorrhagic Shock
Stage	**Class**
Compensated Stage	Class I (<15% blood loss) (up to 750 mL)
Progressive Stage	Class II (15%–30% blood loss) (750–1500 mL)
	Class III (30%–40% blood loss) (1500–2000 mL)
Irreversible Stage	Class IV (>40% blood loss) (>2000 mL)

consciousness; cool, clammy skin that is pale with cyanosis or mottling; delayed capillary return; extended diaphoresis; a noticeably faster heart rate (usually above 100); rapid and shallow respirations, and a falling blood pressure.

Several phenomena occur in response to progressively high levels of hypoxia and ischemia. The "washout" phenomenon appears when postcapillary sphincters finally relax, allowing accumulated waste products to circulate to the core. Hydrogen ions, potassium ions, clustered red blood cells, carbon dioxide, lactic acid, and other acid waste products make the blood highly toxic to surrounding tissue, and cellular membranes begin to break down, releasing harmful enzymes. This is especially evident in the vital organs still being perfused. Cardiac rhythm disturbances may occur as ventricular irritability increases. Eventually, the rhythm slows down, the QRS widens, and an idioventricular rhythm results.

Together, the toxins in the blood contribute to organ failure. Myocardial depressant factor (MDF), a toxic component of the inflammatory process, further interferes with cardiac muscle function. Red blood cell clustering increases, causing widespread obstruction of capillary beds further contributing to tissue ischemia, enzyme release, and cellular death.

Adult respiratory distress syndrome (ARDS), kidney failure, and heart failure are all implicated in this process. The underlying cause of all this tissue destruction and organ failure is hypoxia.

At some point in late shock, patients become unresponsive; the exact point of onset varies considerably. A detectable pulse disappears, the rate slows, the P wave disappears and the QRS widens into an idioventricular rhythm that progresses to asystole. There is no detectable BP, respirations become agonal and the skin appears gray and mottled. The hands and feet may appear waxen or cyanotic. Production of sweat ceases, although the skin will remain clammy if evaporation has not occurred. Even with resuscitation, the mortality rate is very high at this point. The patient often suffers organ failure, with ARDS the most common problem. If the organ systems can be supported long enough for the body to heal itself, however, the patient may recover.

Assessment

Recognition of the patient's status in the shock process is crucial. The sooner the process is recognized and appropriate management begun, the better the patient's chance for survival. The assessment process begins upon approach to the patient. Important components of the physical assessment that apply to the shock cycle include skin color and temperature, level of consciousness, vital signs, and presence of postural hypotension. It is important to keep in mind that the signs and symptoms of the shock cycle change as the process continues, so assessment must be repeated. Table 9-2 lists the clinical responses to different types of shock.

The patient in shock may complain of several symptoms related to compensatory mechanisms. Thirst is a frequent complaint caused by volume deficit, fluid shifts, and blood shunted to the vital organs. Patients may also complain of feeling cold because of peripheral vasoconstriction and of feeling

dizzy upon body movement because of the fall in cardiac output. Vasoconstriction and hypoperfusion of the GI tract can cause nausea and vomiting.

Specific Types of Shock

Any factor that interferes with cardiac function (pump), vascular integrity (vessels), or volume can cause shock (see Table 9-3). When the shock cycle begins, the initial organ system affected will usually determine the specific signs and symptoms. The most concise method of classifying shock uses three general categories—hypovolemic, cardiogenic, and distributive.

Hypovolemic

Hypovolemic shock refers to a loss of fluid volume, either by frank blood loss or plasma loss. Shock caused by blood loss, or hemorrhagic shock, is frequently seen in the field. Traumatic causes of shock may result in obvious bleeding or, in the case of blunt trauma, internal bleeding. Other causes of internal bleeding include ruptured cysts, aortic aneurysms, and GI bleeds.

Shock caused by plasma loss includes dehydration, usually a result of vomiting or diarrhea, excessive sweating and third spacing, as in burn edema and ascites. Burn shock is usually not seen in the field. Ascites is an end result of cirrhosis of the liver and is also uncommon in the field. Dehydration, however, is an acute and common problem encountered in the field.

The elderly and the very young are prone to dehydration. Fluid loss is usually caused by prolonged vomiting, diarrhea, or drug overdoses, especially of diuretics. Patient history is extremely important, especially in determining the events leading up to the incident, such as frequency of vomiting and diarrhea and whether water can be kept down.

Skin vitals can differ somewhat from hemorrhagic shock in that sweating is not always apparent and the skin may have poor turgor. A frequent assessment finding is warm, dry skin with "tenting." Thirst is a common complaint, except in the elderly, who may have impaired thirst mechanisms. Treatment is based on fluid replacement. Ringer's lactate and normal saline are both acceptable methods of treatment. The rate should be titrated to the blood pressure. Oral fluids are avoided because of the tendency to vomit.

Cardiogenic

Cardiogenic shock occurs as a result of abnormal function of the heart. This condition can result from primary causes, such as heart muscle failure because of infarction, valvular insufficiency, or dysrhythmias, or secondary causes, such as pulmonary emboli, cardiac tamponade, or tension pneumothorax.

Of all the causes of cardiogenic shock, heart muscle failure caused by acute myocardial infarction (AMI) is the most common. For cardiogenic shock to occur, at least 40% of the heart muscle must malfunction. Valvular insufficiency and a heart rate inadequate to maintain cardiac output (usually < 50 or >

TABLE 9-2　Clinical Responses to Different Types of Shock

Vital Sign	Cardiogenic	Hypovolemic	Neurogenic	Septic	Anaphylactic
Heart rate	↑ or ↓	↑	↓	↑	↑
Blood pressure					
Early	BP can be maintained	BP can be maintained	BP can be maintained or ↓	BP can be maintained	BP can be maintained
Late	↓	↓	↓	↓	↓
Respiratory rate	↑	↑	↑ or ↓	↑	↑
Skin temperature and condition	Cool and usually moist	Cool and usually moist	Warm and usually dry	Warm and usually dry	Warm and usually dry
Skin color	Pale or cyanotic	Pale or cyanotic (late)	Normal or flushed (early) pale (late)	Flushed (early) pale or cyanotic (late)	Flushed or rash (hives)

TABLE 9-3　Types of Shock with Pathologies

Cardiovascular system components	Type of shock	Pathology
Heart	Cardiogenic	Ineffective pumping due to weak muscle, dysrhythmia, valve dysfunction
Blood volume	Hypovolemic	Inadequate amount of blood or plasma to fill vascular space due to blood loss, dehydration, etc.
	Hemorrhagic	Inadequate amount of blood to fill vascular space due to hemorrhage
Vessels	Distributive	Vascular bed is abnormally dilated, leaky, or both
	Anaphylactic	Increased capillary permeability and vasodilation
	Neurogenic	Vasodilation of vessels
	Septic	Microvasodilation and increased capillary permeability

170 in the adult) result in similar signs and symptoms. Secondary causes of cardiogenic shock are not as common, and recognition of these causes is generally history-dependent.

One common difference between hemorrhagic shock and cardiogenic shock is historical—chest pain is the most common symptom in cardiogenic shock. The physical examination also offers common differentiating factors. Distended neck veins are typical of most forms of cardiogenic shock, and pulmonary edema is characteristic in acute myocardial infarction. Early pulmonary edema may simply present with diminished lung sounds. As the fluid increases, wheezes, and crackles or rales may develop. If fluid fills the alveolar spaces, lung sounds will be absent over that area. The patient will complain of increased difficulty when breathing as this process continues. In late stages, a productive cough of white or pink, foamy sputum can appear.

Patient management is based on correcting the cause. For instance, failure of cardiac muscle may require administration of dopamine or dobutamine, and rate and rhythm correction may indicate lidocaine to correct ventricular tachycardia, adenosine to correct supraventricular tachycardia, or atropine or external pacing to correct bradycardias.

Cardiac tamponade and tension pneumothorax impede the heart's ability to pump effectively, and thus are sometimes included in the cardiogenic shock category. This type of shock is also called mechanical or obstructive shock. Both are typically associated with trauma, although tension pneumothorax is also common in COPD patients when a bleb ruptures. Chest pain is a common complaint in a patient with a ruptured bleb.

Cardiac tamponade and tension pneumothorax are both associated with a paradoxical pulse and a narrowed pulse pressure. A paradoxical pulse occurs as the pressure increases either directly on the aorta (cardiac tamponade) or in the thoracic cavity more generally (tension pneumothorax). Both conditions present with clear lung sounds, but they are unequal in tension pneumothorax. Lung sounds with a pulmonary embolus depend on clot location.

Management of secondary causes of cardiogenic shock depends on the specific cause. Oxygen therapy, IV initiation, and ECG monitoring are standard. Dopamine and dobutamine are both used to support blood pressure in a patient with a pulmonary embolus. Tension pneumothorax calls for chest decompression, and pericardiocentesis, which is usually performed only in a hospital setting, is the treatment for cardiac tamponade.

Distributive

Distributive or low resistance shock occurs when the blood vessels either vasodilate en masse, as they do in neurogenic shock, or vasodilate and become permeable, as in anaphylactic and septic shock. This is also sometimes called capacitance shock or vasogenic shock.

Neurogenic

Neurogenic shock results when the nervous system loses sympathetic control of vascular resistance, or massive stimulation of the parasympathetic system occurs (as in a drug overdose or poisoning). Both mechanisms result in widespread vasodilation. Causes commonly seen in field practice include spine injury (most commonly seen), blunt head trauma to the back of the head, and overdoses of drugs affecting the central nervous system.

Blood vessels normally maintain a certain amount of tone, being neither totally constricted nor dilated. Further, vessels in one tissue will have more or less tone than those in another. This is how the system maintains pressure and satisfies metabolic needs in various areas.

In a spine-injured patient, the point at which neurogenic shock appears depends on when complete cord interruption occurs (Fig. 9-6). It may appear immediately, with physical interruption, or later if cord hypoxia is the cause. When it does occur, loss of vasomotor tone results in widespread vasodilation below the level of cord interruption. The total blood volume remains the same, but the capacity of the vessels is increased. Unlike other types of shock, the process is limited. Blood vessels only vasodilate so far. Blood pressure falls, but because of the fixed diameter of blood vessels at maximum dilation, it rarely falls below 70 systolic. Paradoxically, these patients do not become tachycardic, as would be expected when the blood pressure falls.

The degree of hypoperfusion depends on the level of cord interruption, and results in signs and symptoms that differ from the classic presentation of shock. Immediately after the injury, there is skin flushing because of vasodilation, which can cause loss of body heat. Hypothermia is a very real problem. Blood eventually pools and leaves the upper-most skin surfaces pale. The time in which this occurs is highly individual and depends partly on the level of cord interruption. Sweating does not occur below the level of injury.

As long as the heart receives enough sympathetic stimulation, the body will compensate. However, high cord injuries leave the heart without sympathetic stimulation. With the

parasympathetic system in control, heart rate will drop, further decreasing cardiac output.

High-cord injuries also disrupt intercostal nerve control of rib movement, resulting in abdominal breathing. Phrenic nerve control of the diaphragm may also be affected. This results in shallow, labored, and sometimes irregular breathing. In the worst case, there is no respiratory movement at all.

The biggest difference in the physical examination between neurogenic shock and other types of shock is paralysis below the level of cord interruption. Altered sensation is also associated with the impaired motor function.

High-cord injuries often initially present with unconsciousness, but not all of these patients have an altered mentation level. If the patient is alert, the anxiety level may not seem as high as in the hemorrhagic shock patient because of the lack of norepinephrine and epinephrine release. The stimulus for release of these catecholamines, which pass through the spinal cord, is blocked by the injury.

Management involves spinal immobilization and the use of spinal precautions if intubation is necessary. It is helpful to use a bag-valve-mask to ventilate. Time the ventilations to the patient's own respiratory effort for best results. Because this shock is self-limiting, IV initiation and treatment with fluid boluses is usually sufficient. Occasionally if the patient is bradycardic, it is also necessary to use atropine to inhibit the parasympathetic system and allow the heart's inherent rate to take over and maintain cardiac output.

Anaphylactic

Anaphylactic shock is an exaggerated, potentially lethal allergic reaction. The reaction can occur within seconds or hours after an exposure to an allergen (Fig. 9-7). The speed of the reaction depends on the degree of sensitivity and the route of exposure (e.g., injection, ingestion, absorption, or inhalation). Initial signs and symptoms depend on the speed of the reaction and the target organ. Target organs include the vascular system, lungs, GI tract, and skin.

When contact with an allergen occurs, mast cells (located just outside the small blood vessels) and basophils (in the blood) release histamine, SRSA (slow-reacting substance of anaphylaxis), heparin, and platelet-activating factors. These substances cause widespread vasodilation and increase permeability of the blood vessels. A major loss of fluid into the surrounding tissues occurs, and local smooth muscle contracts. Numerous types of abnormal tissue responses can occur, depending upon the type of tissue affected and the speed of the reaction.

The common skin reaction is hives, caused by local vasodilation. Increased permeability causes swelling, which is especially noticeable in the mucous membranes of the larynx (stridor), trachea and bronchial tree. The permeability change may be extensive enough to cause a fluid shift into the alveoli that leads to rales or frank pulmonary edema. The permeability and microclotting (from platelet activation) may be extensive enough to cause petechiae to form.

Smooth muscle contraction, in combination with vasodilation and increased permeability, can lead to stomach cramps, vomiting, and protracted diarrhea, as well as bronchospasm (wheezing) and laryngospasm (stridor or respiratory arrest). Because increased heart rate cannot compensate

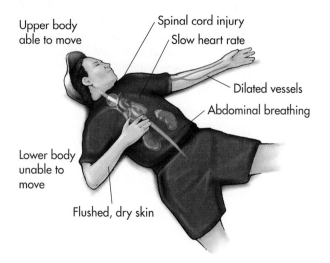

Upper body able to move

Spinal cord injury

Slow heart rate

Dilated vessels

Abdominal breathing

Lower body unable to move

Flushed, dry skin

Figure 9-6

Neurogenic shock does not present with "normal" shock signs and symptoms.

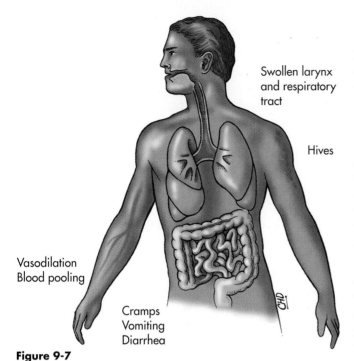

Swollen larynx
and respiratory
tract

Hives

Vasodilation
Blood pooling

Cramps
Vomiting
Diarrhea

Figure 9-7

Anaphylactic shock can have immediate or slow onset of signs and symptoms, the most severe of which result in airway closure and death.

for such widespread vasodilation and fluid shifts, a rapid drop in cardiac output is likely to follow.

Patient management involves removing the allergen source, administering epinephrine (for its vasoconstricting, antihistamine, and membrane stabilizing effects), and infusing a crystalloid such as Ringer's lactate or normal saline. Other medications given include antihistamines, especially Benadryl® (diphenhydramine), and steroids.

Septic

Septic shock is complex; it presents the most confusion and rapidly changing signs and symptoms of all the types of shock. Septic shock begins with an infection of the blood, called septicemia. Because the infection is in the blood, it can easily spread through the body and overwhelm its defense mechanisms. However, septicemia may exist for some time before shock develops. Toxins released by the causative organism inhibit the body's compensatory mechanisms and a combination of increased capillary permeability and vasodilation causes shock. Those prone to developing septic shock include the elderly, patients with depressed immune systems, para- and quadraplegics, neonates, diabetics, and those with long-term, indwelling Foley or IV catheters.

The wide range of responses to septic shock is accounted for by the strength of the immune response and inflammation process, and by the involvement of various tissues and organs as sepsis progresses.[4]

Management of septic shock involves supporting the respiratory and cardiovascular systems. Appropriate oxygen therapy may include high-flow oxygen with positive pressure, fluid boluses, and dopamine or dobutamine administration.

General Management

Management is based on supporting the respiratory and cardiovascular systems. Prevention of hypothermia is an additional treatment priority.

Pitfalls

Several factors that mask or interfere with the body's compensatory mechanisms can confuse the paramedic whose assessment is too focused on the expected signs and symptoms of shock. These factors include age of the patient, hypothermia, pacemakers, and drugs such as beta blockers and alcohol.

Age

The older patient has difficulty tolerating hypotension caused by traumatic hemorrhage. Compensatory mechanisms are not as efficient, and may require a longer time period to take effect. Many older patients have existing medical problems that may also complicate the assessment. For instance, hypotension in the patient with chronic hypertension can go unrecognized because a systolic pressure of 110 may be hypotensive for the patient with a normal pressure of 150. Prolonged hypotension can cause AMI or stroke in the elderly.

In addition to complicating patient assessment, existing medical problems can disrupt the body's normal compensatory mechanisms, and the patient may deteriorate more rapidly as a result.

For a discussion of the variations seen in pediatric patients, see Chapter 22 and Chapter 25.

Hypothermia

Shock predisposes patients to hypothermia. A trauma victim under the influence of alcohol and exposed to cold temperatures is especially vulnerable to hypothermia. Patients suffering from hypothermia and hemorrhagic shock are resistant to appropriate resuscitative measures.[1] Geriatric patients are at particular risk. Research suggests that the elderly multiple-trauma patient with hypotension lasting 15 minutes or longer will have a fatal outcome if allowed to become hypothermic.[6]

Pacemakers

Pacemaker patients are unable to use tachycardia to compensate for blood loss. Although the vessels can still vasoconstrict, this increases only one part of the cardiac output equation (the stroke volume). This may not be enough to maintain adequate tissue perfusion. The fact that the heart rate remains at a steady 70 to 72 beats per minute may be confusing unless the pacer is recognized.

Beta blockers

This class of drugs inhibits beta receptors from responding to sympathetic stimulation. These drugs may be prescribed for hypertension, angina, tachycardias, and migraine headaches, and are taken by people in many age groups.

Beta blockers inhibit the ability of the heart to increase rate (it seldom exceeds 100) or strengthen contractions. Because of this inhibition of cardiac compensation, shock can progress more quickly than usual, and treatment may take longer to have a positive effect.

Alcohol

Several things must be considered when hypotension seems to exceed the severity of the apparent injury. One of them is alcohol use. Alcohol is a peripheral vasodilator; it causes a drop in blood pressure and increases susceptibility to hypothermia. When hypotension is a result of blood loss, peripheral vessels usually constrict well in response to catecholamine release. However, this is not always true in the long-term alcohol user.

Alcohol also clouds mentation. An altered level of consciousness caused by alcohol intoxication is almost impossible to discriminate from head injury, shock, diabetic reactions, and other possible sources. Because alcohol is a body-wide anesthetic, patient complaints of pain may be altered or absent.

Finally, the patient's gag reflex is often impaired, leading to an increased chance of aspiration. The risk is further aggravated by alcohol's tendency to irritate the stomach and induce vomiting.

SUMMARY

Shock is a multifaceted, potentially fatal condition with many possible origins. It is encountered in all age groups and many situations. Prehospital providers can have a direct and lasting impact on the morbidity and mortality of their victims. Factors that have the potential for greatest impact on patient survival include early recognition, early and aggressive airway management, and rapid transport to the appropriate facility.

REFERENCES

1. **American College of Surgeons, Committee on Trauma, Shock:** Advanced Trauma Life Support Course for Physicians Instructor Manual, ed 5, 77-94, 1993.

2. **Guyton AC:** Human Physiology and Mechanisms of Disease, ed 5, Philadelphia, 1992, WB Saunders.

3. **McCaffree DR:** Shock: How to recognize its early stages and what to do about it. *Res Staff Phys,* 27-34, Jan 1980.

4. **McCance KL, Huether SE (ed):** Pathophysiology: the biologic basis for disease in adults and children, St. Louis, 1990, CV Mosby.

5. **Perry AG, Potter PA (ed): Shock:** Comprehensive nursing management, St. Louis, 1983, CV Mosby.

6. **Oreskovich MR, Howard JD, Copass MK,** *et al:* Geriatric trauma: injury patterns and outcome. *J Trauma,* 24:565-572, 1984.

David J. Barillo, MD

Chapter 10

Infection Control

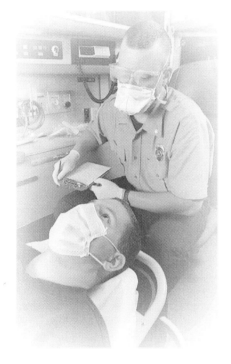

A paramedic should be able to:

OBJECTIVES

1. Define the following terms: antibody, antigen, carrier, host, host resistance, incubation period, microorganism, pathogen, seroconversion, virulence, window phase.
2. Differentiate between a communicable disease and an infectious disease.
3. Differentiate between direct and indirect transmission of a communicable disease.
4. Describe the hazards to paramedics posed by communicable diseases.
5. List common signs and symptoms, high-risk groups, mode(s) of transmission, and precautions specific for tuberculosis, hepatitis B, and acquired immunodeficiency syndrome.
6. Describe Universal Precautions and Body Substance Isolation as they apply to prehospital use.
7. Define legal issues related to treatment or transport of patients with a communicable disease.
8. Identify the precautions that prehospital personnel should take to protect themselves from communicable diseases.
9. Describe the goal, proper selection, use and disposal of personal protective equipment.

KEY TERMS

1. **Antibody**—a protein produced by the body to provide immunity against a specific antigen, pathogen, or other foreign substance. Antibodies can be measured in the blood, and the presence of antibodies indicates previous exposure to a disease. *See also*: seroconversion.
2. **Antigen**—a substance or pathogen that the body recognizes as foreign, causing activation of the immune system.
3. **Body substance isolation (BSI)**—a concept that considers all body fluids and tissues potentially infectious. Applies to bloodborne, foodborne (enteric), and airborne pathogens.
4. **Communicable disease (contagious disease)**—any disease that can be spread from person to person.
5. **Exposure**—contact with blood, body fluids, tissues or airborne droplets through direct or indirect means.
6. **Host**—a person or animal capable of supporting or harboring another organism.
7. **Immune system**—a system that protects the body against pathogens and other foreign bodies.
8. **Incubation period**—the time interval between exposure to a disease and the development of symptoms.
9. **Pathogen**—a microorganism capable of causing disease in a suitable host.
10. **Personal protective equipment**—the equipment used to protect the provider from communicable diseases (e.g., masks, gloves, particulate respirators).
11. **Virulence**—the relative strength of a pathogen; its ability to produce disease.

n 1847, an obstetrician named Semmelweis noticed that the death rate from infection was four times higher when his patients were treated by medical students. Investigation revealed that the students were dissecting human bodies in the anatomy lab and then providing patient care in the hospital without washing their hands.[34] This discovery established the field of infection control and the importance of hand washing to prevent the spread of disease. Rubber gloves were introduced into medical practice in 1890 by a surgeon named William Halstead.[3] The purpose of his inventions was originally to protect the hands of his scrub nurse from the irritation of disinfectants.

Infection control practices were never popular with health care workers, and they fell into general disuse with the discovery of antibiotics. These practices were "reinvented" when antibiotic-resistant bacteria evolved, and the practices have seen more use recently in protecting health care workers from Human Immunodeficiency Virus (HIV) and hepatitis B (HBV) infection.

The occupational hazard of bloodborne pathogens was recognized in the 1980s, resulting in federal legislation developed by the Occupational Safety and Health Administration (OSHA) to protect health care workers, including paramedics and EMTs.[27,28,29]

Historically, infection control techniques were intended for hospital use. The prehospital environment is less predictable and less controlled, and hospital infection control practices are often inadequate or impractical in the field. For these reasons, infection control guidelines specific for emergency responders have been developed. These include a curriculum guide for public safety and emergency response workers, developed by the Centers for Disease Control and Prevention;[16] a standard on infection control written by the National Fire Protection Association;[13] a course offered by the National Fire Academy;[11] and a guide to developing and managing an emergency service infection control program provided by the United States Fire Administration.[21] Although these guidelines are useful, it is important to realize that both the knowledge base and the regulations that govern prehospital infection control are rapidly changing. Refresher training courses are essential to keep up with the latest information and techniques.

The chances of developing a communicable disease following an occupational exposure are small but real. The risks of communicable disease exposure can be further decreased by proper training and the appropriate use of personal protective equipment (PPE).

Infection Control Terms and Concepts

A host is a person or animal capable of supporting or harboring another organism. A microorganism is a life form such as a bacteria, virus, fungus, or parasite that is too small to be seen with the unaided eye. A pathogen is a microorganism that can cause disease in a suitable host. The term etiologic agent refers to a category of hazardous materials containing microorganisms capable of causing human disease.[7] Infection is the growth of an organism in a host, with or without detectable signs of illness.[11] An infectious disease is any disease caused by a pathogen or etiologic agent. A communicable or contagious disease is any disease that can be spread from person to person. Note that the terms *infectious disease* and

communicable disease are not the same. For example, toxic shock syndrome is an infectious disease because it is caused by a bacteria. It is not, however, a communicable disease, because it cannot be transmitted from person to person. The primary concern in emergency response is protection from communicable diseases.

Communicable diseases are classified as airborne, bloodborne, foodborne, or sexually transmitted, depending on the normal method of transmission. Airborne communicable diseases include chickenpox, measles, mumps, rubella, and tuberculosis and are spread by droplets produced by coughing or sneezing. Bloodborne communicable diseases such as HBV, hepatitis C (HCV), or HIV are spread by contact with blood or body fluids that contain disease pathogens. Foodborne diseases such as salmonella, hepatitis A, and staphylococcal food poisoning are spread by improper handling of food or by poor personal hygiene. Sexually transmitted diseases such as Chlamydia and gonorrhea usually pose little occupational hazard to prehospital responders. Several diseases such as syphilis, HBV, and HIV infection may be spread by either blood or sexual contact.

Exposure is defined as contact with infected blood, body fluids, tissues or airborne droplets through either direct (person to person) or indirect means (via a contaminated object).[11] Exposure to a communicable disease does not automatically result in infection. Infection depends on three factors: 1) the dose of the microorganism present; 2) its virulence; and 3) the host resistance.[35] The dose is the number of organisms transmitted during an exposure. The dose necessary to cause infection is different for each disease, but in general, a higher dose or longer exposure results in a greater chance of infection. Virulence is the relative strength of a pathogen, or its ability to produce disease. Highly virulent organisms can survive adverse conditions such as heat or dehydration. Weaker or less virulent organisms are often unable to survive outside of living cells. Host resistance is the ability of the exposed individual to withstand infection.[35] The incubation period is the time interval between exposure to a communicable disease and the development of symptoms (Fig. 10-1). During this

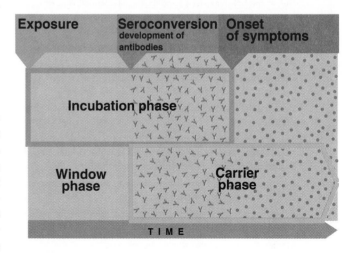

Figure 10-1

The stages of infection. Note that the exposed individual may be capable of spreading the disease prior to the onset of symptoms.

time, the disease organism is multiplying and the patient may be capable of spreading the disease. A carrier is a person who harbors a pathogen but has no current symptoms. For example, a HBV carrier may continue to have the virus present after he or she is cured of symptoms of the disease and thus can still transmit it to others.

The human body has many natural defenses against infection. The barrier protection provided by normal skin is very important; most pathogens cannot cross intact skin. The immune system provides additional protection (Fig. 10-2). It is activated by contact with an antigen, which can be a pathogen or any substance that the body recognizes as foreign. Certain white blood cells provide nonspecific immunity by attacking many antigens. Others provide specific immunity by producing proteins called antibodies to attack a specific pathogen or foreign substance. Antibodies can be measured in the blood, and the presence of antibodies indicates previous exposure to a disease. A person who develops antibodies after disease exposure is said to have seroconverted. The time between exposure to a disease and the development of measurable antibodies is termed the window phase. During the window phase, a person may have the disease and be capable of spreading it, but when tested, produce a negative reading. For this reason, a negative antibody test does not always mean that an individual is disease free.

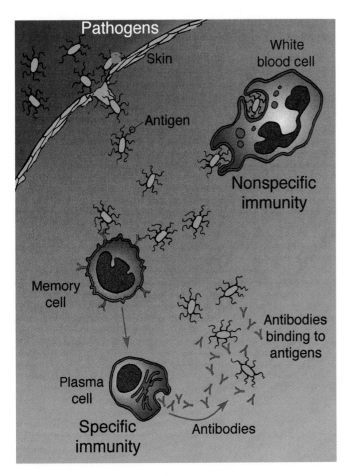

Figure 10-2

The immune system provides specific and nonspecific immunity to fight pathogens that cross the skin.

Diagnosis of Communicable Disease

Paramedics cannot be expected to make an exact diagnosis of a communicable disease because signs and symptoms are frequently subtle, nonspecific, or even absent. In addition, there is little specific therapy that can be provided in the field other than supportive care. Many patients with communicable diseases are completely asymptomatic, particularly during the window phase, incubation phase, and carrier phase. For this reason, it is safest to treat all victims' diseases as potentially communicable.

Key information about common infectious diseases, including causes, methods of transmission, incidence/target population, incubation period, availability of vaccines, and signs and symptoms, is provided in Tables 10-1, 10-2, and 10-3. Hepatitis, tuberculosis, and HIV infection pose the greatest risks to paramedics.

Hepatitis

Hepatitis, or inflammation of the liver, may be caused by toxic chemicals or by a variety of different viruses. Viral hepatitis is communicable, and chemical hepatitis, such as alcoholic hepatitis, is not. Hepatitis A, B, C, D, and E are viral diseases caused by known pathogens. In addition, there are several unidentified viruses that cause foodborne or bloodborne hepatitis; collectively, these are known as Hepatitis Non-A, Non-B (NANB). Hepatitis A (HAV, infectious hepatitis) and hepatitis E are foodborne, or enteric, illnesses and usually pose little risk for prehospital responders. Hepatitis D (HDV, delta hepatitis) is a viral illness that occurs only in victims with current or previous HBV infection.

Hepatitis B (HBV, serum hepatitis) is the major occupational bloodborne pathogen risk to paramedics. There are an estimated 300,000 new cases of HBV infection each year in the United States.[17] More than 50% of these cases demonstrate either minimal symptoms or none at all.[9] An additional 1 million victims are asymptomatic HBV carriers capable of spreading the disease[17] Between 5% and 10% of acute HBV victims[9] and up to 25% of HBV carriers[17] develop chronic hepatitis, which may result in long-term disability, cirrhosis, or liver cancer. Approximately 250 health care workers, including paramedics, die each year as a result of occupationally acquired HBV infection.[18]

Hepatitis B can spread by contact with infected blood or body fluids through open skin or mucous membranes, or by sexual contact. A needlestick exposure from a HBV infected patient will transmit the disease between 6% and 43% of the time, depending on the stage and serologic status of the source patient.[6,11,14] A vaccine is available to protect against HBV infection. Present OSHA regulations mandate that HBV vaccine be made available at no cost to health care workers, including paramedics, EMTs, and firefighters. Vaccination should be complete before assignment to patient care responsibilities. In jurisdictions not covered by OSHA, paramedics and EMTs should insist on this protection from their employer or volunteer organization.

Hepatitis C virus is another health risk for paramedics.

TABLE 10-1   Human Immunodeficiency Disease[1,2,8]

Disease	Cause	Method of Transmission	Incidence*/ Target Population	Incubation Period	Vaccine Available?	Signs and Symptoms
All	HIV 1 or HIV 2 viruses	Bloodborne and sexual	Homosexual/bisexual men, IV drug users, hemophiliacs prostitutes, heterosexual contacts		No	
Acute syndrome (note: most patients do not develop acute syndrome)				2–4 weeks		Fever, rash, muscle pain, "flu-like" symptoms, transient lymphadenopathy
Asymptomatic carrier			Present estimates: up to 7.5 million in US			No symptoms
Persistent Generalized Adenopathy						Lymphadenopathy > 1cm in at least 2 extra-inguinal sites for at least 3 months
Acquired Immunodeficiency Syndrome			Estimates: 1991 approximately 45,500 cases reported 1992 approximately 47,000 cases reported 1993 estimate: 47,000–85,000 new cases 1994 estimate: 43,000–93,000 new cases			Fatigue, lymphadenopathy, weight loss, opportunistic infections and cancers

NOTE: IN 1993 THE CDC EXPANDED THE DEFINITION OF AIDS TO INCLUDE DECREASED CD4+t LYMPHOCYTE COUNTS (WHITE BLOOD CELLS AFFECTED BY HIV). THIS WILL RAISE THE APPARENT NUMBER OF INDIVIDUALS MEETING THE CDC DEFINITION OF AIDS INFECTION.
*Incidence figures are the number of cases reported to the CDC annually. The reported number of cases usually underestimates the actual number of cases.
Copyright David J. Barillo, MD

This virus was first identified in 1989 and a lab test to determine infection was developed and released for screening in late 1990. Prior to this, many cases of transfusion-associated hepatitis caused by HCV were labeled as Non-A-non-B hepatitis. HCV is primarily spread by percutaneous (through the skin) transmission, and currently occurs most frequently among IV drug users.[1] Transfusion recipients, hemodialysis patients, and hemophiliacs are other high risk individuals. Sexual transmission of HCV is possible but uncommon.[1,6] The risk of seroconversion following a needlestick exposure from a HCV patient is unknown, but has been estimated at 2.7%.[6] The incubation period for HCV is shorter than that for HBV, and up to 75% infected individuals are asymptomatic or have minimal and nonspecific complaints including jaundice, abdominal pain, and flu-like symptoms. Despite this, patients with HCV are more likely to develop long-term complications. Chronic active hepatitis develops in 45% to 60% of cases, and cirrhosis develops in approximately 20%.[1] A vaccine is not available, and presently the best protection against HCV infection is the use of barrier protection. HBV vaccination does

TABLE 10-2   Hepatitis[1,2,8]

Disease	Cause	Method of Transmission	Incidence*/ Target Population	Incubation Period	Vaccine Available?	Signs and Symptoms
Hepatitis A (infectious)	Hepatitis A virus	Foodborne/fecal-oral	22,600 cases/year	2–6 weeks	No	Fever, jaundice, nausea, fatigue usually asymptomatic in children
Hepatitis B (serum)	Hepatitis B virus	Bloodborne/sexual	Reported: 16,470 Estimated: 300,000	42–200 days	Yes	Fever, jaundice, nausea, fatigue 55% of cases asymptomatic
Hepatitis C	Hepatitis C virus	Bloodborne, rarely sexual	Approximately 5% of all types of hepatitis. Most cases are intravenous drug users	Up to 6 months	No	Fever, jaundice, nausea, fatigue most are asymptomatic 45%–60% develop chronic hepatitis
Hepatitis D	Delta agent (virus)	Bloodborne	Present/past HBV infection	6–12 weeks	No	Only affects current or previous hepatitis B victims
Hepatitis E	Hepatitis E virus	Foodborne/fecal-oral		Average = 40 days	No	Fever, jaundice, nausea, fatigue
Non A-Non B Hepatitis (NANB)	Unknown viruses (several)	Bloodborne and foodborne/ fecal-oral	Unknown	2–26 weeks	No	Fever, jaundice, nausea, fatigue

NOTES:* Incidence figures are the number of cases reported to the Centers for Disease Control annually. The reported number of cases usually underestimates the actual number of cases.
Copyright David J. Barillo, MD

TABLE 10-3 Other Communicable Diseases

Disease	Cause	Method of Transmission	Incidence*/ Target Population	Incubation Period	Vaccine Available?	Signs and Symptoms
Chickenpox	Varicella-Zoster	Airborne/respiratory secretions childhood disease	Very common	14–21 days	Pending FDA approval	Fever, rash
Diphtheria	Corynebacterium bacteria	Airborne/respiratory secretions	Very rare: 2 cases/year	1–4 days	Yes	Fever, sore throat, cardiac/neurologic damage possible
Gonorrhea	Neisseria gonorrhoeae bacteria	Sexual	Sexually active individuals	2–7 days	No	Male—pain on urination, urethral discharge Female—abdominal pain or asymptomatic
Herpes Simplex (whitlow)	Herpes simplex virus	Contact with respiratory secretions	Dentists, respiratory therapists	2–20 days	No	Skin lesion on fingertips
(fever sores)	Herpes simplex virus	From previous exposure, triggered by sun, stress, etc.	General population	N/A	No	Blisters on lips or mucous membranes
Herpes Zoster	Varicella-zoster (chickenpox) virus	Dormant virus from previous chickenpox triggered by stress	Past chickenpox infection	N/A	No	Painful skin blisters in lines or groups
Herpes Type II (genital)	Herpes Simplex type II	Sexual		4–7 days	No	Painful genital lesions
Measles (rubeola, red or 8-day measles)	Paramyxovirus	Airborne, respiratory secretions	10,000 cases/year	8–13 days	Yes	Fever, conjunctivitis, red blotchy rash, white spots in mouth
Meningitis Bacterial	Neisseria meningitidis, homophilus influenza	Airborne, respiratory secretions	2000 cases/year	2–10 days	No	Fever, headache, stiff neck, nausea, rash on lower trunk
Aseptic (viral)	Several viruses	Oral-fecal	14,000 cases/year	Variable	No	Same: less serious infection
Mononucleosis	Epstein-Barr virus	Airborne, respiratory secretions	Young adults	10–50 days	No	Fatigue, headache, sore throat, lymphadenopathy, splenomegaly
Mumps	Paramyxovirus	Airborne, respiratory secretions	4000 cases/year	12–26 days	Yes	Children—fever, swelling of parotid glands Adults—testicle swelling; infection may cause sterility or deafness
Pertussis (Whooping cough)	Bordetella pertussis bacteria	Airborne, respiratory secretions	2500–4000 cases/year mostly young children	10–16 days	Yes	Severe coughing with "whoop" sound on inspiration, sneezing, fatigue
Rubella or German Measles	Virus	Airborne, respiratory secretions	1400 cases/year	14–21 days	Yes	Children—mild illness with rash, fever Pregnant women—possible birth defects
Syphilis	Treponema pallidum bacteria	Sexual, rarely bloodborne	48,000 cases/year	3 weeks	No	Primary genital lesion Secondary—hand/foot rash adenopathy Tertiary—nerve or cardiac damage
Tuberculosis	Mycobacterium tuberculosis	Airborne, respiratory secretions	26,000 cases/year	4–12 weeks	No	Fever, cough, night sweats, weight loss

NOTES:* Incidence figures are the number of cases reported to the Centers for Disease Control annually. The reported number of cases usually underestimates the actual number of cases.
Copyright David J. Barillo, MD

not protect against HCV or other forms of hepatitis. Recent availability of a screening test for HCV in blood products has lowered the risk of acquiring HCV from transfusion.

Tuberculosis

Tuberculosis (TB) is an airborne transmissible disease caused by the bacteria *Mycobacterium tuberculosis*. TB is normally a pulmonary disease, but can also infect lymph nodes, vertebrae, kidneys, and other organs. TB causes an estimated 1 million deaths annually worldwide.[36] The incidence of TB in developed countries has dramatically decreased during this century, but it has started to increase again as a result of the increase in HIV infection. OSHA has released interim guidelines to protect health care workers from tuberculosis, based on the Centers for Disease Control and Prevention recommendations.[19,20,30,37] Further regulatory action is anticipated.

Pulmonary TB may be asymptomatic or may produce symptoms of cough, weakness, weight loss, and fever with night sweats. TB may become inactive as the lung lesions are sealed off by scar tissue, but these lesions may retain live bacteria for many years. Immunosuppression caused by drugs (steroids or cancer chemotherapy), HIV infection, or other factors that weaken the body may allow recurrence of inactive TB. People at high risk for TB include HIV victims, alcoholics, immigrants from countries with a high prevalence of TB, nursing home or institutionalized patients, and indigent elderly men in urban settings who have a reactivation of childhood-acquired infection. TB is not highly contagious, and transmission usually occurs between household contacts under crowded and poorly ventilated living conditions. Droplets produced by coughing or sneezing are the principal method of spread. Resistant TB strains are appearing in urban areas as a result of patients that discontinue treatment prematurely. At least 16 health care workers are known to have developed multidrug-resistant TB, and at least five health care workers have died from this disease since 1988.[30]

A positive TB skin test (Mantoux or tuberculin test) indicates previous TB exposure and remains positive for many years. A seroconversion following TB exposure indicates recent infection and requires medical evaluation.

The Centers for Disease Control and Prevention guidelines for TB protection include the use of high-efficiency particulate air (HEPA) respirators (also known as particulate respirators or PRs) in certain situations. These include the transport, in a closed vehicle, of a patient with known or suspected TB.[20,30] The commercial availability of disposable respirators meeting this requirement is presently limited. When respirators are used in the workplace, OSHA also requires the establishment of a respiratory protection program, including pulmonary function testing.[30,31]

Paramedics transporting a patient with a known or suspected case of TB should place a surgical mask (not a particulate respirator) on the patient if medically feasible (Fig. 10-3). In addition, the paramedics should wear particulate respirators.[20] The windows should be kept open if possible, and the heating or cooling system operated in a non recycling mode[20] (see Sidebar 1).

HIV Infection

Human Immunodeficiency Viruses type 1 and 2 (HIV-1 and HIV-2) cause a spectrum of disease ranging from an asymptomatic carrier state to the Acquired Immunodeficiency Syndrome (AIDS). Individuals with AIDS have a compromised immune system and consequently are unable to fight off disease. Most HIV infection in the United States is due to the HIV-1 strain, although HIV-2 infection, already common in Africa, is on the increase. Tests for HIV-1 usually do not detect HIV-2.[10]

HIV infection can be either bloodborne or sexually transmitted. Initially reported in homosexual men and IV drug users, HIV infection is also spread by transfusion of contaminated blood products and through heterosexual intercourse. Blood products have been screened for HIV-1 since 1985, reducing the risk from this source. HIV infection occurs in all areas of the country and in all economic and ethnic groups; for this reason, the term high-risk behavior is preferable to high-risk group in determining infection potential. HIV is not trans-

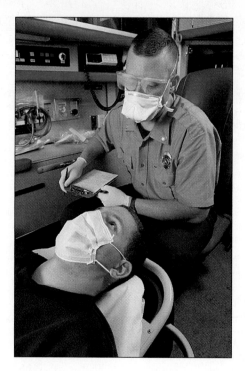

Figure 10-3

To protect the EMS team, patients with airborne infections, like tuberculosis, should be treated and transported while wearing respiratory protections specifically designed to minimize the risk of exposure.

mitted through casual contact, and nonsexual household contacts usually have no detectable evidence of HIV infection (remain seronegative) even after years of cohabitation.[14]

The vast majority of HIV-infected individuals are asymptomatic. Others may display a transient flu-like illness with joint pain, fever, and skin rash occurring several weeks after exposure. Individuals generally seroconvert after this illness. Seroconversion may also occur in the absence of the acute viral illness, usually 6 to 8 weeks following exposure, but occasionally up to 3 years later.[4] Individuals may remain asymptomatic, or may progress to a persistent generalized lymphadenopathy state or to AIDS. It is presently not known why some seropositive individuals remain healthy and others develop AIDS. Once AIDS does develop, the victims usually die of opportunistic infections or cancer such as Kaposi's sarcoma (Fig. 10-4). Opportunistic infections are caused by pathogens that a healthy immune system can usually defeat. Ninety-five percent of AIDS victims die within 4 years of onset of the disease.[9]

The risk of developing HIV infection from a needlestick exposure is estimated at 0.3% to 0.5%, or between 1/200 and 1/330.[4,14,21] This is considerably lower than the risk of HBV from a needlestick exposure (6% to 43%). The higher infection rate from hepatitis exposure is explained by a higher concentration of viral particles in blood. HIV patients typically have 10,000 virus particles per cubic centimeter of blood, while HBV patients may have 10,000,000,000,000 particles.[4]

In the field, it is not possible to predict HIV risks by the presence or absence of high-risk behaviors, or on a social, economic, or ethnic basis. The use of universal precautions or body substance isolation for all victims is the safest course.

- A written TB infection control plan should be developed and revised on a regular basis by the agency responsible for prehospital medical care (hospital, fire department, EMS system, or private employer). Protocols should address the identification and management of patients who may have active TB.
- A risk assessment of the potential for TB exposure should be performed annually.
- EMS personnel should receive appropriate TB training, education, and screening. Postexposure follow-up should be available.
- If risk assessment determines that exposure to TB patients is possible, EMS personnel should be issued appropriate respiratory protection. A respiratory protection program is required by OSHA when respirators are used. Respirators must meet criteria established by theNational Institute of Occupational Safety and Health.
- EMS personnel should have tuberculin testing performed at appropriate intervals (3 months, 6 months, or 1 year) as determined by TB risk assessment. Tuberculin testing should also be performed after unprotected exposure to a patient

with known active TB. Testing is not necessary after exposures where appropriate personal protective equipment was used.
- During transport of a patient with known or active TB:
  -A surgical mask should be placed over the patient's nose and mouth, if medically feasible. The patient should not wear a HEPA respirator with exhalation valve, as this type of mask does not restrict the outflow of TB bacteria.
  -EMS personnel should wear respiratory protection.
  -If possible, the windows of the vehicle should be kept open.
  -The heating and air-conditioning system should be set on a nonrecirculating cycle.
- Under the Ryan White Act, EMS responders must be notified of exposure to patients with infectious pulmonary TB by the medical facility receiving the patient.

From Guidelines for Preventing the Transmission of Mycobacterium Tuberculosis in Health-Care Facilities. *Morb Mort Wkly Rep,* 43:RR–13 October 28, 1994.

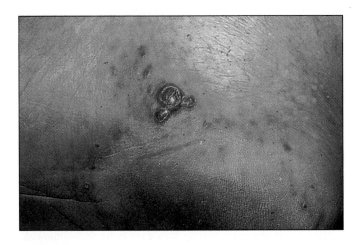

Figure 10-4

Kaposi's sarcoma, a form of skin cancer that is normally treatable, has devastating results for a person who is immunocompromised with AIDS. *From Thibodeau: Structure and Function of the Body, ed 9, St. Louis, 1992, Mosby–Year Book.*

Universal Precautions and Body Substance Isolation

The concept of universal precautions originated as universal blood and body fluid precautions,[5] a hospital system used when a patient had a known or suspected bloodborne disease. Because of the hazards posed by asymptomatic but infected individuals, the Centers for Disease Control and Prevention (CDCP) extended these precautions to all patients in 1987.[22] Universal precautions initially applied only to blood and body fluids containing visible blood, but were expanded in 1988 to include vaginal, seminal, cerebrospinal, synovial, pleural, pericardial, peritoneal, and amniotic fluids, and human tissue.[23] Universal precautions do not apply to tears, nasal secretions, sputum, vomitus, urine, feces, or sweat unless the fluid is contaminated with visible blood or circumstances exist "where it is difficult or impossible to differentiate between body fluids".[27] Most rescue situations fit into the latter category.

Body substance isolation (BSI) is a concept that considers all body fluids and tissues to be potentially infectious. While universal precautions applies to bloodborne pathogens, BSI also provides protection against enteric (foodborne) and airborne pathogens. For this reason, BSI is the preferred protection method for paramedics. OSHA recognizes BSI as an acceptable alternative to universal precautions.[27] Regardless of the name, in the field it is safest to assume that any body tissue or fluid is potentially infectious. Appropriate barrier protection should always be used as well.

Infection Control Legislation

Legislation at the federal, state, and local levels affects prehospital infection control practices, particularly the storage and disposal of infectious or biohazardous waste. This chapter discusses concerns of a global nature and is not intended to provide legal advice or to discuss regulations specific to each jurisdiction. EMS services require local advice.

Refusal to Treat or Transport

Media attention to the HIV epidemic has generated fear of infection among emergency response personnel, and some have developed nonresponse policies for victims with known or suspected communicable diseases. Others have refused to provide on-scene care or transportation to victims exhibiting HIV high-risk behaviors. Such policies are medically unjustified.

An expert panel of medical, legal, EMS, and fire personnel convened by the US Fire Administration in 1988 found that "there is no legal, medical or ethical justification for health care workers to refuse treatment to patients with a proven (confirmed or diagnosed) or perceived existence of communicable disease."[33] Refusal to care for such victims raises issues of patient abandonment and civil rights violations. In addition, the Americans with Disabilities Act (ADA) specifically classifies both HIV infection and TB as disabilities. Failure to provide care for such individuals may constitute discrimination against the disabled.

The Ryan White Act

Subtitle B of the Ryan White Comprehensive AIDS Resources Emergency Act of 1990 is intended to protect prehospital personnel from communicable diseases. The Act allows prehospital responders to determine if they have been exposed to an infectious disease while providing patient care and requires the appointment of a Designated Officer by each employer of emergency response personnel to coordinate communication between hospitals and the emergency organization.

Communicable disease exposure notification may be routine or by request. Under routine notification, a hospital is automatically required to notify the Designated Officer if transportation was provided to a victim with an airborne transmissible disease, including those that die en route or shortly after hospital arrival. Notification must be made within 48 hours of disease determination. Routine notification applies only to airborne transmissible diseases, and only to transport crews. Paramedics and others who provide on-scene care but not transportation, and those exposed to bloodborne diseases, may obtain similar information by request. A notification by request is initiated through the Designated Officer, who reviews and forwards the request to the hospital if disease transmission was possible. If the hospital determines that an expo-

sure took place, the Designated Officer is notified of any infectious disease diagnosis. The local Public Health Officer has the authority to intervene if disagreement exists or if there is insufficient information to determine an exposure hazard (see sidebar).

The Ryan White Act does not mandate HBV or HIV testing if the source patient refuses to give consent.

The OSHA Bloodborne Pathogen Standard

The Department of Labor, OSHA is the branch of federal government responsible for safety in the workplace. Federal law requires all states to follow federal OSHA regulations or develop their own OSHA plans that are at least as stringent. Employees of state or local governments, including paramedics and firefighters, are not covered by federal OSHA regulations, but are usually covered by state regulations where such plans exist. Paramedics employed by private hospitals or organizations are subject to federal OSHA regulations. Volunteer organizations may or may not be subject to OSHA regulation; local legal consultation is advised on this subject.

The OSHA bloodborne pathogen standard requires that employers provide training, personal protective equipment, HBV vaccine, and postexposure medical care to employees occupationally exposed to blood or other potentially infectious materials.[27,29]

Each employer must develop a written exposure control plan to eliminate or minimize bloodborne pathogen exposure through the use of engineering and work practice controls. The plan must be accessible to employees, be revised at least annually, and include detailed SOPs for the use, disposal, and decontamination of all patient care equipment.[27] A Guide to Developing and Managing an Emergency Service Infection Control Program is available from the US Fire Administration, Emmitsburg, Maryland, to assist paramedic services in the development of an exposure control plan.

HBV vaccination must be made available to all employees with occupational blood or body fluid exposure, and medical evaluation and prophylaxis must be made available to all employees who have had an exposure incident. These services must be provided at no cost to the employee and at a reasonable time and place.[27] Employees may refuse vaccination, and may later request vaccination after initially declining.

The employer is responsible for the availability, accessibility, cleaning, laundering, repair, replacement, and disposal of infection control personal protective equipment (PPE). This includes resuscitation bags, pocket masks or other ventilation devices (Fig. 10-5).[27] PPE must be made available at no cost to the employee.

Infection control training must be provided at the time of initial employment and at least annually thereafter. It must occur during normal working hours and at no cost to the employee. Training must include information on the epidemiology, symptoms, and methods of transmission of bloodborne pathogens; the exposure control plan and postexposure follow-up system in use; the availability and proper use of PPE; the risks and benefits of HBV vaccine; and the provision of a personal copy of the OSHA bloodborne pathogen standard for each employee.

by Captain Forrest Dalton Sr.

Every health care organization must have standards for the prevention of transmission of bloodborne and airborne pathogens, as well as other infectious diseases, during work-related activities. These standards exist in the form of protocols, standard operating procedures (SOP) and policies that provide for comprehensive occupational safety and health programs geared toward minimizing the risk of infectious exposures.

If infection control protocols and policies are written but not implemented or managed, the potential exists for long-term or even fatal consequences to patients, responders, or their families. Even when protocols, SOPs, and policies are used properly, unexpected circumstances can always occur. There is an additional burden on those who oversee infectious disease policy and procedure. Rapid changes in laws, discovery of new infectious agents, information updates regarding known infectious agents, and improvements in immunizations demand that policy and procedure be flexible and adaptable to the workplace. Health care workers must be informed of these constant changes. Thus, the need arises for an Infectious Disease Control Officer (IDCO), sometimes referred to as a Designated Officer or DO.

It is the function and responsibility of the IDCO to keep up with the changes. Every health care organization must have an IDCO, to whom every member of the organization has direct, immediate, and confidential access. Depending on the size of the organization, assistant IDCOs may be necessary to ensure 24-hour access by employees.

An IDCO should have a background in health care, with prehospital experience if possible. This person must be educated on infection control standards, laws, regulations, infectious diseases, epidemiology, modes of transmission, and prevention of diseases. The ICDO is responsible for development and implementation of regular infection control training programs. These should include, but not be limited to proper use of personal protective equipment, SOPs for safe work practices regarding infection control, proper methods of disposal of contaminated articles and medical waste, and exposure management, including all necessary medical follow-up. The IDCO must attend conferences and seminars and have access to periodicals to stay abreast of all advances.

To address unusual situations or answer uncommon questions about infection control, an IDCO must also have access to an individual or organization that deals routinely with infection control matters, such as an infection control practitioner at a local medical facility, the CDC (Centers for Disease Control and Prevention), OSHA (Occupational Safety and Health Administration), NFPA (National Fire Protection Association) or NAPSICO (National Association of Public Safety Infection Control Officers).

Because the IDCO functions as an advocate for responders and a liaison between the EMS service and medical community, the IDCO must maintain communication among employees, management, appropriate city officials, involved hospitals, responding departments, and any other entity that will interact in the implementation of infection control policies and procedures.

Because of the 48-hour time frame from notification to beginning postexposure management, the IDCO should be notified immediately of any exposure in the field. The IDCO is responsible for directing the exposed person in the appropriate policies and procedures. The IDCO investigates the incident to determine if proper infection control measures were implemented, if a problem in policy or procedure exists or if there is an equipment, education, or training need. The IDCO also ensures provision of appropriate medical follow-up, completion of necessary documentation, and other appropriate actions were taken.

To properly perform these duties, the IDCO must have enough authority in the organization to accomplish needed tasks without interference or unnecessary delay. If the IDCO has assistants, it is the IDCO's responsibility to keep the assistants informed of laws, education, training, and any changes dealing with infection control.

The IDCO must work closely with the organization's medical director or physician adviser. It may be necessary to counsel a health care worker who develops any limitation because of an infectious exposure, and who in the course of normal duties, would not be able to follow infectious control policy and procedure or would present a risk to coworkers or patients. In addition, the IDCO works with the physician to maintain immunization status of employees, ensure all medical follow-up is completed, and necessary prophylaxis is provided.

REFERENCES

1. IAFF: Infectious Diseases and the Fire and Emergency Services, Washington, 1992, Department of Occupational Health and Safety, International Association of Fire Fighters.

2. NFPA 1500 Standard on Fire Department Occupational Safety and Health Program, Quincy, 1992 National Fire Protection Association.

3. Omaha Fire Department: Standard Operating Procedures: Communicable Disease Infectious Control Police, vol IV, EMS 1.1 Omaha, 1993.

4. Zimmerman L, Neuman M, Jurewicz D: Infection Control for Prehospital Care Providers, ed 2, Grand Rapids, 1993, Mercy Ambulance.

5. West KH: Infectious Disease Handbook for Emergency Care Personnel, ed 2, Cincinnati, 1994, American Conference of Governmental Industrial Hygienists.

Infection Reduction and Prevention

Although emergency response can not be made completely risk free, it is possible to minimize the risk of communicable disease by following some common-sense guidelines. Treat all victims as potentially infectious, always use appropriate PPE when providing medical care, and always wash hands after contact with the victim.

Proper infection control practices begin before the call comes in. All responders should be in a state of good health and have any necessary immunizations completed before being assigned to emergency response duties. The availability of HBV vaccination is an OSHA requirement, but paramedics should also be immunized against tetanus, diphtheria, measles, mumps, rubella, and polio. Mantoux skin testing for TB is required at the time of initial employment and then an-

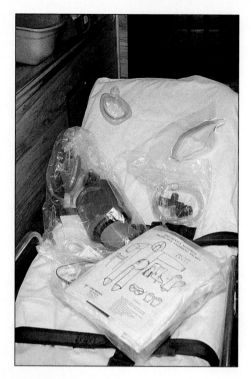

Figure 10-5

Personal protective equipment (PPE) is designed to protect EMS providers and patients from exposure to diseases from a variety of direct or indirect sources.

nually thereafter. Health care workers frequently exposed to TB infection should be retested every 3 to 6 months.[37] Present regulations do not require annual chest radiographs in tuberculin-negative, asymptomatic health care workers.[20,37]

The department or emergency response organization should have a work restriction policy for infection control purposes. A paramedic with a communicable disease should not provide patient care when acutely ill. Work restrictions might also be instituted for a member with dermatitis or large, open-skin lesions.[11,13] Smaller cuts, scratches, or breaks in the skin should be covered with an impervious dressing before a paramedic performs patient care activities.[11,13,27,32]

On-scene, it is easy but dangerous to forget infection control habits. Use the minimum number of rescuers necessary to safely complete each task, keep non involved personnel out of the area where communicable disease exposure is possible, and use appropriate PPE. PPE is appropriate when it prevents body fluids from contacting work or street clothes, undergarments, skin, eyes, mouth or other mucous membranes.[27] There is no universal PPE to cover all situations, and disease-specific PPE is impractical because most communicable diseases cannot be diagnosed in the field. Instead, PPE selection should be based on the potential for disease transmission. Some situations may require PPE for both bloodborne and TB protection. For example, if a patient is coughing, regardless of the diagnosis, a safe maneuver is to place a mask on the patient, and to wear a particulate respirator while providing patient care. A stabbing victim may splash others with blood; in this situation, barrier protection covering the mouth, eyes, hands, and clothing would be appropriate. Recommendations

for the selection of PPE based upon Centers for Disease Control and Prevention and US Fire Administration guidelines are listed in Table 10-4. These recommendations are further simplified in Box 10-1. The goal of PPE selection should be to prevent any contact between the body fluids of the victim and the skin or mucus membranes of the paramedic.[9]

Wearing disposable medical gloves under structural firefighting gloves is controversial. This practice is recommended for any situation in which sharp edges may puncture medical gloves, such as vehicle extrication, but may be hazardous for structural firefighting activities. A second controversy is the appropriate use of gowns in the field. Gowns are intended as barrier protection to cover clothing, but may be hazardous to the wearer during firefighting or extrication procedures. Structural firefighting gear also provides barrier protection, and should be used instead of gowns in these situations. Gowns may be useful in activities such as emergency childbirth where exposure to flame or sharp objects is not anticipated.[11]

Facial protection should consist of a full face shield, or protective eyewear and a protective mask over the mouth and nose (Fig. 10-6). Whenever possible, use disposable patient care equipment, especially for respiratory care. Choices for cardiopulmonary resuscitation (CPR) airway equipment include demand-valve resuscitators with disposable face masks, disposable bag-valve-masks, and face (pocket) masks with one-way valves. Mouth-to-mouth resuscitation should be avoided unless absolutely necessary; to prevent this possibility, prehospital providers should carry personal pocket masks.

Work uniforms contaminated with body fluids should be changed when the run is completed. Clean work clothes should always be available. If clothing is extensively contaminated, the paramedic should shower before returning to duty. Hands should be washed immediately after removing PPE and after completing patient care activities. Waterless hand washes can be used initially at the scene, followed by a complete hand washing with soap and water at the conclusion of the run.

BOX 10-1	**Simplified Field Selection of Personal Protective Equipment**

1. If it's wet, it's infectious—use gloves.

2. If it could splash in your face, wear a full face shield or eye protection and a face mask.

3. If it could splash on your clothes, wear a gown or structural firefighting gear.

4. If the patient has a cough, place a surgical mask on the patient and a particulate respirator on the crew.

5. Proper planning avoids the need for mouth-to-mouth resuscitation. Use disposable airway equipment and carry a pocket mask.

6. When in doubt, use too much, rather than too little, PPE.

7. Always have a change of clothing available.

Modified from: National Fire Academy Infection Control for Emergency Response Personnel: The Supervisor's role. Emmitsburg, Maryland, 1992, The National Fire Academy (#NFA-ICERP-IG).

TABLE 10-4	USFA Guidelines for Prevention of Transmission of HIV and HBV to Emergency Responders Recommended Personal Protective Equipment for Protection Against HIV and HBV Transmission[1] in Prehospital[2] Settings			
Task or activity	**Disposable gloves**	**Gown**	**Mask[3]**	**Protective eyewear[3]**
Bleeding control with spurting blood	Yes	Yes	Yes	Yes
Bleeding control with minimal bleeding	Yes	No	No	No
Emergency childbirth	Yes	Yes	Yes	Yes
Blood drawing	Yes[4]	No	No	No
Starting an intravenous (IV) line	Yes	No	No	No
Endotracheal intubation, esophageal obturator use	Yes	No	Yes	Yes
Oral/nasal suctioning, manually cleaning airway	Yes[5]	Yes	Yes	Yes
Handling and cleaning instruments with possible microbial contamination	Yes	Yes	Yes	Yes
Measuring blood pressure	Yes	No	No	No
Giving an injection	Yes	No	No	No
Measuring temperature	Yes	No	No	No
Rescuing from a fire[6]	Yes	No	No	No
Cleaning back of an ambulance after a medical alarm[7]	Yes	No	No	No

Notes for instructor:
[1]The recommendations for PPE provided in this chart are more stringent than those provided in the CDC Guidelines. The CDC Guidelines are based on application of universal precautions; this chart is based on application of body substance isolation.
[2]Defined as a setting where delivery of emergency health care takes place away from a hospital or other health care facility.
[3]Protective face shields can serve as both mask and eyewear to protect against blood splashes.
[4]Gloves should reduce the incidence of blood contamination of hands during phlebotomy (drawing of blood samples), but they cannot prevent penetrating injuries caused by needles or other sharp instruments.
[5]While not clearly necessary to prevent HIV or HBV transmission unless blood is present, gloves are recommended to prevent transmission of other agents (e.g., Herpes simplex).
[6]To be worn under structural firefighting gloves.
[7]If other than soap and water is used, personal protective equipment recommended on the MSDS should be worn.
*Adapted from the CDC Guidelines, February 1989

Contaminated needles or other sharp objects should not be bent, removed, or recapped (Fig. 10-7). The most common preventable bloodborne pathogen exposure is a puncture injury occurring during needle recapping.[4] The nondominant index finger is the usual needlestick site. A no-recapping policy is an integral part of the department exposure control plan mandated by OSHA; needlestick injuries should alert management to the need for further infection control training. Blunt no-stick needles or needle-free IV connector systems are commercially available for the safe intermittent administration of IV medications. A disposable sharps container that meets applicable OSHA and environmental protection standards

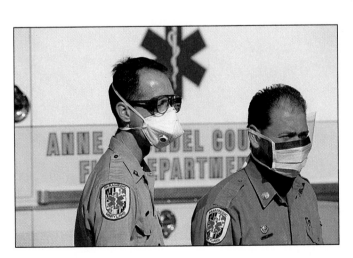

Figure 10-6

The face should be shielded from the danger of splashing blood or bodily fluids such as vomitus.

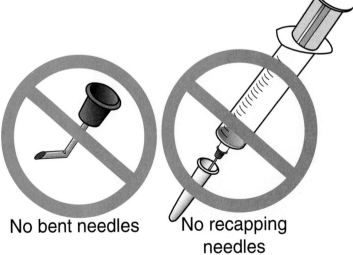

No bent needles

No recapping needles

Figure 10-7

Once used, a needle should be immediately disposed of in the appropriate container, without bending or recapping.

should always be carried along with the IV kit or drug box, and should be immediately accessible when providing emergency care (Fig. 10-8).

After the run, decontaminate patient care equipment in accordance with manufacturers' recommendations. Appropriate PPE should be used during cleaning and decontamination procedures. Usually, the first step is to wash the equipment with soap and water to remove any obvious body fluid or tissue. Disinfection is then performed with an EPA approved hospital disinfectant chemical germicide, or with a solution of chlorine bleach diluted 1:100 with water (see Box 10-2) . The material safety data sheets (MSDS) for any chemical solutions used should be readily available. (Material safety data sheets are discussed in more detail in the hazardous materials chapter.) Commercial disinfectants must be labeled as tuberculocidal. Since TB bacteria are known to be resistant to disinfection, this requirement insures that the disinfectant is also strong enough to kill other pathogens commonly seen in the field. Ambulance surfaces should likewise be washed and disinfected if contaminated with blood, body fluids, or respiratory secretions.

Certain EMS equipment may require sterilization. Other equipment may be damaged by chemical solutions. For example, chlorine bleach will destroy the fire-resistant properties of Nomex® (Aramid fiber, DuPont). The manufacturers' recommendations for cleaning and decontamination should be a part of the Exposure Control Plan.

Linen should be changed after each patient use. Contaminated linen should be placed in labeled, leakproof bags or containers, and not sorted or rinsed prior to laundering (Fig. 10-9).

BOX 10-2 — Bleach as a Germicide

"In addition to commercially available chemical germicides, a solution of sodium hypochlorite (household bleach) prepared daily is an inexpensive and effective germicide. Concentrations ranging from approximately 500 ppm (1:100 dilution of household bleach) sodium hypochlorite to 5000 ppm (1:10 dilution of household bleach) are effective depending on the amount of organic material (e.g., blood, mucus) present on the surface to be cleaned and disinfected. Commercially available chemical germicides may be more compatible with certain medical devices that might be corroded by repeated exposure to sodium hypochlorite, especially to the 1:10 dilution."

—Centers for Disease Control and Prevention, 1987[22]

"All spills of blood and blood-contaminated fluids should be promptly cleaned using an EPA-approved germicide or a 1:100 solution of household bleach . . . Visible material should first be removed."

—Centers for Disease Control and Prevention, 1989[18]

Summary: Lower (1:100) concentrations of bleach appear to be effective if initial soap and water cleaning removes most organic material. Higher concentrations (1:10) may be harmful to certain equipment.

NFPA infection control standards state that "protective clothing, station/work uniforms or other clothing shall not be taken home" for laundering.[13] According to OSHA, if a uniform is "intended to act as PPE," the employer must "provide, clean, repair, replace and/or dispose of it."[29] If a paramedic wishes to maintain his or her own uniform, then he or she must wear additional "employer handled and employer-controlled PPE" in situations where blood or body fluid contact was likely.[29] Many EMS agencies provide laundry service for uniforms or in-station washers and dryers to comply with this requirement.

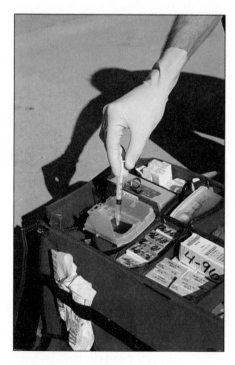

Figure 10-8

A sharps container that conforms to federal safety and infection control standards should be easily accessible.

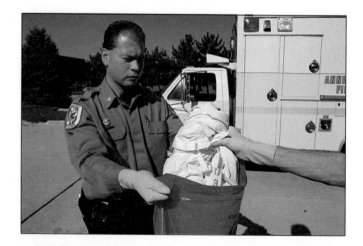

Figure 10-9

While observing proper infection control procedures, paramedics should store contaminated laundry appropriately in clearly identified containers.

SUMMARY

Communicable diseases pose health and safety hazards to pre-hospital providers. As with the other hazards inherent in emergency response, this risk can be minimized by adherence to safe operating practices and the use of PPE. Paramedics should consider all patients as potentially infectious and use appropriate barrier protection.

REFERENCES

1. Aledort LM: Consequences of chronic hepatitis C: a review article for the hematologist. *Am J Hematol* 44:29–37, 1993.

2. Berkow, R (ed): The Merck manual of diagnosis and therapy, ed 15, Rahway, 1987, Merck, Sharpe & Dohme Research Laboratories.

3. Crowe SJ: Halstead of Johns Hopkins, Springfield, 1957, Charles C. Thomas Publishers.

4. Davis JM: Acquired Immunodeficiency Syndrome. In Wilmore D, et al (ed): American College of Surgeons care of the surgical patient, vol 2, New York, 1990, Scientific American.

5. Garner JS, Simmons BP: Guideline for isolation precautions in hospitals, *Infect Control* 4:245–325, 1983.

6. Gerberding JL, Henderson DK: Management of occupational exposures to bloodborne pathogens: hepatitis B virus, hepatitis C virus, and human immunodeficiency virus, *Clin Infect Dis* 12:179–185, 1992.

7. Henry, Martin: Hazardous materials response handbook, Quincy, 1989, National Fire Protection Association.

8. Hoofnagle JH: Type D (Delta) hepatitis, *JAMA,* 261:1321–1325, 1989.

9. Howard RJ: Viral Infection. In Wilmore D, et al, (ed): American College of Surgeons care of the surgical patient, vol 2, New York, 1991, Scientific American.

10. Lucey DR: The first decade of human retroviruses: a nomenclature for the clinician, *Mil Med,* 156:555–557, 1991.

11. National Fire Academy: Infection control for emergency response personnel: the supervisor's role, Emmitsburg, 1992, The National Fire Academy (#NFA-ICERP-IG).

12. National Fire Academy: Student manual: firefighter health and safety: program implementation and management, Emmitsburg, 1988, National Fire Academy.

13. National Fire Protection Association: NFPA 1581: standard on fire department infection control program, Quincy, 1991, National Fire Protection Association.

14. Rapoza N (ed): HIV Infection and disease, Chicago, 1989, American Medical Association.

15. Smedira N, Schecter W: AIDS and the trauma care provider, *Adv Traum,* 4:67–88, 1989.

16. United States Department of Health and Human Services, Centers for Disease Control and Prevention: A curriculum guide for public safety and emergency response workers: prevention of transmission of human immunodeficiency virus and hepatitis B virus. Atlanta, 1989, Centers for Disease Control and Prevention.

17. United States Department of Health and Human Services, Centers for Disease Control and Prevention: Protection against viral hepatitis–recommendations of the immunization practices advisory committee. *Morb Mortal Wkly Rep,* 39: RR-2, 1990.

18. United States Department of Health and Human Services, Centers for Disease Control and Prevention: Guidelines for prevention of transmission of human immunodeficiency virus and hepatitis B virus to health care and public safety workers. *Morb Mortal Wkly Rep,* 38:S6, 1989.

19. United States Department of Health and Human Services, Centers for Disease Control and Prevention: Draft guidelines for preventing the transmission of tuberculosis in health care facilities, second edition: notice of comment period. Federal Register, 52810-52-854, 1993.

20. United States Department of Health and Human Services, Centers for Disease Control and Prevention: Guidelines for Preventing the Transmission of Tuberculosis in Health-Care Settings, with Special Focus on HIV-Related Issues. *Morb Mortal Wkly Rep,* 39:RR-17, 1990.

21. United States Department of Health and Human Services, Centers for Disease Control and Prevention: Recommendations for preventing transmission of human immunodeficiency virus, hepatitis B virus to patients during exposure-prone invasive procedures. *Morb Mortal Wkly Rep,* 40:RR-8, 1991.

22. United States Department of Health and Human Services, Centers for Disease Control and Prevention: Recommendations for prevention of HIV transmission in health-care settings. *Morb Mortal Wkly Rep,* 36:2S, 1987.

23. United States Department of Health and Human Services, Centers for Disease Control and Prevention: Update: universal precautions for prevention of transmission of human immunodeficiency virus, hepatitis B virus, and other bloodborne pathogens in health-care settings. *Morb Mortal Wkly Rep,* 37: 229–234, 1988.

24. United States Department of Health and Human Services, Centers for Disease Control and Prevention: Projection of the number of persons diagnosed with AIDS and the number of immunosuppressed HIV-infected patients—United States, 1992–1994. *Morb Mortal Wkly Rep,* 41:RR–18, 1992.

25. United States Department of Health and Human Services, Centers for Disease Control and Prevention: Update: Acquired Immunodeficiency Syndrome—United States, 1992. *Morb Mortal Wkly Rep,* 42:557–552, 1993.

26. United States Department of Health and Human Services, Centers for Disease Control and Prevention: 1993 Revised classification system for HIV infection and expanded surveillance case definition for AIDS among adolescents and adults. *Morb Mortal Wkly Rep,* 41:RR-17, 1–19, 1992.

27. United States Department of Labor, Occupational Safety and Health Administration: Occupational exposure to bloodborne pathogens: final rule (29 CFR Part 1910.1030) Washington, DC, 1991, Federal Register, 56:235, 1991.

28. United States Department of Labor, Occupational Safety and Health Administration: Enforcement procedures for occupational exposure to hepatitis B virus (HBV) and human immunodeficiency virus (HIV), OSHA instruction CPL 2-2.44B, 1990.

29. United States Department of Labor, Occupational Safety and Health Administration: Enforcement procedures for the occupational exposure to bloodborne pathogens standard, 29 CFR 1910.1030, OSHA Instruction CPL 2-2.44C, 1992.

30. United States Department of Labor, Occupational Safety and Health Administration: Enforcement policy and procedures for occupational exposure to tuberculosis, 1993.

31. United States Department of Labor, Occupational Safety and Health Administration: Respiratory Protection. 29 CFR part 1910.134, 1991.

32. United States Fire Administration: Guide to developing and managing an emergency service infection control program, Washington, 1992, United States Government Printing Office (FA-112).

33. United States Fire Administration. Forum on communicable diseases, Emmitsburg, 1988, United States Fire Administration.

34. Wenzel R: Handbook of hospital acquired infections, Boca Raton, 1981, CRC Press.

35. West K: Infectious disease handbook for emergency care personnel, ed 2, Cincinnati, 1994, American Conference of Governmental Industrial Hygienists.

36. Wolinsky E: Tuberculosis. In Wyngaarden JB, Smith LH (ed): Cecil Textbook of Medicine, ed 18, Philadelphia, 1988, WB Saunders.

37. United States Department of Health and Human Services, Centers for Disease Control and Prevention: Guidlines for Preventing the Transmission of Mycobacterium Tuberculosis in Health-Care Facilities. *Morb Mortal Wkly Rep,* 43:RR–13, 1994.

Mark A. Kirk, MD
S. Rutherfoord Rose, PharmD

Chapter 11

General Pharmacology

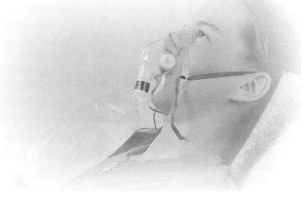

A paramedic should be able to:

1. Describe differences in generic and trade names of medications.
2. Explain the role of government agencies (FDA, DEA) and the laws that affect drug administration in prehospital care.
3. Describe how drugs are absorbed, distributed, metabolized and eliminated.
4. Discuss therapeutic effect and processes that affect absorption and distribution of drugs.
5. Define the following terms: a) receptor b) target tissue c) drug agonist d) drug antagonist e) dose response f) therapeutic window.
6. Describe how drug are related to the autonomic nervous system.
7. Define the following terms:
   A. Contraindication   E. Indication   I. Tolerance
   B. Dependence   F. Precaution   J. Toxicity
   C. Hypersensitivity   G. Side Effects
   D. Idiosyncrasy   H. Therapeutic Action
8. Describe the five "patient rights" of drug administration.
9. Identify the units of measurements and common abbreviations used in the metric system.
10. Convert units of measurement utilized in the metric system.
11. Given a dosage of medication to be administered and how it is supplied, calculate the correct amount of administer.
12. Given a patient's weight in pounds and a dosage of medication in milligrams per kilogram (mg/kg), calculate the volume of a drug to be administered.
13. Given a scenario with a macro (regular) or microdrip infusion set, calculate the IV drip rate per minute.
14. Given an amount of medication and solution for an intravenous infusion, calculate the IV drip rate per minute.
15. Describe the routes of drug administration used in prehospital care and compare their rates of absorption.
16. Describe the therapeutic action, uses, and side effects of general drug categories.
17. List specific examples of drugs in each category.

1. **Adverse drug effect**—undesirable effect of an administered drug.
2. **Contraindication**—a disease process or specific situation in which a drug should absolutely not be given.
3. **Dependence**—the total psychophysical state of a person addicted to drugs or alcohol who must receive increasing amounts of the substance to prevent the onset of craving and withdrawal symptoms.
4. **Distribution**—the process of moving a drug through the body and delivering it to various tissues.
5. **Drug absorption**—the process of a drug moving into the blood from oral, sublingual, transdermal, subcutaneous, intramuscular, or endotracheal administration.
6. **Excretion**—the process of eliminating substances by body organs or tissues, as part of a natural metabolic activity.
7. **Hypersensitivity reaction**—allergic reactions to a drug that are not related to dosage.
8. **Indication**—the specific use of a medication.
9. **Metabolism**—the process of detoxification and conversion of chemicals and drugs so that they are more easily eliminated by the kidney.
10. **Potentiation**—the enhancement of the effects of one drug by the administration of another.
11. **Precaution**—information regarding the handling of a drug that will avoid adverse drug effects.
12. **Receptor**—the basic site of drug interaction, composed of a protein that has a specific shape.
13. **Side effect**—undesirable effect that occurs with routine, therapeutic doses of a drug.
14. **Synergism**—the combined effect of two medications, which is greater than the sum of their individual effects.
15. **Target organ**—the tissue or organ ultimately affected by the drug.
16. **Therapeutic action**—the desired beneficial effect of a drug.
17. **Therapeutic window**—the margin between the level at which a drug in the body acts therapeutically, and the level at which it becomes toxic.
19. **Tolerance**—the tendency of some drugs to lose the intensity of their effect after repeated doses are given.
20. **Toxic effects**—the undesirable and potentially harmful effects from poisoning, overdose, or chronic misuse of a medication.

This chapter covers the principles of safe drug administration in the prehospital field. One of the most important goals of the paramedic is to make a difference in patient outcome, and drugs are among the most powerful tools available to meet this goal. Medications make a difference—between life and death, between long-term disability and a quick return to recovery, and between relief and prolonged suffering.

As you may have already noted, the terms "drug" and "medication" are often used interchangeably; however there is a difference in the terms. The term *drug* refers to any chemical compound that produces an effect on a living organism whereas the term *medication* refers to those drugs that are used in the practice of medicine as a remedy. The study of the action of drugs and their effect on living organisms is called *pharmacology*.

Comprehensive knowledge and understanding of the properties of life-saving medications are critical to the accurate administration of drugs. If improperly used, medications can be dangerous, or even fatal.

Drug Names

Because of the many unfamiliar names, learning pharmacology is much like learning a foreign language. Many drugs are identified by several names, which is confusing for both health care providers and patients. All drugs have a generic name, such as morphine, aspirin, or digoxin, that is unique to that particular chemical. The generic name of a drug often serves as the official name as well. The official names of drugs are listed in the United States government publication, US *Pharmacopeia*. Generic names are often an abbreviated chemical name. Trade, or brand, names are created by manufacturers to identify their specific brand of a generic drug. Drug advertisements are always labeled with copyrighted trade names emphasized for marketing purposes. Many generic drugs have several trade names if more than one manufacturer markets the drug. Examples of generic and brand names are listed in Table 11-1. To avoid confusion, it is generally best to use generic drug names. This name will be standard, regardless of the drug manufacturer. In this text, generic names are used and the trade names follow in parentheses.

TABLE 11-1	Examples of Generic and Trade Names
Generic Name	**Trade Name**
digoxin	Lanoxin
dopamine	Intropin
furosemide	Lasix
ibuprofen	Advil, Motrin, Rufen
meperidine	Demerol
nifedipine	Procardia, Adalat
procainamide	Procan SR, Pronestyl
verapamil	Calan, Isoptin

Regulation of Drugs

Natural sources of drugs include minerals, microorganisms, plants and animals. Other drugs are chemically synthesized in a laboratory. Many new drugs are developed each year. Research and development of a new drug takes years, with only one out of every 10 drugs submitted for marketing.

Testing and marketing of prescription drugs in this country is controlled by the federal Food and Drug Administration (FDA). Prior to FDA approval, drugs are tested in animals, in healthy volunteers, and in clinical studies. These tests must prove that the drug is safe and effective for use in humans. The FDA also controls the availability of drugs, either by prescription ("legend" drugs) or over-the-counter (OTC).

Throughout history, newly discovered drugs were thought to be the cure-all for human suffering until undesired effects were identified. Heroin (opioids) and cocaine were once enthusiastically supported for their medicinal benefits. Over the years, these drugs proved highly addictive and of limited medicinal benefit. Since the early 1900s, legislative acts have been passed to control such drugs. The Comprehensive Drug Abuse Prevention and Control Act (Controlled Substance Act of 1970) classified and regulated drugs based on medicinal benefits and abuse potential and placed restrictions on drugs such as narcotics, stimulants, and sedatives.

Paramedics should be familiar with the federal Drug Enforcement Agency (DEA). The DEA enforces the Controlled Substances Act. Controlled substances are divided into five schedules (I through V), depending on their potential for abuse. The use of controlled substances in an EMS system requires special documentation and accountability to verify legitimate use and to detect theft.

- Schedule I—These drugs have a high abuse potential and no accepted medical uses (e.g., heroin and LSD)
- Schedule II—These are strictly regulated because of their high abuse potential, and include such drugs as codeine, morphine, meperidine, Tylox, Percodan, and amphetamines.
- Schedules III and IV—These drugs have moderate abuse potential and include phenobarbital, diazepam (Valium), Tylenol with codeine, most prescription hypnotics (sleeping pills), and prescription anorectics (appetite suppressants).
- Schedule V—These are drugs with low abuse potential but which still contain small amounts of narcotics or other controlled substances. Examples include some cough preparations and antidiarrheal medications.

Drug Actions and Interactions

The purpose of administering a drug is to create a desired effect (therapeutic effect or pharmacologic effect) on a target organ or tissue. The target organ or tissue is the site ultimately affected by the drug. Several processes occur from the time a drug is administered until the drug produces its effect. All drugs undergo five stages: 1) entry into the body and then bloodstream (absorption); 2) movement through the blood-

by Elizabeth Criss, RN, MEd

The entire process of developing and obtaining approval for a medication is a long, expensive, and sometimes futile process. Each year approximately 2000 investigational new drug (IND) applications are submitted to the FDA for permission of human testing, but only approximately 10% of the applicant drugs become available for general use. It is estimated that it takes approximately 10 to 12 years and millions of dollars to complete all phases of drug testing and evaluation.

There are three required stages in the development of a new drug. The first is the preclinical period, during which the initial research and drug development take place. Then, short- and long-term animal testing projects are conducted to establish preliminary information about side effects, lethal dosage limits, and an effective dosage range. This information is compiled and, based on the results, the pharmaceutical company submits an application to the FDA for an IND. This phase can last from 1 to 3 years.

More than 95% of all drugs are allowed to begin the second stage of evaluation, the clinical period, which is divided into three phases. Phase I is designed to evaluate drug reactions within the body, the toxicological actions found in humans, and drug metabolism. The process involves giving healthy volunteers incrementally larger doses of the drug and observing them for actions and reactions. Because the dosage is titrated slowly, the therapeutic range can be safely and accurately determined. This phase usually involves approximately 100 subjects.

Phase II trials are designed to evaluate drug efficacy in the presence of the actual pathology it was designed to treat. Because the medication being tested has not yet been proven to be effective for the specific pathology, it cannot be offered in place of the current standard of care. The typical patient treated in this phase has, therefore, already received the standard care, but his/her condition has remained unchanged. On average, 200 patients are enrolled in this phase.

Phase III involves multicenter, thousand-patient trials to determine the efficacy of the drug, evaluate safety issues, and profile the specific side effects using a specific treatment protocol that will be followed by all of the chosen investigational sites. Because the drug has been proven effective, it can now be offered in direct comparison to the standard care for a disease or specific pathology. The protocol sets down criteria for the type of patient that can and cannot be included in the study, the conditions of drug administration, the drug dosage, the types of tests, and the physical assessments to be done, as well as the length of time the patient will receive the drug. Ideally, these studies are randomized and controlled so no one is aware of which drug is being given to a patient. This reduces the chance that assessments or other necessary information will be biased by the patient or caregiver.

The entire clinical period ranges from 2 to 10 years depending on the ease in recruiting patients and investigational sites. After this information is compiled and analyzed it is forwarded to the FDA with a new drug application (NDA). The NDA review process can take as little as 2 months or as long as 7 years to complete. Once FDA approval is obtained, the drug is released for general use.

It is possible that a paramedic will be asked to participate in a clinical evaluation. If your agency has been chosen as a clinical site for a Phase III study, it will be essential that you understand the importance of documentation and adherence to treatment protocols. Patient records must be complete and the protocol must be strictly followed.

REFERENCE

Coleman B: The Drug Approval Process: A Primer. *Cal J Hosp Pharm*, 1:4–6, Oct 1989.

stream to the target organ (distribution); 3) production of a desired drug effect; 4) chemical breakdown (metabolism); and 5) removal from the body (elimination).

Absorption

Drugs can be administered by many routes (Table 11-2). The purpose of most administration routes is to get the drug to the bloodstream so that it can be carried to the target organ.

Each medication has unique characteristics that make a particular route of administration more advantageous. Table 11-3 lists common routes of administration for prehospital medications and examples of each. Procedures for administration by these routes appear in the Skills Section at the end of this text.

Medications are frequently administered by the oral route in outpatient and hospital settings. Slow or erratic absorption limits the value of oral drug administration in the emergent situation. On the other hand, because of the rich blood supply to the base of the tongue, sublingual administration of medication results in rapid absorption and can be used in the field.

Some medications have the ability to traverse the skin, allowing the subcutaneous blood vessels to absorb the drug. Administration of medication in this fashion is known as transdermal administration.

Figure 11-1 illustrates injection routes used in prehospital care. Medications may be injected superficially into the skin (subcutaneously) or deeper into the muscle (intramuscular). Intravenous (IV) access allows administration of medications directly into the peripheral circulation and is the mainstay of emergency therapy.[1,11] This is the only route that does not require absorption because all of the dose is immediately available to a patient. Some drugs are administered by rapid IV bolus injection, some are given by slow IV push, and others require a period of time to be infused via an IV drip.

A needle inserted into the marrow cavity of a bone allows for intraosseous infusion of medications (Fig. 11-2). It is a rapid and effective route to use in pediatric emergencies when IV access is difficult or time consuming.[9,10] The rich blood supply to the long bones allows large amounts of fluid and medications to move rapidly into the central circulation. The medial aspect of the proximal tibia is the preferred site of administration. Medications demonstrated to be effective when given by intraosseous infusion are listed in Box 11-1.

TABLE 11-2	Routes for Administration and Time Until Effect
Intracardiac	Approximately 15 seconds
Intravenous	Approximately 30–60 seconds
Intraosseous	Approximately 30–60 seconds
Endotracheal	Approximately 2–3 minutes
Inhalation	Approximately 2–3 minutes
Sublingual	Approximately 3–5 minutes
Intramuscular	Approximately 10–20 minutes
Subcutaneous	Approximately 15–30 minutes
Rectal	Approximately 5–30 minutes
Ingestion	Approximately 30–90 minutes
Transdermal	Varies greatly, minutes to hours

TABLE 11-3	Drug Administration Routes and Examples	
Route	**Example**	
Dermal/topical	Patches: nitroglycerin, clonidine, scopolamine	
	Ointment: nitroglycerin	
Endotracheal	Epinephrine, atropine	
Inhalation	Albuterol inhaler, oxygen	
Intramuscular	Diphenhydramine, phenergan, compazine	
Intraosseous	Epinephrine, atropine	
Intravenous	All advanced cardiac life support medications	
Oral	Most chronic medications	
Oral spray	Nitroglycerin	
Subcutaneous	Epinephrine, terbutaline	
Sublingual	Nitroglycerin	

Intracardiac administration is the direct injection of medication into the left ventricular chamber of the heart, historically used as a last resort in cardiac arrest resuscitations. Because of the availability of other effective routes and the risk of complications associated with intracardiac penetration, this route is considered obsolete.

The concept of "directly medicating" the lung for pulmonary disease was suggested early in this century and is currently the mainstay of asthma therapy. Inhalation of medication is achieved by aerosolizing certain drugs for patients to breathe (Fig. 11-3). In addition, anesthetic gases such as nitrous oxide reach the systemic circulation after inhalation. The large absorptive surface of the lung allows some emergency drugs to be effectively administered by the endotracheal route, which is indicated whenever urgent drug administration is required and rapid vascular access is not possible.[1,2] Box 11-2 lists those drugs recommended for endotracheal administration. Drugs such as epinephrine, atropine, lidocaine, and naloxone have been safely and effectively administered by this route. Diazepam is also effective endotracheally, but pulmonary injury may occur by use of this route.[12] Thus, diazepam is not recommended for routine endotracheal administration until further studies demonstrate its safety.

Drug absorption is the process in which a drug enters the blood. Drug absorption depends on many variables. Food in the stomach will decrease the absorption of some orally administered drugs. Certain drugs are destroyed by digestive enzymes in the stomach and are unlikely to be of any benefit if given orally. The thickness of the absorbing surface also influ-

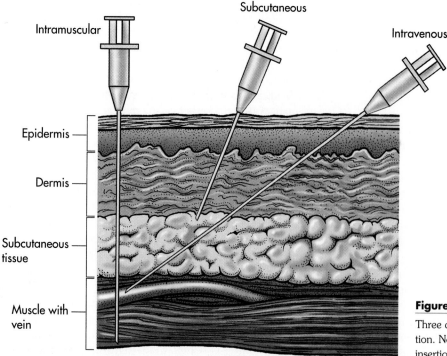

Intramuscular Subcutaneous Intravenous

Epidermis

Dermis

Subcutaneous tissue

Muscle with vein

Figure 11-1

Three common prehospital routes of drug administration. Note that each technique has a different angle of insertion and target organ.

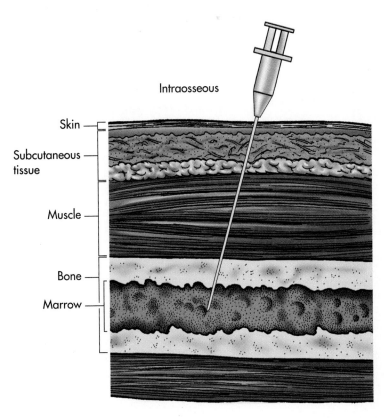

Intraosseous

Skin

Subcutaneous
tissue

Muscle

Bone

Marrow

Figure 11-2

The intraosseous route is rapid and an effective route to use
in pediatric emergencies when IV access is difficult or time
consuming.

ences the rate of drug absorption. Skin has many layers of
cells that a drug must pass through as opposed to the single
layer of cells in the GI tract. Therefore, drugs are more readily
absorbed when given orally than when applied topically. The
large surface area of the lung provides for rapid absorption
when medications are inhaled.

| BOX 11-1 | Drugs That Have Been Safely Administered Via Intraosseous Route |

Crystalloid IV solutions
Dextrose
Whole blood
Plasma
Epinephrine
Sodium bicarbonate
Calcium chloride and gluconate
Lidocaine
Atropine
Dopamine
Diazepam

| BOX 11-2 | Drugs That Can Be Administered Through An Endotracheal Tube |

Epinephrine
Atropine
Naloxone
Lidocaine
Diazepam or lorazepam (controversial)

Drug absorption can also be affected by a patient's physiologic condition. For example, absorption of a subcutaneously
administered drug is much slower in a shock state, because
blood flow to the skin is diminished. Thus, administering subcutaneous epinephrine to a patient in shock will result in a
slower absorption and increased travel time to the bloodstream than would administering IV, intraosseous, or endotracheal epinephrine to the same patient. Thus, the most effective route of administration for a drug needed emergently
(e.g., because of cardiac arrest or shock) is the one which delivers the drug directly into the bloodstream.[6] Drugs injected
IV bypass the process of absorption. Absorption of drugs by
various routes of administration is illustrated in Figure 11-4.

Distribution

The bloodstream acts as a transportation network with rapid
access to virtually all body tissues. Some drugs are dissolved directly into the liquid portion of the blood (serum). Others attach
to carriers, much like a truck loaded with cargo. The carriers
are typically proteins (such as albumin) that unload their cargo
at the target organ. Distribution is the process of moving a drug
through the body and delivering it to various tissues (Fig. 11-5).

Movement of a drug into the tissues from the blood is not
a uniform process. Drugs must pass through barriers to reach
tissues and cells. The cell membrane itself may serve as a barrier to some drugs. Chemical characteristics (e.g., solubility in
fat or water, size of the molecules) and interactions with carrier
proteins in the blood control which tissues the drugs can
reach. Fat-soluble drugs can pass through most cell membranes easily and therefore have access to tissues such as the
brain. Blood flow to certain organs also determines the
amount of drug distributed. More drug-laden blood flows into

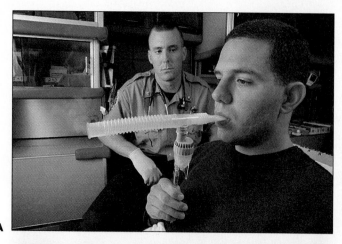

A

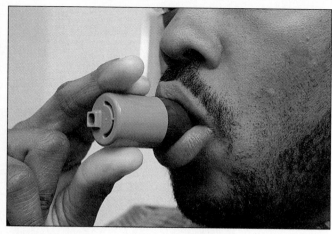

C

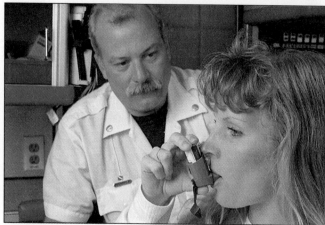

B

Figure 11-3

The technique of aerosolizing a medication allows for delivery of a drug directly to the lungs. A) nebulizer B) metered dose inhaler, and C) roto haler.

the brain, kidneys, and liver than to other tissues, because these organs receive approximately 65% of the total blood flow from the heart. However, low blood flow that results from shock will impair distribution to even these tissues.

The central nervous system is a highly restricted area with regard to drug passage. A specialized capillary membrane system known as the blood-brain barrier prevents the passage of many drugs. Because the brain and cell membranes are composed mostly of fat, fat-soluble drugs pass most easily across this barrier.

In pregnant patients, the placenta is only a minimal barrier to drugs; the fetus is exposed to most drugs given to the mother. In emergency situations, the risk of an adverse outcome of pregnancy must be weighed against the drug's benefit.

Mechanism of Drug Action

Once a drug is distributed to the target tissue, it may produce a desired effect. Drugs can be essential materials that fuel the

Time of Drug Absorption by Routes of Administration

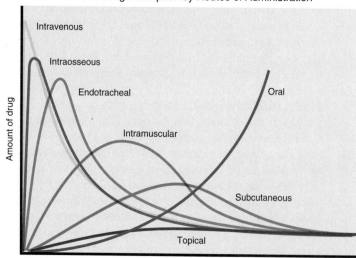

Intravenous

Intraosseous

Endotracheal

Oral

Amount of drug

Intramuscular

Subcutaneous

Topical

Time

Figure 11-4

The amount of time it takes to absorb a drug into the bloodstream depends on the route of administration. The chemical makeup of a drug or potential reactions with the body may determine which route is used. The route selected will be the safest and fastest.

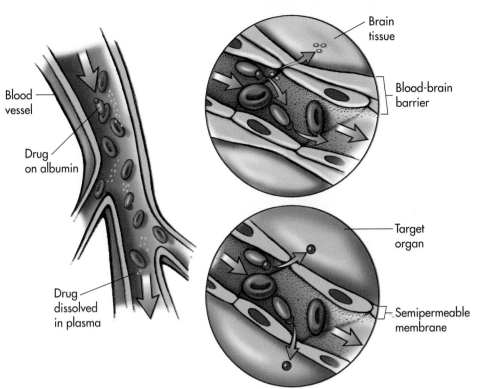

Figure 11-5

Drugs being distributed to the brain and target organs via the bloodstream are dissolved in plasma or bound to proteins. The ability of a drug to cross out of the bloodstream is determined by the permeability of the membrane it is trying to cross.

Blood vessel

Drug on albumin

Drug dissolved in plasma

Brain tissue

Blood-brain barrier

Target organ

Semipermeable membrane

vital functions of cells, such as oxygen or glucose, or they can alter cell function or impulse transmission in tissues that conduct electricity, such as nerve, skeletal, and cardiac tissues.

The basic site of drug interaction is the receptor. A receptor is a protein that has a specific shape and is located on cell membranes, on structures within a cell, at nerve synapses, or on a gland. Receptors can be compared with light switches that can be turned on and off. They regulate normal daily physiologic functions such as digestion and respiration by controlling cellular activity and are stimulated by naturally occurring chemical messengers, such as epinephrine and acetylcholine.

A drug or chemical messenger must have a very specific shape to activate a receptor, just as a key must fit exactly to turn a lock (Fig. 11-6). A drug effect occurs when the drug agonist key fits exactly into the receptor "keyhole" and "turns the lock." Some drugs are shaped so that the key will fit the keyhole, yet fail to turn the lock. When such a drug binds to a receptor, it prevents other chemicals from turning on the receptor. This type of drug is known as an "antagonist." For example, naloxone (Narcan) binds to morphine (opioid) receptors and blocks morphine from turning on its drug effect. Many medications, such as advanced cardiac life support drugs, produce their effects as agonists or antagonists at receptors in the autonomic nervous system (ANS). Therefore, it is essential to understand the basic function of the ANS to understand prehospital pharmacology (see Chapter 8). Familiarity with drug receptor terms and terminology used in describing advanced cardiac life support drugs will also help in understanding prehospital pharmacology.

The binding of a drug to a receptor is a dynamic process that is seldom permanent. The drug or chemical is constantly in motion, binding and then leaving the receptor to bind again at another site. If more than one drug or naturally occurring chemical can bind to the receptor, each will compete for binding to that receptor. The more drug that is available near a receptor, the more chances it has to bind. The overall drug effect seen in a patient is the sum of all receptor interactions in affected cells.

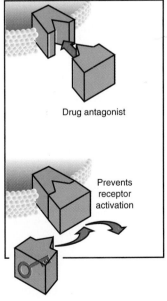

Drug agonist

Activates receptor

Drug antagonist

Prevents receptor activation

Figure 11-6

Both a drug agonist and antagonist must fit into a specific receptor site found on the membrane of the target cell to exhibit an effect. An "agonist" promotes an action, and an "antagonist" prevents an action.

The overall drug effect may not occur until a certain number of cells are affected by the drug; that is, a specific drug dose may be required to produce a desired, or therapeutic, effect. Thus, if only a few cells are stimulated, the drug may not produce the desired response; this is known as a subtherapeutic dose. The amount of drug given will influence the intensity and nature of the drug effect. Consider the person who drinks ethanol. With increasing amounts of ethanol, the effect intensifies. This relationship between dose and effect is known as dose-response and is illustrated in Figure 11-7. As ethanol intake is continued, the pleasant intoxicating effects may become harmful effects. Most drugs have a threshold at which the therapeutic effect is surpassed by harmful or toxic effects.

Consider each drug or medication a potential poison. Too much medication can poison the entire organism. For example, taking two aspirin tablets for a headache is therapeutic; taking 100 aspirin will poison many biological processes, resulting in toxicity and possible death of the organism. Some medications have a narrow margin between therapeutic effect and toxicity. This margin of safety is called the therapeutic window and is illustrated in Figure 11-8. The recommended therapeutic dose of a drug is calculated to fall within this therapeutic window.

Drugs rarely cause a single, specific effect. Although a desired effect is occurring in the target tissue, in most cases the drug is also acting on many other tissues. Adverse drug reactions are undesirable effects that are either expected or unexpected and range from unpleasant to harmful. Side effects are those undesirable but expected effects that occur with usual therapeutic doses. For example, administering an albuterol aerosol treatment to a patient with asthma can produce anxiety and muscle tremors in addition to its therapeutic action of bronchodilation. Hypersensitivity or allergic reactions, and idiosyncratic reactions, are unexpected adverse drug effects. For example, administering lidocaine may produce hives, itching, and wheezing in patients who have been sensitized to the drug.

In some cases, the continued use of a drug will produce less and less effect. Habitual use of opiates such as morphine

or heroin, for instance, will require increasing doses to achieve the same "high." This phenomenon is termed tolerance. When the body develops a drug tolerance, a craving for the drug occurs which results in dependence, or addiction. If the drug is not supplied to the body, unpleasant physical symptoms are often produced, along with the psychological craving. This physiologic response to absence of the "needed" drug is called withdrawal (*see* Chapter 42).

Metabolism and Elimination

Drug effects are temporary because body processes exist that detoxify and eliminate foreign chemicals such as drugs. The kidney has the important role of regulating the internal environment of the body by eliminating (excreting) unnecessary or potentially harmful substances. The kidney's filtering system processes water-soluble substances. Many biologically active drugs are fat-soluble instead, and must be converted to water-soluble compounds before the kidney can eliminate them.

The liver is the great biochemist of the body. A major function of the liver is to detoxify and convert (metabolize) chemicals and drugs so they can be more easily eliminated by the kidney (Fig. 11-9). Other tissues may play a role in metabolism, but the majority of drugs are altered by the liver. Within the liver, drugs are split apart or have substances attached to them to produce a water-soluble chemical. The lifespan of a drug is determined by this process. For example, a single dose of phenobarbital, a sedative-anticonvulsant, would continue its effect for more than 100 years if metabolism did not occur.[4]

Normal function of the liver and kidneys is necessary to adequately remove drugs from the body. When these organs are diseased, drug metabolism and elimination are less efficient. Normal aging also causes both the liver and kidneys to work less efficiently, resulting in slower drug metabolism and excretion. The elderly generally absorb drugs more slowly than adolescents and middle-aged adults. Older patients also tend to have cardiovascular diseases that decrease blood

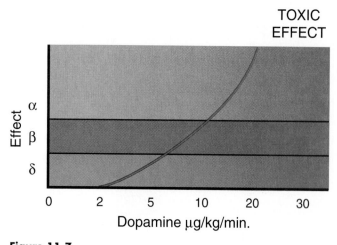

Figure 11-7

Dose response is the relationship between the dose taken and the effect seen. Too little of a drug does not produce the desired effect; too much of a drug may become toxic and harmful.

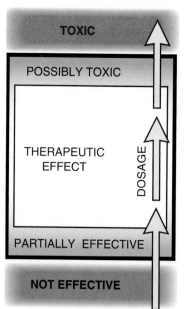

Figure 11-8

The therapeutic window is the balance between the desired therapeutic effect, partially effective or ineffective levels (underdosed), and toxicity (overdosage). Some drugs, such as phenytoin or theophylline, have a very narrow range of therapeutic effect, which means that they are very easy to accidentally or intentionally overdose.

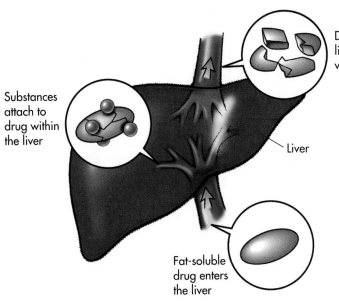

Substances attach to drug within the liver

Drug exits liver as water-soluble

Liver

Fat-soluble drug enters the liver

Figure 11-9

The liver is the site of metabolism of most drugs. Once a drug is made water soluble by the liver, it is available for the body tissues to use or can be excreted by the kidney.

flow to tissues and thus alter drug distribution. In addition, elderly patients frequently receive multiple medications that may interact dangerously with each other. Neonates also eliminate drugs inefficiently because of immature livers and kidneys. Thus, in both the elderly and the very young, doses of some medications must be altered to avoid adverse or toxic reactions.

In some situations, drug elimination may be very rapid and the drug effect short-lived. To maintain a therapeutic effect, the drug must be kept above a certain concentration in the blood, and the drug must be replaced at a rate that matches elimination. A bolus of medication is intended to achieve a concentration that will create a rapid drug effect. To sustain an effective drug level, an IV infusion may be needed (Fig. 11-10). For example, lidocaine must be at a blood concentration of 1 to 5 micrograms per milliliter (μg/mL) to effectively control ventricular ectopy. Giving a bolus of 100 mg of lidocaine will only achieve that level for approximately 20 minutes, because the liver quickly inactivates the drug. To maintain the concentration at an effective level in the blood, the drug lost to metabolism must be replaced by a continuous IV infusion.

Bolus Effect vs Bolus + Continuous Infusion vs Infusion Alone

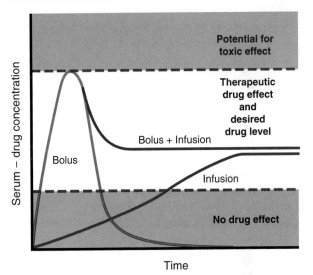

Serum – drug concentration

Potential for toxic effect

Therapeutic drug effect and desired drug level

Bolus + Infusion

Bolus

Infusion

No drug effect

Time

Figure 11-10

The ability to maintain a therapeutic effect involves a delicate balance between the amount of drug available within the bloodstream and the amount being taken away from the blood by the liver or kidneys. Using a combination of bolus and/or continuous infusion of a specific drug will achieve that needed balance and allow a therapeutic effect to take place.

Basics of Medication Administration

The provision of advanced life-saving therapy carries with it a great deal of responsibility; medication dosage errors can have

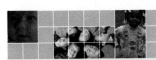

PEDIATRIC PERSPECTIVE

- Medications are administered to infants and children based on their weight. A Broselow tape measures the child's height, estimates the child's weight, and can be used to guide treatment.

- Drug effects are unpredictable in the newborn because of variations in the maturity of the kidneys and liver. Consequently, drug toxicity and higher drug serum levels may occur.

BOX 11-3	The Five Patient Rights of Drug Administration

1. The RIGHT drug
   - Verify orders
   - Check the label
   - Know the indications for the drug
2. The RIGHT patient
3. The RIGHT dosage
   - Verify dosage
   - Use dosage charts for assistance
   - Perform accurate calculations
   - Double check calculations
   - Be familiar with the usual dosages
4. The RIGHT route
   - Verify route
   - Determine urgency of the situation
   - Know the effectiveness of medications by various routes
5. The RIGHT time
   - How rapidly can the drug be administered?
   - What are the time intervals for repeat doses?

BOX 11-4	Examples of Prefixes and Meanings

Prefix	Meaning
kilo-	= 1000
deci-	= 1/10 or 0.1
centi-	= 1/100 or 0.01
milli-	= 1/1000 or 0.001
micro-	= 1/1,000,000 or 0.000001

fatal consequences. The golden rule in drug administration is to check and recheck at every step. Although many situations require rapid action, accuracy and attention to detail must not be compromised. Every paramedic must be thoroughly familiar with the dosage, route of administration, and calculations for all prehospital drugs. Safe and effective drug administration in prehospital care can be summarized by the five patient rights of drug administration in shown Box 11-3.

Communication

When direct radio communication is required, accurate relay of information must be ensured. Particular attention must be paid to names of medications, doses, and routes of administration. Orders should be verified by repeating the drug name, dosage, and route of administration exactly as received. Once confirmed, medication orders must be carried out exactly as ordered. If orders seem inappropriate or potentially harmful to a patient, concerns should be discussed immediately prior to administration of the drug.

Calculations

Drug administration requires accurate calculation of the correct dose. Paramedics must be thoroughly familiar with drug dosage calculations, because these calculations are typically performed during stressful situations. A backup system must be in place, in the form of reference cards or other charts, to guarantee accuracy.

Drugs are most commonly dosed in metric units (grams and milligrams) and fortunately, most medications are packaged and labeled in the same units. The metric system is based on units of 10, which make calculations and conversions relatively straightforward. Weight and fluid volume are the two metric measures used for drug administration. These are expressed in units of grams and liters respectively. Prefixes define the size of each measure relative to the base measure (e.g., liter, gram) (see Box 11-4).

Because units of measure differ from each other in powers of 10, conversion between units is accomplished by simply moving a decimal point.

Some examples of metric conversions are:

1 kilogram (kg) = 1000 grams (g)
1 gram = 1000 milligrams (mg)
1 milligram = 1000 micrograms (mcg)
10 mg = 0.01 g (1 mg = 1/1000 g)
10 g = 10,000 mg (1 g = 1000 mg)
10 μg = 0.010 mg (1 μg = 1/1000 mg)

For volume, replace the word for weight (gram) with that for volume (liter):

1 liter = 1000 milliliters (mL)
1 milliliter = 1000 microliters (μL)

Note: 1 milliliter (mL) = 1 cubic centimeter (cc) for water at 72° F and at sea level; thus, for all practical purposes, mL and cc are interchangeable. A cubic centimeter is the amount of physical space occupied by 1 milliliter of fluid volume. Syringes are frequently marked in cubic centimeters (cc).

Conversion from other systems of measure to the metric system is not as straightforward. Most drug dosages are given as mg of drug per kg of body weight. Since most patients know their weight in pounds, conversion of pounds to kilograms is necessary.

1 kilogram = 2.2 pounds
Example: 150 pound man = 150/2.2 = 68 kg

All drugs are supplied with standard information about the amount of drug available in the container as well as the volume provided. In many cases, for emergency care, drugs are often prepackaged in the usual adult dose. Thus the entire contents would be administered to an adult with no need for performing calculations. In other situations, the amount of drug given will depend on such factors as the desired response to be produced, the size of the patient (particularly important for children), and the packaging or preparation of the medication.

When a drug dosage or volume must be calculated, the following information is required:

- *The dose of the drug to be administered.* This information may be obtained by direct physician order, be a standard adult dose, or be determined by the weight of the patient.
- *The amount of the drug provided in the container.* This information will be found on the label and usually be given in grams, milligrams, or micrograms.

- *The volume of the drug provided in the container.* This will also be found on the label and will likely be expressed in milliliters.

Knowing these three points will allow you to calculate the appropriate volume of drug to be given by using the following formula:

Volume to be given

$$= \frac{(\text{dose to be given})(\text{volume of the drug in the package})}{(\text{amount of drug in the package})}$$

Example #1: an order is received to administer 50 mg of a drug to a patient. The drug is supplied in 5 mL which contains 250 mg. The volume to be administered is calculated as follows:

Volume =

$$\frac{50 \text{ mg (dose ordered)} \times 5 \text{ mL (volume of the drug in the package)}}{250 \text{ mg (amount of drug in the package)}}$$

Thus the volume to be given is:

$$\frac{50 \text{ mg} \times 5 \text{ mL}}{250 \text{ mg}} = \frac{250 \text{ mg/mL}}{250 \text{ mg}} = 1 \text{ mL}$$

Example #2: an order is received to administer 4 mg of a drug to a patient. The drug is supplied in 1 mL which contains 2 mg. The volume to be administered is calculated as follows:

$$\text{Volume} = \frac{(4 \text{ mg}) \times (1 \text{ mL})}{2 \text{ mg}} = 2 \text{ mL}$$

In this case, because the vial only contains 1 mL, it will be necessary to administer two vials.

Example #3: in some cases, a drug dose will be ordered based upon the patient's weight. An order is received to give a child 2 mg/kg of body weight of a particular drug. The patient's weight is determined to be 44 pounds. The drug is supplied in 10 mL which contains 100 mg.

First it is necessary to convert the weight in pounds, to weight in kilograms. Remember that 1 kilogram equals 2.2 pounds. Therefore the conversion calculation is:

$$\frac{44 \text{ pounds}}{2.2 \text{ pounds per kg}} = 20 \text{ kg}$$

The desired dose is 2 mg/kg; therefore, with a weight of 20 kg, the dose is (2 mg/kg) × (20 kg) = 40 mg.

Now using the usual formula:

$$\text{Volume to be given} = \frac{(40 \text{ mg}) \times (10 \text{ mL})}{(100 \text{ mg})} = 4 \text{ mL}$$

Some medications must be administered continuously to maintain a constant drug effect. When medications are continuously infused, time is a factor that must be included in the calculations. The dosage ordered in dose/min or dose/hr must be converted to volume/min or volume/hr. IV solution sets include tubing, a drip chamber, and a clamp control (Fig. 11-11). The drip chamber counts drops of solution, and the clamp control alters the drops/min and alters the flow of medication.

IV tubing is calibrated in drops(gtt)/mL that vary according to setup and manufacturer as follows:

Solution Sets

Minidrip or Microdrip	60 drops = 1 mL
Macrodrip or Standard	10, 15, or 20 drops = 1 mL
Blood Set	10 drops = 1 mL

Example #4: an order is received to administer a drug by IV drip at a rate of 5 mg/min. The IV drip is prepared by mixing 5 g (5000 mg) in a 250 mL IV bag. Using our formula, the volume to be given per minute can be calculated:

Volume to be given

$$= \frac{(5 \text{ mg / min}) \times (250 \text{ mL})}{5000 \text{ mg}} = 0.25 \text{ mL / min}$$

Next, the number of drops per minute can be calculated knowing the volume to be given and the type of drip chamber used. If a minidrip is used, there are 60 drops for each milliliter given. Therefore the number of drops per minute can be calculated as follows:

Number of drops per minute =

(volume per minute to be given) × (number of drops per mL)

In this example, the number of drops per minute = (0.25 mL/min) × (60 drops/mL) = 15 drops/min.

Prehospital medications can be marketed in several different dosage forms (Fig. 11-12). Oral medications are in the form of pills, capsules, or liquids. Parenteral medications are packaged in a variety of single-use ampules, single- and multiple-use vials, and premeasured syringes and cartridges.

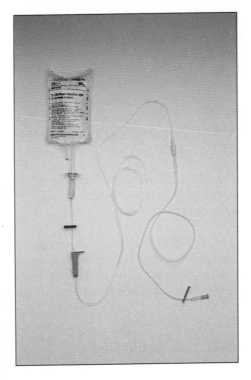

Figure 11-11

A common intravenous solution setup.

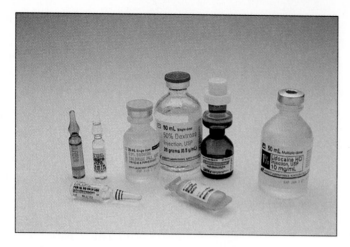

Figure 11-12

Different forms of medications.

Categories of Medications

Thousands of medications are currently in use. Drugs may be classified many ways—by chemical class (e.g., barbiturates, benzodiazepines, cephalosporins, phenothiazines), by mechanism of action (e.g., calcium channel blockers, beta blockers, antihistamines, antimicrobials), or by therapeutic category (e.g., analgesics, antihypertensives, anticonvulsants, anticoagulants). Many drugs fit into more than one classification, so categorizing a drug is somewhat arbitrary. In addition, many medications have multiple actions in the body and can be used to treat more than one disease state. Therefore, it is difficult to assign some drugs to a single classification or therapeutic category.

It is not practical to memorize all the drugs on the market today. It is very important, however, that paramedics be familiar with all drugs that are used in their EMS system. Information on other drugs should be obtained through easily available references. Paramedics should use such references to verify doses, detect drug interactions, and list common adverse reactions. Drugs should be cross-referenced by both generic and brand names, and therapeutic category if possible. Paramedics should attempt to determine the medications (e.g., over-the-counter, prescription, illegal) a patient has taken prior to administering any new drugs. Always consider possible adverse effects or interactions with unfamiliar drugs.

Paramedics are frequently confronted with patients who are unresponsive or unable to communicate, with no medical history available except for medication bottles. Medications may be the best clues to determining a patient's medical problem or diagnosis.

The following is an overview of common drug categories including common characteristics and examples. A variety of categories are used. Some types are found on the ambulance and in emergency departments and others are medications patients have at home.

Cardiovascular Medications

Antidysrhythmics

Therapeutic action: Decrease ventricular irritability; slow conduction through AV node

Uses: Control of ventricular and supraventricular arrhythmias

Side effects: Hypotension, heart block, syncope, nausea

Examples: Oral—quinidine (Quinidex, Quinaglute), procainamide (Pronestyl, Procan SR), mexilitine (Mexitil)
IV—lidocaine, (Bretylium) bretylol
Inhaled—oxygen

Antihypertensives

Many different types of drugs are used to treat hypertension. These include diuretics, angiotensin converting enzyme (ACE) inhibitors, beta blockers, calcium channel blockers, and vasodilators. (These are covered in more detail based upon each class of drugs.)

Angiotensin Converting Enzyme (ACE) Inhibitors

Therapeutic action: Lowers blood pressure (blocks conversion of the hormone angiotensin I to angiotensin II)

Uses: Antihypertensive, congestive heart failure

Side effects: Urticaria, persistent cough, skin rash, hypotension, and hyperkalemia

Examples: benzazepril (Lotensin), captopril (Capoten), enalopril (Vasotec), lisinopril (Prinivil, Zestril)

Beta Blockers

Therapeutic action: Slow heart (sinus) rate; decrease conduction of impulses through AV node; decrease cardiac output; lower blood pressure

Uses: Hypertension, angina, migraine headache, arrhythmias, postmyocardial infarction

Side effects: Bradycardia, hypotension, heart block, fatigue

Examples: propranolol (Inderal), nadolol (Corgard), atenolol (Tenormin), metoprolol (Lopressor), labetalol (Normodyne, Trandate)

Calcium-Channel Blockers

Therapeutic action: Slow conduction through AV node; slow ventricular response with atrial tachydysrhythmias; relax vascular smooth muscle

Uses: (P)SVTs, hypertension, angina

Side effects: Hypotension, nausea, bradycardia, fatigue

Precautions: May cause significant hypotension, bradycardia

Examples: diltiazem (Cardizem), verapamil (Calan, Isoptin), nifedipine (Procardia, Adalat), amlodipine (Norvasc), nicardipine (Cardene)

Cardiac Glycosides

Therapeutic action: Increase force of myocardial contractions; slow conduction through AV node; slow heart rate
Uses: Congestive heart failure; A-fib, A-flutter
Side effects: Nausea, fatigue, cardiac arrhythmias
Precautions: Very narrow range between toxic and therapeutic doses; be alert to potential for toxicity (CNS alterations, bradycardia, arrhythmias)
Examples: digoxin (Lanoxin), digitoxin (Crystodigin)

Coronary Vasodilators

Therapeutic action: Dilate blood vessels, including coronary arteries; decrease myocardial oxygen demand
Uses: Angina, coronary artery disease
Side effects: Headache, nausea, hypotension
Precautions: Must be stored carefully, away from light. May cause significant hypotension.
Examples: nitroglycerin (NTG), isosorbide dinitrate (Isordil), isosorbide mononitrate (Ismo) (Available in tablet, spray, or paste.)

Diuretics

Therapeutic action: Increase urinary output; decrease circulating blood volume; vasodilation
Uses: Congestive heart failure, edema, hypertension
Side effects: Dehydration, electrolyte imbalances, syncope, hypotension
Examples: hydrochlorothiazide (HCTZ) (Hydrodiuril), furosemide (Lasix)

Parasympatholytics (Anticholinergics)

Therapeutic action: Block the action of the parasympathetic nervous system and vagus nerve by blocking the acetylcholine receptors, resulting in increased heart rate
Uses: Symptomatic bradycardia, asystole
Side effects: Blurred vision, dilated pupils, tachycardia, dry mouth, confusion
Examples: IV atropine sulfate

Sympathomimetics

Therapeutic action: Act on the receptors of the sympathetic nervous system to release endogenous catecholamines, resulting in increased blood pressure, heart rate, and force of contraction.
Uses: Cardiac arrest, severe hypotension, shock (cardiogenic, distributive)
Side effects: Can increase myocardial oxygen demand, headache, nausea, vomiting, anxiety, palpitations
Examples: IV-epinephrine, norepinephrine (Levophed), dopamine (Intropin)

Thrombolytics

Therapeutic action: Act with clotting protein to help dissolve blood clots
Uses: Lysis of blood clot with an acute MI or pulmonary embolism
Side effects: Bleeding, stroke
Examples: streptokinase (Streptase), tissue plasminogen activator [TPA] (Activase)

Vasodilators

Therapeutic action: Vasodilation of arterial smooth muscle; decrease arterial pressure
Uses: Hypertension
Side effects: Sedation, headache, hypotension, bradycardia, impotence
Examples: methyldopa (Aldomet), clonidine (Catapres), prazosin (Minipress), minoxidil (Loniten)

Central Nervous System Medications

Anticonvulsants

Therapeutic action: Inhibit seizure activity in the brain
Uses: Epilepsy, seizure disorders, alcohol withdrawal
Side effects: CNS depression, ataxia, confusion
Relevant info: With epilepsy, must be taken on a daily basis to achieve desired effect
Examples: phenobarbital, carbamazepine (Tegretol), phenytoin (Dilantin), valproic acid (Depakene, Depakote), clonazepam (Klonopin)

Antidepressants (Tricyclic and Others)

Therapeutic action: Mood elevator with sedative effects
Uses: Depression, panic disorders, eating disorders, chronic pain syndromes
Side effects: Sedation, syncope
Relevant info: Cause cardiac dysrhythmias and seizures in toxic doses
Examples: amitriptyline (Elavil), imipramine (Tofranil), fluoxetine (Prozac), sertraline

(Zoloft), trazodone (Desyrel), maprotiline (Ludiomil), amoxapine (Ascendin)

Antipsychotics (Major Tranquilizers)

Therapeutic action: Modify thought processes in the brain; some agents inhibit vomiting

Uses: Management of acute and chronic psychosis (schizophrenia), agitation, vomiting

Side effects: Sedation, syncope, movement disorders

Relevant info: May cause acute muscle spasms (dystonic reaction)

Examples: chlorpromazine (Thorazine), thioridazine (Mellaril), prochlorperazine (Compazine), fluphenazine (Prolixin), haloperidol (Haldol)

Sedatives/Hypnotics (Tranquilizers)

Therapeutic action: Dose-dependent depression of the central nervous system

Uses: Insomnia, anxiety, panic attacks, seizure disorders, muscle relaxation

Side effects: Drowsiness, euphoria, confusion, respiratory depression, withdrawal

Relevant info: Long-term use can lead to addiction

Examples: *Barbiturates* - phenobarbital, pentobarbital (Nembutal), secobarbital (Seconal) *Benzodiazepines* - diazepam (Valium), lorazepam (Ativan), flurazepam (Dalmane), triazolam (Halcion), chlordiazepoxide (Librium), alprazolam (Xanax) *Others* - meprobamate (Equanil)

Narcotic Analgesics

Therapeutic action: Alter perception of emotional response to pain

Uses: Severe pain relief

Side effects: Dose-dependent CNS and respiratory depression, constipation, nausea, dizziness, euphoria

Relevant info: Highly addictive, potentiated by other CNS depressants including ethyl alcohol

Examples: morphine, codeine, meperidine (Demerol), propoxyphene (Darvon), hydromorphone (Dilaudid), pentazocine (TalwinNx) Combinations (with aspirin or acetaminophen): Tylox, Percodan, Percocet, Vicodin, Darvocet N-100, Lortab, Lorcet

Stimulants

Therapeutic action: Direct stimulation of the CNS

Uses: Appetite suppression, attention deficit disorders, decongestants

Side effects: Agitation, tachycardia, hypertension, arrhythmias, seizures, sedation (children)

Relevant info: Highly addictive

Examples: amphetamines, cocaine, caffeine, methylphenidate (Ritalin), phenylpropanolamine

Gastrointestinal Medications

Antidiarrheals

Therapeutic action: Inhibit gastrointestinal motility

Uses: Diarrhea

Side effects: Constipation, drowsiness, nausea

Relevant info: Some medications in this category (Lomotil, paregoric) contain narcotics

Examples: paregoric, Lomotil, Donnatal, Imodium A-D

Antiemetics/Antinauseants

Therapeutic action: Inhibit nausea and vomiting

Uses: Nausea, vomiting, motion sickness, vertigo

Side effects: drowsiness, incoordination, blurred vision

Examples: prochlorperazine (Compazine), trimethobenzamide (Tigan), metoclopramide (Reglan), dimenhydrinate (Dramamine), meclizine (Antivert), promethazine (Phenergan)

Appetite Suppressants

Therapeutic action: Suppress appetite

Uses: Dieting, weight loss

Side effects: Nervousness, tremors, dysrhythmias, hypertension

Examples: diethylpropion (Tenuate), amphetamines

Antisecretories (Antiulcers)

Therapeutic action: Inhibit gastric acid secretion

Uses: Peptic ulcer disease, severe indigestion, reflux esophagitis

Side effects: Headache, fatigue, diarrhea, muscular pain

Examples: cimetidine (Tagamet), ranitidine (Zantac), famotidine (Pepcid) Other drugs used to treat ulcers: sucralfate (Carafate), Omeprazole (Prilosec)

Antimicrobial Agents (Antibiotics)

AIDS Drugs

Therapeutic action: Antiviral
Uses: Boost immunity, antiviral, antibacterial
Side effects: Nausea, vomiting, anemia, headache
Examples: AZT, ddC, ddI, Pentamidine

Antibacterials

Therapeutic action: Destroy bacteria
Uses: Bacterial infections
Side effects: Nausea, vomiting, diarrhea, rash, allergic reaction
Relevant info: The entire course of antibiotics must be taken to eliminate recurrence of infection
Examples: penicillins - PenVK, ampicillin, amoxicillin
                      cephalosporins - Ceclor, Keflex
                      tetracyclines - tetracycline, doxycycline
                      erythromycins - erythromycin, clarithromycin (Biaxin), azithromycin (Zithromax)
                      sulfa drugs - Bactrim, Septra
                      others - nitrofurantoin (Macrodantin), metronidazole (Flagyl)

Antituberculosis

Therapeutic action: Antibiotic action, fight bacteria
Uses: Tuberculosis
Side effects: GI upset, liver toxicity (INH)
Examples: isoniazid [INH], rifampin, ethambutol, clofazimine

Miscellaneous Medications

Alkalizing Agents

Therapeutic action: Provide a bicarbonate buffer to help correct metabolic acidosis
Uses: Known hyperkalemia, tricyclic antidepressant overdose, late in cardiac arrest
Side effects: Metabolic alkalosis
Examples: IV-sodium bicarbonate

Anti-inflammatory Analgesics (Over-the-Counter)

Therapeutic action: Diminish inflammatory response
Uses: Mild-to-moderate pain, inflammation (musculoskeletal), arthritis, fever
Side effects: Nausea, abdominal pain
Relevant info: Chronic use in high doses can result in kidney or liver damage
Examples: aspirin, ibuprofen (Motrin, Advil), indomethacin (Indocin), ketorolac (Toradol)

Anti-inflammatories/Steroids

Therapeutic action: Suppress inflammation
Uses: Severe allergic reactions, acute spinal cord injury, severe exacerbation of COPD, asthma, and certain other conditions
Side effects: Headache, restlessness, hypertension, fluid retention
Relevant info: Patients on chronic steroids should be considered to be immunosuppressed and are at high risk for infections
Examples: IV-methylprednisolone (Solu-Medrol), orally-prednisone

Anticoagulants

Therapeutic action: Increase blood clotting time (blood thinners)
Uses: Thromboembolic disease (deep vein thrombosis, pulmonary embolism, cerebral vascular accident), atrial fibrillation
Side effects: Bleeding, bruising
Examples: heparin, warfarin (Coumadin)

Antihistamines

Therapeutic action: Reduce effects of histamine and allergic responses; produce varying degrees of CNS depression
Uses: Allergies/hayfever, colds, rhinitis, insomnia, nausea
Side effects: Drowsiness, dry mouth, headache, constipation, blurred vision
Examples: diphenhydramine (Benadryl), chlorpheniramine (Chlor-Trimeton), hydroxyzine (Atarax, Vistaril), terfenadine (Seldane), astemizole (Hismanal), cyproheptadine (Periactin)

Bronchodilators

Therapeutic action: Relax bronchial smooth muscle and relieve bronchospasm
Uses: Asthma, COPD, bronchitis
Side effects: Tachycardia, tremor, nausea, headache
Relevant info: May be given orally, inhaled, or IV
                      Theophylline may act as respiratory stimulant
Examples: theophylline (Theodur), albuterol (Ventolin, Proventil), terbutaline (Brethine), metaproterenol (Alupent, Metaprel), epinephrine (1:1,000), racemic epinephrine

Diabetic Medications

Oral Hypoglycemics

Therapeutic action:	Stimulate body's production of insulin
Uses:	Diabetes mellitus (adult onset, primarily)
Side effects:	Hypoglycemia, rash, nausea, fatigue
Examples:	glipizide (Glucotrol), glyburide (Micronase, Diabeta), chlorpropamide (Diabinese), tolbutamide (Orinase)

Insulin

Therapeutic action:	Replaces body's insulin; transports glucose across cell membranes
Uses:	Diabetes mellitus (juvenile onset, primarily)
Side effects:	Hypoglycemia
Relevant info:	Injection only; must be carefully administered and adjusted with food intake to achieve desired effect.
Examples:	regular, NPH, lente

Lipid-lowering Drugs

Therapeutic action:	Lower blood cholesterol
Uses:	High blood cholesterol or lipid levels
Side effects:	Nausea, constipation, abdominal pain
Examples:	niacin, clofibrate (AtromidS), gemfibrozil (Lopid), lovastatin (Mevacor)

Skeletal Muscle Relaxers

Therapeutic action:	Depress of the CNS, reduce tonic muscle activity
Uses:	Muscle sprains, strains, and spasms
Side effects:	Sedation, nausea, syncope, dizziness
Examples:	meprobamate (Equanil), carisoprodol (Soma), cyclobenzaprine (Flexeril)

SUMMARY

The principles in this chapter are the foundation for an understanding of prehospital drug therapy. The medications introduced throughout this text will be more easily understood in light of these principles. To make the best use of the "tools of the trade," paramedics must be knowledgeable in the properties of prehospital medications and meticulous with accurate dosage calculations and administration techniques.

REFERENCES

1. Aitkenhead AR: Drug administration during CPR: What route? *Resuscit,* 22:191–195, 1991.

2. Brown DH, Kasuya A, Leikin JB: Endotracheal drug administration in the critical care setting. *J Emerg Med,* 5:407, 1987.

3. Cordon MJ: *Clinical Calculations for Nurses,* Norwalk, 1990, Appleton and Lange Publishing.

4. Correia MA, Castagnoli N: Pharmacokinetics:II. Drug biotansformation. In Katzung BG (ed): *Basic and Clinical Pharmacology,* Los Altos, 1987, Lange Medical Publishers.

5. Curren AM, Munday LD: *Math for Meds: Dosages and Solutions,* ed 6, San Diego, 1990, Wallcur.

6. Emergency Cardiac Care Committee and Subcommittees, American Heart Association: Guidelines for cardiopulmonary resuscitation and emergency cardiac care, III: Adult advanced cardiac life support. *JAMA,* 268:2199–2241, 1992.

7. Gonsoulin SM, Raynovich W: *Prehospital Drug Therapy,* St. Louis, 1993, Mosby Lifeline.

8. Jaffe JH, Martin WR: Opioid analgesics and antagonists. In Gilman AG, Goodman LS, Gilman A (ed): *The Pharmacologic Basis of Therapeutics,* New York, 1980, Macmillan Publishing.

9. McNamara RM, Spivey WH, Unger HD, et al: Emergency applications of intraosseous infusion. *J Emerg Med,* 5:97, 1987.

10. Miner WF, Corneli HM, Bolte RG: Prehospital use of intraosseous infusion by paramedics. *Pediatr Emerg Care,* 5:5, 1989.

11. Orlowski JP, Porembka DT, Gallagher JM, et al: Comparison study of intravenous, central intravenous, and peripheral intravenous infusions of emergency drugs. *Am J Dis Child,* 144:112, 1990.

12. Rusli M, Spivey WH, Bonner H, et al: Endotracheal diazepam: Absorption and pulmonary pathologic effects. *Ann Emerg Med,* 16:314, 1987.

13. Sackheim GI, Robins L: *Programmed Mathematics for Nurses,* ed 7, New York, 1991, Pergamon Press.

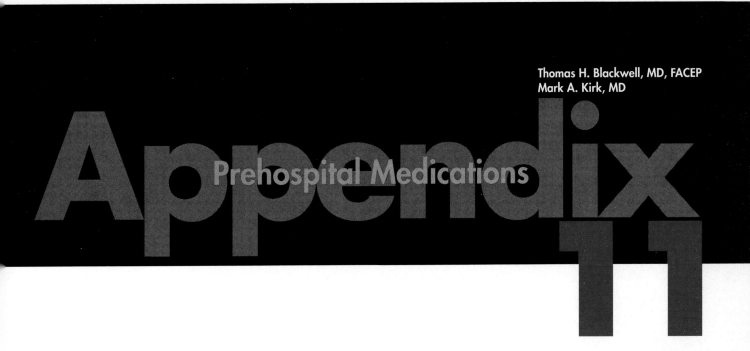

Thomas H. Blackwell, MD, FACEP
Mark A. Kirk, MD

Appendix 11

Prehospital Medications

One of the characteristics that distinguishes paramedics from other prehospital providers is their ability to administer specific medications. Various clinical conditions such as cardiac arrest, congestive heart failure, pulmonary edema, hypoglycemia, and acute bronchospasm may be dramatically improved by early drug administration. To be proficient and competent in this skill, paramedics should be familiar with medications used in the prehospital setting.

The paramedic's scope of practice is clearly dependent on the system in which he or she practices. These medications may be approved by authorities at the state or local levels (i.e., state medical boards, state EMS offices, state or local medical societies or directors). Many states require a minimum medication list that may be expanded by local medical directors. The American College of Emergency Physicians has published a list of medications that have proven beneficial in the field setting. However, further research on these and other medications used by advanced life support (ALS) personnel is necessary to scientifically demonstrate their efficacy.

Lavery and coworkers surveyed 170 EMS systems in 200 cities across the United States to determine which drugs are being used by paramedics. Most ALS systems use the Advanced Cardiac Life Support (ACLS) medications recommended by the American Heart Association (AHA). However, 80 additional medications were reported. Hospital-based services carried the largest number of medications; fire department services carried the least. Government and private services fell in the middle. There appeared to be no correlation between the number of calls answered per year by services, the level of training services required (e.g., ACLS or PALS training), or population of the area served with the number of medications those services carried.

This chapter describes prehospital medications commonly and less frequently used in prehospital patient care. These medications are listed in Box 11-1. These profiles include class, trade name, therapeutic actions, mechanism of action, indications and contraindications, interactions with other drugs, adverse reactions, how they are supplied, and dosages. Dosages are listed for adults (older than 14 years of age) and pediatric patients (under 14 years of age). AHA classification of drugs or therapeutic interventions in emergency cardiac care have also been identified. See Box 11-2 for an explanation of the categories. These profiles may serve as a resource reference for the majority of medications currently used in prehospital care.

BOX 11-1	Prehospital Medication List
Activated charcoal	Lorazepam
Adenosine	Magnesium sulfate
Albuterol	Mannitol
Aminophylline	Meperidine
Aspirin	Metaproterenol
Atropine sulfate	Morphine sulfate
Bretylium tosylate	Naloxone
Calcium chloride	Nitroglycerin
Cyanide antidote kit	Nitrous oxide
Dextrose	Norepinephrine
Diazepam	Oxygen
Diphenhydramine	Oxytocin
Dobutamine	Procainamide
Dopamine	Proparacaine
Droperidol	Propranolol
Epinephrine	Racemic epinephrine
Flumanezil	Sodium bicarbonate
Furosemide	Steroids
Glucagon	Streptokinase
Ipecac (syrup of)	Succinylcholine
Isoetharine	Terbutaline
Isoproterenol	Thiamine
Labetolol	Tissue plasminogen activator
Lidocaine	Verapamil

BOX 11-2   AHA Classifications of Therapeutic Interventions

The 1992 National Conference on CPR and ECG used the following system of classifying interventions, based on the strength of the supporting scientific evidence.

Class I—a therapeutic option that is usually indicated, always acceptable, and considered useful and effective (definitely helpful)

Class II—a therapeutic option that is acceptable, of uncertain efficacy, and may be controversial.

    Class IIa—a therapeutic option for which the weight of evidence is in favor of its usefulness and efficacy (acceptable, probably helpful)

    Class IIb—a therapeutic option that is not well established by evidence but may be helpful and probably not harmful (acceptable, possibly helpful)

Class III—a therapeutic option that is inappropriate, without scientific supporting data, and may be harmful (not indicated, may be harmful)

Source: *The American Heart Association: Textbook of Advanced Cardiac Life Support,* Cummins (ed), 1994.

Activated Charcoal

Class: Adsorbent
Trade Name(s): Acti-Dose, Liqui-Char, Insta-Char
Therapeutic Action: Prevents GI adsorption of various drugs and enhances elimination of particular drugs after adsorption, such as theophylline, phenytoin, carbamazepine, phenobarbital, and aspirin
Mechanism: Binds and adsorbs drugs in GI tract
Indications: Overdose of most ingested medications and poisons
Contraindications: Altered level of consciousness with inability to protect the airway; ingestion of alcohols, heavy metals, or caustics; protracted vomiting; GI bleeding; bowel perforation
Adverse Reactions: Aspiration; nausea; vomiting; diarrhea; constipation
Drug Interactions: None in prehospital setting
How Supplied: Bottles containing 25 or 50 g in powder form or pre-mixed with water or sorbitol
Dosage: Adult and Pediatric: 1 g/kg oral or through gastric tube (doses average 50 to 100 g in adults and 10 to 30 g in pediatrics)

Other Considerations:

Most doses should be diluted with approximately equal volumes of water to increase palatability. Many patients will vomit after charcoal administration, therefore close monitoring is important. If mixed with sorbitol in repeated doses, may cause abdominal cramping and diarrhea. Electrolyte abnormalities and dehydration are a potentially serious problem, especially in children. Charcoal is not effective for toxins absorbed by the inhalational (hydrogen cyanide, carbon monoxide, hydrogen sulfide) or transcutaneous (organophosphates, carbamates) route.

Adenosine

Class: Atrial antidysrhythmic
Trade Name(s): Adenocard
Therapeutic Action: Terminates supraventricular dysrhythmias
Mechanism: Slows conduction of electrical impulses through the sinoatrial (SA) and atrioventricular (AV) node
Indications: Unstable, narrow complex supraventricular tachycardia
Contraindications: Second or third degree heart block; sick sinus syndrome
Adverse Reactions: Transient flushing; dyspnea; chest pain; hemodynamic instability; brief periods of asystole or bradycardia
Drug Interactions: Aminophylline inhibits effects; dipyridamole prolongs effects
How Supplied: 2-mL vials containing 3 mg/mL (6 mg)
Dosage: Adult—6-mg RAPID IV bolus followed by a RAPID 10 mL normal saline flush. If no response in rate noted after 2 minutes, administer 12-mg. If no response in rate noted after 2 minutes, it may be necessary to repeat the 12-mg dose. Each dose is given by rapid IV push at the most proximal port and followed by a 10 mL normal saline flush
Pediatric—Experience is limited, 0.1 mg/kg; may repeat with 0.2 mg/kg up to 12 mg maximum single dose

Other Considerations:

Adenosine is highly effective in terminating acute episodes of paroxysmal supraventricular tachycardia. The drug has similar efficacy as verapamil with fewer adverse reactions. Shortly after adenosine is administered, the cardiac monitor may show a variety of dysrhythmias, including asystole. Due to the short half-life of the drug (5 to 10 seconds), these rhythms are transient and usually do not require intervention. Furthermore, patients who respond may only do so temporarily. Recurrence of the dysrhythmia is common.

Albuterol

Class: Bronchodilator
Trade Name(s): Ventolin, Proventil
Therapeutic Action: Dilates bronchial smooth muscle
Mechanism: Stimulates beta$_2$-adrenergic receptors
Indications: Wheezing due to acute bronchospasm or asthma, COPD exacerbation, Toxic inhalation
Contraindications: None in prehospital setting
Adverse Reactions: Tremor; tachycardia; ventricular ectopy; nervousness; agitation; nausea and vomiting
Drug Interactions: May antagonize beta-adrenergic blockers
How Supplied: For nebulization: solution containing 5 mg/mL or supplied as a unit dose of 2.5 mg in 3 mL normal saline Metered dose inhaler; rotohaler
Dosage: Adult—2.5 mg of 0.5% solution diluted in 2.5 mL normal saline delivered by handheld or mask nebulizer; Metered dose inhaler—2 puffs; Rotohaler—one rotocap
Pediatric—0.01 to 0.03 mL/kg of 0.5% solution diluted in 2 mL normal saline delivered by handheld or mask nebulizer

Other Considerations:

Albuterol may need to be repeated in 10 to 20 minutes when prolonged prehospital times are encountered. Continuous nebulizer therapy should be used when severe bronchospasm is present. Do not withhold in the pregnant asthmatic. Hypoxia is a greater risk to the fetus than the risk of adverse effects from the medication. Small children may respond better to nebulizer.

Aminophylline

Class: Bronchodilator
Trade Name(s): Theophylline
Therapeutic Action: Dilates bronchial smooth muscle and has positive inotropic effects. Cardiac output is increased and peripheral vascular resistance is decreased
Mechanism: Stimulates beta-adrenergic receptors resulting in bronchial wall smooth muscle relaxation and CNS excitation
Indications: Acute COPD exacerbation; asthma
Contraindications: Coronary artery disease; dysrhythmias; peptic ulcer disease; liver or kidney disease; hypersensitivity to xanthene compounds
Adverse Reactions: Cardiac dysrhythmias; tachycardia; hypotension; tremor; nausea; vomiting
Drug Interactions: Will decrease therapeutic effects of propranolol and adenosine
How Supplied: 10-mL ampules and vials containing 25 mg/mL (250 mg)
Dosage: Adult—Loading dose: 4 to 6 mg/kg IV over 20 minutes; Maintenance dose: 0.2 to 0.9 mg/kg per hour
Pediatric—Loading dose: 5 to 7 mg/kg IV over 20 minutes; Maintenance dose: 1 mg/kg per hour

Other Considerations:

All patients receiving aminophylline should have ECG monitoring. Studies have demonstrated that beta-adrenergic agonists (such as albuterol) are safer and more effective than aminophylline in the acute management of asthma. Thus, the popularity of aminophylline use in acute asthma has diminished in recent years. A loading dose should not be given to patients who are currently taking aminophylline or theophylline. If respiratory distress exists and recent drug history is unclear, half the loading dose may be the best option.

Aspirin (Acetylsalicylic Acid [ASA])

Class: Platelet aggregator inhibitor/anti-inflammatory
Trade Name(s): Multiple
Therapeutic Action: Prevents blood clot formation (specifically in coronary arteries), decreases inflammation, controls pain, and decreases fever (antipyretic)
Mechanism: Prevents platelet clumping and blood clot formation by irreversible changes in platelet shape and function. The analgesic, anti-inflammatory, and antipyretic effects are due to blocking prostaglandins. Prostaglandins are chemical messengers that enhance inflammatory responses, enhance pain transmission, and increase body temperature
Indications: Chest pain consistent with acute myocardial infarction
Contraindications: Hypersensitivity to aspirin
Adverse Reactions: Excessive use may cause GI irritation and bleeding
Drug Interactions: Adverse reactions and effects may be increased by concomitant use of other nonsteroidal anti-inflammatory drugs
How Supplied: 325-mg tablets for oral use
Dosage: Adult—160 mg–325 mg by mouth chewed or swallowed with a small amount of water immediately after onset of chest pain
Pediatric—Not recommended

Other Considerations:

Aspirin is also effective as an antipyretic and analgesic although it is not recommended in the prehospital setting for these indications. Aspirin is not used in children because it has been linked to Reye's Syndrome.

Atropine Sulfate

Class: Anticholinergic
Trade Name(s): None
Therapeutic Action: Increases rate of SA node discharge; enhances conduction through the AV junction
Mechanism: Blocks or antagonizes the effects of acetylcholine in the sweat glands, smooth and cardiac muscle
Indications: Symptomatic bradycardia; narrow complex type II 2nd-degree heart block; narrow complex 3rd-degree heart block; slow pulseless electrical activity; asystole; cholinergic poisonings (organophosphates and carbamates)
Contraindications: Wide complex type II 2nd-degree heart block; wide complex 3rd-degree heart block
Adverse Reactions: Tachycardia; dry mouth; dilated pupils; delirium; blurred vision; headache
Drug Interactions: Incompatible with sodium bicarbonate
How Supplied: 10-mL syringe containing 0.1 mg/mL (1 mg)
Dosage: Adult—symptomatic bradycardia: 0.5 to 1.0 mg IV push, repeated every 3 to 5 minutes (maximum dose 0.04 mg/kg or 3 mg)
Adult—pulseless electrical activity and asystole: 1 mg rapid IV push, may repeat dose in 3 to 5 minutes
Adult—cholinergic poisoning: 2 mg IV every 15 minutes
Adult—endotracheal route: 2 to 2.5 times the IV dose, diluted with 1 to 2 mL normal saline or distilled water
Pediatric—symptomatic bradycardia, pulseless electrical activity, and asystole: 0.02 mg/kg rapid IV push (minimum dose 0.1 mg). May repeat dose in 5 minutes (maximum single dose 0.5 mg in child, 1.0 mg in adolescent: maximum total dose of 1.0 mg in child, 2.0 mg in adolescent)
Pediatric—cholinergic poisoning: 2 mg IV every 15 minutes
Pediatric—endotracheal route: 2 times the IV dose, diluted with 1 to 2 mL normal saline or distilled water

Other Considerations:
Administration should be rapid IV push to prevent a reflex bradycardia. In patients experiencing acute myocardial ischemia or infarction, atropine therapy may result in an increase in oxygen demand, thus worsening the ischemia or infarction size.

Bretylium Tosylate

Class: Ventricular Antidysrhythmic
Trade Name(s): Bretylol
Therapeutic Action: Prolongs refractory time and increases conduction in ventricular myocardium, and elevates threshold for ventricular fibrillation
Mechanism: Initially causes a transient increase, then inhibition of norepinephrine release in adrenergic neurons
Indications: Ventricular fibrillation or pulseless ventricular tachycardia, unresponsive to defibrillation, epinephrine, and lidocaine; ventricular tachycardia with a pulse, unresponsive to lidocaine and procainamide; wide complex tachycardia unresponsive to lidocaine and adenosine
Contraindications: None when used for treating life-threatening ventricular dysrhythmias
Adverse Reactions: Hypotension; bradycardia; nausea; vomiting
Drug Interactions: Should not be used in patients taking digoxin
How Supplied: 10-mL vials containing 50 mg/ml (500 mg)
Dosage: Adult—ventricular tachycardia with a pulse: 5 to 10 mg/kg diluted with D_5W to 50 mL administered IV over 8 to 10 minutes; a continuous infusion may be given at 1 to 2 mg per minute
Adult—ventricular fibrillation (or pulseless v.tach): 5 mg/kg IV push. If no response after defibrillation, administer 10 mg/kg; may repeat dose every 5 minutes (maximum dose 30 to 35 mg/kg)
Pediatric—ventricular fibrillation (or pulseless v.tach): 5 mg/kg IV push; if no response after defibrillation, administer 10 mg/kg

Other Considerations:
Bretylium should never be used as a first-line antidysrhythmic agent, but should be used in refractory ventricular tachycardia and ventricular fibrillation unresponsive to defibrillation, epinephrine, and lidocaine. Antidysrhythmic effect for ventricular ectopy is 20 minutes; that plus the hypotensive effect is why bretylium is not frequently used for conscious ventricular tachycardia or suppression of PVCs in the field. Data supporting the use in the pediatric population is unavailable, but may be considered if defibrillation, epinephrine, and lidocaine are ineffective in suppressing ventricular fibrillation.

Calcium Chloride

Class: Electrolyte
Trade Name(s): None
Therapeutic Action: Facilitates conduction in tissues such as nerves, muscles, and cardiac tissue
Mechanism: Increases calcium concentration in blood and tissues
Indications: Hyperkalemia (e.g. renal failure with cardiovascular compromise); hypotension and cardiac dysrhythmias resulting from calcium channel blocker overdose; hypocalcemia (e.g. after multiple blood transfusions); black widow spider envenomations
Contraindications: Digitalis toxicity
Adverse Reactions: Rapid administration may result in bradycardia, hypotension, and syncope
Drug Interactions: Do not mix with sodium bicarbonate, aminophylline
How Supplied: 10-mL vials and prefilled syringes containing 100 mg/mL (1 g)
Dosage: Adult—2 to 4 mg/kg of a 10% solution of calcium chloride slow IV push; may repeat dose every 10 minutes
Pediatric—20 to 25 mg/kg of c 10% solution up to 500 mg slow IV push

Other Considerations:
Calcium is no longer recommended for resuscitation of routine cardiac arrest. Several studies have demonstrated minimal benefit from its use in this setting. Calcium chloride is only recommended for specific circumstances and presently has little or no use in the prehospital setting, except as above.

Cyanide Antidote Kit

Class: Poison antidote
Trade Name(s): Lilly Cyanide Antidote Kit
Therapeutic Action: Detoxifies and eliminates cyanide from the body
Mechanism: Antidote (sodium nitrite) converts hemoglobin into methemoglobin, a form that can bind cyanide. The remaining antidote (sodium thiosulfate) facilitates detoxification and excretion of cyanide
Indications: Any patient with suspected cyanide exposure and signs of toxicity (e.g. industrial accidents, suicide attempts). Signs of cyanide toxicity include unresponsiveness, cardiovascular collapse, and seizures
Contraindications: Sodium nitrite should not be given to patients with suspected cyanide poisoning that are hypotensive or to patients with possible exposure to carbon monoxide
Adverse Reactions: Adverse reactions only to the sodium nitrite portion of the cyanide antidote kit. With rapid administration, it can cause severe hypotension and an increase in methemoglobinemia, a form of hemoglobin that cannot carry oxygen
Drug Interactions: None in prehospital setting
How Supplied: Each kit contains: Two amyl nitrite pearls; sodium nitrite: 10-mL vial of 3% solution (300 mg); sodium thiosulfate: 50-mL vial of 25% solution (12.5 g)
Dosage: Amyl nitrite pearls—Break and inhale for 30 seconds each minute until an IV line is started for the remaining antidotes. Amyl nitrite is unnecessary if an IV line is already established

Sodium nitrite, Adult—300 mg (10-mL) IV over 20 minutes
Pediatric—0.2 mL/kg IV over 20 minutes
Sodium thiosulfate, Adult—12.5 gm (50-mL) IV over 20 minutes
Pediatric—1-mL/kg IV over 20 minutes

Other Considerations:

Antidotes are effective if given separately but work synergistically when administered together. Sodium nitrite may cause hypotension and must be used with caution. Sodium thiosulfate has relatively few side effects and may be given empirically with smoke inhalation when cyanide toxicity is suspected. May be useful in the prehospital setting in areas with a large industrial use of cyanide. A safer cyanide antidote, hydroxocobalamin, is currently undergoing clinical trials in the United States.

Dextrose

Class: Carbohydrate
Trade Name(s): None
Therapeutic Action: Increases serum glucose concentration
Mechanism: Primary energy source distributed by blood to all tissues in the body.
Indications: Hypoglycemia; altered mental status or unresponsiveness; status epilepticus in children
Contraindications: Cerebrovascular accident in presence of normal blood sugar
Adverse Reactions: Tissue damage if extravasation occurs
Drug Interactions: None in prehospital setting
How Supplied: 50 mL syringe 50% dextrose solution (25 g)
Dosage: Adult—25 g (50 mL) IV push
Pediatric greater than 8 years of age—D50% 1 g/kg (2 ml/kg) IV push
Pediatric between 1 year and 8 years—
D25% 0.5–1g/kg (2–4 ml/kg) IV push
D25% produced by diluting 1 part D50% with 1 part sterile water (resulting solution is D25%)
Neonate—
D10% 3–4 ml/kg
D10% produced by diluting 1 part D50% with 4 parts sterile water

Other Considerations:

If available, evaluate blood sugar using a rapid blood glucose test prior to administration of D50%. Otherwise, treat empirically with D50%. Administering glucose will not produce adverse effects if hyperglycemia or diabetic ketoacidosis is present. If no response occurs after an initial bolus, other causes of unresponsiveness should be considered. Hyperglycemia may, however, exacerbate a cerebrovascular accident. Therefore, rapid blood glucose determination should be made on patients with a possible CVA, and D50% withheld if blood glucose is normal or elevated. D50% may precipitate Wernicke-Korsakoff syndrome in thiamine deficient patients, often alcoholics. Consider thiamine administration before dextrose infusion in malnourished or alcoholic patients.

Diazepam

Class: Benzodiazepine
Trade Name(s): Valium
Therapeutic Action: Causes CNS slowing to provide sedation, anticonvulsant effects, and skeletal muscle relaxation
Mechanism: Binds to a specific benzodiazepine receptor in the CNS which inhibits neuronal transmission
Indications: Status epilepticus; severe agitation; alcohol withdrawal syndrome; sedation before cardioversion or external transthoracic pacing
Contraindications: Shock; decreased level of consciousness or unconsciousness; CNS depression from other mind-altering drugs
Adverse Reactions: Respiratory depression or arrest; periods of excitement; hypotension; confusion; prolonged coma
Drug Interactions: Barbiturates or alcohol may worsen CNS and respiratory depression
How Supplied: 2-mL ampules and prefilled syringe containing 5 mg/mL (10 mg)
10 mL ampules containing 5 mg/ml (50 mg)
Dosage: Adult—2 to 5 mg slow IV push; may repeat dose as needed
Pediatric—0.1 mg/kg to 0.3 mg/kg slow IV push (maximum dose 5 mg in the infant, 15 mg in the child)
0.5 mg/kg rectally every 10–15 minutes, up to 3 doses

Other Considerations:

Some physicians prefer valium (0.3 mg/kg to 0.5 mg/kg) to be given rectally in the pediatric patient. Diazepam has an active metabolite that may accumulate and lead to a higher incidence of side effects, specifically respiratory depression. Therefore, emergent airway support must be available following drug administration. Dosage should be reduced in the elderly to prevent severe CNS depression. IV Diazepam reacts with other drugs and therefore should be given alone through a thoroughly flushed line, and close to the IV insertion site.

Diphenhydramine

Class: Antihistamine
Trade Name(s): Benadryl
Therapeutic Action: Prevents responses mediated by histamine such as vasodilatation, bronchospasm, capillary permeability, and edema
Mechanism: Blocks cellular histamine response
Indications: Allergic reactions; anaphylactic shock; drug-induced dystonic reactions
Contraindications: Patients exhibiting anticholinergic syndrome (hot flushed skin, dilated pupils, dry mucous membranes, and hallucinations); asthma (will thicken the bronchial secretions); narrow angle glaucoma
Adverse Reactions: Dizziness; sedation; anticholinergic syndrome; blurred vision; wheezing
Drug Interactions: Ethanol, anticholinergic drugs

How Supplied: 10-mL vials and prefilled syringe containing 10 mg/mL (100 mg)

30-mL vials containing 10 mg/mL (300 mg)

25- and 50-mg capsules

Dosage: Adults—25 to 50 mg IM, IV, or orally

Pediatrics—1 to 2 mg/kg IM or IV

Other Considerations:

Patients presenting with life-threatening anaphylactic reactions should be given epinephrine as a first-line medication. Diphenhydramine may subsequently be used if signs and symptoms of shock improve.

Dobutamine

Class: Catecholamine

Trade Name(s): Dobutrex

Therapeutic Action: Increases the Contractile force of the heart and dilates peripheral vasculature

Mechanism: Stimulates beta-adrenergic receptors

Indications: Cardiogenic shock; congestive heart failure

Contraindications: Known idiopathic hypertrophic subaortic stenosis (IHSS); prior hypersensitivity reaction

Adverse Reactions: Dysrhythmias; tachycardia; hypotension; headache; nausea; tremors

Drug Interactions: Incompatible with aminophylline, calcium chloride, and epinephrine

How Supplied: 20-mL vials containing 12.5 mg/mL (250 mg)

Dosage: Adult and Pediatric—prepared by diluting 500 mg in 500 mL D$_5$W to achieve 500 mcg/mL: 2 to 20 mcg/kg per minute IV infusion

Other Considerations:

Dobutamine may produce peripheral vasodilatation resulting in hypotension. It has a limited role, if any, in the prehospital setting. It may be used with caution in patients experiencing an MI due to the possibility of aggravating myocardial injury. Doses should be titrated to avoid significant increases in heart rate in these patients.

Dopamine

Class: Sympathomimetic amine

Trade Name(s): Dopastat, Intropin

Therapeutic Action: At lower doses (1 to 2 mcg/kg per minute), causes dilation of renal and mesenteric vasculature; at moderate doses (2 to 10 mcg/kg per minute), causes increase in heart rate and myocardial contractility; at high doses (greater than 10 mcg/kg per minute), causes peripheral vasoconstriction and hypertension

Mechanism: Alpha-, beta-, and dopaminergic receptor stimulation

Indications: Cardiogenic shock; hypotension associated with congestive heart failure; hypotension unresponsive to fluid therapy

Contraindications: Hypovolemic shock

Adverse Reactions: Chest pain; palpitations; tachycardia; dyspnea; headache; nausea; vomiting; tissue damage may occur with extravasation

Drug Interactions: Incompatible with sodium bicarbonate

How Supplied: 5-mL ampules containing 40 mg/mL (200 mg) or 80 mg/mL (400 mg)

Dosage: Adult and Pediatric prepared in one of the following concentrations:

1. 200 mg diluted in 250 mL of D$_5$W = 800 micrograms/mL
2. 400 mg diluted in 250 mL of D$_5$W = 1600 micrograms/mL
3. 800 mg diluted in 500 mL of D$_5$W = 1600 micrograms/mL
4. 800 mg diluted in 250 mL of D$_5$W = 3200 micrograms/mL; 2 to 20 mcg/kg per minute IV infusion: dose is titrated until desired effect is achieved

Other Considerations:

In hypovolemic shock states, intravascular volume expansion with IV fluid must be the first-line treatment. Dopamine should be considered early in patients presenting with symptoms of congestive heart failure and hypotension (cardiogenic shock). Dosage should be reduced ten fold for patients receiving MAO inhibitors.

Droperidol

Class: Neuroleptic

Trade Name(s): Inapsine

Therapeutic Action: sedation, tranquilization, anti-emetic

Mechanism: Dopaminergic and mild alpha-adrenergic blockade

Indications: chemical restraint, intractable vomiting

Contraindications: Systolic BP less than 100 mmHg; suspected acute MI; known liver or kidney disease; known Parkinson's disease; respiratory depression

Adverse Reactions: hypotension, tachycardia, extrapyramidal reactions, neuroleptic malignant syndrome (high fever, muscle rigidity); laryngospasm; bronchospasm

Drug Interactions: may have additive effects with sedatives, tranquilizers, or narcotics

How Supplied: 2 ml vials containing 2.5 mg/ml (5 mg)

Dosage: Adult—Chemical restraint; 5 mg slow IV push (may be repeated once in 10–15 minutes, if desired effect is not achieved)

Anti-emetic: 1.25 mg slow IV push

Pediatric—Anti-emetic: 0.05–0.1 mg/kg slow IV push

Other Considerations:

Although extra-pyramidal reactions are uncommon (<1%), if the reaction occurs, diphenhydramine (benadryl) will usually rapidly reverse the side effect. Hypotension and tachycardia are usually self-limited and correctable by placing the patient supine and administering fluid.

Epinephrine

Class: Catecholamine
Trade Name(s): Adrenalin
Therapeutic Action: Vasoconstriction, bronchodilatation, increase in heart rate, and force of myocardial contraction
Mechanism: Sympathomimetic that stimulates alpha- and beta-adrenergic receptors
Indications: Cardiac arrest: Pulseless ventricular tachycardia; ventricular fibrillation; pulseless electrical activity; asystole; anaphylactic reactions; bronchospasm
Contraindications: Suspected intracranial hemorrhage; bronchospasm in patients with coronary artery disease
Adverse Reactions: Palpitations; tachycardia; ventricular ectopy; hypotension; tremors; anxiety; headache; cerebral hemorrhage; nausea; vomiting
Drug Interactions: Antagonizes the effects of vasodilators, adrenergic blockers, and antidiabetic medications. Inactivated by aminophylline, calcium chloride and gluconate, diazepam, and sodium bicarbonate.
How Supplied: 1-mL ampules containing 1 mg/mL of 1:1000 concentration (1 mg)
10-mL vials containing 0.1 mg/mL of 1:10,000 concentration (1 mg)
Dosage: Adult, cardiac arrest (pulseless ventricular tachycardia, ventricular fibrillation, pulseless electrical activity, asystole)—1 mg (10 mL) 1:10,000 IV push; may repeat dose every 3 to 5 minutes
Adult, anaphylaxis, bronchospasm—0.1 to 0.5 mg (0.1 to 0.5 mL, respectively) 1:1000 SQ; may repeat dose in 5 minutes; if no response noted and patient is rapidly deteriorating, administer 0.25 to 0.5 mg (2.5 to 5 mL, respectively) 1:10,000 slow IV push; may repeat dose in 5 minutes
Adult endotracheal route—2 mg 1:1,000 diluted with 10 ml normal saline (2 to 2.5 times the IV dose)
Pediatric cardiac arrest: (pulseless ventricular tachycardia, ventricular fibrillation, pulseless electrical activity, asystole)—First dose: 0.01 mg/kg (0.1 mL/kg) 1:10,000 IV push or intraosseous; subsequent doses: 0.1 mg/kg (0.1 ml/kg) 1:1,000 IV push; may repeat dose every 5 minutes if patient remains pulseless
Pediatric, anaphylaxis, bronchospasm—0.01 to 0.03 mg/kg (0.01 to 0.03 mL/kg, respectively) 1:1,000 SQ (maximum dose 0.3 mg)
Pediatric, endotracheal route—0.1 mg/kg (0.1 mL/kg) 1:1000 diluted 1:1 with normal saline

Other Considerations:

Recent studies suggest outcome from cardiac arrest is not affected by administering higher doses of epinephrine and is considered Class IIb for use after the initial dose. Further studies are needed to fully evaluate this modality. Use extreme caution in administering epinephrine to patients with coronary artery disease in nonarrest situations.

Flumanzenil

Class: Benzodiazepine antagonist
Trade Name(s): Romazicon, Mazicon
Therapeutic Action: Reverses the CNS depressant effects of benzodiazepines
Mechanism: Acts at central nervous system receptors to block (antagonize) the effects of benzodiazepines
Indications: Benzodiazepine toxicity
Contraindications: Seizure disorder; ingestion of seizure inducing toxins; ingestion of cyclic antidepressants; benzodiazepine dependency
Adverse Reactions: Seizures; benzodiazepine withdrawal; agitation; nausea; vomiting; dizziness
Drug Interactions: None in prehospital setting
How Supplied: 5-mL vials containing 0.1mg/mL (0.5 mg)
10-mL vials containing 0.1 mg/mL (1 mg)
Dosage: Adult—0.2 mg IV over 30 seconds. After 30 seconds, administer 0.3 mg over 30 seconds; may repeat dose at 0.5 mg every minute (maximum dose 3 mg)
Pediatric—10 mg/kg IV (maximum 2 doses)

Other Considerations:

Unlike naloxone, flumazenil has a very limited role in the prehospital setting. May precipitate life-threatening benzodiazepine withdrawal in some patients. Contraindicated in overdoses where tricyclic antidepressants are involved because seizures may be precipitated. Effects of drug are short lived and repeated doses are usually necessary. If there is potential for patient to have seizures (result of overdose, head injury, seizure disorder), then flumazenil should not be used because benzodiazepines will then be ineffective for treating the seizure.

Furosemide

Class: Diuretic
Trade Name(s): Lasix
Therapeutic Action: Increases water excretion and venous dilatation
Mechanism: Inhibits sodium and chloride reabsorption in the kidney
Indications: Pulmonary edema; congestive heart failure; hypertension
Contraindications: Hypotension; pregnancy; history of no urine production
Adverse Reactions: Volume depletion; hypotension; electrolyte disturbances (especially potassium depletion); rash; headache; deafness; cardiac dysrhythmias
Drug Interactions: Incompatible with diazepam, diphenhydramine, and thiamine
How Supplied: 2-mL ampules and prefilled syringes containing 10 mg/mL (20 mg)
4-mL ampules and prefilled syringes containing 10 mg/mL (40 mg)
10-mL ampules containing 10 mg/mL (100 mg)
Dosage: Adult—20 to 40 mg slow IV push (0.5 to 1.0 mg/kg) given over 1–2 minutes
Pediatric—1 to 2 mg/kg slow IV push (maximum dose 6 mg/kg)

Other Considerations:

Patients taking furosemide as an outpatient may require a larger dose to achieve the desired effect in the acute setting. Cardiac monitoring should be performed due to potential electrolyte disturbances. The onset of venous dilation is 5 minutes and the onset of urine production is 15 to 20 minutes.

Glucagon

Class: Hormone
Trade Name(s): None
Therapeutic Action: Stimulates the release of glucose from the liver, muscle, and adipose tissue into the bloodstream.
Mechanism: Directly binds to target cells in the liver and counteracts the effects of insulin
Indications: Hypoglycemic reactions
Contraindications: Pregnancy; pheochromocytoma (adrenal gland tumor)
Adverse Reactions: Headache; allergic reactions; nausea
Drug Interactions: None in prehospital setting
How Supplied: 1-mL vials containing 1 mg/mL (1 mg) 10-mL vials containing 1 mg/mL (10 mg)
Dosage: Adult—0.5 to 1 mg SQ, IM, or IV; may repeat dose in 20 minutes.
Pediatric—0.1 to 0.3 mg/kg SQ, IM, or IV

Other Considerations:

Glucagon allows an additional method of treating hypoglycemia, especially when unable to obtain IV access. Its effects are not immediate. It is recommended that a rapid blood glucose determination be done prior to administration, although the drug may be given empirically if this test is not available. Glucagon improves cardiac contractility and increases heart rate in beta-adrenergic blocker and calcium channel blocker toxicity. Do not mix with saline.

(Syrup Of) Ipecac

Class: Emetic
Trade Name(s): None
Therapeutic Action: Promotes vomiting to evacuate stomach contents
Mechanism: Stimulates the vomiting center in the CNS and acts locally as an irritant on gastric mucosa
Indications: Induction of vomiting in conscious patients with acute, potentially toxic ingestions
Contraindications: Decreased level of consciousness or coma; seizures; caustics (acids and alkalis); hydrocarbons; nontoxic ingestions
Adverse Reactions: Persistent vomiting; lethargy; aspiration
Drug Interactions: Activated charcoal may bind ipecac and decrease its efficacy
How Supplied: 15- and 30-mL unit doses as a syrup
Dosage: Adult—30 mL PO

Pediatric—6 months to 1 year: 10-mL po; 1 to 5 years: 15-mL po; greater than 5 years: 30-mL po; all doses should be followed by 1 to 2 glasses of water; may repeat dose in 30 minutes if emesis has not occurred

Other Considerations:

Should not be administered to patients who have taken a drug which has the potential to produce altered levels of consciousness or seizures. Syrup of Ipecac has an important role in the home management of poisoning. It should have a limited role in prehospital poisoning management because studies have shown activated charcoal to be more effective in preventing toxin absorption.

Isoetharine

Class: Bronchodilator
Trade Name(s): Bronkosol, Bronkometer
Therapeutic Action: Dilates bronchial smooth muscle
Mechanism: Stimulates beta$_2$-adrenergic receptors
Indications: Wheezing due to acute bronchospasm or asthma; COPD exacerbation; toxic inhalation
Contraindications: Hypersensitivity to the drug; use with caution in patients with hypertension and coronary artery disease
Adverse Reactions: Tremor; tachycardia; nervousness; agitation; nausea; vomiting; headache
Drug Interactions: May antagonize beta-adrenergic blockers
How Supplied: For nebulization—assorted vials containing assorted percentage solutions (most common: 2.5-mg and 5-mg vials)
Metered dose inhaler
Dosage: Adult—0.5 mL of 1% solution diluted in 2.5 mL normal saline delivered by hand held or mask nebulizer; metered dose inhaler: 2 puffs
Pediatric—0.01 to 0.03 mL/kg diluted in 2 mL normal saline delivered by hand held or mask nebulizer

Other Considerations:

Isoetharine may need to be repeated in 30 minutes when prolonged prehospital times are encountered. Continuous nebulizer therapy should be used when severe bronchospasm is present. Do not withhold in the pregnant asthmatic. Hypoxia is a greater risk to the fetus than the risk of adverse effects from the medication. Small children may respond better to nebulizer.

Isoproterenol

Class: Sympathomimetic
Trade Name(s): Isuprel
Therapeutic Action: Produces bronchodilatation, increase in heart rate, and decrease in peripheral vascular resistance
Mechanism: Stimulates beta-adrenergic receptors

Indications: Complete heart block; symptomatic bradycardia unresponsive to atropine; refractory Torsades de Pointes (a rare variation of ventricular tachycardia); bronchospasm

Contraindications: Dysrhythmias; coronary artery disease

Adverse Reactions: Tachycardia; palpitations; restlessness; tremor; nausea; vomiting; ventricular irritability; hypotension

Drug Interactions: Increases potential dysrhythmic effect of epinephrine and digitalis

How Supplied: 1-mL ampules containing 0.2 mg/mL (0.2 mg)

5-mL ampules containing 0.2 mg/mL (1 mg)

Dosage: Adult—2.0 to 10 mcg per minute IV infusion. Preparation: mix 1 mg in 500 mL D$_5$W or 2 mg in 1000 mL (2 mcg/mL); titrate to heart rate and rhythm response. Avoid heart rates greater than 130 beats per minute. Higher doses may lead to ventricular tachycardia or ventricular fibrillation Pediatric—0.1 mcg/kg per minute IV infusion (maximum dose 1.0 mcg/kg per minute)

Other Considerations:

No longer a first-line drug according to ACLS protocols. Instead of isoproterenol, epinephrine has been suggested for severe bradycardia unresponsive to usual therapies. It is only indicated in the unusual setting of the bradycardia patient with a heart transplant. It is only to be used as a temporary treatment until transcutaneous or IV pacing can be accomplished. Isoproterenol is considered a Class IIb intervention in low doses; at higher doses it is considered a Class III intervention. When titrating dose, avoid heart rates greater than 130 beats per minute. May induce myocardial ischemia or dysrhythmias (especially ventricular). It has little, if any role in the prehospital setting.

Labetolol

Class: Alpha- and beta-adrenergic blocker

Trade Name(s): Normodyne, Trandate

Therapeutic Action: Decreases heart rate and blood pressure

Mechanism: Competes for alpha- and beta-adrenergic receptors

Indications: Hypertensive emergencies; accelerated hypertension in acute myocardial infarction; hypertensive encephalopathy; unstable angina; acute renal failure

Contraindications: Hypotension; congestive heart failure; heart block; asthma/COPD; pheochromocytoma (adrenal gland tumor)

Adverse Reactions: Orthostatic hypotension; ventricular dysrhythmias; bradycardia; heartblock; bronchospasm; pulmonary edema

Drug Interactions: Decreases the effect of beta-adrenergic bronchodilators

How Supplied: 4-mL syringes containing 5 mg/mL (20 mg) 8-mL syringes containing 5 mg/mL (40 mg)

20- or 40-mL vials containing 5 mg/mL (100 mg and 200 mg, respectively)

Dosage: Adult—Do not recommend infusions in field; initial bolus of 20 mg IV over 2 minutes; may repeat dose at 40 mg in 10 minutes, then 80-mg in another 10 minutes until desired blood pressure is obtained; may repeat 80-mg dose until a maximum dose of 300 mg is administered

Other Considerations:

Labetolol is rarely used in the prehospital setting due to significant side effects. The onset of action is 5 to 10 minutes with maximum decrease in blood pressure noted within 30 minutes. The advantage of using this IV agent is that it can be changed to oral therapy after initial control of blood pressure. The patient must be closely monitored for cardiovascular and respiratory changes during administration. Patient must be supine during and for at least 3 hours after administration due to orthostatic hypotension.

Lidocaine

Class: Ventricular antidysrhythmic

Trade Name(s): Xylocaine

Therapeutic Action: Suppresses ventricular ectopy and increases fibrillation threshold

Mechanism: Decreases automaticity and refractory period in cardiac tissue

Indications: Pulseless ventricular tachycardia; stable ventricular tachycardia; ventricular fibrillation; ventricular ectopy in the presence of acute myocardial infarction; wide complex tachycardia of undetermined origin

Contraindications: Allergies to amide anesthetics (bupivicaine); ventricular escape rhythm

Adverse Reactions: Drowsiness; numbness and tingling; disorientation; convulsions; coma; respiratory arrest

Drug Interactions: None in prehospital setting

How Supplied: 5-mL prefilled syringe containing 20 mg/mL (100 mg) for IV push

50-mL prefilled syringe containing 1 or 2 g for infusion

Dosage: Adult—1.0 to 1.5 mg/kg IV over 2 to 3 minutes; may repeat dose at 0.5 to 1.5 mg/kg every 5 to 10 minutes (maximum dose 3 mg/kg); when dysrhythmia is controlled, a continuous infusion may be used to prevent recurrence. Prepare for continuous infusion by adding 2 g of lidocaine to 500 mL D$_5$W

Adult continuous infusion—2 to 4 mg per minute

Adult endotracheal route—2 mg/kg diluted with 10 mL normal saline

Pediatric—1.0 mg/kg IV over 2 to 3 minutes (maximum dose 1.5 mg/kg)

Pediatric continuous infusion—20 to 50 mcg/kg per minute

Pediatric endotracheal route—2 mg/kg diluted 1:1 with normal saline

Other Considerations:

Lidocaine reduces the incidence of ventricular fibrillation in the setting of acute myocardial infarction; however, lidocaine administration is no longer recommended in uncomplicated myocardial infarction without associated ventricular ectopy. Ventricular escape rhythms associated with bradycardia or high-grade heart block should not be treated with lidocaine.

Suppressing a ventricular escape rhythm may be fatal. The use of bolus lidocaine therapy to achieve therapeutic levels during cardiac arrest is now considered a standard approach (Class IIa). Once the dysrhythmia is controlled and perfusion restored, a continuous infusion may be used. Dosage may need to be decreased in the elderly patient as well as those with liver disease and CHF.

Lorazepam

Class: Benzodiazepine
Trade Name(s): Ativan
Therapeutic Action: Causes CNS slowing to provide sedation, anticonvulsant effects, and skeletal muscle relaxation
Mechanism: Binds to a specific benzodiazepine receptor in the CNS which inhibits neuronal transmission
Indications: Status epilepticus; severe agitation; alcohol withdrawal syndrome; sedation before cardioversion or external transthoracic pacing
Contraindications: Shock; decreased level of consciousness or unconsciousness; CNS depression from other mind-altering drugs; acute narrow angle glaucoma
Adverse Reactions: Respiratory depression or arrest; dizziness; periods of excitement; hypotension; confusion; prolonged coma
Drug Interactions: Additive effects with alcohol, barbiturates, antidepressants phenothiazines, and narcotics may worsen CNS and respiratory depression
How Supplied: 1-mL or 10-mL vials and prefilled syringe containing 2 mg/mL or 4 mg/mL, respectively
Dosage: Adult—2 to 4 mg slow IV push or IM; may be repeated every 15 to 20 minutes
Pediatric—0.05 mg/kg to maximum of 2.0 mg/kg dose slow IV push

Other Considerations:
Lorazepam is as effective as diazepam in stopping seizure activity and controlling agitation. Lorazepam has no active metabolite but has a duration of action longer than diazepam in controlling seizures.

Magnesium Sulfate

Class: Electrolyte
Trade Name(s): None
Therapeutic Action: Stops convulsive seizures associated with preeclampsia; CNS depressant
Mechanism: Increases intracellular potassium and alters calcium's effect on conduction
Indications: Seizures associated with toxemia of pregnancy (eclampsia); Torsades de Pointes (a rare variation of ventricular tachycardia); asthma
Contraindications: Kidney failure; heart block; respiratory depression
Adverse Reactions: Hypotension, respiratory depression or arrest

Drug Interactions: May interfere with effects of neuromuscular blocking agents and calcium
How Supplied: Vials containing 10% or 50% solutions Syringes containing 50% solutions
Dosage: Adult—Eclamptic seizures: 1 g per minute IV (maximum dose 4 g); Cardiac dysrhythmias: 1 to 2 g in 100 mL D_5W over 1 to 2 minutes; Asthma: 1 to 2 gms in 100 mL D_5W over 1 to 2 minutes
Pediatric—25 to 50 mg/kg IV over 3 to 5 minutes

Other Considerations:
Prehospital indications are typically limited to toxemia associated seizures. It may be used for asthma not responsive to three nebulizers during long transports. Despite enthusiasm for the use of magnesium in the treatment of myocardial ischemia, myocardial infarction, and cardiac dysrhythmias, data is inadequate to support its use as a first-line agent. Therefore, its role in the prehospital setting is limited. Calcium chloride should be available as an antidote if respiratory depression occurs.

Mannitol

Class: Diuretic
Trade Name(s): Osmitrol
Therapeutic Action: Decreases cerebral edema and intracranial pressure
Mechanism: Causes osmotic diuresis by drawing water from tissues and elimination through the kidneys
Indications: Cerebral edema resulting from head trauma
Contraindications: Hypovolemia; congestive heart failure; use with caution in patients with renal failure
Adverse Reactions: Produces hypovolemia by increasing water excretion from kidneys; may cause fluid overload, pulmonary edema; hypotension
Drug Interactions: Incompatible with sodium chloride
How Supplied: 50-mL vials and syringes containing 25% solution (12.5 g)
Dosage: Adult—1 to 2 g/kg of 25% solution IV over 5 to 10 minutes
Pediatric—0.25 gm/kg of 25% solution IV

Other Considerations:
The role of mannitol in cerebral edema is to dehydrate the brain. Cerebral edema is initially due to dilated blood vessels and not cellular edema, therefore the primary treatment should be intubation and hyperventilation.

Meperidine

Class: Narcotic analgesic
Trade Name(s): Demerol
Therapeutic Action: Produces analgesia, euphoria, and sedation

Mechanism: Binds opioid receptors in the CNS which results in a decrease in pain transmission

Indications: Severe pain from etiologies such as fractures, kidney stones, or burns

Contraindications: Respiratory depression or respiratory distress; head trauma; acute bronchospasm or asthma; hypovolemia; shock; abdominal pain of unknown etiology; sickle cell anemia; patients taking MAO inhibitors

Adverse Reactions: CNS depression; respiratory depression; bronchospasm; hypotension; nausea; vomiting

Drug Interactions: Other respiratory depressants; patients taking MAO inhibitor drugs

How Supplied: Ampules and vials containing various volumes of either 25, 50, or 100 mg/mL

Dosage: Adult—50 to 100 mg IM; 25 to 50 mg IV
Pediatric—1 to 1.5 mg/kg IM; 1 mg/kg IV

Other Considerations:

Meperidine is highly addictive; however, this alone is not a contraindication for its use in the prehospital setting. Analgesia resulting from trauma is indicated if the injury only involves an isolated extremity, because meperidine may potentially mask pain associated with chest or abdominal trauma. When meperidine is used, the patient's respiratory status must be carefully monitored. Toxicity from overadministration responds to naloxone.

Metaproterenol

Class: Bronchodilator

Trade Name(s): Alupent, Metaprel

Therapeutic Action: Dilates bronchial smooth muscle

Mechanism: Stimulates beta$_2$-adrenergic receptors

Indications: Wheezing due to acute bronchospasm or asthma; COPD exacerbation; toxic inhalation

Contraindications: tachydysrhythmias

Adverse Reactions: Tremor; tachycardia; nervousness; agitation; nausea; vomiting; ventricular ectopy

Drug Interactions: May antagonize beta-adrenergic blockers

How Supplied: For nebulization—10-mL vial containing 5% solution (500 mg)
Metered dose inhaler

Dosage: Adult—0.3 mL of 5% solution diluted in 2.5 mL normal saline delivered by handheld or mask nebulizer; Metered dose inhaler: 2 puffs
Pediatric—0.1 mL diluted in normal saline to 3 mL total volume, delivered by handheld or mask nebulizer

Other Considerations:

Metaproterenol may need to be repeated in 30 minutes when prolonged prehospital times are encountered. Continuous nebulizer therapy should be used when severe bronchospasm is present. Do not withhold in the pregnant asthmatic. Hypoxia is a greater risk to the fetus than the risk of adverse effects from the medication. Small children may respond better to nebulizer.

Morphine Sulfate

Class: Narcotic analgesic

Trade Name(s): Duramorph, Astramorph

Therapeutic Action: Analgesic, CNS depressant. Also causes peripheral venous dilatation which may decrease pulmonary edema and myocardial oxygen requirements

Mechanism: Binds opioid receptors in the CNS which results in a decrease in pain transmission

Indications: Pulmonary edema; pain relief from acute myocardial infarction; pain from etiologies such as isolated fractures, kidney stones, or burns

Contraindications: Respiratory depression or respiratory distress; head injury; acute bronchospasm or asthma; hypovolemia; shock; acute abdominal pain of unknown etiology

Adverse Reactions: CNS depression; respiratory depression or arrest; bronchospasm; hypotension; nausea; vomiting

Drug Interactions: Other respiratory depressants

How Supplied: 10 mL ampules and vials containing 0.5 mg/mL (5 mg)
10 mL ampules and vials containing 1.0 mg/mL (10 mg)

Dosage: Adult—2 to 10 mg IV push slowly; may repeat at smaller doses every 5 to 10 minutes to titrate for pain relief
Pediatric—0.1 to 0.2 mg/kg IV push slowly every 2 to 4 hours for pain relief (maximum dose 15 mg)

Other Considerations:

Morphine is highly addictive; however, this alone is not a contraindication for its use in the prehospital setting. Analgesia resulting from trauma is indicated if the injury only involves an isolated extremity because morphine may potentially mask pain associated with chest or abdominal trauma. When morphine is used, the patient's respiratory status must be carefully monitored. Toxicity from overadministration responds to naloxone.

Naloxone

Class: Narcotic antagonist

Trade Name(s): Narcan

Therapeutic Action: Reverses the effects of narcotics

Mechanism: Blocks opioid receptors which prevents narcotics from binding

Indications: Narcotic overdose; unresponsiveness of unknown etiology

Contraindications: Known hypersensitivity to naloxone

Adverse Reactions: May precipitate opioid withdrawal syndrome (anxiety, agitation, gastrointestinal distress, and yawning); pulmonary edema, severe agitation; hypertension have been reported

Drug Interactions: None in prehospital setting

How Supplied: 1-mL ampules or prefilled syringe containing 0.4 mg/L (0.4 mg)
2-mL ampules or prefilled syringe containing 1 mg/mL (2 mg)

Dosage: Adult—2 mg IV, IM, or SQ. May repeat dose every 2 to 3 minutes (maximum dose 10 mg)

Adult endotracheal route (less effective than other routes)—4 mg diluted with 10 mL normal saline

Pediatric—0.01 mg/kg IV, IM, or SQ; may repeat dose at 0.1 mg/kg if initial dose is ineffective

Pediatric endotracheal route—0.2 mg/kg diluted 1:1 with normal saline

Other Considerations:

Naloxone administration for an overdose associated with heroin or other narcotic analgesics may precipitate acute agitation or violent behavior and should be administered slowly while observing patient's level of consciousness and respiratory status. Personal safety is a consideration in this setting. Naloxone will remain effective in the body for only 30 to 60 minutes, therefore repeat doses may be required during prolonged transport times.

Nitroglycerin

Class: Vasodilator

Trade Name(s): Nitrostat, Nitrolingual

Therapeutic Action: Systemic arterial and venous dilatation which reduces work and oxygen demand on the heart

Mechanism: Relaxes vascular smooth muscle

Indications: Chest pain suspected to be of myocardial origin; congestive heart failure; pulmonary edema; hypertension

Contraindications: Hypotension; CNS hemorrhage

Adverse Reactions: Hypotension; headache; syncope; facial flushing; and nausea

Drug Interactions: Must be used with caution when combined with other medications that potentially cause hypotension

How Supplied: Sublingual aerosol canister delivers 0.4 mg/spray

Sublingual tablets—0.15, 0.3, 0.4, and 0.6 mg

Intravenous: 5-mL ampules containing 5 mg/mL (25 mg); 10-mL ampules containing 0.5 mg/mL (5 mg); 10-mL ampules containing 5 mg/mL (50 mg)

Dosage: Adults—1 to 2 sprays sublingual every 3 to 5 minutes or 1 tablet sublingual every 5 minutes, maximum 3 administrations

Continuous infusion: 5 mcg per minute IV, titrating for pain relief or adverse effects (predominantly hypotension); the infusion may be increased 5 mcg per minute every 3–5 minutes to achieve the desired effect

Pediatric—Not recommended

Other Considerations:

Sublingual administration is highly recommended by some for acute pain relief from angina. Sublingual spray has advantages of stability, ease of use, and more rapid onset of action. The IV route is recommended in the hospital for minute-to-minute control of pain from myocardial ischemia, although much less practical in the field. Nitroglycerin tablets should be protected from light; deterioration results from repeated exposure to light, air, and temperature extremes. A bitter taste and subsequent headache usually indicates that the tablet is still effective.

Nitrous Oxide

Class: Inhaled analgesic and anesthetic

Trade Name(s): Nitronox

Therapeutic Action: Pain relief and sedation

Mechanism: CNS anesthetic and analgesic

Indications: Pain associated with isolated fractures, burns, acute myocardial infarction, kidney stones, or labor

Contraindications: Shock; COPD; altered mental status; head injury; diving accidents; uncooperative patients or patients incapable of administering the medication to themselves; any injury or disease process where the potential for pneumothorax or bowel obstruction exists

Adverse Reactions: Hypotension and bradycardia in patients with coronary artery disease; junctional rhythm; increased intracranial pressure; excessive sedation; nausea; vomiting

Drug Interactions: None in prehospital setting

How Supplied: Cylinders containing 50:50 mixture of O_2 and N_2O with a patient-regulated demand valve; mixtures may vary depending on altitude

Dosage: Adult and Pediatric—The patient controls the amount of gas administered by a patient-regulated demand valve. The paramedic should not attempt to hold the mask in place. Dosing is totally dependent on the patient who may choose to stop at any time. The end-point of administration is subjective relief of pain

Other Considerations:

Nitrous oxide should not be used for pain associated with trauma if the chest or abdomen is involved. Due to potential effects on personnel, the ambulance should be well ventilated when using this medication. Because the gas only lasts 2 to 5 minutes, this is an effective prehospital analgesic for some patients.

Norepinephrine

Class: Vasoactive catecholamine

Trade Name(s): Levophed

Therapeutic Action: Increases blood pressure, heart rate, and produces peripheral vasoconstriction

Mechanism: Primarily stimulates alpha receptors with some beta-adrenergic receptor stimulation

Indications: Severe hypotension, refractory to high dose dopamine therapy; post-cardiac arrest hypotension

Contraindications: Hypovolemia

Adverse Reactions: Increases myocardial oxygen demand and produces myocardial ischemia; extravasation results in ischemic necrosis and sloughing of tissue

Drug Interactions: Additive effect when used with other vasopressors; incompatible with aminophylline, phenytoin, and sodium bicarbonate

How Supplied: 4-mL ampules containing 1 mg/mL (4 mg)

Dosage: Adult—prepared by mixing 4 mg norephinephrine in 500 mL D_5W

Continuous IV infusion: 0.5 to 1.0 mcg per minute IV, titrating to a desired effect
Pediatric—0.1 to 1.0 mcg/kg per minute IV

Other Considerations:
Norepinephrine causes vasoconstriction of kidney and mesenteric blood vessels as opposed to dopamine, which dilates kidney and mesenteric vessels at low doses. Alkaline solutions, such as sodium bicarbonate, in the same IV line may inactivate norepinephrine.

Oxygen

Class: Gas
Trade Name(s): None
Therapeutic Action: Adjunct for cellular respiration and function
Mechanism: Distributed and directly used by all tissues
Indications: Any patient complaining of chest pain or shortness of breath; hypoxemia from any cause (e.g., shock and cardiac or respiratory arrest); respiratory emergencies (e.g., asthma, COPD exacerbation, pulmonary edema, or toxic inhalation); cardiovascular emergencies (e.g., myocardial infarction, shock, or congestive heart failure); neurologic diseases (e.g., coma, status seizures, or head trauma); multiple trauma; suspected carbon monoxide toxicity
Contraindications: None in prehospital setting
Adverse Reactions: None
Drug Interactions: None
How Supplied: Cylinder
Dosage: Adult and Pediatric—Nasal cannula: 1 to 15 liters per minute provides 24 to 44% O_2; Simple face mask: 10 to 12 liters per minute provides 40 to 60% O_2; Nonrebreathing mask with reservoir: 10 to 15 liters per minute provides 60 to 100% O_2; Venturi mask: Available to provide 24%, 28%, 35%, and 40% O_2

Other Considerations:
Consider oxygen administration in any emergency situation. Oxygen should not be withheld or minimally administered to patients with COPD for fear of blocking the hypoxic ventilatory drive. Patients with exacerbated COPD require oxygen, and when provided in the prehospital setting, will seldom depress respiratory drive.

Oxytocin

Class: Hormone
Trade Name(s): Pitocin
Therapeutic Action: Stimulates contraction of uterine smooth muscle to decrease bleeding from uterine vessels
Mechanism: Acts directly on uterine smooth muscle
Indications: Postpartum hemorrhage
Contraindications: Do not use prior to delivery of the baby and placenta; multiple gestations

Adverse Reactions: Cardiac dysrhythmia; uterine rupture; anaphylaxis; nausea; vomiting; water retention; subarachnoid hemorrhage
Drug Interactions: Severe hypertension may result from coadministration of vasopressors
How Supplied: Ampules containing 10 units/mL
Dosage: Adult—10 units in 1 liter of IV fluid; begin at 20–40 milliunits per minute IV and titrate to desired effect (hemorrhage control)
Pediatric—Not recommended

Other Considerations:
Oxytocin is used to produce uterine contractions during the last stage of labor, but this is not an indication for use in the prehospital or emergency department setting for a pregnant patient. When used to control postpartum hemorrhage, it should be used in conjunction with uterine massage, and placing the baby at the mother's breast. Baby's sucking stimulates the natural secretion of oxytocin.

Procainamide

Class: Antidysrhythmic
Trade Name(s): Procan, Pronestyl
Therapeutic Action: Decreases ectopy in ischemic cardiac tissue
Mechanism: Acts directly to slow conduction and excitability in ischemic cardiac tissue
Indications: Ventricular dysrhythmias unresponsive to lidocaine; wide-complex tachycardias unresponsive to lidocaine; wide-complex tachycardias in which the origin cannot be distinguished between ventricular and supraventricular
Contraindications: Patients on digitalis; second- and third-degree AV blocks; Torsades de Pointes; lupus; myasthenia gravis
Adverse Reactions: Hypotension; heart block; exacerbation of ventricular dysrhythmias; widening of QRS complex; anorexia; nausea; vomiting
Drug Interactions: Enhances bradycardia produced by atropine; imcompatible with bretylium, phenytoin
How Supplied: 2-mL vials containing 500 mg/mL (1 g)
10-mL vials containing 100 mg/mL (1 g)
Dosage: Adult—25 to 50 mg per minute IV until dysrhythmia suppressed, hypotension occurs, the QRS complex widens by 50%, or total of 17 mg/kg administered.
Continuous infusion (adult only): 1 to 4 mg per minute
Pediatric—2 to 6 mg/kg/dose given over 5 minutes IV

Other Considerations:
Useful for treatment of those ventricular dysrhythmias that are unresponsive to lidocaine. Safe to use for wide complex tachycardias when the origin of the tachycardia is unclear (supraventricular tachycardia with aberrancy or ventricular tachycardia). Avoid use of procainamide if the dysrhythmia is due to drug toxicity from quinidine or similar type antidysrhythmics, digitalis, or cyclic antidepressants. Close blood pressure and cardiac monitoring is required during drug administration.

Proparacaine

Class: Topical anesthetic
Trade Name(s): Alcaine, Ophthaine
Therapeutic Action: Provides pain relief to corneal surface of eye
Mechanism: Reversibly blocks nerve conduction to pain
Indications: Foreign body or chemical irritation to eye
Contraindications: Ruptured globe
Adverse Reactions: Occasional hypersensitivity reaction
Drug Interactions: None in prehospital setting
How Supplied: Bottle containing 0.5% solution
Dosage: Adult and Pediatric—1 to 2 drops, instilled into affected eye

Other Considerations:

Proparacaine is useful prior to irrigating eyes. Visual acuity (light perception and finger counting) should be tested prior to instillation of drops. Prolonged use of these drops may delay corneal healing and produce corneal ulcerations.

Propranolol

Class: Beta-adrenergic receptor blocker
Trade Name(s): Inderal
Therapeutic Action: Decreases heart rate and blood pressure
Mechanism: Competes for beta-adrenergic receptors
Indications: Angina; antidysrhythmic following acute myocardial infarction; aortic dissection; supraventricular tachycardia; administered with thrombolytics
Contraindications: Congestive heart failure; heart block; conduction delays; hypotension; asthma/COPD
Adverse Reactions: Bronchospasm; bradydysrhythmias; heart failure; hypoglycemia
Drug Interactions: Effects enhanced by calcium channel blockers
How Supplied: 1-mL ampules containing 1 mg/mL (1 mg)
Dosage: Adult—1 mg IV diluted in 10 mL D_5W over 1 minute; may repeat dose every 5 minutes until desired heart rate is achieved
Pediatric—0.01 to 0.015 mg/kg IV over 3 to 5 minutes

Other Considerations:

Other agents such as adenosine and verapamil have become first-line agents for supraventricular tachycardias. Beta-blockers have a limited role in the prehospital setting as their side effects can be life-threatening.

Racemic Epinephrine

Class: Catecholamine
Trade Name(s): Vaponefrin, MicroNEFRIN
Therapeutic Action: Decreases mucosal edema in respiratory tract and produces bronchodilatation

Mechanism: Stimulates adrenergic receptors causing mucosal vasoconstriction and beta-adrenergic bronchodilatation
Indications: Croup
Contraindications: Upper airway obstruction due to epiglottitis
Adverse Reactions: Tachycardia; tremor; agitation; headache
Drug Interactions: Cardiovascular side effects are exacerbated by albuterol and SQ epinephrine
How Supplied: For nebulization—2.25% solution
Dosage: Adult and Pediatric—0.05 mL/kg of 2.25% solution diluted in 3-mL normal saline delivered by handheld or mask nebulizer (maximum dose 0.5 mL)

Other Considerations:

May cause a "rebound" or pronounced bronchospastic effect, clinically manifested by a worsening of the initial condition being treated. It is difficult at times to distinguish epiglottitis from croup. An anxious, toxic-appearing child with stridor, drooling, and refusal to drink liquids should be regarded as having epiglottitis. In such cases, the child should be kept upright and calm using only humidified oxygen. Be prepared for complete airway obstruction. In cases where the diagnosis is unclear, racemic epinephrine should not be administered. It is indicated in the stable, cooperative child who likely has croup.

Sodium Bicarbonate

Class: Alkalizing agent
Trade Name(s): None
Therapeutic Action: Increases pH (alkalinization) in blood and urine. Acts as a buffering (neutralizing) agent for acids in the blood and interstitial fluid
Mechanism: Acts as source of bicarbonate ions
Indications: Documented metabolic acidosis; prolonged resuscitation efforts; tricyclic antidepressant; overdose hyperkalemia
Contraindications: Congestive heart failure; kidney failure
Adverse Reactions: Decreases oxygen delivery at the tissue level; paradoxical CNS acidosis; metabolic alkalosis; hypernatremia
Drug Interactions: May precipitate when given with atropine, calcium chloride and gluconate, morphine sulfate, aminophylline, and magnesium. Epinephrine, dopamine, and isoproterenol are inactivated when given with sodium bicarbonate
How Supplied: Ampules containing 4.3%, 7.5%, or 8.4% solution
Dosage: Adult—1 mEq/kg slow IV push; may repeat dose at 0.5 mEq/kg every 10 minutes
Pediatric—1 mEq/kg of 8.4% solution slow IV push; may repeat dose of 0.5 mEq/kg every 10 minutes during cardiac arrest

Other Considerations:

Adequate ventilation is the mainstay of acid-base balance in cardiac arrest. Sodium bicarbonate was once used as a standard ACLS medication. Currently it is reserved for patients with severe acidosis (pH less than 7.1), or empirically when prolonged resuscitation efforts after ventilation, oxygenation, perfusion is established. Sodium Bicarbonate is Class IIa agent used to alkalinize the serum in severe tricyclic overdose and other overdoses.

Steroids

Class: Steroid
Trade Name(s): (Decadron) Dexamethasone
(Solu-Medrol) Methylprednisolone
Therapeutic Action: Decreases inflammatory response and reduces edema in many tissues
Mechanism: Has strong anti-inflammatory and cell membrane stabilizing effects
Indications: Severe anaphylactic and hypersensitivity reactions; acute asthma exacerbation; acute spinal cord injury
Contraindications: None for single dose therapy in prehospital setting
Adverse Reactions: Side effects are commonly seen with prolonged administration but are not seen with single doses
Drug Interactions: None in prehospital setting
How Supplied: Dexamethasone and Methylprednisolone are dispensed as elixirs, tablets, aerosols, topical ointment, and injectable forms
Decadron— 1-mL vials containing 4 mg/mL (4 mg)
5-mL vials containing 4 mg/mL (20 mg)
25-mL vials containing 4 mg/mL (100 mg)
Solu-Medrol— vials containing 500 mg, 1 and 2 g
Dosage: Adult and Pediatric asthma—Dexamethasone: 0.25 mg/kg IV; Methylprednisolone—2 mg/kg IV
Adult and Pediatric spinal cord injury—Methylprednisolone: 30 mg/kg IV over 1 hour, then 5.4 mg/kg per hour for the next 23 hours

Other Considerations:
Steroids have been shown to have little effect on cerebral edema associated with head trauma and are not recommended in the prehospital setting for this reason. Corticosteroids should be avoided in burn or smoke-inhalation patients with wheezing because studies have shown an increased risk of infection and mortality. Although their beneficial effects are not seen for several hours, corticosteroids are recommended early in the treatment of severe asthma. Corticosteroids are used simultaneously with antihistamines (diphenhydramine) and epinephrine in the treatment of severe allergic and anaphylactic reactions.

Streptokinase

Class: Thrombolytic agent
Trade Name(s): Streptase
Therapeutic Action: Breaks down blood clots, thus restoring blood flow
Mechanism: Activates enzymes involved with dissolving blood clots
Indications: Acute myocardial infarction
Contraindications: Absolute—Prolonged (more than 5 to 10 minutes) CPR; severe hypotension; suspected aortic dissection; active internal bleeding; a history of stroke in the past 6 months; recent head trauma or known intracranial tumor; severe trauma or major surgery within the past 2 weeks; pregnancy
Relative—Initial blood pressure greater than 180 mm Hg systolic or greater than 110 mmHg diastolic; known bleeding disorder or current use of anticoagulants; history of stroke, tumor, head injury, or brain surgery; recent trauma or major surgery in the past 2 months; active peptic ulcer disease or blood in stools; significant liver or kidney disease
Adverse Reactions: Peripheral or systemic bleeding; intracranial hemorrhage; reperfusion dysrhythmias; and bleeding from invasive procedures; allergic reactions are seen in up to 5% of cases, manifested as bronchospasm, urticarial skin changes; pruritis; nausea
Drug Interactions: Additional risks of bleeding complications when administered to patients already taking oral anticoagulants
How Supplied: Vials containing 250,000, 750,000, or 1,500,000 IU
Dosage: Adult—Myocardial infarction: 1.5 million units IV over 1 hour
Pediatric—Not recommended

Other Considerations:
Thrombolytic agents should be administered as soon as possible following acute myocardial infarction to reduce morbidity and mortality. The time of initiating therapy after onset of myocardial infarction is critical to the drug's effectiveness. Because of the urgency to initiate this drug, it has been proposed that it should be administered in the prehospital setting; however, this requires the use of a 12-lead ECG. Studies are ongoing, but presently have not shown any significant advantages for initiating therapy in the field. Prehospital administration of thrombolytic therapy may only be useful in systems where transportation times are relatively long.

Succinylcholine

Class: Skeletal muscle relaxant
Trade Name(s): Anectine
Therapeutic Action: Skeletal muscle and diaphragmatic paralyzation
Mechanism: Combines with cholinergic receptors on the muscle motor-end plate which causes depolarization
Indications: Adjunct to endotracheal intubation
Contraindications: Airway anatomy makes intubation unlikely; absence of surgical airway skills; penetrating eye injury; acute narrow angle glaucoma
Adverse Reactions: Produces apnea and hyperkalemia (not an acute problem, but may occur several days after burns or crush injury)

Drug Interactions: None in prehospital setting
How Supplied: 10-mL vials containing 20 mg/mL (200 mg)
Dosage: Adult and Pediatric—1 to 1.5 mg/kg IV

Other Considerations:

This drug has limited use in the prehospital setting. Rapid sequence induction for intubation requires expertise in airway management and surgical airway skills. When an airway needs to be emergently secured and rapid sequence induction is required, several medications are administered simultaneously (including succinylcholine and sedative or anesthetic agents). The duration of action of this drug is approximately 4 to 6 minutes; therefore, if the patient is unable to be intubated, spontaneous respirations will resume in approximately 5 to 10 minutes. A thorough neurologic examination noting movement of extremities should be done prior to administering the drug.

Terbutaline

Class: Bronchodilator
Trade Name(s): Brethine, Bricanyl, Brethaire
Therapeutic Action: Dilates bronchial smooth muscle. Relaxes uterine smooth muscle
Mechanism: Stimulates beta$_2$-adrenergic receptors
Indications: Wheezing due to acute bronchospasm or asthma; COPD exacerbation; toxic inhalation; Tocolysis (inhibition of contractions) for premature labor
Contraindications: Known hypersensitivity to sympathomimetic amines
Adverse Reactions: Tachycardia; palpitations; tremor; nervousness; agitation; nausea; vomiting; may cause hypoglycemia in the expectant mother and neonate when used during labor
Drug Interactions: May antagonize beta-adrenergic blockers
How Supplied: For nebulization: 1-mL ampule containing 1 mg/mL (1 mg)
Metered dose inhaler
Dosage: Adult—0.25 mg subcutaneous; may repeat dose in 15 to 30 minutes for bronchospasm only; Metered dose inhaler: 2 puffs; nebulized 0.5–1.0 mg in 25 ml saline
Pediatric—0.01 mg/kg subcutaneous; (maximum dose 0.25 mg)

Other Considerations:

Preterm labor may be defined as that occurring between 20 and 37 weeks gestation. Tocolysis should only be considered with an uncomplicated pregnancy, regular uterine contractions, intact membranes, cervical dilatation of no greater than 4 cm, and after consultation with a physician.

Thiamine

Class: Vitamin
Trade Name(s): None

Therapeutic Action: Thiamine is typically obtained in a normal diet; administration of thiamine replenishes depleted thiamine stores in malnourished states
Mechanism: Vitamin that plays an essential role in creating and using cellular energy
Indications: Treatment and prevention of Wernicke's encephalopathy; replacement therapy for malnutrition associated with alcoholism or chemotherapy; delirium tremens
Contraindications: None in prehospital setting
Adverse Reactions: Hypotension; anaphylactoid and hypersensitivity reactions
Drug Interactions: Incompatible with aminophylline, furosemide, corticosteroid, morphine sulfate, phenytoin, and sodium bicarbonate
How Supplied: 1-mL vials containing 100 mg/mL (100 mg)
Dosage: Adult—100 mg IV or IM
Pediatric—Not recommended

Other Considerations:

Thiamine should be given prior to or as soon as possible after administration of IV glucose to the potentially thiamine deficient patient to prevent the development of Wernicke's encephalopathy. This is a severe neurologic condition that presents as confusion, ataxia, and paralysis of eye muscles.

Tissue Plasminogen Activator

Class: Thrombolytic agent
Trade Name(s): Activase
Therapeutic Action: Breaks down blood clots thus restoring blood flow
Mechanism: Activates enzymes involved with dissolving blood clots
Indications: Evolving acute myocardial infarction documented by 12-lead ECG and no contraindications to thrombolytic therapy (see below); the time of onset of symptoms should be no longer than 6 to 12 hours
Contraindications: Absolute—Prolonged (more than 5 to 10 minutes) CPR; severe hypotension; suspected aortic dissection; active internal bleeding; a history of stroke in the past 6 months; recent head trauma or known intracranial tumor; severe trauma or major surgery within the past 2 weeks; pregnancy
Relative—Initial blood pressure greater than 180 mm Hg systolic or greater than 110 mm Hg diastolic; known bleeding disorder or current use of anticoagulants; history of stroke, tumor, head injury, or brain surgery; recent trauma or major surgery in the past 2 months; active peptic ulcer disease or blood in stools; significant liver or kidney disease
Adverse Reactions: Peripheral or systemic bleeding; intracranial hemorrhage; reperfusion dysrhythmias; bleeding from invasive procedures; allergic reactions are seen in up to 5% of cases, manifested as bronchospasm, urticarial skin changes; pruritis; nausea
Drug Interactions: Additional risks of bleeding complications when administered to patients already taking oral anticoagulants

How Supplied: Vials containing 20, 50, and 100 mg
Dosage: Adult—recent studies suggest a 15-mg bolus IV followed by 0.75 mg/kg up to 50 mg maximum over 30 minutes, then 0.5 mg/kg up to 35 mg maximum over 60 minutes (total dose less or equal to 100 mg); various institutions use alternate dosing regimens
Pediatric—Not recommended

Other Considerations:

Thrombolytic agents should be administered as soon as possible following acute myocardial infarction to reduce morbidity and mortality. The time of initiating the therapy after onset of myocardial infarction is critical to the drug's effectiveness. Because of the urgency to initiate this drug, it has been proposed that it should be administered in the prehospital setting; however, this requires the use of a 12-lead ECG. Studies are ongoing, but presently have not shown any significant advantages for initiating therapy in the field. Prehospital administration of thrombolytic therapy may only be useful in systems where transportation times are relatively long.

Verapamil

Class: Calcium channel blocker
Trade Name(s): Calan, Isoptin
Therapeutic Action: Delays atrioventricular (AV) nodal conduction and inhibits atrial dysrhythmias

Mechanism: Selectively inhibits slow calcium channels in cardiac tissue
Indications: Narrow complex paroxysmal supraventricular tachycardia; atrial fibrillation/flutter with rapid ventricular response
Contraindications: Hypotension or wide complex tachycardia; congestive heart failure in patients with left ventricular dysfunction; patients on beta-adrenergic blockers or digitalis; sick sinus syndrome or AV conduction disturbances; Wolff-Parkinson-White syndrome
Adverse Reactions: Bradycardia; hypotension; headache; dizziness
Drug Interactions: Potentiates the cardiovascular effects of beta-adrenergic blockers
How Supplied: 2-mL ampules containing 2.5 mg/mL (5 mg)
Dosage: Adult—2.5 to 5 mg IV over 2 minutes; may repeat dose at 5 to 10 mg every 15 to 30 minutes (maximum dose 30 mg)
Pediatric—Not recommended

Other Considerations:

Verapamil slows the ventricular response to atrial fibrillation and flutter; however, conversion to normal sinus rhythm is unlikely. In the prehospital setting, verapamil is contraindicated for paroxysmal supraventricular tachycardia in patients with Wolff-Parkinson-White syndrome because the ventricular response may increase. Asystole or AV block may occur as a result of the slowed AV conduction. In the middle-aged or older patient, the IV dose should be given over a minimum of 3 minutes.

BIBLIOGRAPHY

Adenosine. *Med Let,* 32 (821):63-64, 1990.

Anderson HV, Willerson JT: Thrombolysis in acute myocardial infarction. *N Engl J Med,* 329:703-709, 1993.

Barsan WG: Respiratory Drugs. In Barsan WE, Jastremski MS, Syverud SA (ed): Emergency Drug Therapy, Philadelphia, 1991, WB Saunders.

Bertel O, Conen D, Radu EW, *et al:* Nifedipine in hypertensive emergencies. *Br Med J,* 286:19-21, 1983.

Bracken MB, Shepard MJ, Collins WF, *et al:* A randomized control trial of methylprednisolone or naloxone in the treatment of acute spinal cord injury. *N Engl J Med,* 322:1405-1411, 1990.

Browning RG, Olson DW, Stueven HA, *et al:* 50% Dextrose: antidote or toxin? *Ann Emerg Med,* 19:683-687, 1990.

Burkhart KK, Kulig KW: The diagnostic utility of flumazenil (a benzodiasepine antagonist) a coma of unknown etiology. *Ann Emerg Med,* 19:319-321, 1990.

Calhoun DA, Oparil S: Treatment of hypertensive crisis. *N Engl J Med,* 323:1177-1183, 1990.

Carter E, Cruz M, Chesrown S, *et al:* Efficacy of intravenously administered theophylline in children hospitalized with severe asthma. *J Pediatr,* 122:470-476, 1993.

Curtis RA, Barone J, Giacona N, *et al:* Efficacy of ipecac and activated charcoal/cathartic prevention of salicylate absorption in a simulated overdose. *Arch Intern Med,* 144:48-52, 1984.

Derlet RW, Albertson TE: Activated charcoal—past, present, and future. *West J Med,* 145:493-496, 1986.

DiGiulio GA, Kercsmar CM, Krug SE, *et al:* Hospital treatment of asthma: lack of benefit from theophylline given in addition to nebulized albuterol and intravenously administered corticosteroid. *J Pediatr,* 122:464-469, 1993.

Drugs for cardiac arrhythmias. *Med Let,* 28 (727):111-116, 1986.

Drugs for epilepsy. *Med Let,* 28 (723):91-94, 1986.

Drugs for hypertension. *Med Let,* 29 (730):1-6, 1987.

Drugs for asthma. *Med Let,* 29 (732):11-16, 1987.

Dunmire SM, Paris PM: Analgesics. In Barsan WE, Jastremski MS, Syverud SA (ed): Emergency Drug Therapy. Philadelphia, 1991, W.B. Saunders.

Eisenberg MS, Aghababian RV, Bossaert L, *et al:* Thrombolytic therapy. *Ann Emerg Med,* 22:417-417, 1993.

Elliott JP: Magnesium sulfate as a tocolytic agent. *Am J Obstet Gynecol,* 147:277-284, 1983.

Emergency Cardiac Care Committee and Subcommittees: American Heart Association Guidelines for Cardiopulmonary Resuscitation and Emergency Cardiac Care. *JAMA,* 268:2171, 2206, 2207, 2208, 2209-2210, 2211, 2226, 2267-2268, 2269-2270, 2302, 1992.

Evand D, Hoepner J: Ophthalmologic Agents. In Barsan WE, Jastremski MS, Syverud SA (ed): Emergency Drug Therapy. Philadelphia, 1991; WB Saunders.

Fanta C, Rossing TH, McFadden ER; Glucocorticords in acute asthma, a critical control trial. *Am J Med,* 74:845-851, 1983.

Flomenbaum N, Gallagher EJ, Eagen K, *et al:* Self administered nitrous oxide: An adjunct analgesic. *J Am Coll Emerg Physicians,* 8:95-97, 1979.

Garrison MG, Benson NM, Whitley TW, *et al:* Paramedic skills and medications: practice options utilized by local advanced life support medical directors. *Prehosp Dis Med,* 6:29-34, 1991.

Greenberger PA, Patterson R: Management of asthma during pregnancy. *N Engl J Med,* 312:897-902, 1985.

Hall AH, Rumack BH: Clinical toxicology of cyanide. *Ann Emerg Med,* 915:1067-1074, 1986.

Hall AH, Rumack BH: Hydroxocobalamin/sodium thiosulfate as a cyanide antidote. *J Emerg Med,* 5:115-121, 1987.

Haynes BE, Niemann JT, Haynes KS: Supraventricular tachyarrhythmias and rate-related hypotension: cardiovascular effects and efficacy of intravenous verapamil. *Ann Emerg Med,* 19:861-864, 1990.

Hedges JR, Dronen SC, Feero S, et al: Succinylcholine-assigned intubations in prehospital care. *Ann Emerg Med,* 17:469-472, 1988.

Herbert WN, Sefalo RC: Management of post-partum hemorrhage. *Clin Obstet Gyneco,* 27:139-147, 1984.

Hoffman JR, Schriger DL, Votey SR, *et al:* The empiric use of hypertonic dextrose in patients with altered mental status: a reappraisal. *Ann Emerg Med,* 21:20, 1992.

Jolly SR, Kipnis JN, Lucchesi BR: Cardiovascular depression by verapamil: reversal by glucagon and interactions with propranolol. *Pharmacol,* 35:249-255, 1987.

Kette F, Weil MH, Gazmuri RJ: Buffer solutions may compromise cardiac resuscitation by reducing coronary perfusion pressure. *JAMA,* 266:2121-2126, 1991.

Kulig K, Bar-Or D, Cantrill SV, *et al:* Management of acutely poisoned patients without gastric emptying. *Ann Emerg Med,* 14:562-567, 1985.

Lavery RF, Doran J, Tortella BJ, *et al:* A survey of advanced life support practices in the United States. *Prehos Dis Med,* 7:144-150, 1992.

Lehr CV, Heban PT, Huss P, *et al:* Comparative systemic and regional hemodynamic effects of dopamine and dobutamine in patients with cardiomyopathic heart failure. *Circulation,* 58:466-475, 1978.

Littenberg B: Aminophylline treatment in severe asthma: a mega analysis. *JAMA,* 259:1678-1684, 1989.

Littenberg B, Gluck EH: A control trial of methylprednisolone in the emergency treatment of acute asthma. *N Engl J Med,* 314:150, 1986.

Marshal LF, Smith RW, Rausher LA, *et al:* Mannitol dose requirements in brain-injured patients. *J Neurosurg,* 48:169-172, 1978.

Meltzer EO. Antihistamine- and decongestant-induced performance decrements. *J Occup Med,* 32:327-334, 1990.

Murphy-Macabobby M, Marshall WJ, Schneider C, *et al:* Neuromuscular blockade in aeromedical airway management. *Ann Emerg Med,* 21:664-668, 1992.

Norris RM, Barnaby PF, Brown MA, *et al:* Prevention of ventricular fibrillation during acute myocardial infarction by intravenous propranolol. *Lancet,* 2:883-886, 1984.

O'Toole KS, Heller MB, Menegazzi JJ, *et al:* Intravenous verapamil in the prehospital treatment of paroxysmal supraventricular tachycardia. *Ann Emerg Med,* 10:291-294, 1990.

Rossing TH, Fanta CH, Goldstein DH, *et al:* Emergency therapy of asthma: comparison of the acute effects of parenteral and inhaled sympathomimetics and infused aminophylline. *Am Rev Respir Dis,* 122:365-371, 1980.

Sharma AD, Klein GJ, Yee R: Intravenous adenosine triphosphate during wide QRS complex tachycardia: safety, therapeutic efficacy, and diagnostic utility. *Am J Med,* 88:337-343, 1990.

Sheets CA: Emetics and antiemetics. In Barsan WG, Jastremski MS, Syverud SA (ed): Emergency Drug Therapy. Philadelphia, 1991, WB Saunders.

Shuster M, Chong J: Pharmacologic intervention in prehospital care: a critical appraisal. *Ann Emerg Med,* 18:192-196, 1989.

Stueven HA, Thompson BM, Aprahamian C, *et al:* Calcium chloride: reassessment of use in asystole. *Ann Emerg Med,* 1984; 13:844-845, 1984.

Tafuri J, Roberts J. Organophosphate poisoning. *Ann Emerg Med,* 16:193-202, 1987.

Tanssig LM, Castro C, Beaudry PH, *et al:* Treatment of laryngotracheitis (croup). *Am J Dis Child,* 129:790-793, 1975.

Vandenburg MJ, Griffiths GK, Brandman S: Sublingual nitroglycerin or spray in the treatment of angina. *Br J Clin Pract,* 40:524-527, 1986.

Vidt DG: Intravenous labetalol in the emergency treatment of hypertension. *J Clin Hypertens,* 2:179-186, 1985.

Votey SR, Bosse GM, Bayer MJ, *et al:* Flumazenil: a new benzodiazepine, an antagonist. *Ann Emerg Med,* 20:181-188, 1991.

Vukmir RB, Paris BM, Yealy DM: Glucagon: prehospital therapy for hypoglycemia. *Ann Emerg Med,* 20:375-379, 1991.

Watson P: Postpartum hemorrhage and shock. *Clin Obstet Gynecol,* 23:985-1001, 1980.

Weaver WD, Eisenberg MS, Martin JS, *et al:* Myocardial Infarction Triage and Intervention project, phase I: patient characteristics and feasibility of prehospital initiation of thrombolytic therapy. *J Am Coll Cardiol,* 15:925-931, 1990.

Weaver WD, Cerqueira M, Hallstrom AP, *et al:* Prehospital initiated vs hospital initiated thrombolytic therapy. The Myocardial Infarction Triage and Intervention trial. *JAMA,* 270:1211-1216, 1993.

Weiss TA, Fine DG, Applebaum D, *et al:* Prehospital coronary thrombolysis: a new strategy in acute myocardial infarction. *Chest,* 92:124-128, 1987.

Woods KL, Fletcher S, Roffe C, *et al:* Intravenous magnesium sulphate in suspected acute myocardial infarction: results of the second Leicester Intravenous Magnesium Intervention Trial (LIMIT-2). *Lancet,* 339:1553-1558, 1992.

Wrenn KD, Murphy F, Slovis CM: A toxicity study of parenteral thiamine hydrochloride. *Ann Emerg Med,* 18:867-870, 1989.

James M. Atkins, MD

Chapter 12

Basic Rhythm Interpretation

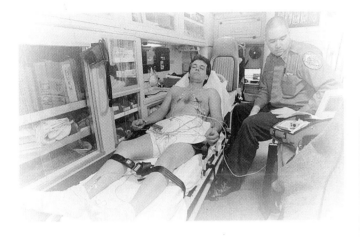

A paramedic should be able to:

1. Describe the normal electrical activity in the heart.
2. Describe the relationship between the electrical activity in the heart and the electrocardiogram.
3. Define the standard leads and special monitor leads.
4. Describe the five basic blocks to determine rhythm.
5. Describe the major methods to determine rate of rhythm.
6. Describe the six different patterns of rhythm.
7. Describe and explain aberrant conduction.
8. Describe the three relationships where the atrium can cause the ventricle to fire.
9. Define the four sites that can originate an impulse to the heart.
10. Define and describe the four rhythms that begin in the sinus node.
11. Define and describe the three types of premature complexes.
12. Define and describe atrial fibrillation and atrial flutter.
13. Define and describe the four variations of block in the AV node.
14. Describe the function of pacemakers and implanted defibrillators.
15. Describe the four different rhythms that must be associated with a cardiac arrest.

1. **AV node (atrioventricular node)**—the AV node (atrioventricular node or junction in the lower right atrium) delays impulses from the atrium so that the atrium can contract and fill the ventricles before the ventricles contract. The AV node also limits the maximum rate at which the atrium can cause the ventricles to be depolarized.
2. **Atria**—the two upper chambers of the heart.
3. **Bradycardia**—a slow heart rate; usually defined as less than 60 beats per minute.
4. **Bundle branches**—the two subdivisions from the bundle of His that connect to the Purkinje fibers.
5. **Bundle of His**—the part of the conduction pathway that connects the AV node to the bundle branches.
6. **Depolarization**—the electrical discharge of a cardiac working cell or an electrical system cell.

7. **Electrocardiogram**—graphic display of the electrical activity of the heart generated by the depolarization and repolarization of the atria and ventricles.
8. **Electrodes**—the wires and patches that connect the patient to the ECG machine or monitor and sense the flow of electrical current within the heart.
9. **Fibrillation**—the chaotic, uncoordinated firing of cardiac muscle cells; although it generates electrical activity, it cannot cause organized contraction of the chamber involved, and cardiac output decreases or ceases.
10. **Junction**—*see* AV node.
11. **Lead**—a combination of three or more electrodes that make up a single channel of the ECG.
12. **P wave**—the ECG wave representing atrial depolarization.
13. **R-R interval**—section of the ECG between the onset of one QRS complex and the onset of an adjacent QRS complex or the distance between two adjacent R waves.
14. **Pacemaker**—the cell that initiates a cardiac impulse; it is usually the sinus node but can be any cell of the atrium, AV node, or ventricle; a pacemaker can also be an artificial electronic device implanted in the heart to stimulate the formation of an electrical conduction.
15. **Paroxysmal**—sudden onset.
16. **Purkinje fibers**—fibers that line the inside of both ventricles, they conduct impulses from the bundle branches and fascicles to the ventricular muscle.
17. **Q wave**—a negative deflection from the baseline that precedes the R wave; it may not be present at all times.
18. **QRS complex**—a ventricular depolarization wave.
19. **QRS interval**—the width of the QRS from the start of the Q wave to the end of the S wave; if one or more portions are not present, it is measured from the beginning deviation above or below the isoelectric line to the end of whatever waves are present.
20. **R wave**—the first positive deflection of the QRS complex.
21. **R' wave (R prime wave)**—the second positive deflection of the QRS complex; this wave is seen occasionally.
22. **Repolarization**—recharging of cardiac cells after they have been depolarized. This phase allows the cell to accept and transfer the next electrical impulse.
23. **S wave**—a negative origin deflection that returns to the baseline that follows the R wave; it may not be present in all cases.
24. **ST segment**—the segment between the end of the QRS complex and the beginning of the T wave.
25. **Sinus node**—the primary pacemaker of the heart, located in the high right atrium below the opening for the superior vena cava.
26. **Supraventricular**—impulse origin from above the ventricle; the term is used to describe an impulse or rhythm that begins in the sinus node, the atrium, or the AV node.
27. **T wave**—the wave representing repolarization of the ventricle.
28. **Tachycardia**—a heart rate faster than 100 beats per minute.
29. **U wave**—although the origin is uncertain, it is believed to represent repolarization of the Purkinje fibers.
30. **Ventricle**—the lower chambers of the heart that pump blood to the lungs and the body.

The electrocardiogram (ECG) is a recording of the electrical activation of the heart muscle. The electrocardiogram was a German invention, and "cardio" in German is spelled "kardio." Hence, the term is sometimes abbreviated as EKG. The English abbreviation, ECG, is also acceptable and is used in this text.

The chief purpose of the ECG in prehospital care is to identify abnormal rhythms that might require management. The ECG is thus an adjunct to observation of the patient's symptoms. The symptoms establish the need for treatment, and the ECG helps to determine what that treatment should be. Although ECG monitoring is an important prehospital tool, it does not replace thorough patient assessment.

The Normal Electrical Heart

There are two different types of cells within the heart. The first is the working myocardial cell that actually does the contracting which makes the heart pump blood. These cells tend to maintain an electrical charge across the cell wall, by a condition called polarization. When the cells are stimulated by an electric current, they electrically discharge, or depolarize.

Depolarization makes the muscle filaments contract, shortening the cell length and causing the heart to contract and pump blood. After contraction, the cell relaxes and its wall returns to the polarized state. The process begins again as the next electrical wave passes through (Fig. 12-1).

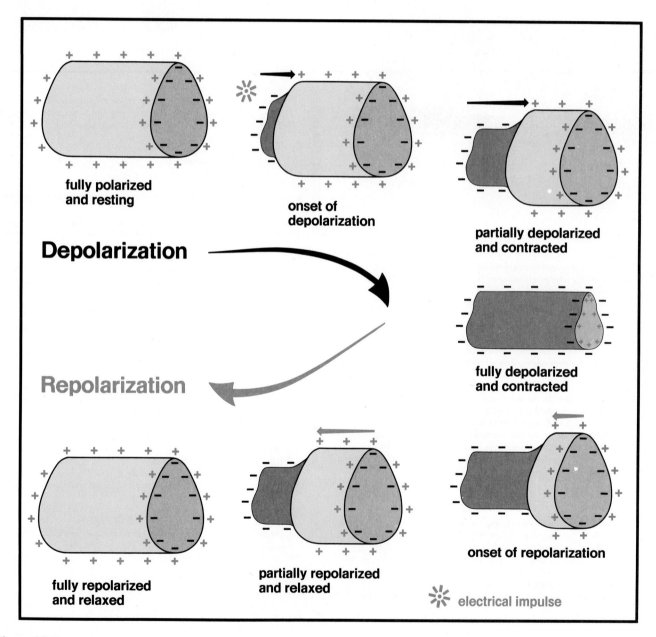

Figure 12-1

Cardiac cell depolarization/repolarization. *From Huszar: Basic dysrhythmias, second edition, 1994, Mosby Lifeline.*

The second type of cardiac cell is the electrical system cells, which can function as pacemakers. A pacemaker can initiate an electrical discharge on its own and then recharge. This property is called "automaticity." These cells are also specialized to conduct electrical current from one portion of the heart to another through the electrical conduction system. The function of these electrical system cells is two-fold: they originate electrical activity and they transmit it to the working cells to trigger their discharge and contraction. The ability to transmit an electrical impulse is called "conductivity."

The electrical activity normally begins in the sinus, or sinoatrial (SA), node (Fig. 12-2). The SA node is located in the right atrium, at its junction with the superior vena cava. The sinus node will discharge, or fire, automatically at approximately 60–100 times per minute. The sinus node is affected by two sets of nerves, the vagus nerve (parasympathetic nervous system) that slows the rate of sinus discharge, and sympathetic nerves that speed its rate of firing. Thus, when a person at rest has a pulse of 55 beats per minute, the parasympathetic sys-

tem is slowing the sinus node to conserve energy. When exercise increases the rate to 145 beats per minute, the sympathetic system is speeding the heart to pump more blood and maintain cardiac output and perfusion.

Once the sinus node has depolarized, the impulse is conducted down four pathways. Three internodal pathways within the right atrium conduct the impulse to the atrioventicular (AV) node, and the fourth conducts the impulse from the right atrium to the left. As the impulses are conducted through these pathways, atrial muscle tissue depolarizes in a wave from top right to bottom left (Fig. 12-3). Atrial muscle then contracts and pumps blood into the ventricles through the mitral and tricuspid values.

The electrical impulse is delayed when it reaches the AV node. The AV node is located in the right atrium, near the point where the atria and ventricles meet. Its function is to create a pause between atrial depolarization and ventricular depolarization that alllows the ventricles to fill before they contract. The delay at the AV node is normally 0.12 to 0.20

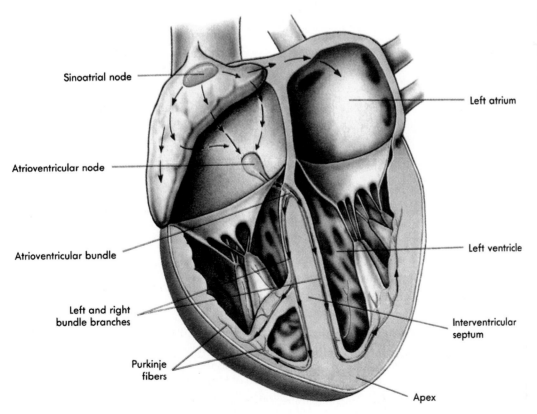

Figure 12-2

The electrical conduction system of the heart. *From Sanders: Mosby's paramedic textbook, 1994, Mosby Lifeline. Illustrator: Ronald J. Ervin.*

Sinoatrial node

Left atrium

Atrioventricular node

Atrioventricular bundle

Left ventricle

Left and right bundle branches

Interventricular septum

Purkinje fibers

Apex

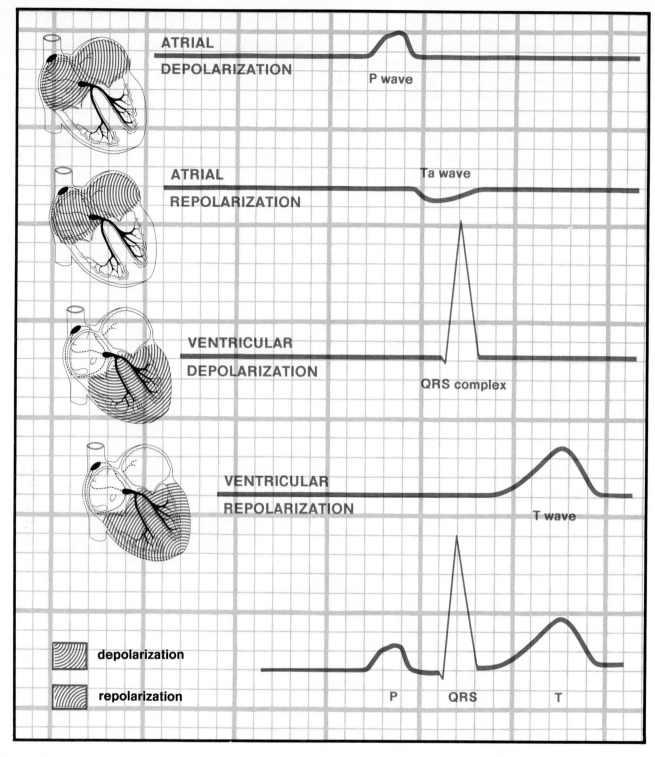

Figure 12-3

Depolarization and repolarization. *From Huszar: Basic dysrhythmias, second edition, 1994, Mosby Lifeline.*

seconds. Diastole (relaxation) and systole (contraction) of the ventricle are shown in Fig. 12-4.

The AV node also limits how many beats per minute can be conducted to the ventricles. If the atria were firing at 400 beats per minute, the AV node would not allow all of the beats through to the ventricles. In most circumstances, the AV node will only allow passage of 200 beats per minute, although on rare occasions it may conduct up to 300 beats per minute.

After the delay in the AV node, the impulse is conducted down the bundle of His, a conducting path or "wire" that connects the atria to the ventricles. The bundle of His divides into the right and left bundle branches, each leading to the ventri-

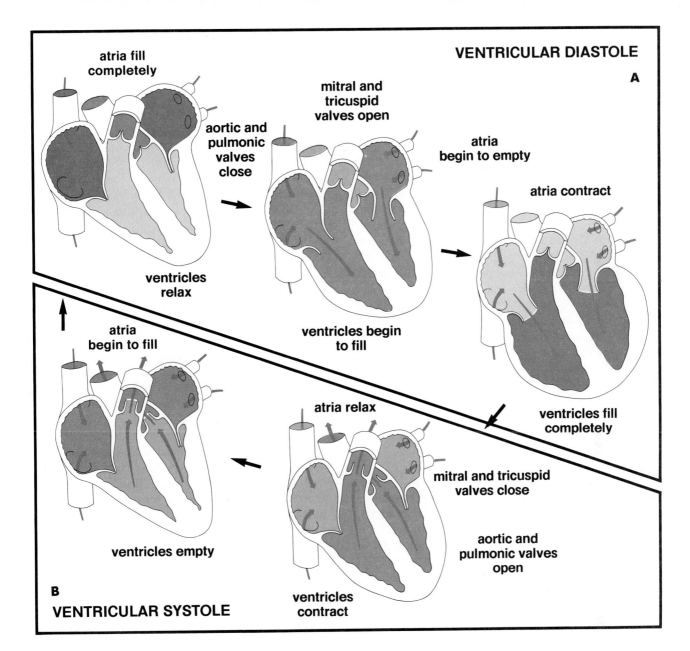

VENTRICULAR DIASTOLE

A

atria fill completely

aortic and pulmonic valves close

ventricles relax

mitral and tricuspid valves open

atria begin to empty

ventricles begin to fill

atria contract

ventricles fill completely

B

VENTRICULAR SYSTOLE

atria begin to fill

ventricles empty

atria relax

ventricles contract

mitral and tricuspid valves close

aortic and pulmonic valves open

Figure 12-4

Diastole (relaxation) and systole (contraction) of the ventricle. *From Huszar: Basic dysrhythmias, second edition, 1994, Mosby Lifeline.*

cle on its respective side. The left bundle branch divides into the anterior and posterior divisions or fascicles. From the right bundle branch and the two fascicles of the left bundle branch, the impulses are conducted to the Purkinje fibers that line the inside of both ventricular walls.

Finally, the Purkinje fibers conduct the impulses to the ventricular working cells. The ventricles depolarize simultaneously from the inside out, unlike the atria, which fire in a wave. As the working cells contract, the ventricles pump blood out through the aortic and pulmonic valves. Each area of the conducting tissue and the muscle cells then recharges or repolarizes. Cardiac cells will not function properly while repolarizing. They will not fire at all early in the process; they may fire later, but more slowly, causing slower and possibly aberrant conduction.

There are four different sites in the heart that routinely generate impulses (Table 12-1). The usual pacemaker is the sinus (SA) node, because it is the fastest firing rate and has the highest

TABLE 12-1	Intrinsic Rate of Pacemakers
Pacemaker	**Normal Rate**
Sinus node	60–100/min
Atrium	40–60/min
AV node (junction)	40–60/min
Ventricle	30–40/ min

level of automaticity. It tends to fire between 60 and 100 beats per minute at rest. This is known as the inherent rate. It can accelerate to 200 beats per minute in an adult (220 in an infant) and slow to less than 40. The vagus nerve has a variable influence on the sinus node; respiration alters vagal tone, and this causes the sinus node to speed and slow with breathing.

If the sinus (SA) node fails, three other sites known as escape pacemakers can originate impulses: the atrium, the AV node or "junction," and the ventricles. These other pacemakers are suppressed and do not generate the impulse; however, if the sinus node fails to fire or the impulse fails to be conducted after one to three seconds, one of these other sites will take over. Some diseases and drugs can cause these pacemakers to discharge at other than their normal rates, or to turn on inappropriately. The junction may fire inappropriately slow (10 to 40 beats per minute) or inappropriately fast (60 to 200 beats per minute). The electrical and muscle cells of the atrium and ventricle can also fire at inappropriate rates. The muscle in the atrium and ventricle can fire at extremely rapid rates (up to 700 times per minute). Except for fibrillation of the atrium or ventricle, each of these pacemakers tends to fire very regularly, if the pacemaker is providing all of the impulses and generating the rhythm.

The ECG Cycle

The ECG records the electrical activity of the heart. Mechanical activity, which is a response to the electrical stimulus, is confirmed by the presence of a pulse. The ECG shows a broad picture of electrical activity in major areas of the heart, primarily atrial and ventricular depolarization and ventricular repolarization. Figure 12-5 shows the components of the ECG. Atrial depolarization causes the P wave, ventricular depolarization causes the QRS complex, and ventricular repolarization is responsible for the T and U waves. The atrial repolarization wave is normally hidden in the QRS complex.

The best starting point in analyzing a rhythm is the QRS complex (see Box 12-1). Because it usually has the highest voltage and is the sharpest portion of the ECG, it is usually also the easiest to identify. The baseline of the ECG is called the isoelectric line, or what would be left if all of the waves

were removed from the ECG. The isoelectric line can usually be identified by looking at the flat portion of the tracing just before the P wave, or the area between the P wave and the QRS complex.

The QRS complex is defined in relation to the isoelectric line. The R wave is the first portion of the QRS complex that rises above the isoelectric line (a positive deflection). The Q wave is anything before the R wave that extends below the isoelectric line (as negative deflection). The S wave is any negative deflection that follows the R wave. If there is a second positive deflection, it is called an R′ (R prime) wave. The T wave always follows a QRS and is a slower and broader wave than the QRS. A U wave may follow the T wave.

The ST segment is the flat portion between the end of the QRS complex and the beginning of the T wave (Fig. 12-6). It can be "elevated" above the isoelectric line in patients with an acute myocardial infarction or pericarditis, and in some normal individuals in their teens through 30 years of age. The ST segment may be "depressed" below the isoelectric line in patients who are taking digitalis or in patients who have angina, thickened cardiac muscle, or damage to the muscle. Although these conditions can cause abnormalities in the ST segment, diagnosis can only be made with a 12-lead ECG. A single monitor lead cannot be used to make any diagnosis other than rhythm.

The ECG paper is usually run through the machine at 25 mm/second. Thus, each millimeter is 0.04 seconds. The small boxes on the paper are 1 mm long by 1 mm high (Fig. 12-7). Each large square is 5 mm, or 0.20 seconds. To properly interpret the ECG, there are two intervals that are important to calculate: the P-R interval and the QRS interval. The P-R interval is measured from the start of the P wave to the start of

---

BOX 12-1	Definitions of the ECG Complex

P wave—atrial depolarization

QRS complex—ventricular depolarization

Q wave—a part of ventricular depolarization, it is a negative deflection and precedes the R wave. It may not be present in all cases.

R wave—It is the first positive deflection of the QRS complex

S wave—a negative deflection from the baseline that follows the R wave. It may not be present in all cases.

T wave—repolarization of the ventricle. It follows the QRS complex, and at times may be difficult to see in a single lead

U wave—part of the final repolarization of the ventricle, at the end of or just after a T wave. These are sometimes confused with P waves.

PR interval—the interval (length of time) from the onset of the P wave to the onset of the QRS complex.

QRS interval—the width of the QRS from the start of the Q wave to the end of the S wave, or from the beginning to the end of whatever waves are present.

ST segment—the segment between the end of the QRS complex and the beginning of the T wave

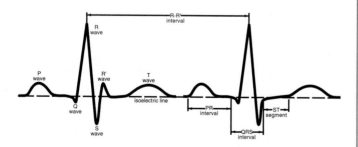

Figure 12-5

ECG waves, segments, and intervals.

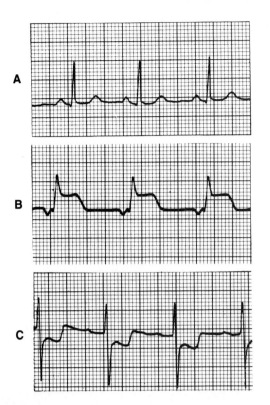

Figure 12-6

ST Segments (A) Normal (B) Elevated (C) Depressed below the isoelectric line. *From Goldberger, et al: Clinical electrocardiography, fifth edition, 1994, St. Louis, Mosby-Year Book, Inc.*

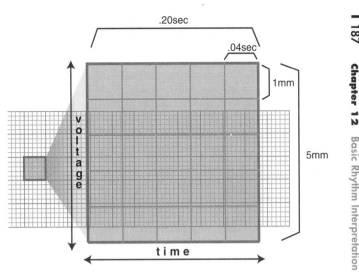

Figure 12-7

ECG graph paper. *From Phalen: The 12-lead ECG in acute myocardial infarction, 1994, Mosby Lifeline.*

Many times, the QRS does not return to the baseline. Look at the last portion of the QRS and beginning of the ST segment and try to determine the corner between the two.

ECG Application

To obtain an ECG, electrodes are attached to the patient. An electrode is an electrical connection between the patient and the machine; it is composed of a patch, paddle or metal contact that is placed on the patient's skin, and the cable or wire that runs from that skin contact to the machine. These leads provide a view of the heart from a specific angle. Standardized 12-lead ECGs require precise positioning of electrodes. Monitoring electrodes do not require such precision and are often placed in modified positions for convenience.

the QRS complex (Fig. 12-8A). It correlates with the pause that occurs in the AV node. This interval should be 0.20 seconds or less.

The width of the QRS is measured from the onset to the end of the complex (Fig. 12-8B). A normal QRS complex is less than 0.12 seconds wide. Measuring the QRS may be difficult. Recognizing the beginning of the complex is usually easy, but its end is sometimes more difficult to determine.

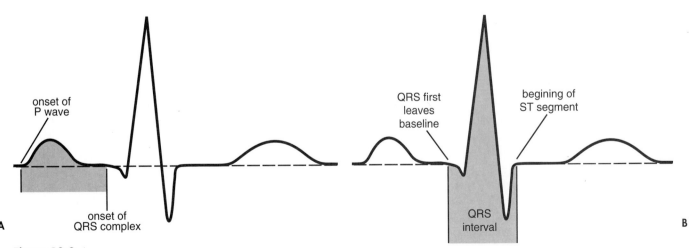

Figure 12-8

Measurement of (A) PR Interval and (B) QRS Interval.

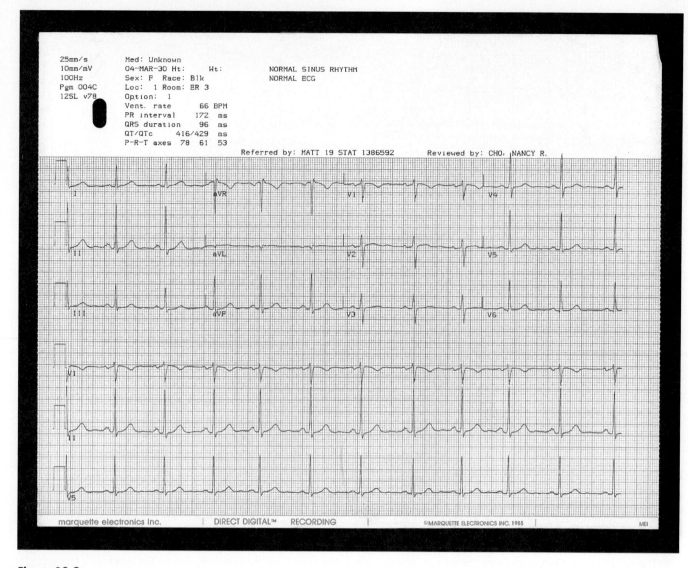

```
25mm/s          Med: Unknown
10mm/mV         04-MAR-30 Ht:     Wt:          NORMAL SINUS RHYTHM
100Hz           Sex: F  Race: Blk              NORMAL ECG
Pgm 004C        Loc:  1 Room: ER 3
12SL v78        Option:  1
                Vent. rate      66 BPM
                PR interval    172  ms
                QRS duration    96  ms
                QT/QTc     416/429  ms
                P-R-T axes  78  61  53
                     Referred by: MATT 19 STAT 1386592        Reviewed by: CHO, NANCY R.
```

marquette electronics inc. | DIRECT DIGITAL™   RECORDING | ©MARQUETTE ELECTRONICS INC. 1985 | MEI

Figure 12-9

A 12 lead ECG tracing. *From Phalen: The 12-lead ECG in acute myocardial infarction, 1994, Mosby Lifeline.*

Classically for a 12-lead ECG, electrodes are attached to each wrist, each ankle, and six chest locations. The electrodes are connected to the ECG machine and processed by an amplifier (Fig. 12-9). A lead is a combination of electrodes that are connected to the amplifier. The electrode attached to the right ankle is always a ground electrode.

Standard limb lead placement is shown in Figure 12-10. Lead I uses the right wrist electrode as a negative electrode

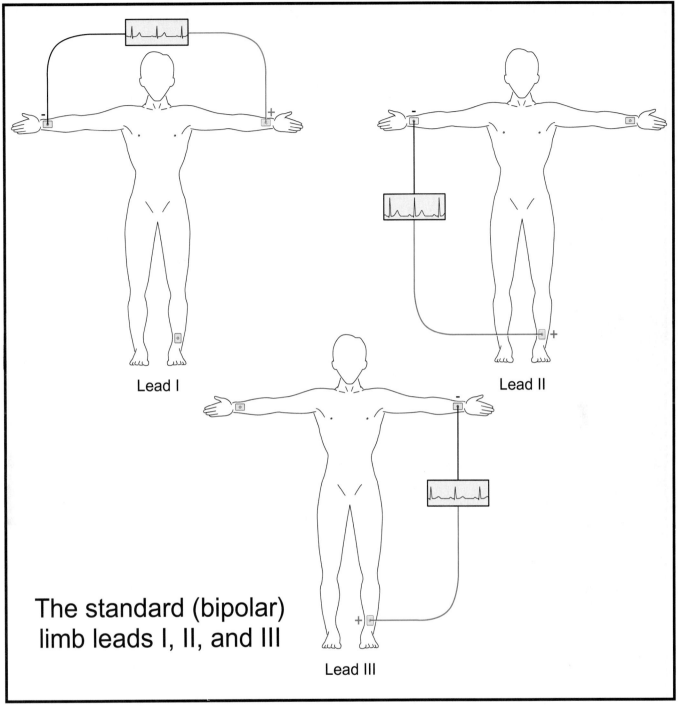

Lead I

Lead II

The standard (bipolar) limb leads I, II, and III

Lead III

Figure 12-10

Standard limb lead placement. *From Huszar: Basic dysrhythmias, second edition, 1994, Mosby Lifeline.*

and the left wrist as positive. Lead II uses the right wrist as negative and the left ankle as positive. Lead III uses the left wrist as negative and the left ankle as positive.

The augmented lead ties two electrodes together as a common negative. Augmented limb lead placement is shown in Figure 12-11. Lead AVR uses the left ankle and the left wrist as common negative and the right wrist as positive. Lead AVL uses the left ankle and the right wrist as common negative and the left wrist as positive. Lead AVF uses both wrists as common negative and the left ankle as positive.

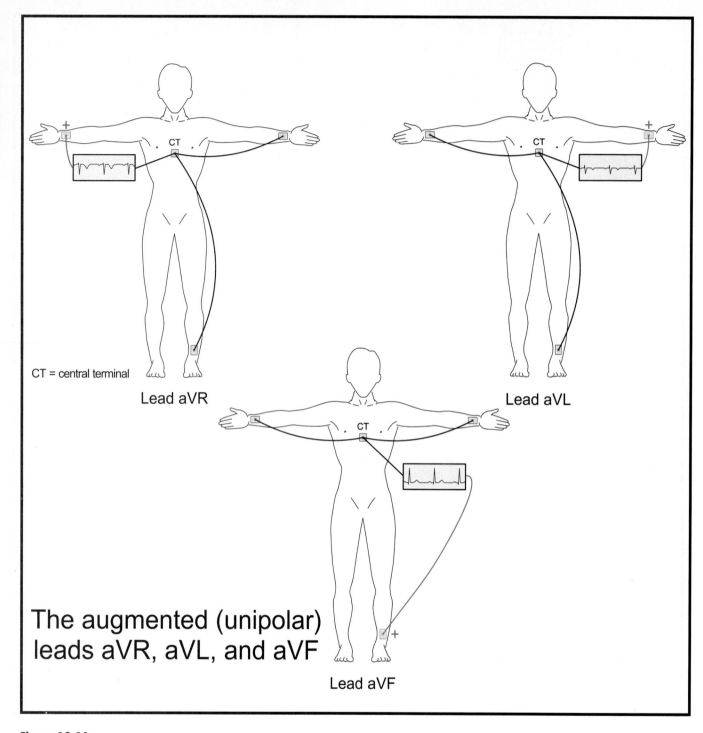

CT = central terminal

Lead aVR

Lead aVL

The augmented (unipolar) leads aVR, aVL, and aVF

Lead aVF

Figure 12-11

Augmented limb lead placement. *From Huszar: Basic dysrhythmias, second edition, 1994, Mosby Lifeline.*

The chest leads are named as V_1-V_6 leads (Fig. 12-12). The chest leads tie all of the limb electrodes together as a common ground and use a single positive electrode to go across the chest over the heart.

A few EMS systems use standardized 12-lead ECG machines with computer interpretation. Use of these machines can determine the need for specialized treatment in some car-diac patients, such as thrombolytic, or clot dissolving, therapy. However, many systems are more interested in determining abnormal rhythms than in making definitive diagnoses. Thus, single leads that have been modified are often used for pre-hospital cardiac monitoring (Figure 12-13).

Because standard electrode placements are very sensitive to patient motion and ambulance vibration, they are not prac-

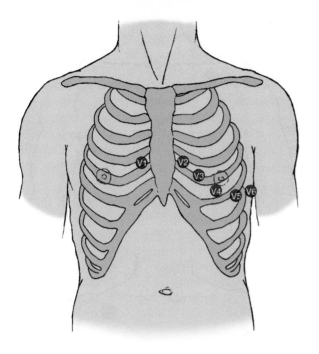
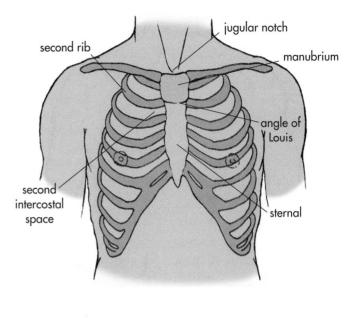

Figure 12-12

Precordial leads. *From Phalen: The 12-lead ECG in acute myocardial infarction, 1994, Mosby Lifeline.*

tical for field monitoring. The solution involves using only three electrodes, and moving them to positions on the chest (Fig. 12-14). This method is called a "modified lead."

Distortion of the ECG tracing, or artifact, can be caused in numerous ways. In addition to patient movement, a dry or disconnected electrode can also cause problems. Other

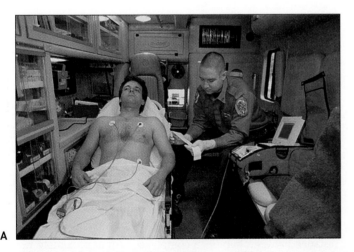

Figure 12-13

(A) Monitoring a patient with 3 leads (B) Lead tracing (Lead II) with 3 lead monitoring. *From Sanders: Mosby's paramedic texbook, 1994, Mosby Lifeline.*

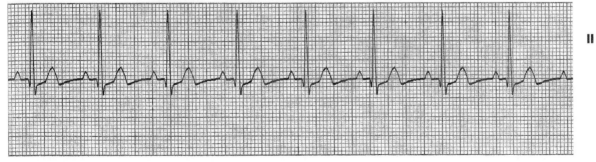

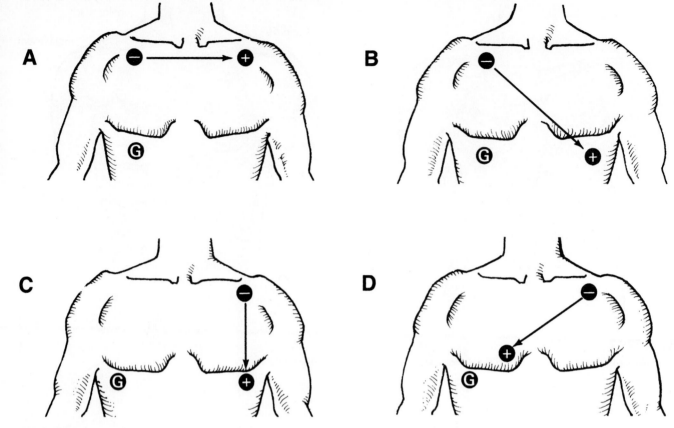

Figure 12-14

Placement for modified leads (A) Lead I (B) Lead II (C) Lead III (D) MCL1. *Reproduced with permission.*
©Textbook of Advanced Cardiac Life Support, 1994, Copyright American Heart Association.

sources include electrical interference (60-cycle), a broken wire, excessive patient chest hair, and problems with the amplifier. Figure 12-15 shows some examples of artifacts. When possible, the cause of the artifact should be determined and corrected.

Determining Cardiac Rhythm

There are five basic steps in determining a rhythm:

1. Rate: What is the rate?
2. Pattern: Is the rhythm regular or irregular? If irregular, is there pattern? (Called regularly irregular.)
3. QRS Width: Is it normal (less than 0.12 seconds) or abnormal?
4. Atrial Activity: Is there atrial activity? If so, what is it?
5. Relationship: Is there a relationship between the atrial activity and the QRS complexes?

Rate Calculation

There are many different methods that can be used to determine a patient's heart rate on the ECG. Each QRS typically causes the ventricle to contract, thus causing the heart to pump blood. The paramedic should never assume, however, that a QRS complex on the ECG monitor indicates the presence of a pulse. This reading should be verified by feeling a pulse at the wrist or other appropriate area for pulse assessment.

The most accurate method of calculating rate is to count the number of complexes occurring in 1 minute. However, if the rhythm is regular, this degree of accuracy is generally not needed. Most ECG paper has 3-second marks above or below the grid. The rate can be quickly approximated by counting the number of QRS complexes within two adjacent 3-second intervals (a 6-second strip) and multiplying by 10 (Fig. 12-16). Another method is to base the rate on one cardiac cycle (the distance between two QRS complexes). An approximate rate can be determined by counting the number of large, 5-mm boxes from one QRS complex to the next and dividing that number into 300 (Fig. 12-17). A more accurate method is to count the number of small 1-mm boxes and divide that result into 1500. The dividing method requires that the heart rate be regular to get an accurate reading.

A normal heart rate is defined as 60 to 100 beats per minute. A heart rate of less than 60 is defined as bradycardia. A rate greater than 100 beats per minute is defined as a tachycardia.

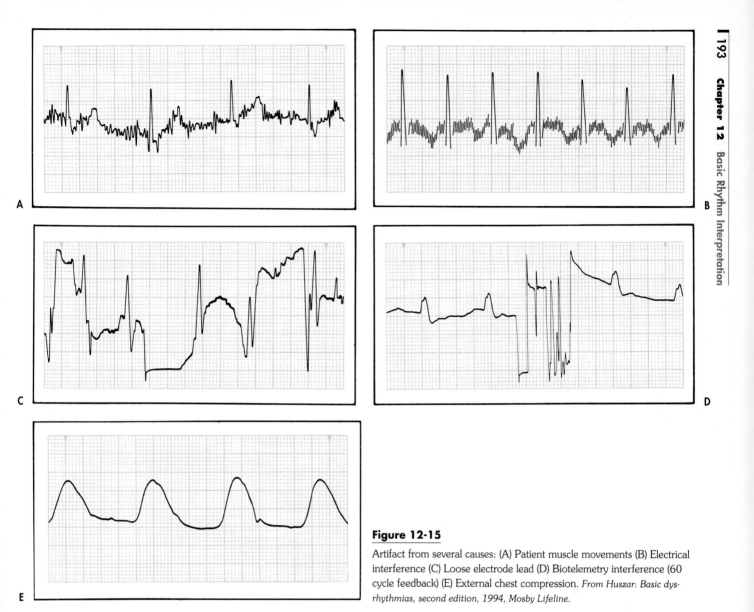

Figure 12-15

Artifact from several causes: (A) Patient muscle movements (B) Electrical interference (C) Loose electrode lead (D) Biotelemetry interference (60 cycle feedback) (E) External chest compression. *From Huszar: Basic dysrhythmias, second edition, 1994, Mosby Lifeline.*

Pattern Recognition

Six basic patterns appear in ECG rhythms (Fig. 12-18).

1. A regular rhythm means that the time between each beat is the same. The pulse felt with this rhythm would be reg-

ular, as would the distances between QRS complexes on the strip. P waves can be analyzed in the same manner. All pacemaker sites (e.g., sinus, atrial, junctional (nodal) and ventricular) can produce a regular rhythm.

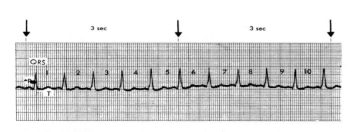

Figure 12-16

Six second strip method for counting minute heart rate. *From Goldberger, et al: Clinical electrocardiography, fifth edition, 1994, St. Louis, Mosby-Year Book, Inc.*

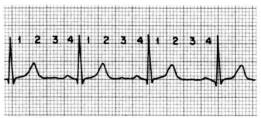

Figure 12-17

Box method. With a regular rhythm, count the number of large boxes (0.2 seconds) between two adjacent QRS complexes and divide into 300. *From Goldberger, et al: Clinical electrocardiography, fifth edition, 1994, St. Louis, Mosby-Year Book, Inc.*

2. Another common pattern is one that has a premature beat, one that comes earlier than expected. Premature beats can come from the atrium, the junction (node) or the ventricle. The underlying rhythm remains regular.

3. The rhythm can speed or slow gradually over several beats, without a sudden change. This is a function of the sinus (SA) mode.

4. A pause is the absence of a beat when it is supposed to occur; the rhythm pauses, then continues. A pause is usually caused by a blocked beat.

5. "Grouped" beats can appear, separated by pauses; grouped beats are usually indicative of a block at the AV node, or of frequent premature beats in a repetitive pattern.

6. The final type is a chaotic one in which the rhythm is irregular, lacking any pattern. This usually represents atrial fibrillation, though it can also be seen when several different types of premature beats are present.

QRS Width

The width of the QRS complex is important in determining whether the ventricles depolarized simultaneously. The conducting system allows this simultaneous depolarization. Impulses arising in the AV node, atrium, or sinus (SA) node are conducted through the bundle of His and the bundle branches to the Purkinje fibers. This is the fastest route to depolarize the ventricle. Once the Purkinje fibers are activated, both ventricles depolarize from the inside out at almost the same time. This simultaneous activation causes a narrow QRS complex (less than 0.12 seconds). Supraventricular generation of impulses uses this pathway.

Impulses beginning in the ventricles cannot use this conduction system. They conduct more slowly through working cells, and are therefore wider on the ECG. QRS complexes can also be wide if there is abnormal, or aberrant, conduction through one of the bundle branches resulting in a slower conduction along one bundle branch. So, a narrow QRS complex means that the impulse originated at or above the AV node; this is often referred to as a supraventricular focus (site of origin). Wide QRS complexes (≥0.12 seconds) either originate in

the ventricles or are aberrantly conducted through one of the bundles. Figure 12-19 shows abnormal QRS complexes.

Atrial Activity

Atrial activity can take several forms. Normally, the impulse begins in the sinus (SA) node. Because the sinus node is high in the right atrium, the atrium is depolarized in a wave from the top right to bottom left. Because lead II points from the right shoulder to the left leg, exactly the direction in which the atrium is being depolarized, an atrial impulse originating in the sinus (SA) node will be seen as an upright, or positive, P wave. The P wave is usually positive in leads I, III, and AVF, The P wave from a sinus beat may be positive or negative in other leads. Most EMS systems use a modified lead II for monitoring.

A negative P wave occurring close to the QRS or after the QRS in lead II usually comes from the AV node, indicating that the atrium is being depolarized from the bottom to top.

A third type of atrial activity is a flutter pattern. This pattern looks like a picket fence or sawtooth, with both a positive and a negative component.

The fourth form of atrial activity is fibrillation. This is often characterized as an irregular waviness to the baseline. At times, this can look like a positive or negative P wave or a sawtooth, but it is never consistent. It is also possible that there will be no atrial activity at all. Abnormal P waves are illustrated in Figure 12-20. The atrial pattern can switch between fibrillation and flutter.

The paramedic should look for evidence of atrial activity by searching for each of these types. Look between the end of a T wave and the start of the following QRS complex for this electrical activity. Occasionally, this atrial activity is on top of

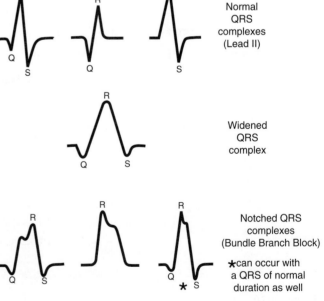

Figure 12-19

Abnormal QRS complexes.

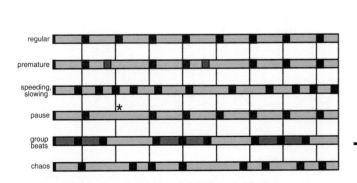

Figure 12-18

All rhythms follow into one if six basic patterns.

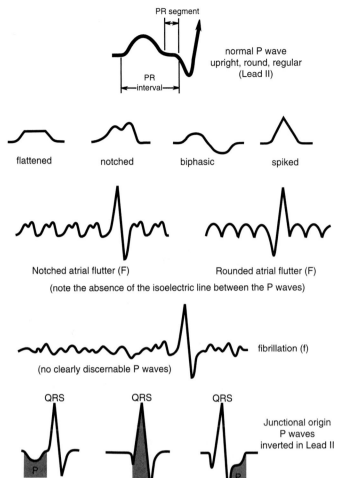

Figure 12-20

Abnormal P waves.

A fixed, 1:1, normal relationship means that every P wave is followed by a QRS complex (1:1), the PR interval is constant or unchanging (fixed), and the PR interval is 0.20 seconds in duration or less (normal). In a fixed, 1:1, prolonged relationship, every P wave is followed by a QRS complex (1:1), and the PR interval is constant or unchanged (fixed), but the PR interval is longer than 0.20 seconds (prolonged). If there are more P waves than QRS complexes, then the P waves may not be causing the QRS complexes. Other criteria have to be used to make this determination. See second- and third-degree block, discussed below. If none of these three relationships exists, the P waves did not cause the QRS complexes, even if P waves are visible on the tracing.

Sources of Impulses

After the five steps have been determined, the rhythm is undefined. To determine whether it acts similar to a given rhythm, certain characteristics must be understood about each of the four pacemaker sites previously mentioned.

- *Sinus (SA) Node.* The sinus (SA) node tends to pace in a regular pattern. Because this node is influenced by the vagus and sympathetic nerves, it can speed or slow gradually over several beats. Its rate can vary from 35 to 200 in adults and can also vary with respiration.
- *Atrium.* The atrium can fire regularly, but it is also the most erratic of the pacemakers and can be extremely irregular. Although the atrium can produce rhythms with its own intrinsic escape mechanisms, this is unusual and hard to differentiate in a single lead. The more common pattern is atrial rhythms involving either single premature beats or groups of beats. The atrium shifts suddenly into one of these types of rhythms, unlike the gradual changes in the sinus (SA) node. Atrial flutter is present when there is a picket fence or sawtooth appearance to the atrial activity. The sawtooth of atrial flutter is very regular and very fast. Atrial fibrillation is a chaotic firing of atrial muscle with no organization to the pattern. This is the most chaotic of the rhythms that can pump blood, and it leads to a very irregular pulse and ECG.
- *Junction (AV Node).* The junction, or AV node, or junction, tends to discharge in an extremely regular manner. The junction can cause premature beats alone or in groups. If the node is causing most of the beats on a tracing, the tracing will be very regular in pattern. The junction can vary in slow and regular rates from 30 to nearly 240.
- *Ventricle.* The ventricle can also fire at both extremely slow and very rapid rates. The rhythms are usually regular in nature, but can be irregular. When impulses begin in the ventricles, the QRS is always abnormally wide (0.12 seconds or greater). In addition to causing regular rhythms of varying rates, the ventricle can produce premature beats, either alone or in groups, and ventricular fibrillation, a chaotic pattern that cannot pump blood.

the previous T wave. The normal T wave from many cycles can be compared with the T wave in the cycle in question to see if there is an increased size, notching, or "hat" that suggests a P wave.

Relationship Between P Waves and QRS Complexes

Impulses initiating in the sinus (SA) node or atrium usually continue on to cause a ventricular depolarization. If the impulse conducts through the AV node to the ventricles, then the P wave must precede the QRS complex it caused. The AV node can be a two-way path. Occasionally, an impulse beginning in the ventricle can follow a retrograde conduction path back up to the atrium. This will cause a P wave that follows the QRS complex.

There are three basic ways in which atrial activity can cause a QRS complex:

1. A fixed, 1:1, normal relationship
2. A fixed, 1:1, prolonged relationship
3. More P waves than QRS complexes.

BOX 12-2	Sinus Rhythm
Rate	60–100 beats/min
Pattern	Regular
QRS width	Usually normal (can be abnormal)
Atrial activity	Positive P waves in lead II
Relationship	Usually 1:1, fixed, normal (PR 0.20 sec or less), but may be fixed, prolonged (1° AV block), or have more Ps than QRSs (2° or 3° AV block)

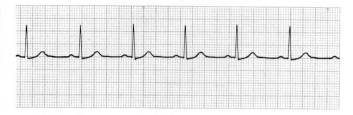

Figure 12-21

Normal sinus rhythm. *From Huszar: Basic dysrhythmias, second edition, 1994, Mosby Lifeline.*

Identifying the Basic Rhythm

The first step in identifying the rhythm strip is to identify the underlying or basic rhythm. This is the rhythm that is causing the majority of beats when no abnormal rhythm is present. To identify the underlying rhythm, the paramedic must use the five basic steps described previously, and use logic to determine the nature of the rhythm. The following section will use lead II to identify the dysrhythmia, because it is the simplest and most common lead used to differentiate dysrhythmias.

Sinus Rhythm

Sinus rhythm begins in the sinus (SA) node and is regular with a rate between 60 and 100 beats per minute (*see* Box 12-2 and Fig. 12-21). Because the sinus (SA) node is high in the right atrium, the P wave will be positive in lead II. The pattern of the rhythm will be regular, because the sinus (SA) node is regular. The P waves, and usually the QRS complexes, are equal distances apart. The sinus (SA) node may gradually speed up or slow down. The atrial activity results in a positive P wave before each QRS, and the P waves are regular. For sinus rhythm, the width of the QRS was not used to make the final determination; therefore, the width of the QRS could either be normal or abnormal. In most patients, the QRS width will be normal. Any of these three relationships in which a P wave causes a QRS complex could exist. By convention, if the QRS width and the relationship are normal, they are not mentioned. Hence, if the rhythm is called normal sinus rhythm, the rate should be 60 to 100, regular, start with normal P waves, and have normal PR intervals and normal QRS complexes. If the PR interval is prolonged, then there is an AV nodal block.

If the QRS complex is wide, then there is aberrant conduction (bundle branch block).

Sinus Bradycardia

Sinus bradycardia begins in the sinus (SA) node and is regular with a rate less than 60 beats per minute (*see* Box 12-3 and Fig. 12-22). Because the sinus (SA) node is high in the right atrium, the P wave will be positive in lead II. The pattern of the rhythm will be regular because the sinus (SA) node is regular. A slight irregularity of the R-R interval can be seen with bradycardia and still be considered normal. The P waves, and usually the QRS complexes, are equal distances apart. In most patients, the QRS width will be normal. Any of the three relationships could exist in which a P wave causes a QRS complex.

Sinus Tachycardia

Sinus tachycardia begins in the sinus (SA) node and is regular with a rate greater than 100 beats per minute (*see* Box 12-4 and Fig. 12-23). Because the sinus (SA) node is high in the right atrium, the P wave will be positive in lead II. The pattern of the rhythm will be regular, because the sinus (SA) node is regular. The P waves, and usually the QRS complexes, are equal distances apart. Any of the three relationships could exist here as well in which a P wave causes a QRS complex.

Sinus Dysrhythmia

Sinus disrhythmia begins in the sinus (SA) node and is irregular (*see* Box 12-5 and Fig. 12-24). Sinus dysrhythmia is caused

BOX 12-3	Sinus Bradycardia
Rate	Less than 60 beats/min
Pattern	Regular
QRS width	Usually normal (can be abnormal)
Atrial activity	Positive P waves in lead II
Relationship	Usually 1:1, fixed, normal (PR 0.20 sec or less); but may be fixed, prolonged (1° AV block) or have more Ps than QRSs (2° or 3° AV block)

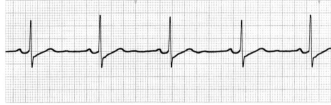

Figure 12-22

Sinus bradycardia. *From Huszar: Basic dysrhythmias, second edition, 1994, Mosby Lifeline.*

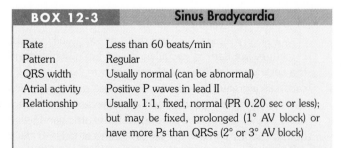

BOX 12-4	Sinus Tachycardia
Rate	More than 100 beats/min
Pattern	Regular
QRS width	Usually normal (can be abnormal)
Atrial activity	Positive P waves in lead II
Relationship	Usually 1:1, fixed, normal (PR 0.20 sec or less); but may be fixed, prolonged (1° AV block) or have more Ps than QRSs (2° or 3° AV block)

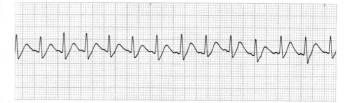

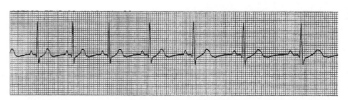

Figure 12-23

Sinus tachycardia. *From Huszar: Basic dysrhythmias, second edition, 1994, Mosby Lifeline.*

BOX 12-5	Sinus Disrhythmia
Rate	Variable; usually between 40 and 100 beats/min
Pattern	Varies with respiration: speeds with inspiration and slows upon expiration
QRS width	Usually normal (can be abnormal)
Atrial activity	Positive P waves in lead II
Relationship	Usually 1:1, fixed, normal (PR 0.20 sec or less); but may be fixed, prolonged (1° AV block) or have more Ps than QRSs (2° or 3° AV block)

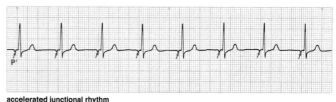

Figure 12-24

Sinus dysrhythmia. *From Sanders: Mosby's paramedic textbook, 1994, Mosby Lifeline.*

BOX 12-6	Junctional Rhythm (Accelerated)
Rate	60–100 beats/min
Pattern	Regular
QRS width	Normal (<0.12 sec)
Atrial activity	Negative P waves in lead II before or after QRS, or no P wave associated with the QRS.
Relationship	1:1 before or after QRS, or no relationship; P-R interval, when present, should be abnormally short (<0.12 sec)

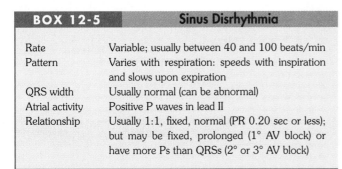

accelerated junctional rhythm

Figure 12-25

Accelerated junctional rhythm. *From Huszar: Basic dysrhythmias, second edition, 1994, Mosby Lifeline.*

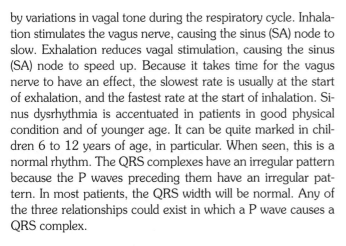

by variations in vagal tone during the respiratory cycle. Inhalation stimulates the vagus nerve, causing the sinus (SA) node to slow. Exhalation reduces vagal stimulation, causing the sinus (SA) node to speed up. Because it takes time for the vagus nerve to have an effect, the slowest rate is usually at the start of exhalation, and the fastest rate at the start of inhalation. Sinus dysrhythmia is accentuated in patients in good physical condition and of younger age. It can be quite marked in children 6 to 12 years of age, in particular. When seen, this is a normal rhythm. The QRS complexes have an irregular pattern because the P waves preceding them have an irregular pattern. In most patients, the QRS width will be normal. Any of the three relationships could exist in which a P wave causes a QRS complex.

Junctional Rhythm (Accelerated)

Junctional rhythm begins in the AV node, or junction, and is regular with a rate between 60 and 100 beats per minute (*see* Box 12-6 and Fig. 12-25). (Some authorities define junctional rhythm by the intrinsic rate of the AV node [*40 to 60 beats per minute*]. They define a junctional rate of 60 to 100 beats

per minute as an "accelerated" junctional rhythm, and a rate below 40 beats per minute as a junctional bradycardia. Because treatment decisions are partially based upon whether the rate is less than or greater than 60 beats per minute, junctional rhythm is defined here as being between 60 and 100 beats per minute, and bradycardia (or escape) as less than 60 beats per minute.) Junctional rhythms may have a negative P wave that occurs before or after the QRS or no P waves at all. On occasion there may be a positive P wave, but it has no relationship to the QRS complex. The QRS complexes are usually normal, and the R-R interval of each of the QRS complexes is an equal distance apart.

Junctional Bradycardia (Escape)

Junctional bradycardia begins in the AV node, or junction, and is regular with a rate less than 60 beats per minute (*see* Box 12-7 and Fig. 12-26). Junctional rhythms may have a negative P wave before or after the QRS, or no P wave at all. On occasion there may be a positive P wave, but it has no relationship to the QRS complex. The QRS complex is usually normal.

BOX 12-7	Junctional Bradycardia (Escape)
Rate	Less than 60 beats/min
Pattern	Regular
QRS width	Normal (<0.12 sec)
Atrial activity	Negative P waves in lead II before or after QRS, or no P wave associated with the QRS
Relationship	1:1 before or after QRS or no relationship; P-R interval, when present, should be abnormally short (<0.12 sec)

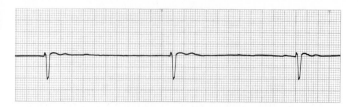

Figure 12-26

Junctional bradycardia. *From Huszar: Basic dysrhythmias, second edition, 1994, Mosby Lifeline.*

BOX 12-8	Junctional Tachycardia
Rate	More than 100 beats/min
Pattern	Regular
QRS width	Normal (<0.12 sec)
Atrial activity	Negative P waves in lead II before or after QRS, or no P wave associated with the QRS
Relationship	1:1 before or after QRS or no relationship; P-R interval, when present, should be abnormally short (<0.12 sec)

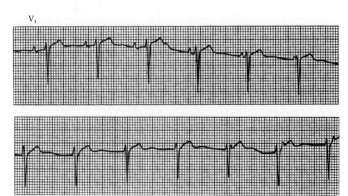

Figure 12-27

Junctional tachycardia. *From Aehlert: ACLS quick review study guide, 1994, Mosby Lifeline.*

BOX 12-9	Ventricular Rhythm (Accelerated Idioventricular Rhythm, Slow Ventricular Tachycardia)
Rate	60–100 beats/min
Pattern	Usually regular
QRS width	Abnormal (0.12 sec or wider)
Atrial activity	Positive or negative P waves in lead II after QRS, but more likely none at all
Relationship	Usually no relationship, but may be 1:1 after QRS

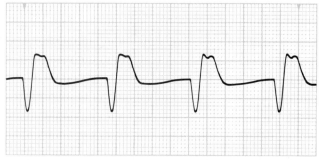

Figure 12-28

AIVR (Accelerated idioventricular rhythm). *From Huszar: Basic dysrhythmias, second edition, 1994, Mosby Lifeline.*

Junctional Tachycardia

Junctional tachycardia begins in the AV node or junction and is regular, with a rate more than 100 beats per minute (*see* Box 12-8 and Fig. 12-27). Junctional rhythms may have a negative P wave before or after the QRS or no P waves at all. On occasion there may be positive P waves, but they have no relationship to the QRS complexes. The QRS complexes are usually normal.

Ventricular Rhythm

Ventricular rhythm (e.g., accelerated idioventricular rhythm, slow ventricular tachycardia) begins in the ventricle and is usually regular, with a rate between 60 and 100 beats per minute (*see* Box 12-9 and Fig. 12-28). Some authorities define ventricular rhythm by the intrinsic rate of the ventricle (30 to 40 beats per minute). They define a ventricular rate of 60 to 100 beats per minute as an accelerated ventricular rhythm or slow ventricular tachycardia, and a rate below 40 beats per minute as an idioventricular rhythm. Because treatment decisions are partially based upon whether the rate is less than or greater than 60, ventricular rhythm is defined here as being between 60 and 100 beats per minute, and bradycardia as less than 60 beats per minute. Ventricular rhythms may have a negative P wave after the QRS or no P waves at all. On occasion there may be a positive P wave, but this has no relationship to the QRS complex. The QRS complex is always at 0.12 seconds or wider.

Ventricular Bradycardia

Ventricular bradycardia (e.g., idioventricular rhythm or ventricular escape) begins in the ventricle and is usually regular, with a rate less than 60 beats per minute (*see* Box 12-10 and

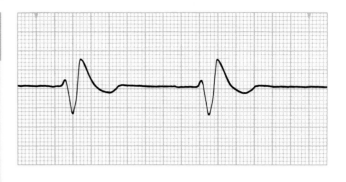

BOX 12-10	**Ventricular Bradycardia (Idioventricular Rhythm or Ventricular Escape)**
Rate	Less than 60 beats/min
Pattern	Usually regular
QRS width	Abnormal (0.12 sec or wider)
Atrial activity	Positive or negative P waves in lead II after QRS, but more likely none at all
Relationship	Usually no relationship, but may be 1:1 after QRS

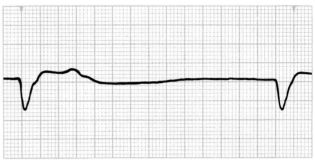

Fig. 12-29). (See ventricular rhythm for other definitions of ventricular rhythm and bradycardia.) Ventricular rhythm may have a negative P wave after the QRS or no P wave at all. On occasion there may be positive P waves seen on the tracing, but they have no relationship to the QRS complexes. The QRS complexes are always abnormal at 0.12 seconds wider.

Figure 12-29

Slow ventricular rhythm like that seen with idioventricular rhythm or ventricular escape. *From Huszar: Basic dysrhythmias, second edition, 1994, Mosby Lifeline.*

Ventricular Tachycardia

Ventricular tachycardia begins in the ventricle and is usually regular, with a rate greater than 100 beats per minute (*see* Box 12-11 and Fig. 12-30). Ventricular rhythms may have a negative P wave after the QRS or no P wave at all. On occasion there may be positive P waves, but they have no relationship to the QRS complexes. The QRS complexes are always abnormal at 0.12 seconds wider.

Premature Complexes

Premature complexes may arise in the atrium, the AV node, or the ventricle. As a premature beat is a sudden change in rate, it does not originate in the sinus (SA) node. The sinus node can speed or slow, but it cannot suddenly change rates. A premature beat is relative to the rate of the basic rhythm, which can be slow, fast or normal. A premature beat is early compared with the underlying rhythm beats. To define a premature beat, the paramedic must determine two additional characteristics. The first is the presence of a positive P wave before the complex. If there is not, the second factor is to use the width of the QRS to determine the site of origin of the impulse. The algorithm shown in Figure 12-31 should be used to differentiate premature beats in lead II.

Premature atrial complexes (PACs) have two characteristics: 1) they are early, and 2) they start with a positive P wave (*see* Box 12-12 and Fig. 12-32). Because premature atrial complexes may not give the AV node or bundle branches adequate time to repolarize, the impulses may not conduct properly. If the AV node does not conduct properly, the PR interval could be prolonged or the AV node may not conduct (called AV block). If the bundle branch does not conduct normally, the QRS may be wide (called bundle branch block).

Premature Junctional Complexes

Premature junctional complexes (PJCs) have three characteristics: 1) they are early, 2) they do not start with a positive P

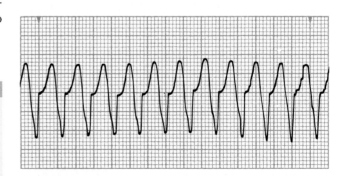

Figure 12-30

Ventricular tachycardia. *From Huszar: Basic dysrhythmias, second edition, 1994, Mosby Lifeline.*

BOX 12-11	**Ventricular Tachycardia**
Rate	More than 100 beats/min
Pattern	Usually regular
QRS width	Abnormal (0.12 sec or wider)
Atrial activity	Positive or negative P waves in lead II after QRS, but more likely none at all
Relationship	Usually no relationship, but may be 1:1 after QRS

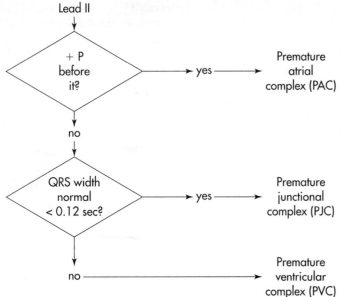

Figure 12-31

Differentiation of premature complexes.

BOX 12-12   **Premature Atrial Complexes**

Rate	Rate of underlying rhythm
Pattern	Sudden and premature
QRS width	Normal or abnormal
Atrial activity	Positive P wave in lead II
Relationship	Normal, prolonged, or blocked

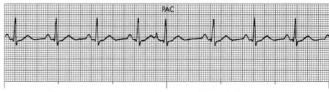

Figure 12-32

PACs (Premature atrial complexes). *From Aehlert: ECGs made easy, 1995, Mosby Lifeline.*

wave, and 3) they have a normal QRS width (*see* Box 12-13 and Fig. 12-33). Premature junctional complexes may have a negative P wave immediately before the complex (PR interval less than 0.12 sec), a negative P wave after the complex, or no P wave associated with the QRS complex at all.

Premature Ventricular Complexes

Premature ventricular complexes (PVCs) have three characteristics: 1) they are early, 2) they do not start with a positive P wave, and 3) they have an abnormal QRS width (*see* Box 12-14 and Fig. 12-34). Premature ventricular complexes may have a negative P wave after the complex or no P wave associated with the QRS complex at all. PVCs frequently appear with the wide QRS deflected one direction and the T wave deflected the opposite direction.

Couplets and Paroxysmal Tachycardias

A couplet is merely two premature beats of any origin in a row. A paroxysmal tachycardia is three or more premature complexes in a row. When a rhythm suddenly changes into a tachycardia, particular attention should be paid to the first pre-

mature complex. This complex is usually the easiest in which to detect a preceding, positive P wave.

Paroxysmal Atrial Tachycardia

A paroxysmal atrial tachycardia is merely three or more premature atrial complexes in a row; the beats are early and begin with positive P waves (*see* Box 12-15 and Fig. 12-35). At times, the P wave may have different configurations and be irregular. Frequently, it is difficult to see P waves during the run of the tachycardia; pay particular attention to the first beat of a string. Occasionally, the word *paroxysmal* is dropped and it is called simply *atrial tachycardia*.

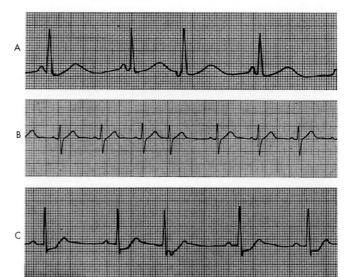

Figure 12-33

PJCs (Premature junctional complexes). *From Conover: Understanding electrocardiography, seventh edition, 1996, St. Louis, Mosby-Year Book, Inc.*

BOX 12-13   **Premature Junctional Complexes**

Rate	Rate of underlying rhythm
Pattern	Sudden and premature
QRS width	Normal (<0.12 sec)
Atrial activity	Negative P waves in lead II before or after QRS, or no P wave associated with the QRS
Relationship	1:1 before or after QRS or no relationship; P-R interval, when present should be abnormally short (< 0.12 sec)

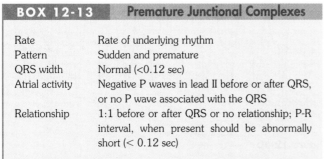

<table>
<tr><td colspan="2">BOX 12-14   Premature Ventricular Complexes</td></tr>
<tr><td>Rate</td><td>Rate of underlying rhythm</td></tr>
<tr><td>Pattern</td><td>Sudden and premature</td></tr>
<tr><td>QRS width</td><td>Abnormal (0.12 sec wider)</td></tr>
<tr><td>Atrial activity</td><td>Negative P waves in lead II after QRS, or no P wave associated with the QRS</td></tr>
<tr><td>Relationship</td><td>Usually no relationship, but may be 1:1 after QRS</td></tr>
</table>

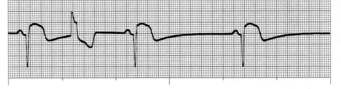

Figure 12-34

PVCs occurring during sinus bradycardia. *From Aehlert: ECGs made easy, 1995, Mosby Lifeline.*

<table>
<tr><td colspan="2">BOX 12-15   Paroxysmal Atrial Tachycardia</td></tr>
<tr><td>Rate</td><td>Greater than 100 (usually 150 to 240 beats/min)</td></tr>
<tr><td>Pattern</td><td>Starts suddenly, usually regular</td></tr>
<tr><td>QRS width</td><td>Normal or abnormal</td></tr>
<tr><td>Atrial activity</td><td>Positive P wave in lead II</td></tr>
<tr><td>Relationship</td><td>Normal, prolonged, or blocked</td></tr>
</table>

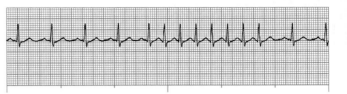

Figure 12-35

Atrial tachycardia. *From Aehlert: ECGs made easy, 1995, Mosby Lifeline.*

Paroxysmal Junction Tachycardia

A paroxysmal junctional tachycardia is merely three or more premature junctional beats in a row (*see* Box 12-16 and Fig. 12-36). The premature beats do not have positive P waves before them, but do have narrow QRS complexes. Premature junctional beats are usually very regular; the negative P waves look the same. The word *paroxysmal* is often dropped, and it is called a *junctional* or nodal *tachycardia.*

Paroxysmal Supraventricular Tachycardia (PSVT)

This term is used to include both paroxysmal atrial tachycardia and paroxysmal junctional tachycardia. Because the complexes are so close together, it is difficult to tell whether there is a positive P wave, or any P wave, before the complex (*see* Box 12-17 and Fig. 12-37). Because the treatments for paroxysmal atrial tachycardia and paroxysmal junctional tachycardia are the same, most people use the term paroxysmal supraventricular tachycardia (PSVT) to include both. A

narrow, sudden tachycardia with a narrow QRS can simply be called paroxysmal supraventricular tachycardia (or just PSVT) without further differentiation.

Paroxysmal Ventricular Tachycardia

A paroxysmal ventricular tachycardia is merely three or more premature ventricular complexes (PVCs) in a row (*see* Box 12-18 and Fig. 12-38). The premature ventricular complexes do not have positive P waves before them and have wide QRS complexes. Ventricular tachycardia is occasionally called paroxysmal ventricular tachycardia when it is not sustained but occurs suddenly and lasts for only a few beats or a short time.

Atrial Flutter

Atrial flutter is a circus movement within the atrium; this means that the impulse is being conducted around a circuit or

<table>
<tr><td colspan="2">BOX 12-16   Paroxysmal Junctional Tachycardia</td></tr>
<tr><td>Rate</td><td>Greater than 100 (usually 150 to 240 beats/min)</td></tr>
<tr><td>Pattern</td><td>Starts suddenly; regular</td></tr>
<tr><td>QRS width</td><td>Normal (<0.12 sec)</td></tr>
<tr><td>Atrial activity</td><td>Negative P waves in lead II before or after QRS or no P wave associated with the QRS</td></tr>
<tr><td>Relationship</td><td>1:1 before or after QRS or no relationship; P-R intervals, when present, are likely to be abnormally short (<0.12 sec)</td></tr>
</table>

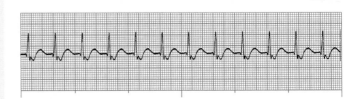

Figure 12-36

Junctional tachycardia. *From Aehlert: ECGs made easy, 1995, Mosby Lifeline.*

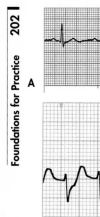

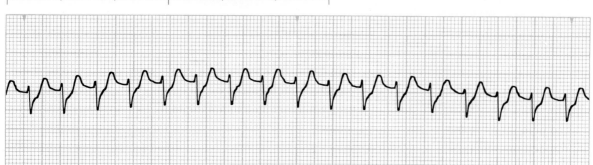

A

B

Figure 12-37

Supraventricular tachycardia. *A) From Aehlert: ECGs made easy, 1995, Mosby Lifeline. B) From Huszar: Basic dysrhythmias, second edition, 1994, Mosby Lifeline.*

loop, reproducing itself as it goes (*see* Box 12-19 and Fig. 12-39). Part of the time the atrium is depolarized from the top to the bottom, causing a positive P wave, and part of the time the atrium is depolarized from the bottom to the top, causing a negative P wave. There is a slight pause between the positive and negative P waves, causing a notch. The atrial activity is very regular. The AV node frequently blocks some of the impulses, causing the ventricular rate to be slower and sometimes irregular. The regular portion of atrial flutter is the atrial component.

Atrial Fibrillation

Atrial fibrillation is a chaotic firing of the atrial muscle (*see* Box 12-20 and Fig. 12-40). The atrial activity can resemble a positive P wave, a negative P or a sawtooth, but more often it is a

flat line or hash (signal noise). None of these patterns is consistent. Some of the activity is conducted through the AV node, but because it is chaotic, the formation of the QRS complexes are totally irregular. This rhythm is irregularly irregular or is even grossly irregular. It may mimic other rhythms for a beat or two, but it is never consistent. The hallmark of atrial fibrillation is irregularly irregular firing of the QRS complexes that do not fit an identifiable pattern. Because the AV junction is generally responsible for the formation of the QRS, the QRS width is generally normal.

Ventricular Fibrillation

Ventricular fibrillation is a lethal rhythm that results in an inability of the heart to pump blood. There are no QRS complexes or P waves detectable, only a wavy baseline that re-

BOX 12-17	**Paroxysmal Supraventricular Tachycardia ([PSVT] Combination of Paroxysmal Atrial Tachycardia and Paroxysmal Junctional Tachycardia)**
Rate	Greater than 100 (usually 150 to 240 beats/min)
Pattern	Starts suddenly; regular
QRS width	Usually normal (<0.12 sec)
Atrial activity	Not defined
Relationship	Not defined

BOX 12-18	**Paroxysmal Ventricular Tachycardia**
Rate	Rate of underlying rhythm
Pattern	Sudden and premature
QRS width	Abnormal (0.12 sec or wider)
Atrial activity	Negative P waves in lead II after QRS or no P wave associated with the QRS
Relationship	Usually no relationship, but may be 1:1 after QRS

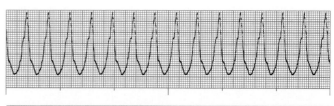

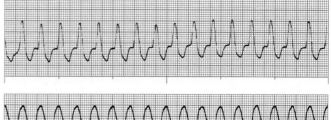

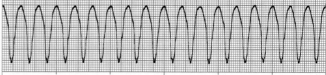

Figure 12-38

Ventricular tachycardia. *From Aehlert: ECGs made easy, 1995, Mosby Lifeline.*

BOX 12-19 — Atrial Flutter

Rate	Atrial rate 240 to 320 beats/min; ventricular rate usually less
Pattern	Atrial regular, ventricular usually slower and may be regular or irregular
QRS width	Normal or abnormal
Atrial activity	Sawtooth or picket fence appearance in lead II
Relationship	Usually more flutter waves than QRS, but may be 1:1

BOX 12-20 — Atrial Fibrillation

Rate	Atrial rate > 350 beats/min, if a rate can be determined at all; ventricular rate less
Pattern	Atrial irregular, ventricular slower and very irregular
QRS width	Normal or abnormal
Atrial activity	Irregular; occasionally may look like positive or negative P wave or sawtooth/picket fence appearance in lead II, but never consistent
Relationship	More fibrillation waves than QRSs; exact relationship impossible to determine

BOX 12-21 — Ventricular Fibrillation

Rate	Ventricle >.350 beats/min, if a rate can be determined at all
Pattern	Ventricular very irregular
QRS width	Not seen
Atrial activity	Not seen
Relationship	Not seen

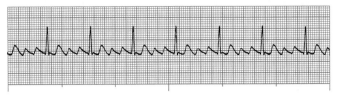

Figure 12-39

Atrial flutter. *From Aehlert: ECGs made easy, 1995, Mosby Lifeline.*

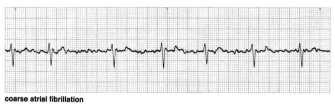

coarse atrial fibrillation

Figure 12-40

Atrial fibrillation. *From Huszar: Basic dysrhythmias, second edition, 1994, Mosby Lifeline.*

sembles signal noise (*see* Box 12-21 and Fig. 12-41). Often, other obstacles can mimic the pattern, such as a loose or defective electrode, a bad wire or connector, or patient movement or seizures, resulting in a signal noise that resembles ventricular fibrillation. Therefore, the rhythm must also be recognized through clinical assessment. Ventricular fibrillation produces no pulse, and the patient will be unresponsive within 12 to 15 seconds after onset of the rhythm. When a patient goes into ventricular fibrillation, it is usually coarse in nature with great fluctuations in the baseline. As time goes by, it becomes finer in appearance.

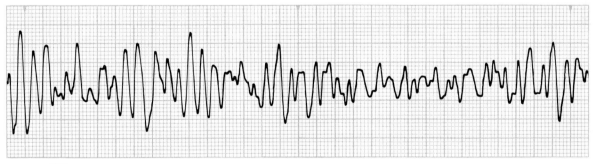

A

coarse VF

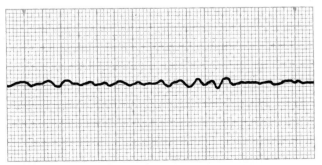

fine VF

B

Figure 12-41

Coarse (A) and fine (B) ventricular fibrillation. *From Huszar: Basic dysrhythmias, second edition, 1994, Mosby Lifeline.*

BOX 12-22	Asystole
Rate	0
Pattern	None
QRS width	Not seen
Atrial activity	Not seen
Relationship	Not seen

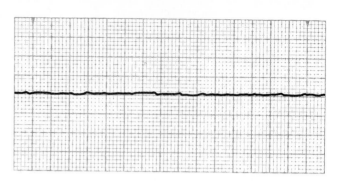

Asystole

Asystole is another form of cardiac arrest; no rhythm is present at all, only a flat line (*see* Box 12-22 and Fig. 12-42). The paramedic must be sure that the electrodes are connected and that the machine is turned on to the proper lead; asystole should be verified in a second lead. The patient will be pulseless and unresponsive. Asystole may be difficult to distinguish from fine ventricular fibrillation.

Figure 12-42

Asystole. *From Huszar: Basic dysrhythmias, second edition, 1994, Mosby Lifeline.*

Escape Rhythms

An escape beat is one that occurs after a pause and is seen on the ECG as an abnormally long R-R interval (Fig. 12-43). Escapes are named similarly to premature beats. The atrium does not normally cause an escape, although the sinus (SA) node can. If the beat after a pause has a positive P wave in front of it, it is a sinus escape. If the beat after a pause does not have a positive P wave in front of it and has a normal QRS width, then it is likely a junctional escape. The late beat with a wide QRS and absent P wave is probably a ventricular escape. Sometimes the sinus (SA) node fails to fire and is replaced by a junctional or ventricular escape rhythm. This is a protective mechanism, preventing cardiac arrest from failure of the conduction system. Remember that the intrinsic rate of the junction is 40 to 60 beats per minute, and that of the ventricles is 30 to 40 beats per minute. A junctional bradycardia occurring as a result of conduction system failure is also called junctional escape. For the same reason, ventricular bradycardia could be called ventricular escape.

Figure 12-43

(A) Junctional escape beat (B) Sinus escape beat (C) Junctional escape rhythm (D) Ventricular escape rhythm. *From Goldberger, et al: Clinical electrocardiography, fifth edition, 1994, St. Louis, Mosby-Year Book, Inc.*

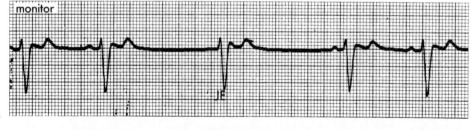

A

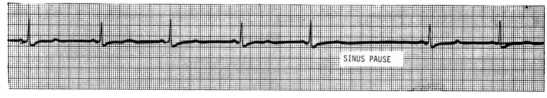

B

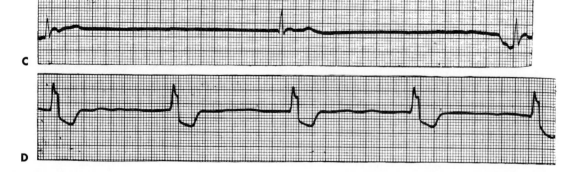

C

D

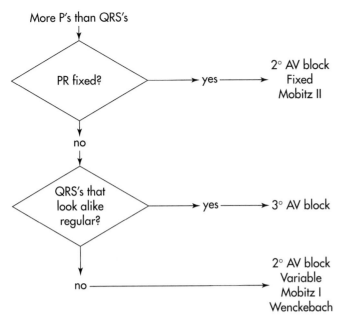

Figure 12-44

Differentiation of second- and third-degree AV blocks.

AV Blocks

Conduction of the impulses through the AV node can be delayed at times. These delayed conduction patterns are called blocks. Blocks within the AV node can be divided into three types. In first-degree block, every P wave is conducted through the AV node and is delayed; the PR interval is consistently prolonged for every beat. In second-degree block, the AV node conducts some but not all of the P waves. In third-degree AV block, none of the P waves are conducted through the AV node; the QRS complexes are either junctional or ventricular escape beats that have no relationship to the P waves.

Differentiation between second- and third-degree AV blocks can be difficult. A simple algorithm for differentiation is shown in Figure 12-44. Whenever there are more P waves than QRS complexes on the tracing, the paramedic must suspect a second- or third-degree block. Either flutter wave in atrial flutter can be considered as if it were a P wave (sometimes called F waves). Each fibrillation wave in atrial fibrillation can also be considered as if it were a P wave (sometimes called F waves). The paramedic should look at the P wave that precedes each QRS complex. If the P wave has a constant PR interval, then the block is second-degree. This type of second-

degree block is referred to as a fixed second-degree AV block, a Type II second-degree block, or a Mobitz II block.

If the PR interval is variable, the paramedic should look at the QRS complexes that look alike, and determine if they are regular or irregular in pattern. If the PR interval is variable and the QRS complexes have an irregular pattern, this is the variable form of second-degree AV block.

Look-alike QRS complexes that are regular suggest a third-degree AV block, also called complete heart block; a variable PR interval cannot cause a regular pattern. The reason for analyzing only QRS complexes that look alike is to determine if there is more than one escape site operating. There may be both junctional and ventricular escapes, for instance, which will have different appearances. At times, multiple escape focuses may be active in the ventricles, and they can have different rates. Patients with third-degree heart block can also have premature ventricular complexes.

Fixed second-degree AV has two characteristics: 1) there are more P waves than QRS complexes; and 2) there is a constant PR interval. The variable form of second-degree AV block has three characteristics: 1) there are more P waves than QRS complexes; 2) there is a variable PR interval; and 3) the QRS complexes that look alike have an irregular pattern. Third-degree AV block has three characteristics: 1) there are more P waves than QRS complexes; 2) there is a variable PR interval (no relationship between P waves and QRS complexes); and 3) the QRS complexes that look alike have a regular pattern. There is usually a regular R-R interval and often a regular P-P interval present with third-degree block, because they are functioning independently but often regularly.

First-Degree AV Block

First-degree AV block may be seen in patients with sinus rhythm, sinus bradycardia, sinus tachycardia or sinus dysrhythmia and also sometimes appears after premature atrial complexes (see Box 12-23 and Fig. 12-45). When the origin of the rhythm is sinus, the long PR interval (greater than 0.20 sec) is seen with every beat and is constant. When the beat is a premature atrial complex, it may be the only beat with a long PR interval. This occurs when a premature beat does not give sufficient time for the AV node to repolarize.

BOX 12-23	First-Degree AV Block
Rate	Variable
Pattern	Regular or irregular
QRS width	Usually normal (can be abnormal)
Atrial activity	Positive P waves in lead II
Relationship	1:1, fixed, prolonged relationship

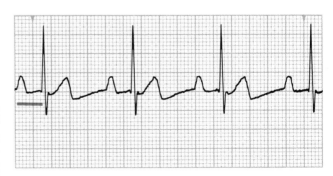

Figure 12-45

First-degree AV heart block. *From Huszar: Basic dysrhythmias, second edition, 1994, Mosby Lifeline.*

Second-Degree Variable AV Block

Second-degree variable AV block is also called Wenckebach block or Mobitz I (Type I) second-degree block. Each successive P wave is delayed longer than the previous one, until the block occurs (see Box 12-24 and Fig. 12-46). The first PR interval in a group is usually normal, the next PR interval is longer and so on. When a P wave is finally blocked, a P wave is seen with no QRS after it and the AV node resets itself to the first PR interval. Because the PR varies, the QRS complexes have an irregular pattern. The block is usually in the AV node, which is not as dangerous as one that occurs lower on the conduction pathway. For this reason, second-degree variable block is usually stable and rarely progresses to more dangerous rhythms.

Second-Degree Fixed AV Block

Second-degree fixed AV block is also called Type II or Mobitz II block. Frequently, there is a repeated ratio of 2:1 or 3:1 block. With these ratios, every other P wave, or every third, fails to conduct and produce a QRS complex (see Box 12-25 and Fig. 12-47). The PR interval of the beat that conducts may be either normal or prolonged, but it is constant. If there is a fixed ratio, such as 2:1, the QRS complexes will occur in a regular pattern, with one missing at predictable intervals. However, many times the conduction rate varies, making the QRS pattern irregular. The QRS width may be normal if the

BOX 12-24	Second-Degree Variable AV Block (Wenckebach or Mobitz I)
Rate	Variable
Pattern	Irregular
QRS width	Usually normal (can be abnormal)
Atrial activity	Positive P waves in lead II
Relationship	More P waves than QRS complexes; the PR interval is variable

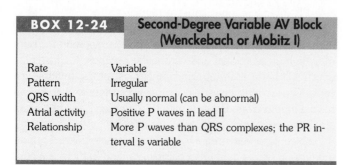

Figure 12-46

Second-degree AV heart block—Type I (Wenchebach or Mobitz I). *From Huszar: Basic dysrhythmias, second edition, 1994, Mosby Lifeline.*

BOX 12-25	Second-Degree Fixed AV Block (Mobitz II)
Rate	Variable
Pattern	Regular or irregular
QRS width	Usually abnormal (can be normal)
Atrial activity	Positive P waves in lead II
Relationship	More P waves than QRS complexes; the PR interval is constant

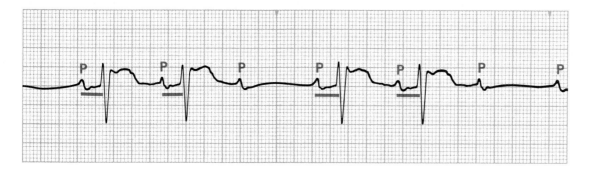

Figure 12-47

Second-degree AV heart block—Type II (Classic or Mobitz II). *From Huszar: Basic dysrhythmias, second edition, 1994, Mosby Lifeline.*

block is in the AV node. In this case, the risk to the patient is similar to the variable form of second-degree block described earlier. The more common form of fixed second-degree block, which has a wide QRS complex, occurs in the bundle branch, (below the bundle of His). Fixed second-degree block with a wide QRS complex can suddenly and unpredictably change to asystole, causing cardiac arrest. This form of block, therefore, is ominous, and the paramedic must be prepared to handle the block quickly.

Third-Degree AV Block

In this form of block, all atrial activity is blocked from conduction to the ventricle and the QRS complexes arise from junctional or ventricular escape activity (see Box 12-26 and Fig. 12-48). The PR interval appears to be completely variable, although there is no actual PR relationship. As both junctional and ventricular escapes are regular, QRS complexes that look alike are regular. On a single strip more than a single escape may occur.

Patients with third-degree AV block can also have premature ventricular complexes, which add irregularity to the pattern. Thus, it is important to compare QRS complexes that look alike and determine regularity. Junctional escape beats usually have a normal QRS width, and ventricular escape beats are wide.

Bundle Branch Blocks

The bundle branches may not depolarize properly, or may not conduct at all. As they must conduct normally for a narrow QRS complex to occur, block will cause the QRS complex to be wide. Remember, a beat is ventricular in origin only if the QRS complex is wide and there is no atrial activity evident that could have caused it.

Pacemakers and Implanted Defibrillators

Artificial pacemakers can be implanted in the heart to provide a rhythm when normal conduction mechanisms fail to provide an adequate heart rate. These devices are usually implanted under the skin on the chest wall below the clavicle. An electrode wire is floated down the subclavian vein to the right atrium or ventricle. A battery box, usually about 3 mm thick and 3 cm in diameter, is connected to the electrode and implanted under the skin. On occasions, the battery box can be implanted in the abdominal wall with the wires connected via a tunnel to the external surface of the heart.

A pacemaker has a circuit that looks either for a QRS complex or P wave, depending on where the electrode is implanted. If the pacemaker is set at a rate of 60 beats per minute and attached to the ventricle, it waits for 1 second for a QRS complex. If there is no QRS complex within 1 second, the pacemaker fires, causing an abnormally wide QRS complex. When a pacemaker causes a QRS complex, this is called capture. If the patient produces a QRS complex within the 1 second, then the pacemaker resets its 1-second time and begins waiting again. This pause for the patient's own QRS complex is called sensing. Therefore, when the patient has his or her own beat, the pacemaker should sense the beat, and when the patient does not have his or her own beat, the pacemaker should fire and capture the ventricle (Fig. 12-49).

Pacemakers are often placed only in the ventricle. These provide a QRS complex when the patient does not initiate one. Pacemakers can also be placed in the atrium, to generate a P wave when the patient does not. Atrial pacemakers are very uncommon. An AV-sequential pacemaker can pace the atrium, pause (like the AV node) and then pace the ventricle (Fig. 12-50). Newer pacemakers can speed up when they detect patient movement, and some pacemakers are designed to speed up to 130 or 140 beats per minute when the patient exercises.

Another new type of pacemaker is the antitachycardia pacer, which can detect when the patient is in paroxysmal supraventricular tachycardia or ventricular tachycardia. When the tachycardia is detected, the device fires quickly, up to eight times, to break the rhythm.

Some pacemakers can be analyzed over the telephone. A small box can be connected to the patient and then to the tele-

BOX 12-26	Third-Degree AV Block (Complete Heart Block)
Rate	Variable
Pattern	Regular for QRS complexes that look alike
QRS width	Normal or abnormal
Atrial activity	Positive P waves in lead II
Relationship	No relation between P waves and QRS complexes

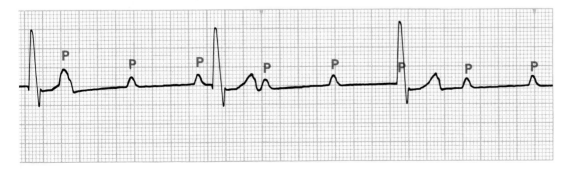

Figure 12-48

Third-degree (complete) AV heart block. *From Huszar: Basic dysrhythmias, second edition, 1994, Mosby Lifeline.*

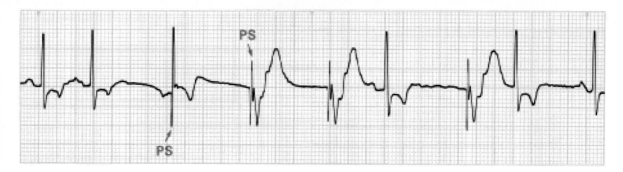

Figure 12-49

Ventricular demand pacemaker. *From Huszar: Basic dysrhythmias, second edition, 1994, Mosby Lifeline.*

phone. These devices transmit rhythm and internal circuitry information from the pacemaker, such as how much battery power is left.

Another artificial device is an automatic internal cardioverter-defibrillator (AICD) (Fig. 12-51). This device can detect ventricular fibrillation and shock the patient. These battery boxes are much larger than those for pacemakers, frequently 5 cm in diameter and nearly 1 cm thick. They may be placed in the abdominal wall or under the clavicle and will automatically shock the patient up to eight times, depending on how they are programmed. The paramedic may feel a slight shock if touching the patient at the time of firing, but this is not dangerous. The paramedic should treat the patient in a normal manner when one of these devices is present, including defibrillating if the patient is in ventricular fibrillation.

Both implanted pacemakers and automatic internal cardiovertor-defibrillators present one special consideration. If the need arises to defibrillate a patient with one of these devices, keep the defibrillator paddles or pads at least 2 inches and preferably 5 inches away from the battery box. Defibrillation over the metal battery box can cause serious burns around the battery box and could damage the circuitry inside it. Otherwise, treat a patient with a pacemaker or AICD like any other patient.

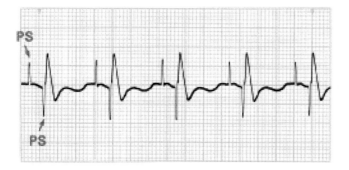

Figure 12-50

AV Sequential pacemaker. Note the presence of two pacemaker spikes. *From Huszar: Basic dysrhythmias, second edition, 1994, Mosby Lifeline.*

Critical Rhythms

Knowing the exact mechanism of a rhythm is not essential for most field treatment decisions made by the paramedic. The paramedic should look at the clinical situation and determine what to do.

If a patient is in cardiac arrest, CPR should be initiated while a manual or automated external defibrillator (AED) is attached. Defibrillation should then proceed as quickly as possible if the patient is in ventricular fibrillation. The most common pattern seen in cardiac arrest is ventricular fibrillation.

Ventricular fibrillation and pulseless ventricular tachycardia are both managed with defibrillation. In each case, the patient should be shocked with 200 joules (abbreviated J), 200 to 300 J, and 360 J of electricity. If defibrillation fails, the patient should be given epinephrine and defibrillated again at 360 J. Another common arrest rhythm, asystole, is treated with CPR, transcutaneous pacing, epinephrine and atropine (*see* Chapter 19 for ACLS treatment algorithms).

The final pattern that can be seen in a cardiac arrest is the presence of a QRS pattern on the ECG without a pulse; this is called pulseless electrical activity (PEA). PEA is divided into QRS rates that are less than 60 beats per minute and those with rates of 60 beats per minute or above. If the rate is less than 60, epinephrine and atropine are given. If the heart rate is 60 beats per minute or greater, epinephrine is the primary drug to use.

In patients with a pulse, another serious abnormality that can appear on the ECG is the presence of bradycardia or a slow rate. Low heart rates are important only if the slow rate causes symptoms. If a patient shows signs of dyspnea, heart failure, chest pain, bursts of ventricular tachycardia, or altered mental status with a low or low to normal blood pressure, the bradycardia must be treated. Initial therapies include atropine and transcutaneous pacing. Further treatment could include IV drips of dopamine, epinephrine or, less frequently, isoproterenol.

The patient with ventricular tachycardia is treated on the basis of symptoms. The asymptomatic patient is treated with drugs such as lidocaine and procainamide. If the patient has symptoms such as shock, dyspnea, chest pain, acute myocardial infarction, altered mental status, or heart failure, synchronized electrical cardioversion is indicated before the use of

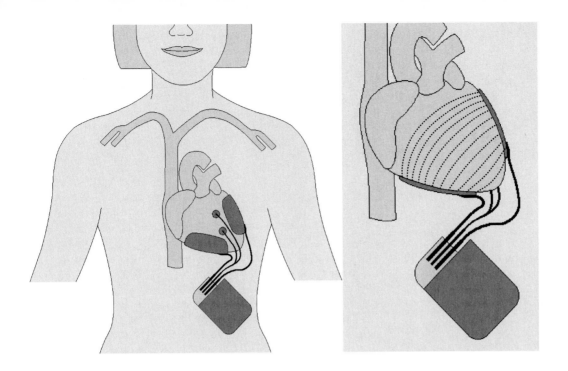

Figure 12-51

An automatic implantable cardioverter defibrillator (AICD). *From Conover: Understanding electrocardiography, seventh edition, 1996, St. Louis, Mosby-Year Book, Inc.*

medications. The use of sedation should be considered in the responsive patient.

SUMMARY

The ECG is an adjunct that can be used by the paramedic to assess and treat certain patients, particularly cardiac patients. It is a helpful tool that, along with sound clinical assessment skills, enables the paramedic to more thoroughly manage the patient.

SUGGESTED READINGS

1. **Aehlert, B.** *ECG, Made Easy,* Mosby, St. Louis, 1995.

2. **Conover, MB.** *Understanding Electrocardiography,* 7th ed., Mosby, St. Louis, 1995.

3. **Huszar, RJ,** *Basic Dysrhythmias,* 2nd ed., Mosby Lifeline, St. Louis, 1994.

4. **Loebs, S.** *ECG Interpretation Clinical Skillbuilders,* Springhouse, Springhouse, Pennsylvania, 1990.

5. **Norman, AE.** *Rapid ECG Interpretations, A Self Teaching Manual,* McGraw Hill, New York, 1993.

6. **Phillips, RE, Freeney, MK.** *The Cardiac Rhythms: A Systematic Approach to Interpretation,* W.B. Saunders, Philadelphia, 1990.

7. **Scheidt, S,** *Basic Electrocardiography,* CIBA-GEIGY Pharmaceuticals, 1986.

8. **Stein, E,** *Rapid Analysis of Arrhythmias,* 2nd ed., Lea & Febiger, Philadelphia, 1992.

9. **Walraven, AS,** *Basic Arrhythmias,* 4th ed., Brady/Prentice Hall, Englewood Cliffs, New Jersey, 1995.

Kate Dernocoeur, EMT-P

Chapter 13

Interpersonal Communication Skills

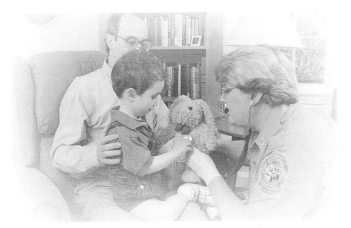

KEY TERMS

Communication—the transmission and reception of information, resulting in common understanding.

Compassion—a feeling of deep sympathy and sorrow for another who is stricken by misfortune, accompanied by a strong desire to alleviate the suffering.

Rapport—connection, especially harmonious or sympathetic relation.

Respect—esteem for, or a sense of the worth or excellence of, a person or a personal quality or ability.

A paramedic should be able to:

OBJECTIVES

1. Describe the importance of effective interpersonal communication skills.

2. Describe the three coping mechanisms that people may exhibit in response to stress.

3. Describe how the following factors can enhance or inhibit communication in an emergency situation:
   a. introductions and first impressions
   b. voice dynamics
   c. eye contact
   d. facial expression
   e. body stance and posture
   f. positioning
   g. touching
   h. good listening

4. Describe specific tactics for establishing trust and rapport.

5. Explain special communication techniques to employ when dealing with the following types of patients:
   a. pediatric according to age range
   b. geriatric
   c. mentally impaired
   d. foreign language speaking
   e. hearing impaired
   f. obstinate or potentially violent persons

6. Discuss appropriate communication methods to use with families and bystanders.

7. Discuss the need for effective communication with professional colleagues.

The paramedic faces many medical and logistical challenges in the course of his or her career. Hours of education, training, and practice provide the paramedic with the skills and judgment necessary to handle nearly any situation. For example, the paramedic spends hours learning about childbirth, and may deliver a few babies over the course of his or her career. Yet most paramedic students receive little instruction in the one skill required in every prehospital situation: interpersonal communication.

It is difficult to adequately emphasize the impact of effective interpersonal communication. People have a wide range of needs, from straightforward interfacility transfers to rapid, life-saving action. Gaining trust by rapidly building rapport with the people at each scene is imperative. When paramedics can assess each individual's specific needs and use effective interpersonal skills to meet those needs, prehospital situations tend to be safer (because of increased trust), more cooperative (because of improved rapport), and more rewarding.

Achieving effective interpersonal communication is not always possible because of the nature of the crisis. A crisis is an unplanned event, usually viewed negatively. People's personalities change in crisis, and this change creates special circumstances for the paramedic. Humans by nature dislike change and disruption, and emergencies bring both. Surging adrenalin, the fight-or-flight hormone, creates high (and sometimes explosive) levels of excitement. Other powerful emotions such as anger, fear, frustration, and grief are also common. In this world of instant gratification, people want everything resolved on the spot so that their normal lives may resume.

People cope with stress and crisis in a variety of ways. As stated in Chapter 58, people communicate differently when they are depressed, angry, irritated, or irrational. The following are examples of types of coping mechanisms:

- *Depression.* An emotional closing up, with the hope that the threatening feeling will blow over without causing too much harm. This response is similar to the way an armadillo curls up as a defense against its predators.
- *Regression.* The use of behaviors that were successful during earlier stages of development, even as early as toddler age. The adult version of a "temper tantrum" is relatively common in times of crisis.
- *Aggression.* The striking out, either verbally or physically, against personal threats. Verbal aggression may be relatively harmless, but physical aggression is definitely not. Many potentially explosive scenes can be defused with calm, professional, interpersonal communications strategies. Obviously, dangerous circumstances should be handled by law enforcement personnel.
- *No obvious change.* Fortunately, many people recognize that paramedics can work best when the scene and surroundings remain calm and cooperative.

General Principles

Paramedics routinely enter strangers' lives, ask intimately personal questions, touch the patient's body, and provide medical care. This approach works best when the patient is trusting and cooperative. Bystanders, too, must often be helpful and adopt these attributes. The paramedic can shape the emotional climate of most calls with effective interpersonal communication. Building trust, establishing rapport, increasing cooperation, and making a crisis situation as agreeable as possible are all important skills. Without these skills, necessary medical assistance can be difficult to deliver.

Consider the complexity of establishing a working relationship with strangers in crisis. The paramedic has expectations, opinions, assumptions—as does everyone else at the scene. These expectations seldom match up, especially since paramedics are quite accustomed to crisis, and those who called for help usually are not. As a human, the paramedic is subject to moods, exhaustion, prejudices and so on, but the professional paramedic is aware of how to keep personal feelings in check. For example, it is important for the paramedic not to allow feelings generated by one call to carry over to the next. To prevent this, the paramedic must develop methods of self-awareness and monitor his or her own responses to the stress of emergency care.

Everyone also has a natural presence. A person's stance, gait, posture, word choices, and facial expressions all relay an impression to others. Presence can range on a spectrum from meek and mild to powerful and intimidating. Each point on this spectrum is an effective interpersonal style at times. For example, a gentle and mild presence is often most effective when interacting with children and older people, while a tougher demeanor can be successful in other settings. Each person has a place on this soft-to-hard spectrum that could be considered his or her natural or typical interpersonal style. This serves as a starting point for changing one's interpersonal style as circumstances change. The paramedic essentially becomes an actor. The mild-mannered person can learn the tougher postures, facial expressions, and word choices needed to work effectively in tough settings, and the naturally intimidating individual can learn what it takes to appear soft and gentle when necessary.

The paramedic must quickly decide which demeanor will be most effective in different situations. Trying to impose an unchanging interpersonal style across all situations can lead to problems. Sometimes, the paramedic must take on different roles for different people at the same scene; a child may require a gentle demeanor, while the parent requires a firmer disposition. Or, the same patient may respond to one style initially, but require a different demeanor later. The more adept the paramedic becomes at alternating roles, the more effective the communication will be. This practice is an ongoing effort but a rewarding one.

To determine how a person is coping with a crisis, it may be necessary to "read" the patient during the period of introductions and first impressions. Look for behavioral clues, remembering the four typical responses to crisis. It is best to begin with a gentle, calm approach with depressive patients. For regressive patients, a parental or authoritative approach may be necessary until the tantrum passes; then it is usually possible to revert to a gentler, interpersonal style. A tough style may work with some aggressive people but it not always. The aim is to discover which tactics work best to defuse the situation safely. Fortunately, in the majority of prehospital cases, there is no need for the paramedic to move far from his or her natural style.

Once people at the scene see that the paramedic will meet their medical and emotional needs, good rapport is usually quick to develop. Honesty, mutual respect, a nonjudgmental approach, and preservation of the patient's sense of dignity all contribute to good rapport. When these principles are ignored, trouble results.

Methods of Communication

Paramedics use specific techniques to implement these general principles. Because each situation is unique, the paramedic will discover many strategies.

Introductions and First Impressions

From the onset of each situation, seek the cues that indicate which interpersonal approach will lead to the best rapport. The patient and bystanders will also be absorbing cues from responders, so first impressions are vital.[1] A person can form an opinion of someone else within the first 15 seconds. The more professional the paramedic appears, the more positive that impression will be (Fig. 13-1). An introduction is helpful in making the encounter specific. To a patient, hearing, "Hi, my name is Syd, and I'm the paramedic who will be helping you today," begins an emotional transition from the general "911 is coming" to the more personal "Syd is here."

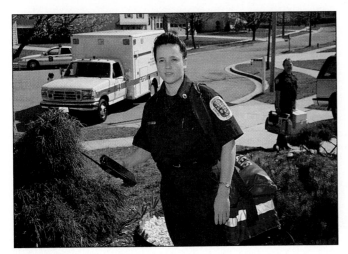

Figure 13-1

Professionalism is expressed in appearance and attitude.

Vocal Dynamics

Certain physical dynamics help facilitate good communication, beginning with the ability of the patient to hear the paramedic. The crucial vocal elements are volume, pitch, rate, and clear pronunciation. Adjust volume first, then rate; people who are overwhelmed during a crisis cannot absorb information as rapidly as usual. Clear pronunciation is especially important when there is background noise. People with high-pitched voices must also be aware that certain people have pitch-related deafness.

Tone of voice, too, carries many specific (sometimes negative) emotional messages. Use voice tone carefully. Notice how a voice—regardless of the words being said—can impart friendliness, disdain and condescension, or support and caring. The paramedic should become adept at using various tones of voice. For example, the paramedic can test how many ways the three words "How are you?" can sound just by changing the tone of his or her voice.

Eye Contact

Eye contact can demonstrate everything from compassion and gentleness to take-charge authority. Eye contact is an uncomfortable skill for many people because of the direct interpersonal link that is created. One way paramedics can learn this skill is to practice by looking at the other person's nose, right between the eyes. When ready, he or she should look directly into one eye of the other person. If this begins to feel uncomfortable, the paramedic can return to the "safe" point on the bridge of the nose until the skill becomes second nature. However, one situation in which direct eye contact may be too threatening is when interacting with agitated or violent patients.

Nonverbal communication includes other elements, such as facial expression, body stance and posture, and several aspects of positioning (e.g., distance, relative height, open and closed angles). To send a convincing overall message, the paramedic must keep these factors consistent with the choice of words. It is unwise for the paramedic to go into a notoriously rough bar with the powerful words, "Everyone listen! Help is here, so settle down!" if he or she is backed up by a frightened expression and a meek physical presence. Putting all of these elements together requires the "actor" to be aware of them all at once, in addition to the medical demands of the situation.

Facial Expression and Body Stance

Many paramedics have failed in their efforts to communicate because they unconsciously adopted authoritative expressions and postures. They stand with square shoulders and hips, arms crossed, and a confrontational expression, regardless of the situation (Fig. 13-2A). There are times to use this posture, but not many. This pose is safer if one foot is placed ahead of the other, allowing for a "fall-back" stance if needed (Fig. 13-2B). It is often better to demonstrate flexibility by opening the stance. He or she may stand to the side or change the angle of the shoulders and hips (Fig. 13-2C). For safety purposes,

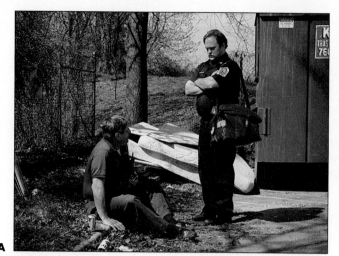

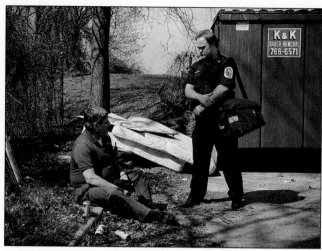

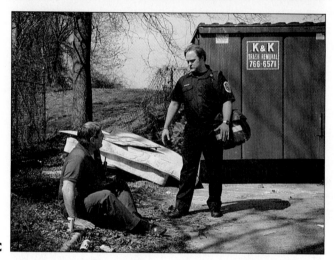

A

B

C

Figure 13-2

Choose the posture appropriate for the situation you are in. Usually, an open stance is the most friendly and will enhance communications.

Positioning

Positioning is another important consideration. The paramedic must quickly judge the need for safety, effective communication, and medical care, because they overlap when considering the options for positioning. Judgment includes deciding how close to get to the patient and how quickly to get there. Relative height is another factor. In some cases, it is best to tower authoritatively over the patient; at other times, standing either at or below the patient's eye level is best (Fig. 13-3). Likewise, distancing decisions are variable. Some patients need the paramedic to keep away until a certain degree of rapport has been achieved; fortunately, natural trust of EMS personnel usually allows the paramedic to come into the intimate zone rapidly (Fig. 13-4).

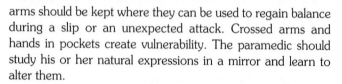

arms should be kept where they can be used to regain balance during a slip or an unexpected attack. Crossed arms and hands in pockets create vulnerability. The paramedic should study his or her natural expressions in a mirror and learn to alter them.

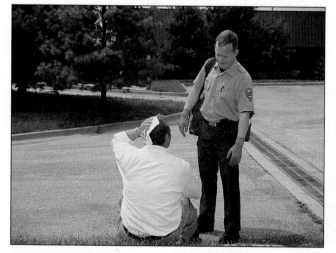

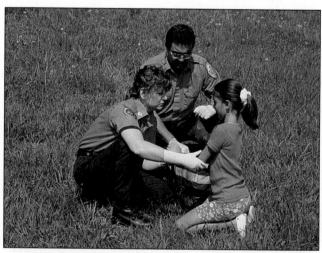

Figure 13-3

Choose a position appropriate for the situation. An authoritarian stance is sometimes needed to control a situation, but eye level is best for enhanced communications.

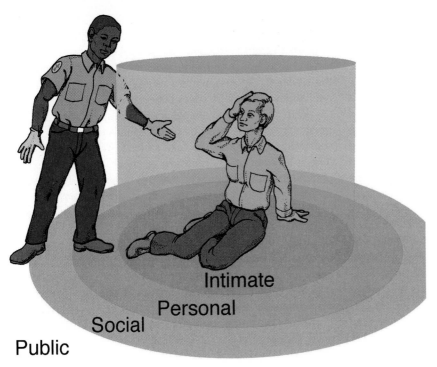

Intimate

Personal

Social

Public

Touching

In nonaggressive situations, a touch is one of the most powerful tools available. In addition to an assessment technique, touching is a sign that communicates caring and support. Hand holding and similar therapeutic touch methods are nonessential skills but are very effective when used appropriately (Fig. 13-5). The best paramedics know how to touch a patient's elbow, knee, or shoulder, or even give a hug in appropriate circumstances. Some paramedics are naturals at touching for compassion; others must make a conscious effort to work through the initial sense of awkwardness. Before touching a patient, the paramedic should consider how the patient will likely respond. Touching can be imposing; touching the patient because it was recommended in a book will not work with every encounter.

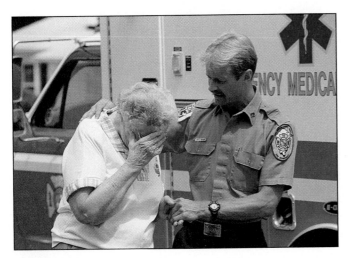

Figure 13-5

A gentle, appropriate touch can offer a great deal of reassurance and comfort to an ill or injured person.

Good Listening Skills

Another means of demonstrating support, which also improves with the accuracy of the medical history, is good listening. Because paramedics tend to be fast moving and oriented toward action and control, their listening skills can be weak. By listening, the paramedic allows the patient to re-establish a sense of control, which can help calm the situation. Not listening may make the patient feel disregarded, increasing the chance of a negative reaction. There are specific ways to improve listening skills. Many people have a bad habit of finishing others' sentences for them. Improvement of this habit may only come with conscious effort. Efforts to improve this habit can be to bite the tongue or hold the lips closed—anything to avoid interrupting.

Because it is often necessary to perform other duties while asking questions, the paramedic should be sure to say, "I am listening, please go ahead." Or the paramedic may reflect something the patient said in the next question: "You said you had taken your nitroglycerin medication. How many pills did you take?" The patient's words should be attended to. By avoiding assumptions and preconceived notions, the all-important history may lead the medical team down unexpected pathways and ultimately to a more accurate assessment.

Aspects of Professionalism

The paramedic should try to understand what is happening from the patient's point of view. When an interaction is not progressing well, he or she should consider if the patient is perceiving it differently. Remember the adage about walking a mile in another person's shoes. For example, paramedics are accustomed to seeing bodies; however, most people are not used to being undressed in front of an audience. The patient's right to both physical and emotional privacy should be respected at all times.

Patients remember the quality of the interpersonal interaction far longer than the quality of the actual hands-on medical care. Laypersons do not recognize a good IV nearly as easily as they do a sense of caring and support. The traits of patience, tolerance, and respect must be constantly communicated and refined. Again, the paramedic can be compared with the professional actor. An actor may play one part a thousand times, with the same lines, the same stage, and the same set. Yet, he or she makes the role appear fresh, exciting, and interesting at each performance. There is nothing artificial or insincere about it. Similarly, the paramedic may handle a thousand chest pain situations in his or her career. Those who have become cynical may administer oxygen, start an IV, set up a cardiac monitor, and feel cheated if there are no arrhythmias to interpret. But the professional senses the subtle changes that can keep each interaction unique: the time of day, how the patient and family are coping, the different setting ("stage"), the paramedic's own changing moods, and the level of experience.

Special Communications Challenges

Pediatric Patients

Children are a less familiar patient population than adults, and can be intimidating in their own ways. The following are basic suggestions for situations that can be very complex (also see Chapter 25). As paramedics mature in the profession, they must learn much more about working with children (Sidebar). First, the paramedic must examine his or her own feelings about caring for children. Most medical professionals view this as the most challenging population of all because of the intense emotional component. No one likes to see children hurting; everyone wants to make things better, and sometimes it is impossible. Tragedy seems more profound when children are involved. It may help the paramedic to recognize that most people feel this way and to make a special commitment to studying pediatric medicine. It boosts the paramedic's confidence to learn about normal, healthy children of all ages and how to establish rapport with them. Volunteering in a day care setting is a good opportunity to do so.

Very small infants are surprisingly hardy and do not break as long as the head is supported to prevent it from falling backward. Infants do not differentiate familiar from unfamiliar arms, and tend to go willingly to strangers. Within a few months (approximately 7 to 9 months is typical), they may prefer to stay in the arms of a trusted caregiver. In noncritical cases, the paramedic may elect to establish rapport by speaking with the parent for some time and establishing friendly eye contact before trying to touch the child. Gradually, the child's natural curiosity overcomes the shyness, especially if the stethoscope is made to seem like a toy (Fig. 13-6). Avoid speaking as if the child is a third party; choose words that indicate that the child is included.

The paramedic should move and speak slowly; children need extra time to take in information. Each child should be read for clues to ease communication. For example, examining a child either from head-to-toe or toe-to-head depends on the situation. Adolescents are usually shy about physical examinations and require special efforts to respect privacy.

With children who are old enough to understand, be careful of word choices. Imagine how it sounds to naive ears when someone says they plan to *take* a blood pressure or temperature; it is better to say *measure* or *check*. Pain hurts, so the paramedic should not understate this by saying, "It's just a little touchy." The honest approach will build more trust. If a child cries, it is not because the paramedic failed, but because children are honest about their feelings.

Children with less life experience may seem too unruffled by serious medical emergencies or overly sensitive to minor ones. Often, they take cues for reaction from their caregivers. A pediatric situation naturally implies at least two patients for the paramedic: the child and the child's caregiver. The paramedic must be emotionally prepared to handle more than one needy person.

Geriatric Patients

Paramedics spend a great deal of time with geriatric patients. It is especially important for the paramedic to remain respectful and provide for the dignity of these patients. Some older people have cognitive or functional impairments, such as incontinence or mental debilitation caused by aging. These are causes for compassion, not condescension.

The paramedic should avoid assuming that an elderly person's faltering mentation is chronic. That person may be suffering from hypoxia, hypovolemia, hypoglycemia, cardiac decompensation, or another treatable condition. When establishing rapport, the paramedic should use an older pa-

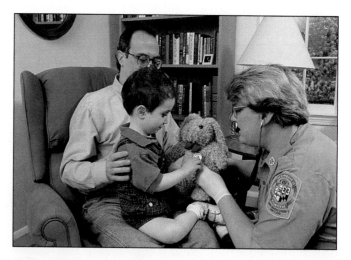

Figure 13-6

Use your medical equipment as a "toy" to help gain the confidence of your pediatric patients. Once they are allowed to play with it, the equipment becomes less threatening. You can also use your equipment as a distraction so you can examine the patient.

By Kate Dernocoeur, EMT-P

Children are individuals. It is the paramedic's task to determine what each child will tolerate, in terms of handling and interacting. The following age breakdowns are approximate, and are presented from oldest to youngest for the purpose of emphasizing the full range of changes that occur as a person develops:

- *Adolescents.* Remember that adolescents are still not considered fully mature, regardless of their "savvy." Privacy is an intensely important issue, especially regarding their bodies. Anything the paramedic can do to educate an adolescent about body function, such as pulse range and location, may help. The paramedic should be matter-of-fact and avoid presuming to understand the adolescent's feelings.
- *Ages 6 to 12.* Children in this age group are usually somewhat familiar with medical procedures, such as blood pressure and pulse measurement. The paramedic can begin with these assessments to build rapport with the child. The paramedic should engage the child with relevant questions and remain calm and matter-of-fact. A frightened child may be challenging, but will often settle down with rapport and be able to help with his or her own medical care (e.g., holding a bandage).
- *Ages 4 to 5.* These children are generally cooperative and willing to help, (e.g., helping uncover the area to be examined). With a gentle and honest approach, these children are often delightfully curious and open to explanations of what has happened and what to expect.

- *Ages 2 to 3.* These children are variable in their degree of clinginess to a familiar adult. Some are curious and helpful, others require more effort to gain rapport. One way for the paramedic to build trust is to play with tools such as the stethoscope, or to have the adult handle the equipment to demonstrate it as a safe thing. The child should be spoken to and not around; a child of this age can understand much of what is said.
- *Ages 18 to 24 months.* The child may express resistance to exposing or touching the area to be examined. The paramedic should take time to build rapport and trust with children of this age. When approching the child, the paramedic should avoid appearing timid, yet not be too "hard." A calm, understanding, and straightforward tone of voice is helpful. A singsong cadence and a constant banter may also help.
- *Ages 9 to 17 months.* A child of this age may be particularly anxious about being separated from a familiar adult. Examine the child in the lap of the adult, if possible. If an examination of the entire body is indicated, it may help to remove one section of clothing at a time. Examine the child from toe to head.
- *Infancy.* The baby's head should be supported when picking up or holding the baby. Undressing and examination is usually tolerated well, as long as the child is warm and dry. The child should be examined from toe to head.

From Dernocoeur: Streetsense: Communication, Safety, and Control, 3rd edition, Redmond, WA, 1996, Laing Communications.

tient's formal name (e.g., "Mrs. Jones"). This is more respectful than assuming that the patient would prefer intereaction on a first name basis or that the patient will tolerate belittling endearments ("sweetie," "honey," or "pal"). The paramedic should speak slowly and clearly.

Death is life's final rite of passage. Death plays a more important, even daily, role in the lives of geriatric patients. They lose good friends and relatives more frequently than younger people, and are thus likely to be in various stages of the grief process on a nearly continual basis (see Chapter 57). The emotional response to this may play a part in the patient's physical complaint.

Older people know that they have a higher chance than most of dying when they go to the hospital. Thus, many older people present communications challenges because they resist medical help. Their fears include loss of control and independence and the cost of medical care. The paramedic may find better rapport by slowing down, when possible, and checking the house to be sure the cat is fed, the appliances are off, the doors and windows are locked, and the patient has the belongings needed. There may not be someone to stop by later for forgotten items. In particular, gather the patient's wallet, teeth, eyeglasses, hearing aid, medications, robe and slippers, something to wear home, and keys. The patient's address book may be particularly helpful to the hospital staff. The paramedic should note which of the patient's personal items are packed and be sure they are properly inventoried during hand-off at the hospital.

Family members who will not be going to the hospital should have the chance to say goodbye if time allows. For some, it may be the last chance to do so. If the paramedic is honestly optimistic that the patient will be home in a few hours or days, it can be very reassuring, especially to children, to hear this.

Non–English-speaking Patients

When people at the scene do not share the same language, the result may be frustrating. Nonverbal communication becomes the only means of communication, and therefore an even more important skill for the paramedic. Non–English-speaking people may tend to be very anxious. The paramedic must display tolerance, patience, and compassion—all quite easy to do nonverbally.

Cultural differences may make hands-on medicine challenging. For example, in some cultures it is considered threatening or offensive to make eye contact or touch a member of the opposite gender. This section of the text is meant to raise awareness and cannot be comprehensive; each paramedic is well-advised to learn about local foreign cultures and their customs. An effective rapport-building tactic is to learn common words or phrases of typical foreign languages in your area and the culture and customs that go with them.

If an interpreter is available, the paramedic may be able to obtain some medical information, but the paramedic must understand the limitations of using an interpreter. This person is often a child who has learned English in school. Questions should be phrased slowly and one at a time, using words common to the interpreter's level of comprehension, and the paramedic should wait for an answer. Cultural differences of perception should also be accounted for, for example, regarding the intensity or characteristics of the pain. The paramedic should be patient and try to help the interpreter, who is also reacting to the crisis.

Interpreters are sometimes available through the hospital, and also through certain long-distance telephone companies. The local emergency medical dispatcher may know a resource for establishing verbal communication with a non–English-speaking patient.

Hearing Impaired Patients

People who cannot hear often have other excellent resources for sending and receiving messages. The best strategy is to ask the patient what will work best. Someone at the scene may know sign language, or the patient may be able to write notes. Some hearing impaired people can hear some sounds or read lips (speech read). If the paramedic shouts or exaggerates lip movements, this will distort the words. The person speaking must be visible to the speech reader, be sure there is enough light on the face of the person speaking for the patient to see, and be sure that no other lights are blinding the patient. A heavy mustache or beard may also interfere with a hearing impaired patient's ability to speech read.

The speech of some hearing impaired people sometimes sounds strained or distorted. Speaking without hearing one's own words is not easy. The manner in which a hearing impaired person speaks is not a reflection of mental acuity.

Mentally Challenged Patients

There are numerous causes of mental handicaps. People whose mental challenges require full-time assistance are usually with someone who knows them and can assist the paramedic in communicating. In some cases, a person may appear mentally handicapped when the challenge is actually physical. Avoid making assumptions; it is better to ask, "What is the nature of your disability?" and "What is the best way we can work together?" before deciding communication is impossible.

In the unlikely case there is no one familiar with the patient to assist, the paramedic must use basic communication strategies that demonstrate a reason for the patient to trust him. Be gentle and consistent. It may be impossible to detect a response, but the effort alone has value.

Obstinate and Potentially Volatile Patients

Safety issues cannot be ignored, although it is not always possible to have law enforcement assistance at the scene. Communicating effectively with obstinate and potentially volatile patients is almost always possible if the paramedic remains self-aware enough to avoid being drawn into verbal battle. The goal is not to lock horns but to deliver appropriate prehospital care. There is usually a way around perceived communications obstacles. The exceptions are organically impaired people: those who are hypoglycemic, hypoxic, drug impaired, or have known organic brain syndrome.

If a patient demonstrates potentially volatile behavior (e.g., clenched fists, verbal threats, and angry appearance), the paramedic can try to defuse the emotions with nonverbal messages. These must demonstrate enough toughness to control the situation, but still leave room for the patient to cooperate.

If a patient is obstinate, the paramedic should try to find out the cause. People stalling departure to the hospital are often frightened about leaving familiar territory. Many are concerned about their bills. Pat reassurances about, "It'll be OK" or "They won't make you pay" are not acceptable. The paramedic should focus on the patient's medical needs; sometimes it helps for the paramedic to remind the patient that coping with these problems improves with restored health.

Communications with Family and Bystanders

Interaction with other people at the incident scene is too often ignored in prehospital care, and it can spell the difference between success and failure for the paramedic's communication efforts. As does the professional actor, the paramedic often has an audience, with its share of critics and hecklers. Bystanders and relatives are an unavoidable element of most scenes. In the theater, it works best to play to a friendly crowd; in EMS, it is also safer.

All the elements of effective communication previously mentioned also apply to bystanders. The paramedic should keep bystanders in peripheral vision, relate to them as needed,

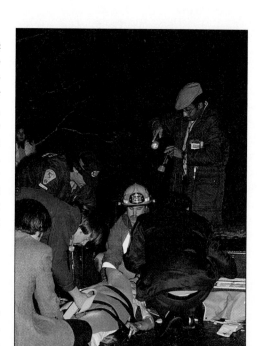

Figure 13-7

Bystanders may be called upon to assist in some situations. Make sure they are helping in a safe, appropriate manner.

and let them help when it is practical (Fig. 13-7). Bystanders should not be treated with disdain or contempt for being naturally curious, as long as their actions do not interfere with the paramedic's duty to perform.

With large (but calm) groups, the paramedic may assign crowd control to the neighborhood's natural leader. A definite boundary such as a curb should be defined; The paramedic should use *eye* contact, and say, "Could you keep these folks back on the curb so we can work? That would be very helpful."

In critical situations, such as cardiac arrests, the family deserves frequent updates and a chance to understand that bad news may be coming (see Chapter 57). The behavior of the bystanders may range from apparent self-control to hysteria; the more bystanders trust the EMS providers and understand their actions, the more they are likely to let paramedics do their work. Update bystanders frequently on what is happening and why. Most people have very low levels of medical sophistication, so paramedics should keep their vocabulary simple.

Professional Communication

Paramedics must communicate as effectively with their colleagues as they do with their patients. Whether working with auxiliary personnel at the scene of an accident or interacting with supervisors, effective communication will enhance job motivation and performance. Communication with coworkers in the ambulance is particularly important to optimizing patient care. The principles of *effective communication* should also be used when working in administrative, legislative (political), or hospital environments.

SUMMARY

Paramedics who have been in the patient's shoes know what it is like to be at the mercy of the helpers. Those who have been bystanders know the helpless feelings and difficulty of that role. Paramedics who have participated in prehospital care only from the caregiver's point of view must work hard to imagine the importance of effective communication in a time of crisis. No other skill will be as frequently used, tested, varied, or rewarding when the job is done well.

For the paramedic, mastering the art of effective interpersonal communication is a continuing endeavor. Something new can be learned from every EMS call, regardless of its nature or intensity.

SUGGESTED READINGS

1. **Bradley S:** The Signs of Silence. *JEMS* 16(8):26 32, 1991.
2. **Cormier LS, Cormier WH, Weisser RJ:** Interviewing and Helping Skills for Health Professionals, Boston, 1986, Jones and Bartlett Publishers.
3. **Dernocoeur KB:** Streetsense: Communication, Safety, and Control, ed 3, Redmond, WA, 1996, Laing Communications.
4. **Dick T:** Street Talk: Notes from a Rescuer, Solana Beach, 1988, JEMS Publishing.
5. **Purtilo R:** Health Professional and Patient Interaction, ed 4, Philadelphia, 1990, WB Saunders.
6. **Thompson GJ, Stroud MJ:** Verbal Judo: Redirecting Behavior with Words, Albuquerque, 1984, The Verbal Judo Institute.

Walt A. Stoy, PhD, EMT-P
Debra Lejeune, NREMT-P
Gregg S. Margolis, MS, NREMT-P
Thomas E. Platt, NREMT-P

Chapter 14

Communication and Documentation

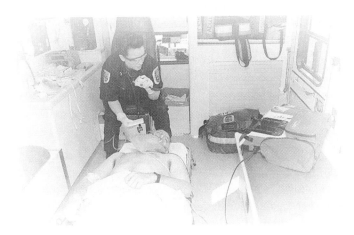

A paramedic should be able to:

1. Describe the overall significance of accurate communication of patient data in the prehospital setting.

2. Describe the two types of verbal reports and the goals and purposes of each.

3. List and discuss three general principles that should be utilized when presenting patient data.

4. Define "SOAP" format and describe its use in communication of patient data.

5. Describe pertinent findings (positive and negative) and their importance in the verbal report.

6. Given a patient scenario, list the 11 components of a standard radio report and the order of presentation.

7. Discuss the techniques that contribute to effective radio communication.

8. List the purposes of the patient care report (PCR).

9. List and describe the components to include on a PCR.

10. Describe three important characteristics of a PCR.

11. Discuss three major pitfalls associated with the preparation of PCRs.

12. List ten cases in the prehospital setting that are more likely to result in an inquiry or litigation.

OBJECTIVES

he art of effective communication of patient information is an important aspect of prehospital care. Failure to appropriately communicate with the patient, coworkers, medical direction, or other medical professionals may result in confusion and complications in the timely delivery of patient care. Paramedics are responsible for rapidly and accurately gathering information from the patient and scene. They must then determine which aspects are important to report to other personnel involved in the chain of patient care. Hospitals often need time to prepare for patients, particularly those who are in critical condition, because additional personnel or certain resources may need to be activated or mobilized. Communication of patient data is first reported verbally and then documented on the patient care report (PCR).

The key component in all aspects of communication is an accurate description of the patient condition. As with many paramedic skills, this requires practice to become proficient. Observing experienced colleagues and seeking frequent feedback will aid in refinement of this essential skill. Diligent efforts not only benefit the patient, but also contribute to the paramedic's respect as a medical professional.

Verbal Reports

Paramedics function as the eyes, ears, and hands of physicians. In the early years of EMS, paramedics were linked closely to on-line medical direction (OLMD). Before beginning any patient care, paramedic contact with OLMD was required in most systems. As EMS evolved and training standards increased, the paramedic became a more integral part of the team approach to patient care. Today, many paramedics provide patient care under physician-directed protocols. Some advanced care for the patient frequently begins before contact is established. Protocols increase the likelihood of correcting a life-threatening condition quickly. Once these procedures have been performed, however, paramedic contact with OLMD for further orders or consultation may be helpful, and informing OLMD of the patient's condition, the care provided, and the estimated time of arrival is still important.

If direct contact with the receiving facility or OLMD is not available, the dispatch center will usually contact the facility to relay the information. Stable patients that only require transport are not necessarily a reason for contacting OLMD. Typically, information about such patients is communicated en route to the hospital.

Although some systems find it useful to use various codes (such as "10-4") for dispatch communications, these codes should not be used when communicating to OLMD or the receiving hospital. The use of codes can result in miscommunication of vital medical information, although standard abbreviations can save time and are frequently used (see Chapter 6). Medical direction typically approves the list of abbreviations to be used in the local system.

Types of Verbal Reports

There are two distinct types of verbal reports in EMS, each with its own purpose. The first is provided by radio or telephone to OLMD from the scene or during transport; the second is given in person at the receiving hospital as patient care is transferred (Fig. 14-1). The following discussion focuses on key aspects of the radio report, although most of the general principles discussed also apply to the report given at the hospital.

The goal of radio reporting is to provide a visual image of the patient and situation to the physician who is not on scene. A clear and accurate description will assist OLMD in evaluating the patient's condition and medical needs.

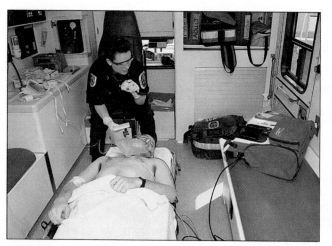
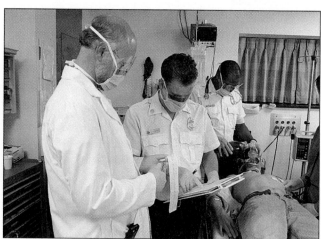

A   B

Figure 14-1

A, Communication between the EMT-P and the hospital is a crucial part of the chain of total patient care. B, Verbal reports given in the hospital to the receiving medical team mean a speedy resumption of patient care services for the sick or injured patient.

SOAP is an acronym that is used to help remember what information should be obtained for written and verbal communication, and to organize the reports themselves.

S—Subjective This area includes all patient symptoms including chief complaint, associated symptoms (pertinent negatives and positives), past history, current medications and allergies. Bystanders and family information are also included in this area.

O—Objective This area includes all patient signs and physical examination information, such as vital signs, level of consciousness, head-to-toe examination, ECG findings, pulse oximetry, rapid blood glucose determination, etc.

A—Assessment This area includes the conclusion or clinical impression based on the subjective and objective data obtained.

P—Plan of patient management This area includes treatment that has already occurred (such as cervical spine stabilized, oxygen administered) and plans for additional treatment items with OLMD permission.

Patient data should be presented in a logical and organized format, and a standard presentation is preferred. Some systems use the SOAP format to obtain and report relevant patient information (see Box 14-1). This format organizes patient data for both verbal reports and PCRs. Standardization minimizes the chance of omitting or repeating important facts. An orderly report is time efficient, and the OLMD need not ask questions to fill in gaps.

Components of The Report

Although many components of the verbal report are common throughout the country, there are acceptable variations. For most EMS systems, OLMD will dictate the standard report that is desired. The common theme in all verbal reporting is that the information be pertinent. For example, a report about a patient who is very unstable typically need only be a brief list of relevant information, so that treatment can be expedited. Other patient reports may require more detailed information.

The type of information given is an important factor. When performing a patient history and physical examination, data is collected in support of the chief complaint. A positive finding is the presence of a sign or symptom, such as abdominal tenderness in a patient with abdominal pain. A negative finding is the denial of a sign or symptom, such as bloody stools by the same patient. Both of these findings are important.

The crew calling medical direction should identify itself by name and number. A short explanation for seeking OLMD should be included. For example: "Pittsburgh Medical Command, this is Pittsburgh Medic Five. We would like to speak

with a physician regarding a patient with chest pain." A report to OLMD typically includes the following components, although the sequence may vary according to the situation:

- Description of the scene
- Level of consciousness, age, gender, and weight (if pertinent)
- Chief complaint
- Vital signs
- Brief history of the present illness or injury
- SAMPLE history (see Box 14-2)
- Associated signs and symptoms
- Physical examination findings
- Treatment already provided
- Results of treatment (if any)
- Patient destination and estimated time of patient arrival

See Box 14-3 for an example of radio communication to an online medical director regarding a patient who sustained injury in an automobile collision.

All orders received from the OLMD should be repeated by the paramedic to verify accurate reception. Any orders that are unclear or that deviate from standard protocol should be clarified. Each system should identify how these situations will be handled. Once the procedure has been performed, OLMD

BOX 14-2 SAMPLE History

A useful acronym to assist in the gathering of pertinent patient information.

S = Signs and Symptoms
A = Allergies
M = Medications
P = Past pertinent history
L = Last oral intake, solid or liquid
E = Events leading to the illness or injury

BOX 14-3 Example of Radio Communication

"Pittsburgh Medical Command, this is Pittsburgh Medic Five. We are on the scene of an auto collision with a 45-year-old conscious woman, weighing approximately 130 lbs. The patient's vehicle struck a side rail traveling approximately 30 miles per hour. She is alert, oriented, and complaining of shortness of breath. The patient did hit the steering wheel but states she did not hit the windshield. Vital signs are as follows: B/P: 120/70, Pulse: 110, Regular Respirations: 24 and somewhat shallow. The patient has bruising on her left chest, although the chest moves evenly and breath sounds are clear and equal. On head-to-toe examination, the abdomen is soft, there are no obvious fractures, and the only apparent injury is a 2-inch head laceration. ECG shows sinus tachycardia. We have extricated the patient with a C-collar and backboard, started an IV Ringer's lactate TKO and are administering oxygen. The patient's shortness of breath seems improved at this time. We are preparing for transport, and should arrive at your facility in approximately 7 minutes."

should be notified. Any response to the treatment provided or a change in the patient's condition en route should also be reported.

Radio Communication Techniques

The following 12 techniques will contribute to effective radio communication:

1. *Listening to the channel prior to beginning.* This will reduce the chance of transmitting while others are also trying.
2. *Pressing the transmit button and waiting momentarily before speaking so that the first word will not be cut off.* Minimize background noise such as sirens, open windows, and crew conversations.
3. *Holding the microphone at a slight angle to the mouth and at a distance of 2 to 3 inches.* Experience and feedback from dispatchers will help establish the ideal distance for clear transmission.
4. *Pronouncing each word clearly and speaking slowly.*
5. *Speaking in a calm tone of voice.* Voice tone is dramatically amplified over the radio.
6. *Using unit identifiers rather than proper names when referring to other persons or units in the system.*
7. *Protecting patient privacy.* Airwaves are easily monitored by the public; do not refer to the patient by name.
8. *Breaking the transmission every 30 seconds to recheck the signal.* If transmission is poor, it can be improved by moving the portable unit to an outside wall. If transmission is still not possible, establish contact by telephone. At the scene, communication can be improved by using the radio in the ambulance, which usually has greater power than a portable radio.
9. *In general, the higher the antenna, the greater the clarity of transmission.* Remember the antenna is designed to function in an upright position.
10. *When in the basement of a patient's home or a low-lying geographical area, transmission can usually be improved by moving to a higher point.*
11. *Spelling words that medical direction may have difficulty understanding.* The International Phonetic Alphabet can be used to optimize communication. If the International Phonetic alphabet is not known, use simple words that assist in the spelling (D=Dog, R=Rain, U=Under, and G=Good).
12. *At the end of transmission, obtaining confirmation that communication was received by the medical direction.* Using the term *over* when completing a simplex transmission to which a response is expected.

The paramedic should avoid:

- *Words that are difficult to hear.* "Yes" or "No" should be stated as "Affirmative" and "Negative."
- *The use of slang or profanity.* Profane language is forbidden by the Federal Communications Commission (FCC) regulations.
- *Phrases such as "Please" or "Thank you."* Courtesy is implied, and these words are unnecessary.

Reporting to the Receiving Hospital

The second type of verbal report is given to the hospital personnel who are receiving the patient. The goal of this report is to ensure the continuity of patient care. The information provided should be consistent with the data given to OLMD. Typically, this includes a brief summary of the pertinent findings, including significant findings about the scene and changes in the patient's status which can only be provided by paramedics. If the receiving facility was contacted initially, the report at the hospital should focus on treatment given since that contact, response to treatment, and any other change in patient status. A copy of the PCR should be left with the receiving hospital to clarify any questions about the patient or the prehospital care.

Written Patient Care Reports

As the saying goes, "No job is complete until the paperwork is done." Although paperwork is often a chore, responsible documentation is essential and patient care cannot be considered complete until it is thoroughly documented. A written report should be made for every patient seen in the field, including those who refuse care or transport against medical advice. If the patient's condition is stable, the report may be started at the scene or en route to the hospital. If the patient is unstable, it is more practical to complete it after transfer to the receiving facility. Without this documentation, there is a risk of improper management or duplication of treatment.

The Purposes of the Patient Care Report

Written reports have additional important purposes beyond their vital role in patient care. These can be divided into three categories: 1) legal; 2) system; and 3) reimbursement. The copy of the PCR that remains at the hospital becomes part of the patient's permanent record, and thus is a legal record of patient care. The legal purposes of the PCR include both prevention of a claim or lawsuit and defense if there is civil or criminal action against the prehospital service or employee. Although criminal charges are rarely a problem, civil suits claiming malpractice are on the increase (see Chapter 5). In addition, state and federal authorities may have specific documentation requirements.

The EMS system often benefits from data obtained from PCRs. Data are used in medical audits and quality improvement measures. For example, evaluating the amount of time spent on scene for critical trauma patients enables a system to take measures to minimize the time. Or, a review of reports on patients complaining of shortness of breath might reveal a lack of prehospital patient improvement and influence a medical director's decision to add a new drug to the inventory. Response times, placement of ambulances, and patient population data are also important aspects of system information obtained from the reports.

Most EMS system administrators would agree that reimbursement is an important function of the PCR. Revenue collection often depends on data gathered by paramedics.

Types of Written PCRs

The type and format of the prehospital care report vary among EMS systems. Most systems use a standardized set of reports for documentation of prehospital care. There are two primary methods of recording a written report:

- A traditional, hand-written hard copy
- A computer-generated report

Hard-Copy PCRs

Most written reports are designed to allow EMS personnel to record information by means of circling items or checking appropriate boxes, marking a body diagram, or filling in blanks (Fig. 14-2). This is an effective and expedient means of gathering general types of demographic or routine information. Since this method is unlikely to tell the complete story, a written narrative is often required to document information more specific to the individual patient (Fig. 14-3).

Computer-Generated PCRs

Some EMS systems use optical scan PCRs for the collection of all objective information regarding the run. Patient information and treatment are recorded by darkening small circles with a pencil. The report is then scanned into a computer and a summary is generated (Fig. 14-4). As noted above, some written (in this case, typed) information is also likely to be needed.

Some EMS systems combine the written hard copy with the computer-generated report. A written hard copy is created and a copy left at the hospital. The information from the written report is later entered into a computer.

The more sophisticated computer systems presently used in health care include such devices as the notebook computer (Fig. 14-5). The notebook computer converts the handwritten information into typed words.

In addition to these reports, some systems also use other adjuncts, such as ECG tracings and Polaroid photographs of motor vehicle collisions, to add to the documentation of patient care.

BOX 14-4   Patient Care Report Components

Run Data
- Location of call
- Date of call
- Time of call*
- Time of dispatch
- Time of response to dispatch*
- Time of arrival at scene
- Time of departure from scene
- Time of arrival at hospital
- Names of crew members
- Unit responding
- Service
- Other responding EMS, fire, or police units
- Reason for arrival delay, if applicable

Patient Data
- Patient's name, address, date of birth, and gender
- Chief complaint or nature of illness
- Mechanism of injury or illness
- Location of the patient when first encountered
- Rescue and treatment by first responders or bystanders
- Patient history including medications taken, allergies, and all pertinent information
- Physical examination including vital signs and all pertinent information
- Name of patient's physician, if available

Treatment Data
- BLS provided
- ALS provided
- Response to therapy
- Time of drug and procedure
- Transport code
- Hospital destination
- Receiving medical personnel signature

Although this information is not typically part of the PCR, it is important information for system performance and accountability.

Components of the PCR

Regardless of the method of documenting information, each PCR should include run data, patient data, and treatment data. Box 14-4 lists the standard elements for each of these components.

Run Data

The information typically considered run data includes the date and all pertinent times, locations, and names of responders, unit, and service. Some systems document times in the dispatch center or through a computer system rather than on the PCR. The data are important, however, and should be easily retrievable either way. Pertinent information should also be included for any incident with unusual or extenuating circumstances. If arrival was delayed, for instance, the reason should be documented. Hazards such as traffic, weather, and fire should also be described.

Patient Data

A major portion of the PCR contains information about the patient. The data are obtained from the patient, family members or bystanders, or from the scene. Patient information includes demographics, history and physical examination data.

Some EMS systems document patient assessment and management information in a SOAP format similar to the one presented above for verbal reports. Another technique for recording patient assessment information is in head-to-toe order (Box 14-5). A standardized format improves consistency and accuracy.

Because a patient's condition may change from minute to minute, the PCR must have space to record serial assessments. Serial neurological and vital signs are of particular importance.

Treatment Data

Every PCR should contain documentation of the treatment provided. The chronological (start-to-finish) method is an effective way to document treatment (Box 14-6). Again, an

DESOTO FIRE RESCUE EMERGENCY MEDICAL SERVICES — PATIENT FORM

DESOTO FIRE RESCUE

DATE	RECEIVED	ENROUTE	ON SCENE	TO HOSPITAL	AT HOSPITAL	AVAILABLE	IN QUARTERS

Location _____ Apt./Suite No. _____

Incident # _____ 3703

TYPE CALL:

- ☐ 42 Allergic Reaction
- ☐ 41 Aggravated Assault
- ☐ 12 Breathing Difficulty
- ☐ 06 Burns
- ☐ 22 Cardiac Arrest CPR
- ☐ 22 Chest Pain
- ☐ 34 CVA - Stroke
- ☐ 09 Diabetic
- ☐ 10 Drowning
- ☐ 14 Emergency Transfer
- ☐ 27 Electrocution
- ☐ 27 Fall - Traumatic
- ☐ 42 Fall - Medical
- ☐ 21 GSW
- ☐ 20 Abdominal Pain
- ☐ 22 Hypertension
- ☐ 27 Injured Person
- ☐ 42 Medical Emergency
- ☐ 04 MVA
- ☐ 25 OB/GYN
- ☐ 28 Overdose
- ☐ 30 Psychiatric
- ☐ 42 POPTA
- ☐ 29 Poison
- ☐ 07 Seizure
- ☐ 33 Stab Wound
- ☐ 40 Unresponsive
- ☐ 42 Weak & Dizzy

EMS Unit _____ Shift _____

Fire Co. # _____

Environment _____

Last Name _____ First _____ MI ____ DOB __/__/__ Age ____

Race
- ☐ 0 Race / Origin Undetermined
- ☐ 1 American Indian / Eskimo / Aleut
- ☐ 2 Asian / Pacific Islander
- ☐ 3 African / American
- ☐ 4 Hispanic
- ☐ 5 Caucasian
- ☐ 6 Other
- ☐ 7 Unknown
- ☐ 9 Race / Origin Not Classified

Sex
- ☐ 1 Male
- ☐ 2 Female
- ☐ 0 Sex Undetermined

Patient's Address _____ Apt. # _____

City _____ State _____ Zip _____ Telephone _____

Responsible Adult _____ Relation to Patient _____

Pt. Medicate/Medicaid/SSN _____ DL # _____ Resp. Adult SSN _____

Chief Complaint _____

Past History _____

Patient Medications _____

Allergies: ☐ 1 NKDA   ☐ 2 Codeine   ☐ 3 Caine Drugs   ☐ 4 Penicillin   ☐ 5 Sulfa   ☐ 6 Other _____

Vital Signs:
- Time: __:__ B/P __/__ P ___ Reg: ☐ Y ☐ N Resp: ___ Position: ☐ Lying ☐ Sitting
- Time: __:__ B/P __/__ P ___ Reg: ☐ Y ☐ N Resp: ___ Position: ☐ Lying ☐ Sitting
- Time: __:__ B/P __/__ P ___ Reg: ☐ Y ☐ N Resp: ___ Position: ☐ Lying ☐ Sitting

TILT TEST: B/P __/__ P ____   B/P __/__ P ____   **POS or NEG**

Dextrostix _____   Temp _____   Pulse Oximeter _____

Role in Incident (if MVA)
- ☐ 51 Bicycle Rider
- ☐ 52 Driver
- ☐ 55 In Back of Pick-Up
- ☐ 56 Motorbike Driver
- ☐ 57 Motorbike Passenger
- ☐ 53 Passenger, Front Seat
- ☐ 54 Passenger Rear Seat
- ☐ 58 Pedestrian

Restraint/Protection (if MVA)
- ☐ 61 Air Bag
- ☐ 62 Child Restraint
- ☐ 63 Helmet
- ☐ 64 No Lap, But Shoulder
- ☐ 65 No Shoulder, But Lap
- ☐ 68 None Available
- ☐ 69 Not Used
- ☐ 67 Protective Padding
- ☐ 66 Lap / Shoulder
- ☐ 70 Use Undeter.

Personnel	ID #	NARRATIVE

RESPIRATIONS
- ☐ 1 Normal
- ☐ 2 Absent Left
- ☐ 3 Absent Right
- ☐ 4 Apnea
- ☐ 5 Bilateral Sounds Clear
- ☐ 6 COPD
- ☐ 7 Decreased on Left Side
- ☐ 8 Decreased on Rt. Side
- ☐ 9 Denies Dyspnea
- ☐ 10 Dyspnea
- ☐ 11 Hemomptysis
- ☐ 12 Hyperpnea
- ☐ 13 Hyperventilation
- ☐ 14 Labored
- ☐ 15 No Spontaneous
- ☐ 16 PND
- ☐ 17 Rales
- ☐ 18 Undetermined
- ☐ 19 Ronchi
- ☐ 20 Shallow
- ☐ 21 Stridor
- ☐ 22 Tachypnea
- ☐ 23 Wheezes
- ☐ 24 Refused Assess.

PUPILS
- ☐ 1 Perla
- ☐ 2 Blind
- ☐ 3 Blind, Left
- ☐ 4 Blind, Right
- ☐ 5 Cataract (Left)
- ☐ 6 Cataract (Right)
- ☐ 7 Chronic Eye Hist.
- ☐ 8 Constricted
- ☐ 9 Constricted Left
- ☐ 10 Constricted Right
- ☐ 11 Dilated
- ☐ 12 Dilated Left
- ☐ 13 Dilated Right
- ☐ 14 False Left
- ☐ 15 False Right
- ☐ 16 Irregular
- ☐ 17 Nonreactive
- ☐ 18 Reactive
- ☐ 19 Ref. Assess.

CARDIAC
- ☐ 1 Not App / No Complaint
- ☐ 2 Denies Chest Pain
- ☐ 3 Edema
- ☐ 4 Mid-Sternum
- ☐ 5 Nitro. Relieved
- ☐ 6 Radiates, Left
- ☐ 7 Radiates, Right
- ☐ 8 Radiates, Other
- ☐ 9 Refused Assessment
- ☐ 10 Unremarkable/Undef.

NEUROLOGICAL
- ☐ 1 A & 0 x 3
- ☐ 2 A & 0 x 2
- ☐ 3 A & 0 x 1
- ☐ 4 Decreased Motor Function
- ☐ 5 Disoriented
- ☐ 6 Moves All Extremities
- ☐ 7 No Purposeful Movements
- ☐ 8 Posturing, Decerebrate
- ☐ 9 Posturing, Decorticate
- ☐ 10 Responds to Pain
- ☐ 11 Responds to Verbal
- ☐ 12 Seizures
- ☐ 13 Unconscious
- ☐ 14 Refused Assessment

SKIN
- ☐ 1 Normal
- ☐ 2 Ashen
- ☐ 3 Clammy
- ☐ 4 Cool
- ☐ 5 Cyanotic
- ☐ 6 Dermatological
- ☐ 7 Diaphoretic
- ☐ 8 Dry
- ☐ 9 Flushed
- ☐ 10 Frostbite
- ☐ 11 Hot
- ☐ 12 Pale / Pallor
- ☐ 13 Turgor, Good
- ☐ 14 Turgor, Poor
- ☐ 15 Undetermined
- ☐ 16 Warm
- ☐ 17 Refused Assess.

ABDOMEN
- ☐ 1 Unremarkable, No Complaint
- ☐ 2 Distended
- ☐ 3 Guarding
- ☐ 4 Nausea Vomiting
- ☐ 5 Pain
- ☐ 6 Pulsating Mass
- ☐ 7 Quadrant, LU
- ☐ 8 Quadrant, LL
- ☐ 9 Quadrant, RU
- ☐ 10 Quadrant, RL
- ☐ 11 Rebound
- ☐ 12 Rigidity
- ☐ 13 Soft
- ☐ 14 Tender
- ☐ 15 Trauma
- ☐ 16 Ref. Assess.

BLEEDING
- ☐ 1 No Bleeding
- ☐ 2 Arterial
- ☐ 3 Minimal
- ☐ 4 Moderate
- ☐ 5 Severe
- ☐ 6 Stop PTA
- ☐ 7 Venous

EMESIS
- ☐ 1 Not Applicable
- ☐ 2 Blood Clots
- ☐ 3 Bright Blood
- ☐ 4 Clear
- ☐ 5 Coffee Ground
- ☐ 6 Food
- ☐ 7 Green
- ☐ 8 White
- ☐ 9 Yellow

GI / GU
- ☐ 1 Unremarkable, No Complaint
- ☐ 2 Diarrhea
- ☐ 3 Dysuria
- ☐ 4 Hematemesis
- ☐ 5 Hematuria
- ☐ 6 Melena
- ☐ 7 Rectal Bleed

SIGNAL 27
- ☐ 1 Arm Band
- ☐ 2 Decapitation
- ☐ 3 Decomposition
- ☐ 4 Dependent Lividity
- ☐ 5 Injuries Non Comp w/ Life
- ☐ 6 Rigor Mortis
- ☐ 7 Trauma Body
- ☐ 8 Trauma Head

Figure 14-2

Patient care reports (PCRs) vary from jurisdiction to jurisdiction. What are the common elements noted in this report that your jurisdiction uses? *Courtesy Desoto Fire Rescue Emergency Medical Services.*

_____(Last)_____ _____(First)_____ _____(MI)_____

PREGNANCY INFORMATION

No. of Months _____ G: _____

P: _____ AB: _____

Contractions (Y N) every _____ minutes

Lasting _____ minutes each

Birth: BOWI _____ BOWR _____

Delivery Time _____ : _____

APGAR, 1 min. _____ APGAR, 5 min. _____

LNMP _____

OB/GYN

- ☐ 1 No App/ No Complaint
- ☐ 2 Abortion / Miscarriage
- ☐ 3 Assisted Delivery
- ☐ 4 Birth PTA
- ☐ 5 Discharge
- ☐ 6 False Labor
- ☐ 7 OB
- ☐ 8 Pain / Discomfort
- ☐ 9 Vaginal Bleeding

AID PROVIDED

- ☐ 1 Airway EOA
- ☐ 2 Airway ET
- ☐ 3 Airway Nasal
- ☐ 4 Airway Oral
- ☐ 5 Assessment
- ☐ 6 Assessment & Vitals
- ☐ 7 Assisted Ventilation
- ☐ 8 Attended, Extra
- ☐ 9 Backboard / C-Collar / H.J.D.
- ☐ 10 Bandaging
- ☐ 11 Burn Sheet
- ☐ 12 BVM
- ☐ 13 Cardioversion
- ☐ 14 Chest Decomp.
- ☐ 15 Cold Packs
- ☐ 16 Control Bleed
- ☐ 17 CPR
- ☐ 18 CPR By Citizen
- ☐ 19 Defibrillation
- ☐ 20 D-Stick
- ☐ 21 EKG
- ☐ 22 12 Lead
- ☐ 23 Emot. Sup-Talking
- ☐ 24 Extrication
- ☐ 25 Gray Top Col Tube
- ☐ 26 Intraosseous Infusion
- ☐ 27 Invalid Assist
- ☐ 28 IV, Admin Set / Fluid
- ☐ 29 KED
- ☐ 30 MAST PANTS
- ☐ 31 Other
- ☐ 32 Oxygen
- ☐ 33 Pacing, External
- ☐ 34 _____ / _____ MA.
- ☐ 35 Search & Rescue
- ☐ 36 Scoop
- ☐ 37 Splint, Traction
- ☐ 38 Splinting, Not Tract.
- ☐ 39 Sterile Water
- ☐ 40 Stretcher
- ☐ 41 Stuffed Animal / Toy
- ☐ 42 Suction
- ☐ 43 Thumper
- ☐ 44 Transport
- ☐ _____
- ☐ _____
- ☐ _____
- ☐ _____

Therapy Given

TIME	EKG Drug Type Cardioversion Pacing, Defib	Rate, Rhythm MG WS	Result (if any) / PMT ID #
1.			
2.			
3.			
4.			
5.			
6.			
7.			
8.			
9.			
10.			
11.			
12.			
13.			
14.			

DRUGS

- ☐ F D-5W
- ☐ F Normal Saline
- ☐ F Ringers Lactate
- ☐ 1 Activated Charcoal 50gms
- ☐ Z Adenosine
- ☐ T Albuterol
- ☐ S A S A
- ☐ C Benadryl
- ☐ 2 Bretyiol
- ☐ U Calcium Chloride
- ☐ G D-50
- ☐ D Dopamine
- ☐ E Epinephrine 1:1.000
- ☐ E Epinephrine 1:10.000
- ☐ X Furocemide
- ☐ 3 Insta Glucose
- ☐ P Levophed
- ☐ L Lidocaine 2%
- ☐ L Lidocaine 20%
- ☐ 4 Lido Jelly

- ☐ M Morphine
- ☐ 5 Narcan
- ☐ N Nitroglycerin Spray
- ☐ 6 Saline Irr
- ☐ C Sodium Bicarbonate
- ☐ 7 Syrup of Ipecac
- ☐ V Valium
- ☐ T Ventolin
- ☐ _____
- ☐ _____
- ☐ _____
- ☐ _____
- ☐ _____

Biotel Nurse # _____

Biotel Doctor _____

TRAUMA / COMPLAINT

- ☐ 1 Abrasion
- ☐ 2 Amputation
- ☐ 3 Asphyxiation
- ☐ 4 Avulsion
- ☐ 5 Battles Signs
- ☐ 6 Burn: Chemical
- ☐ 7 Burn: Electrical
- ☐ 8 Burn: Thermal
- ☐ 9 Burn: Scald
- ☐ 10 Contusion / Minor Trauma
- ☐ 11 Crushing
- ☐ 12 Dislocation 13
- ☐ 13 Distal Pulse Absent
- ☐ 14 Drowning
- ☐ 15 Drowning, Near
- ☐ 16 Edema
- ☐ 17 Electrical Shock
- ☐ 18 Evisceration
- ☐ 19 Eye Trauma R L
- ☐ 20 Flail Chest R L
- ☐ 21 Frostbite Possible
- ☐ 22 FX / Augulated Poss.
- ☐ 23 FX / Closed Poss.
- ☐ 24 FX / Depressed Poss.
- ☐ 25 FX / Open Poss.
- ☐ 26 FX / Spine / Possible
- ☐ 27 Gunshot
- ☐ 28 Hematoma
- ☐ 29 Hemorrhaging
- ☐ 30 Laceration
- ☐ 31 Mechanism of Injury
- ☐ 32 Obstructed Airway
- ☐ 33 Pain
- ☐ 34 Pain in Joint
- ☐ 35 Pain in Muscle
- ☐ 36 Penetration
- ☐ 37 Puncture: No Stab
- ☐ 38 Puncture: Stabbing
- ☐ 39 Smoke Inhalation
- ☐ 40 Sprain / Strain
- ☐ 41 Targeting
- ☐ 42 Trauma, Blunt
- ☐ 43 Other

AFFECTED LOCATION

- ☐ 1 Undeter. / No Comp.
- ☐ 2 Head Not Face
- ☐ 3 Face Not Eyes, Nose, Mouth, Ears
- ☐ 4 Both Eyes
- ☐ 5 Eye, Right
- ☐ 6 Eye, Left
- ☐ 7 Nose, Exterior Trauma
- ☐ 8 Nose Bleed Ant Post
- ☐ 9 Mouth - Lips
- ☐ 10 Mouth - Inside
- ☐ 11 Ear, Right
- ☐ 12 Ear, Left
- ☐ 13 Tongue
- ☐ 14 Teeth
- ☐ 15 Neck - No Airway Involved
- ☐ 16 Neck - Airway Involved
- ☐ 17 Back - No Spine Involved
- ☐ 18 Back - Spine Involved
- ☐ 19 Chest - External Only
- ☐ 20 Chest - Internal Incl.
- ☐ 21 Abdomen - External Only
- ☐ 22 Abdomen - Internal Incl.
- ☐ 23 Buttocks
- ☐ 24 Genitals
- ☐ 25 Pelvis - GU Not Incl.
- ☐ 26 Pelvis - GU Incl.
- ☐ 27 Upper Body, All
- ☐ 28 Up Extremity Rt Hand
- ☐ 29 Up Extremity Rt Wrist
- ☐ 30 Up Extrenity Rt Forearm
- ☐ 31 Up Extremity Rt Elbow
- ☐ 32 Up Extremity Rt Arm
- ☐ 33 Up Extremity Rt Shoulder
- ☐ 34 Up Extremity Rt All
- ☐ 35 Up Extremity Lt Hand
- ☐ 36 Up Extremity Lt Wrist
- ☐ 37 Up Extremity Lt Forearm
- ☐ 38 Up Extremity Lt Elbow
- ☐ 39 Up Extremity Lt Arm
- ☐ 40 Up Extremity Lt Shoulder
- ☐ 41 Up Extremity Lt All
- ☐ 42 Lower Body, All
- ☐ 43 Lower Extremity Rt Foot
- ☐ 44 Lower Extremity Rt Ankle
- ☐ 45 Lower Extremity Rt leg
- ☐ 46 Lower Extremity Rt Knee
- ☐ 47 Lower Extremity Rt Thigh
- ☐ 48 Lower Extremity Rt Hip
- ☐ 49 Lower Extremity Rt All
- ☐ 50 Lower Extremity Lt Foot
- ☐ 51 Lower Extremity Lt Ankle
- ☐ 52 Lower Extremity Lt Leg
- ☐ 53 Lower Extremity Lt Knee
- ☐ 54 Lower Extremity Lt Thigh
- ☐ 55 Lower Extremity Lt Hip
- ☐ 56 Lower Extremity Lt All
- ☐ 57 Respir. - Not Chest Related
- ☐ 58 Cardiac - Not Chest Related
- ☐ 59 Neuro - Not Head Related
- ☐ 60 Neuro - Head Related
- ☐ 61 Entire Body
- ☐ 62 Other

TRAUMA SCORE

Eye Opening	Spontaneous	4	To calculate the Trauma Score, the Glascow Coma Scale must first be calculated.
	To Voice	3	
	To Pain	2	
	None	1	
Motor Response	Obeys Commands	6	Circle the appropriate point value in each category
	Localizes to Pain	5	
	Withdraws to Pain	4	
	Flexion (pain)	3	
	Extension (pain)	2	
	None	1	
Verbal Response	Oriented	5	Add the points circled in these three categories to obtain the Glascow Coma Scale.
	Confused	4	
	Inappropriate Sounds	3	
	Incomprehensible Sounds	2	
	None	1	

GLASGOW COMA SCALE TOTAL

The Glascow Coma Scale must be converted as shown:	Converted Glascow Coma Scale	13 - 15 = 4 9 - 12 = 3 6 - 8 = 2 4 - 5 = 1 3 = 0
Add the points circled in these three categories to obtain the Trauma Score	Respiratory Rate	10 - 29 = 4 Over 29 = 3 6 - 9 = 2 1 - 5 = 1 0 = 0
Under 10 transport to trauma center	Systolic Blood Pressure	Over 89 = 4 76 - 89 = 3 50 - 75 = 2 1 - 49 = 1 0 = 0
	REVISED TRAUMA SCORE	

O₂ Device _____ LPM _____

GA _____ ☐ RL ☐ D5W site: _____ by _____ # attempts _____ successful ☐ Y ☐ N

GA _____ ☐ RL ☐ D5W site: _____ by _____ # attempts _____ successful ☐ Y ☐ N

ET size _____ by _____ # attempts _____ successful ☐ Y ☐ N

TRANSPORTED BY: Code ( )1 ( )3 Pt Priority ( )3 ( )2 ( )1

- ☐ 1 Desoto F R
- ☐ 2 CareFlight
- ☐ 3 Priv. Veh.
- ☐ 4 Police
- ☐ 5 NO SICK OR INJURED
- ☐ 6 Left Scene
- ☐ 7 FD Refused
- ☐ 8 PT Refused
- ☐ 9 Respons. Ref.

Patient Condition Upon Arrival at Hospital

☐ 01 Same ☐ 02 Improved ☐ 03 Deteriorated

BP: _____ / _____ P _____ Irreg. ☐ Y ☐ N

Resp. _____

TRANSPORTED TO: Accepting Signature: _____ ☐ PM Choice ☐ PT Choice ☐ Biotel Choice

- ☐ 2 Baylor of Dallas
- ☐ 99 Baylor of Waxahachie
- ☐ 41 Charlton Methodist
- ☐ 11 Childrens Medical
- ☐ 47 Columbia Dallas SW
- ☐ 14 Doctors Hospital
- ☐ 43 Medical City of Dallas
- ☐ 3 Methodist Central Hosp.
- ☐ 46 Columbia Lancaster
- ☐ 1 Parkland Memorial
- ☐ 4 Presbyterian Hospital
- ☐ 5 St. Paul Hospital
- ☐ 8 R.H. Dedman
- ☐ 38 Veterans Hospital
- ☐ _____

I refuse transport and/or treatment _____ Time _____

Yo me he negado ha aceptar transportacion en ambulancia hoy _____ Time _____

Figure 14-2

(continued)

DENVER HEALTH AND HOSPITALS
PARAMEDIC TRIP REPORT

Report # ____ of ____ Total Reports due for this Ambulance's Trip

TRIP #	DATE	TIME	CODE OUT 10 - 9	DRIVER		I.D. #	ATTENDANT		I.D. #

LOCATION		ASSISTED BY FD - PD	RIDER		SPONSOR	AMB #

LAST NAME	FIRST NAME	M.I.	AGE	SEX M F	DOB	SOC. SEC. #

ADDRESS	CITY	STATE	ZIP CODE	PHONE

INSURANCE (Type & #)	DHH #

DGH KSR APH ARMC CNL ETT — Immobilization
UH PMH RMC LMC FAL - GOA EKG — Restraints
SAH SMC PSL NND - AST IV X ___ — Single
SJH TCH FAMC DPT - DTX O₂ — Shared
Rx X ___ — Trtmnt/No Txpt

PATIENT VALUABLES

VALUABLES LEFT WITH

ASSESSMENT

_____ OTHER DESTINATION

ICD9 (Office Use Only)

Base Contact   RFD - PIR - POV - PAT - TNR - MEC

AUTHORIZING PHYSICIAN (Office Use Only)

_____ M.D.   CODE IN 10 - 9 - N/A   END MILEAGE - START MILEAGE = TOTAL MILES ____ ____ ____

TIME	PULSE	B/P	RESP	PUPILS	CARDIAC RHYTHM	SaO₂	EYES +	VERBAL +	MOTOR =	GCS
							4 3 2 1	5 4 3 2 1	6 5 4 3 2 1	
							4 3 2 1	5 4 3 2 1	6 5 4 3 2 1	
							4 3 2 1	5 4 3 2 1.	6 5 4 3 2 1	
							4 3 2 1	5 4 3 2 1	6 5 4 3 2 1	

CHIEF COMPLAINT	MECHANISM OF INJURY / ILLNESS

HISTORY, PHYSICAL, MANAGEMENT, COURSE

PMHx ☐ CARDIAC ☐ RESPIRATORY ☐ SEIZURE ☐ DIABETES ☐ OTHER:

MEDICATIONS

Author's Signature

ALLERGIES

F06-010 (8/95) DHH

Figure 14-3

The narrative is a written part of the patient's permanent medical record and can include information that is not easily put on other fill-in-the-blank reports. *Courtesy Denver Health and Hospitals.*

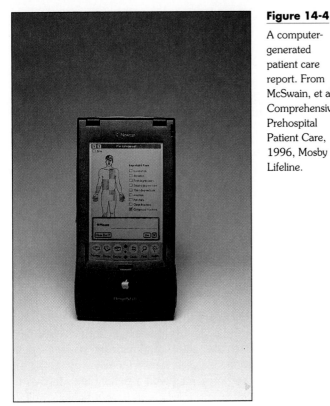

Figure 14-4

A computer-generated patient care report. From McSwain, et al. Comprehensive Prehospital Patient Care, 1996, Mosby Lifeline.

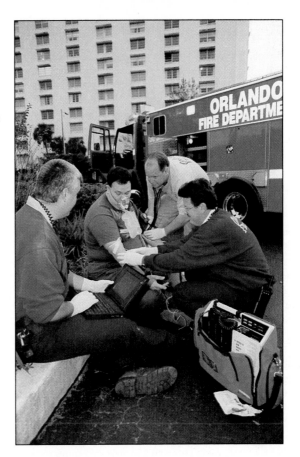

Figure 14-5

The notebook computer converts handwritten information into typed words. *Photographed by Craig Jackson.*

organized, consistent approach reduces errors. Although PCRs may allow treatment information to be coded or entered in check boxes, a narrative is also beneficial. All advanced life support (ALS) treatment should be accompanied by the time administered and notes on the patient's response to treatment.

Characteristics of the PCR

The prehospital care provider is wise to develop the habit of complete, accurate, and legible record keeping. Good documentation takes time, but it is time well spent if it later prevents a lawsuit or provides a sound defense against one. The report should be free from prejudiced or unrelated material and should avoid assumptions or judgments. Facts, findings, and observations are most appropriate. For example, rather than writing, "The patient is intoxicated," describe the behaviors observed: "The patient was slurring his words, had an ataxic gait, and had the smell of alcohol on his breath." Direct quotes from the patient are often helpful, particularly regarding possible drug abuse.

Pitfalls to Avoid

When completing the PCR, the paramedic should keep in mind the purposes of the report. The importance of patient information to hospital personnel and the potential legal defense the report may provide can help the paramedic avoid pitfalls.

Inadequate Documentation

Regardless of the nature of the call or the condition of the patient, the paramedic should document all related information.

BOX 14-5	Sample Report—Head to Toe Format of Objective Findings

HEENT:	Head:	2" laceration L occiput with dried blood in hair
	Eyes:	PEARL
	Ears:	Negative for discharge or Battle's sign
	Nose:	Negative for discharge or S/S of injury
	Mouth:	Intact, no missing teeth or bleeding noted
	Throat:	Neck: soft, nontender to palpation
CHEST:		Fist-sized bruise noted left lateral chest over ribs 7–10, chest wall intact, no crepitus or unstable segments noted on palpation. Breath sounds: clear & equal bilateral with equal chest rise
ABDOMEN:		Soft, nontender, negative for guarding on palpation
PELVIS:		Intact with no pain on palpation
GENITALIA:		Intact with no discharge noted
LOWER EX:		FROM, no pain on palpation, = pulses, CRT 2 seconds, = sensory & motor responses
UPPER EX:		FROM, no pain on palpation, = pulses, CRT 2 seconds, = grips
BACK:		No tenderness or deformity noted on examination

| **BOX 14-6** | **Chronological Format** |

The chronological format follows through the care of the patient by identifying the steps taken in the order in which they were performed (all abbreviations used are officially defined and approved for that organization).

1725: 45 y/o restrained female driver in a single-vehicle collision found AAOx4 with CC of SOB. Per bystanders, pt. struck guardrail, travelling estimated 30 MPH. Pt. states she impacted steering wheel with anterior chest. Steering wheel is not bent. No airbag is present in vehicle. Head & neck stabilized in neutral in-line position by FF in back seat of vehicle.

1726: Assess ABC, Pt C/O dyspnea. O2 10 LPM via NRB mask applied. Lungs sounds clear & equal, expansion of chest noted upon visual examination.

1732: Cervical collar applied following palpation of posterior & anterior neck. No tenderness or pain noted upon examination. No JVD, neck veins flat.

1734: Physical exam conducted: abdomen soft, nontender, no fractures noted to extremities, equal pulses and +neuro to all extremities. Pt. noted to have a 2″ laceration to L occiput. No free bleeding noted. Bandaged by FF.

1738: Rapid extrication to long BB accomplished without incident. Pt. Immobilized with 9 ft straps, 2″ tape, CID. Moved to unit to begin transport.

1746: Continued assessment performed enroute to PTC. No other injuries noted during examination. VS: Resp. 24/regular lungs: clear to auscultation, P: 110/reg. ECG: sinus tachycardia without ectopy, BP: 120/100.

1748: IV LR R antecubital, TKO with 14g angiocath & macrodrip tubing.

1752: Patient notes an improvement to dyspnea.

1753: Consult with Dr. Joyner at PMC, no orders or interventions given.

1758: Patient at PTC without incident, no further information.

Failure to complete information concerning the run data will make it difficult for the EMS system to document the frequency and types of calls. Incomplete information regarding the patient's condition or treatment can result in inappropriate care at the receiving facility.

If legal action is initiated, an incomplete PCR may contribute to a court decision in favor of the patient; poor documentation may be viewed as a reflection of poor patient care. It is wise to adopt the philosophy that "if it isn't written down, it wasn't done."

Every patient encounter should result in a PCR with at least one set of vital signs documented. The frequency of vital sign evaluation is governed by patient condition and local protocols. The more severe the patient condition, the more frequently vital signs should be obtained and documented. It is particularly important to check and record vital signs after giving medications or other advanced therapies.

Abbreviations are helpful in minimizing the time required to write reports. The abbreviations used, however, should be standardized within a system and approved by medical direction, so that they lead to understanding rather than confusion.

Some cases are more likely than others to result in an inquiry or litigation. When involved in any of these situations, the paramedic should pay particular attention to writing a thorough report. These situations include: 1) patients with possible spinal cord injures; 2) angry, hostile family members or a friend; 3) combative or confused patients; 4) restrained patients; 5) possible criminal activity; 6) patients whose conditions deteriorate en route; 7) long transport times; 8) breakdown of equipment or the ambulance; 9) deviations from known standards or protocols; and 10) refusals of treatment or transportation.

Patient Refusals

Any competent adult patient has the right to refuse care (*see* Chapter 5). When the paramedic faces this situation, PCR documentation should include the following:

- Complete patient assessment, including mental status examination
- Treatment the paramedic desired to provide to the patient
- Explanation given to the patient regarding possible results of refusal of medical care

If the patient still refuses to be transported, the paramedic should then read the patient refusal statement (which should be on every PCR) to the patient, and have the patient sign it. This should be witnessed by a family member, bystander, or police officer. When presented with a patient who refuses to sign the refusal statement, it is best to have a family member sign on his or her behalf. Whether the patient is willing to sign the patient refusal sheet or not, patient refusals should involve communication with medical direction.

Correction of Errors Made While Writing on the PCR

Most PCRs have multiple copies. Corrections made on the top sheet may not be legible on the additional pages. When making a correction, the provider should place a single line through the incorrect information, write the correct information beside it, and then initial the corrections. The paramedic should take care not to "black out" the mistake, since this could be viewed as trying to hide information.

If corrections are made to the PCR following a quality improvement audit, each correction should be initialed and dated.

SUMMARY

There are two major areas of EMS communication: the verbal report and the written report. Both methods of reporting are essential for quality patient care. Good reporting lessens the likelihood of errors occurring in the patient care chain.

Legal concerns are continually an issue in the health care arena. An accurate, complete report will be valuable if future legal action arises. Failure to document treatment can result in speculation about the quality of the provided care.

REFERENCES

1. **American Academy of Orthopaedic Surgeons:** Emergency Care and Transportation of the Sick and Injured, ed 4, Park Ridge, 1987, American Academy of Orthopaedic Surgeons.

2. **Bledsoe BE, Porter RS, Sade BR:** Paramedic Emergency Care, Englewood Cliffs, 1991, Brady Prentice Hall.

3. **Grant HD, Murray Jr RH, Bergeron JD:** Emergency Care, ed 5, Englewood Cliffs, 1990, Brady Prentice Hall.

4. **Hafen BQ, Karren KJ:** Prehospital Emergency Care and Crisis Intervention, ed 4, Englewood Cliffs, 1992, Brady Morton Prentice Hall.

5. **Henry MC, Stapleton ER:** EMT Prehospital Care, Philadelphia, 1992, WB Saunders.

6. **Jones SA, Weigel A, White RD, McSwain NE, Breiter M:** Advanced Emergency Care for Paramedic Practice, Philadelphia, 1992, JB Lippincott.

7. **National Association of EMS Physicians:** Prehospital Systems and Medical Oversight, ed 2, St. Louis, 1994, Mosby Lifeline.

8. **Yvorra JG:** Mosby's Emergency Dictionary: Quick Reference for Emergency Responders, St. Louis, 1989, The CV Mosby Company.

Section

Scene and Patient Assessment

3A

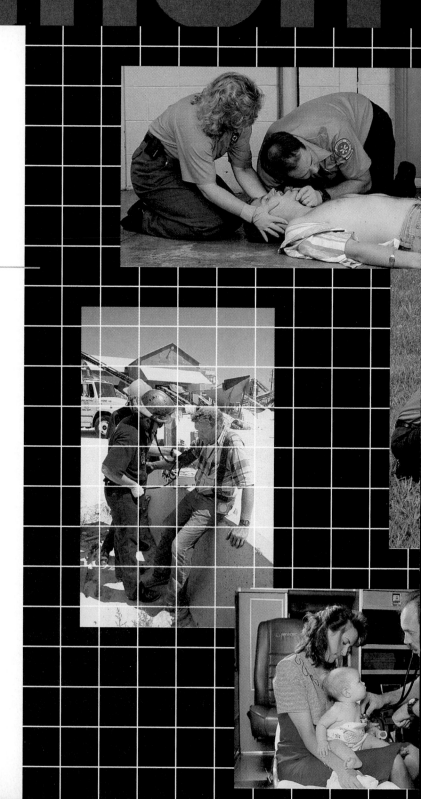

Included In This Section:

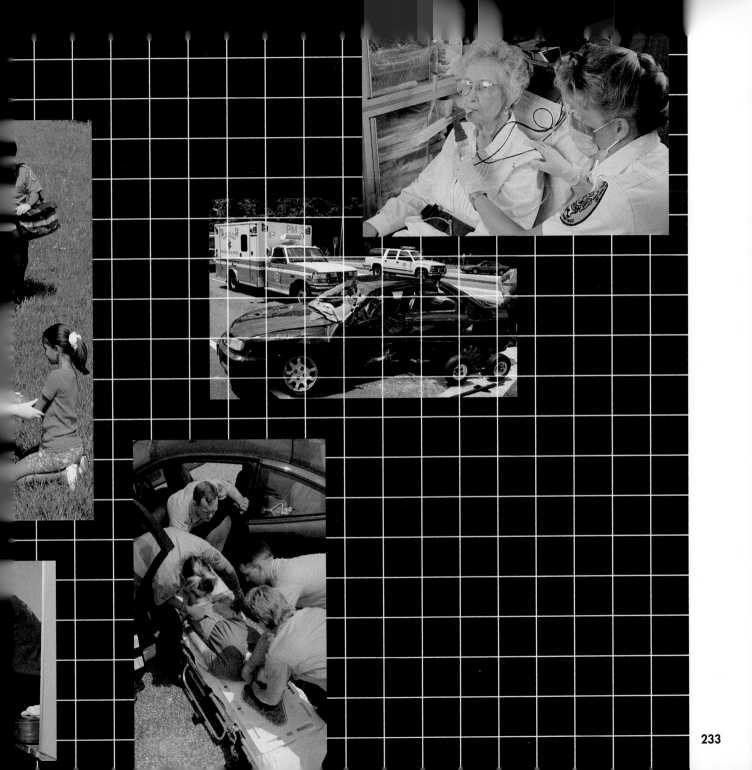

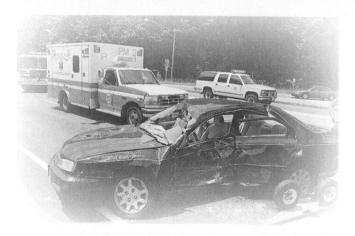

A paramedic should be able to:

OBJECTIVES

> **Scene Survey**
>
> **Initial Assessment**
> **Focused History**
> **and Physical Exam**
>
> **Continued Assessment**

One of the critical variables in prehospital care is the setting in which the patient is found. Because the emergency scene can be different on every call, paramedics must have a flexible approach that allows them to adapt to the special situations they encounter. Taking care of a boy hit in the head with a baseball during a game is different from taking care of a man hit in the head with a beer bottle during a bar fight. Although the mechanism of injury is similar, the sequence and location of patient care will differ. The child may be treated by home plate where he fell, whereas care may have to be delayed for the man in the bar fight until the scene is brought under control or until he can be brought outside to the paramedics. The bottle may have broken and caused lacerations requiring bleeding control. The presence of blood increases the danger of disease transmission at the scene.

If any aspect of the emergency setting is altered, the entire plan of action may be changed. For example, in a simple vehicle collision with a tree, what happens to the scene with the addition of pouring rain, fog, or high winds? What about a cliff or total darkness? One of the most important attributes of the streetwise paramedic is having the ability to evaluate and control the emergency scene when coordinating patient care.

This chapter focuses on developing the following skills:

- Identifying and managing safety hazards
- Evaluating the scene to obtain essential information
- Coordinating the scene to the advantage of the provider and the patient

Dispatch Information

When the dispatch for a call comes in, ask the basic question: Does this dispatch make sense? Being dispatched to a grade school for a heroin overdose doesn't make sense, at least during school hours. It is more likely to be accurate in the evening, however, especially if there are secluded areas on school property where drug-related problems may occur.

Although priority dispatch and prearrival instructions have made dispatchers better able to contribute to the quality of emergency care, they still can only act on the limited information they receive. The public's general lack of medical knowledge can easily lead to a basic life support response to a more serious call. It's up to responders to read between the lines.

Know the Response Area

Many times, the location of a call provides clues to the situation paramedics are about to encounter. At 2:30 A.M. in a tavern district, it is a safe bet that the emergency scene will be fueled with alcohol. When the possibility for violence is high, an early call for police backup is important. If it turns out that police aren't needed, it will be easy to cancel their response. Walking into a violent situation without police assistance, however, can be a more difficult mistake to recover from.

Is the location of the call in an area known for gang activity? It is worth the effort to learn to identify the graffiti that marks gang turf. There is usually no better resource than local law enforcement personnel, who deal with this on a daily basis. It is essential to have a good working relationship with police agencies, especially when it comes to dealing with gangs. Be aware that a dark blue shirt, badge, and shoulder patch can easily result in a case of mistaken identity. Being misidentified as a police officer can be deadly in a gang environment (Fig. 15-1).

Scene Size-Up

The scene size-up is the first and most important part of patient assessment. Size-up requires the paramedic to evaluate the situation quickly. It is essential to ensure the safety of the crew and the patient. Information may be obtained as part of dispatch, but should always be confirmed upon arrival at the scene.

During scene size-up, the paramedic should determine:

- the safety of the scene
- the mechanism of injury or nature of illness
- the need for additional help
- the personal protective equipment required, including that for infectious disease protection

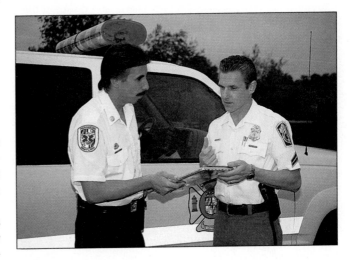

Figure 15-1

For purposes of safety, many EMS jurisdictions are moving away from a formal, public safety style appearance. Be aware of how your appearance is perceived, especially when dealing with a potentially hostile situation.

by William K. Atkinson, MPH, MPA, EMT-P

Once considered the good guys who assisted others and saved lives, EMS providers—like police officers and other symbols of authority—are now often viewed as scapegoats for the anger of the disenfranchised, including gang members.

Gangs are no longer an urban phenomena. Because of the interstate highway system, gang members travel swiftly to new markets where they peddle drugs, recruit new members, and use incendiary devices, semiautomatic and automatic weapons to dispatch their rivals and claim new turf. For example, in suburban areas like Aurora, Colorado, a city southeast of Denver and the state's third largest city, gang membership exploded by 83% between 1988 and 1991.

Gangs now cross all racial, social, and economic groups encompassing black, Hispanic, Asian, motorcycle, and white gangs, as well as skinheads and other hate groups. The psychological cement that holds gangs together is the sense of belonging that members receive from the group, which defines itself through continually evolving hand signals, language, graffiti, styles of dress, and behavior. However, for EMS providers responding to a call involving gang-related activity, identifying gangs is not as important as being alert, recognizing the potential for violence, and guarding their own safety and their patients.

Different types of gangs exhibit different types of behavior and criminal activity. In street gang–infested areas, EMS personnel are likely to treat victims of gang-related prostitution scams, drug users, victims of violent gang initiation rites and gang members and bystanders felled by firearms. Asian gang members use violence to extort money and property from members of their own ethnic group or subcontract with organized crime groups. Motorcycle gangs involved in drug manufacturing tend to booby-trap their clubhouses and use extremely volatile chemicals. HazMat support may be required in responding to a call. Even yuppie gangs, although not fitting the street gang stereotype, can be just as prone to violent behavior as any other gang, skinhead or hate group.

Whatever the type of gang and activity involved, EMS providers must be street smart and make sure their approach to rendering care protects them from becoming victims of their own good intentions. Street survival techniques used by police can be adapted to EMS practice. For courses and information, contact your local police academy. In the meantime, here are some key commonsense guidelines:

- *Expect the unexpected and be alert to sudden happenings.* Make sure to get enough information from dispatch to determine if body armor or police escort is required or recommended.
- *Work with police to be aware of all potentially dangerous neighborhoods and situations.* If necessary or appropriate, wait for police to secure an area before proceeding directly to the scene.
- *If called to a hostile or dangerous gang area, plan the entrance, exit, and escape route in advance.* To avoid drawing unnecessary attention to you and your crew, enter the area with lights and siren off if appropriate.
- *Keep an eye on the surrounding area, not only the patient.* It is best to have one person in charge of the scene.

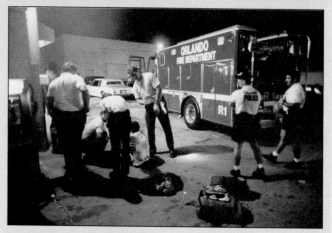

Photographed by Craig Jackson.

Make sure all personnel responding to the call are monitoring their radios and are alert to changing conditions. Park your vehicle for your own and your patient's safety as well as a quick exit. Also, consider the source of the injury. If the injury is a gunshot or stab wound, the perpetrator could be close by waiting for an opportunity to finish off the victim.

- *Be especially careful when entering a building; use the buddy system.* Get a sense of the layout of the structure, the other residents, and possible traps. It is better to use the stairs than the elevator. Knock, wait, and look before entering a residence. Be aware of tight spaces with no exits, other rooms, and the potential for hidden weapons. If the situation appears dangerous, use preplanned code words with your partner. Leave together to get a fictitious piece of equipment. That way, you won't raise suspicions or compromise your safety.
- *Constantly monitor your vehicle and equipment; otherwise, they may disappear into the wrong hands.* Be extra cautious about letting others ride with the patient. Their intentions may not be honorable. In some cases, it may be best to load the patient and leave the scene immediately. Resume patient care when you're in a safe area or go immediately to the nearest appropriate hospital.

Although street smarts are essential in dealing with gang-related calls, proactive activities can help trigger a long-term solution to curb gang activity. EMS providers throughout the country are making an effort to strengthen their ties with the community they serve through adopting schools, teaching students how EMS personnel serve their community, mentoring select students, helping expand and develop recreational opportunities and alternatives for at-risk youth and getting involved in gang prevention organizations.

At worst, today's proliferation of gang violence may mean a lengthening of time on scene or a delay in delivering assistance to those in need, situations that counter what most EMS providers have been trained to do. At best, acknowledging gang violence and applying street-smart skills to EMS practice may actually mean providing help and hope to gang members who see only hopelessness.

Scene size-up is an ongoing process. As additional information is obtained, the paramedic modifies the assessment of both patient and scene requirements.

Scene Safety

Once on the scene, take a few seconds to look around. A car sitting in a driveway with its engine running is either a sign that someone was attempting to leave (perhaps for the hospital), or that someone has recently arrived in response to a call for help. While not immediately dangerous, the vehicle should be placed in park and turned off, with the emergency brake engaged so that it does not pose a threat to others arriving or departing. Another example is an open front door with the lights out inside. Even in rural America, most people aren't this trusting anymore. This type of scenario should be approached cautiously.

Suppose that a trail of blood leads from the front of the house to the back. It might be easy for a paramedic to be entrapped by the urge to follow the blood trail. However, consider, that it may lead either to the victim or the assailant. Once again, having law enforcement at any potentially dangerous scene is crucial. The paramedic should also look in windows of houses and vehicles on approach. When knocking on a door, stand off to the side, rather than in front of the door to avoid being struck by any subjects.

In the classroom, it is impossible to recreate all of the safety issues than can surface at an emergency scene. On real responses, the paramedic has to be observant and think through the possibilities. The following sections describe some of the most obvious situations.

Violent and Hostile Environments

The single most volatile aspect of any call can be summed up in one word—people. When emotions run high and judgment runs low, the result is often trouble. Scenes that will commonly produce hostile situations include:

- *Family disturbances.* Lovers' quarrels, child or elder abuse or neglect, and drug or alcohol problems are frequent causes.
- *Bars and taverns.* Excessive alcohol consumption usually leads to one of two events: the person either passes out or gets violent. Either situation can prompt a call for medical aid. Impaired judgment goes hand-in-hand with alcohol consumption; it's always a good idea to watch for signs of impending violence, such as loud, argumentative voices or increasing physical contact.
- *Gang territory.* Any trip into gang territory is dangerous, from turf battles to drug deals to senseless violence. In some gangs, prospective members have to perform an act of violence, such as a drive-by shooting, as an initiation. Drugs and alcohol are usually involved in these encounters.

Other Dangerous Environments

While not violent, the following patient situations may also prove dangerous to the rescue crew or the patient:

- *Hazardous materials.* Assume that any emergency call at an industrial scene involves some form of hazardous material exposure or noxious environment (Fig. 15-2). There are literally thousands of chemicals used in industrial processes. Eye, ear, or breathing protection may be required before it is safe to approach the patient. A foreman or safety specialist may be a valuable resource when information is needed regarding the type of substances involved (see Chapter 52, Hazardous Materials and Radiation Incidents).
- *Radiation.* Any setting where radioactive materials are present poses special threats, because radiation is odorless and colorless. Thorough knowledge of what the rescue team may be exposed to is essential so the necessary precautions can be taken prior to entering the scene.
- *Farm emergencies.* Any call for EMS assistance in a farm setting is potentially dangerous for a number of reasons (Fig. 15-3). Many of the machines used in the business of agriculture are large and powerful. A careless paramedic can quickly become entrapped along with the patient if

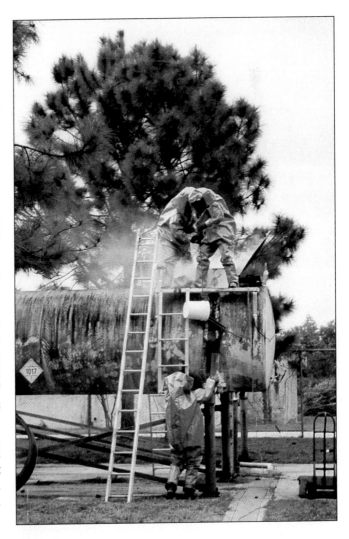

Figure 15-2

Hazardous materials can appear on any scene. Be especially alert for them during any response in an industrial setting. Photograph by Craig Jackson.

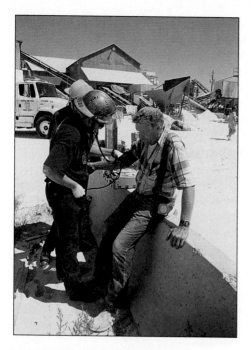

Figure 15-3

Farm machinery, chemicals, and situations can create a hazardous scene for EMS providers. Photographed by Colin Williams.

the machine is not turned off and secured prior to initiating rescue activities. Agriculture also relies on countless chemicals to enhance the growth of crops and protect them from weeds and pests, and many of these substances are toxic. The storage, handling, and application of agricultural chemicals are frequent causes of and dangers in emergency calls.

In addition, the farm setting may be the scene of a confined-space rescue involving a silo, a grain entrapment, or the toxic environment of a manure pit or hog confinement. A response area that includes any agricultural operations should be surveyed and preplanned to identify any unusual risks that may be encountered.

Freeway and Transportation Incidents

Motor vehicle collisions are everyday occurrences, and EMS is called to respond to them on a regular basis. Once on scene, the paramedic should expect to find at least two hazards—bystanders and traffic. Of the two, traffic is a more lethal threat.

On a side street with minimal traffic flow, the traffic hazard can be addressed by simply rerouting traffic. If that is not an option, position the ambulance between oncoming traffic and the emergency scene. The position should offer maximum protection while still allowing quick access for equipment (Fig. 15-4).

Some of the collisions that require an EMS response occur in the more dangerous setting of a freeway. Providing patient care in the middle of high-speed traffic is risky and should be avoided if possible. Again, proper ambulance placement is essential, as is working with law enforcement to provide traffic

control. If there is fire and smoke, it is wise to park upwind at least 100 yards. Keep in mind that any transportation incident can potentially involve hazardous material. It doesn't have to be a large semitrailer or tanker truck to produce toxicity. Should there be hazardous materials involved, it may be necessary to remain at a staging area and proceed to the scene only after it is secured by the Hazmat team.

Learning from the Scene

First, consider the environment the patient is in. If the patient has collapsed in a hot factory, does his physical presentation match the physical setting? Is he hot? Is his skin flushed or sweaty? If not, why? It is essential to look at the additive effect of the environment on the condition of a patient who is already compromised.

Aside from considering the dangers a scene presents, look to the scene for valuable information about how the incident occurred. Consider the physical surroundings where the patient is found. Be alert for:

- Drug paraphernalia
- Beer cans or liquor bottles
- Medication bottles
- Cult or gang literature or markings
- Items that can be used as weapons against the rescue team

Some pieces of information are only available at the emergency scene from bystanders and can be very important to the physician who is treating the patient later in the emergency department.

Trauma Patients

In trauma situations, evaluate how the incident occurred, or the *mechanism of injury*. Taking a few moments to deter-

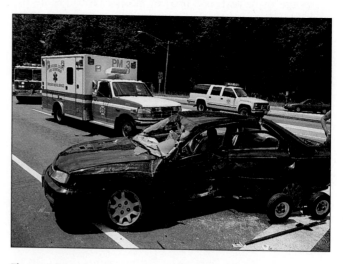

Figure 15-4

Positioning of the ambulance between oncoming traffic and the emergency scene provides a barrier of safety for the EMS and rescue team.

mine how an accident unfolded can improve the paramedic's awareness of what injuries may have occurred. Look to bystanders as a source of information. Considering the forces involved in the incident can provide a clearer picture of the extent of possible injury to the patient. Chapter 16 provides an extensive overview of the mechanism of injury.

Medical Patients

The medical emergency scene is also filled with valuable information. Compared with the often highly visible clues at trauma scenes, the clues pertaining to medical patients are more subtle. As with trauma patients, look to bystanders to provide information about facts as how a patient was feeling prior to losing consciousness.

Scene Control

Learning to manage a scene is not a simple matter. Depending on where the patient is located, there are often distractions that make focusing on the patient's needs more difficult. Any aspect of the physical environment that compromises the emergency care efforts should be addressed. For example, traffic can be stopped or rerouted while the patient is immobilized and moved out of the street. The stereo or TV can be turned down so the rescue team can communicate more effectively. The family dog can be confined to a bedroom. Furniture and toys can be moved to make room for transferring a patient from a house to an ambulance. These distractions can often be eliminated quickly by other support personnel or bystanders.

Friends, Family, and Bystanders

Properly managed, friends, family, and bystanders can be valuable resources at an emergency scene. Although they usually mean well, these people can cause some difficulties. First, they may have an emotional investment in the patient's well-being, and often feel they must ensure that their loved one is well cared for. Although the paramedic has the same agenda, a conflict can develop if friendship interferes with patient care.

If someone is being unruly or is agitating other people at the scene, it is essential to control them or have them removed as quickly as possible. It is always more desirable to work with people when possible. Conflict detracts from the real focus of the call. When friends or family try to direct patient care, a brief explanation of the patient's status and the medical control system can help lessen their anxiety. Often, giving the family or friends simple tasks to perform will also help them feel useful and make the scene easier to control.

Infectious Disease Exposure

High on the list of safety checks is taking infection-control precautions (see Chapter 10). When indicated, protective equipment should be in place before entering the scene. This includes wearing gloves, masks, and gowns to avoid exposure to airborne and bloodborne pathogens. Special masks, such as HEPA masks, may be needed for some airborne pathogens, such as those causing tuberculosis. Some safety issues can be assessed prior to arrival, some while en route, and still others may be managed during the call itself. Identifying risks is the crucial first step. If safety issues are not identified, they are unlikely to be managed, and unmanaged safety factors compromise all other aspects of an emergency response.

SUMMARY

The paramedic's ability to assess and manage the scene is a critical skill. It is also a difficult skill, because it must occur at the same time the paramedic is gathering information and preparing to treat the patient. Even when patient care is well under way, the scene control often continues to demand attention. Lastly, clues to the medical condition that are provided by the scene assessment should be documented and reported at the time of patient handoff.

Mike Smith, REMT-P

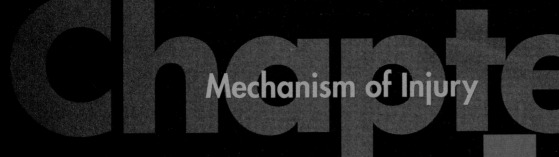

chapter 16

Mechanism of Injury

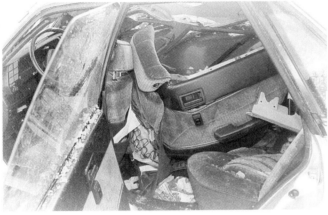

A paramedic should be able to:

OBJECTIVES

1. Describe the relationship between a high index of suspicion and mechanism of injury.

2. List the three time "phases" of a traumatic incident and the historical information included in each one.

3. Explain the significance of minimizing on-scene time in prehospital trauma care.

4. Explain how the three basic physics laws of force and energy relate to trauma and injury potential.

5. Name three types of collisions that can occur during change of speed impact.

6. Describe shear and compression forces and the types of injuries each can cause.

7. List important historical information to consider when evaluating mechanism of injury in motor vehicle collisions.

8. Describe the injury patterns produced by the following types of collisions:
   a. Head-on
   b. Side/lateral
   c. Rear-end
   d. Rollover

9. Explain the advantages and potential disadvantages of seat belts and airbags.

10. Describe the forces, mechanisms, and injury patterns most often involved in vehicle-pedestrian accidents, falls, hangings, and explosions.

11. List important historical information to gather in penetrating trauma incidents and explain their relationship to potential injuries.

KEY TERMS

1. **Blunt trauma**—an injury produced by the wounding forces of compression and change of speed, both of which may disrupt tissue.

2. **Kinematics**—the study of energy transfer from one source or object to another.

3. **Kinetic energy**—the energy that involves motion.

4. **Mass**—the physical property of matter that gives it weight and inertia.

5. **Mechanism of injury**—the physical manner and forces in which an injury occurred; a criterion for assessment in which the potential for the severity of trauma is estimated by analyzing the physical forces which caused the injury.

6. **Penetrating trauma**—an injury or wound affecting the interior of an organ or cavity.

7. **Trauma**—an injury caused by transfer of energy from some external source to the human body.

8. **Velocity**—the rate of change in the position of a body moving in a particular direction.

Scene Survey

Initial Assessment

Focused History
and Physical Exam

Continued Assessment

Despite efforts to prevent trauma, it is still the leading cause of death in the United States for individuals between the ages of 1 and 37, and it is the fifth leading cause of death for individuals of all ages.[1]

In addition to the high death toll of America's youth, traumatic injuries disable millions of people and cost our society billions of dollars. An understanding of the behavior of force and energy, types of collisions, and likely mechanisms of injury will help paramedics best care for trauma victims and reduce their death and disability.

Concepts of Trauma Care

Traumatic injuries are often very graphic and can visually trap prehospital providers. When this happens, serious injuries can be overlooked, and less serious, but more graphic, injuries are treated first. Maintaining a high index of suspicion is the key to countering the trapping effect of the more visual injuries.

The index of suspicion can be raised by several factors, such as:

- *Pattern recognition.* Certain types of accidents have the potential to produce specific kinds of injuries.
- *Logical thinking.* Begin with a premise and think forward to possible outcomes. Or, start with a conclusion (a man was shot) and think backward (the type of gun and distance from assailant to the victim), which can also point to potential injuries and their severity.
- *Intuition.* This "sixth sense" can lead to important treatment even in the absence of obvious medical findings.

Each traumatic incident has three distinct phases: preoccurrence, occurrence and postoccurrence. Each of these phases contains valuable information to be gathered by the paramedic.

Important ways to optimize prehospital trauma care include information relative to the patient's immediate needs, providing meaningful intervention, and trying to limit the scene time to 10 minutes or less. The following factors in each phase affect patient outcome and should be determined whenever possible:

Preoccurrence phase

- Age and physical condition of the victim
- Past medical history
- Current medications
- Alcohol or substance abuse

- Position of victim
- What the victim was doing

Occurrence phase

- Was victim wearing seat belt?
- Structural integrity of vehicle
- Energy transfer (to patient or elsewhere)
- Motion of victim (thrown, fell, crushed)

Postoccurrence phase

- Time from occurrence of incident until delivery to definitive care
- Type and level of prehospital care rendered

Examples of information that can be obtained about each phase are given in Box 16-1.

The Time Factor

Once a traumatic event has occurred, the survival clock begins ticking. The longer it takes to deliver a seriously injured patient to definitive care at the hospital, the less likely the patient's survival becomes.[1] The time that passes during on-scene care is irreplaceable; whenever possible, it should be limited to 10 minutes or less. The following ideas will make optimal use of time:

- Only employ ALS therapies and interventions that can improve the patient condition in less time than the ETA.
- Limit scene time on trauma calls to 10 minutes or less, although some situations (e.g., entrapment and cribbing unstable vehicles) can extend scene time.
- Perform only essential care at the scene. All other procedures should be provided en route.
- Know what a dying patient looks like. As the severity of the patient's condition increases, so does the importance of limiting scene time. Remember to assess and reassess for life-threatening conditions.
- Plan and prepare so that the right equipment arrives at the patient's side as soon as possible.
- End *every* assessment and reassessment with a patient status decision.

BOX 16-1	Phases of Traumatic Incidents
Phase	**Sample Information Obtained**
Preoccurrence	Passenger states 42-year-old, otherwise healthy driver clutched chest, gasped for breath, and fainted. According to the passenger, the driver was not taking any medications and was not under the influence of alcohol.
Occurrence	Car ran off road, fell down embankment, and impacted tree on driver side. Driver and passenger wore 3-point restraint seatbelt.
Postoccurrence	Bystander pulled driver and passenger from vehicle.

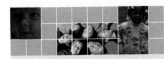

PEDIATRIC PERSPECTIVE

- Blunt trauma remains the leading cause of injuries in children.[2]
- Following blunt chest trauma in children, pulmonary contusions are more common than skeletal injuries. This is due to the greater elasticity of the child's chest wall. Energy is therefore transmitted to internal organs causing "hidden" injuries.[1,2]
- Motor vehicle accidents, falls, as well as domestic violence such as child abuse and assaults, are the most common "mechanisms" of head trauma in infants and children.[2]
- Children who are struck by a vehicle often show a triad of injuries involving the legs (hit by the bumper), the chest and abdomen (hit by the front of the vehicle) and the head (striking the hood).

- The larger size of the infant and child's head may contribute to a high incidence of head trauma.
- A child unrestrained in a motor vehicle involved in a front-end collision traveling a speed of 30 mph will hit the dashboard with approximately the same force applied and energy transferred as from a three story fall.[2]

REFERENCES

1. Barkin R et al. Pediatric emergency medicine, concepts and clinical practice. St. Louis, 1992, Mosby-Year Book, Inc.

2. Eichelberger M. Pediatric trauma. Prevention, acute care, rehabilitation. St. Louis, 1993, Mosby-Year Book, Inc.

The Laws of Physics Applied to Trauma

Consider these situations:

- A man slips off a ladder while cleaning his gutters and falls 25 feet to the ground.
- A young boy steps into the batter's box and is struck in the face with a fastball.
- A woman backs her car out of the driveway into the path of an oncoming motorcycle, which collides with the car, ejecting the biker over the car and onto the ground.

Each of the above mechanisms of injury is very different, yet each involves three basic components (Fig. 16-1):

1. Energy in motion
2. Deceleration
3. Transfer or transformation of energy

Newton's Laws of Motion

To better understand how to evaluate an incident and predict what types of injuries may have been produced, it is necessary to understand some of the laws of physics as described by Sir Isaac Newton:

- An object at rest will remain at rest unless acted upon by an outside force.
- An object in motion will remain in motion in a straight line unless acted upon by an outside force.

How might these laws apply to the previous scenarios? The man cleaning on the ladder was an "object at rest" until he slipped and became an object in motion. The fastball was an "object in motion" that acted upon an object at rest as it struck the young boy. The same law applies in the case of the motorcycle striking the car. In each case, there is a transfer of energy that results in injury to the patient.

These are all examples of objects that were either put into motion or stopped from moving when an outside force acted upon them. To further explore this, one needs to apply another law of physics:

- Energy cannot be created or destroyed, but it can be changed in form.

The interactions described in the above scenarios each represent energy in motion that was changed in form. These are good examples of the significance of looking beyond the obvious external signs of trauma to assess the subtle, but potentially more lethal, internal injuries that can occur as energy is changed in form.

Kinetic Energy

To evaluate the process of energy transfer, it is necessary to have a basic understanding of kinetic energy (the energy of motion). This is tied directly to the evaluation of velocity (speed). Although mass is an important concept as well, velocity is more significant. To put this into perspective, consider the following equation for determining kinetic energy (KE):

$$KE = Mass/2 \times Velocity^2$$

For a practical application of this equation, consider a 200-pound man involved a car wreck at 55 mph:

$$KE = 200/2 \times 55^2 = 302,500$$

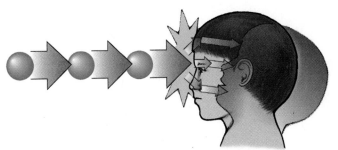

Figure 16-1

The physics of trauma: energy in motion, deceleration, and transfer or transformation of energy.

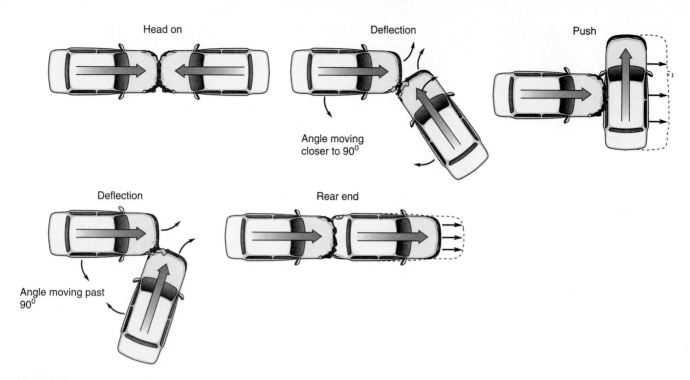

Figure 16-2

The angle of impact has bearing on the overall force involved in an accident.

Add 40 lbs to his weight and see what happens now.

$$KE = 240/2 \times 55^2 = 363,000$$

As you can see, a weight change of 40 pounds only produced an increase of about 60,000 kinetic units (or approximately 20%). However, if we take the original man at 200 pounds and increase his velocity by 10 mph, we get a much different outcome:

$$KE = 200/2 \times 65^2 = 422,500$$

In this case, there is almost a 40% increase in the amount of energy that is transferred.

The Mechanism of Blunt Trauma

When a moving object is acted upon by an outside force, a collision or impact occurs. In the most severe form of impact, the outside force meets the moving object straightaway, or what is

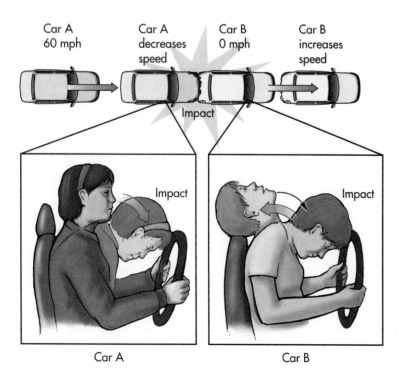

Figure 16-3

As a rear-end impact occurs, energy is transferred from the moving car to the stationary car.

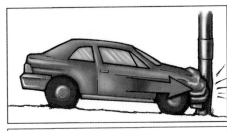

Collision #1

Auto hits pole

A

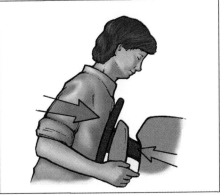

B

Collision #2

Body hits steering wheel, causing broken ribs

Figure 16-4

Collisions that occur during a motor vehicle accident. A) The car strikes an object. B) The occupant impacts the car.

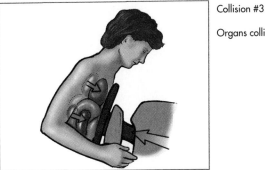

Collision #3

Organs collide internally

Figure 16-5

Third collision that occurs during a motor vehicle accident. The soft, flexible organs within the body collide with the body's structures.

commonly called head-on (Fig. 16-2). If the outside force's angle of impact moves away from head-on, the force of the collision is reduced. As the angle of the impact moves toward 90°, or perpendicular, the collision becomes more of a deflection. And, as it gets closer to 90° it becomes more of a push and less of a deflection. As the angle moves past 90°, it again becomes more of a deflection, until it approaches 180°, when it becomes a rear-end impact. In a head on collision, the momentum of two vehicles striking each other at 60 mph is additive—the same as a moving car hitting a stationary one at 120 mph.

Change-of-Speed Injuries

With any impact, there is either deceleration or acceleration. With some collisions, there is both, as in a rear-end collision in which a moving vehicle hits a motionless one. As the moving vehicle makes contact, it immediately begins to decelerate, and the stationary vehicle begins to accelerate (Fig. 16-3). Regardless of which mechanism occurs, any change-of-speed impact will produce shear and compression forces (described below) on the occupants. There are actually three possible collisions that can occur during an impact (Fig. 16-4 and 16-5). Take, for example, a car and driver hitting a tree:

- The car strikes tree
- The driver hits the steering wheel or dashboard
- The driver's organs collide internally

Shear

Because of their ligamentous attachments and anatomic positions in the body, a number of organs are at risk for shear injuries. Shear injury occurs in organs that are relatively free to move about inside the body but are held in place at one or two points by a restraining ligament. The aorta, liver, spleen, and kidneys are examples. Shear injury occurs when the organ tears at or near the point of attachment. When the aorta is involved in a shear injury, it is most commonly torn at its point of attachment at the ligamentum arteriosum, just beyond the left subclavian artery (see Chapter 46). If a total shear injury occurs, the aorta is completely torn and the victim will internally bleed to death almost immediately. However, when the aortic shear is partial, there is a good possibility of survival if surgical intervention is rapid.

The liver is also highly susceptible to shear. In a serious deceleration, its connection to the ligamentum teres can literally cut the liver in half. Shear injuries to either the aorta or liver can lead to serious, possibly fatal, outcomes because they produce occult (hidden) bleeds. It is easy to remain at ease with a patient who appears stable—until signs and symptoms of **shock** suddenly develop. At this point, the paramedic has lost valuable time and must make up lost ground. It is essential to maintain a high index of suspicion when the mechanism of injury points toward the possibility of shear injuries.

Compression

The other major force involved in blunt trauma is direct pressure, or compression (Fig. 16-5). The organs most susceptible to this force are the heart, lungs, diaphragm, liver, spleen, and bladder. In addition, compression injuries to the head can produce **skull fractures** and brain injuries, and spinal compression can cause vertebral fractures and **spinal cord injury**. When chest trauma is present, there is a possibility of **fractured ribs**, **flail chest**, **pneumothorax**, **hemothorax**, and **pulmonary contusions**. Whenever a bent steering wheel is noted, there should be a high index of suspicion for both compression and shear. Even with properly worn seat belts, high-speed deceleration can produce both these mechanisms and their corresponding injuries.

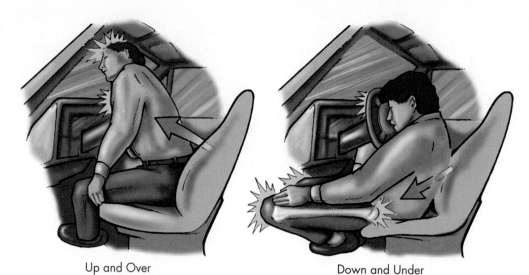

Figure 16-6

Patterns of injury seen in unrestrained occupants of motor vehicle accidents.

Up and Over   Down and Under

Motor Vehicle Collisions

There are a number of different types of motor vehicle collisions that a paramedic may encounter. They can be as simple as a car running off the road into a tree or as complex as an incident involving multiple collisions and cars off the roadway or rolled over. A number of clues can enhance the assessment and management of trauma patients involved in those collisions. The paramedic should evaluate:

- *Estimated speed.* Eyewitnesses may supply this information. High velocity increases injury potential.
- *Skid marks.* Their presence indicates that the driver attempted to slow down prior to the collision, which reduces the kinetic energy involved.
- *Number of collisions.* Areas of impact may help to identify where energy was directly transferred to the occupants.
- *Seat belts.* Were they worn, and worn properly? Unbelted occupants have a much higher potential for injuries, especially to the head.

- *Airbags.* Were they deployed?
- *Starred windshield.* This indicates a direct hit from an occupant and the possibility of c-spine and head injury.
- *Wrinkled metal with no visible point of impact.* This suggests a vehicle rollover.

Types of Collisions

The type of motor vehicle collision can give the paramedic valuable information about the victim's mechanism of injury and the types of potential injuries.

Head-On Collisions

For every 1 inch of metal or fiberglass body that is bent or destroyed, there was approximately 1 mph deceleration. Unbelted occupants will follow one of two different paths: down-and-under the steering wheel or up-and-over the steering wheel (Fig. 16-6). Victims who fall down-and-under the steering wheel have the potential for serious orthopedic trauma

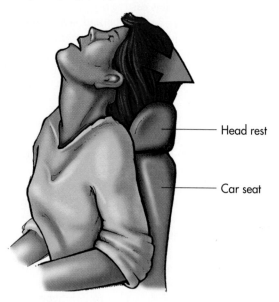

Figure 16-7

Hyperextension occurs from an improperly placed headrest.

Head rest

Car seat

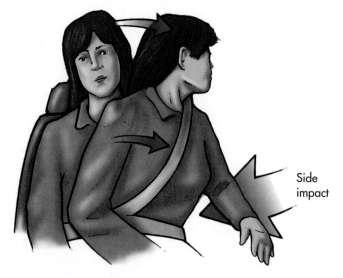

Side impact

Figure 16-8

Even when the occupant is properly restrained, a side impact can result in twisting of the body.

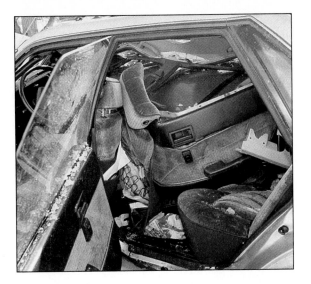

Figure 16-9

Cars are designed to withstand great force in the passenger compartment. Anticipate severe injuries when this compartment is damaged. Photographed by Craig Jackson.

because they can fracture any of the long bones of the leg, dislocate the knee, or fracture or dislocate the head of the femur at the acetabulum. Occupants who follow the up-and-over path first collide with the steering wheel, then continue into the windshield. Head, brain, face, and cervical trauma are very likely with this path of movement, as is serious chest injury. In either case, the vehicle may also roll over or be involved in another collision, and the unbelted participants may be thrown in any direction. If both vehicles are moving at full speed at the time of the collision, the force of the impact equals the sum of the two speeds.

Rear-End Collisions

Occupants in a car that was struck in the rear move backwards

after the initial impact. After this movement occurs, passengers also have the potential to rebound forward and follow one of the two paths described previously in "Head-on Collisions." If the headrest in the car is too low, the victim's cervical spine can undergo extreme hyperextension (Fig. 16-7). Possible areas of injury include head, brain, and cervical spine, and if the rebound movement is severe enough, chest, abdomen, long bone, and soft tissue injuries can occur as well.

Side-Impact or Rotational Collisions

Even if the passenger is seat-belted, there is a high probability of lateral-medial (sideways) or rotational (twisting) motion of the head and cervical spine (Fig. 16-8). This can be lethal because there is little to no protection for the occupants. If unbelted occupants collide with other occupants, they can produce internal injuries that are very difficult to assess because there may be little visible evidence. If there is passenger compartment intrusion, the likelihood of serious injuries rises (Fig. 16-9). Some vehicles are now equipped with side-impact airbags.

Rollovers

The possibility of head and cervical spine injuries is very likely in this type of collsion. Unbelted occupants may also do serious damage to each other as the vehicle rolls.

Seat Belts and Airbags

Despite the occasional story about some lucky soul who survived a horrible collision by being thrown clear of the car, the fact remains that seat belts save lives. An unrestrained occupant is much more likely to suffer serious head trauma and other injuries. Head injuries are a leading cause of death from motor vehicle collisions. The reason that properly used seat belts have improved survival rates is that the belt prevents the

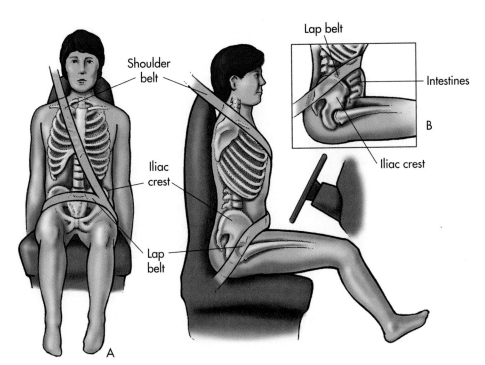

Figure 16-10

A) The three-point restraint restrains the upper torso and the pelvis. B) When lap belts are positioned too high, compression injuries to the abdominal organs can occur, as well as injuries to the thoracic and lumbar spine.

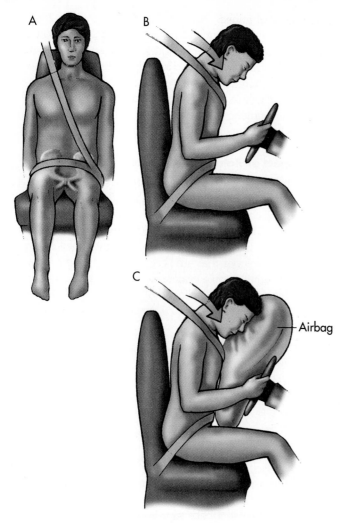

Figure 16-11

Injury can occur even with three-point restraints and airbags. A snugly and properly worn three-point system (A) reduces the likelihood of injury from the body impacting with (B) the restraints or (C) an airbag.

"second collision"—the occupant's body striking the inside of the car. In addition, seatbelts keep victims from being ejected from the vehicle. Once the victim is airborne, the likelihood of fatal injuries increases significantly.

When seat belts were initially introduced, there were only lap belts. The belts were designed to fit low and tight across the iliac crests, and they did in fact prevent ejection. However, the victim could still flex forward at the waist and have the potential of striking either the steering wheel, dashboard, or the back of the seat. With lap belts, head, face, and cervical trauma are still common. When lap belts are worn but positioned too high, compression injuries to the abdominal organs occur, as well as injuries to the thoracic and lumbar spine (Fig. 16-10).

The newer combination of lap belt and shoulder harness, commonly known as a three-point restraint, restrains the upper torso as well as the pelvis. With this configuration, not only is ejection eliminated, but forward motion is also greatly reduced. Despite their improved performance, three-point restraints still leave the head unrestrained, and therefore the potential for head and cervical spine trauma still exists (Fig. 16-11). Again, there is the problem of wearing the devices im-

properly. Some people apply the three-point restraint and tuck the shoulder harness under their arm, which can produce liver shear at speeds under 30 mph. A shoulder harness worn without a lap belt can allow the victim to slip down-and-under the steering wheel, and create a hangman effect that produces spine injury or carotid artery damage. Even when properly applied, three-point restraints still cannot prevent the "third collision" as organs move inside the body.

The current device in occupant restraint is the airbag, which is designed to deploy in the first seconds after a frontal collision. Sodium azide, a solid, receives an electrical charge and turns into a gas that inflates the bag. The airbag cushions the head, face, and chest remarkably well and is used in conjunction with a three-point restraint. It is designed to deflate immediately; if there is another collision after the initial impact, the airbag will not offer protection, because it will not inflate a second time.

There are several important points worth remembering about airbags. 1) The cylinder housing for the airbag is quite hot immediately after deployment, and care should be taken when working around it. In fact, the accident victim may have suffered minor burns if he or she contacted the airbag soon after the crash. There have also been reported cases of patients complaining of respiratory difficulties as a result of inhaling the powder used on the surface of the airbag when it is packed. 2) It is worth taking a moment to push the airbag aside to see if the steering wheel has been bent. Airbags do not completely eliminate the possibility of significant injuries. Airbags for side impact collisions are available on a few car models. 3) Children and small adults in the passenger seat have been fatally injured after airbag deployment; the public is cautioned to place child safety seats in the back seat of these cars.

Motorcycle Collisions

As with automobile occupants, motorcycle riders who are involved in collisions have predictable patterns of injury. Be-

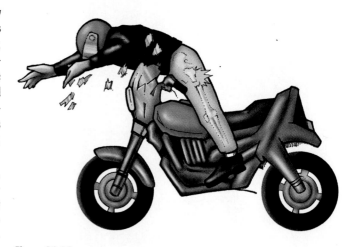

Figure 16-12

Injuries are often seen when a motorcycle driver is thrown over the handlebars.

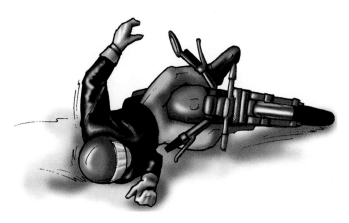

Figure 16-13
Motorcycles can entrap the driver, causing severe injuries to trapped body parts and tissues.

cause seat belts are not a factor, victims from a motorcycle collision are turned into missiles unless the motorcycle driver has to "lay the bike down." Skid marks and estimated speed are once again important considerations. The paramedic should also be alert to:

- *Helmets.* Head injuries are more likely if not worn. Even when worn, they may contribute to cervical spine injuries from the rider bouncing on the pavement. Be alert for scratches, indentations, or cracks in or on the victim's body, which may indicate a very serious impact.
- *Leather or vinyl clothing.* There is an increase in abrasion potential if these materials are not worn by the victim.
- *Bike size.* Bigger motorcycles are heavier and more powerful, both of which increase injury potential.

Types of Collisions

The type of collision can give the paramedic important information about the victim's mechanism of injury and potential injuries.

Head-On Collisions

Victims traveling up-and-over the handlebars can present with bilateral femur fractures with serious soft-tissue injuries and blood loss (Fig. 16-12). Head, face and cervical trauma are likely to occur upon landing. If the motorcycle has a windshield and the victim is propelled into it, serious head, facial, and cervical spine injury can result from this as well.

Once the victim is airborne, possibilities of collision include: bouncing off the hood or windshield of a car, hitting a fixed object such as a signpost or trees, or being run over by a following vehicle. Virtually any injury can be caused by these mechanisms.

Side- or Lateral-Impact Collisions

The driver's or passenger's legs or pelvis may be crushed as a car hits them laterally. The motorcycle and its passengers may be pushed into the path of an oncoming vehicle.

Ejection

Injury severity depends both on how the victim lands and the nature of the object struck.

Laying the Bike Down

If the operator or passenger can get away from the bike, injuries may still involve soft tissue, head, and c-spine. If the occupants slide while still "attached" to the bike there is a high probability of entrapment, and almost any injury is possible. At a minimum, an extremity that is trapped under the bike as it slides is almost certain to be severely injured (Fig. 16-13).

All-Terrain Vehicle Collisions

All-terrain vehicles (ATVs) are common, especially in rural America, and are popular as both recreational and work vehicles. The most dangerous type of vehicle, because of its instability, is the three-wheel ATV, which has been taken off the

Side overturns

Rear overturns

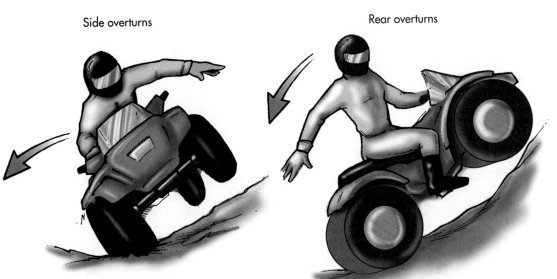

Figure 16-14
All-terrain vehicles (ATVs) are prone to rollovers because of their high center of gravity and oversized wheels.

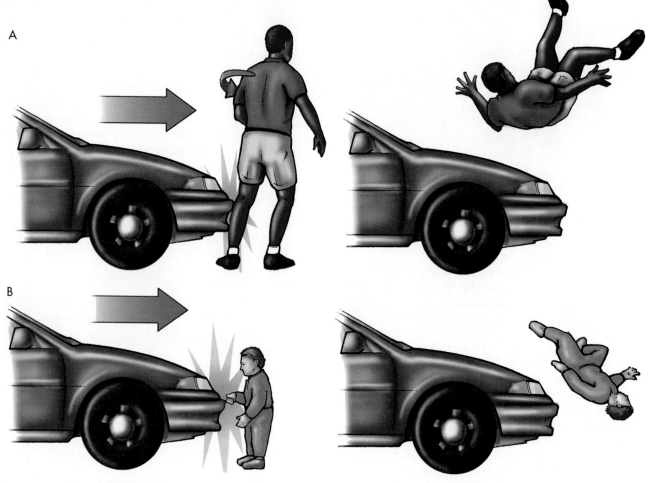

A

B

Figure 16-15

A, When an adult pedestrian is struck, he or she often turns, is struck on the side of the body, and tumbles end over end to the ground. B, Because of immature reflexes, children usually turn and look at what is hitting them and then fall to the ground head first.

market. Depending on how it crashes, an ATV can produce minor to very serious injuries. When an ATV is moving sideways up an incline and begins to tip over, the operator frequently steps off, and the vehicle drives over the driver's leg, resulting in ankle and lower leg trauma. If an ATV flips over backward, the operator is often sandwiched between the vehicle and ground, which can cause chest, abdominal, soft tissue, spinal or orthopedic trauma (Fig. 16-14). Face, head, and neck trauma should all be suspected following a head-on collision.

Tractor Rollovers

Tractor rollovers are one of the leading causes of death in farming accidents. Side rollovers are the most frequent type; often the operator is either thrown clear or can crawl clear and avoid being crushed. Rear rollovers occur less frequently but produce fatalities in almost all cases. As with ATVs, the operator involved in a rear rollover is crushed between the seat and

the ground. The difference is size. An ATV may weigh several hundred pounds, but a large tractor can weigh 25,000 pounds or more.

Pedestrians

When a pedestrian is struck by a motor vehicle, the pedestrian is often severely injured, as the weight and velocity of the vehicle transfers significant energy to the body. When approaching the scene, look for skid marks. A long skid mark indicates that the vehicle was traveling at a high rate of speed, and that the energy of motion was being transformed by the brakes. However, to the paramedic, skid marks do not necessarily indicate minor injuries. The vehicle could have struck the pedestrian without slowing at all, and produced the skid after the fact. In this situation, long skid marks point to a serious outcome, because the vehicle had to be travelling quite fast at the time of the impact.

The age of the pedestrian can also influence injury pattern

by John Barron

America's fascination with fitness has brought about a significant increase in the sales of bicycles and in-line skates, commonly referred to as rollerblades. Paramedics may encounter patients of any age with a broad range of injuries caused by these activities. The highest rate of injuries from bicycle accidents still occurs in the pediatric population (ages 5 through 15). However, adult injuries and death rates have increased substantially in recent years.[7] Injuries can range from simple "road rash" to life-threatening head injuries.

The mountain bike has replaced the 10-speed street bike as the most popular form of bicycle, carrying riders into areas never before accessible by bicycles. Along with this new accessibility comes potential for special types of injuries and rescue requirements. In the same way the mountain bike has revolutionized the bicycle industry, in-line skates have changed roller skating. New designs, improved materials, and advanced technology have contributed to increased speeds and increased dangers.

Injuries associated with bicycles and in-line skates are predictable according to the rules of physics. The most basic rule still applies: The faster you go, the harder you hit. Most bikers soon realize that when they fall over the handlebars, the bike will run them over before it stops. As Newton observed, objects in motion stay in motion in the same direction until they encounter a force that changes their direction or stops them. Bicyclists who ride on the roads face different dangers, especially collisions with cars. Head injuries top the list of fatal injuries, especially when bicycle helmets are not worn.[1-6] Orthopedic injuries of all types are also possible, and with high-speed impacts, internal injuries can lead to shock. Paramedics must perform a thorough **kinematics** assessment and ask witnesses for information. Trail riding mountain bikers face their own share of dangerous obstacles, but injuries are usually minor.

The most serious cycling injuries occur when riders fail to wear properly fitted helmets. Approximately 1000 bicycle-related fatalities are reported each year in the United States, and more than 70% of all these are caused by critical head injuries.[1,7] All research articles cited conclude that the use of helmets can significantly decrease injury and deaths associated with bicycle accidents. One study[7] also provides the following figures on head injuries related to bicycling:

1. Bicyclists hospitalized with head injuries are 20 times as likely to die as those cyclists without head injuries.
2. Bicycle injury rates are highest in riders between the ages 5 and 15.
3. Among fatally injured bicyclists, 50% are 20 years of age or older.
4. Death rates for men bicyclists ages 20 to 54 have substantially increased in recent years.

Bicycle and in-line skate accidents are usually low-speed when compared with most automobile accidents, and therefore produce low-energy impact injuries. However, these injuries can still be devastating, especially head injuries. Other injuries common to bicyclists are orthopedic injuries, such as broken collar bones, extremity fractures, broken and cracked ribs, and spinal injuries. "Road rashes," eye injuries, cuts, scrapes, bumps, and bruises are also common to bicycle injury lists.

Most serious trail riders wear some form of eye protection. Those who don't are subject to eye trauma from branches, thorn bushes, flying insects, and flying mud and debris.

In-line skaters have similar injury patterns from their falls, but don't have to worry about their bike running over them. Skaters stay mainly on smooth, hard surfaces, which contribute to their injuries. A person's natural reaction to a fall is to break the fall using hands. Special wrist protectors are commonly sold along with the skates to help decrease orthopedic injuries to the wrists. Here, too, helmets are invaluable in the prevention of serious head injuries.

Mountain bikers who become injured when riding remote mountain trails can create unique rescue problems for paramedics. Extrication from these situations often requires specialized personnel and equipment and can be more efficient if the service area implements a preplan for access and practices with simulated extrications. Some services train paramedics to ride mountain bikes to increase the speed of response to remote sites.

Dehydration is another concern for bicyclists and skaters who exercise for long periods of time without proper fluid and electrolyte replacement. This concern is amplified at races, where competitive spirit often drives people beyond the limit of their physical tolerance. Experienced cyclists know the value of fluid and electrolyte replacement, and the limits of their endurance. However, even experienced cyclists can make mistakes and underestimate a course. Dehydration is a key element in fatigue, and fatigue often results in poor decisions when riding.

Finally, never overlook the possibility of conditions associated with exposure to heat and cold. Heat stroke and hypothermia are both real possibilities for any biker who has been out too long in extreme weather. Improper clothing can lead to a rider's lower body temperature even in relatively cool temperatures. These exposure illnesses often cloud the rider's ability to make rational decisions. As with dehydration, this can lead to mistakes and additional injuries.

Bicycles and in-line skates are still a major source of injuries in the pediatric population, these injuries are no longer restricted to this age group. More and more adults are riding bicycles and using skates for fitness and recreation. Paramedics must be ready and able to assess and manage a victim of any age with injuries resulting from these sports.

REFERENCES

1. Bicycle related head injuries and death in the United States. *JAMA*, 266(21):3016, 1991.

2. Fatal bicycle injuries in children: a plea for prevention. *JAMA*, 270(15):1801, 1993.

3. Mandatory Helmet Use. *JAMA*, 269(23):2967, 1993.

4. Fatal Bike Injuries. *Pub Health Rep*, 108(2):212, 1993.

5. Injuries Associated with Bicycles. Am Family Phys, 48(8):1544, 1993.

6. Haigh G: The Perils of Pedal Power. *Times Edu Suppl*, 3893:39, 1991.

7. Johns Hopkins Helmet Safety (national research study) conducted and sponsored by the Snell Memorial Foundation, PO Box 493, St. James, New York 11780.

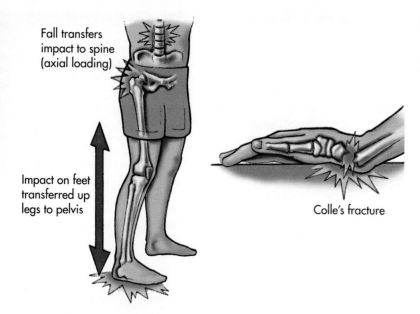

Fall transfers impact to spine (axial loading)

Impact on feet transferred up legs to pelvis

Colle's fracture

Figure 16-16

Energy is transferred inside the body, creating predictable injury patterns. Make note of the surface that the victim has landed on, because this may add to injuries.

(Fig. 16-15). Adults tend to turn and avoid the collision, so the point of impact may be on the victim's side. Because of the higher center of gravity, the adult may also go through an "end over end" motion prior to landing on the ground. Children, on the other hand, often become transfixed as the vehicle approaches, and many times are struck while looking directly at the car. When this occurs, the child may suffer bilateral tibia, fibula, or femur fractures from the bumper, chest trauma from striking the hood, and head and face injuries from striking the hood or windshield. If the child is thrown from the vehicle, the relatively large head size of a child increases the risk of the child landing on it.

Falls and Hangings

For victims of falls and hangings, it is important to note four main points:

1. The distance of the fall
2. The surface on which the victim landed
3. The anatomical areas struck
4. Whether it was a free fall

Did the patient slip and fall off a roof or was it a controlled, low-speed fall such as a hanging? During a free fall, the victim can increase velocity quickly; falls from over three times the victim's height should be considered serious. The way in which the victim landed, what objects (if any) were struck on the way down, and what surface was landed on, are all important considerations as well (Fig. 16-16). Adults who have jumped rather than fallen tend to land on their feet, and then fall onto their buttocks or outstretched hands. This mechanism can produce compression injuries of the spine, lower extremity trauma, and fractures of the upper extremities. When young children fall, they often land on their heads because of disproportionate weight of their heads in relation to the rest of their bodies; serious face and cervical trauma are thus common.

In hangings there are two distinct patterns. If the victim falls slowly or only a short distance, as is common in a suicide in the home, strangulation and asphyxiation are likely. If the victim falls quickly, or for a greater distance, the chance of spinal injury is greater. The paramedic should also be aware of airway compromise resulting from a crushed trachea, or the possibility of hypoxic brain injury resulting from compression of blood vessels.

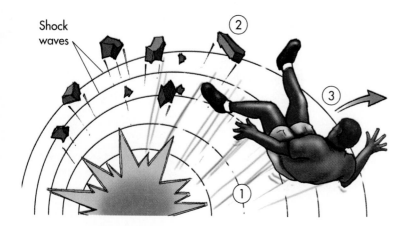

Shock waves

Figure 16-17

Three mechanisms of injury act upon the body during an explosion.

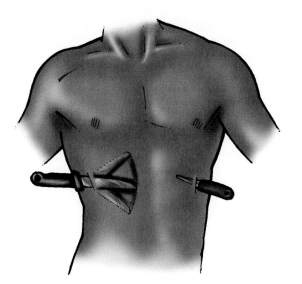

Figure 16-18

With penetrations to the body, consider the length of the blade as well as the motion applied to the blade itself.

Explosions

Although explosions are a relatively infrequent occurrence in the United States, they can produce a wide variety of injuries. During an explosion, victims may be injured by any or all of three primary mechanisms of injury (Fig. 16-17):

1. Shock waves from the blast can produce serious internal injuries.
2. Debris can be blown into the victim, producing soft tissue and internal injuries.
3. The victim may become a "projectile" and be thrown into fixed objects, resulting in almost any type of injury.

Any patient who has been involved in an explosion requires careful assessment and reassessment. Close attention should be paid to ongoing status, as injuries unnoticed initially may become more apparent as time goes on. Assessment may be hampered because of hearing difficulties produced by the explosion. Explosions in a confined space can be especially devastating as the explosive force is concentrated.

Penetrating Trauma

Accidents in rural settings often have a high incidence of blunt trauma, whereas urban-centered accidents usually produce more penetrating trauma. Each of these mechanisms produces unique injuries. Assessing the victim of penetrating trauma, such as a gunshot wound or a stabbing, is a challenging matter. A small entry wound may be all that is visible to the naked eye, but it does not reveal what has happened internally. To complicate matters, the paramedic must consider several other key issues.

- *The apparent direction of travel of the penetrating object.* Although it is not always possible to tell, sometimes the trajectory of the object can be determined and provide clues to the organs injured.
- *The weapon itself.* Was the weapon sharp or dull? Sharp weapons sometimes produce bloodless injuries. A dull weapon can rip and tear as it enters, resulting in serious bleeding that is difficult to control.
- *The speed of entry.* A sharp object entering quickly may transect a vessel and cause little or no bleeding. The slow application of a dull weapon can produce devastating effects.
- *Type of knife and length of blade* (Fig. 16-18). Serrated blades rip more than cut.
- *Movement of the object during or after entering the body.* A knife with a 6-inch blade is by no means a large knife, but it can easily kill someone if it is inserted in the right location, particularly if it is moved back and forth.

Low-energy weapons include hand-driven weapons, such as knives, needles, and ice picks. These weapons produce damage only with their sharp edges and less secondary trauma is usually associated with them.[2] These injuries can usually be predicted by the path of the weapon into the body.

Figure 16-19

Penetrating projectiles can damage the body in many ways.

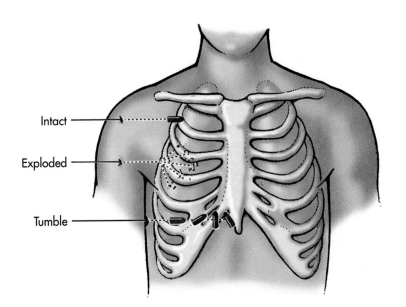

Intact

Exploded

Tumble

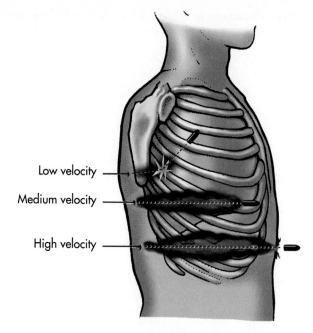

Figure 16-20

The higher the velocity, the greater the likelihood that the penetrating object exits the body. The highest velocity projectiles produce a shock-wave type of force, called cavitation, as it travels through the body.

Medium-energy weapons include handguns and some rifles. As the amount of gunpowder in the cartridge increases, the speed of the bullet increases. These weapons damage the tissue directly in the path of the missile, as well as the tissue on each side of the missile's path.

High-energy weapons include assault rifles, hunting rifles, and other weapons that discharge high-velocity missiles. The tissue damage is far more extensive with a high-energy penetrating object.

Although a low-velocity bullet may not produce a through-and-through injury, it can still "tumble" and produce serious, possibly life-threatening, injuries. For example, the autopsy of a young man who had been shot in the neck with a 22-caliber handgun showed that the bullet had deflected down the cervical spine and through the chest, tearing the aorta and left ventricle in the process. It continued through the abdomen and spiraled down the victim's left femur, coming to rest just proximal to the left ankle.

Key points the paramedic should consider when trying to estimate injury potential include (Fig. 16-19):

- *Projectile size.* The larger the bullet, the greater the mass, the higher the resistance or "drag," and the larger the path of travel.
- *Projectile characteristics.* Bullets, such as hollow points, mushroom and flatten out on contact, increasing the amount of surface area that contacts the body. Bullets that are designed to tumble will also increase the surface area of the bullet and increase injury size accordingly.

Punctures produced by a low-velocity weapon, such as a knife, usually cause injuries to tissue and organs directly in line with the path of entry. As mentioned earlier, low-velocity bullets can tumble once they enter the body and can come to rest

nearly anywhere. The patient or an eyewitnesses may be able to provide some insight about the location or angle of the attacker and the gun. However, for understandable reasons, victims often cannot offer much of this information.

As the velocity of the weapon increases, the projectile is more likely to go entirely through the victim than to tumble about (Fig. 16-20). However, with increased velocity comes an increase in cavitation. Cavitation is the development of pressure waves that push the surrounding organs and tissues out of place. These pressure waves form, collapse, and reform, until all the energy is dissipated. There have also been specialty weapons developed that have armor-piercing capabilities and will penetrate so-called bulletproof vests. For all practical purposes, it is best to assume that anyone shot with a high-velocity weapon, including many rifles, has serious injuries regardless of what is seen at the surface.

SUMMARY

The ability to assess the mechanism of injury quickly is a valuable skill for the street-smart paramedic. Applying the basic laws of physics helps with that assessment, as does associating the patterns of injuries with specific types of collisions and assaults. Being able to look beyond the obvious to consider possible additional underlying injuries is an important part of the paramedic's role. Minimizing on-scene time will maximize the likelihood of a positive outcome for the patient.

REFERENCES

1. **National Safety Council:** Accident Facts, 1995 edition; Itasca, 1995, National Safety Council.

2. **McSwain, et al:** The basic EMT: Comprehensive Prehospital patient Care, St. Louis, Mosby-Year Book Inc, 1997

SUGGESTED READINGS

1. **Blacksin MF:** Patterns of Fracture After Air Bag Deployment. J Trauma, 35(6), 1993.

2. **Bone LB, et al:** Mortality in Multiple Trauma Patients with Fractures, J Trauma 37(2), 1994.

3. **Davis JW, et al:** The Etiology of Missed Cervical Spine Injuries, J Trauma 34(3), 1993.

4. **Dischinger PC, Cushing BM, Kerns TJ:** Injury Patterns Associated with Direction of Impact: Drivers Admitted to Trauma Centers, J Trauma 35(3), 1993.

5. **Hendey GW, Votey SR:** Injuries in Restrained Motor Vehicle Accident Victims, Ann Emerg Med 24:1, 1994.

6. **Kluger Y, et al:** Diving Injuries: A Preventable Catastrophe, J Trauma 36(3), 1994.

7. **Lane PL, McClafferty KU, Nowak ES:** Pedestrians in Real World Collisions, J Trauma 36(2), 1994.

8. **McDermott FT, et al:** The Effectiveness of Bicyclist Helmets: A Study of 1710 Casualties, J Trauma 34(6), 1993.

9. **Orsay EM, et al:** Motorcycle Helmets and Spinal Injuries: Dispelling the Myth, Ann Emerg Med 23:4, 1994.

10. **Seigel JH, et al:** Safety Belt Restraints and Compartment Intrusions in Frontal and Lateral Motor Vehicle Crashes: Mechanism of Injuries, Complications, and Acute Care Costs, J Trauma 5(34), 1993.

11. **Shatney CH, Sensaki K:** Trauma Team Activation for "Mechanism of Injury" Blunt Trauma Victims: Time for a Change? J Trauma 37(2), 1994.

12. **Swierzewski MJ, et al:** Deaths From Motor Vehicle Crashes: Patterns of Injury in Restrained and Unrestrained Victims, J Trauma 37(3), 1994.

13. **Weesner CL, et al:** Fatal Childhood Injury Patterns in an Urban Setting, Ann Emerg Med 23(2), 1994.

14. **Williams J, et al:** Head, Facial, and Clavicular Trauma as a Predictor of Cervical Spine Injury, Ann Emerg Med 21:6, 1992.

Section

Assessment of the Critical Patient

3B

Included In This Section:

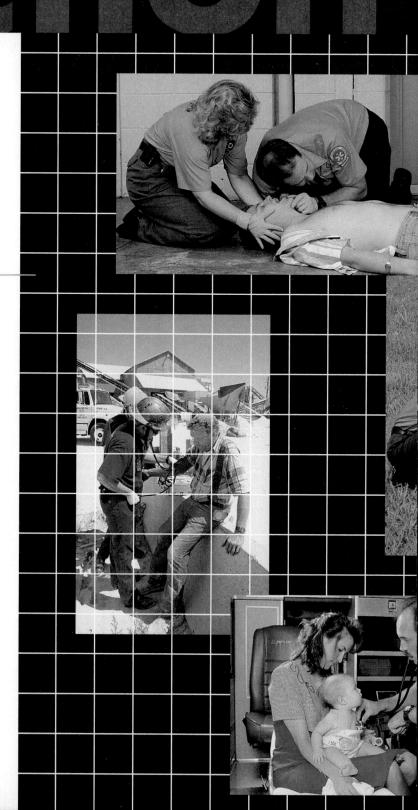

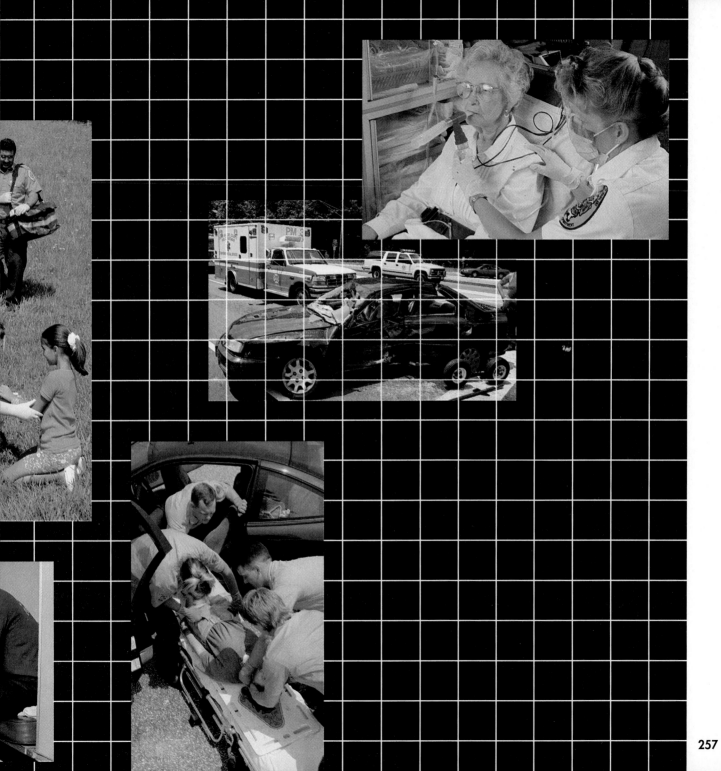

Introduction to Assessment

Patient assessment is one of the most critical skills performed by the paramedic. It requires a thorough understanding of each step involved and skillful decision-making. This introduction provides an overview of the patient assessment process.

```
                      ┌─────────────────────┐
                      │    Scene Survey     │
                      └─────────────────────┘
  YES                                              NO

                    Is the scene safe?  ──────▶  Take appropriate
                           │                     precautions
                           ▼                     Determine
                  ┌─────────────────────┐        mechanism of
                  │ Initial Assessment  │        injury or nature of
                  └─────────────────────┘        illness

  Protect spine  ◀──  Is head/neck
                      trauma suspected?
                           │
                           ▼
  Evaluate level of  ◀──  Is patient responsive?
  responsiveness
                           │
                           ▼
                    Is the airway open?  ──────▶  Reposition,
                           │                      suction/remove
                           │                      foreign material/
                           │                      (Heimlich)
                           ▼
  O₂ (if indicated)  ◀──  Is the patient  ──────▶  O₂, BVM
                          breathing?               ventilation,
                           │                       intubation
                           ▼
                    Does the patient  ──────▶  CPR, quick-look,
                    have a pulse?               defib
                           │
                           ▼
  Control  ◀──  Is there severe
  hemorrhage     bleeding?
                           │
                           ▼
                    Is circulation normal? ──▶  Rhythm vs.
                           │                     volume (meds,
                           ▼                     pacing, fluids)
  ┌──────────────────────────────────────────────┐
  │  Focused History and Physical Examination    │
  └──────────────────────────────────────────────┘
                 Conduct focused history
                 and physical examination
                      ↙         ↘
           Medical              Trauma
           Nature of illness    Mechanism of injury
           Medical history      Rapid focused exam
           Focused examination  History
                      │
                      ▼
          ┌─────────────────────────┐
          │  Continued Assessment   │
          └─────────────────────────┘
            Detailed physical examination
            Ongoing assessment
```

Every patient encounter begins with the scene survey. If a quick, accurate scene survey is not performed, a potentially dangerous situation can result in further injury to the patient and rescue personnel. The scene survey is performed to determine the safety of the scene, the patient's mechanism of injury or nature of illness, and the need for additional resources.

Scene survey is followed by the initial patient assessment. During the initial patient assessment, the paramedic identifies and corrects immediate life threats that involve problems with the patient's level of responsiveness, airway, breathing, and circulation. Patients with immediate life-threatening conditions can die within minutes without rapid recognition and correction of their problems. Determining the type of the patient's condition (i.e., medical or trauma related) is also part of the initial assessment.

The focused history and physical examination follows the initial assessment. Some patients can appear to be stable initially, but then rapidly deteriorate. A closer, focused assessment can reveal information that will assist in identifying the illness or injury and its severity, as well as appropriate management that will prevent progression to a life-threatening condition.

Once the patient's most serious conditions have been managed (or if none can be determined), the continued assessment is performed. This assessment is a more detailed examination and in every case includes continued reevaluation of the patient while in the paramedic's care. In patients with serious conditions, this evaluation is usually performed en route to the hospital. This more complete physical assessment of the patient may reveal additional secondary injuries or other information that will assist in diagnosis and treatment at the hospital. All patients must be continually observed and reevaluated during transport to prevent or manage emerging conditions.

The following section begins by discussing the first steps in the assessment process, which involve a scene survey and evaluation of the patient's mechanism of injury or nature of illness. The following chapters provide an overview of the initial assessment process; detailed life threat assessment and management; and critical trauma and critical pediatric patients.

After a close look at the clinical significance of vital signs, the focused history and physical examination, as well as the continued assessment, are explored. Pediatric and geriatric assessment are also thoroughly covered in this section.

More thorough and detailed assessment information is provided in the Patient Presentation and Trauma sections specific to the patient's chief complaint or area of injury.

S. Scott Polsky, MD, FACEP
Phil Fontanarosa, MD, FACEP

Chapter 17

Initial Assessment

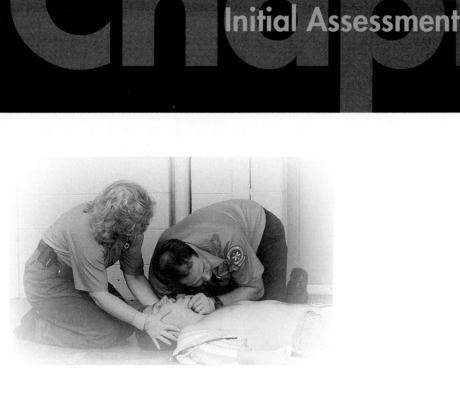

A paramedic should be able to:

1. Describe the purpose of the initial patient assessment.

2. List the steps of the initial assessment in sequential order and describe how each is performed.

3. Describe how to use one's senses to help recognize immediately life-threatening conditions.

4. Explain the acronym AVPU.

5. Describe how the initial assessment of a patient's airway differs between trauma and medical patients.

6. Describe the signs and symptoms and management of the following life-threatening conditions:
   - Unresponsiveness
   - Airway Obstruction
   - Absent Breathing
   - Absent Pulse
   - Severe Bleeding

Scene Survey

↘ **Initial Assessment**

Focused History and Physical Exam

Continued Assessment

O nce the scene has been quickly surveyed and found to be or made safe, the paramedic can arrive at the patient's side and begin the initial assessment (Box 17-1).

The objective of initial patient assessment is to determine if there are life-threatening problems present that require rapid intervention. This assessment involves evaluation of the patient's level of responsiveness, airway, breathing, and circulation and is a systematic process that should not be altered (Box 17-2). This assessment usually requires less than 30 seconds to complete but the process may last longer if intervention is required at any point. At this stage, the patient's problem will most likely be identified as medical or trauma.

Recognizing and Managing Immediate Threats to Life

To be most effective, the paramedic must rapidly analyze all available patient information, condense it into pertinent facts, and make quick decisions regarding the care needed. The paramedic relies on the senses of sight, speech, hearing, and smell in this approach to the patient. The initial impression of the patient will reveal obvious ill appearance, external bleeding, vomiting, sweating, convulsions, and flushed or pale skin.

By speaking and listening to the patient, the paramedic will determine the level of responsiveness, presence or absence of breathing, the degree of breathing difficulty, and the degree of pain. The paramedic's sense of smell can also identify odors such as vomit, loss of bowel control, or the acetone (fruity) breath sometimes noted in diabetic emergencies.

The paramedic must determine if the patient's signs and symptoms are consistent with the mechanism of the injury noticed upon arrival at the scene or consistent with the nature of the illness mentioned in the dispatch. The paramedic should then decide if the patient's problem is medical or traumatic. Although the general approach to the initial assessment is the same, there are variations in the way the steps are performed (e.g., the technique for opening the airway for an unresponsive patient). Decisions regarding transportation of the patient also depend upon the nature of the patient's problem.

Responsiveness

Upon arrival at the patient's side, the paramedic should begin the initial assessment with a check for responsiveness (Box 17-3). If there is a possibility of trauma to the patient's head or neck, another EMS team member may hold the patient's head to minimize movement and avoid causing further damage (Fig. 17-1).

Level of consciousness (LOC) or responsiveness is one of the most important indicators of the patient's overall condition. LOC can vary from fully alert to unresponsive. The AVPU scale is used to describe the spectrum of LOC from the highest level of responsiveness to the lowest (Table 17-1).

TABLE 17-1	AVPU Scale
A	Alert and aware
V	Responds to verbal stimuli
P	Responds to painful stimuli
U	Unresponsive

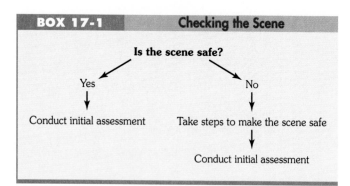

BOX 17-1 — Checking the Scene

Is the scene safe?

Yes → Conduct initial assessment

No → Take steps to make the scene safe → Conduct initial assessment

BOX 17-2 — Steps in the Initial Patient Assessment

1. Consider the mechanism of injury or nature of illness to determine if the patient's condition is a medical or trauma problem.
2. Check the patient's **L**evel **O**f **C**onsciousness.
3. Check the patient's **A**irway.
4. Check the patient's **B**reathing.
5. Check the patient's **C**irculation (pulses and severe bleeding).

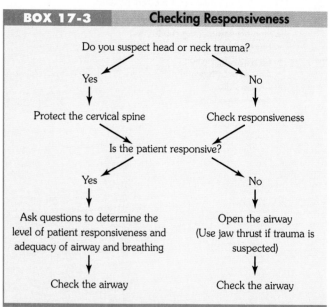

BOX 17-3 — Checking Responsiveness

Do you suspect head or neck trauma?

Yes → Protect the cervical spine

No → Check responsiveness

Is the patient responsive?

Yes → Ask questions to determine the level of patient responsiveness and adequacy of airway and breathing → Check the airway

No → Open the airway (Use jaw thrust if trauma is suspected) → Check the airway

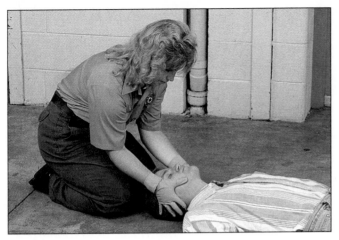

Figure 17-1

In-line immobilization of the head and neck is an immediate priority if trauma is suspected.

Alert implies that the patient is aware of his or her identity and the surroundings and is able to respond appropriately to questions. A patient who is oriented to person, place, time, and event is said to be "alert and oriented times four." A patient who is unable to respond correctly or is slow to respond is considered "disoriented."

Verbal refers to a patient who must be stimulated by sound, such as a voice, in order to respond. This patient may appear to be lapsing in and out of responsiveness. Patients who only respond to verbal prodding are unlikely to provide complete and accurate answers.

Painful means that the patient responds only to a painful stimulus. This assessment is often performed by pinching the skin on the earlobe or above the collarbone, or rubbing the sternum (Fig. 17-2).

Unresponsive refers to a patient who does not respond to any stimuli, verbal or painful. This patient is also described as unresponsive or unconscious. This is the most severe of the four levels of responsiveness.

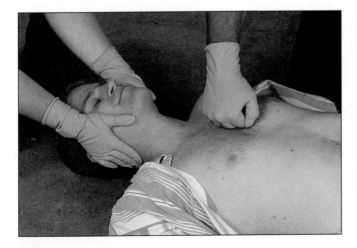

Figure 17-2

Brisk rubbing on an intact chest wall will determine the patient's level of responsiveness. (Be prepared for a potentially rapid, violent response.)

The paramedic should begin the LOC check by speaking to the patient. If the patient can converse, breathing and heartbeat are considered present. If the patient does not respond immediately to voice, the paramedic should tap the patient's shoulder and speak loudly to the patient, asking "Are you okay?" The patient who responds at this point is considered responsive to some degree. If there is no response, the paramedic should try a painful stimulus. If this attempt is unsuccessful, the patient is considered to be unresponsive.

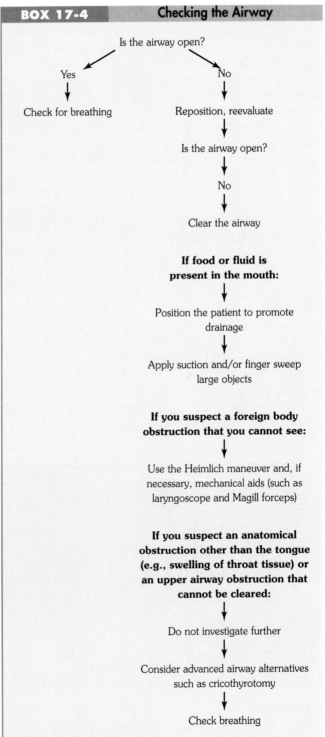

BOX 17-4 **Checking the Airway**

Is the airway open?

Yes → Check for breathing

No → Reposition, reevaluate

Is the airway open?

No

Clear the airway

If food or fluid is present in the mouth:

Position the patient to promote drainage

Apply suction and/or finger sweep large objects

If you suspect a foreign body obstruction that you cannot see:

Use the Heimlich maneuver and, if necessary, mechanical aids (such as laryngoscope and Magill forceps)

If you suspect an anatomical obstruction other than the tongue (e.g., swelling of throat tissue) or an upper airway obstruction that cannot be cleared:

Do not investigate further

Consider advanced airway alternatives such as cricothyrotomy

Check breathing

Airway

For a patient to breathe adequately, the airway must be open. This means that the airway must be free of obstructions, both anatomical (i.e., the tongue) and mechanical (e.g., food, fluid, vomitus, or other objects). In an alert patient, airway assessment is easily performed. If the patient is speaking clearly or crying loudly, the airway is clear of obstruction. If the patient cannot talk, cry, or cough forcefully, then the airway is likely obstructed and must be reevaluated and cleared (Box 17-4). At this point, the Heimlich maneuver is the appropriate method to clear an obstructed airway in the adult responsive patient. Obstructed airway problems are discussed and illustrated in greater detail in Chapter 18.

In an unresponsive patient lying supine, the most frequent obstruction is the tongue. This is often made evident by snoring respirations. Repositioning the airway to remove the obstruction is usually all that is needed. If there is no suspicion of head or neck trauma, the airway should be repositioned using the head-tilt/chin-lift method. If head or neck trauma is a possibility, the jaw-thrust technique should be used to prevent further injury.

If the patient's airway is obviously obstructed by food or fluid in the mouth, the obstruction should be removed with suction. A laryngoscope and Magill forceps are effective tools to clear larger objects from the back of the throat (*see* Skill 11 in the Skills Section). Once the patient's airway is clear of obstruction, the initial assessment can be continued.

Breathing

If the patient is obviously breathing, the paramedic should determine whether the breathing is sufficient to support life (Box 17-5). A patient speaking in full sentences is rarely in serious respiratory distress. However, the patient who struggles to answer and can only say a word or two between breaths is in severe respiratory distress and may stop breathing.

Patients breathing at a rate between 12 and 20 times per minute and moving adequate air volume may not require in-

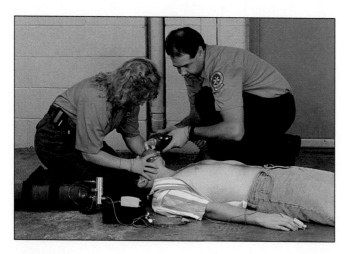

Figure 17-3

Ventilatory assistance is required if the patient has inadequate ventilation rate or volume.

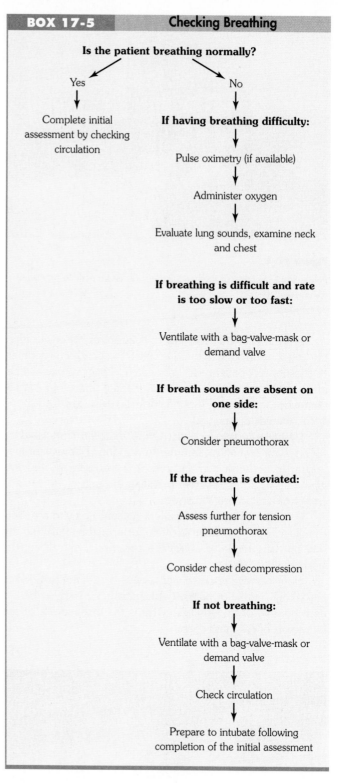

tervention other than oxygen through a nasal cannula or non-rebreathing mask. Patients having difficulty moving air and breathing less than 8 times per minute or more than 24 times per minute require ventilatory assistance with a bag-valve-mask (BVM) or demand valve (Fig. 17-3).

If the patient is unresponsive and the airway has been opened, breathing should be assessed. This is performed by the paramedic looking at the patient's chest while placing his or her ear next to the patient's mouth. In this manner, the paramedic can "look, listen, and feel" for approximately 5 sec-

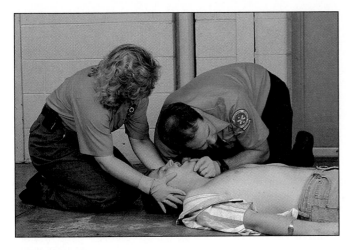

Figure 17-4

The paramedic should examine the patient's chest, listen for air movement from the mouth, and lean close to the patient's body to feel air movement on his or her cheek.

onds to determine if the patient is breathing (Fig. 17-4). If the patient is not breathing, an oropharyngeal airway should be placed in the mouth to keep the tongue from blocking the airway and the patient should be ventilated between 12 and 20

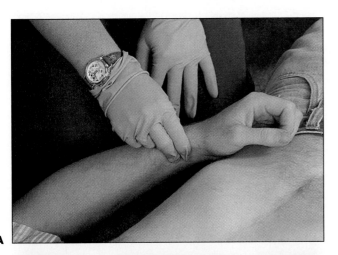

A

times per minute (1 breath every 3 to 5 seconds) using a BVM or demand valve. A resuscitation mask can be used initially to provide rescue breathing for the patient until the aforementioned equipment is available.

To maintain a patent airway and provide efficient ventilation, the patient should be intubated, but only after the initial assessment is complete and the patient is adequately hyperventilated. More information about caring for the dyspneic or apneic patient appears in Chapters 18 and 27.

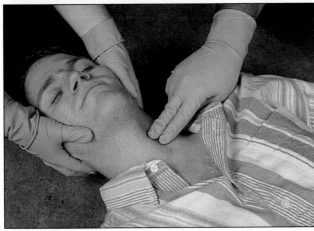

B

Figure 17-5

Pulses should be monitored at the wrist and neck when initially assessing a patient.

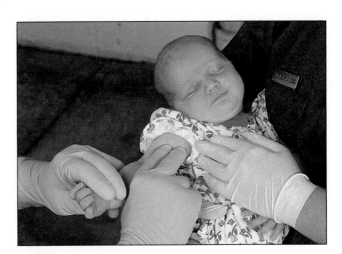

Figure 17-6

The brachial artery should be used when assessing pulse in an infant.

Circulation

After airway and breathing problems are assessed and corrected, the adequacy of the patient's circulation should be evaluated (Box 17-6). "Circulation" implies assessment of the patient's pulse and skin, and the search for severe bleeding.

Pulse

To check the pulse, the appropriate artery should be located and felt for approximately 10 seconds. In a responsive patient, the radial artery should be used (Fig. 17-5A). For infants, the brachial artery can be checked (Fig. 17-6). A normal adult pulse beats regularly at a rate of 60 to 90 times per minute. An abnormal pulse is one that is weak, irregular, too fast or too slow in respect to the patient's preceding activity level and other pertinent factors, such as medications and age.

If the patient is unresponsive, the carotid artery can be checked (Fig. 17-5B). If the patient does not have a pulse, CPR must be started until a monitor-defibrillator can be applied to determine the rhythm. If the monitor-defibrillator can be quickly applied, that should be done first. CPR should be continued and the patient treated according to the appropriate ACLS algorithm. This often involves both electrical and pharmacological therapy. Chapter 19 provides more detailed information.

Cardiac arrest is not the only possible life-threatening circulation problem. Inadequate blood flow, caused by loss of blood volume or heart failure, is also a possible problem.

A rapid, weak pulse often indicates insufficient blood or fluid volume and results in poor perfusion. This is also true if a carotid pulse is present, but the radial pulses are absent. Intervention for this condition may include oxygen, fluid resuscitation, medication administration, and rapid transport.

A rapid evaluation of the patient's skin can provide additional information about the circulatory status. While feeling the pulse, the paramedic can also assess skin temperature, color, and condition (e.g., moist, dry, hives), and the speed of capillary refill. Patients with cool, pale, and moist skin must be presumed to have a serious problem, often associated with hypoperfusion.

Severe Bleeding

Another problem associated with deficient circulatory status is severe bleeding (Box 17-7). Severe external bleeding includes blood that is spurting from a wound or flowing heavily and uncontrollably. Signs of internal bleeding are not as obvious and are often not seen until after the initial assessment.

If external bleeding is present, it should be controlled with pressure. Rapid transportation is extremely important for the patient who has suffered severe blood loss, and fluid resuscitation should begin during transport.

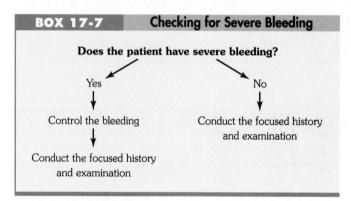

BOX 17-7   Checking for Severe Bleeding

Does the patient have severe bleeding?

Yes → Control the bleeding → Conduct the focused history and examination

No → Conduct the focused history and examination

SUMMARY

Patients with immediate life-threatening conditions may die within minutes without rapid recognition and correction of the problem. In such situations, there will be no time or real need for a lengthy physical examination; the first few steps of the patient assessment process will identify the most critical conditions. Although this information is part of every first aid or EMT course, the importance of using a systematic approach to patient assessment cannot be overstated.

S. Scott Polsky, MD, FACEP
Phil Fontanarosa, MD, FACEP

Chapter 18

The Patient With Airway and Breathing Compromise

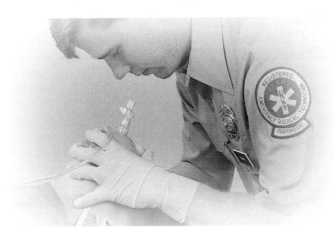

A paramedic should be able to:

OBJECTIVES

1. Describe the normal anatomy of the respiratory system.
2. Describe the normal physiology of breathing.
3. List the various causes of respiratory distress.
4. Describe the history and assessment of the patient experiencing respiratory distress.
5. Describe various abnormal breath sounds and their significance.
6. List signs and symptoms of respiratory distress.
7. Describe the management of various patient conditions that present with respiratory distress.
8. Identify normal and abnormal values for tidal volume, respiratory rate, blood gases, and pulse oximetry.

KEY TERMS

1. **Accessory respiratory muscles**—supplementary muscles used to aid in difficulty when breathing.
2. **Airway obstruction**—a blockage of the airway as a result of a foreign body, such as food or vomitus, or as a result of an anatomical problem such as tongue displacement or tissue swelling.
3. **Apnea**—absence of breathing; respiratory arrest.
4. **Dyspnea**—difficulty breathing.
5. **Heimlich maneuver**—a technique used to help dislodge a foreign body airway obstruction.
6. **Rescue breathing**—the process of breathing for a patient who is in respiratory arrest.
7. **Respiratory arrest**—the cessation of breathing as a result of illness or injury.
8. **Stridor**—a shrill, high-pitched respiratory sound indicating upper airway obstruction.

Scene Survey

Initial Assessment

Focused History
and Physical Exam

Continued Assessment

A patient who is experiencing severe difficulty breathing poses one of the greatest challenges the paramedic will face. Because of the devastating effects that hypoxia can have on the circulatory and nervous systems, rapid, appropriate intervention is essential. For problems such as foreign body airway obstruction in a responsive patient, the steps for care are simple and the patient outcome is often immediately positive. However, when patients have been without oxygen for a long period of time, the intervention skills required can be more complex, and the outcome is not always immediately clear.

The patient assessment steps discussed in Chapter 17 help the paramedic to quickly identify a breathing problem. This chapter provides the basic information needed to better understand critical airway and breathing problems and how to correct those problems. Patient complaints of "shortness of breath" are addressed in Chapter 27.

Review of the Respiratory System

The respiratory system is responsible for providing the body with oxygen and removing waste products, such as carbon dioxide. To accomplish this, the airway must be clear of obstructions that prevent gas exchange. The respiratory system also relies on adequate pulmonary blood flow for the exchange of oxygen and carbon dioxide and the use of respiratory muscles to attain a sufficient volume of air exchange.

The respiratory system is commonly divided into the upper and lower airways (see Chapter 7 for illustrations). The upper airway structures begin with the cavities of the mouth and nose and extend past the pharynx to the larynx. The larynx joins the pharynx to the trachea and houses the vocal cords.

The lower airway begins just beneath the larynx and extends to the alveoli, where respiratory gas exchange takes place. Air enters the lower airway through the trachea, which divides into the two main bronchi entering the lungs. These divide into secondary bronchi and then into the smallest air passages (bronchioles) and finally terminate in the alveoli.

The pleura are the connective tissues that cover the lungs. They consist of two layers, the visceral pleura (innermost, covering the lungs) and the parietal pleura (outermost, lining the thoracic cavity). Pleural fluid lies between these two layers in the pleural space, to allow the lungs to freely slide against the chest wall during the process of inspiration and expiration.

The process of respiration occurs when there is an exchange of oxygen and carbon dioxide between the blood and the environment. During inspiration, muscle movement involving the diaphragm and intercostal muscles makes the chest wall expand, increasing the size of the thoracic cavity

and slightly lowering intrapulmonic pressure. This pressure reduction causes air to flow into the lungs from outside the body. During expiration, muscle movement reduces lung volume, thereby increasing intrapulmonary pressure and forcing air out. A healthy adult breathes 12 to 20 times a minute at rest and has a tidal volume of approximately 500 mL.

The medulla is the primary center that regulates breathing. Chemoreceptors of the medulla continuously monitor changes in pH and the concentration of oxygen and carbon dioxide in the blood. The partial pressure of carbon dioxide (pCO_2) plays the most important role in controlling respiration; pCO_2 is closely related to hydrogen ion concentration (pH). If pCO_2 increases, the resulting drop in pH (respiratory acidosis) adversely affects cellular metabolism. The medulla responds by increasing respiratory rate and depth, in an attempt to maintain pCO_2 in the range of 35 to 45 mm Hg.

Arterial oxygen concentration (pO_2) normally plays a smaller role in regulating respiration. Chemoreceptors in the medulla, carotid arteries, and aorta monitor the pO_2 level. If the pCO_2 level and pH remain constant but pO_2 decreases, the medulla responds by increasing ventilation. Patients with chronic obstructive pulmonary disease rely more on pO_2 than pCO_2. These patients normally have an elevated pCO_2 level, which reduces chemoreceptor sensitivity to changes in pCO_2 levels. As a result, these patients have a hypoxic drive as their main stimulus for ventilation; the medulla relies on the pO_2 level to regulate breathing, rather than pCO_2.

Common Causes of Breathing Emergencies

Respiratory distress often results from injury or illness, but can also be a product of stress, anxiety, or excitement. Anatomical causes include conditions that narrow airway passages and foreign objects that occlude the airway. Specific medical conditions and traumatic injuries that can result in breathing emergencies are listed in Box 18-1.

BOX 18-1	Causes of Breathing Emergencies
Medical Conditions	**Traumatic Injuries**
Asthma	Rib fractures
Emphysema	Pneumothorax
Chronic bronchitis	Burns to the face, neck, and
Pleurisy	airway
Pneumonia	Cervical spine injury
Anaphylaxis	Laryngeal fracture
Croup	Tracheal fracture
Epiglottitis	Any condition resulting in
Hyperventilation syndrome	shock
Pulmonary embolism	
Airway obstruction	
Heart conditions (e.g., congestive heart failure and pulmonary edema)	

Assessing a Patient for Breathing Difficulty

Breathing should be an effortless task. Whether responsive or unresponsive, the patient experiencing difficulty breathing will usually display obvious signs (Table 18-1). Some of these signs involve respiratory rate and quality. The respiratory rate may be unusually fast or slow, and the depth of the respirations can be shallow or deep and labored. The patient may make unusual sounds indicating airway obstruction, including wheezing, gurgling, and stridor. The paramedic should consider whether the patient is straining to breathe, and look to see if the patient is using accessory muscles to breathe, if the patient's intercostal muscles are retracting, or if cyanosis is present. The paramedic should also look for nasal flaring. In children, lung assessment includes auscultating breath sounds. Some of the more common terms used to describe abnormal breath sounds are found in Box 18-2.

Assessing the Responsive Patient

At the scene, the paramedic should approach the patient from the front and conduct an initial assessment, as detailed in Chapter 17. The initial patient assessment is directed toward discovering life-threatening problems that require rapid intervention. This involves checking the ABCs. Although the patient is responsive, there still may be a serious problem involving the airway or breathing.

Recognizing Airway Obstruction

The first breathing emergency that warrants immediate attention is foreign body airway obstruction. Whether the result of illness or injury, foreign body airway obstruction is a significant problem that affects the ability to breathe. The most common source of obstruction is food, but fluids such as vomitus, saliva, blood, and water can also block the airway. Elderly patients are the most frequent victims of foreign body airway obstruction. When examining a responsive patient who may have difficulty breathing, the airway is the first thing the paramedic must check. When the airway of a responsive person is obstructed by a foreign object, the patient is typically choking. There are many different causes of choking, including:

TABLE 18-1	Normal and Abnormal Breathing	
	Normal	**Abnormal**
Rate	Adult: 12–20 Child: 15–30 Infant: 25–50	Above or below the ranges indicated
Quality • Effort	Effortless, natural	Labored, use of accessory muscles, intercostal retraction, nasal flaring, stridor
• Rhythm	Regular	Irregular
• Lung Sounds	Present and equal	Absent, diminished, unequal
• Chest Expansion	Equal, normal	Unequal, inadequate

BOX 18-2	Terms Describing Abnormal Lung Sounds

Rales or crackles—Intermittent high-pitched "crackling" sounds usually indicating the presence of fluid in the small airways or alveoli. Often heard in patients with acute pulmonary edema. They can be heard anywhere in the lungs but often start in the bases of the lungs as gravity draws fluid downward.
Rhonchi—Harsh, low-pitched, continuous, rattling sounds; more prominent than rales, that indicate the presence of mucous or secretions in the larger airways. Frequently heard in patients with chronic bronchitis or pneumonia.
Wheezing—High-pitched "whistling" sounds produced by air moving through narrowed passages. Often associated with patients experiencing asthma.
Friction Rub—Harsh sounds like pieces of dried leather being rubbed together, created by inflammation of the pleura.
Stridor—Harsh, high-pitched, "crowing" sound indicating a narrowing or obstruction of the upper airway. This sound is heard in patients experiencing croup, anaphylaxis, or a foreign body obstruction and can be heard without the use of a stethoscope.
Snoring—Snoring often indicates upper airway obstruction, usually when the tongue obstructs the airway of an unconscious, supine patient.

- Excessive use of alcohol while eating
- Failing to chew food properly
- Eating too fast
- Running or playing with food or objects in the mouth

If the patient is coughing, talking clearly, or crying loudly, the airway is clear of obstructions. If the patient cannot talk or cough forcefully or is making stridorous sounds, the airway is likely obstructed and must be cleared before further treatment. The choking patient may also clutch at the throat in what is called the universal distress sign.

Managing Airway Obstruction in the Responsive Patient

The Heimlich maneuver is used to clear an obstructed airway in a responsive patient more than 1 year of age. This technique has been effective at dislodging solid foreign bodies. The Heimlich maneuver is a thrust that compresses the abdomen (Fig. 18-1). This movement increases pressure in the lower airway, simulating a cough, and forces trapped intrapulmonary air to push the object out of the airway. It usually requires only a few thrusts to expel the object. If the patient is so large that the rescuer cannot reach around the patient's waist, or if the patient is noticeably pregnant, chest thrusts are performed instead of abdominal thrusts (Fig. 18-2). The force used to provide these thrusts should be less when rescuing small children. Because these thrusts are performed in a forceful manner, there is a chance of injury to the patient. For this reason, all patients who require the use of the Heimlich maneuver should be further evaluated by a physician.

Choking is a common emergency in children and infants, but clearing the obstruction with the use of abdominal thrusts poses an increased risk of injury. If the responsive patient is an infant (less than 1 year of age), back blows and chest thrusts

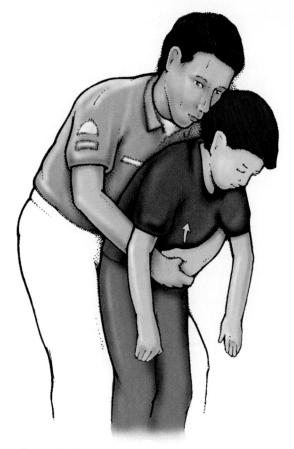

Figure 18-1

The Heimlich maneuver is effective in removing airway foreign body obstructions.

should be used to clear the obstruction (Fig. 18-3). The cycle of back blows and chest thrusts can be repeated until the object is dislodged.

Recognizing Respiratory Distress in the Responsive Patient

When the paramedic is certain that the patient's airway is clear, he or she should check for any other breathing difficulty (see Chapter 27). The paramedic should continue to talk to the patient and consider whether the patient is straining to breathe while answering. Patients who can speak in full sentences are not likely to be experiencing severe breathing problems. The patient's face should be checked for cyanotic lips. If cyanosis is present, the tissues are not properly oxygenated. If the patient is breathing through "pursed lips," there is likely to be a history of a chronic obstructive pulmonary disease such as emphysema. In children, the paramedic should look at the nostrils. Widening of the nostrils (nasal flaring) is a good indication that the child is having breathing difficulty.

The rescuer should continue to examine the patient's body, checking the outline of the trachea to see that it is midline. Lateral displacement is most likely an indication of a tension pneumothorax.

Next, the patient's chest should be examined. Whenever possible, the patient's chest should be inspected for symmetrical movement, the use of accessory muscles, and retraction of the intercostal muscles. Any tenderness, crepitus, or air leakage that may present as subcutaneous emphysema should be noted.

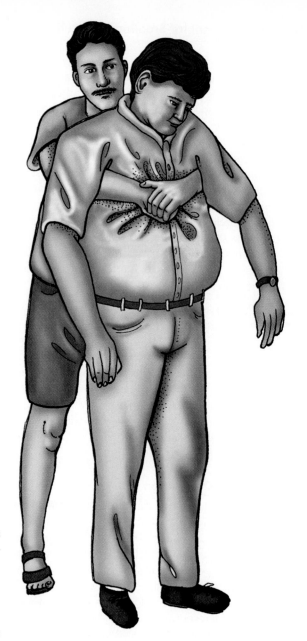

Figure 18-2

If the patient is too large to perform an abdominal thrust, a chest thrust may be used instead.

Breath sounds should be auscultated with the patient in a seated position whenever possible. This should be done in a symmetrical pattern, allowing the time to check all fields. This usually means one to two respiratory cycles for each area that is examined.

The patient's breathing rate and quality of the respirations should be determined and recorded as part of the baseline vital sign measurements. If available, pulse oximetry should be used to provide a baseline oxygen saturation (see Sidebar).

Managing Respiratory Distress

The steps for managing a patient in respiratory distress are:

1. Place the patient in the position of comfort. This is usually a seated position, unless the problem involves trauma to the head, thorax or pelvis.
2. Administer oxygen by nonrebreather mask at a rate of 10 to 15 L/min.

by Robert Carter, NREMT-P

Pulse oximetry is rapidly becoming a widely used and simple noninvasive monitoring device for the evaluation of adequate oxygenation in a patient. When properly used and interpreted, the device can be very helpful in alerting the paramedic of a patient's impending deterioration and hypoxia.

Pulse oximetry indirectly measures the amount of oxygen bound to hemoglobin by the transmission of both red and infrared light through the blood flow of arterial beds. The light is transmitted via a specially designed probe which consists of two light-emitting sensors. Infrared light is absorbed by hemoglobin bound with oxygen (oxyhemoglobin) and red light is absorbed by hemoglobin that is bound to something other than oxygen (methemoglobin). The oximeter measures the differences and reveals the saturation of oxyhemoglobin.

Pulse oximetry has many useful applications in the prehospital setting, including monitoring of patients during intubation, extubation, and suctioning. In certain cases, intubation attempts take longer than expected and patient goes too long without adequate oxygenation. The oximeter's low saturation limit alarm (preferably 94%) can alert the paramedic to interrupt the intubation attempt so that the patient can be reoxygenated through appropriate ventilations. The pulse oximeter also can monitor possible deterioration of a wide variety of patients, including trauma and cardiac patients. For example, a progressively lowering saturation in a patient with chest trauma can be the first clue of an impending problem. This can also be the case in cardiac patients and asthmatics. Another application in trauma situations could include using the pulse oximeter in the assessment of pulses and perfusion distal to a fracture site in an extremity. Often times, inadvertent movement of a fractured bone may cause arterial occlusion or diminished perfusion. A dropping saturation or inability of the oximeter to find a reading may alert the paramedic to impending problems.

Carbon monoxide will bind with hemoglobin more rapidly than oxygen; therefore, pulse oximeter readings of carboxyhemoglobin and methemoglobin will not accurately reveal the "real" oxygen saturation. The oximeter cannot distinguish between hemoglobin bound with oxygen or bound with carbon monoxide. A high saturation (> 95%) may be shown when the patient is actually hypoxic. The paramedic should be alert in cases of carbon monoxide poisoning and smoke inhalation. Inaccurate readings may also be present in the presence of shock, hypoperfusion, hypothermia, and excessive movement, which is common in infants and children.

To ensure a proper and accurate reading, the heart rate shown on the oximeter should correlate with the palpable heart rate. The visual correlation indicator would associate as well. If

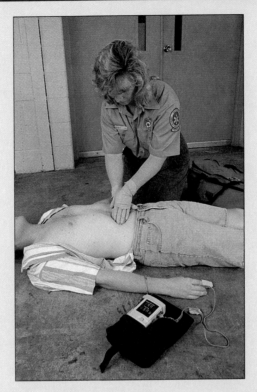

all readings are consistent, the oxygen saturation reading will be correct. A normal oxygen saturation level is 95% to 100%. Saturation levels below 94% may indicate respiratory distress or respiratory deterioration. Saturation levels below 91% indicate the need for aggressive respiratory management (e.g., oxygenation, ventilation, and ensurance of airway patency).

Sensors are commonly found as either a reusable finger probe or disposable sensors which can be placed on a finger, toe, earlobe, and even the bridge of the nose. Sensors come in both adult and child sizes. In the infant or neonate, the adult probe can be placed around the palm of the hand or around the foot.

Pulse oximetry is an important and useful prehospital tool. However, it should never be relied upon alone, but only in conjunction with the proper assessment of the patient's clinical appearance, level of responsiveness, skin color and temperature, and breath sounds.

REFERENCES

American Heart Association, American Academy of Pediatrics: Textbook of pediatric advanced life support, 1995.

Koff P, Eitzman D, Neu J: Neonatal and pediatric respiratory care, St. Louis, 1993, Mosby–Year Book.

3. Establish baseline vital signs, including breath sounds and pulse oximetry when available.
4. Determine the need for rapid transport.
5. Establish an IV of normal saline or lactated Ringer's at a TKO rate.
6. Determine the need for pharmacologic intervention.

If the patient is having difficulty breathing, the paramedic must act quickly to provide care. In some cases, this means determining the exact nature of the breathing problem, but this is not always necessary. For example, a patient experiencing severe wheezing may be having an asthma attack or an allergic reaction. In either case, the condition requires high-concentration oxygen and IV access. With all other vital signs being equal, the patient could benefit from a bronchodilator such as epinephrine 1:1000 or nebulized albuterol. Patients having difficulty moving air, breathing less than eight times per minute, or breathing more than 24 times per minute should receive ventilatory assistance with a bag-valve-mask (BVM) or demand valve.

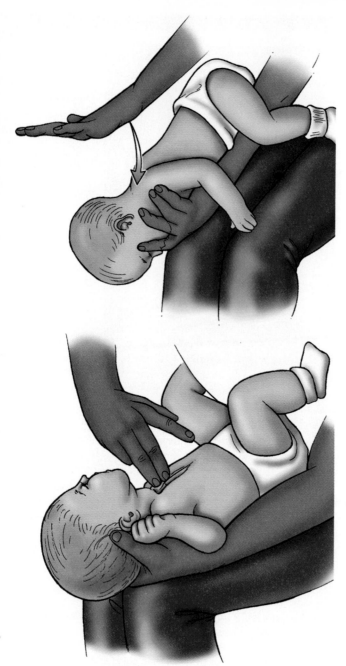

Figure 18-3

Back blows and chest thrusts are used to clear a blocked airway in an infant.

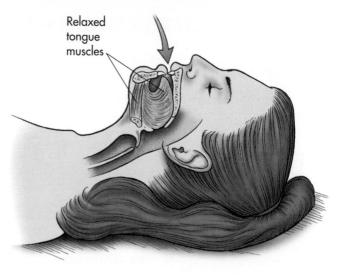

Relaxed tongue muscles

Figure 18-4

The most common cause of airway obstruction in an unresponsive patient is from the tongue.

If the patient's airway is obviously obstructed by food or fluid in the mouth, the obstruction can be removed by suctioning the airway, rolling the patient onto the side and using a finger sweep, a laryngoscope, or Magill forceps to remove large objects. With the airway clear of obstructions, the initial assessment can be continued, focusing on the patient's breathing.

Breathing should be monitored for approximately 5 seconds. The paramedic should look, listen, and feel for air movement. If the patient is breathing, the paramedic should check circulation and move on to the focused history and examination. At this point, the patient's breathing efforts can be evaluated. The head, neck, and chest should be examined and lung sounds auscultated.

Assessing the Unresponsive Patient

When initial assessment indicates an unresponsive patient, the paramedic should continue with the ABCs. In a supine unresponsive patient, the most frequent airway problem is obstruction, resulting from the relaxation of the muscles controlling the tongue (Fig. 18-4). Opening the airway relieves this anatomical obstruction. For patients without head or neck trauma, the airway can be opened using the head-tilt/chin-lift method (Fig. 18-5). When **head** or **spinal cord injury** is suspected, the airway should be opened using the jaw-thrust technique to avoid moving the neck (Fig. 18-6).

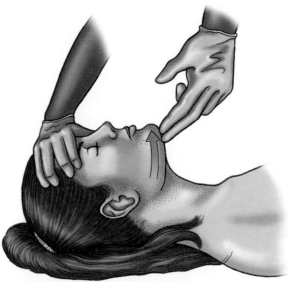

Figure 18-5

The head-tilt/chin-lift method is used for patients who are not suspected of having neck trauma.

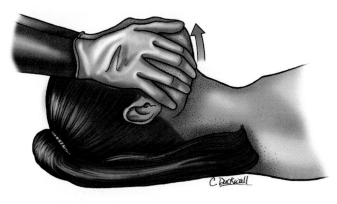

Figure 18-6

The jaw-thrust method allows the rescuer to open the airway, while maintaining a neutral alignment of the neck.

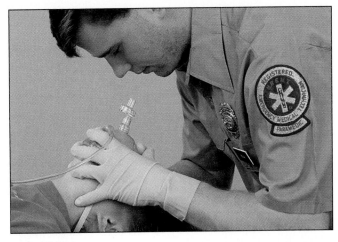

Figure 18-7

A pocket mask provides some protection during mouth-to-mask ventilation.

Managing Patients in Respiratory Arrest

The patient who is not breathing is in respiratory arrest. In this case, the paramedic must breathe for the patient. Rescue breathing involves ventilating the patient at a rate and depth that approximates normal breathing; this attempt can be done using various methods of ventilation including:

- Mouth-to-mouth
- Mouth-to-nose
- Mouth-to-stoma
- Mouth-to-mask
- Bag-valve-mask
- Demand valve

The most common practices today involve the use of a barrier between rescuer and patient during ventilation, typically with a resuscitation mask, BVM, or demand valve. Unprotected rescue breathing should only be performed as a last resort.

In the absence of more advanced equipment, a resuscitation mask can be used initially to provide immediate rescue breathing and reduce the chance of disease transmission. Any valves that filter airflow to or from the patient should be checked to ensure attachment. A one-way valve enables the rescuer's air to freely enter the patient and then diverts the patient's exhaled air away from the rescuer. The newer two-way valves are designed to filter both the rescuer's and patient's exhaled air to further reduce the likelihood of disease transmission. With the valve attached, position the mask and use both hands to maintain a good seal (Fig. 18-7).

Regardless of the patient's age and the means of ventilation, it is always important to ventilate the patient slowly. One of the most significant problems encountered during ventilation is gastric distention. This occurs when the patient is ventilated too quickly and with too great a volume of air; pharyngeal pressures exceed esophageal opening pressures, forcing air into the stomach. This air restricts the ability of the diaphragm to contract, reducing the lung volume available during ventilations and making vomiting more likely.

To minimize the chance of gastric distention, the paramedic should provide ventilations that last 1.5 to 2 seconds.

The rescuer should give between 12 and 20 ventilations per minute (one breath every 3 to 5 seconds). This allows for adequate inspiration and expiration time. When using the bag-valve-mask, the paramedic should squeeze the bag smoothly, not forcefully. Recent evidence suggests that when multiple rescuers are available, one rescuer should hold the mask in place while another squeezes the bag; this technique results in a better mask seal and more effective ventilation.

There is no question that endotracheal intubation is the most effective means of maintaining a patent airway. However, the patient must be adequately oxygenated prior to intubating. Intubation should also not occur before completing the initial assessment. Management of the patient's airway with an oropharyngeal airway and BVM will enable the paramedic to complete the initial assessment and determine circulatory status. For example, a patient who is apneic may also be pulseless. In this case, the priority would be to start CPR, evaluate the heart rhythm, and defibrillate if necessary, before attempting intubation.

Oral endotracheal intubation is the most common method (see Skills #4 and # 5 in the Skills Section) of ventilating a patient. The laryngoscope permits easy visualization of the upper airway, including the glottic opening. When attempting to intubate a patient with no suspected spinal injuries, the paramedic should have another rescuer hyperventilate the patient for approximately 1 minute while checking and assembling the equipment. The patient's head should be positioned appropriately and then the paramedic can insert the laryngoscope and visualize the vocal cords. If the paramedic is unable to adequately visualize the cords, another rescuer should apply cricoid pressure (the Sellick maneuver). After this, the endotracheal tube can be inserted and the cuff inflated. Proper tube placement should be checked by auscultating the lung fields for bilateral, equal breath sounds and listening at the epigastrium for the absence of sounds. The paramedic should then secure the tube, noting the depth of insertion and ventilate the patient. If trauma is possible, the head and neck should be immobilized during the intubation attempt (see Skill 37 in the Skills Section).

Managing the Patient with Airway Obstruction

Air often will not enter the lungs if the airway is blocked as a result of inadequate head-tilt or chin-lift method. After repositioning the airway, the paramedic should reattempt to ventilate the patient. If the chest will still not rise or ventilation force meets resistance, the airway is still obstructed. In a child or adult, the Heimlich maneuver should be performed (Fig. 18-8).

If unable to dislodge the object after repeated attempts, the rescuer may use a laryngoscope to examine the upper airway and Magill forceps to remove or dislodge anything found (*see* Skill #11 in Skills Section). Once the object is removed or at least partially dislodged, ventilation should be possible.

If an upper airway obstruction cannot be relieved by conventional methods, it may be necessary to create an artificial airway below the vocal cords. Cricothrotomy is an invasive airway procedure that involves using a large-gauge catheter or a scalpel to puncture the cricoid membrane (*see* Skills #9 and #10 in the Skills Section). Local protocols will dictate patient age restrictions for performing this skill.

A Closer Look at Breathing Emergencies

One main purpose of gathering pertinent patient history is to determine the patient's chief complaint. Most patients experience difficulty breathing as a result of a medical condition and will be responsive and able to provide information about that condition. As part of the SAMPLE history, the paramedic should ask key questions about medical history such as, "Do you have any medical problems?" If so, he or she should ask if the patient takes medication for those conditions and if the medication has been taken recently.

There are also patients whose dyspnea results from trauma. Here, too, the focused history and examination will help determine the nature of the problem. It is not always nec-

essary to identify the exact nature of the breathing problem, but the examination must attend to several critical signs:

- Abnormal chest motion
- Abnormal sounds
- Tracheal deviation
- Engorged neck veins
- Deformities or other abnormal findings upon palpation

Traumatic Conditions

Abnormal chest motion, such as paradoxical movement, often occurs with a **flail chest.** A flail chest exists when at least three ribs are broken in two places, allowing a segment of the chest to move independently. This creates movement in the opposite direction from that of the rest of the chest. When the patient inhales, the flail segment moves inward, compromising the ability of the lung on the affected side to expand. The segment moves outward during exhalation, reducing the volume of exhaled air. The patient with a flail chest should have the segment stabilized with a pillow or towels. Positive pressure ventilation will help ensure an adequate ventilation volume.

Decreased chest motion can occur on one or both sides. Diminished movement on one side can indicate **pneumothorax, hemothorax,** or **tension pneumothorax.** Subcutaneous emphysema indicates that air is leaking into the pleura, which is sometimes found with a tension pneumothorax. Although it is a late sign that can be difficult to spot, a deviated trachea is also a good indication of a tension pneumothorax. Lung sounds will help confirm this finding (*also see* Chapter 46).

The definitive care for tension pneumothorax is chest decompression (*see* Skill #36 in Skills Section). This is done by inserting a large-gauge, 2.25-inch catheter into the second intercostal space at the midclavicular line. Inserting the catheter through the cut-off finger of a latex glove prior to inserting it into the chest creates a one-way or "flutter" valve that prevents air from entering the chest through the catheter. A syringe attached to the hub of the catheter once the stylet has been withdrawn will accomplish the same.

Abnormal sounds heard during inspiration or expiration help provide additional critical information. An audible sucking sound should prompt a search for an opening in the chest that has created a sucking chest wound. This type of wound can be covered with an occlusive dressing that is taped down on three sides (Fig. 18-9). This provides a valvelike action that enables air to escape during expiration, preventing tension pneumothorax. It also prevents air from entering the wound during inspiration. A patient with a sucking chest wound requires high-flow oxygen and, based on the degree of difficulty and the rate of inspiration, may require positive pressure ventilation.

In addition to the obvious breath sounds heard without a stethoscope, some subtler sounds can only be heard upon auscultation. All fields should be carefully auscultated to determine bilateral sounds and adequacy of breathing.

Medical Problems

Chronic obstructive pulmonary disease (COPD) is a term generally used to cover a variety of lung diseases that in-

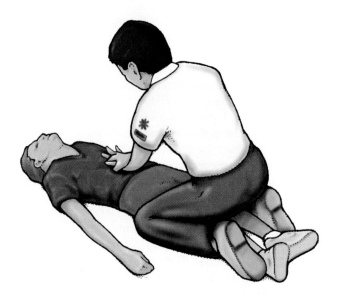

Figure 18-8

The Heimlich maneuver applied to an unresponsive patient.

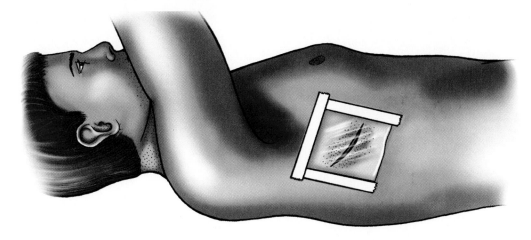

Figure 18-9

An open pneumothorax requires immediate treatment with an occlusive dressing.

273 **Chapter 18** The Patient With Airway and Breathing Compromise

clude **emphysema, chronic bronchitis,** and **asthma.** Each of these conditions results in restricted air movement in the lower airway that can be heard during auscultation. Other conditions that restrict air flow include wheezing caused by **allergic reaction** and rales secondary to **pulmonary edema** in **congestive heart failure.** These patients should all receive oxygen initially to help ease the difficulty breathing (*also see* Chapter 27).

Wheezing and limited air movement are caused by spasm, obstruction, or fluids in the lower airway. Even when fluid obstruction is present, spasm is usually part of the problem. Beta adrenergic aerosols such as albuterol are used to control the problem because they reverse the spasm without much effect on the heart. For patients less than 35 years of age, subcutaneous epinephrine 1:1000 may also be appropriate.

If there is no history of COPD or allergy, consider the possibility that the wheezing or rales is of a cardiac origin. **Hypertension,** especially a diastolic pressure above 120 mm Hg, can cause fluid buildup in the lungs. Nitroglycerin or nifedipine can help lower the blood pressure and thus treat the breathing difficulty.

If rales are present with chest pain, the pulmonary edema is probably secondary to congestive heart failure. Under these circumstances, a diuretic such as Lasix can be given. Morphine and nitroglycerin can also be used as vasodilators to reduce the heart's oxygen demand.

Children less than 7 years of age experience two common airway problems that can be serious: **croup** and **epiglottitis.**

Both of these problems are caused by infections that can obstruct the airway and awaken children at night with respiratory distress. These problems are explained in detail in Chapters 22 and 25.

SUMMARY

Rapid assessment and correction of airway and breathing problems is critically important. Assessment at the scene and en route to the hospital will enable the paramedic to detect and manage both medical and traumatic problems resulting in breathing emergencies. The paramedic should look, listen, and feel to identify any immediately obvious problems such as **apnea** or severe respiratory distress. Any airway and breathing problems should be corrected as they appear. With the assessment completed, and at least the general nature of the problem more clear, decisions can be made about more definitive treatments such as medications, intubation, or invasive procedures (e.g., cricothyrotomy and chest decompression).

REFERENCES

1. **Jersudian MC, Harrison RR, Keenan RL, Maull KI:** Bag-valve-mask ventilation: two rescuers are better than one. *Crit Care Med* 13:122—123, 1985.

2. **Melker RJ:** Recommendations for ventilation during cardiopulmonary resuscitation: time for a change? *Crit Care Med* 13(part 2):882—883, 1985.

Peter Maningas, MD, FACEP

Chapter 19

The Patient Without a Pulse

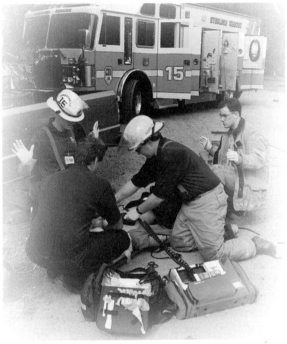

KEY TERMS

1. **Asystole**—a life-threatening cardiac condition characterized by the absence of electrical and mechanical activity in the heart. Clinical signs include absent pulse and breathing.

2. **Cardiac output**—the amount of blood the heart pumps in 1 minute.

3. **Cardiopulmonary resuscitation (CPR)**—the basic emergency procedure for life support, consisting of artificial respiration and manual external cardiac massage.

4. **Defibrillation**—the termination of ventricular fibrillation, by delivering an electric shock to the patient's precordium.

5. **Pulseless ventricular tachycardia**—regular, rapid, wide-complex cardiac contractions which do not produce a palpable pulse. *See Conditions by Diagnosis Section.*

6. **Pulseless electrical activity (PEA)**—organized electrical activity, without a palpable pulse, observed on a cardiac monitor (other than VT or VF).

7. **Ventricular fibrillation (VF)**—a cardiac dysrhythmia marked by rapid, disorganized depolarizations of the ventricular myocardium.

A paramedic should be able to:

OBJECTIVES

1. Describe the anatomy and physiology of the cardiovascular system.

2. Define the following terms: systole, diastole, cardiac output, stroke volume, preload, afterload, depolarization, repolarization, automaticity, and contractility.

3. Describe the normal sequence of electrical conduction in the heart.

4. Identify the assessment steps in determining that a patient is in cardiac arrest.

5. Describe the purpose and significance of early CPR and defibrillation.

6. Identify the critical findings, including cardiac rhythms, in pulseless patients from various causes.

7. Describe the different management approaches to various patient conditions that present with pulselessness.

8. Identify medications commonly used to correct ventricular fibrillation or pulseless ventricular tachycardia, pulseless electrical activity, and asystole.

9. Describe how the general management approach may vary in a patient who is pulseless as a result of associated trauma, electric shock, near-drowning, or hypothermia.

Scene Survey

Initial Assessment

Focused History
and Physical Exam

Continued Assessment

Cardiovascular disease accounts for approximately 1 million deaths each year in the United States. Nearly 50% of these deaths are the result of coronary disease, most of which are sudden deaths outside of the hospital setting.[11] Rapid intervention by bystanders, dispatchers, and EMS providers can make a difference in the outcome of a large percentage of these sudden deaths.

This chapter provides a brief review of the role of the circulatory system, focusing on its mechanical and electrical aspects. It also reviews the initial patient assessment steps that determine when a patient is pulseless and discusses several unique situations that can cause cardiac arrest.

The Cardiovascular System

Working in conjunction with the respiratory system, the cardiovascular system distributes oxygen and other nutrients throughout the body and removes waste products. The components of the cardiac system are illustrated in Chapter 7.

This system is composed of three principal components: the heart, blood vessels, and blood. The heart has several layers of tissue. The outermost protective sac is known as the pericardium. Between the pericardium and the heart is pericardial fluid, which acts as a lubricant during its contraction.

The cells of the myocardium have unique electrical properties similar to those of smooth muscles. These properties permit the rapid transmission and reception of electrical impulses between cells and ensure coordinated contraction of the entire heart.

The heart has two superior chambers (the atria) and two inferior chambers (the ventricles). Each of these pairs is divided right from left by a septum made of connective tissue and muscle. Deoxygenated blood flows into the right atrium from the superior and inferior vena cavas. This blood passes through a series of one-way valves in the heart; the first is the tricuspid valve, which is located between the right atrium and the right ventricle. The blood then passes through the pulmonary valve to the pulmonary arteries and the lungs, where carbon dioxide and other waste products are removed and oxygen is absorbed.

The oxygenated blood returns to the left atrium through the pulmonary veins and then passes through the mitral valve and into the left ventricle. Blood exits through the aortic valve into the aorta for distribution to the body. The heart takes the nutrients it needs to supply the myocardial muscle from the two main coronary arteries, right and left. They originate in the aorta, just outside the aortic valve. These vessels have the unique ability to develop collateral circulation, which is an alternate pathway for blood flow in the event that one or more arteries become occluded. Deoxygenated blood is removed from the heart muscle by means of the coronary veins, which drain into the right atrium.

Blood flow requires the force generated by the coordinated, cyclic efforts of the atria and ventricles. The right and left atria contract together, filling the ventricles. This period when the ventricles are at rest and filling is known as diastole. The ventricles then contract together, ejecting blood into the pulmonary arteries and the aorta. This contraction-ejection phase is called systole. This entire sequence, from the beginning of one contraction to the beginning of another, is the cardiac cycle.

The amount of blood ejected from each of the ventricles is the same and is referred to as the stroke volume. Because the left ventricle must pump against the resistance of the entire arterial system, it is more muscular and capable of more forcefully ejecting blood. It is a high pressure system, whereas the right ventricle generates less pressure. The average stroke volume is approximately 70 mL, and depends on three elements:

1. **Preload**—the pressure in the ventricles after diastole, when the atria have completed filling the ventricles
2. **Contractility**—the force of ventricular contraction
3. **Afterload**—the pressure against which the ventricles must pump

As the return of venous blood to the right atrium increases, so does the amount of blood available to the ventricles (preload), the stretch of the myocardial muscle, the force of contraction (contractility), and the stroke volume. Cardiac output is the amount of blood pumped in 1 minute, a quantity calculated by multiplying stroke volume by heart rate. Given an average heart that beats approximately 70 times per minute and has a stroke volume of 70 mL, the cardiac output would be 4900 mL (nearly 5 L, or the entire blood volume) per minute.

The Conduction System

The heart can contract in a coordinated manner because of the rapid transmission of impulses through electrically excitable cells. The conduction system is illustrated in Chapter 12. Significant electrical changes take place across cell membranes, and sodium and potassium play major roles in the process. Sodium is a positive ion that normally remains outside of the cell. Potassium is a positive ion that to a lesser degree remains inside the cell. The result is a cell that is negatively charged inside, relative to its external environment.

When stimulated, the cell membrane allows sodium to enter the cell rapidly, followed more slowly by calcium. These positive ions change the cell's internal charge from negative to positive. This depolarization process continues until the entire muscle mass is depolarized, resulting in muscle contraction. Once the influx of sodium and calcium cease, they are actively pumped out of the cell. This repolarization returns the cell to its normal resting (negative) state.

Cells in the cardiac conduction system share a property known as automaticity or the ability to self-depolarize. Those cells with the fastest rate of discharge at any given moment tend to serve as the pacemakers. Three groups of cells commonly act as pacemakers, each with its own intrinsic rate of discharge. The primary pacemaker is the sinoatrial (SA) node, located in the right atrium. This node is connected to the atrioventricular (AV) node or "junction," by internodal pathways. As an electrical impulse from the SA node nears the AV node, it slows at the AV junction to allow the ventricles to fill. The impulse continues into the ventricles through a band of fibers known as the bundle of His, which subdivides into the right and left bundle branches before delivering the impulse to the ventricular purkinje's fibers. Here, the impulse results in depolarization of the ventricles.

Causes of Cardiac Arrest

Disease and trauma can both impair either the normal transmission of cardiac electrical impulses or the heart's mechanical ability to pump blood. Therefore, there may be occasions when the electrical activity of the heart is normal but the pump fails, or vice versa.

Cardiovascular disease is the number one cause of death in the United States.11 A major form of cardiovascular disease, atherosclerosis, affects the heart's ability to maintain adequate blood flow. Over time, atherosclerosis causes formation of calcium deposits, or plaque, on arterial walls, which can result in restricted blood flow or even complete occlusion.

When the coronary arteries cannot meet cardiac oxygen demand, the heart becomes ischemic and several problems can occur, including myocardial infarction (MI) (heart attack), heart failure, cardiogenic shock and cardiac arrest.

Chest pain is often the major symptom of cardiac ischemia (also see Chapter 31). This pain may be transient, as it is in individuals who experience angina pectoris, or constant when a patient suffers an MI. An MI occurs when the demand for oxygen exceeds supply over an extended period of time. Frequently, a blood clot (thrombus) forms in a coronary artery that is already narrowed by atherosclerosis. Most MIs affect the left coronary artery, and thus the left ventricle. An infarction can destroy various layers of the myocardial muscle. If the blockage is not relieved and collateral circulation is inadequate, the tissue will die, become necrotic, and form scar tissue.

The tissue immediately surrounding the site of the infarction is often the origin of dysrhythmias. If the infarction is extensive, it can cause lethal dysrhythmias and sudden death, commonly called cardiac arrest. Other conditions that can lead to cardiac arrest include electrocution, drowning, suffocation, foreign body airway obstruction, and chest trauma.

Patient Assessment

Responding to the Call

Prior to rescuers' arrival at the scene, dispatchers will try to determine the amount of time since the patient's pulseless collapse, and whether bystanders have started cardiopulmonary resuscitation (CPR). If CPR has not been started, the dispatcher should provide prearrival instructions for CPR. While en route, the paramedic should consider the possible need to have additional personnel dispatched, the equipment that will be required on scene and the tasks that must be performed. The major tasks when caring for a pulseless patient are:

- Vital sign assessment
- CPR
- Cardiac monitoring and defibrillation
- Airway management
- IV access
- Medication administration

Approaching the Patient

Upon arrival at the scene, the paramedic should assess the environment and consider the possible cause of the problem.

Upon reaching the patient, the paramedic should note any efforts that are underway, such as bystander CPR. The rescuer should ask bystanders to stop the activity they may be engaged in and assess the patient's vital signs, including responsiveness, airway patency, breathing and pulse.

Recognizing Cardiac Arrest

The paramedic should tap the patient's shoulder and shout in an effort to arouse the patient. If the patient does not respond, the airway can be opened using the appropriate maneuver, depending on the likelihood of trauma. If trauma is not suspected, the airway should be opened using the head-tilt/chin-lift method. The patient's mouth should be visually examined for obstructions and breathing should be checked for 3 to 5 seconds. If the patient is not breathing, someone (bystander, rescuer) should provide two slow initial ventilations, making certain that the chest rises. A pulse can be assessed by locating the carotid arteries and monitoring for approximately 10 seconds. Pulselessness indicates cardiac arrest.

Managing the Patient in Cardiac Arrest

After confirming that the patient is pulseless, the paramedic must quickly determine that there is no severe external bleeding. Most cardiac arrest situations are of a medical nature. However, if the cardiac arrest has occurred as a result of trauma, there will not be any spurting or heavy bleeding. However, there may still be a significant injury, such as a chest or abdominal wound, resulting from an assault or suicide attempt. If a significant wound is present, a pressure bandage should be applied quickly before beginning CPR.

Mechanical Therapy

Without a pulse, the heart ceases pumping adequately to sustain life. CPR provides a mechanical pump to supplement the failed heart function. By supplying oxygen, ventilating, and compressing the chest, oxygenated blood can be circulated to the vital organs, particularly the heart and brain. Effective CPR can help prolong ventricular fibrillation until a defibrillator can be applied, but CPR generates at most one third of normal cardiac output.[11] The resulting hypoxia will adversely affect the brain within 4 to 6 minutes. Therefore, CPR is only one form of treatment needed by the pulseless patient.

Electrical Therapy

Approximately 85% of all adult patients who suffer medical cardiac arrest have an underlying rhythm of ventricular fibrillation (VF) or ventricular tachycardia (VT).[11] Because these rhythms can be corrected with early defibrillation, it is important to immediately assess the patient's underlying rhythm and prepare for defibrillation (Fig. 19-1). The success of defibrillation is directly related to the delay until it is performed. The longer the downtime, the less chance that defibrillation will be successful. Initiation of CPR should not delay defibrillation, although CPR is certainly appropriate until defibrillation can be achieved.

Pharmacological Therapy

In addition to CPR and defibrillation, the administration of certain medications can improve cardiac output and tissue oxygenation. Other medications work to control heart rhythm and rate. It is important to remember, however, that pharmacolog-

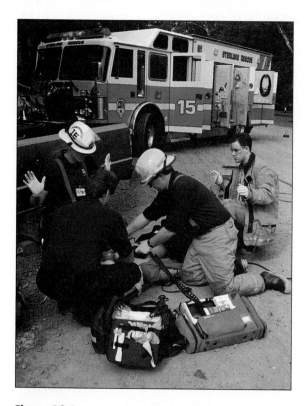

Figure 19-1

Early defibrillation improves a patient's chance of survival. From Cummins: ACLS Scenarios: Core Concepts for Case-Based Learning, St. Louis, 1996, Mosby–Year Book.

ical therapy is secondary to other efforts, especially airway management.

The highest possible oxygen concentration should be administered quickly to a pulseless patient. The administration of 100% oxygen through a bag-valve-mask with reservoir or a demand valve improves hemoglobin saturation and tissue oxygenation. IV access provides a route for the rapid introduction of medications into the circulatory system. The fluids of choice are crystalloid solutions such as normal saline and lactated Ringer's. Although D_5W is also an acceptable fluid, hyperglycemia in patients who survive cardiac arrest is associated with a poor neurological outcome.[11] These fluids are usually run at a keep-open rate, although volume expansion is appropriate for patients who may be volume depleted.

Epinephrine is the principal medication used to treat pulseless patients. It produces several beneficial effects, most notably an increase in blood flow to the heart and brain during CPR. The correct dose of epinephrine during cardiac arrest has been studied extensively. Animal studies demonstrated that high doses caused increased blood flow[5,6,16,17], but human studies failed to show improved outcomes.[7,9,15,22]

The recommended initial dose of epinephrine is 1 mg every 3 to 5 minutes, with alternative high-dose regimens available as options. It is important for paramedics to stay abreast of current American Heart Association guidelines for drug dosages.

Antidysrhythmic agents such as lidocaine and bretylium are also commonly used in the prehospital cardiac arrest setting when the patient is in ventricular fibrillation or pulseless ventricular tachycardia. These agents will usually not convert a fibrillating heart to a sinus rhythm, but may prevent the immediate recurrence of ventricular fibrillation or ventricular tachycardia after successful defibrillation. Neither is clearly superior as an antidysrhythmic agent, but lidocaine is the first medication to be administered because bretylium can cause hypotension.[13,18] Lidocaine is administered 1.5 mg/kg, which can be repeated once, to a maximum total dose of 3.0 mg/kg. Bretylium is administered at 5 mg/kg initially, with subsequent doses at 10 mg/kg to a maximum of 35 mg/kg.

Other medications that may be used include sodium bicarbonate, atropine, and magnesium sulfate. Magnesium deficiency can lead to cardiac arrest, and can cause ventricular fibrillation to recur. Magnesium sulfate is administered by diluting 1 to 2 grams in 10 mL of D_5W, rapidly infused over 1 to 2 minutes. Atropine may be beneficial in the presence of asystole and pulseless electrical activity. The dose for atropine is 1 mg every 3 to 5 minutes to a maximum of 0.04 mg/kg. Sodium bicarbonate may be helpful in cardiac arrest patients with preexisting metabolic acidosis, hyperkalemia, or tricyclic antidepressant overdose, or in prolonged resuscitations. The dose is 1 mEq/kg, preferably guided by laboratory determination of blood pH. Because blood pH determination is not possible in the field, repeat doses are generally not recommended.

Restoring Circulation

After a successful resuscitation, the paramedic must determine accurate vital signs and modify treatment as the patient's condition changes. Atropine can be used to increase cardiac rate, and if the blood pressure fails to respond to the rate increase, dopamine may be useful. Lidocaine can be used as a maintenance infusion to prevent the recurrence of ventricular fibrillation. The key point to remember is that the job is far from done once the patient has a pulse and a viable rhythm.

Managing Specific Cardiac Arrest Conditions

The paramedic should be familiar with common conditions associated with pulselessness (see Fig. 19-2):

- Ventricular fibrillation and pulseless ventricular tachycardia
- Pulseless electrical activity
- Asystole

Effective management of these conditions depends on rapid recall of treatment algorithms, avoidance of complications, such as misplaced endotracheal tubes, and the help available from other EMS personnel.

Ventricular Fibrillation and Pulseless Ventricular Tachycardia

In the sudden cardiac arrest patient, VF and VT are the most common dysrhythmias. In these rhythms, immediate defibrillation is critical to patient outcome and should be followed by the administration of medications. This pattern continues until the rhythm is corrected or changes to another rhythm. Figure 19-3 outlines the energy settings for defibrillation, the types of medications and their proper dosages, and the order of treatments.

Pulseless Electrical Activity

Pulseless electrical activity (PEA) indicates the presence of an organized cardiac rhythm when a pulse cannot be detected. PEA includes narrow and wide complex rhythms previously grouped under the term electromechanical dissociation (EMD). EMD has been commonly used to describe organized electrical activity without mechanical (pumping) function. More recently, the term PEA was adopted when research showed that some patients do have cardiac wall motion that is not sufficient to generate a pulse.[11]

Because PEA is not an electrical disturbance that produces an uncoordinated rhythm, as VF does, the treatment is to detect and correct the underlying causes, rather than to defibrillate. Figure 19-4 includes these causes and the steps for treating PEA.

Asystole

Asystole is the absence of electrical activity in the heart. Unfortunately, this is more often a confirmation of death, than a rhythm that can be treated. However, there are some underlying causes similar to those in PEA, which if corrected increase the chances of survival. Treatment is also similar to PEA. The steps for treating asystole appear in Figure 19-5.

In the past, asystole was sometimes thought to be fine VF, and treated with defibrillation. Because defibrillation can worsen the situation, it is no longer performed when a check of at least two ECG leads confirms asystole.

Transcutaneous pacing, although recognized as the definitive treatment for bradycardia, rarely changes asystole and does not improve survival rates.[10] Because this lack of success may be caused by delays in beginning pacing, it must be initiated early, in conjunction with the administration of epinephrine and atropine, if it is done at all.

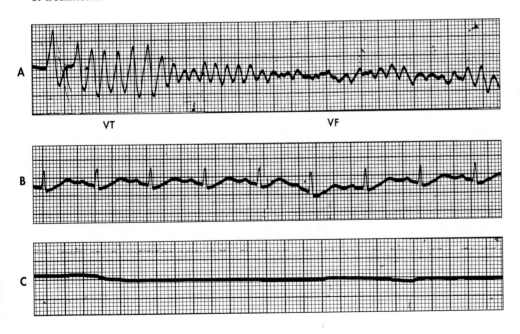

Figure 19-2

Rhythm disturbances and inadequate pumping of the heart muscle can result in pulselessness. A, Pulseless ventricular tachycardia and ventricular fibrillation recorded during a cardiac arrest. B, Pulseless electrical activity. Although the ECG shows sinus rhythm, the patient had no pulse or blood pressure. C, Asystole producing a straight-line pattern during cardiac arrest. From Goldberger: Clinical Electrocardiography: A Simplified Approach, ed 5, 1994, St. Louis, Mosby-Year Book.

Ventricular Fibrillation and Pulseless Ventricular Tachycardia Algorithm

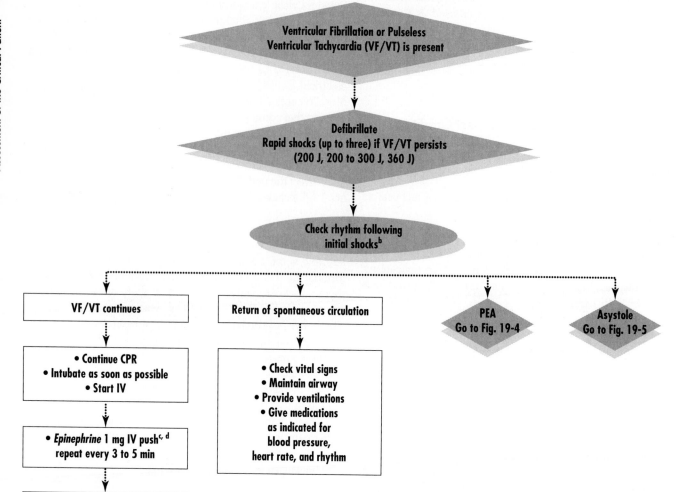

Ventricular Fibrillation or Pulseless Ventricular Tachycardia (VF/VT) is present

Defibrillate
Rapid shocks (up to three) if VF/VT persists
(200 J, 200 to 300 J, 360 J)

Check rhythm following initial shocks[b]

VF/VT continues

- Continue CPR
- Intubate as soon as possible
- Start IV

- *Epinephrine* 1 mg IV push[c, d]
  repeat every 3 to 5 min

- Defibrillate
  360 J within 30 to 60 sec[e]

- Add antiarrhythmics if
  VF/VT continues or recurs[f, g]

- Defibrillate
  360 J, 30 to 60 sec
  after each medication[f]
- Sequence should be drug-shock,
  drug-shock

Return of spontaneous circulation

- Check vital signs
- Maintain airway
- Provide ventilations
- Give medications
  as indicated for
  blood pressure,
  heart rate, and rhythm

PEA
Go to Fig. 19-4

Asystole
Go to Fig. 19-5

Class I: Definitely helpful

Class IIa: Acceptable, probably helpful

Class IIb: Acceptable, possibly helpful

Class III: Not indicated, may be harmful

[b] Hypothermic cardiac arrest is treated differently after this point.

[c] The recommended dose of **epinephrine** is 1 mg IV push every 3-5 min. If spontaneous circulation does not return consider several Class IIb dosing regimens:

- Intermediate: **Epinephrine** 2-5 mg IV push, every 3-5 min.
- Escalating: **Epinephrine** 1 mg-3 mg-5 mg IV push, 3 min apart.
- High: **Epinephrine** 0.1 mg/kg IV push, every 3-5 min.

[d] **Sodium bicarbonate** (1 mEq/kg) is Class I if patient has known preexisting hyperkalemia.

[e] Continued delivery of shocks is acceptable here (Class I), especially when medications are delayed.

[f] Medications sequence:

- **Lidocaine** 1.0-1.5 mg/kg IV push. Repeat in 3-5 min to maximum dose of 3 mg/kg. A single 1.5 mg/kg dose in cardiac arrest is also acceptable.
- **Bretylium** 5 mg/kg IV push. Repeat in 5 min at 10 mg/kg.
- **Magnesium** sulfate 1-2 g IV in torsades de pointes, suspected hypomagnesemic state, or refractory VF.
- **Procainamide** 30 mg/min in recurrent VF (maximum total dose 17 mg/kg).

[g] **Sodium bicarbonate** (1 mEq/kg IV). Follow these indications:

Class IIa
- If overdose with tricyclic antidepressant
- To alkalinize the urine in drug overdoses
- If known preexisting bicarbonate-responsive acidosis

Class IIb
- If patient is intubated and arrest continues for long intervals
- If circulation restored after prolonged arrest

Class III
- Hypoxic lactic acidosis

Figure 19-3

The algorithm for ventricular fibrillation and pulseless ventricular tachycardia. Adapted from Cummins: ACLS Scenarios: Care Concepts for Case-Based Learning, St. Louis, 1996, Mosby–Year Book. Adapted with permission, Journal of American Medical Association, 1992, Vol. 268, Guidelines for Cardiopulmonary Resuscitation and Emergency Cardiac Care, 1992, American Medical Association.

Pulseless Electrical Activity Algorithm

The term pulseless electrical activity (PEA) includes the following:
- Electromechanical dissociation (EMD)
- Pseudo-EMD
- Idioventricular rhythms
- Ventricular escape rhythms
- Bradyasystolic rhythms
- Post-defibrillation idioventricular rhythms

Continue Basic Life Support
Perform focused history and physical examination
- Intubate if needed
- Access ventilations
- Obtain IV access

Consider the differential diagnosis:
(Possible treatments shown in parenthesis)

Five H's:
- Hypovolemia, includes anaphylaxis (volume infusion)
- Hypoxia (oxygen and ventilation)
- Hypothermia (see Figure 19-6)
- Hyper-/hypokalemia (and other electrolyte abnormalities)
- Hydrogen ion (acidosis)

Five T's:
- Tension pneumothorax (needle decompression)
- Tamponade, cardiac (pericardiocentesis)
- Thrombosis, pulmonary (surgery, thrombolytics)
- Thrombosis, acute myocardial (thrombolytics)
- Tablets, drug overdoses (drug-specific interventions)

- *Epinephrine* 1 mg IV push[a-c]
- Repeat every 3 to 5 min

- If rate of electrical activity is slow (<60 beats/min), give *atropine* 1 mg IV
- Repeat every 3 to 5 min to a total of 0.03 to 0.04 mg/kg[d]

Class I: Definitely helpful

Class IIa: Acceptable, probably helpful

Class IIb: Acceptable, possibly helpful

Class III: Not indicated, may be harmful

(a) **Sodium bicarbonate** 1 mEq/kg is Class I if patient has known preexisting hyperkalemia.

(b) **Sodium bicarbonate** (1 mEq/kg) is given as follows:

Class IIa
- If known preexisting bicarbonate-responsive acidosis

- If overdose with tricyclic antidepressants
- To alkalinize the urine in drug overdoses

Class IIb
- If patient is intubated and arrest continues for long intervals
- If circulation is restored after prolonged arrest

Class III
- Hypoxic lactic acidosis (unventilated patient)

(c) The recommended dose of **epinephrine** is 1 mg IV push every 3 to 5 min. If spontaneous circulation does not return, consider several Class IIb dosing regimens:

- Intermediate: **Epinephrine** 2-5 mg IV push, every 3 to 5 min.
- Escalating: **Epinephrine** 1 mg-3 mg-5 mg IV push, 3 min apart.
- High: **Epinephrine** 0.1 mg/kg IV push, every 3 to 5 min.

(d) The shorter atropine dosing interval (3 minutes) is possibly helpful in cardiac arrest (Class IIb).

Figure 19-4

The algorithm for pulseless electrical activity. Adapted from Cummins: ACLS Scenarios: Core Concepts for Case-Based Learning, St. Louis, 1996, Mosby–Year Book. Adapted with permission, Journal of the American Medical Association, Guidelines for Cardiopulmonary Resuscitation and Emergency Cardiac Care, vol 268, 1992, American Medical Association.

Asystole Treatment Algorithm

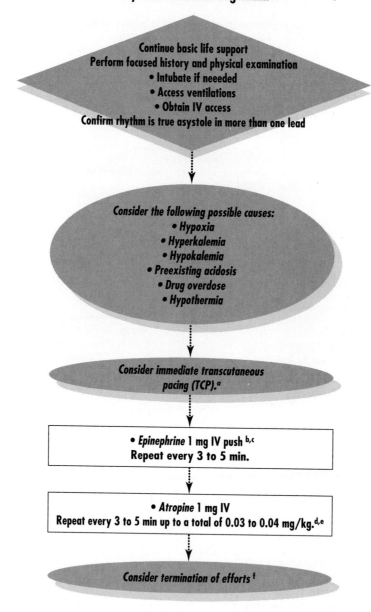

Continue basic life support
Perform focused history and physical examination
- **Intubate if neeeded**
- **Access ventilations**
- **Obtain IV access**
Confirm rhythm is true asystole in more than one lead

Consider the following possible causes:
- *Hypoxia*
- *Hyperkalemia*
- *Hypokalemia*
- *Preexisting acidosis*
- *Drug overdose*
- *Hypothermia*

Consider immediate transcutaneous pacing (TCP).[a]

- *Epinephrine* 1 mg IV push [b,c]
Repeat every 3 to 5 min.

- *Atropine* 1 mg IV
Repeat every 3 to 5 min up to a total of 0.03 to 0.04 mg/kg.[d,e]

Consider termination of efforts [f]

Class I: Definitely helpful

Class IIa: Acceptable, probably helpful

Class IIb: Acceptable, possibly helpful

Class III: Not indicated, may be harmful

[a] Pacing is an acceptable intervention (Class IIb). Perform TCP as early as possible, without waiting for the effects of medications. Not recommended as routine treatment for asystole.

[b] The recommended dose of **epinephrine** is 1 mg IV push every 3 to 5 min. If spontaneous circulation does not return, consider several Class IIb dosing regimens:

- Intermediate: **Epinephrine** 2 to 5 mg IV push, every 3 to 5 min

- Escalating: **Epinephrine** 1 mg – 3 mg – 5 mg IV push, 3 min apart
- High: **Epinephrine** 0.1 mg/kg IV push, every 3 to 5 min

[c] **Sodium bicarbonate** 1 mEq/kg is definitely indicated (Class I) if patient has known preexisting hyperkalemia.

[d] The shorter **atropine** dosing interval (3 min) is Class IIb in asystolic arrest.

[e] **Sodium bicarbonate** (1 mEq/kg) follow these indications:

Class IIa
- If known preexisting bicarbonate-responsive acidosis
- If overdose with tricyclic antidepressants
- To alkalinize the urine in drug overdoses

Class IIb
- If patient intubated and arrest continues for long intervals

Class III
- Hypoxic acidosis (unventilated patient)

[f] Consider stopping resuscitative efforts when patient remains in documented asystole or other agonal rhythms for more than 10 minutes *after:*

- Patient successfully intubated
- Initial IV medications given
- No reversible causes identified
- Physician concurs

Figure 19-5

The algorithm for asystole. Adapted from Cummins: ACLS Scenarios: Core Concepts for Case-Based Learning, St. Louis, 1996, Mosby–Year Book. Adapted with permission, Journal of the American Medical Association, Guidelines for Cardiopulmonary Resuscitation and Emergency Cardiac Care, vol 268, 1992, American Medical Association.

Special Considerations

Numerous special situations can lead to cardiac arrest or complicate resuscitation efforts. Awareness of the more common situations enables the paramedic to adapt management efforts accordingly. In addition, resuscitative attempts fail even after extensive efforts in some patients. Local protocol will dictate when it is appropriate to stop resuscitative efforts in these situations.

Traumatic Arrest

The approach to the patient in traumatic cardiac arrest differs from medical arrest because traumatic arrest is usually a result of massive internal hemorrhage. Restoration of blood volume and control of ongoing bleeding can only be accomplished at the hospital. The likelihood of a patient surviving a traumatic cardiac arrest is extremely rare, unless transport is rapid and an immediate emergency department thoracotomy is performed. There have been few reports of neurologically intact survivors of blunt trauma resulting in cardiac arrest in the usual prehospital setting or during transport.[1,3,8] One possible exception may be the young patient who sustains a direct blow over the precordium with subsequent cardiac arrest. The prognosis for cardiac arrest secondary to penetrating chest trauma is somewhat more favorable, but still worse than in medical arrest.[1,3,8]

Resuscitation should begin in all patients who appear to have some potential for survival, such as the patient who arrests while en route to the hospital. On the other hand, resuscitation is not appropriate in patients with obvious, severe blunt trauma who are without vital signs, pupillary response, or any organized or shockable rhythm at the scene.

Electric Shock

Electric shock can cause a wide range of injuries including sudden death. The magnitude of the energy delivered, type of current, voltage, duration of contact, resistance, and anatomical pathway are all factors that determine the severity of the trauma. Ventricular fibrillation, ventricular tachycardia and asystole are common presenting rhythms for patients experiencing immediate death, including those struck by lightning.

The paramedic should follow current ACLS guidelines for treating dysrhythmias associated with electric shock. If electrical burns occur on the mouth or neck, extensive soft tissue swelling can complicate airway management, including endotracheal intubation. Volume replacement will be necessary for patients with significant tissue destruction from burns (see Chapter 49).

With lightning strikes involving several patients, standard triage priorities may be altered somewhat. Normally, a patient found in cardiac arrest at the scene of an MCI would be a low treatment priority. But in this situation, the arrested patient can be saved if the underlying dysrhythmia is corrected quickly and ventilatory support provided. Those who survive a lightning strike are not likely to suffer cardiac arrest later, and so do not need immediate attention. The patient in cardiac or respiratory arrest is thus the highest priority patient.

Near Drowning

Near-drowning is normally associated with a dismal outcome. The lack of oxygenation will result in hypoxemia, requiring aggressive efforts to restore ventilation and perfusion. Submersion accident victims are often found with an agonal rhythm or asystole. Management of the airway can be complicated by water or debris in the mouth, which must be suctioned out. In addition, CPR often results in continuing obstruction of the airway with water and vomitus. Intubation is extremely important to prevent further airway compromise. Although survival is unlikely in patients who have been submerged for an extensive period of time, there are two special factors: water temperature and patient age. Younger patients submerged in cold water have been known to recover fully, even after being submerged for longer than 30 minutes.

Hypothermia

The old adage, "They're not dead until they're warm and dead," is important to remember when attempting to resuscitate a hypothermic patient. The patient may appear dead because deep depression of brain and cardiovascular functions makes peripheral pulses and respiratory effort difficult to detect. Initial clinical findings should thus not cause a rescuer to withhold resuscitation efforts.

The paramedic should follow these steps to provide care (also see Fig. 19-6) for a patient suffering from hypothermia:

- Remove any wet clothing and dry the patient.
- Insulate against additional heat loss by applying a blanket.
- Monitor the cardiac rhythm.
- Start CPR, ventilate with warm, humidified oxygen if available.
- Defibrillate up to three times if indicated by the rhythm.
- Establish an IV of normal saline.
- If possible, monitor core temperature with a rectal thermometer.
- If the body temperature is lower than 86° F, withhold additional shocks and cardiac medications. If greater than 86° F, administer medications and repeat defibrillations according to ACLS protocol.
- Transport to a hospital for active internal rewarming.

Transport

Transporting a cardiac arrest patient to the hospital can be an especially difficult task, requiring a coordinated effort among EMS personnel while moving the patient (Fig. 19-7) and providing care in the back of a moving ambulance. The endotracheal tube and IV lines should be secured. If an automatic transport ventilator is available, it should be set up at this point. This is also the time to apply an automatic compression and ventilation device if it will not complicate movement of the patient to the ambulance.

The decision about when to transport is made case by case, and according to system protocols. Generally, transport is appropriate whenever:

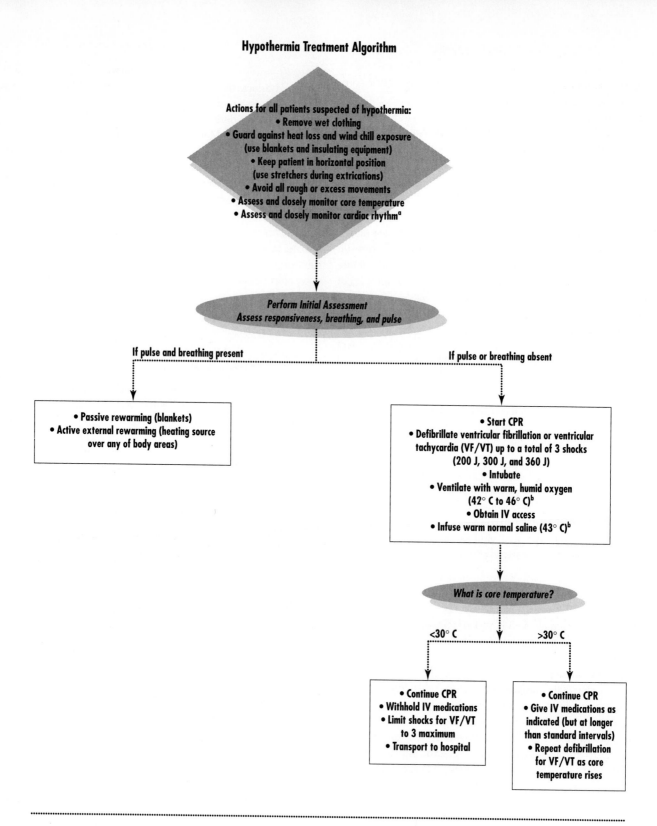

Hypothermia Treatment Algorithm

Actions for all patients suspected of hypothermia:
- Remove wet clothing
- Guard against heat loss and wind chill exposure (use blankets and insulating equipment)
- Keep patient in horizontal position (use stretchers during extrications)
- Avoid all rough or excess movements
- Assess and closely monitor core temperature
- Assess and closely monitor cardiac rhythm[a]

Perform Initial Assessment
Assess responsiveness, breathing, and pulse

If pulse and breathing present

- Passive rewarming (blankets)
- Active external rewarming (heating source over any of body areas)

If pulse or breathing absent

- Start CPR
- Defibrillate ventricular fibrillation or ventricular tachycardia (VF/VT) up to a total of 3 shocks (200 J, 300 J, and 360 J)
- Intubate
- Ventilate with warm, humid oxygen (42° C to 46° C)[b]
- Obtain IV access
- Infuse warm normal saline (43° C)[b]

What is core temperature?

<30° C

- Continue CPR
- Withhold IV medications
- Limit shocks for VF/VT to 3 maximum
- Transport to hospital

>30° C

- Continue CPR
- Give IV medications as indicated (but at longer than standard intervals)
- Repeat defibrillation for VF/VT as core temperature rises

[a] This may require needle electrodes through the skin.
[b] A few experts think these interventions should be done only in-hospital, especially with minimally trained rescuers.

Figure 19-6

The algorithm for hypothermia. Adapted from Cummins: ACLS Scenarios: Core Concepts for Case-Based Learning, St. Louis, 1996, Mosby–Year Book. Adapted with permission, Journal of the American Medical Association, Guidelines for Cardiopulmonary Resuscitation and Emergency Cardiac Care, vol 268, 1992, American Medical Association.

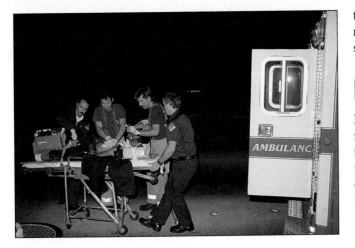

Figure 19-7

Moving a patient while maintaining proper care during a cardiac arrest event is difficult. Photographed by Colin C. Williams.

- The patient is temporarily stabilized
- Adequate personnel are available to move the patient safely
- The treatment sequence reaches a point identified by local protocols (i.e., following intubation, IV access, and administration of epinephrine).

Hospital transport times and the strength of the ALS system will play a role in protocol decisions made by the medical director regarding the extent of treatment provided before transport.

Terminating Efforts

During some resuscitation efforts, a decision must be made about whether to terminate resuscitation efforts. Unlike trauma, the outcome in medical cardiac arrest depends on prehospital care. Rapid response, early defibrillation, aggressive airway management, and proper administration of cardiac medications enable the paramedic to provide the same level of initial care that the patient would receive in an emergency department. Patients who fail to respond to aggressive prehospital care are unlikely to respond later in the hospital, and even less likely to survive until hospital discharge.

Because of growing understanding of the chance of successful resuscitation in some settings, increasing numbers of EMS systems are developing guidelines for terminating resuscitation efforts in the field.[4,12,14] These guidelines often include patients in whom:

- Endotracheal intubation has been accomplished
- ACLS measures, including defibrillation and medication administration have been unsuccessful
- Asystole persists without an identifiable, reversible cause
- Hypothermia is not a consideration

The decision to discontinue resuscitation in the prehospital setting must be made in accordance with local protocols. If the patient does not respond to ACLS efforts in the field and no protocols exist for terminating medical efforts, the patient should be transported to the hospital.

SUMMARY

No other medical emergency is as time-critical as cardiac arrest. Defibrillation, CPR, airway management, IV access, and medication administration are the components of ACLS care for the pulseless patient. By integrating these skills with knowledge of the patient's condition, the paramedic may restore life to a patient without a pulse.

REFERENCES

1. **Baker CC, Thomas AN, Trunkey DD:** The role of emergency room thoracotomy in trauma. *J Trauma* 20:848–854, 1980.

2. **Barton C, et al:** High-dose epinephrine improves the return of spontaneous circulation rates in human victims of cardiac arrest. *Ann Emerg Med* 20:722, 1991.

3. **Bodai BI, et al:** Emergency thoracotomy in the management of trauma. *JAMA* 249: 1891–1896, 1983.

4. **Bonnin MJ, et al:** Distinct criteria for termination of resuscitation in the out-of-hospital setting. *JAMA* 270:1457, 1471, 1993.

5. **Brown CG, et al:** Effect of standard doses of epinephrine on myocardial oxygen delivery and utilization during cardiopulmonary resuscitation. *Crit Care Med* 16:536–539, 1988.

6. **Brown CG, et al:** Comparative effect of graded doses of epinephrine on regional brain blood flow during CPR in a swine model. *Ann Emerg Med* 15:1138–1144, 1986.

7. **Brown CG, et al:** A comparison of standard-dose and high-dose epinephrine in cardiac arrest outside the hospital. *New Engl J Med* 327:1051–1055, 1992.

8. **Cogbill TH, et al:** Rationale for selective application of emergency department thoracotomy in trauma. *J Trauma* 23:453–438, 1983.

9. **Callaham M, et al:** A randomized clinical trial of high-dose epinephrine and norepinephrine versus standard-dose epinephrine in prehospital cardiac arrest. *Ann Emerg Med* 21:606–607(abstract), 1992.

10. **Dalsey WC, et al:** Emergency department use of transcutaneous pacing for cardiac arrest. *Crit Care Med* 13:399, 1985.

11. **Emergency Cardiac Care Committee and Subcommittees,** American Heart Association. Guidelines for cardiopulmonary resuscitation and emergency cardiac care, *JAMA* 268:2172–2301, 1992.

12. **Gray WA, Capone RJ, Most AS:** Unsuccessful emergency medical resuscitation—are continued efforts in the emergency department justified? *New Eng J Med* 325(20):1393–1398, 1991.

13. **Haynes RE, et al:** Comparison of bretylium tosylate and lidocaine in management of out of hospital ventricular fibrillation: a randomized clinical trial. *Am J Cardiol* 48:353–356, 1981.

14. **Kellermann AL, Hackman BB, Somes G:** Predicting the outcome of unsuccessful prehospital advanced cardiac life support. *JAMA* 270(12):1433, 1993.

15. **Koscove EM, et al:** Successful resuscitation from cardiac arrest using high-dose epinephrine therapy: report of two cases. *JAMA* 259(20):3031, 1988.

16. **Lindner KH, Ahnefeld FW, Bowdler IM:** Comparison of different doses of epinephrine on myocardial perfusion and resuscitation success during cardiopulmonary resuscitation in a pig model. *Am J Emerg Med* 9:27–31, 1991.

17. **Lindner KH, Ahnefeld FW, Prengel AW:** Comparison of standard and high-dose adrenaline in the resuscitation of asystole and electromechanical dissociation. *Acta Anaesthesiol Scand* 35:253–256, 1991.

18. **Olson DW, et al:** A randomized comparison study of bretylium tosylate and lidocaine in resuscitation of patients from out-of-hospital ventricular fibrillation in a paramedic system. *Ann Emerg Med* 13(9, part 2):807–810, 1984.

19. **Stiell IG, et al:** High-dose epinephrine in adult cardiac arrest. *New Engl J Med* 327:1045–1050, 1992.

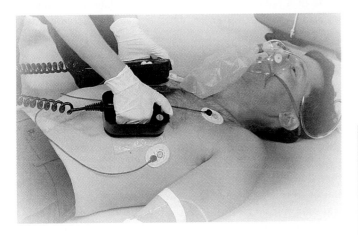

A paramedic should be able to:

1. Explain the pathophysiology of compromised circulation.

2. Given a patient with assessment findings of compromised circulation, explain the importance of rapid recognition and treatment.

3. Identify signs and symptoms of compromised circulation from various causes.

4. Describe the history and assessment of the patient with compromised circulation.

5. Explain the relationship of vital signs to circulation and perfusion.

6. Describe and differentiate among the various causes of compromised circulation in the prehospital setting.

7. Describe the management approaches to various patient conditions that present with compromised circulation.

8. List the therapeutic effects, indications, contraindications, potential side effects, and correct dosages of various medications used to treat specific causes of compromised circulation.

1. **Anaphylactic shock**—shock due to a severe, rapid onset of an allergic reaction that results in widespread vasodilation and tissue permeability. *See Conditions by Diagnosis section.*

2. **Cardiogenic shock**—compromised circulation resulting from the inability of the heart to pump adequately.

3. **Crystalloid**—solution formed by a solute which is in crystal form when dry.

4. **Distributive shock**—compromised circulation resulting from loss of vascular tone leading to dilation of blood vessels and decreased perfusion. Causes include sepsis, anaphylaxis, drugs, toxins, and spinal cord injury.

5. **Hypoperfusion**—the insufficient delivery of oxygen and nutrients necessary for normal tissue and cellular function.

6. **Hypovolemic shock**—the most common cause of compromised circulation in trauma and nontrauma patients, hypovolemic shock is caused by decreased circulating blood volume.

7. **Neurogenic shock**—a type of distributive shock that results when sympathetic control of the vascular system is lost.

8. **Septic shock**—type of hypoperfusion that occurs when toxins are released from certain bacteria into the blood that cause decreased vascular resistance and increased capillary permeability.

9. **Shock**—a state of inadequate tissue perfusion that will result in cell death if not corrected.

Scene Survey

↘ Initial Assessment

Focused History
and Physical Exam

Continued Assessment

Comprised circulation, including cardiac arrest, is an emergency condition that enables the paramedic to have a major impact on the life of a patient. In this situation, rapid intervention must begin before the exact cause has been determined. By understanding the mechanics of compromised circulation and its clinical features, the paramedic can intervene rapidly and increase the patient's chance for survival. Information provided in Chapter 9 will assist the reader in understanding this chapter and applying shock principles to patient assessment.

Regardless of the exact type of shock or its underlying cause, the result is insufficient delivery of the oxygen and nutrients necessary for normal tissue and cellular function, a condition known as hypoperfusion. The body responds in an attempt to preserve circulation to vital organs such as the heart and brain. In the early stages of shock, compensatory mechanisms include measures to increase cardiac output (heart rate and contractility) and divert blood flow away from noncritical organs such as the skin, skeletal muscles, and abdominal organs. These efforts initially maintain adequate blood pressure and perfusion of vital organs. As shock progresses, however, the compensatory mechanisms begin to fail. Cardiac output and blood pressure decrease, resulting in inadequate vital organ perfusion.

Timely intervention may dramatically change the outcome of a patient with compromised circulation. Damage to organ systems begins quickly when circulation decreases. The sooner the underlying cause of inadequate perfusion is corrected, the greater the likelihood that the patient will recover. If the initiation of proper treatment is delayed until hospital arrival, intervention may be too late to reverse the process.

Understanding Circulatory Compromise

The cardiovascular system is composed of three natural divisions: blood, vessels, and the heart. If any of these three components is malfunctioning, the system is disrupted and hypoperfusion or shock occurs.

A disruption in the blood or intravascular volume results in hypovolemic shock. Disruption in the heart results in cardiogenic shock. Disruption in the vessels, either from loss of tone and vasodilation or increased capillary permeability, results in what is called distributive shock, or low resistance shock. Distributive shock includes anaphylactic shock, septic shock, and the neurogenic causes of shock such as spinal cord injury, overdose, and vagal stimulation. A review of these types of shock and their common causes is found in Table 20-1.

Recognizing Circulatory Compromise

Circulatory compromise can arise from many underlying causes, but regardless of the cause, there are common signs and symptoms (Fig. 20-1).

These manifestations become more noticeable as circulatory compromise progresses and represent the body's attempt to compensate for the disruption or its failure to compensate. Without intervention, failed compensation results in irreversible shock. Table 20-2 shows the progression of circulatory compromise in terms of signs and symptoms by examining the three stages of shock: compensated, uncompensated, and irreversible.

TABLE 20-1	Comparison of the Causes of Three Types of Shock	
Hypovolemic Shock	**Distributive Shock**	**Cardiogenic Shock**
Hemorrhage	Septic	Myocardial Infarction
Trauma		Hypoxia
GI bleeding		
Dehydration	Allergic	Bradycardia
Prolonged vomiting		Tachycardia
Diarrhea	Neurogenic	Secondary causes
	Spinal trauma	Heart valve damage
Third-Spacing	Vasovagal stimulation	Tension pneumothorax
Burns	Drugs	pericardial tamponade
Ascites	Toxins	

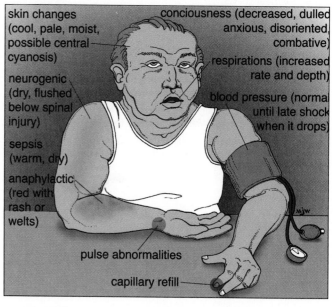

Figure 20-1

Common findings in patients with circulatory compromise.

TABLE 20-2	Signs and Symptoms of Three Stages of Shock		
Signs/Symptoms	**Stage 1:** **Compensated** **Shock**	**Stage 2:** **Uncompensated** **Shock**	**Stage 3:** **Irreversible** **Shock**
Responsiveness	Agitation, anxiety	Confusion, unresponsive	Comatose
Pulse	Rapid, strong	Rapid, weakening	Slow, with dysrhythmias
Respirations	Rapid	Rapid	Varies—irregular, rapid, agonal, absent
Skin	Cool	Cool, cyanotic	Pale, cool, moist
Capillary Refill	Delayed	Delayed	Delayed; undetectable
Blood Pressure	Normal—elevated	Decreased	Significantly Hypotensive

Approaching the Patient

Consider the information provided in the initial dispatch. When dispatched for calls involving patients with chest pain, heart attack, unresponsiveness, or some form of significant trauma, the paramedic must think about the patient's condition and possible presentation, and the immediate treatment that may be required upon arrival. Who will gather patient history, handle the patient's airway and breathing problems, and perform other critical procedures? When these roles and responsibilities are determined en route, care at the scene proceeds more smoothly.

Assessing the Patient

The process of identifying compromised circulation follows the standard patient assessment steps (Box 20-1). The first step is to start with the initial assessment to check for and correct any immediately life-threatening problems, such as absence of breathing or a pulse. Once this check is complete, the paramedic can conduct the focused history and examination. This involves SAMPLE history, baseline vital signs, and a rapid physical assessment. Once en route to the receiving facility, there may be time to do a continued physical examination.

Initial Assessment

Level of responsiveness, airway and breathing adequacy, adequacy of pulse, and the presence of severe bleeding can be assessed rapidly in the responsive patient. A patient who can give an appropriate verbal response to the question, "What seems to be the problem?" is responsive, has an open airway, is breathing, and has a pulse. This does not necessarily mean that the patient's circulation is adequate, however. A patient suffering a **myocardial infarction** or losing blood can present in this manner, but the pulse may be inadequate to perfuse the tissues.

A number of factors can contribute to a diminished level of responsiveness in patients with compromised circulation. Depending on the underlying cause, diminished responsiveness may result from hypoxia, toxins, or structural damage to the brain. In the early stages of shock, patients often appear anxious because of the effects of compensatory catecholamine release. As cerebral perfusion decreases and cerebral hypoxia

occurs, confusion, agitation, and combativeness may occur. As shock progresses further, the patient can become unresponsive or deeply comatose.

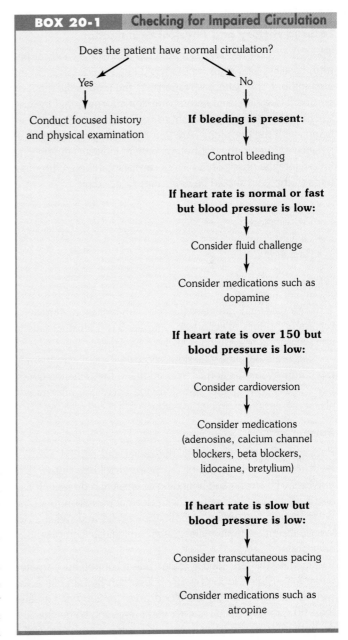

BOX 20-1   Checking for Impaired Circulation

Does the patient have normal circulation?

Yes → Conduct focused history and physical examination

No →

If bleeding is present:
↓
Control bleeding

If heart rate is normal or fast but blood pressure is low:
↓
Consider fluid challenge
↓
Consider medications such as dopamine

If heart rate is over 150 but blood pressure is low:
↓
Consider cardioversion
↓
Consider medications (adenosine, calcium channel blockers, beta blockers, lidocaine, bretylium)

If heart rate is slow but blood pressure is low:
↓
Consider transcutaneous pacing
↓
Consider medications such as atropine

For an unresponsive patient, the paramedic should tap the patient's shoulder and shout to elicit a response. If the patient does not respond, the paramedic should then assess the adequacy of the airway and breathing. The cervical spine should be protected if there is any possibility of trauma. Next, the patient's carotid and radial pulses should be assessed and if found to be apneic and pulseless, CPR and advanced life support procedures should be initiated. If the patient has a pulse, its rate and quality should be determined. Finally, the patient's body should be quickly examined for severe bleeding.

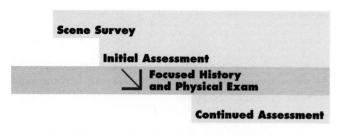

Focused History and Physical Examination

The focused history and examination includes a medical history, baseline vital signs, and a rapid head-to-toe physical examination. If the patient is responsive, the paramedic may ask pertinent questions and gather vital sign information. One critical line of questioning relevant to the present medical history begins with the question, "Are you having any chest pain?" A positive answer in the nontrauma patient indicates the need to investigate the possibility of a myocardial infarction. Other features of the pain should be determined, including:

- Onset
- Provocation
- Quality
- Radiation
- Severity
- Time

The type and extent of the pain can indicate a cardiac or respiratory origin of pain (*see* Chapter 31). Pain that fails to change during respiration is likely to be cardiac.

Accurate baseline vital signs allow the health care team to track improvements and deteriorations in the patient's condition. The following vital signs provide necessary information about the patient's circulatory status.

Pulse

Pulses should be palpated at the radial and carotid arteries. Both the rate and quality of the pulse should be noted. The pulse may be strong and bounding or weak and thready. It can also be irregular. In a patient with normal perfusion, a strong pulse is easy to palpate at both the carotid and radial sites. Weak, absent, or rapid radial pulses can indicate compromised circulation.

In general, an adult's radial pulse cannot be palpated when the systolic blood pressure is less than 80 mm Hg. If the carotid pulse is present, the blood pressure is usually greater than 60 mm Hg. Radial and carotid pulses should be checked on both sides of the body in case the pulse abnormality is the result of a more localized problem with blood flow, such as arterial occlusion or restriction in the arm or neck. The pulse rate may also help indicate compromised circulation.

There are two principal reasons why a patient with compromised circulation can still have a normal heart rate. The first is a primary cardiac problem. Any disease that decreases the ability of the heart to pump, including myocardial infarction, can present this way. The second reason is fluid loss in a patient taking medication that suppresses the heart rate, such as a beta blocker.

Tachycardia usually represents the compensatory response to compromised circulation; in patients experiencing severe tachycardia (greater than 150/min) the compromised circulation is more likely to be the result of the rapid rate itself. During normal compensatory responses, the heart beats more rapidly and forcefully to maintain perfusion, but this response works only to a certain point. As the rate exceeds 150/min, there is less time for the atria to fill, less blood is ejected during each contraction, and the blood pressure begins to fall. A young, healthy heart can maintain an adequate blood pressure at rates greater than 180/min, but an older heart often begins to lose efficiency around 150/min. Compromised circulation caused by severe tachycardia is often treated with synchronized cardioversion, which is discussed later in this chapter.

An accurate patient history and careful evaluation of the cardiac rhythm strip will determine if an electrical conduction abnormality is contributing to compromised circulation. If bleeding or fluid loss accompanies sinus tachycardia, then the volume deficiency is causing the tachycardia. Evidence of **paroxysmal supraventricular tachycardia,** rapid **atrial fibrillation, atrial flutter,** or **ventricular tachycardia** suggest that the underlying dysrhythmia is causing or contributing to circulatory compromise.

Respirations

As the patient's condition worsens, changes in respiratory rate and pattern often appear. Rate and depth increase to compensate for increased myocardial oxygen demand, and to help remove increased metabolic acids by excreting carbon dioxide. As circulatory compromise continues, the breathing rate overrides the depth, and respirations become rapid and shallow. As cerebral hypoxia occurs, respirations can slow, become irregular or cease altogether.

Skin

Skin color, temperature, and moisture are important indicators of compromised circulation. Cool or pale skin results from arteriole constriction that is part of a compensatory response to redistribute blood to the body's core. Delayed capillary filling (> 2 seconds) in the skin or nail bed is a similar sign. Although delayed capillary refill often reflects compensation for shock, it also depends on the ambient temperature; in a cold environment, it may not be an accurate indicator of perfusion status. Because hypoperfused skin will attain the temperature of the environment, hypothermia is a very real threat to the patient in shock. Likewise, if the temperature is hot, the patient is likely to feel warm to the touch.

Pallor, or loss of normal skin color, is most noticeable in the conjunctiva, the mucous membranes, and the earlobes.

Pallor usually results from a combination of vasoconstriction and blood loss. Cyanosis often appears in the fingers, toes, and lips. Cyanosis has two primary causes, hypoxia and hypoperfusion. Cyanosis involving only the fingers and toes is called peripheral cyanosis, which usually represents decreased blood flow to the extremities and is indicative of hypoperfusion. Cyanosis at the lips and mouth is called central cyanosis and may indicate either hypoxia or hypoperfusion. In general, oxygen-deficient blood must be present in the skin capillaries for cyanosis to be evident. When acute blood loss occurs with respiratory compromise, the patient may appear pale but is usually not cyanotic.

Sweat is produced in response to heat, or to the stimulation of alpha receptor sites that occurs during shock with the release of epinephrine and norepinephrine. Sweat tends to appear initially in the same places that patients become pale—the upper lip, nose, and hairline. As the level of hormones increases, sweating and pallor spread to other areas of the body.

Blood Pressure

Compensatory mechanisms may keep the blood pressure relatively normal in the early stages of shock. In patients without significant underlying medical conditions, such as heart disease or diabetes, systolic blood pressure may be maintained until cardiac output decreases significantly, or until about one quarter of the blood volume is lost. Even though hypotension may not appear until late in the process, the paramedic should obtain a blood pressure reading early in the evaluation. For adults, a systolic blood pressure of 90 mm Hg or less, or of 30 mm Hg less than the patient's normal pressure, is a significant indication of compromised circulation.

The paramedic must consider whether normal pulse and blood pressure measurements taken while the person is supine differ from those taken in a seated or standing position. This is known as taking orthostatic vital signs, or a tilt test, and is used to determine if the patient has lost a significant volume of blood or body fluid. If blood pressure and pulse do not change significantly (by 20 or more) when the patient changes position, blood volume is probably normal. Orthostatic measurements should not be conducted if the supine patient is already showing signs of compromised circulation or if the patient has significant trauma.

Bleeding

Patients should be evaluated for bleeding and ongoing fluid loss, either of which can be visible or hidden (see Chapter 28). Visible bleeding includes external blood loss from trauma, vomited blood, vaginal bleeding, and bloody stools. Traumatic bleeding can usually be controlled with direct pressure or by pressing firmly over arterial pressure points proximal to the bleeding site. Visible causes of fluid loss, including severe vomiting and diarrhea, can result in dehydration. Fluid loss can also occur as a result of burn injuries.

Gastrointestinal (GI) bleeding is a major cause of hidden blood loss. Most patients with active GI bleeding present with characteristic signs such as bloody or brownish ("coffee ground") emesis, produced by the mixture of blood with stom-

ach acids or with black, tarry stools ("melena") created by partial digestion of blood as it passes through the GI tract. Internal bleeding also can result from blunt abdominal trauma, ectopic pregnancy, ruptured abdominal aortic aneurysm, or splenic rupture. Hidden fluid loss can occur in patients with various medical problems including cancer, liver disease, kidney disease, and diabetes.

Major fractures such as pelvis or femur fractures can result in 1 to 2 L of hidden blood loss, as well as damage to other organs and structures that maintain adequate circulation. This amount of blood loss can easily result in hypovolemic shock. A fractured rib could result in a laceration to the liver or spleen. Because both of these organs have a rich blood supply, significant internal blood loss is likely. Although it is not always possible to diagnose the underlying organs involved, by maintaining a high degree of suspicion, the paramedic can begin prompt treatment to minimize blood loss and its effects.

Managing Compromised Circulation

An assessment that indicates possible circulatory compromise requires rapid intervention. Begin with basic life support skills. Body temperature should be kept normal to decrease energy needs. Place the patient in the position of comfort. Whenever possible, this position should be the supine with legs elevated 8–12″ or Trendelenburg position, to minimize blood pooling in the lower part of the body. The patient with respiratory distress may be kept in an upright position to make breathing easier. Oxygen should always be administered.

Oxygenation

As the heart works harder, the demand for oxygen increases. Besides satisfying myocardial oxygen demand, supplemental oxygen helps meet the increased needs of other organs and tissues. Administering the highest concentration of oxygen possible usually means 15 L/min through a nonrebreather mask. If the patient has significant difficulty breathing, as evidenced by respiratory rate and quality, the paramedic should assist breathing efforts with positive pressure ventilation. This can be done with a bag-valve-mask and oxygen reservoir or with a demand valve.

Some EMS personnel use pulse oximetry to help assess oxygen saturation and determine the need for supplemental oxygenation (see Sidebar in Chapter 18). The pulse oximeter reading will often indicate compromised circulation before the blood pressure drops. Pulse oximetry should not be solely relied upon because it is inaccurate in situations involving high systemic vascular resistance, hypothermia, and carbon monoxide poisoning, among other situations.

Controlling Blood Loss

Serious blood loss will result in hypovolemic shock and must be rapidly corrected. Bleeding can be controlled by applying pressure to the site of a wound or a nearby pressure point, or using the pneumatic antishock garment (PASG). Although the PASG has been shown to be beneficial in splinting long bone and pelvic fractures and in tamponading certain types of bleeding, inappropriate use may worsen thoracic bleeding and complicate pulmonary edema and head injury conditions (*see* Chapter 46).

Fluid Administration

An IV line of a crystalloid solution should be established, preferably with a large-bore IV cannula. If history suggests the likelihood of internal bleeding, the patient should be prepared for immediate transport to the hospital; these patients will require therapy beyond what can be provided in the prehospital setting. Whenever such a patient is a candidate for urgent transport, weigh the value of performing a procedure, such as initiating an IV, at the scene against the time lost by delaying transport. It may be appropriate to do less when transport times are short than when they will be prolonged. Whenever possible, it is preferable to establish IV lines en route to the hospital.

The majority of patients in shock require fluid replacement with either normal saline or lactated Ringer's solution. The initial infusion is administered at a wide open rate until the blood pressure is above 90 systolic. In some situations, fluid may be administered in a series of 250 to 500 cc boluses, or through multiple lines. There are limitations to the amount of fluid that is appropriate. Since high-volume fluid replacement can contribute to **adult respiratory distress syndrome** (ARDS) and cerebral edema, fluid requirements in excess of 3 L in an adult usually mean blood must be transfused to keep up with ongoing losses. Pediatric patients can receive a 20 mL/kg bolus that can be repeated. In elderly patients, 200 to 300 mL of fluid is given initially. All of these administrations should be accompanied by an assessment for the development of pulmonary edema. If signs such as rales or neck vein distention do appear, the IV should be decreased to a TKO rate.

In the patient with possible pulmonary edema, left-sided congestive heart failure and cardiogenic shock should also be suspected. This patient will not tolerate aggressive fluid administration. Treatment should be directed toward improving the heart's pumping action and correcting dysrhythmias. Fluid replacement should begin with a 100- to 200-mL fluid challenge. If the patient's condition improves, fluid administration can continue until blood pressure is stabilized. The presence of rales in both lungs, particularly if there is a history of heart failure, makes a fluid bolus inappropriate. Administer a vasopressor agent, such as dopamine, to increase blood pressure.

Continuous cardiac monitoring and pulse oximetry should be instituted. The paramedic should monitor the patient closely during transport, repeating assessments at 5- to 10-minute intervals.

Pharmacological Therapy

Pharmacological therapy can be used in a variety of situations involving patients with compromised circulation. The use of pharmacological agents can:

- Reduce myocardial oxygen demand
- Correct dysrhythmias
- Increase blood pressure
- Correct bronchospasm
- Reduce anxiety

The choice of medication to control the pain associated with chest pain or cardioversion depends on what local protocols permit. For cardioversion, it is best to combine a sedative, such as diazepam (Valium®) or midazolam (Versed®), with an analgesic such as morphine or meperidine (Demerol®). Any of these agents can also be used alone. However, they can cause respiratory depression or respiratory arrest, particularly when combining midazolam with either morphine or meperidine.

Aside from its excellent pain relief effect, morphine's ability to decrease preload and afterload can result in decreased myocardial workload and oxygen demand. This is also true of nitroglycerin.

In cardiogenic shock, the blood pressure does not always respond to efforts to increase the heart rate or replace fluids. Medications such as dopamine and epinephrine can be used for their sympathomimetic effect. By stimulating alpha- and beta-adrenergic receptors in a dose-related manner, these medications can help resolve hypotension. Dopamine is commonly used to treat hypotension associated with cardiogenic shock; epinephrine is used for distributive shock caused by anaphylaxis (Boxes 20-2 and 20-3). Norepinephrine (Levophed) is used for postresuscitation persistent hypotension. *See* the Appendix to Chapter 11 to reinforce key drug information.

When **dysrhythmias** compromise circulation, medications can be used. Atropine, adenosine, calcium channel

---

BOX 20-2   Dopamine (Intropin, Dopastat)

Therapeutic Action

- At lower doses (1 to 2 μg/kg per minute), causes dilation of renal and mesenteric vasculature
- At moderate doses (2 to 10 μg/kg per minute), causes increase in heart rate and myocardial contractility
- At high doses (greater than 10 μg/kg per minute), causes peripheral vasoconstriction and hypertension

Indications

- Cardiogenic shock
- Hypotension associated with congestive heart failure
- Hypotension unresponsive to fluid therapy

Contraindications

- Hypovolemic shock

Adverse Reactions

- Chest pain
- Palpitations
- Tachycardia
- Dyspnea
- Headache
- Nausea and vomiting
- Tissue damage may occur with extravasation

BOX 20-3 Epinephrine (Adrenalin)

Therapeutic Action

- Vasoconstriction, increased heart rate and force of myocardial contraction

Indications

- Cardiac arrest:
    Pulseless ventricular tachycardia
    Ventricular fibrillation
    Pulseless electrical activity
    Asystole
- Anaphylactic reactions
- Bronchospasm

Contraindications

- Suspected intracranial bleed
- Bronchospasm in patients with coronary artery disease

Adverse Reactions

- Palpitations
- Tachycardia
- Ventricular ectopy
- Hypotension
- Tremors
- Anxiety
- Headache
- Cerebral hemorrhage
- Nausea and vomiting

blockers (such as verapamil), lidocaine, procainamide, and bretylium are examples. These medications are discussed later in this chapter.

Electrical Therapy

Dysrhythmias that do not respond to medications may require electrical therapy. In perfusing patients, this includes synchronized cardioversion and transcutaneous pacing. Defibrillation is usually used only in the pulseless patient.

Synchronized Cardioversion

Synchronized cardioversion is used to terminate ventricular and supraventricular wide- and narrow-complex tachycardias that include atrial fibrillation, atrial flutter, paroxysmal supraventricular tachycardia, and perfusing ventricular tachycardia (see Fig. 20-2 and Skill #16 in Skills Section).

Synchronized cardioversion differs from defibrillation in the timing of the energy delivery. In defibrillation, the current is delivered when the operator discharges the paddles, with no concern for the phase of the cardiac cycle. Synchronized cardioversion delivers the shock just after the peak of the R wave, avoiding the vulnerable relative refractory period, which could induce ventricular fibrillation. Because of this efficiency in delivering the shock, synchronized cardioversion may require less energy to terminate the dysrhythmia, and reduce the chance of developing new, problematic rhythms.

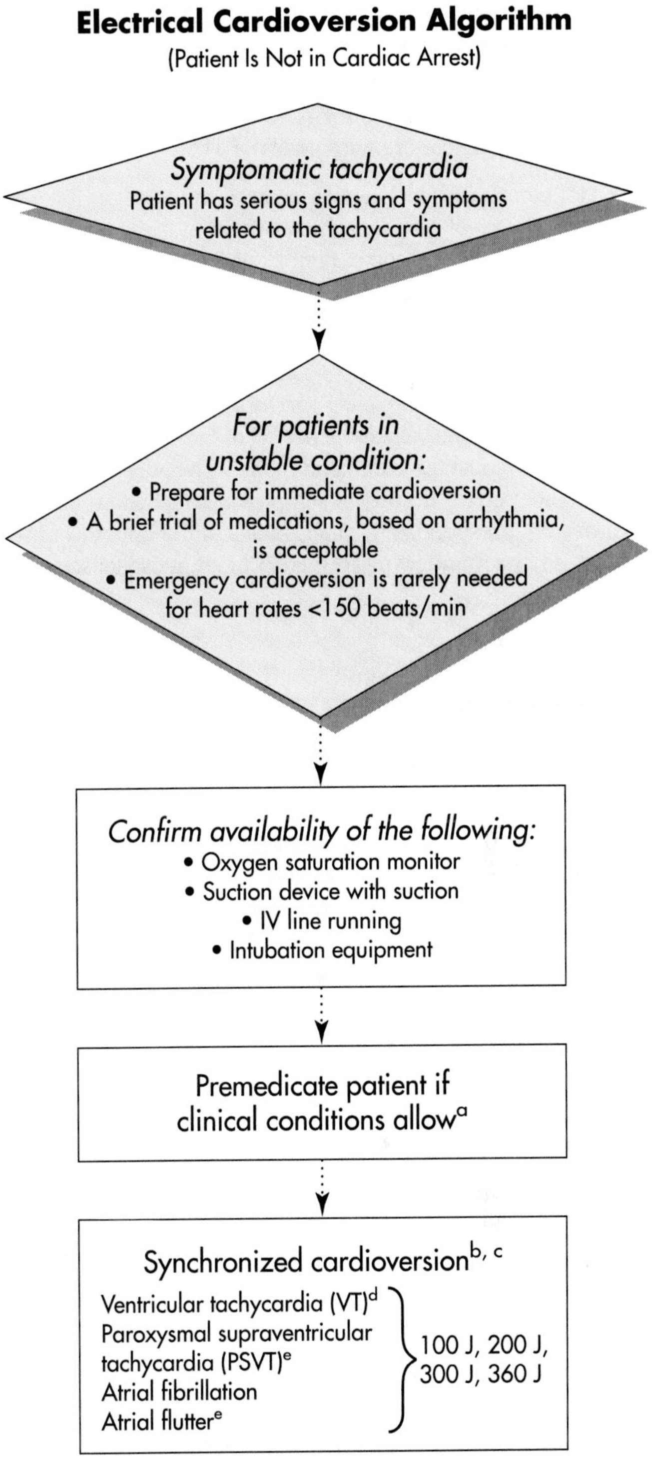

Electrical Cardioversion Algorithm
(Patient Is Not in Cardiac Arrest)

Symptomatic tachycardia
Patient has serious signs and symptoms related to the tachycardia

For patients in unstable condition:
- Prepare for immediate cardioversion
- A brief trial of medications, based on arrhythmia, is acceptable
- Emergency cardioversion is rarely needed for heart rates <150 beats/min

Confirm availability of the following:
- Oxygen saturation monitor
- Suction device with suction
- IV line running
- Intubation equipment

Premedicate patient if clinical conditions allow[a]

Synchronized cardioversion[b, c]
Ventricular tachycardia (VT)[d]
Paroxysmal supraventricular tachycardia (PSVT)[e]
Atrial fibrillation
Atrial flutter[e] } 100 J, 200 J, 300 J, 360 J

[a] Effective premedication regimens have included a sedative (e.g., diazepam, midazolam) with or without an analgesic agent (e.g., fentanyl, morphine, meperidine).
[b] You often need to resynchronize the defibrillator after each cardioversion.
[c] If synchronization is delayed and clinical conditions are critical, perform unsynchronized shocks.
[d] Treat polymorphic VT (irregular form and rate) like ventricular fibrillation: 200 J, 200 to 300 J, 360 J.
[e] PSVT and atrial flutter often respond to lower energy levels (start with 50 J).

Figure 20-2

The algorithm for electrical cardioversion. Adapted from Cummins: ACLS Scenarios: Core Concepts for Case-Based Learning, St. Louis, 1996, Mosby-Year Book. Adapted with permission, Journal of the American Medical Association: Guidelines for Cardiopulmonary Resuscitation and Emergency Cardiac Care, vol 268, ©1992, American Medical Association.

Transcutaneous Pacing

Transcutaneous pacing (TCP), also called external pacing, is an electrical therapy used primarily to treat bradycardia dysrhythmias such as complete heart block (*see* Skill #17 in Skills Section). There are two modes of TCP:

- Nondemand (asynchronous or fixed-rate) pacing involves the delivery of timed electrical stimuli at a predetermined rate, regardless of the patient's own cardiac activity.
- Demand (synchronous) pacing senses the patient's intrinsic QRS complex and delivers electrical stimuli only when needed.

Because of the possibility that nondemand pacing could discharge during the vulnerable period of the cardiac cycle, it is not used as frequently as demand mode is. Nondemand pacing can also be used to "overdrive" symptomatic tachydysrhythmias that have not responded to other means of therapy. Overdrive pacing is not commonly performed in the prehospital setting.

Managing Select Conditions

Symptomatic Bradycardia

When there is a pulse of less than 60 in an adult with evidence of compromised circulation, the pulse rate itself may be the cause of the problem. There are several reasons that the pulse may be slow, including cardiac disease, stimulation of the vagus nerve, and medications such as beta blockers. An athlete may normally have a heart rate in the 45 to 60 range, but the pulses will be strong and there will not be signs of compromised circulation.

A patient with bradycardia in the presence of compromised circulation requires rapid treatment (Fig. 20-3). The first line of treatment is atropine IV or by endotracheal tube (Box 20-4). Atropine acts by decreasing the effect of the vagus nerve. It does not always work, and when it does, its effect often only lasts for a few minutes.

BOX 20-4	Atropine

Therapeutic Action

- Increases heart rate and atrioventricular nodal conduction

Indications

- Symptomatic bradycardia
- Narrow-complex Mobitz type II second-degree heart block
- Narrow-complex third-degree heart block
- Slow pulseless electrical activity
- Asystole
- Cholinergic poisonings (organophosphates and carbamates)

Contraindications

- Wide-complex Mobitz type II second-degree heart block
- Wide-complex third-degree heart block

Adverse Reactions

- Tachycardia
- Dry mouth
- Dilated pupils
- Delirium

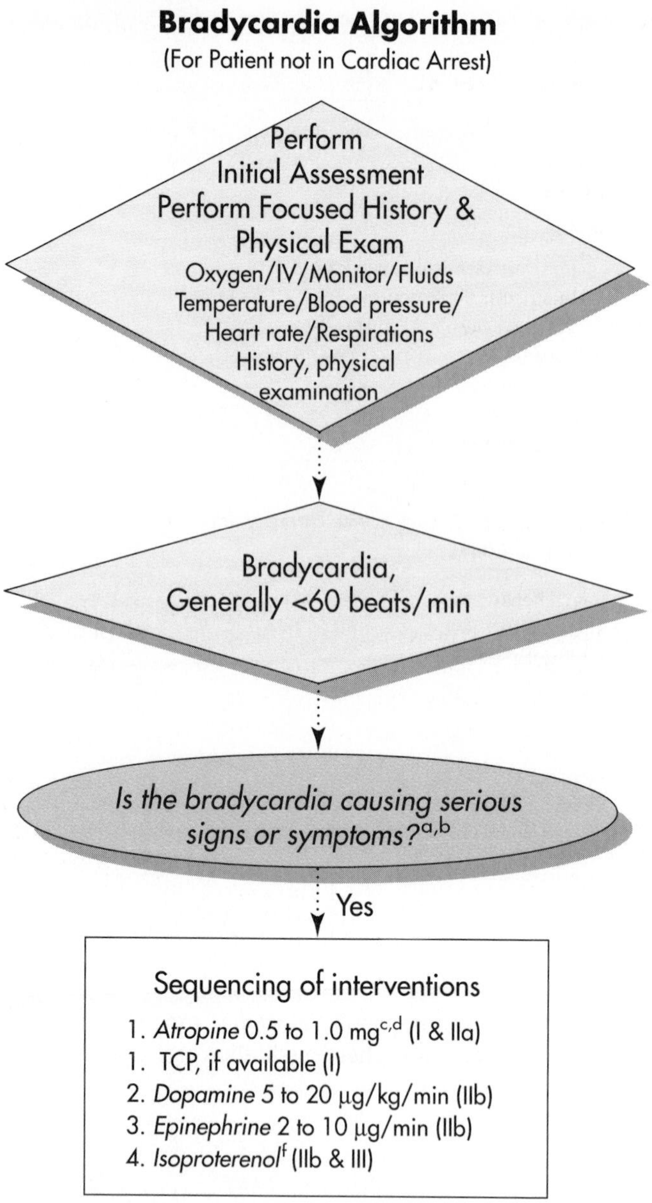

Bradycardia Algorithm

(For Patient not in Cardiac Arrest)

Perform
Initial Assessment
Perform Focused History &
Physical Exam
Oxygen/IV/Monitor/Fluids
Temperature/Blood pressure/
Heart rate/Respirations
History, physical
examination

Bradycardia,
Generally <60 beats/min

Is the bradycardia causing serious signs or symptoms?[a,b]

Yes

Sequencing of interventions

1. *Atropine* 0.5 to 1.0 mg[c,d] (I & IIa)
1. TCP, if available (I)
2. *Dopamine* 5 to 20 µg/kg/min (IIb)
3. *Epinephrine* 2 to 10 µg/min (IIb)
4. *Isoproterenol*[f] (IIb & III)

[a] The clinical signs or symptoms must be related to the slow rate. Clinical manifestations include the following.
- Symptoms (chest pain, shortness of breath, decreased level of consciousness)
- Signs (low blood pressure, shock, pulmonary congestion, congestive heart failure, AMI)

[b] Start TCP before atropine takes effect if patient is symptomatic.

[c] Transplanted hearts will not respond to *atropine*. Go at once to pacing, *catecholamine infusion*, or both.

[d] *Atropine* should be given in repeat doses every 3 to 5 minutes up to total of 0.03 to 0.04 mg/kg. Use the shorter dosing interval (3 min) in severe clinical conditions. *Atropine* is seldom effective in atrioventricular (AV) block at the His-Purkinje level (type II AV block and new third-degree block with wide QRS complexes) (Class IIb).

[e] A potentially fatal error is to treat third-degree heart block plus ventricular escape beats with lidocaine.

[f] Only use *isoproterenol* with extreme caution. At low doses it is Class IIb (possibly helpful); at higher doses it is Class III (harmful).

Figure 20-3

The algorithm for bradycardia. Adapted from Cummins: ACLS Scenarios: Core Concepts for Case-Based Learning, St. Louis, 1996, Mosby-Year Book. Adapted with permission, Journal of the American Medical Association: Guidelines for Cardiopulmonary Resuscitation and Emergency Cardiac Care, vol 268, ©1992, American Medical Association.

Atropine must be thought of as temporary help. Preparations for transcutaneous pacing should be started immediately. Placing the pads on the patient while waiting to see if the atropine is effective decreases the time required to start the pacing. Pulses should be palpable at the same rate as the pacer to assure that there is capture by the heart. This can be challenging. As the current passes through the chest, the body will twitch, making it difficult to determine the presence of a pulse. If pacing is not available, immediate transport to an emergency department is warranted.

If the blood pressure and other signs of compromised circulation do not respond to these interventions, or a pacemaker is not available, the patient can be treated with dopamine. Although useful in wide-complex tachycardias, lidocaine is contraindicated in bradycardias. The drug may be lethal in these patients, because it could suppress critical ventricular escape activity.

Symptomatic Tachycardia

Tachycardia may have wide or narrow QRS complexes. Severe tachycardia (> 150 beats/min) in a patient with weak or absent radial pulses is likely to be the cause rather than the result of compromised circulation. The treatment for tachycardia is outlined in Figure 20-4.

Synchronized cardioversion can be painful. If the patient is awake and is not deteriorating rapidly, the patient should be premedicated with a sedative or pain control medication, or a combination of the two. While waiting for the medication to take full effect, there may be time for a brief trial of adenosine.

Wide-Complex Tachycardia

Lidocaine is the first-line medication for wide-complex tachycardia (Box 20-5). If there is no time for a trial of lidocaine or pain medication, the paramedic should prepare for immediate synchronized cardioversion.

If the rhythm is a wide-complex tachycardia (QRS ≥ 0.12 seconds) or atrial fibrillation, synchronized cardioversion should begin at an energy setting of 100 joules. If unsuccessful, the paramedic can increase the energy to 200, 300, and then 360 joules. If still unsuccessful, the underlying rhythm should be reassessed for further treatment.

If the complexes remain wide, the rhythm is usually ventricular tachycardia and is treated with lidocaine, if it has not already been administered. In the patient with compromised circulation, synchronized cardioversion at 360 joules should be attempted after each dose of lidocaine.

Some EMS services carry procainamide, which can be used for narrow- and wide-complex tachycardias that have not responded to lidocaine (Box 20-6). The major disadvantage of procainamide in field use is that it is administered very slowly. For this reason, the second medication used to correct wide-complex tachycardia is usually bretylium (Box 20-7). Each dose of bretylium is followed by synchronized cardioversion.

Narrow-Complex Tachycardia

Atrial flutter, atrial fibrillation and paroxysmal supraventricular tachycardia (PSVT) are the common narrow-complex rhythms (QRS < 0.12 seconds). The medications used to treat the stable patient with these rhythms include adenosine and verapamil. Adenosine may be used in a patient who has mild hypotension, because of its rapid metabolism. Verapamil should not be used in a patient who is hypotensive, because it may exacerbate the hypotension. Atrial fibrillation with rapid ventricular response and hypotension is treated with synchronized cardioversion beginning at 100 joules, as previously discussed for wide complex tachycardia. PSVT and atrial flutter may respond to synchronized cardioversion at lower energy levels, beginning with 50 joules.

BOX 20-5   **Lidocaine (Xylocaine)**

Therapeutic Action

- Suppresses ventricular ectopy and increases fibrillation threshold

Indications

- Pulseless ventricular tachycardia unresponsive to defibrillation and epinephrine
- Ventricular fibrillation unresponsive to defibrillation and epinephrine
- Ventricular ectopy in the presence of acute myocardial infarction
- Wide-complex paroxysmal supraventricular tachycardia

Contraindications

- Allergy to amide anaesthetics (bupivicaine)
- Ventricular escape rhythm

Adverse Reactions

- Drowsiness
- Numbness and tingling
- Disorientation
- Convulsions
- Coma
- Respiratory arrest

BOX 20-6   **Procainamide (Procan, Pronestyl)**

Therapeutic Action

- Decreases ectopy in ischemic cardiac tissue

Indications

- Ventricular dysrhythmias unresponsive to lidocaine
- Wide-complex tachycardias unresponsive to lidocaine
- Wide-complex tachycardias in which the origin cannot be distinguished between ventricular and supraventricular

Contraindications

- Patients on digitalis or antidepressants
- Second- and third-degree AV blocks

Adverse Reactions

- Hypotension
- Heart block
- Exacerbation of ventricular dysrhythmias
- Widening of QRS complex
- Anorexia
- Nausea and vomiting

Tachycardia Algorithm

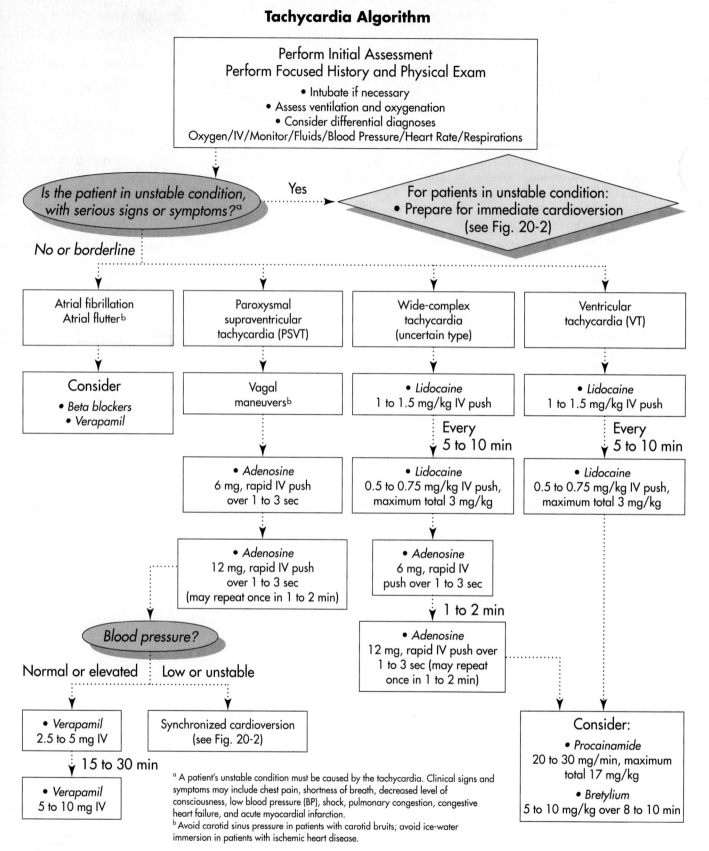

Perform Initial Assessment
Perform Focused History and Physical Exam

- Intubate if necessary
- Assess ventilation and oxygenation
- Consider differential diagnoses
Oxygen/IV/Monitor/Fluids/Blood Pressure/Heart Rate/Respirations

*Is the patient in unstable condition,
with serious signs or symptoms?*[a]

Yes →

For patients in unstable condition:
- Prepare for immediate cardioversion
(see Fig. 20-2)

No or borderline

| Atrial fibrillation
Atrial flutter[b] | Paroxysmal
supraventricular
tachycardia (PSVT) | Wide-complex
tachycardia
(uncertain type) | Ventricular
tachycardia (VT) |

Consider
- *Beta blockers*
- *Verapamil*

Vagal
maneuvers[b]

- *Lidocaine*
1 to 1.5 mg/kg IV push

- *Lidocaine*
1 to 1.5 mg/kg IV push

Every
5 to 10 min

Every
5 to 10 min

- *Adenosine*
6 mg, rapid IV push
over 1 to 3 sec

- *Lidocaine*
0.5 to 0.75 mg/kg IV push,
maximum total 3 mg/kg

- *Lidocaine*
0.5 to 0.75 mg/kg IV push,
maximum total 3 mg/kg

- *Adenosine*
12 mg, rapid IV push
over 1 to 3 sec
(may repeat once in 1 to 2 min)

- *Adenosine*
6 mg, rapid IV
push over 1 to 3 sec

1 to 2 min

Blood pressure?

- *Adenosine*
12 mg, rapid IV push over
1 to 3 sec (may repeat
once in 1 to 2 min)

Normal or elevated   Low or unstable

- *Verapamil*
2.5 to 5 mg IV

Synchronized cardioversion
(see Fig. 20-2)

15 to 30 min

- *Verapamil*
5 to 10 mg IV

Consider:
- *Procainamide*
20 to 30 mg/min, maximum
total 17 mg/kg

- *Bretylium*
5 to 10 mg/kg over 8 to 10 min

[a] A patient's unstable condition must be caused by the tachycardia. Clinical signs and symptoms may include chest pain, shortness of breath, decreased level of consciousness, low blood pressure (BP), shock, pulmonary congestion, congestive heart failure, and acute myocardial infarction.
[b] Avoid carotid sinus pressure in patients with carotid bruits; avoid ice-water immersion in patients with ischemic heart disease.

Figure 20-4

The algorithm for tachycardia. Adapted from Cummins: ACLS Scenarios: Core Concepts for Case-Based Learning, St. Louis, 1996, Mosby-Year Book. Adapted with permission, Journal of the American Medical Association: Guidelines for Cardiopulmonary Resuscitation and Emergency Cardiac Care, vol 268, ©1992, American Medical Association.

BOX 20-7	Bretylium Tosylate-(Bretylol)

Therapeutic Action

- Prolongs refractory time and increases conduction in ventricular myocardium. Elevates threshold for ventricular fibrillation.

Indications

- Ventricular fibrillation or pulseless ventricular tachycardia, unresponsive to defibrillation, epinephrine, and lidocaine.
- Ventricular tachycardia with a pulse, unresponsive to lidocaine and procainamide.
- Wide complex tachycardia unresponsive to lidocaine and adenosine.

Contraindications

None when used for treating ventricular dysrhythmias

Adverse Reactions

- Hypotension
- Bradycardia
- Nausea and vomiting

Congestive Heart Failure

The presence of left-sided congestive heart failure (CHF) means that the patient will not tolerate fluids. The presence of rales in both lungs, particularly if there is a history of heart failure, requires careful fluid administration. The IV should be maintained at a TKO rate and administer a dopamine drip.

Anaphylaxis

Anaphylaxis is the only common cause of hypoperfusion in which the heart rate is *not* helpful in deciding the proper treatment. For this reason, a rapid examination should be performed, looking for signs of an allergic reaction. Usually there will be a history of a recent bite or sting, use of a new medicine, or ingestion of food, especially shellfish. Upon physical examination, the patient may have hives, facial swelling, swelling inside the mouth or mucous membranes, or wheezing.

In a severe anaphylactic reaction with hypoperfusion, the appropriate medication to administer is epinephrine. If an IV has been established and the patient is unconscious, 0.3 mg epinephrine should be administered by slow IV push. If IV access cannot be obtained or if the patient is responsive, 0.3 mg (0.3 mL of 1:1000 for the adult) of epinephrine should be administered subcutaneously. Epinephrine can cause severe elevations in blood pressure, dysrhythmias such as ventricular tachycardia and spasm of the coronary arteries, particularly in the elderly and in patients with a history of cardiac disease.

The paramedic must be sure that there is evidence of hypoperfusion before using epinephrine. The subcutaneous route should be used, except in severe shock with unresponsiveness.

Scene Survey

Initial Assessment

Focused History and Physical Exam

Continued Assessment

Continued Assessment

The keys to managing the patient with compromised circulation are rapid assessment, appropriate and timely treatment, early transport, and reassessment. The worst mistakes occur after initiating the proper treatment, when the rescuer fails to recognize a change in patient condition that requires a change in therapy. The patient with compromised circulation requires reassessment at least *every* 5 minutes and whenever the cardiac rhythm changes. Although it is difficult to obtain an accurate blood pressure in the back of an ambulance, a strengthening or weakening pulse, or a change in pulse rate, gives a clear indication of a change in circulatory status. Reassessment of the patient's respiratory status, including repeated auscultation of breath sounds, will reveal CHF if it develops.

SUMMARY

The initial assessment, focused history, and examination of the medical patient provide the information necessary to identify circulatory compromise. The strength of the radial pulse is a simple indicator of perfusion status. By assessing other vital signs, gathering patient information and looking for possible causes such as dysrhythmias, blood loss caused by trauma, fluid loss resulting in dehydration, congestive heart failure and anaphylaxis, the paramedic can provide specific treatment needed to save the patient's life.

SUGGESTED READINGS

American Heart Association: Textbook of Advanced Cardiac Life Support, 1994, Dallas, American Heart Association.

Cummins: ACLS Scenarios: Core Concepts for Case-Based Learnings, 1996, St. Louis, Mosby Year Book.

Jim Hayes, MD, FACEP

Chapter 21

The Critical Trauma Patient

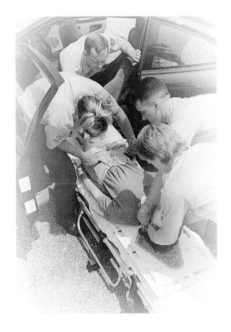

KEY TERMS

1. **Glasgow Coma Scale (GCS)** — a standardized rating system used to evaulate the degree of responsiveness impairment based on eye opening, motor response, and verbal response.

3. **Mechanism of injury** — the event or forces that caused the patient's injury.

4. **Revised Trauma Score (RTS)** — a standardized injury severity index that incorporates the Glasgow Coma Scale and measurements for the systolic blood pressure and respiratory rate.

5. **Trauma center** — a hospital specially equipped and staffed to handle trauma patients.

A paramedic should be able to:

OBJECTIVES

1. Describe the relationship of time (the Golden Hour) to the care of the critical trauma patient.

2. Discuss the goals of trauma assessment in the prehospital setting.

3. Discuss the relevance of trauma scoring systems in the prehospital setting.

4. Given a scenario involving a trauma patient, calculate the Glasgow Coma Score and the Revised Trauma Score.

5. Describe the systematic process used to rapidly assess and manage trauma during:
   a. Initial assessment
   b. Focused history and physical examination
   c. Continued assessment

6. Explain why it is important to re-evaluate the critical patient.

7. Identify "load and go" trauma emergencies, and describe patient management in these situations.

8. Discuss assessment factors to consider for the critically injured pediatric patient.

9. Discuss assessment factors to consider for the critically injured pregnant patient.

10. Identify two specific traumatic conditions that can occur in the last trimester of pregnancy and the appropriate field management of them.

Trauma is the leading cause of death in the first 40 years of life in the United States, and is surpassed only by cancer and cardiovascular disease as a cause of death in all age groups. In patients under 34 years of age, trauma accounts for more deaths than all diseases combined. The total cost for trauma care in the United States is estimated at more than $100 billion annually.[2] Beyond the impact of lethal trauma injuries, survivors may have disabilities that last for months to years. To reduce the mortality and morbidity associated with trauma, greater emphasis must be placed on prevention, prehospital intervention, entry into the trauma system, definitive care, and rehabilitation.

This chapter provides an overview of the role that the mechanisms of force and energy play in the severity of a patient's injuries. The discussion in this chapter leads to an understanding of the types of situations that require rapid transport to a trauma center, the rapid assessment needed to make this determination and the type of care necessary for the critical trauma patient.

Causes of Critical Trauma

Trauma means injury, and critical trauma refers to a life-threatening injury caused either by blunt or penetrating force. Critical trauma results from a variety of mechanisms that include:

- Motor vehicle collisions involving other vehicles or pedestrians
- Falling from a height
- Work-related accidents
- Blast injuries
- Firearms
- Fire

These critical injuries occur as a result of the transfer of energy from some external source to the body. The type of energy transferred, the location of the energy transfer and the speed at which it occurs are all factors in the extent of the injury. *See* Chapter 16 for a comprehensive discussion of mechanism of injury.

Let's consider what happens when an unrestrained, 200-pound person strikes a utility pole while driving a vehicle at 65 mph. One law of motion states that the vehicle would stay in motion until acted upon by an outside force, such as the pole. The law of energy conversation dictates that energy cannot be created or destroyed; it only changes form. In this case, mechanical energy is immediately absorbed by the pole, vehicle, and driver. Severe tissue destruction occurs as the driver continues moving forward into the steering column and dashboard, and as the remainder of the car moves forward onto the driver. Considering the patient's size, the velocity of the vehicle, and the rate of deceleration, the body will be exposed to tremendous force and will transfer an incredible amount of energy. Because this impact exceeds the normal parameters the body can withstand, critical lethal injury is inevitable.

The Golden Hour

A patient may die within seconds to minutes following a critical injury, usually from major injury to the brain or cardiovascular system. If the patient survives the initial trauma, however, the next 60 minutes are critical. This time from initial trauma event until arrival of definitive care is commonly referred to as the "golden hour" of trauma care (Fig. 21-1). Patients who die in this time period often have airway problems, major internal injuries, hemorrhagic shock or a combination of injuries referred to as multisystem trauma. The paramedic plays a crucial role during this hour by maintaining the airway, providing oxygen, limiting hemorrhage, stabilizing major fractures, and beginning fluid replacement while transporting the patient rapidly to the hospital, where definitive care often takes place in the operating room.

Because the window of opportunity is so small, the goals of trauma assessment are to rapidly assess the scene and the patient, identify the patient as a high priority, enter the patient into the trauma system, and begin transport within 10 minutes of arrival on scene. Speed is especially important for agencies with long transport times. There are few exceptions to these goals; only situations such as extended extrication and hazards at the scene should prolong scene time. Optimum use of scene and transport time may mean summoning air medical support when extrication or long distance is involved.

The Trauma System

More than 800 of the approximately 6400 hospitals with emergency departments in the United States have a designated specialty in trauma.[1] These trauma centers are prepared to handle patients with varying degrees of injury (Fig. 21-2). There are four different levels of trauma centers. Levels I and II are the most advanced, with surgery teams on hand 24 hours a day. Trauma centers at these levels can handle the most complicated injuries such as gunshot and stab wounds, serious motor vehicle collisions, and severe burns. Patients

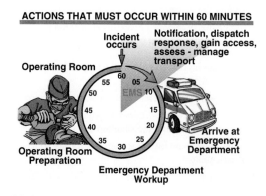

Figure 21-1

The greatest chance of survival occurs when the patient arrives in surgery within 60 minutes from the initial time of injury.

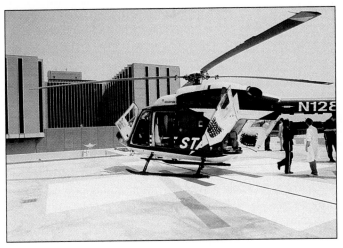

Figure 21-2

For a critically injured patient, definitive care is best provided by a trauma center. *From McSwain, et al: The Basic EMT, 1996, Mosby Lifeline.*

Prearrival Considerations

A number of elements of trauma care should be in place before a call for an EMS ambulance occurs. Local policies should address transport destinations for critical trauma patients. Although most emergency departments accept noncritical patients, there may be specialized facilities in an area that are designated for critical trauma patients. Some EMS systems have transport policies that call for transport directly to a trauma center, bypassing other hospitals. If transport times are long, such as in rural areas, stabilization may be achieved at a community hospital, with subsequent transfer to a trauma center.

An EMS system that uses a trauma center for critical patients usually has a protocol for identifying eligible patients. This avoids transporting critical patients to less capable hospitals and also minimizes the chance of transporting a noncritical patient to a trauma center.

with less severe injuries can be adequately cared for in level III and IV trauma centers. All of these facilities and out-of-hospital agencies work together closely to provide care in a coordinated trauma system.

Many trauma centers use air medical services to transport patients from areas where ground transport is not possible, or would delay the necessary care. Always consider air transport if environmental conditions allow for it and the patient's care would be enhanced.

Local protocols should define the process of:

1. Identifying a critical trauma patient.
2. Entering the patient into the trauma system.
3. Providing rapid ground or air transport to the level of trauma care appropriate to the patient's condition.

Trauma Scoring Systems

A number of scoring systems exist to evaluate which patients are best cared for in a trauma center. Although these systems can identify trauma patients who are clearly at high risk, none are as accurate in identifying less obviously injured patients who may have life-threatening injuries. Two examples of these scoring systems are the Glasgow Coma Scale and the Revised Trauma Score.[4] The Glasgow Coma Scale uses a 15-point system that evaluates eye opening, verbal response and motor response (Table 21-1). The Revised Trauma Score calls for an assessment of the patient's respiratory rate, systolic blood pressure, and Glasgow Coma Scale Score (Table 21-2).

Several studies have demonstrated that the paramedic can effectively determine which patients should be transported to a trauma center based on the patient assessment.[5,6,9,10] Other studies have identified a beneficial role in making the determination for on-line medical direction physicians working closely with EMS personnel.[3,8]

TABLE 21-1	Glasgow Coma Scale
Response	**Score**
Eye Opening	
Spontaneous	4
To voice	3
To pain	2
None	1
Verbal Response	
Oriented	5
Confused	4
Inappropriate words	3
Incomprehensible	2
None	1
Motor Response	
Obeys command	6
Localizes pain	5
Withdrawn (pain)	4
Flexion (pain)	3
Extension (pain)	2
None	1
Total GCS	1–15

TABLE 21-2	Revised Trauma Score		
Glasgow Coma Scale	**Systolic BP**	**Respiratory Rate**	**Points Assigned**
13–15	>89	10–29	4
9–12	76–89	<29	3
6–8	50–75	6–9	2
4–5	1–49	1–5	1
3	0	0	0

Note: The number of points in each of the three categories is assigned based on the observed measurement and then totaled. The lower the total score, the greater the likelihood for significant injury.

↘ **Scene Survey**

      Initial Assessment

        **Focused History
        and Physical Exam**

            Continued Assessment

Scene Survey

There are several items the paramedic must consider when approaching the trauma scene. The two most important are scene safety and mechanism of the injury.

Safety

The paramedic should always approach the scene in a manner that ensures rescuer safety. The presence of weapons, fire, unstable structures or vehicles, violent individuals or hazardous materials requires caution and consideration of the possible need for other resources. Making the scene safe can include summoning additional support, properly positioning the ambulance, placing flares or reflective warning devices, diverting traffic, and stabilizing damaged vehicles (*see* Chapter 15).

Mechanism of Critical Injury

Upon arriving at the scene, the rescuer should review the entire scene while looking at the mechanism of the injury. Generally, this means considering the external forces that could have caused injuries. For example, an overturned vehicle on an interstate highway is substantially different from a minor "fender bender" involving a car that backed out of a driveway and struck another vehicle. The first example has a much greater likelihood for serious injury because of the higher speed and rotational forces involved. Chapter 16 provides a thorough explanation of mechanism of injury, including distinct types of trauma that can result in critical injuries.

Scene Survey

   ↘ **Initial Assessment**

        **Focused History
        and Physical Exam**

            Continued Assessment

Initial Assessment and Management

The systematic approach to patient assessment described in previous chapters also applies to the critical trauma patient. The focus of this assessment is recognition and management of immediate life threats (Table 21-3). This process does not require a lengthy examination. The examination should be focused on identifying and correcting problems such as:

- Patient unresponsiveness resulting in the inability to maintain an open airway
- Airway compromise.
- Breathing compromise resulting from a flail chest or tension pneumothorax.
- Circulatory compromise caused by internal or external bleeding.

The determination of a trauma patient's level of consciousness (LOC) is one of the most important indicators of the patient's overall condition, especially in the presence of a head injury. The AVPU scale can be used to determine the patient's level of responsiveness (*see* Chapter 17).

The jaw-thrust technique should always be used when opening the airway of a patient believed to have head or neck trauma. After the airway is opened, the head should be maintained in-line with the body. If the airway is not patent, standard procedures for relieving an obstructed airway should be employed. If necessary, a laryngoscope can be used to visualize the larynx directly and remove any foreign body, while maintaining in-line stabilization. Oral or nasal airways may be appropriate to help maintain an open airway, but should be used cautiously in patients with severe facial, nasal, or oral trauma.

With an adequate airway ensured, the paramedic should check for the presence of breathing, as well as breathing rate and quality. If the patient is having difficulty breathing, oxygen can be proivded through a nonrebreathing mask at 15 L/min. If breathing rate and effort are abnormal or if the patient is not breathing, the paramedic should assist ventilations with a bag-

TABLE 21-3 Initial Evaluation of the Critical Trauma Patient

Critical Observations	Critical Actions
Alertness	
What happened?	Check response to stimulation
Can you speak?	
Airway	
Can patient talk?	Protect C-spine
Airflow?	Jaw thrust
	Clear airway
	Clear obstruction
	Consider oral or nasal airway
	Endotracheal intubation
	Needle cricothyrotomy
Breathing	
Rate of respirations?	Assist ventilations
Quality of breath sounds?	Apply oxygen
	Chest decompression
Circulation	
Carotid pulse present?	CPR if pulseless
	Control hemorrhage
Radial pulse present?	Vascular access
Capillary refill <2 seconds?	PASG
	Fluid replacement

valve-mask or demand valve. In-line cervical stabilization should be maintained at all times while ventilating the patient. If the patient cannot be ventilated, endotracheal intubation should be performed (*see* Skill #37 in Skills Section).

Patient circulation can be checked by examining the pulse at the carotid and radial artery sites. Distal pulses could be diminished or absent as a result of injury to the extremity; if this is suspected, the other extremity should be checked as well. A pulse present in the radial arteries indicates a systolic blood pressure of approximately 80 mm Hg. If the pulse is only present at the carotid arteries, the systolic blood pressure is closer to 60 mm Hg. In both cases, the pulse is only one indicator of possible compromised circulation.

A rapid evaluation of the patient's skin provides additional information about circulatory status. While feeling the pulse, the paramedic can also determine the patient's skin temperature, color, condition, and the rate of capillary refill. Patients with cool, pale, and moist skin, and patients with slow capillary refill must be presumed to have a serious problem associated with **hypoperfusion.** Any severe external bleeding discovered should be controlled. Rapid transportation is important for the patient who has suffered severe blood loss, especially when internal bleeding is likely.

In the presence of shock, the patient requires rapid transport to a trauma center. The paramedic can apply the PASG according to local protocols (*see* Skill #35 in Skills Section). Fluid resuscitation can be initiated with normal saline or lactated Ringer's en route to the receiving facility or on scene while awaiting extrication or air transport. Whenever possible, this intervention should be initiated with a large-bore IV catheter. Transportation should not be delayed to start an IV line.

The initial assessment steps usually take less than 30 seconds to complete, unless the need arises to intervene along the way. The focused history and examination of the trauma patient will cover the head, neck, and chest in more detail, and reconsider the mechanism of the injury, looking for causes of airway, breathing, and circulation problems.

Scene Survey

Initial Assessment

Focused History and Physical Exam

Continued Assessment

Focused History and Physical Examination

The focused history and examination determines additional problems that the patient may have and may also reveal information about the severity of the patient's condition. This process involves a rapid physical examination and brief patient history. Although the medical history is important for a patient with a sudden illness, it is less likely to be pertinent to the

trauma patient's condition, unless the trauma was the direct result of a medical condition. In trauma, mechanism of injury is the more critical aspect of history.

It is important for the paramedic to record a baseline set of vital signs, including respirations, lung sounds, pulse, blood pressure, skin, heart rhythm, and pupil status. When assessing vital signs, the paramedic must consider the average parameters for patients of different ages. Any abnormalities in these areas should be noted and further explored after determining pertinent transport. Initially, it is enough to recognize problems that require intervention.

During the physical examination, the paramedic should look and feel for abnormalities in the patient's body. The most significant problems associated with trauma are those affecting the head, neck, back, chest, abdomen, pelvis, and femur. The acronym DCAP—BTLS is a useful way to remember the areas to assess (*see* Box 21-1).

The patient's head and neck can be examined while another rescuer maintains in-line stabilization. The rescuer should look and feel for obvious deformities and also for bleeding from the patient's head or ears. Blood-tinged fluid seeping from the patient's ears could be cerebrospinal fluid, which would indicate a skull fracture. The neck should be examined for abnormalities, such as a deviated trachea, which would indicate a possible tension pneumothorax. After completing the neck examination, the paramedic should apply a cervical collar to the patient.

The patient's chest should be examined by palpating the sternum and ribs and auscultating breath and heart sounds. The presence of pain could mean anything from a bruise to flail chest. Distant or muffled heart sounds may indicate pericardial tamponade. The absence of lung sounds on one side of the chest can signify a lung injury, such as a tension pneumothorax.

The four quadrants of the abdomen should be assessed for discoloration, pain, tenderness, distention, and rigidity. Organs in the abdomen can easily be injured, and some organs may bleed profusely.

The paramedic should examine the pelvis by first checking for pain. If the patient is not in obvious pain, gentle compression can be applied to the pelvis to verify that it is intact.

This phase of the patient assessment should only last 1 to 2 minutes. At this point, there is enough information to determine the severity of the patient's injuries, the level of trauma care required, the speed of transport indicated, and the need for additional care en route.

BOX 21-1	DCAP-BTLS Acronym for Evaluating Injuries

Deformities
Contusions
Abrasions
Punctures
Burns
Tenderness
Lacerations
Swelling

Scene Survey

Initial Assessment

Focused History
and Physical Exam

Continued Assessment

Continued Assessment

The final phase of patient assessment, the detailed examination, can be completed en route to the hospital, unless critical therapy prevents it. A more thorough physical assessment may uncover additional injuries, although these findings will usually not change care required for the most serious injuries.

Some signs may only appear upon closer examination. The paramedic should look for emerging signs of bruising in the area of the patient's eyes (raccoon's eyes) and behind the ears (Battle's Sign). The pupils can be examined for size and reactivity to light. Pupils that are unequal or that fail to react to light in the presence of head trauma, indicate a significant head injury.

Reevaluation of the trauma patient is vital. The patient may appear stable at one moment and quickly deteriorate as internal injuries take their toll. The critical trauma patient should be reevaluated every 3 to 5 minutes during transport.

When the patient has any one of these conditions, he or she should be transferred to a backboard, given oxygen, and loaded and transported to the nearest appropriate hospital. Some critical life support procedures are performed at the scene, such as managing the airway, controlling severe bleeding, sealing a sucking chest wound, decompressing a tension pneumothorax, applying a traction splint or PASG, and initiating CPR. Before starting other treatment, however, the paramedic must weigh the time that it will take to perform the procedure against the benefit to the patient.

IV access and fluid replacement can be accomplished en route with large-bore IV catheters and liter bags of lactated Ringer's or normal saline. The necessary amount of fluid to administer remains controversial. At present, crystalloid solutions are replaced at a rate of 20 mL/kg body weight up to 3 L in an adult. After this, blood must be given to keep up with ongoing hemorrhage. However, some physicians believe that the absence of blood clotting elements in crystalloid solutions and the increase in blood pressure actually cause more rapid blood loss in a patient.

Further controversy exists in regard to the use of the PASG. Although this garment has been shown to be effective as a splint for pelvic fractures, many physicians now believe this is its only true benefit, and that the garment should not be inflated in the presence of closed head or chest injury or with eviscerations or impaled penetrating objects. Local protocols should be followed regarding application of the PASG (*see* Chapter 46).

Managing the Critical Trauma Patient

Load and Go Situations

Critical trauma patients require rapid transport, with additional intervention performed en route. Perfect immobilization techniques are inappropriate if they require 15 to 20 minutes to complete. In critical "load and go" situations, the paramedic bypasses certain procedures that would be performed for less critical patients. For example, a paramedic should not take the time to apply a KED or similar immobilization device to a critical trauma patient inside a motor vehicle. Instead, with the help of other EMS personnel, apply a cervical collar, place the backboard at an angle and slide the patient out of the vehicle (*see* Fig. 21-3). This patient likely needs surgical intervention, not perfect immobilization. This means rapid identification of critical conditions and transport to a trauma center.

Load and go situations include any trauma patient with:

- Decreased level of responsiveness
- Airway or breathing difficulty
- Compromised circulation (shock, hypoperfusion)
- Unequal pupils
- Tender, rigid, distended abdomen
- Unstable pelvis
- Bilateral femur fractures

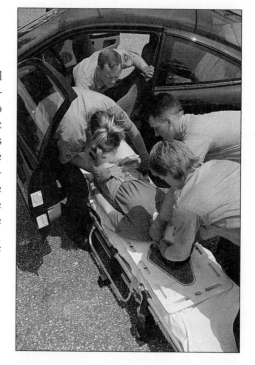

Figure 21-3

Rapid extrication is required whenever a trauma patient is critically injured.

Special Considerations

Pediatric Trauma

Although children are susceptible to the same injury mechanisms as adults, a child's anatomic, physiologic, and psychologic responses to trauma are unique. These responses are covered in detail in Chapter 22. Blunt trauma accounts for 87% of childhood trauma; penetrating injuries comprise only 10%, and the remaining 3% are related to drowning.[7] Falls and vehicle collisions cause nearly 80% of all pediatric injuries. Nonaccidental trauma or child abuse must always be a consideration as well. Multisystem injury is the rule rather than the exception, so all organ systems must be assumed to be injured until proven otherwise. Sadly, many pediatric injuries could be prevented with wider use of devices such as child restraint seats in automobiles.

Because children are smaller than adults, blunt trauma usually results in forces and impacts distributed over a larger portion of the body. Whereas an adult might sustain a leg fracture from an automobile-pedestrian collision, the small child may have chest, abdominal, and head injuries from the same mechanism. Growing bones that are not yet fully calcified may not break. Ribs may not be fractured, for example, but a pulmonary contusion can still be present.

Because children's heads are proportionally larger and heavier when compared with the rest of their bodies, head injuries occur with greater frequency, especially when sustaining multiple injuries.

Additionally, the proportionately large head size means that placing the patient supine on a flat surface is likely to flex the neck. This poses two potential problems: aggravation of a spinal injury secondary to flexion of cervical vertebrae and partial airway obstruction caused by tongue position and "kinking" of the flexible trachea. Figure 21-4 illustrates proper immobilization of a pediatric trauma patient. The smaller size of pediatric airways, combined with a tendency for children to produce more airway secretions than adults do, further prioritizes two factors early in the assessment process: attention to possible obstruction and readiness to provide suction when needed.

The large surface area relative to body weight means that a child is more prone to hypothermia; extra care must be taken to preserve the injured child's body temperature.

In the pediatric patient, shock is not defined by any specific blood pressure value. Because a child is better able to tolerate rapid heart rates and to increase peripheral vascular resistance than the adult, the child is more capable of maintaining normal blood pressures in the face of hemorrhagic shock. Normal systolic blood pressure for a child can be estimated with the following formula:

Systolic blood pressure = 80 mm Hg + (2 × age in years). Any blood pressure that is more than 10 mm Hg lower than this value should raise the concern about possible occult hemorrhage.

The child's heart rate should be monitored closely; tachycardia is the earliest manifestation of shock. Capillary refill should also be monitored in the infant and child.

Chest injuries in a child are similar to those in an adult, including pneumothorax, hemothorax, pulmonary contusion, pericardial tamponade, and cardiac contusion. Because of the elasticity of growing bones, children have a relatively low incidence of rib and sternal fractures and flail chest. Yet, pulmonary contusions are the most common serious injury resulting from blunt chest trauma. A large hemothorax may cause deadly hemorrhagic shock in a child. It is important for the paramedic to be suspicious of internal chest injuries based on signs of trauma, such as bruising or even the mechanism of injury itself. The child's abdominal organs lie close together in a small space and have less protection from injury than those of an adult. Consequently, the abdominal organs are at increased risk of injury. The spleen is the most commonly injured organ, followed by the liver, in blunt trauma.

Accidental falls and child abuse are also among the sources of pediatric blunt trauma that are seen most often. Special categories of frequent injury include burns, drowning, and penetrating trauma; gunshot wounds are also surprisingly common.

Extremity injuries require special awareness in several areas. Femur fractures can easily be overlooked during hasty surveys. Also, closed fractures can account for more serious blood loss in children than those in adults. This is especially true of femur fractures but also can be true at other sites.

Damage to epiphyseal (growth) plates in long bone fractures is of particular significance. The growth plates lie in the rounded "bulbs" at both ends of long bones. Special caution is needed to avoid aggravation of suspected fractures at or near the joints. Fracture damage and careless movement during emergency care can damage the epiphysis or separate it from the bone shaft, compromising later bone growth. For this reason, pediatric long bone fractures are splinted as found when possible and repositioning of dislocations is discouraged.

The Pediatric Trauma Score (Table 21-4) and the Children's Modified Glasgow Coma Scale (Table 21-5) can assist paramedics with patient management and communication of information to the receiving facility.

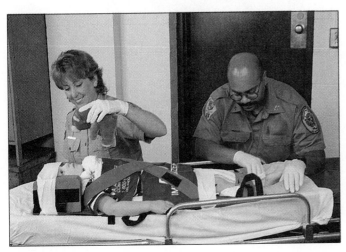

Figure 21-4

Proper pediatric immobilization requires that padding be placed under the shoulders and along the spine to allow the airway to remain open in the "sniffing" position.

TABLE 21-4	Pediatric Trauma Score		
Component	**+2**	**+1**	**−1**
Size	>20 kg	10–20 kg	<10 kg
Airway	Normal	Maintainable	Unmaintainable
Systolic BP	>90 mm Hg	90–50 mm Hg	>50 mm Hg
CNS (LOC)	Awake	Obtunded/LOC	Coma/decerebrate
Open wound	None	Minor	Major/penetrating
Skeletal	None	Closed	Open/multiple fractures

A sum of less than eight = transport to trauma center.

TABLE 21-5	Children's Modified Glasgow Coma Scale	
	Infants	**Children/Adults**
Eye Opening		
4	Spontaneous	Spontaneous
3	To speech	To verbal stimuli
2	To pain	To pain
1	No response	No response
Best Motor Response		
6	Normal spontaneous movement	Follows commands
5	Withdraws to touch	Localizes pain
4	Withdraws to pain	Withdraws to pain
3	Abnormal flexion	Abnormal flexion to pain
2	Abnormal extension	Abnormal extension to pain
1	No response	No response
Best Verbal Response		
5	Coos and babbles	Oriented
4	Irritable cries	Confused
3	Cries to pain	Inappropriate words
2	Moans to pain	Incomprehensible words
1	No response	No response

Vascular access may involve peripheral sites or, if they are unobtainable, the intraosseous route (*see* Skill #25 in Skills Section). Treatment of shock involves infusing 20 mL/kg of lactated Ringer's solution or normal saline as a fluid bolus. This can be repeated up to two times, depending on the clinical response.

Trauma During Pregnancy

Critical trauma in a patient who is pregnant creates special challenges that arise out of two key areas:

- The remarkable anatomic and physiologic changes that occur with pregnancy (*see* Chapter 37).
- The automatic presence of two patients: the mother and the fetus.

Although injury patterns and severity may vary because of pregnancy, the treatment priorities are the same as those used to treat other patients. Survival of mother and fetus is influenced by the extent of injuries. Fetal survival is dramatically influenced by the presence of shock and hypoxia.

During pregnancy, the mother's cardiac output increases by approximately 40% by the tenth week of gestation and remains elevated until delivery. Heart rate increases gradually until the third trimester, during which it increases by another 10 to 15 beats/min. Systolic and diastolic blood pressures typically decrease by 5 to 15 mm Hg by the second trimester and return to normal near the time of birth.

When the pregnant patient is in a supine position, the enlarged uterus exerts enough pressure on the vena cava to cause hypotension by decreasing venous return and cardiac output. Once the patient is secured to the backboard, elevating the right side of the backboard will relieve the vena cava compression and improve venous return (Fig. 21-5).

Depth of respirations increases during pregnancy. Because of the upward pressure of the enlarging uterus on the diaphragm and several other physiologic changes, the pregnant patient also has less respiratory reserve, or the ability to compensate for respiratory problems. This can be important for the pregnant patient who has a chest injury or who is in shock.

The uterus grows up to 20 times its original size by the final days of pregnancy. As it assumes a prominent position in the abdomen and rises out of the pelvis, the uterus becomes more susceptible to injury.

As a result of these anatomical and physiological changes, the evaluation of the pregnant trauma victim can be difficult.

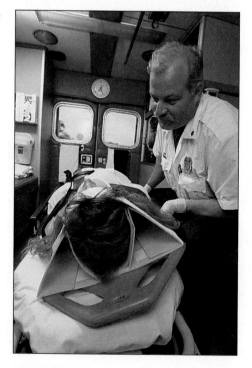

Figure 21-5

Vena cava compression is relieved by placing the immobilized patient in the left lateral recumbent position. This promotes venous return from the lower extremities and improves fetal circulation.

When catecholamines are produced in response to shock, uterine blood flow decreases to shunt blood to vital organs. Because the uterus has no means of regulating blood flow, the mother can appear clinically stable, while the fetus is in shock.

Treatment priorities do not change for critical trauma in a patient who is pregnant. An initial assessment is followed by a focused history and examination, and appropriate actions are based on the clinical findings. Liberal use of oxygen and aggressive treatment of shock are of primary importance. If a pregnant patient sustains blunt trauma, complains of severe abdominal pain and is hypotensive, the paramedic should consider the possibility of a ruptured uterus. This is a catastrophic injury that can be lethal for both mother and fetus. Occasionally, this patient may present with minimal signs and symptoms. Treatment is the same as for other critical trauma patients, with emphasis on minimizing scene time and transporting rapidly to a hospital where definitive care can be provided. Unfortunately, fetal survival is rare with uterine rupture.

A complication that occurs more often than a ruptured uterus is placenta abruptio, in which the placenta tears away from the uterine wall. This complication is the most common cause of fetal death in mothers who survive their injuries. The patient complains of abdominal pain and may have vaginal bleeding. The pregnant patient should be transported positioned on her left side or supine with the right side of the spine board elevated to approximately 15° to avoid hypotension associated with uterine compression of the vena cava.

Although two patients are being treated, it is important for the paramedic to remember that the best treatment for the fetus is appropriate assessment and treatment of the mother.

SUMMARY

Systematic patient assessment skills provide the most effective means of determining the critical trauma patient's problems and deciding if transport is warranted. A consistent approach should be employed, whether the patient is adult, pediatric, or pregnant, to ensure that the patient receives the best possible care. That care is aimed at intervening in life-threatening processes and limiting potential disability from injuries.

REFERENCES

1. **American Hospital Association:** Hospital Statistics 1994—1995, American Hospital Association, 1994.

2. **American College of Surgeons:** Textbook for advanced trauma life support program, 1993.

3. **Champion HR, Sacco WJ, Gainer PS, et al:** The effect of medical direction on trauma triage. *J Trauma* 28:235—239, 1988.

4. **Champion HR, Sacco WJ, Copes WS, Gann DS, Gennarelli TA, Flanagan ME:** A revision of the trauma score. *J Trauma* 29:623—629, 1989.

5. **Emerman CL, Shade B, Kubuncanek J, et al:** A comparison of EMT judgment and prehospital trauma triage instruments. *J Trauma* 31:1369—1375, 1991.

6. **Hedges JR, Feero S, Moore B, Haver DW, Shultz B:** Comparison of prehospital trauma triage instruments in a semirural population. *J Emerg Med* 5:197—208, 1987.

7. **Inaba AS, Seward PN:** An approach to pediatric trauma. In Burkle FM, Wiebe RA, (eds): Pediatric Emergencies. *Emerg Med Clin North Am* 9:523—548, 1991.

8. **Neely KW, Norton R, Bartkus E, et al:** The effect of base station contact on ambulance destination. *Ann Emerg Med* 19:906—909, 1990.

9. **Ornata J, Mlinek EJ JR, Craren EJ, et al:** Ineffectiveness of the trauma score and the CRAMS scale for accurately triaging patient to trauma centers. *Ann Emerg Med* 14:1061—1064, 1985.

10. **Sloan EP, Koenigsberg M, Nolan J, et al:** EMS field trauma triage criteria in an urban trauma system. *Ann Emerg Med* 17(abstract):426, 1988.

Norman Christopher, MD
Loren Marshall, MA, EMT-P

Chapter 22

The Critical Pediatric Patient

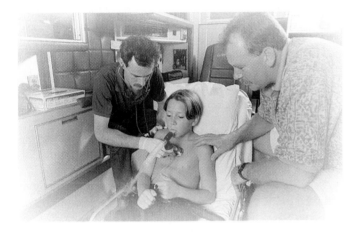

Pediatric emergency response presents special challenges, both emotional and behavioral. The complex relationships and dependencies that exist between children and caregivers can modify expected patient behavior. EMS providers sometimes feel that they are caring for two patients: the child and the guardian. A paramedic's sensitivity to the needs of both parties is necessary in this setting, although the paramedic's primary responsibility is to the child.

Another challenge in caring for critically ill children is the low number of life-threatening illnesses occuring in this population. Because it is unusual for a pediatric patient to require advanced life support, the assessment and treatment skills can be difficult to maintain. Consequently, it is very important for EMS providers to develop a systematic approach to the pediatric patient. This chapter primarily discusses the challenges of a critically ill pediatric patient. Traumatic injuries to the infant and child are discussed in Chapter 21.

Epidemiology of Critical illness and Trauma

Pediatric emergencies make up 10% or less of most EMS service call volumes. Many of the calls involve children in the first few years of life or adolescence, and the incidents often occur when unstructured play and outdoor activities are common. This time of occurance is frequently during the afternoon and early evening, on weekends, and in the summer months.[11]

Less than 5% of all prehospital pediatric calls involve life- or limb- threatening illness or injury.[5] When a serious injury does occur, EMS response may be too late to reverse the outcome. Morbidity is high among patients who do survive, leaving family members with significant emotional burdens.

Pre-existing conditions, birth defects, and sudden infant death syndrome (SIDS) account for most patient deaths in the first 12 months of life, although infection, injury, and respiratory failure also contribute significantly. Approximately 80% of all nontraumatic cardiopulmonary arrests in children occur within the first year of life; more than 50% of these occur within the first 3 months, when clinical assessment and treatment procedures are the most difficult.[7] After the first year of life, trauma is the leading cause of death in pediatric patients.[4]

Preparing for Pediatric Response

Equipment

A full range of age- and size-appropriate equipment must be readily available for use in pediatric emergencies (see Table 22-1). Unlike adult patients, for whom standard equipment sizes and doses of medication are conveniently available, the child's size will determine equipment needs and medication doses. The supplies needed can be estimated quickly by a length-based resuscitation device used to measure the child's height (see Fig. 22-1).

For basic life support procedures, such as CPR and airway clearing, patient age has long been the criterion for deciding what procedures are performed. For the purposes of CPR, a patient less than 1 year of age is considered an infant, and patients from 1 to 8 years of age are considered children.

Charts and special adjuncts such as the Broselow® tape are helpful, but published guidelines are only estimates. Paramedics should have a wide variety of equipment available and should be ready to use judgment at the time of assessment and treatment. In addition to equipment for managing airway, breathing, and circulation problems, pediatric immobilization equipment should be near at hand.

TABLE 22-1	Equipment Needs for Pediatric Resuscitation			
Age	Endotracheal tube ID (mm)	Laryngoscopy blade	Chest tube (Fr)	Nasogastric tube/Foley (Fr)
Newborn (1 kg)	2.5	0 st	8–10	5 (feeding)
Newborn (2–3 kg)	3.0	1 st	10–12	5–8 (feeding)
1 month	3.5			
6 months	3.5			8
1 year	4.0	1 st	16–20	
2–3 years	4.5		20–24	10
4–5 years	5.0	2	20–28	
6–8 years	6.0			10–12
10–12 years	6.5	2–3	28–32	12
> 14 years	7.0–8.5	3	32–42	>12

Vascular Access:

Age	Intracatheter Gauge
< 1 year	22, 24
1–12 years	18, 20
> 12 years	16, 18

Adapted from Barkin-Rosen: Emergency Pediatrics, ed 4, St. Louis, 1994, Mosby—Year Book.

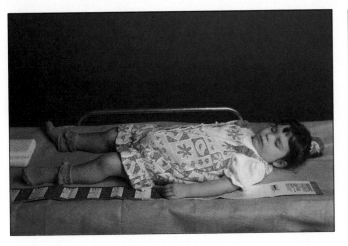

Figure 22-1

The Broselow resuscitation tape is used to quickly estimate a child's height and determine equipment needs and medication doses. *From Aehlert, B. Pediatric Advanced Life Support Study Guide, Hanover, 1994, Mosby Lifeline.*

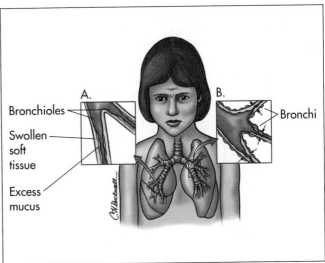

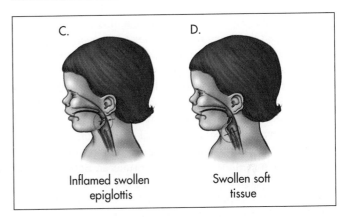

Figure 22-2

A, Bronchiolitis is caused by inflammation of distal aiways, which causes swelling and mucus secretion. B, Asthma is caused by constriction of the bronchi and viscus mucoid bronchial secretions. C, Croup is caused by an infection of the upper and lower airways, which causes soft-tissue swelling, particularly around the level of the cricoid cartilage. D, Epiglottitis is caused by the rapid swelling of the epiglottis, which can cause airway obstruction.

Managing Critical Conditions

Airway and Breathing Compromise

Respiratory failure is a condition characterized by inadequate oxygenation and ventilation. Although pulse oximetry now makes it possible to directly assess oxygenation, blood gas values such as carbon dioxide levels—an indicator of ventilatory adequacy—are not commonly used in the prehospital setting.

The paramedic relies on historical indicators and the physical examination to identify and treat respiratory distress in patients before it progresses to respiratory failure and subsequent circulatory compromise. It is critically important for the paramedic to recognize early signs and symptoms of respiratory distress and to anticipate the required interventions (*see* Chapter 25).

Anatomic airway obstruction

Children are more likely to have anatomic airway obstructions than adults. Infections can cause swelling in the posterior pharynx, and other factors can constrict air passages and reduce air flow. The child's large tongue, relative to the size of the oropharynx, can also cause obstruction, especially in the supine, unresponsive child. Four diseases that commonly cause airway obstruction problems are discussed in the following paragraphs.

Bronchiolitis

Bronchiolitis is an obstructive lower airway process that may present much similar to asthma (tachypnea, wheezing, prolonged expiration), but the primary cause of bronchiolitis is different. Bronchiolitis is caused by inflammation of distal airways (the bronchioles) which then causes swelling and mucus secretion (Fig. 22-2A). The result is a narrowing airway which obstructs expiration and leads to air trapping. The inflammation can be the result of viral infection, especially with the virus known as RSV (respiratory syncytial virus) or of allergic reaction.

Differentiation from asthma can be difficult, but several distinguishing factors may be present. Bronchiolitis is seasonal, occurring most frequently in the winter and spring months, and appears primarily in the age group under 18 months of age. Asthma is rare in children less than 1 year of age. Bronchiolitis also often accompanies upper respiratory tract infection (URI), so typical URI symptoms such as mild fever, runny nose, and a cough may be present.

Bronchiolitis is quite common and seldom dangerous, but occasionally it progresses to the point of severe hypoxia, progressive respiratory failure, and even respiratory arrest. It may also accompany or lead to dehydration or pneumonia, so an examination that covers all systems, and focuses especially on signs of hypoxia and respiratory distress is important.

Patients' treatment is focused on correcting hypoxia and assisting ventilations when necessary. The latter, as usual, must begin with the paramedic's detection of early signs of patient respiratory failure, before the progression into dire, later stages. Humidified, high-concentration oxygen by mask is ideal if tolerated by the patient. Placing the patient in a position of comfort and allowing the patient close parental contact are likely to be important in obtaining cooperation.

Nebulized bronchodilators, such as albuterol, are sometimes recommended for patients with severe conditions. These medications do not directly treat the cause of the disease as they do with asthma, but they may cause enough dilation to briefly ease respiratory distress and improve oxygenation. Effective, long-term therapy for the infectious or allergic cause involves hospital treatment.

Asthma

Asthma, or reactive airway disease, is a common inflammatory disorder of the airways, characterized by bronchoconstriction and bronchial edema (Fig. 22-2B). Dyspnea, tachypnea, orthopnea, audible expiratory wheezes, and use of accessory respiratory muscles are also typically present in cases of asthma. Absence of wheezing in this setting can be a grave sign; airways may have progressed to nearly total constriction, in which air movement is inadequate even to produce wheezing. Common trigger factors for asthma attacks are food, exercise, cold air, emotional stress, drugs such as aspirin, and allergens such as dust, pollen, and lint.

Management of an acute asthma attack includes administration of humidified oxygen, reversal of the bronchoconstriction, and rapid transport (Fig. 22-3). A calm, reassuring caregiver is also important to the asthma sufferer. Severe asthma attacks may require airway and ventilatory assistance and circulatory support. Nebulized albuterol and terbutaline are medications often used, and subcutaneous epinephrine may be necessary in severe asthma cases. A steroid preparation may be called for when transport time will be prolonged (*see* Box 22-1).

Status asthmaticus is a prolonged, severe attack that is unresponsive to therapy. This condition is a medical emergency in which responders should anticipate the possibility of respiratory arrest. The child in status asthmaticus is typically exhausted, acidotic, and dehydrated, and has a distended chest caused by trapped air that cannot be exhaled through constricted airways. Airway control, IV fluids, and rapid transport are essential in this condition.

Croup

The technical term for croup, laryngotracheobronchitis, suggests an infection that can involve nearly the entire length of the airway system. In its severest form, it is primarily a problem of upper airway obstruction caused by swelling of the soft tissue around the trachea. This condition can significantly narrow the tracheal lumen, particularly around the level of the cricoid cartilage below the glottis (Fig. 22-2C).

Croup is a viral infection that most commonly occurs in the late fall and early winter months and in children no more than 3 years of age. The condition is often preceded by the gradual onset (over several days) of mild fever or signs of upper respiratory tract illness. Development of inspiratory stridor signifies tracheal narrowing, and swelling of the vocal cords may also cause a barking cough. Lower respiratory involvement sometimes adds wheezing to the symptoms. The most severe episodes can lead to respiratory distress with all of its classic signs.

Symptoms of croup are usually worse at night and are often relieved by cool, humidified air. Keeping the patient outdoors for a moment before transport or opening an ambulance window can also help provide the cool air that often reduces respiratory distress. Allowing the child to inhale the mist produced by running a shower in a closed bathroom for a few minutes is also sometimes helpful.

Although airway obstruction may be significant, intubation is usually not required. Prehospital therapy includes cool, humidified oxygen and a position of comfort. "Comfort" extends to anything that reduces patient anxiety; crying aggravates swelling and breathing difficulty. Some EMS systems use nebulized racemic epinephrine to help reduce swelling. The effects of epinephrine may wear off shortly, however, so immediate hospital transport is mandatory.

Epiglottitis

Epiglottitis is a less common condition but considerably more life threatening than croup. Epiglottitis is characterized

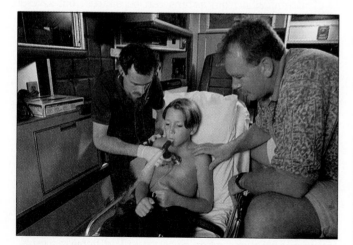

Figure 22-3

Management of an acute asthma attack includes humidified oxygen, reversal of the bronchoconstriction, and rapid patient transport.

BOX 22-1	Pediatric Asthma Pharmacology

- Oxygen
  Humidified, nonrebreather mask
- Albuterol
  Metered Dose Inhaler (MDI)—1 to 2 inhalations every 4 to 6 hours
  Rotohaler—1200 mg Rotocap, may repeat × 1
  Solution—0.03 mL/kg up to 0.5 mL total in 2 mL NS in nebulizer
- Terbutaline
  Metered Dose Inhaler (MDI)—2 inhalations every 4 to 6 hours
  Solution—0.03 mL/kg up to 0.5 mL NS in nebulizer
- Epinephrine 1:1000
  SQ 0.01 mg/kg to maximum of 0.3 mg
- Methylpredisolone
  1 to 2 mg/kg IV push

by the rapid onset of swelling of the epiglottis and subsequent respiratory distress, usually without recognizable earlier illness (Fig. 22-2D). The condition typically occurs in patients between 3 and 7 years of age. Sore throat, pain when swallowing, muffled voice, and drooling are also typical symptoms. The swelling may progress to complete airway obstruction, particularly if the child is agitated or anxious, or if the throat is stimulated.

The patient often presents sitting, sometimes with his or her head extended and tongue protruding, and the patient usually still and quiet—all are indications of the struggle to pass air and the patient's anxiety about progressive obstruction. The possibility of inspiratory stridor and the general signs of respiratory distress can make epiglottitis difficult to differentiate from croup. Patient age and history (e.g., rapidity of onset, absence of preceding illness) may help, and the presence of drooling and throat pain are likely indicators of epiglottitis.

When caring for this patient, the paramedic should withhold all anxiety– provoking procedures, including airway visualization, IV initiation, and removal of the child from parents. Sudden and complete airway obstruction can occur if the child becomes agitated. If complete obstruction does develop, bag-valve-mask ventilation may force air around the obstruction.

Intubation is very difficult and requires insertion of a small endotracheal tube; however, this procedure should not be attempted in the field, short of the occurrence of total airway obstruction and apnea. Swelling may make intubation impossible; paramedics must also be ready for needle cricothyrotomy, and ventilation with transtracheal jet insufflation if supported in local protocol (see Skills #9 and #10 in Skills Section).

Foreign body airway obstruction

Children with **foreign–body airway obstructions** can present either dramatically or subtly. A high index of suspicion may be required for the paramedic to spot the condition quickly. Aspiration is most common in young children who are just becoming mobile and whose curiosity leads them to place small objects in the mouth. Because this incident may not have been noticed by a parent, the expected history of choking or gagging may be absent. A patient's repeated coughing can indicate an effort to expel the object.

The paramedic should attempt to relieve the object if it causes complete obstruction or near-total obstruction as indicated by stridor or a weak, ineffective cough. However, the paramedic should avoid blind finger sweeps of the oropharynx, because this action may push the object further into the airway. When indicated, a series of five abdominal thrusts (for older children) or an alternating cycle of five back blows and five chest thrusts (for infants) should be used to relieve the obstruction (also see Chapter 18 for illustrations). If repeated attempts fail, direct visualization of the upper airway with a laryngoscope, and manual removal of the object with Magill forceps may be necessary (see Skill #11 in Skills Section).

Respiratory distress and failure

All patients showing signs of respiratory distress should be assumed to be oxygen deficient (Fig. 22-4). Basic respiratory treatment, such as supplemental oxygen administration,

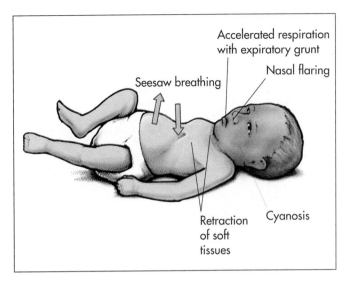

Figure 22-4

Common signs of respiratory distress include seesaw breathing, accelerated respiration with expiratory grunt, nasal flaring, cyanosis, and retraction of soft tissues.

should be performed in a nonthreatening manner to avoid causing anxiety to the child who is alert and responsive. Whenever possible, the patient should be allowed to assume a position of greatest comfort.

Simple maneuvers to open the airway should be initiated before more invasive techniques. A basic chin-lift or jaw-thrust maneuver is sometimes all that is required to reopen an obstructed airway in a child with a depressed level of responsiveness. Secretions, including vomit and blood, may need to be cleared when they interfere with the patient's respirations. An oral airway is appropriate in the patient at risk for obstruction because of a reduced level of responsiveness.

Failure to manage the airway is one of the most important causes of morbidity and mortality in otherwise salvageable patients. Aggressive patient airway management does not always require intubation. Although this is not a difficult procedure for the experienced paramedic, complications with endotracheal intubation in children are common.[8] Proper positioning and ventilatory assistance with 100% oxygen may be adequate. Before attempting invasive maneuvers, the paramedic should be thoroughly familiar with the anatomic and physiologic features unique to the pediatric airway (see Chapter 25).

Significant gastric distention may cause upward pressure on the diaphragm and restrict the effectiveness of ventilation. Placement of an orogastric or nasogastric tube will often increase the effectiveness of ventilation and decrease the risk of the patient vomiting and aspiration (see Fig. 22-5). The success of gastric decompression with this method is limited by the size of tube that the pharynx and proximal gastrointestinal tract will accept.

If prolonged ventilatory assistance is required in the patient, external compression of the esophagus (Sellick's maneuver) may further limit the risk of gastric distention, vomiting, and aspiration. In a supine child, gentle pressure placed downward over the trachea compresses the esophagus between the trachea and the spinal column. The procedure

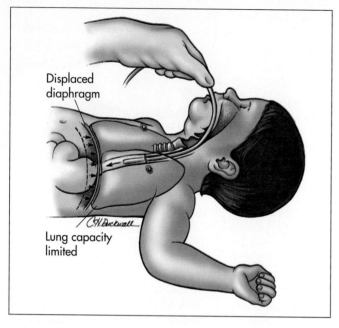

Figure 22-5

Gastric distention, which interferes with ventilation by causing pressure on the diaphragm, can be relieved by placement of an orogastric tube passed into the stomach.

requires caution in the very young child; the trachea is extremely compliant, and undue pressure can also result in airway compression or tracheal injury.

The anterior and cephalad position of the glottis in children makes blind nasotracheal intubation difficult. This technique is best reserved for patients older than 8 years of age. Because the tracheal rings are poorly developed and easily damaged in young children, cuffed endotracheal tubes should not be used in patients younger than 8 years of age. The normal subglottic narrowing in the pediatric airway serves as an anatomic cuff in younger children, which helps to secure the endotracheal tube and provides some protection against aspiration.

Surgical cricothyrotomy is contraindicated in children less than 12 years of age because of the difficulty in locating landmarks in these patients and the increased risk of severe bleeding. The surgical airway of choice in these patients, when needed, is needle cricothyrotomy with a large-bore catheter placed through the cricothyroid membrane (also see Skill 9 in Skills Section). Although this technique has several limitations, such as the need for specialized ventilation equipment, adequate oxygenation can usually be maintained in the patient until a tracheostomy can be performed at the hospital.

Once a patent airway is obtained, its monitoring and care should be the responsibility of a designated member of the resuscitation team. A displaced endotracheal tube can lead to rapid deterioration. Other complications include advancing the tube into a mainstem bronchus (usually the right side), major air leakage around the tube, loss of the oxygen source, development of a **pneumothorax,** and tube obstruction by a foreign body or mucous plug. If it is not possible to confirm the airway by physical examination or by direct visualization of the

tube passing through the cords, it should be assumed to be misplaced, and be removed. Respirations can be supported with bag-valve-mask ventilation until a new tube can be placed.

After securing the patient's airway, the rescuer should maximize oxygenation and ventilation, remembering that a patent airway alone does not guarantee adequate gas exchange. Because a relatively small pressure change results in a large change in lung volume, it is easy to confirm adequacy of ventilation by observing full and symmetric chest rise with each ventilation. Pulse oximetry is an excellent way to verify the paramedic's clinical assessment of a child's respiratory status, although the technology has limitations.[2]

Circulatory Compromise

Shock

Children with evidence of circulatory compromise require aggressive care. In these cases, the paramedic must secure a patent airway, maximize oxygenation and ventilation, and control serious external blood loss. IV access and fluid resuscitation should be initiated promptly.

Fluid replacement

Establishing IV access in a critical pediatric patient can be difficult, even for the experienced practitioner (see Skills #22–25 in Skills Section). Priority sites for IV access include the brachial and saphenous veins, because these veins generally maintain their diameter.

Although the external jugular vessels are large, they can be a difficult target in the child with a short, fat neck. Access is further complicated when a cervical collar is required, or when other advanced life support interventions limit the ability to maneuver near the patient's head and neck.

Intraosseous infusion is a safe, rapid, and effective means of administering fluids and medications when venous access is not available in pediatric patients[6]. Access sites are usually restricted to the proximal tibia and the distal tibia at the medial malleolus. The insertion site and surrounding tissues require careful monitoring for extravasation of fluid into soft tissue.[6]

Fluid therapy should be aggressively initiated in the prehospital environment when a child presents with clinical evidence of shock. The amount of fluid given depends upon the weight of the patient. The rescuer should administer a rapid fluid bolus of 20 mL/kg of normal saline or lactated Ringer's solution, followed by reassessment and additional infusions if necessary. Children with significant volume depletion may require repeat boluses to restore normal circulatory volume and function. Successful fluid resuscitation is indicated by the return of central and peripheral perfusion signs and by improved mental status.

Glucose-containing fluids should not be used for resuscitation, although boluses of a 10% or 25% glucose solution are given if **hypoglycemia** is documented or suspected. Using glucose-containing fluids for repeated volume doses can produce complications associated with **hyperglycemia,** such as intravascular fluid shifts.

Fluid overload can occur quickly in the pediatric patient, so the fluid administration rate must be monitored closely. A mini-drip IV set is used to minimize consequences of a "runaway" IV. Rales and "cardiac wheezing" are less common in children than in adults with congestive heart failure (CHF) and should be thought of as late findings when present in the pediatric patient with possible fluid overload. Peripheral edema and jugular venous distention, very useful findings in adults, are rarely present in children even with advanced heart failure. Pulmonary edema and CHF initially appear in children as tachypnea and tachycardia.

Hypothermia

When treating a critically ill or injured child, the paramedic should pay careful attention to maintaining core temperature. Infants and young children have a relatively large ratio of body surface area to volume and a relatively low subcutaneous fat content. Both of these factors predispose children to rapid heat loss. The thermoregulatory mechanisms of children are also underdeveloped. Compensatory responses that generate and conserve heat are only partially effective, resulting in a rapid decline in temperature if left exposed for even a short time. In addition, heat maintenance mechanisms are metabolically costly; these mechanisms lead to early development of fluid, electrolyte, and acid-base abnormalities. Cool IV fluids can also be a problem.

Hypothermia is often hard to differentiate from sepsis and shock. An initial catecholamine release results in tachycardia and redistribution of blood flow from the peripheral to the central circulation. In this early stage, physical signs include:

- Decreased perfusion caused by increased vascular resistance
- Normal or elevated blood pressure
- Mottled or cyanotic skin
- Early signs of decreasing level of consciousness

As hypothermia worsens, respiratory distress and even apnea may appear in the patient, and myocardial depression (bradycardia and other dysrhythmias) develops. Medications are not effective in a significantly hypothermic patient (<90° F or 32° C), making resuscitation difficult until rewarming has taken place.

Use passive external rewarming techniques to gradually improve the patient's temperature, bundling or covering the child during assessment and transport, especially when the environmental temperature is low. Because a significant amount of heat is lost through the scalp in newborns and infants, the patient's head should also be covered. Drying and passive external warming are simple but often neglected components of resuscitation in a newborn, infant, or young child.

Cardiac arrest

Although out-of-hospital cardiac arrest is unusual in children, outcomes are poor when this situation does occur. The expected mortality rate of pediatric prehospital cardiac arrest is 90%.[3] Often, the only children who survive are those whose arrest occurs in the presence of paramedics.[10] Cardiac arrest is rarely a sudden event and even less often is it caused by a primary cardiac problem; it is more likely the result of pro-

gressive deterioration in respiratory or circulatory function.[1] Therefore, the primary action in these cases is to establish an airway and ventilate the patient. Initiation of CPR, IV access, and pharmacologic treatment follow.

Children do not often present in ventricular fibrillation, so pediatric defibrillation is a rare occurrence. Bradydysrhythmias usually indicate significant respiratory or circulatory compromise and call more for direct attention to causes than for medication administration. If the patient's heart rate becomes too low to sustain life, CPR and other ACLS measures are indicated (see Figures 22-6 and 22-7).

CPR rates for children are faster than those of adults. For an infant, the paramedic should compress the patient's chest using two or three fingers at a rate of 100 or more times per minute. For a child, the paramedic should use the heel of one hand and compress the chest at 100 times per minute. Five compressions are given for each breath. The exception to this ratio is neonates, in whom the ratio is 3:1.

Vascular access can be gained through the IV or Intraosseous routes. The patient should be intubated and ventilated with high-concentration oxygen. Medications often include epinephrine, atropine and dopamine. Dosages are calculated by patient weight; some medications can be given

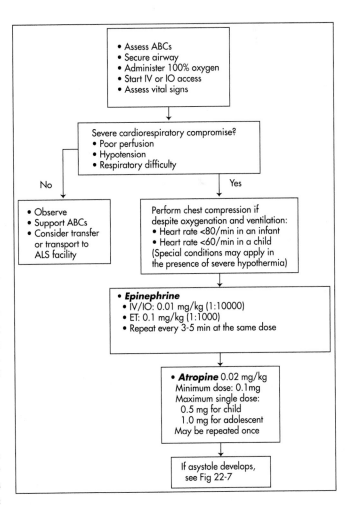

Figure 22-6

The bradycardia decision tree. *From JAMA, October 28, 1992, Vol. 268, No. 16, Copyright American Medical Association.*

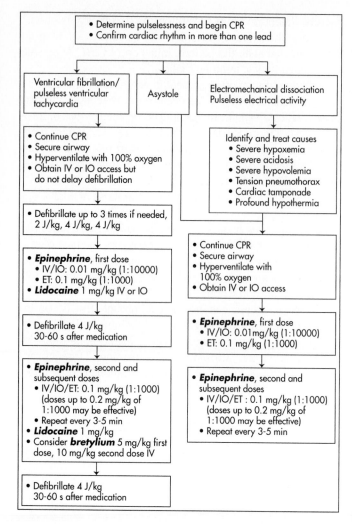

Figure 22-7

The asystole and pulseless arrest decision tree. *From JAMA, October 28, 1992, Vol. 268, No. 16, Copyright American Medical Association.*

through the endotracheal tube (*see* Table 22-2 for information on the drugs used in pediatric advanced life support).

Sudden Infant Death Syndrome (SIDS) Despite the common assumption among responders that an infant resuscitation is a SIDS response, prehospital caregivers cannot be certain during the response. SIDS is a diagnosis of exclusion, applied only when an autopsy and a full consideration of the child's history do not produce a clear cause of death.

By definition, a SIDS death is an unexpected event involving a healthy child. The huge majority of cases occur in the first 6 months of life, and a few cases occur between 6 months and the end of the first year. The incidence of SIDS deaths is highest during the cooler half of the year and during the late night or early morning hours while the infant is sleeping. Extensive research has identified general risk factors but no studies have proven any value in predicting or preventing the problem.

The issue of beginning infant resuscitation is a delicate one. Of course, any patient who is potentially viable should receive full resuscitative efforts. The emotional impact of infant death on families is so devastating that some EMS systems

have protocols that include at least limited resuscitations in situations when adult patients would not be treated (e.g., rigor mortis). Local protocols created in agreement with law enforcement and court officials must address this topic in detail.

Statistics on infant resuscitation in these cases are grim. The fact that few cardiac arrest patients survive underscores the primary role that paramedics play in providing emotional support to parents. As is the case with older children who are ill or injured, parents often feel guilt where none is warranted. They need complete support from prehospital responders, who must refrain from any speculation or advice that might imply negligence or wrongdoing.

This support is particularly important in view of the fact that some innocent infant deaths look suspiciously like abuse cases. Bloody froth from pulmonary edema that occurs in the final moments of life often appears in the baby's mouth, for instance. Paramedics must observe and document scene findings objectively and must report obvious signs of potential abuse, but their demeanor with parents should not vary from positive and supportive.

The other major service that responders can perform for parents and other family members is activation of support resources. One reason many services transport nonviable infants is the tremendous need for assistance that most parents have, and that need can be met at least initially through hospital social services and the contacts with support groups that hospital staff can provide. When the patient is not transported, paramedics may also be able to help by explaining police and coroner's procedures and contacting relatives or clergy for follow-up support.

Parents display the full spectrum of feelings and emotional intensity during pediatric emergencies, from numbness and disbelief to guilt and rage. Infant deaths are among the most stressful of responses for many public safety workers, who must look after their own feelings, those of their partners and colleagues, and those of the families involved. Counseling, formal debriefing or just one-on-one discussion with close friends can all be helpful, just as denial and isolation may be harmful (*see* Chapter 58).

Altered Level of Responsiveness

An altered level of responsiveness in an infant or child can have many causes. Box 22-2 identifies causes to consider. When caring for a child with a diminished level of responsiveness, the paramedic must monitor the patient's ability to protect the airway from aspiration and provide adequate oxygenation and ventilation. The airway is normally protected by both voluntary and involuntary mechanisms, such as the gag and swallowing reflexes, and normal muscle function and tone in the pharynx, mandible, and neck.

Neurologic injury and a depression in the level of responsiveness can affect any of these mechanisms, placing the child at increased risk of aspiration. Intubation and assisted ventilation should be considered when the child may not be able to protect the airway, when respiratory efforts are insufficient enough to support normal oxygenation and ventilation, and when increased intracranial pressure is suspected.

TABLE 22-2   Drugs Used in Pediatric Advanced Life Support

Drugs	Dosage (Pediatric)	Remarks
Adenosine	0.1–0.2 mg/kg Maximum single dose: 12 mg	Rapid IV bolus
Atropine sulfate*	0.02 mg/kg	Minimum dose: 0.1 mg Maximum single dose: 0.5 mg in child, 1.0 mg in adolescent
Bretylium	5 mg/kg; may be increased to 10 mg/kg	Rapid IV
Calcium chloride 10%	20 mg/kg	Give slowly.
Dopamine hydrochloride	2-20 μg/kg per min	α-Adrenergic action dominates at $\geq$ 15–20 μg/kg per min.
Dobutamine hydrochloride	2-20 μg/kg per min	Titrate to desired effect.
Epinephrine for bradycardia*	IV/IO: 0.01 mg/kg (1:10 000, 0.1 mL/kg) ET: 0.1 mg/kg (1:1000, 0.1 mL/kg)	Be aware of total dose of preservative administered (if preservatives are present in epinephrine preparation) when high doses are used.
Epinephrine for asystolic or pulseless arrest*	**First dose:** IV/IO: 0.01 mg/kg (1:10 000, 0.1 mL/kg) ET: 0.1 mg/kg (1:1000, 0.1 mL/kg) IV/IO doses as high as 0.2 mg/kg of 1:1000 may be effective. **Subsequent doses:** IV/IO/ET: 0.1 mg/kg (1:1000, 0.1 mL/kg) • Repeat every 3–5 min. IV/IO doses as high as 0.2 mg/kg of 1:1000 may be effective.	Be aware of total dose of preservative administered (if preservatives are present in epinephrine preparation) when high doses are used.
Epinephrine infusion	Initial at 0.1 μg/kg per min Higher infusion dose used if asystole present	Titrate to desired effect (0.1–1.0 μg/kg per min).
Lidocaine*	1 mg/kg	
Lidocaine infusion	20-50 μg/kg per min	
Naloxone*	If $\leq$ 5 years old or $\leq$ 20 kg: 0.1 mg/kg If > 5 years old or > 20 kg: 2.0 mg	Titrate to desired effect.
Sodium bicarbonate	1 mEq/kg per dose or 0.3 $\times$ kg $\times$ base deficit	Infuse slowly and only if ventilation is adequate.

*For ET administration dilute medication with normal saline to a volume of 3 to 5 mL and follow with several positive-pressure ventialtions. Reproduced with permission. Textbook of Pediatric Advanced Life Support, 1994. Copyright American Heart Association.

Assessment of perfusion and other indicators of cardiovascular and circulatory status should be performed, with fluid resuscitation initiated as necessary to maintain cerebral perfusion. The fluid volume should be limited when increasing intracranial pressure is a possibility.

The paramedic should maintain core temperature, gain IV access, and gather baseline (pretreatment) blood samples as indicated. If opiate toxicity is suggested either by history or examination (respiratory depression, pinpoint pupils), administration of IV naloxone is appropriate. If hypoglycemia is documented, or if immediate determination of the serum glucose is impossible and history suggests hypoglycemia, administration of IV or IO dextrose is indicated.

When trauma is suspected, the full spine should be immobilized with a backboard and the head maintained in line with the body, using a cervical collar and head immobilization device. Hyperventilation is useful to control rising intracranial pressure in the patient with cerebral edema, but the method has limits. The paramedic must avoid overaggressive hyperventilation that could cause an extreme drop in the patient's serum carbon dioxide level and actually lead to cerebral vasospasm and further reduction of blood flow. A rough guideline can be to bag ventilate the patient at a rate 1.5 to 2 times the normal respiratory rate. Depending on local protocols, the use of an osmotic diuretic, such as IV mannitol, may be indicated to reduce cerebral swelling when neurologic examination reveals posturing or dilated and unreactive pupils in the patient.

Hypoglycemia

Hypoglycemia is especially important to identify and treat in children with diminished responsiveness. Because of a child's inability to store large quantities of glucose and to mobilize rapidly what they can store, hypoglycemia is common in metabolically stressed children. Clinical evidence of low blood glucose is very nonspecific and can include lethargy, seizures, apnea and refractory dysrhythmias, such as bradycardia and asystole. This presentation makes blood testing especially useful. Resuscitation of an infant or child will be unsuccessful without correction of hypoglycemia.

BOX 22-2   Causes of Altered Level of Consciousness in Children

- Acute hydrocephalus
- Environmental causes
- Hypoxemia
- Infection
  Meningitis, encephalitis
  Cerebral abcess
- Mass lesions (neoplasm, abscess)
- Metabolic disease
  Electrolyte abnormalities
  Acid-base abnormalities
  Hypoglycemia
  Diabetic ketoacidosis
  Uremia
- Migraine headache
- Primary cardiac event
  Hypertensive crisis
  Dysrhythmia
- Seizures, postictal state
- Shock (hypovolemic, septic, anaphylactic)
- Toxic ingestion or exposure
- Trauma
  Subarachnoid hemorrhage
  Subdural hematoma
  Epidural hematoma
  Cerebral contusion
- Vascular disorders
  Spontaneous subarachnoid hemorrhage
  Venous or arterial thrombosis
  Vasculitis
  Cerebral embolism

A single IV dose of 25% dextrose should be given in a symptomatic child with a serum glucose below approximately 60 mg/dL. A normal newborn may have a serum glucose as low as 40 mg/dL, and if otherwise asymptomatic, does not require emergent glucose replacement. Local protocol should dictate the exact level below which dextrose must be administered; some systems may not order treatment until the level is below 45 mg/dL. Children usually receive dextrose in a 25% solution and newborns in a 10% solution; protocol must also address the age at which administration of adult-strength 50% dextrose is appropriate. Some systems advocate the use of 50% dextrose with patients over 2 years of age.

Seizures

In addition to all of the reasons that adults seize, pediatric patients have a category of their own: febrile (fever-related) seizures. Seizures are quite common in childhood, and they account for a significant fraction of EMS calls.

Most grand mal seizures (febrile seizures included) are self-limiting, require no intervention beyond protecting the patient from injury, and pose no serious threat. Paramedics see actual seizure activity rather infrequently; it is usually over with well before their arrival at the scene. Febrile seizures are most likely to occur when the patient's temperature rises quickly. Most seizures occur in children younger than school age, particularly in children younger than 2 years of age.

Determining the cause of a seizure requires careful history and often cannot be done with certainty in the field. Important points in the patient's history include the following:

- Previous seizures, including febrile seizures, or a diagnosis of epilepsy
- Medications taken, including compliance with any for known seizure problems
- Possibility of toxic ingestion or exposure
- Vomiting and possible aspiration during the seizure
- Recent trauma, particularly head injury
- Current fever or other signs of illness, especially headache or stiff neck (possible meningitis)
- Description of the seizure activity

The examination should focus initially on ABCs, particularly airway positioning and the need for suction, adequacy of respirations (accounting for both rate and depth), and oxygenation. Other factors include assessment of temperature, dehydration status, blood glucose level, and any trauma incurred during the seizure. The examination will often be performed on a postictal patient. If the patient is still seizing, attention to airway, breathing, and oxygenation is even more central. Most patients breathe during seizures, but rate and depth of respirations may not be adequate enough to provide the pulmonary circulation with the oxygen required during a period of extreme physical stress.

Management often involves no more than general support and transport for further evaluation. Most EMS protocols call for transport of all pediatric seizure patients, to ensure full evaluation of patients with first-time seizures or changes in their seizure patterns, and to ensure that cases of meningitis, for instance, are not left untreated. The rarer, major problems can present subtly, and it is easy for the paramedic index of suspicion to be dulled by the sheer volume of calls to febrile seizures.

Local protocol may call for cooling of febrile, postseizure patients above a certain body temperature. This procedure should be performed gradually with tepid water to avoid overcooling, which is a real risk in small patients who give up heat quickly. Protocols usually state a slightly febrile point at which to stop, such as 102° F (39° C), because the patient's body temperature is likely to continue to drop after active cooling is discontinued. Cooling can be completed in the ambulance and should not delay transport unnecessarily.

Testing the patient's blood sugar level is also a good idea; seizure activity burns unusual amounts of metabolic fuel. Dextrose administration is indicated without blood testing when patient history strongly suggests hypoglycemia.

Status epilepticus is the true emergency among seizure patients. It is defined as two or more seizures without a lucid interval (responsive, oriented period) in between, or continuous seizure activity for a period of more than 20 to 30 minutes. Brain damage, severe dehydration, hypoxia, and hypoglycemia can result if the patient's condition remains untreated.

Paramedics may need to assist ventilations and provide oxygen for the status epilepticus patient and are faced with the challenge of initiating an IV for administration of anticonvulsant medications in the seizing patient. Diazepam, lorazepam, phenytoin, and phenobarbital are all used in these situations. Some of these medications can also be administered intramuscularly or rectally, a fact that provides important backup possibilities for situations in which IV access is not possible. Most of the anticonvulsant medications also have serious possible side effects, such as respiratory depression and hypotension, that require cautious administration and close patient monitoring.

Infectious Processes

Sepsis

The general term sepsis is sometimes used in place of the more specific term *septicemia* which is a body-wide infection in the bloodstream. Among pediatric patients, neonates are most vulnerable to this condition. The condition may arise from a localized infection, such as **pneumonia,** but at other times may occur without an obvious point of origin.

General signs include lowered level of responsiveness, irritability and vomiting. Fever may be present initially, but septic children often become hypothermic later. Septic shock is the most common life threat that sepsis poses.

As with adults, the shock presentation differs somewhat from the more common hypovolemic forms. In children, differences are even more pronounced; the early flush of peripheral vasodilation resembles that in adults, but the hypothermia that sometimes follows can be confusing unless paramedics know that it may specifically indicate sepsis. The combination of infectious signs and hypoperfusion indicators will usually emerge in a thorough patient history and examination. Tachypnea, tachycardia, and patient history or evidence of existing infection are among the most reliable signs.

Field treatment for sepsis is supportive, focusing on airway maintenance, ventilation, oxygenation and fluid administration. Definitive treatment involves antibiotic therapy.

Meningitis

Meningitis, or inflammation of the membranes that cover the brain and spinal cord (meninges), most often arises from bacterial or viral infection. Viral meningitis usually runs its course without threatening the patient, but bacterial forms can be much more severe. Complications such as seizures, septic shock, and cerebral edema can pose life threats if the disease is not identified and treated.

The identification of meningitis can be difficult in infants and small children. They typically present with general signs of illness, such as irritability and fever. Slightly taut fontanelles are a possible indicator in this patient group but not a consistent one. Older children are more likely to show (and be able to communicate) the classic signs often seen in adults: headache, stiff neck, and altered mentation. Pain upon fully straightening the legs (which stretches the tender meninges) is also a strongly suggestive sign.

Treatment of suspected meningitis is supportive with rapid transport for definitive diagnosis and aggressive treatment with antibiotics at the hospital. As well as being more dangerous, bacterial meningitis is more communicable than the viral form. Transmission of the disease is most common by nasal or oral secretions emitted during coughing and sneezing. When meningitis is suspected, placing a mask on the patient is the ideal means of preventing cross infection. When this method is not possible, providers should wear masks and plan to disinfect the transport vehicle thoroughly afterward. Caregivers who have been exposed to certain types of meningitis may have to take precautionary antibiotics afterward.

Reye's Syndrome

Reye's syndrome is a poorly understood process that causes damage to numerous vital organ systems. This condition most commonly occurs in winter months, often in association with flu outbreaks or chickenpox, and has also been linked to the use of aspirin and other salicylate-containing substances in children. This syndrome occurs in patients of all ages, but most frequently in the pediatric age ranges from preschool age to adolescence.

The syndrome (it is not a distinct disease) can present with a wide variety of signs and symptoms. Common presentations include sudden or excessive vomiting, signs of increasing intracranial pressure, respiratory failure, altered mentation, and right upper quadrant pain caused by liver inflammation.

As most of these signs are not very specific, paramedics will do well simply to suspect Reye's syndrome when one or more of these symptoms is present. There is often a patient history of viral illness or **gastroenteritis.** The syndrome is easily mistaken for other conditions. Mentation changes may appear to be caused by alcohol or drug ingestion. Meningitis and sepsis can also present with similar signs and symptoms.

Reye's syndrome is rare and usually responds well if recognized and treated early enough. Cerebral edema poses the most immediate threat to severely ill patients. Brain stem herniation is a common cause of death, so airway control and ventilatory support are the mainstays of field treatment. Testing the patient for hypoglycemia and treating with dextrose, as indicated, are also important.

Neonatal Resuscitation

Signs of distress that indicate the need for resuscitation in the newborn will be evident early in the initial patient assessment that begins immediately after every delivery (see Chapter 37). The essentials of care will also begin immediately for each baby, regardless of the need for extensive resuscitation. These essentials include drying and heat conservation (including covering the head), airway clearing, proper positioning to maintain the airway and encourage fluid drainage, and physical stimulation to promote breathing. Only a small number of neonates will require care beyond these basics. The "Inverted Pyramid" for resuscitation of the newborn illustrates the importance of these basics (Fig. 22-8).

This routine care also includes APGAR score evaluations at 1 and 5 minutes after birth (see Chapter 37). APGAR scores of seven and above are normal for children who will need no more than the standard steps listed above. Scores below seven indicate the likely need for some additional level of care, most often just oxygen and brief ventilatory support.

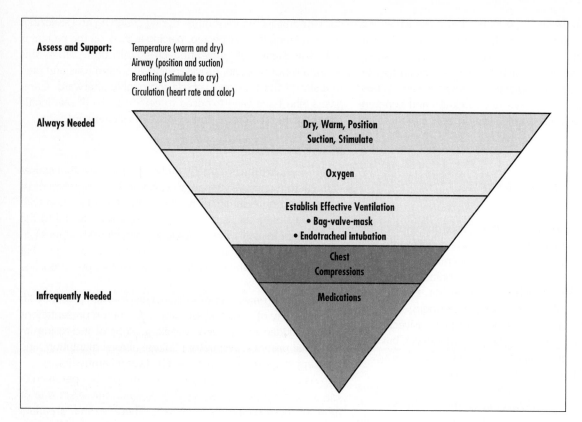

Assess and Support: Temperature (warm and dry)
Airway (position and suction)
Breathing (stimulate to cry)
Circulation (heart rate and color)

Always Needed

Dry, Warm, Position
Suction, Stimulate

Oxygen

Establish Effective Ventilation
• Bag-valve-mask
• Endotracheal intubation

Chest
Compressions

Infrequently Needed

Medications

Figure 22-8

The inverted pyramid reflecting relative frequencies of neonatal resuscitation efforts for the newborn who does not have meconium-stained amniotic fluid. A majority of newborns respond to simple measures. *Reproduced with permission, American Heart Association: Textbook of Pediatric Advanced Life Support, 1994, © American Heart Association.*

However, APGAR scoring is not the primary determining factor in initiating resuscitation, and early resuscitative measures cannot be delayed for scoring.

Evaluating the Need for Resuscitation

Evaluating the need for resuscitation of the distressed newborn includes skin color, respiratory status, and heart rate. (*Note*: all references to oxygen therapy and assisted ventilation in this section assume administration of high-concentration oxygen.)

- *Color.* Peripheral cyanosis and sometimes mottling are normal immediately after delivery. Central cyanosis is a more significant sign, indicating the need for immediate oxygen therapy.
- *Respirations.* After opening and suctioning the airway, the paramedic should check the newborn's breathing. Respiratory rate should be rapid (> 30; preferably 40 per minute), and inspiratory efforts should be deep enough to cause good chest rise. If the respiratory rate is slow or depth is shallow, the paramedic should attempt a brief period of tactile stimulation and oxygen administration. Assisted ventilation is necessary if these measures do not lead to lead to quick improvement in the patient. Other patient indications for bag-valve-mask ventilation include: gasping respirations, heart rate less than 100 per minute, and central cyanosis that does not resolve with passive oxygen administration.

- *Heart rate.* Heart rate is the best single sign of oxygenation and perfusion in the neonate. A rate of more than 100 per minute is normal. Lower rates call for immediate ventilation. Rates below 60 and rates in the 60 to 80 range that do not improve quickly with assisted ventilation, require initiation of chest compressions. Pulse can be palpated at the brachial or femoral arteries or the base of the umbilical vein, or the pulse can be auscultated over the apex.

Specifics of Resuscitation

Table 22-3 outlines the CPR rates, intubation equipment, and medications used in neonatal resuscitation.

Airway and ventilation

Oxygen administered to neonates should ideally be warmed and humidified. Room-temperature oxygen will suffice when warming is not possible, but responders should be careful not to use tanks that have been stored in unheated compartments during cool or cold weather.

Bag-valve-mask ventilation will be adequate for all but a few neonates who require ventilatory assistance; endotracheal intubation is seldom required. Chest wall movement is the best sign to monitor for adequacy of assisted ventilations. Absent or inadequate movement should lead first to repositioning of the airway, and if that does not help, to further suctioning and

TABLE 22-3   Neonatal Resuscitation Card

Initial cardiopulmonary resuscitation	Term neonatal vital signs (first 12 h of life)[3]
Ventilation rate: 40–60/min when performed without compression Compression rate: 120/min (performed with ventilations) Compression:ventilation ratio: 3:1 (pause for ventilation) Medications: Indicated if heart rate remains <80 bpm despite adequate ventilations with 100% O_2 and chest compressions	Heart rate (awake): 100–180 bpm Respiratory rate: 30–60/min. Systolic blood pressure: 39–59 mm Hg Diastolic blood pressure: 16–36 mm Hg

Intubation Equipment

Weight	ET Tube Size (mm)/Catheter Size	Laryngoscope Blade
1 kg	2.5/5F	0
2 kg	3.0/6F	0
3 kg	3.5/8F	0–1
4 kg	3.5/8F	1

Medications

Medications	Dose/Route	Concentration	Wt (kg)	Total (mL)	Precautions
Epinephrine	0.01–0.03 mg/kg IV or ET*	1:10 000	1 2 3 4	0.1–0.3 0.2–0.6 0.3–0.9 0.4–1.2	Give rapidly Repeat every 3–5 min
Volume Expanders — 5% Albumin — Blood — Normal saline — Ringer's lactate	10 mL/kg IV		1 2 3 4	10 20 30 40	Reassess after each bolus
Naloxone	0.1 mg/kg IV, IM, SQ, ET	0.4 mg/mL	1 2 3 4	0.25 0.50 0.75 1.0	Give rapidly Repeat every 2–3 min
		1.0 mg/mL	1 2 3 4	0.1 0.2 0.3 0.4	

IM indicates intramuscular; ET, endotracheal tube; IV, intravenous; SQ, subcutaneous.

*Note: ET dose may not result in effective plasma concentration of drug, so IV access should be established as soon as possible. ET drugs should be diluted to volume of 3 to 5 mL before instillation.

Reproduced with permission. Textbook of Pediatric Advanced Life Support, 1994. Copyright American Heart Association.

an increase in ventilatory pressure. If this sequence fails to produce good chest rise on ventilation, intubation is indicated.

Neonates have stiffer lungs than infants and children. This reduced compliance can make bagging a patient difficult. It may be impossible to ventilate properly with bags that have functional pop-off valves, which are generally not recommended for prehospital pediatric care. If present, the valve will most likely have to be disabled (taped or held down).

Prematurity and meconium staining are two complications that further reduce the already low pulmonary compliance in neonates and make it more difficult to ventilate a neonate effectively. Gastric distention can also cause resistance to ventilation. Paramedics should place an orogastric tube and aspirate it occasionally with a syringe when distention is obvious or the need for ventilatory assistance continues beyond a few minutes.

It is desirable to let the patient's lungs take over when possible. The paramedic should monitor the patient's sponta-

neous respiratory effort closely and try "weaning" the patient by slowing the rate of ventilation and lowering inspiratory pressure gradually. Increasing heart rate is a good sign that this weaning may work and should be attempted.

Mask size and fit are important equipment considerations in effective ventilation. Paramedic kits should include several equipment sizes and shapes for neonates and infants. Seal can be difficult (cuffed or cushioned rims help) and the mask should be the smallest possible size to minimize the dead space that will receive air but not circulate it to the alveoli.

Endotracheal intubation is necessary when correct bagging is ineffective, thick meconium is present, or ventilation will be necessary for an extended period of time. The procedure requires special equipment sizes and mandates close attention to confirming correct tube placement. Multiple checks can be performed to make the confirmation: auscultation of lateral lung fields and the area over the stomach and observation of chest wall rise, skin color, and heart rate.

CPR and advanced life support

Chest compressions in the neonate can be performed with the thumbs (with fingers wrapped around the back) or with two fingertips (Fig. 22-9). Both methods require care in exact compression position to avoid rib injuries or pressure on the xiphoid that could damage the liver.

Chest compressions are performed at a rate of 120 per minute in a 3:1 ratio with ventilations, with brief pauses for the ventilations. The targets for actual delivery are 90 compressions and 30 ventilations per minute. Pulse checks should be made after 1 minute of CPR and every few minutes thereafter, and compressions discontinued when the patient's spontaneous heart rate rises above 80 beats per minute.

The need for fluid therapy in neonates can arise when there has been maternal bleeding during or just before delivery, or loss of fetal blood through the umbilical cord during or just after delivery. For paramedics trained in umbilical vein access, this site is ideal for both fluid and medication administration, because it is readily available and noninvasive (*see* Skill #26 in Skills Section).

Peripheral IV sites are also possibilities, although the most commonly available locations have drawbacks: scalp veins are very small and difficult to maintain once entered, for instance, and the saphenous vein's distance from the central circulation slows drug action and raises the need to follow medications with fluid flushes.

Endotracheal administration is a good option for epinephrine and is acceptable with naloxone, the two most commonly used medications, when a tube is in place. The regular IV doses can be used diluted in 3 to 5 mL of fluid. Intraosseous infusion is also available for both fluid and drug administration. IO therapy is less well researched in neonates than in older pediatric groups, but this therapy method is at least an important

last resort for venous access during resuscitation and may be listed in some local protocols as an earlier consideration.

Fluid boluses of 10 mL/kg are indicated for the neonate in several circumstances: 1) presence of good heart rate but weak pulses; 2) generally poor response to resuscitation in which ventilatory effectiveness has been confirmed; and 3) the patient whose skin color remains pale after aggressive oxygen therapy. None of these circumstances is an exact, specific indication; careful follow-up monitoring is required to avoid overhydration of the patient and to confirm that fluid is the correct treatment. The bolus is administered slowly over 5 to 10 minutes. Repeat boluses can be given, with the preceding caution in mind.

Epinephrine is used in asystole or for bradycardias (rate < 80) unresponsive to chest compression and aggressive ventilation and oxygen therapy over several minutes. The dose is 0.01/0.03 mg/kg when given IV or IO and 0.1mg/kg when given via endotracheal tube. The 1:10:000 solution is used for IV or IO administration, whereas the 1:1000 solution is used for the ET route.

Naloxone can be administered for apnea resulting from narcotics given to the mother shortly before birth, including possible drug addiction. The latter setting predisposes the infant to withdrawal problems, however; naloxone should be titrated carefully to minimum respiratory response. The dose is 0.1 mg/kg, and as with the adult patient, the paramedic should observe the patient for return of respiratory depression as the relatively short-acting drug wears off.

Special Neonatal Settings

Two relatively common categories of newborns raise special concerns for short-term management: newborns who are delivered prematurely and newborns with meconium staining in the amniotic fluid. These patients require additional attention to the basics of neonatal care.

Prematurity

Prematurity, defined as delivery before 38 weeks of gestation, places the infant at special risk for hypothermia, hypovolemia, and respiratory problems. Quick and effective conservation of body temperature is doubly important in these patients, as is effective cord clamping to avoid depletion of the small circulating blood volume.

Paramedics should expect pulmonary compliance to be even lower than usual in neonates and the pressures necessary to ventilate correspondingly high. Incomplete lung development and its effect on oxygen exchange also account for the tendency of premature infants to respond slowly to resuscitation. These patients are likely to present with lower APGAR scores than scores seen in full-term newborns. The paramedic should consider transporting the premature neonate to a facility with a neonatal intensive care unit if possible.

Meconium staining

Meconium staining threatens the baby in proportion to its thickness in the amniotic fluid and the amount aspirated. Visible presence of meconium in the fluid when the bag breaks

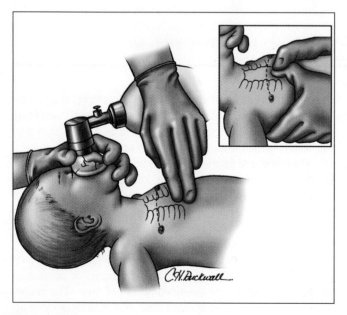

Figure 22-9

Proper placement of chest compression in the neonate is one finger width below the nipple line. The compressor can use two thumbs, one on top of the other, or two fingers in line along the length of the sternum.

alerts responders to the need for aggressive suctioning as soon as the head presents. Fluid still in the newborn's airway will be inhaled upon chest presentation–a critical but preventable complication. Some services use "meconium trap" suction devices to suction the oropharynx and pharynx when meconium is present. Because improper use of the device can lead to further complications and communicable disease exposure to the rescuer, local training and protocol govern the use of this equipment.

The neonate who does aspirate meconium require endotracheal intubation, aggressive oxygen and ventilatory therapy, and expedient transport to definitive care in the hospital. These lungs may be the most difficult of all to inflate with a bag, especially if the meconium is thick and particulate in nature. Meconium staining carries a further message about the importance of oxygenation and ventilation: because the condition arises from prenatal hypoxia, the patient is assumed to be oxygen deficient even before any meconium is aspirated.

SUMMARY

Critical pediatric responses require thorough paramedic preparation and a knowledge of the differences between pediatric care and adult patient care. The low frequency of advanced life support procedures in the young population underscores the importance of regular refresher training and the paramedic's commitment to thorough pediatric care expertise over the course of a career.

REFERENCES

1. **American Heart Association, Emergency Cardiac Care Committee and Subcommittees:** Guidelines for cardiopulmonary resuscitation and emergency cardiac care. Part VI. Pediatric Advanced Life Support. *JAMA* 268:2262–2275, 1992.

2. **Anderson, AB, Zwerdling RG, Dewitt TG:** The clinical utility of pulse oximetry in the pediatric emergency department setting. *Pediatr Emerg Care* 7:263–266, 1991.

3. **Applebaum D:** Advanced prehospital care for pediatric emergencies. *Ann Emerg Med* 14:656–659, 1985.

4. **Barkin RM, Luten RC:** Emergencies in pediatrics and the child in the emergency medical services system. *Pediatr Ann* 19:571–577, 1990.

5. **Foltin G, Fuchs S:** Advances in pediatric emergency medical service systems. *Emerg Med Clin North Am* 9:459–474, 1991.

6. **Fuchs S, LaCovey D, Paris P:** A prehospital model of Intraosseous infusion. *Ann Emerg Med* 20:371–374, 1991.

7. **Ludwig S, Kettrick RG, Parker M:** Pediatric cardiopulmonary resuscitation: a review of 130 cases. *Clin Pediatr* 23:71–76, 1984.

8. **Rivera R, Ribballs J:** Complications of endotracheal intubation and mechanical ventilation in infants and children. *Crit Care Med* 20:193–199, 1992.

9. **Rosetti V, Thompson BM, Aprahamian C, et al:** Difficulty and delay in intravascular access in pediatric arrests. *Ann Emerg Med* 13:406, 1984.

10. **Torphy DE, Minter MG, Thompson BM:** Cardiorespiratory arrest and resuscitation in children. *Am J Dis Child* 138:1099, 1984.

11. **Tsai A, Kallsen G:** Epidemiology of pediatric prehospital care. *Ann Emerg Med* 16:284–292, 1987.

Section

Continued Patient Assessment

3c

Included In This Section:

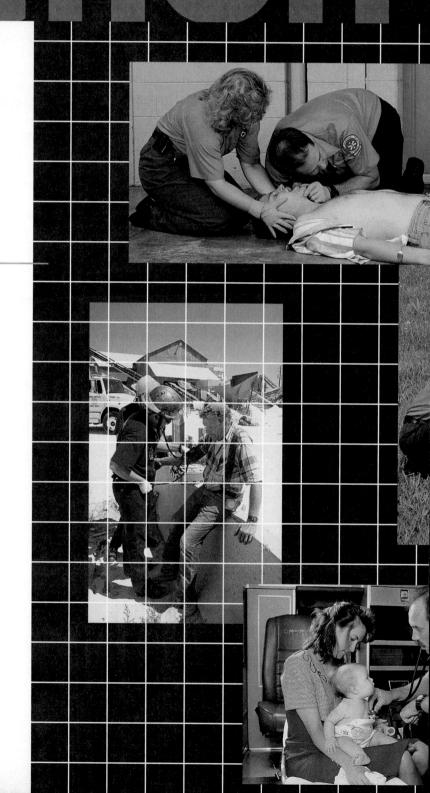

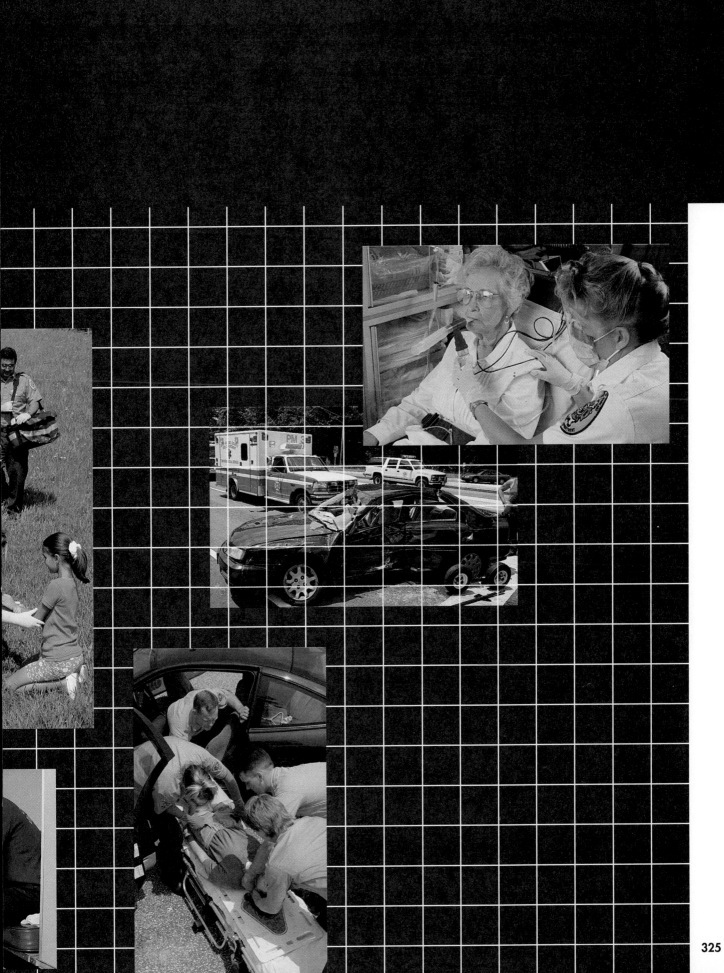

Vince J. Markovchick, MD, FACEP

Chapter 23

Clinical Significance of Vital Signs

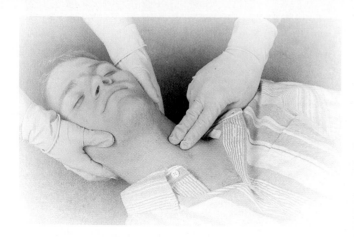

1. **Bradycardia**—abnormally slow heartbeat (pulse rate < 60 beats per minute in an adult patient)
2. **Bradypnea**—abnormally slow breathing.
3. **Hypotension**—abnormally low blood pressure.
4. **Tachycardia**—abnormally fast heartbeat (pulse rate > 100 beats per minute in an adult patient).
5. **Tachypnea**—abnormally rapid breathing.

A paramedic should be able to:

1. Identify normal and abnormal vital signs in patients of varying ages.
2. Describe how age, physical conditioning, the use of medications, and the patient's medical condition can affect vital sign measurements.
3. State ways in which pulse, respiration, and blood pressure measurements can aid in determining the probable cause of a patient's problem.
4. Describe how vital signs can help to identify a patient in shock.
5. Explain how the size of a blood pressure cuff can produce false blood pressure readings.

Any significant illness or injury will alter basic human physiology. Acute illness and injury cause stress on the human organism, and there are predicted patterns of response. The alterations in physiology are most often reflected in changes in vital signs, including mental status and skin changes. This chapter discusses physiologic responses to stress and how they can be recognized by the paramedic through vital sign measurement.

Vital Signs

To appreciate abnormal vital signs, the paramedic must be able to recognize normal vital signs (Table 23-1). Normal ranges for vital signs change with age, physical condition, and use of medications. When differentiating the origins of abnormal vital signs, it is most important to begin with the most serious possibility and proceed toward less-threatening conditions.

There are instances when "normal" vital signs are distinctly abnormal, just as there are specific conditions in which vital signs are expected to vary from accepted normal values. This situation makes it necessary to combine the chief complaint with a critical interpretation of vital signs if the paramedic is to identify patients with life-threatening conditions. For example, the expected respiratory rate for an asthma patient in mild-to-moderate distress is 20 to 30 breaths per minute. An asthmatic patient who is wheezing and has a respiratory rate of 12 to 16 per minute may be assessed incorrectly as being stable because the vital signs appear "normal." In reality, this patient is tiring, losing the ability to move air, retaining CO_2, and approaching respiratory arrest. This is a classic example of how abnormal vital signs can be misinterpreted as normal. In the context of a specific disease state, this vital sign indicates a potential life threat that may go unrecognized until it is too late. The paramedic must understand what the standard vital signs are for patients with specific chief complaints and clinical presentations. When actual vital signs differ significantly from the expectation, suspicion about the patient's risk level should quickly increase.

Vital signs vary dramatically with age; the variations are highest in infants and young children up to 6 years of age. A respiratory rate of 30 breaths per minute is normal for a 1-month-old infant, but clearly abnormal for an older child or adult. Likewise, a blood pressure of 110/70 may be indicative of hypotension in a 70-year-old man, but normal for a young adult. Systolic blood pressure normally increases with age because of decreasing elasticity of the arterial walls.

Pulse

The primary determinant of pulse is overall physical conditioning. For example, the normal resting pulse of a 21-year-old marathon runner would be expected to be in the 40 to 50 beats per minute range. If this individual sustains a traumatic injury, a supine pulse rate of 72 beats per minute would constitute notable tachycardia. In contrast, a poorly conditioned 50-year-old patient could be expected to have a normal resting pulse rate as high as 84 beats per minute. Elderly patients may not show these expected alterations in pulse at all. A 70-year-old patient with a medical condition, such as acute abdomen, may present with a normal pulse rate, although a 20-year-old patient with the same condition nearly always develops tachycardia.

The pulse rate can be affected by many factors, including the use of medications or drugs. It is important to obtain a history of medication or drug use to determine if any of these factors may be altering vital signs, particularly the pulse rate. Beta blockers (drugs that inhibit the stimulation of beta adrenergic receptors to the heart), such as propranolol, may prevent a patient from developing a normal tachycardic response. Other sympathomimetic medications (i.e., those that stimulate the adrenergic, or sympathetic, nervous system and drugs such as amphetamines, cocaine, and over-the-counter cold preparations containing ephedrine) may cause a tachycardia. Tachycardia is associated with some acute overdoses and poisonings. This is particularly true of tricyclic antidepressant toxicity, which is first manifested as sinus tachycardia.

Tachycardia

When a patient presents with a tachycardia, the primary consideration must be given to shock. Regardless of its cause, shock usually presents with tachycardia. A rapid assessment of the pulse, in conjunction with the determination of the type of injury sustained and an assessment of skin characteristics, will help the paramedic to pinpoint the possible causes of shock. A patient who is hypotensive and tachycardiac and has

TABLE 23-1	**Weight and Vital Signs by Age Group**			
Age	**Weight, kg (lb)**	**Respirations**	**Pulse**	**Systolic Blood Pressure**
Newborn	3–4 kg (6–9 lb)	30–50	120–160	60–80
6 mo–1 yr	8–10 kg (16–22 lb)	30–40	120–140	70–80
2–4 yr	12–16 kg (24–34 lb)	20–30	100–110	80–95
5–8 yr	18–26 kg (36–55 lb)	14–20	90–100	90–100
8–12 yr	26–50 kg (55–110 lb)	12–20	80–100	100–110
> 12 yr	> 50 kg (110 lb)	12–20	60–90	100–120

warm, dry skin, represents shock from **sepsis, anaphylaxis,** or spinal trauma. In contrast, if the patient is hypotensive and tachycardiac and has pale, cool, moist skin, the condition is most likely hypovolemic or cardiogenic shock. Cardiogenic shock usually accompanies conditions of acute chest pain.

Another cause of tachycardia is fever. The paramedic should expect the patient to have a gradually increasing pulse with a rising temperature. Because temperatures may not routinely be assessed in the field, this condition will not always be clear during initial assessment.

A primary cardiac etiology must be considered if the patient's pulse rate is above 150 (i.e., paroxysmal atrial tachycardia or atrial flutter with 1:1 or 2:1 conduction). If the QRS complex is widened and the patient's heart rate is above 150, it is likely that the rhythm seen is ventricular tachycardia. When determining if a patient is experiencing atrial fibrillation, the paramedic should visualize the monitor and assess the patient's pulse. It is nearly impossible to read atrial fibrillation at a rate in excess of 150. Atrial fibrillation is the only rhythm that is irregularly irregular with varying pulse strength and deficit (defined as fewer beats being palpable when taking the pulse, in comparison with visualizing the cardiac activity on a monitor or auscultating the activity with a stethoscope). In this situation, circulation is being compromised.

Certain disease states will result in a tachycardia: **heat stroke, hyperthyroidism,** and **thyroid storm, pulmonary embolism,** and hypoxia. Finally, anxiety and pain usually cause a mild degree of tachycardia, although attributing tachycardia to anxiety or pain alone can only be done after excluding the more serious potential causes.

Bradycardia

Bradycardia is much less common than tachycardia; there are several origins for the paramedic to consider. In working from the more serious to the more benign causes, the paramedic should begin with cardiac conditions such as **second- and third-degree heart block. Hypothermia** can also cause a profound bradycardia in which the pulse may not be palpable, and the rhythm can only be detected on a cardiac monitor. Certain medications, primarily beta blockers, can result in significant bradycardias, especially if taken in excessive amounts. Stimulation of the vagus nerve will also result in bradycardias (sometimes enough to cause hypotension or syncope), as do cholinergic poisoning agents such as organophosphate insecticides. Increased intracranial pressure can result in bradycardia as part of Cushing's reflex.

Blood Pressure

Blood pressure is determined by cardiac output (CO) and total peripheral resistance (TPR). Cardiac output is the amount of blood ejected from the heart in 1 minute, and the evaluation is calculated by multiplying stroke volume (i.e., the amount of blood ejected from the heart with each beat) by heart rate (equation: $CO = SV \times HR$). As stroke volume and cardiac out-

put decrease, tachycardia is the normal compensatory response. As cardiac output and blood pressure decrease further, total peripheral resistance increases. Resistance can increase only if the sympathetic nervous system is intact. This increase will not occur in spinal cord injury, which results in the loss of sympathetic innervation necessary to produce vasoconstriction. The patient who is maximally vasoconstricted appears to have an ashen, pale skin color and cool, diaphoretic skin.

Blood pressure is determined through the use of a sphygmomanometer. It is important that the correct cuff size is used for the patient. The width of the cuff should be two thirds the size of the patient's upper arm. An inappropriate cuff size will result in an inaccurate blood pressure reading. If the cuff is too large, it will cause a falsely low reading; if the cuff is too small, it will result in a falsely elevated blood pressure. Severe vasoconstriction makes it difficult for the paramedic to palpate or auscultate peripheral pulses in the patient, and thus can cause an inaccurately low reading or make the reading unobtainable.

Hypotension does not appear in the patient until a significant volume of blood is lost (Table 23-2). A 10% loss (approximately 500 mL in an adult) will result in a minimal change in vital signs, or no change at all. When enough blood volume has been lost to affect vital signs, the first vital sign to change will be the pulse. Once 15% to 25% of the normal blood volume is lost, the patient may manifest orthostatic changes—a pulse increase of greater than 20 beats per minute, or a blood pressure drop of greater than 20 mm Hg—when moved from the supine to the upright position (*see also* Chapter 29). Once there is a loss greater than 25% of intravascular blood volume, the patient will likely begin to exhibit abnormal vital signs, even when placed in the supine position. As the blood loss continues, the magnitude of hypotension and tachycardia will grow.

Respirations

Respiratory rate is frequently estimated, and consequently, is one of the most inaccurately assessed vital signs. If the patient is in obvious respiratory distress, the rate is often accurately taken and recognized as abnormal. However, if the patient is quietly tachypneic for any reason, the tachypnea can sometimes be overlooked. It is very important for the paramedic to assess the respiratory rate accurately in all patients. The normal respiratory rate is approximately 12–20 breaths per minute in an adult.

TABLE 23-2	Hypovolemia
Fluid Loss, %	**Changes**
10% (adult 500 mL)	None or minimal
10%–15%	Pulse rate
15%–25%	Orthostatic changes
25% +	Changes in supine position

Respiratory drive in healthy individuals is determined by the level of CO_2 in arterial blood (pCO_2). As the patient begins to retain CO_2 (hypercapnia), the compensatory response is an increased respiratory rate, or tachypnea. One exception to this normal physiology occurs in some patients with chronic obstructive pulmonary disease (COPD), who retain CO_2 chronically. In these individuals, respiratory drive is determined by the level of oxygen in the blood (pO_2). A decreased pO_2 (hypoxemia) will result in an increased respiratory drive. If too much oxygen is administered, a patient's hypoxic drive may be weakened. However, this situation is rarely seen in the field, because the patient's exposure time to oxygen therapy is normally a contributing factor.

The other determinant of respiratory drive is the acid-base status of the blood. As the blood becomes acidic (pH drops below 7.40), the body compensates by hyperventilating to decrease the pCO_2, which in turn, will raise the pH toward the normal 7.40. Therefore, most patients with shock or other causes of metabolic acidosis will present with compensatory tachypnea. Such is the case with the Kussmaul respiratory pattern that is seen in patients with diabetic ketoacidosis. The tachypnea is accompanied by an abnormal deep respiratory pattern.

Common respiratory causes of tachypnea include conditions in which ventilation is compromised by fluid or pus in the alveoli, such as pulmonary edema and pneumonia. Pulmonary embolus will also usually cause tachypnea. Traumatic causes include pulmonary contusion and pneumothorax. Additional benign causes of tachypnea are chest wall injuries (rib fractures) and infectious conditions (pleurisy). These cause tachypnea because of pleuritic pain and the patient's reluctance to breathe normally. Patients with pleuritic pain compensate for the decrease in tidal volume (i.e., amount of air exchanged with each breath) by increasing their respiratory rate.

An injury or illness that affects the central nervous system can also result in tachypnea. Fever is another cause of tachypnea, as are anxiety and pain. However, attributing tachypnea to anxiety can be dangerous, especially if the problem is believed to be hyperventilation syndrome but is actually a more threatening condition, such as a pulmonary embolus. It is extremely dangerous for a patient with profound hypoxia, misdiagnosed as having hyperventilation syndrome, to rebreathe into a paper bag.

Pharmacologic causes of bradypnea, or a decreased respiratory rate, include all medications that are central nervous system (CNS) depressants. The classic examples are narcotics (e.g., heroin, morphine) and sedative hypnotics (e.g., barbiturates). These drugs will decrease the normal respiratory drive, which is initiated in the brain stem. CNS disease resulting in intracranial lesions secondary to trauma or bleeding can cause a decreased respiratory rate or even apnea. Finally, hypothermia may cause a decreased respiratory rate so profound that the patient may not appear to be breathing at all.

Central nervous system injury or illness can cause abnormal respiratory patterns as well. Lesions within the brain, particularly those affecting the brain stem, may cause the classic abnormal breathing pattern known as Cheyne-Stokes respirations. Biot's breathing, or ataxic breathing, is an unpredictable, irregular pattern that is also associated with compression of the respiratory center. Figure 23-1 illustrates abnormal breathing rates and patterns.

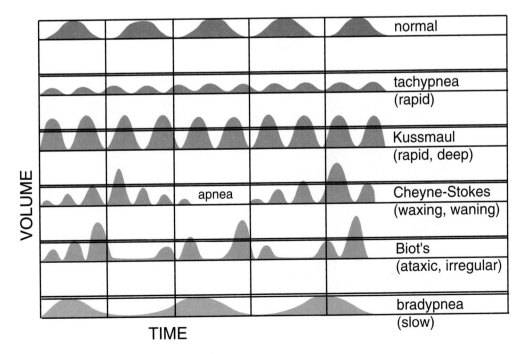

Figure 23-1

Abnormal breathing rates and patterns.

SUMMARY

Nearly all patients with acute life-threatening conditions can be identified in the field by an observant paramedic. The process begins with the chief complaint and continues with a critical interpretation of vital signs, visual observation of the patient, and assessment of skin signs. The vast majority of life-threatening conditions will reveal themselves in this sequence, as will necessary clues about how to initiate treatment.

REFERENCES

1. **Rosen P, Barkin R (eds):** Emergency Medicine: Concepts and Clinical Practice, ed 3, vol II, St. Louis, Mosby-Year Book.

Carol Goodykoontz, RN, MS, EMT-P
and Sandy Race, RN, BSN, CEN

Chapter 24

Focused and Continued Assessment

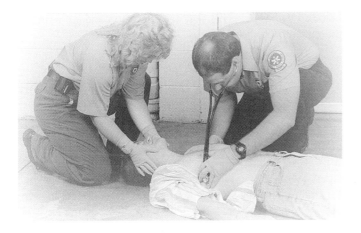

A paramedic should be able to:

The initial assessment is followed by the focused history and physical examination (or focused exam). The focused history and physical exam focuses on the patient's chief complaint, whether it is a medical or trauma condition. The focused exam also identifies other conditions that could be life-threatening if not attended to promptly, and determines the severity of the condition without unnecessarily delaying transportation. The final step in patient assessment is continued assessment, which continues until patient care is turned over to the receiving facility. The continued assessment includes a detailed physical examination and continued reevaluation of potential life threats.

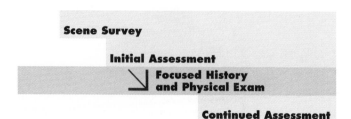

Focused History and Physical Examination: Overview

Up to this point, the initial assessment has been the same for medical and trauma patients, except for the difference in the methods of opening the airway. Whether the patient has a traumatic or a medical problem, the procedural steps in the focused history and examination are similar. The four main steps in the focused history and physical examination are:

1. Assessing the patient's history
   a. Chief complaint
   b. History of the present illness or event (OPQRST)
   c. Pertinent past medical history
   d. Current health status
2. Performing a physical examination, focusing on the area of the patient's chief complaint
3. Obtaining baseline vital signs
4. Providing emergency care based on signs and symptoms in consultation with medical direction

The sequence of the steps of the focused history and physical examination and emphasis placed on each step are different for medical and trauma patients. In the medical patient, emphasis is placed on the patient's medical history. In the trauma patient, emphasis is placed on the mechanism of the injury.

Focused History and Physical Examination: Medical

For the medical patient, the focused examination requires evaluating the patient's responsiveness first. Mental status is assessed during the initial assessment and is reevaluated during the focused physical examination. Communicate any changes in mental status to medical personnel at the receiving facility, and document any changes in mental status in the prehospital care report. Documentation should include the patient's response to a specific stimulus. For example, "The

patient responded to a painful stimulus by arching his back and pulling both arms toward his chest," or "The patient knows his name but does not know the date, where he is, or what happened."

Do not jump to conclusions regarding a patient's behavior. An abusive or combative patient who has ingested alcohol may be suffering from a serious head injury, hypoxia, or hypoglycemia. Be careful not to convey suspicions to other healthcare providers as if they were facts. Assumptions are often incorrect and can lead to inappropriate care.

In the responsive medical patient, the patient's medical history is gathered first and is followed by a physical examination focused on the patient's chief complaint, signs, and symptoms. In the unresponsive medical patient, a rapid physical examination (medical assessment) is performed first and is followed by baseline vital sign determination and gathering of the patient's medical history.

Responsive Medical Patient

Assess Patient History

In the responsive medical patient, gathering information about the patient's medical history is performed before the physical examination. The information obtained from the medical history helps guide the steps of the focused physical examination. However, a change in the patient's condition or the environment may alter how the examination is performed. The patient should be the primary source of information; however, additional sources of information include what is visualized at the scene, first responders, family members, friends, and bystanders.

History taking involves conversing with the patient in an organized manner and gathering information about how the patient feels in relation to what has happened to him or her. The importance of obtaining a history cannot be overemphasized. Much of the paramedic's treatment of a patient is based on the information obtained in the medical history. The focus of the history in the prehospital setting is directed toward the discovery of critical observations that will affect prehospital intervention or will need to be communicated to the receiving facility.

A skillful interviewer can employ various techniques to obtain the patient's medical history. A team approach is useful when two EMS providers are available on a call. One person should interview the patient while the other talks with the family or bystanders. The information obtained should be corroborated to reach accurate conclusions about the patient's condition. Patient confidentiality must be maintained throughout the interview.

Effective communication skills are essential. The use of clear and simple terminology will aid the interview process. Asking the patient one question at a time and allowing time for a response is also an important principle.

The medical history can be obtained by using either direct (closed-ended) or open-ended questions. Direct questions can be answered with a "yes" or "no." In a situation that is not urgent, the paramedic may use open-ended questions to obtain a better description of what happened. (Box 24-1)

The four basic components of the medical history are:

1. Chief complaint
2. History of the present illness or event
3. Pertinent past medical history
4. Current health status

Chief Complaint

The chief complaint is the reason EMS was called, usually in the patient's own words. The patient's statement is not a diagnosis but the reason he or she is seeking medical treatment. Exercise care in not interpreting the reason for the call. Allow the patient to express the reason in his or her own words. For example, "I cannot breathe," or "I feel sick to my stomach."

Patients or family members usually relay the chief complaint when paramedics arrive on the scene. On some calls, however, the patient may not state his or her chief complaint. In these situations, the paramedic must encourage the patient to explain what is wrong. Asking the patient, "Why did you call us today?," will usually elicit this information.

History of Present Illness or Event

The history of the present illness or event (HPI) is a further detailed exploration of the chief complaint. This part of the patient's medical history focuses on determining the factors related to the patient's call for assistance. Allowing the patient to tell his or her "story," followed by specific questions from the interviewer, will provide the most accurate information. For example, "Tell me more about your dizziness," or, "Explain what you mean when you say your stomach hurts."

The specific chronology leading to the current illness, as well as associated or aggravating factors should be discussed. What the patient says is considered subjective findings, or symptoms. These are things the patient perceives about his or her illness. Objective findings are signs of illness that the paramedic uncovers in the interview and/or physical examination. These findings may or may not support the chief complaint, but will assist the examiner in determining the acuity of the sit-

BOX 24-1

Direct Questions	Open-Ended Questions
Does the pain go anywhere else?	How would you describe your pain?
Is this the worst pain you have ever experienced?	How does the pain feel to you?
Are you short of breath or nauseated?	What other symptoms are you having?

uation. The OPQRST acronym is used to help remember the pertinent questions to ask when obtaining the history of the present illness or event (Table 24-1).

The presence or absence of specific signs and symptoms is particularly relevant to the focused history and physical examination. Findings verified by the history or physical exam are called "pertinent positives," while those not found are "pertinent negatives." For example, consider a patient complaining of abdominal pain. The patient complains of right lower quadrant pain (pertinent positive). The patient denies vomiting or diarrhea (pertinent negatives).

Pertinent Past Medical History

Gathering the patient's pertinent past medical history and information about his or her current health status is important. The patient's past medical history may relate to the patient's present illness and affect his or her treatment. The patient may not know what is or is not relevant regarding his or her medical history, so the paramedic should ask several questions to elicit this information. The SAMPLE acronym is used to recall the pertinent questions to ask regarding the patient's medical history (Table 24-2).

Documenting allergies to medications is as important as determining what medications the patient takes. There are times when this information is not available because of the patient's condition, but usually the patient will be able to provide it. If the medications are known, but their exact purpose is unclear, medical direction may be able to use the available infor-

---

TABLE 24-1   OPQRST Acronym for Eliciting History of Present Illness or Event

Description	Definition	Sample Questions
O = Onset	When the pain or illness began	"What were you doing when the problem began?" "When did this begin?"
P = Provocation/Palliative	What actions or situations bring on the symptoms, or make the pain better?	"Did anything bring on the pain?" "Does anything make the pain better or worse?"
Q = Quality	How the patient perceives the pain	"How would you describe your pain?"
R = Region/Radiation/Referral	Where the pain is located and where it goes	"Where is the pain?" (Ask the patient to point to it) "Does it go anywhere else?"
S = Severity	The degree of pain the patient feels	"On a scale of 1 to 10, with 1 being the least and 10 being the worst, what number would you assign your pain or discomfort?" "Is it comparable to something you can describe?"
T = Timing	How long and how often this has affected the patient	"What time of day does the pain occur?" "How often? How long does it last? Does it come and go, or is it a steady pain?"

TABLE 24-2	SAMPLE Acronym for Eliciting Pertinent Past Medical History
Decription	**Sample Questions**
S = Signs/Symptoms	"Have you had any other symptoms such as dizziness, nausea, vomiting, diarrhea?"
A = Allergies	"Are you allergic to anything?"
M = Medications	"Are you taking any medications? What are they for?"
P = Past medical history	"Have you had this problem before? Do you have other medical problems?" (diabetes, hypertension, heart disease, cancer, seizure disorder)
L = Least oral intake	"When did you last eat or drink anything?"
E = Events leading up to the illness or injury	"How had you been feeling before this problem began?" "Have you been doing anything different from your ordinary routine?"

mation to determine the probable medical conditions and help develop an appropriate treatment plan.

Find out if the patient is taking any medications, both prescription and over-the-counter, including laxatives, vitamins, nasal spray, birth control pills, aspirin, and antacids. Knowledge about patient medications can assist healthcare providers in determining previously diagnosed medical illnesses. Ask the patient if he or she has any known sensitivity or allergy to medication, food, or environmental agents (e.g., dust, pollen). Evaluating the patient's compliance in taking medications, his or her response to them (including any untoward reactions), and any recent change in medications (additions, deletions, or change in dosages) are important. Provide all information obtained to the receiving facility for continuity of care.

Last oral intake includes solids and liquids as well as the time and amount ingested. This information is important if surgery is later required and should be of concern to the paramedic if the patient vomits and cannot protect his or her airway. Events leading to the illness or injury can be helpful in determining the patient's illness or injury (e.g., loss of consciousness after the injury, dizziness before a fall, exertion before onset of chest pain).

Family/Social History

In some situations, information regarding the patient's family and social history may be relevant. The family history may reveal risk factors for certain diseases. For example, in a patient complaining of chest pain, it would be helpful to know if there is a history of heart disease or high blood pressure in the patient's family. Particular attention should be given to disorders such as diabetes, heart disease, tuberculosis, cancer, hypertension, and bleeding disorders.

Evaluation of the patient's social history may also be important. The patient's housing and economic conditions (lack of heating or cooling, inadequate diet), travel history (exposure to contaminated water, communicable disease), and occupation (hours, physical or mental stress, heat or cold exposure, exposure to toxins) may be relevant in some situations.

Current Health Status

It is important to determine the patient's state of wellness just before the onset of the present problem. If time permits, determine if the patient regularly sees a physician. Ask the patient about patterns of eating and sleeping, exercise, and quantity of alcohol, tobacco, coffee, and tea ingestion.

Perform a Focused Physical Examination

In addition to the history, an important part of the assessment is the physical examination. The examination should be geared toward identification of factors that may affect decisions regarding immediate treatment. For a responsive medical patient, a focused examination is performed based on the patient's chief complaint and signs and symptoms. For example, if the patient's complaint is abdominal pain, the physical exam is focused on that area.

After the focused assessment, obtain the patient's baseline vital signs and provide emergency medical care based on the patient's signs and symptoms, as per protocol or in consultation with medical direction.

Unresponsive Medical Patient—Perform a Rapid Medical Assessment

The focused history and physical examination of the unresponsive medical patient is performed in a systematic (head-to-toes) manner in order to avoid missing valuable clues about the patient's condition. The paramedic should demonstrate sensitivity regarding the patient's privacy and comfort. When possible, the examination should be conducted in a private setting. A blanket or sheet may be used to cover the patient if this is impractical. The unresponsive patient should be positioned to protect his or her airway.

Assess the Head

Inspect facial features (eyelids, eyebrows, mouth) for symmetry (Fig. 24-1). If asymmetry is present, observe whether all fea-

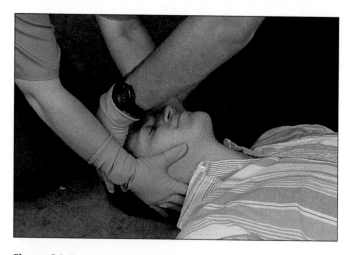

Figure 24-1

Assessment of the head.

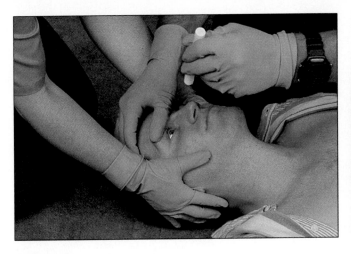

Figure 24-2

Assess the pupils for size, equality and reactivity to light.

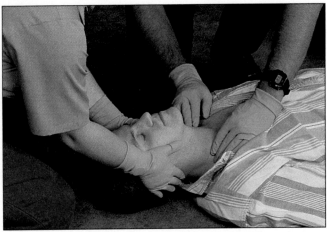

Figure 24-3

Inspect the neck for JVD.

tures on one side of the face are affected, suggesting facial nerve paralysis, or only part of the face such as the forehead, lower face, or mouth, suggesting facial nerve weakness. Look at the color of the face and note the presence of any swelling or excessive perspiration.

Many disorders cause a change in the shape or condition of the face. Overactivity of the thyroid (hyperthyroidism) can cause protrusion of the eyeballs. Underactivity of the thyroid (hypothyroidism) can cause thinning of the scalp hair and eyebrows, and a dry, puffy face with dry skin. Dehydration and prolonged illness can result in sunken eyes, cheeks, and temples.

Assess the pupils and observe their size, equality, and reactivity to light (Fig. 24-2). The pupils are normally black, round, and equal in size. Cloudy pupils often indicate cataracts, which tend to occur in patients more than 65 years of age. Dilated pupils can result from injury, glaucoma, neurological disorders, or drugs (such as atropine). Constricted pupils may indicate inflammation of the iris or may result from narcotic drugs such as morphine.

Note the color of the sclerae (whites of the eyes). The sclerae may become yellow in color (jaundice) if liver disease is present. (It is important not to confuse jaundice with the normal yellow pigmentation in the sclera of a dark-skinned patient). Inspect the color of the conjunctivae by pulling the lower eyelid down. A pale color is often associated with anemia, whereas a bright red color is associated with inflammation (conjunctivitis).

Assess the Neck

Inspect the neck for jugular venous distention (Fig. 24-3). Jugular venous distention occurs in chronic illnesses where the heart is attempting to compensate for an increased workload, such as in congestive heart failure. These veins are normally mildly distended when the patient is supine and flattened when he or she is in a sitting position. Distention observed above the clavicles with the patient sitting at a 45-degree angle is a significant finding. Definitive determination of this finding requires more extensive evaluation at the hospital.

Observe the suprasternal area for retractions or use of accessory muscles. Palpate the anterior neck, noting the position of the trachea. The trachea is normally palpated in the midline of the neck, directly above the suprasternal notch.

Auscultate the carotid arteries of the middle-aged and older adults and patients with suspected cerebrovascular disease (Fig. 24-4). Normally, no sound is heard when auscultating the carotid arteries. If the vessel is narrowed or occluded, blood flowing through the affected portion of the vessel creates turbulence. The turbulence created produces a blowing or swishing sound, called a bruit. If a bruit is heard, gently palpate the artery to determine the presence of a thrill (palpable bruit). A thrill is a vibrating sensation similar to that of a purring cat.

Assess the Chest

Expose the chest. It is important to note that men exhibit primarily abdominal movement with respiration, whereas women exhibit mostly costal movement. The presence of asymmetrical chest movement, a barrel chest (increased anterior-posterior di-

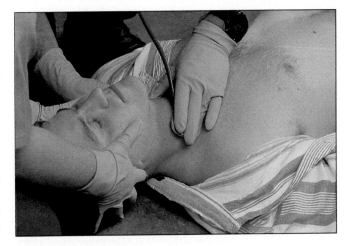

Figure 24-4

Bruits can be assessed by listening over the carotid arteries with a stethoscope. No pressure should be placed on the artery, and only one side of the neck should be touched at a time.

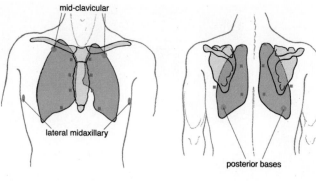

Figure 24-5

Sites for chest auscultation. Using the midclavicular, lateral axillary, and posterior bases allows the paramedic to listen to all lobes of the patient's lungs.

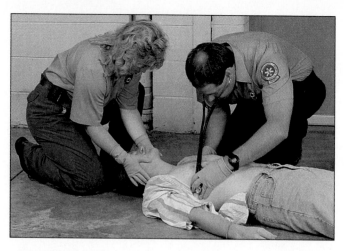

Figure 24-6

Auscultate for breath sounds.

ameter of the chest, often seen in patients with **chronic obstructive pulmonary disease**), retractions, or use of accessory muscles during breathing should be noted. Look for scars that could indicate surgery and a bulging pocket of skin that may contain an implantable defibrillator or pacemaker.

Auscultate for breath sounds over the apex and base of each lung and on the lateral aspects of the chest in the midaxillary line (Fig. 24-5). Determine if breath sounds are present, diminished, or absent and are equal or unequal and are clear or noisy (Fig. 24-6). See Chapter 18 for additional information about abnormal breath sounds.

Heart sounds are often difficult to hear, especially in a noisy environment. The apical heart rate can be auscultated for rate and regularity. To find the apical area, the paramedic must first find the fifth intercostal space just to the left of the sternum. The fingers are then moved laterally to the left midclavicular line.

Normal heart sounds are called S_1 and S_2. Closure of the mitral and tricuspid valves produces the first heart sound (S_1), "lub." The second heart sound, S_2, is produced by closure of the aortic and pulmonic valves, "dub." A third heart sound, S_3, is an extra heart sound associated with rapid ventricular filling that is common in children, athletes, and young adults. The presence of a third heart sound is considered abnormal in persons over age 30.

A pericardial friction rub may be heard as a result of inflamed pericardial layers rubbing against one another. **Myocardial infarction** and **pericarditis** (infection of the pericardium) can predispose a patient to inflammation of the tissues surrounding the heart.

Assess the Abdomen

Assessment of the abdomen is performed with the patient in a supine position. Inspect the abdomen for the presence of scars, bruising, or ascites. Feel all four abdominal quadrants using the pads of the fingers (Fig. 24-7). Palpate the abdomen to evaluate for pain, tenderness, guarding, pulsations, masses, distention, and rigidity. While examining the patient's abdomen, the

examiner's eyes should be kept on the patient's face for clues regarding the quality and degree of pain or tenderness.

Assess the Pelvis

In the pregnant patient, visually examine the perineum if the bag of waters has ruptured. In males and females, inspect the pelvic area for evidence of bowel or bladder incontinence.

Assess the Extremities

Inspect and palpate the entire length of girth of each extremity. compare one upper or lower extremity to the other, noting length, circumference, temperature, pulses, and color of the skin.

Look for swelling in the lower extremities. Dependent edema around the area of the feet and ankles is commonly observed in the elderly and in individuals who stand for long periods. Dependent edema may be a sign of right-sided heart failure and/or venous insufficiency. To assess for edema, press firmly over the medial malleolus or shin for 5 seconds. Edema is present if an impression is left in the skin.

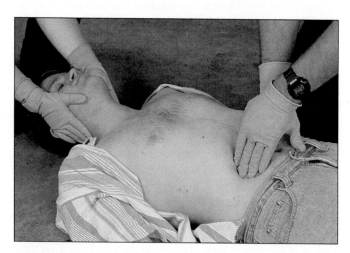

Figure 24-7

Inspect and palpate the abdomen.

Inspect the peripheral leg veins for signs of phlebitis. Signs of phlebitis include warmth and redness over a vein and/or swelling of one calf or leg.

Assess distal pulses in each extremity. Absence of pulsation in one extremity suggests arterial spasm or occlusion. Decreased, weak, or thready pulses suggests impaired cardiac output. Increased pulse strength (volume) may be due to circulatory overload or hypertension.

Evaluate capillary refill in infants and children less than six years of age. Also look for medical identification devices that can help provide clues to the nature of the patient's problem (Fig. 24-8).

Assess the Posterior Body

Inspect and palpate the back for any obvious deformity. In patients who are confined to bed, note the presence of any edema in the sacral region due to poor circulation and fluid retention.

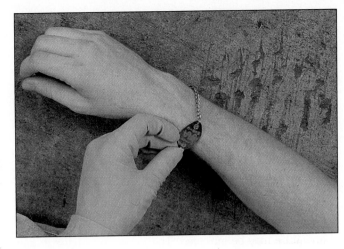

Figure 24-8

The presence of medical identification devices can give the paramedic additional information about the patient's problem.

Assess Baseline Vital Signs and Obtain Medical History

After the rapid medical assessment, obtain the patient's baseline vital signs and gather the patient's medical history from family members, friends, or bystanders as discussed earlier in this chapter.

An initial set of vital signs provides a baseline against which subsequent findings can be compared. Some of this information may have been obtained during initial assessment. There are several vital signs to record, including:

- Respiratory rate, depth and equality, and rhythm (pattern)
- Pulse rate and quality (strength, rhythm, equality)
- Skin color, temperature, and condition (moisture)
- Temperature
- Capillary refill in infants and children less than six years of age
- Pupils
- Blood pressure

Any vital sign abnormalities should be noted and explored further once a transport decision is made. Initially, it is enough to recognize that there is a problem that requires intervention. Baseline vital signs provide data regarding the patient's overall status and how he or she is compensating for the current condition. When assessing vital signs, consider the averages for different ages and focus on abnormal findings. (See Chapter 23)

Respiratory Rate, Depth, and Rhythm

Respiratory problems and/or obstruction can be associated with a variety of illnesses. The patient's respiratory rate should be assessed and documented. Respiratory depth and equality is assessed by observing the amount of movement of the chest wall. With normal breathing, average chest wall motion is observed and the chest expands symmetrically. With shallow breathing, a small volume of air is exchanged and ventilatory movement is difficult to see. Breathing may involve only slight chest or abdominal wall motion. With deep breathing, there is full expansion of the lungs and a large volume of air is exchanged.

Normal breathing is quiet, relaxed, and effortless. Labored breathing is often associated with the use of accessory muscles. Abnormal respiratory sounds heard during auscultation of the lungs are cause for concern.

Pulse Rate and Quality

The patient's pulse rate and quality should be assessed and documented. Evaluation of pulse quality includes evaluation of pulse strength, rhythm, and equality. Pulse strength (volume) refers to the force of the pressure wave as blood is pumped through the body and is described as absent, weak, strong, or bounding.

An absent pulse is not discernible. A weak pulse is difficult to feel and may be called a "feeble" pulse. A weak, rapid pulse is called a "thready" pulse. A normal pulse is readily detected, obliterated by strong pressure, and the pressure is equal for each beat. A normal pulse is called a "strong" or "full" pulse. An extremely strong pulse that is difficult to obliterate with pressure is called a "bounding" pulse. Pulses on both sides of the body should be assessed and compared. Pulses are normally equal bilaterally but may be unequal in strength due to extremity injury, clot formation, or other causes.

Skin Color, Temperature, and Condition

The adult patient's skin color may be assessed in the nailbeds, oral mucosa (mucous membranes of the mouth), and conjunctiva (mucous membrane that lines the inner surface of the eyelid). The nailbeds are the least reliable site to assess skin color because the nailbeds are easily affected by cold, smoking, and many chronic medical conditions. Skin color in infants and children should be assessed in the palms of the hands and the soles of the feet.

Relative skin temperature is assessed by placing the back of the examiner's hands or fingers against the patient's skin. The back surface of the hands and fingers are most sensitive to temperature. The skin is normally warm to the touch.

Assess the patient's skin condition (moisture). The skin is normally dry to the touch. Wet or moist skin may indicate shock (hypoperfusion), a heat-related illness, or diabetic emergency. Excessively dry skin may indicate dehydration.

Temperature

Extreme environmental conditions can cause a rapid change in the body's internal temperature. In areas of the country where this occurs, and/or the patient history warrants, the body temperature reading is an important vital sign to obtain.

Additionally, in the medical patient with vague symptoms, particularly malaise, or a history of chills, an evaluation of the temperature may be indicated. The presence of fever in any patient may indicate an infectious process that requires medical evaluation (see Chapter 38).

Capillary Refill

Capillary refill should be assessed in infants and children less than six years of age. Capillary refill is assessed by pressing on the patient's skin or nailbeds and determining the time for return to initial color. Normal capillary refill is less than 2 seconds. Delayed (greater than 2 seconds) capillary refill suggests circulatory compromise.

Pupils

The pupils are assessed by briefly shining a light into the patient's eyes and assessing size, equality, and reactivity. The pupils are normally equal in size, round, and equally reactive to light. Dilated pupils can result from hypoxia, trauma, eye medications, neurologic disorders, glaucoma, or other conditions. Constricted pupils may be caused by medications, inflammation of the iris, or other causes. A few patients normally have pupils of unequal sizes.

Reactivity refers to whether or not the pupils change in response to light. Normally, a light shown into the pupil of one eye will cause pupil constriction of both eyes (consensual response). Nonreactive pupils do not change when exposed to light and may occur because of medications, cardiac arrest, or central nervous system injury. Unequally reactive pupils (one pupil reacts but the other does not) may occur because of a head injury or stroke. Causes of abnormal pupils are found in Box 24-2.

Blood Pressure

Many factors can affect a blood pressure reading, such as anxiety, stress, trauma, or an inappropriate blood pressure cuff size. A single reading is used as a baseline against which to evaluate subsequent readings. Coupled with assessment of the patient's level of consciousness, pulse and skin signs, the blood pressure can help confirm suspected circulatory problems.

Focused History and Physical Examination: Trauma

While many medical conditions can be corrected at the scene, a patient with significant trauma needs surgical intervention. This requires rapid identification of critical conditions, both actual and potential, and transport to an appropriate receiving facility. The term "load and go" has been used to reinforce the importance of rapid evacuation and patient outcome. The goal is to spend no more than 10 minutes on scene for a patient with serious trauma, unless the patient is entrapped. Since many severe injuries are internal and not easily identified, the mechanism of injury plays an important role in determining time spent on scene.

Reevaluation of Mechanism of Injury

For the trauma patient, the focused examination begins with reevaluation of the mechanism of injury. This helps identify priority patients and helps guide the patient assessment. Significant mechanisms of injury include:

- Ejection from a vehicle
- Death in the same passenger compartment
- Falls from more than 20 feet (or three times body height)
- Rollover of a vehicle
- High-speed vehicle collision
- Vehicle–pedestrian collision
- Motorcycle crash
- Unresponsive or altered mental status
- Penetrations of the head, chest, or abdomen
- Hidden injuries from seat belts or airbags

Infant and child considerations:

- Falls from more than 10 feet in infants and children (or three times body height)
- Bicycle collision
- Vehicle collision at a medium speed
- Any vehicle collision where the infant or child was unrestrained

A rapid trauma assessment should be performed on all patients with a significant mechanism of injury. The rapid trauma assessment is a head-to-toes physical examination performed to detect the presence of life threatening injuries. In the responsive patient, symptoms should be sought before and during the trauma assessment.

BOX 24-2	Causes of Abnormal Pupils	
Dilated	**Pinpoint**	**Unequal**
Fright	Narcotics	May be normal
Drugs	Bright light (normal)	Head injury
Pain	Hemorrhage in the	Stroke
Hypoxia	pons area of the	Cataracts
Glaucoma	brain	
Brain injury (bilateral hemorrhage or swelling)		

Trauma Patient with Significant Mechanism of Injury

Inline spinal stabilization, begun during the initial assessment, should be continued throughout the focused physical examination. After reevaluation of the mechanism of injury, reconsider the transport decision made at the end of the initial assessment. Determine if the patient requires immediate transport with continued assessment and care performed en route to the hospital or on scene stabilization

Rapid Trauma Assessment

Throughout the physical examination, the paramedic should look (inspect), listen (auscultate), and feel (palpate) for injuries or signs of injury. The DCAP-BTLS acronym is used to assist the paramedic in remembering what to assess (see Chapter 21).

During the physical exam, the patient's privacy should be protected as much as possible. Talk to the patient to obtain information about his general condition and whether there is pain on palpation of any areas. Document any abnormal findings. Keep in mind that a painful injury in one area often overrides pain elsewhere.

Assess the Head

When assessing the head and neck of a trauma patient, ensure that someone is maintaining inline spinal stabilization. Look and feel for deformities, contusions, abrasions, penetrations, burns, lacerations, and swelling. Be alert for sharp bony fragments, shards of glass, or other foreign objects. These objects may worsen injuries if they are pressed too firmly.

Assess the periorbital area around the eyes, the nose, maxilla, and mandible. Look for leakage of blood or fluid from the nose or ears. Look for the presence of raccoon's eyes (bruising around the eyes), a sign suggesting basilar skull fracture that often does not appear immediately. If present early, it more likely suggests direct trauma to the face, not the skull. Look for discoloration over the mastoid process (Battle's sign) behind the ear. Battle's sign suggests the presence of a skull fracture but is usually not seen until hours after the injury. Look for burns of the face, nasal hairs, and mouth.

Feel the entire facial bone structure, beginning at the bridge of the nose and extending laterally toward the ears (Fig. 24-9). Note the presence of any tenderness, instability, or crepitation.

Look at each eye individually, and note whether the eyes are working together. Assess the pupils and observe their size, equality, and reactivity to light. Sluggish pupil response can reflect hypoxia, hypercarbia, or the use of depressant substances. Note if there is blood visible in the anterior chamber (hyphema).

Look in the mouth and observe the color of the mucous membranes. Look for blood, vomitus, absent or broken teeth, and a lacerated or swollen tongue. This is especiallly important if the patient is to be immobilized with a cervical spine immobilization collar (CSIC) and a backboard. Have suction ready, as swallowed blood can cause vomiting (Fig. 24-10).

Assess the Neck

When examining the neck, look and feel for deformities, contusions, abrasions, penetrations, burns, lacerations, swelling, and jugular venous distention. Palpate the cervical vertebrae for tenderness and deformity. Palpate the anterior and posterior neck for subcutaneous emphysema. Subcutaneous emphysema occurs when air from the lungs or a tracheal tear leaks into the tissue on the upper chest and neck. The patient with subcutaneous emphysema may appear bloated. The affected tissue feels like small air bubbles under the skin and crackles under the fingertips when palpated.

Palpate the anterior neck for tracheal deviation. Ask the patient if he or she feels any neck pain, tightness, numbness, tingling, or a burning sensation in the shoulders, arms, or legs. A trauma victim with a significant mechanism of injury needs immobilization with a cervical spine immobilization collar, long backboard, and head immobilization device.

Assess the Chest

Palpate the entire chest, including the length of the clavicles, the sternum, and the rib cage including as much of the posterior chest as can safely be reached (Fig. 24-11). Look and feel for deformities, contusions, abrasions, penetrations, paradoxical motion, burns, lacerations, and swelling.

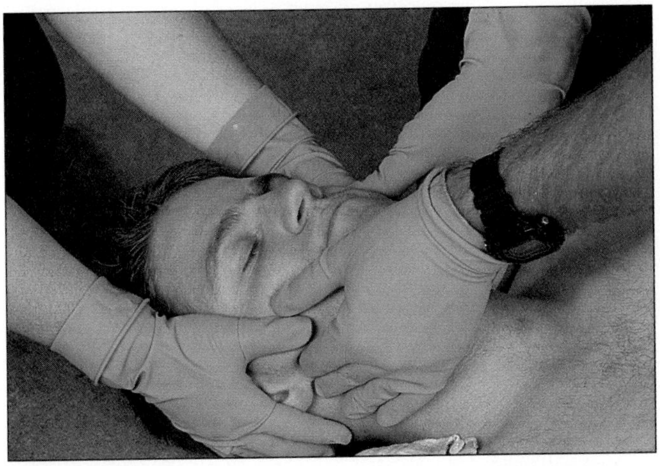

Figure 24-9
A gentle touch should be used when assessing the patient's face.

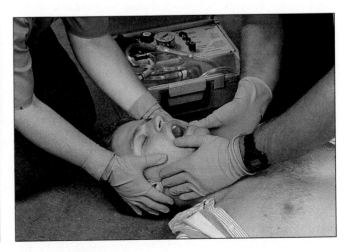

Figure 24-10
Inspect the patient's mouth, with suction readily available.

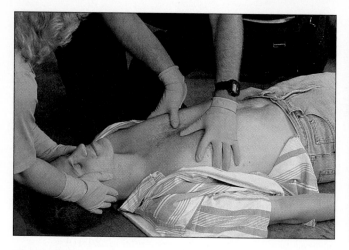

Figure 24-11

Palpate the entire chest.

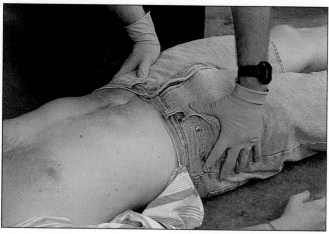

Figure 24-12

Gently compress the pelvis.

Look for open chest wounds and use of accessory muscles during breathing. An open wound of the chest should be covered immediately with an occlusive dressing. Feel for crepitus, instability, tenderness, guarding, and subcutaneous emphysema.

Auscultate for breath sounds over the apex and base of each lung and on the lateral aspects of the chest in the midaxillary line. Determine if breath sounds are present, diminished, or absent, or are equal or unequal, or are clear or noisy. If breath sounds are unequal, evaluate for a **tension pneumothorax** and **hemothorax**. If the patient has been intubated, reassess endotracheal tube placement.

Assess the Abdomen

Unlike the chest, many abdominal organs lack bony protection. Only the upper abdominal quadrants, which contain the liver, spleen, and stomach, are provided some protection by the lower ribs. Because of the general lack of protection, abdominal organs can easily be injured; some, such as the liver and spleen, tend to bleed profusely. If the injury is internal, a rapid assessment will produce only a general idea of the possible organs involved, but this is enough to identify a potentially life threatening condition and the need for rapid transport. Bowel sounds are rarely auscultated in the field because of the need for a quiet environment and the lengthy time needed to detect the presence or absence of sounds in all four quadrants. Transport should not be delayed to evaluate bowel sounds.

For examination purposes, the xiphoid process (tip of the sternum) marks the upper boundary of the abdomen, and the symphysis pubis the lower boundary. The abdomen is divided into four imaginary quadrants for reference. Assessment of the abdomen is performed with the patient in a supine position.

Look for deformities, contusions, abrasions, penetrations, burns, lacerations, swelling, and evisceration. Palpate all four abdominal quadrants using the pads of the fingers. If the patient is complaining of pain in a particular area, ask the patient to point to it and palpate that area last. Assess for rigidity,

masses, and tenderness. A tender, rigid abdomen is considered a threat to life. If the patient develops this finding, reconsider the transport decision and reevaluate the care being provided.

Assess the Pelvis

When assessing the pelvis, consider the patient's age and overall condition. Elderly patients sometimes suffer significant hip and pelvic injuries from what might otherwise be considered a minor fall. A pelvic fracture can result in significant blood loss or a ruptured bladder.

Look and feel for deformities, contusions, abrasions, penetrations, burns, lacerations, and swelling. Do not "rock" the pelvis. Gently compress directly over the symphysis pubis and push in laterally over the iliac crests to assess tenderness, instability, and crepitation (Fig. 24-12). If the patient complains of pain in the pelvic region, or obvious deformity is present, do not palpate the pelvis.

Evaluate the genital region for injury, and note if the patient has lost bladder or bowel control. Loss of bladder or bowel control is called incontinence and can result from coma, **seizures**, stroke, or **spinal injury**.

Assess the Extremities

Inspect and palpate the entire length and girth of each extremity (Fig. 24-13). Look and feel for deformities, contusions, abrasions, penetrations, burns, lacerations, and swelling. Note the temperature and color of the skin. Assess distal pulses, motor function, and sensation in each extremity. To assess motor function, ask the patient to wiggle his or her fingers and toes and squeeze or push against your hand (Fig. 24-14). To evaluate sensation, ask the patient if he or she can feel your touch and identify where you are touching.

Compare one upper or lower extremity to the other, noting length, circumference, temperature, strength, and pulse. Evaluate capillary refill in infants and children less than six years of age. Also look for medical identification devices that can help provide clues to the nature of the patient's problem.

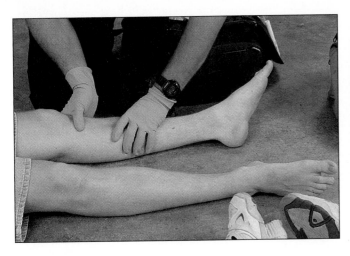

Figure 24-13

Inspect and palpate each extremity.

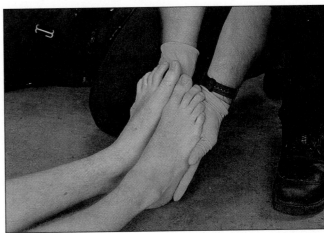

Figure 24-14

Assess motor function.

Assess the Posterior Body

If the patient is not yet immobilized on a backboard, logroll the patient with spinal precautions and assess the posterior body (Fig. 24-15). Look for deformities, contusions, abrasions, penetrations, burns, lacerations, and swelling. Palpate the entire length of the vertebral column for tenderness, instability, and crepitation.

Trauma Patient with No Significant Mechanism of Injury

For a trauma patient with no significant mechanism of injury, a focused assessment is performed on the area the patient states is painful or the paramedic suspects may be injured as a result of the mechanism of injury. For example, if the patient's complaint is a painful wrist, the physical exam is focused on that area. After the focused assessment, obtain the patient's baseline vital signs and gather the patient's medical history as discussed earlier in this chapter.

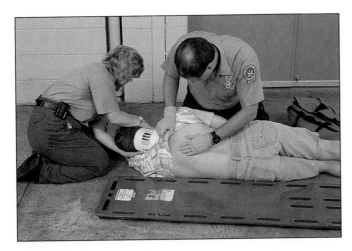

Figure 24-15

Logroll the patient and examine the back.

Remember, the presence or absence of specific signs and symptoms is particularly relevant to the focused history and physical examination. Document pertinent positives as well as pertinent negatives.

> **Scene Survey**
>> **Initial Assessment**
>>> **Focused History and Physical Exam**
>>>> **Continued Assessment**

Continued Assessment

The initial assessment and focused history and physical examinations are completed rapidly so that serious illness or injury can be identified, intervention provided, and transport initiated without delay. Once the patient's most serious conditions have been managed (or if none can be determined), the continued assessment is performed. The continued assessment is a more detailed examination and always includes continued reevaluation of the patient while in the paramedic's care. With serious conditions, this is usually performed en route to the hospital.

The continued assessment is performed to:

- Identify any missed injuries or conditions, particularly those that are life-threatening
- Assess the patient's response to care
- Adjust the patient management as necessary

The detailed physical examination is specific to the patient and injury. Not all patients require a detailed physical exam. For example, a patient with an isolated injury such as a laceration of the hand would not require a detailed physical exam. A trauma patient with a significant mechanism of injury and an unconscious patient should have a detailed physical examination as part of his or her continued assessment. However, depending on the severity of the patient's injury or illness, the detailed physical exam may not be completed because treatment of life-threats takes precedence over performance of the exam.

When performed, the detailed exam begins at the head and ends with the extremities, repeating in more depth the many steps accomplished in the rapid trauma and medical assessments. The detailed exam may reveal additional injuries or other information that will assist in determining the patient's diagnosis at the receiving facility.

To ensure appropriate care, the paramedic must continually observe and reevaluate the patient frequently during transport to prevent or manage emerging conditions. If the patient complains of a new symptom or there is a change in a symptom previously identified, perform a focused examination for the area of the complaint.

Reassess and record the patient's mental status, airway, breathing, circulation, vital signs, and effectiveness of interventions at least every 15 minutes in a stable patient and at least every 5 minutes in an unresponsive or unstable patient. Findings obtained during the continued assessment should be compared with baseline findings obtained during the focused assessment.

Effective assessment techniques at the scene and en route to the hospital make it possible to detect and manage medical and trauma emergencies. By systematically following the steps of the patient assessment process, the paramedic can ensure that critical patients receive early, appropriate intervention.

SUMMARY

The focused history and physical examination follows the initial assessment and consists of four main steps:

1. Assessing the patient's medical history
2. Performing a physical examination, focusing on the area of the patient's chief complaint
3. Obtaining baseline vital signs
4. Providing emergency care based on signs and symptoms in consultation with medical direction

The sequence of the steps of the focused history and physical examination and emphasis placed on each step are different for trauma and medical patients. In the medical patient, emphasis is placed on the patient's medical history. In the trauma patient, emphasis is placed on the mechanism of the injury.

The initial assessment and focused history and physical examinations are completed rapidly so that serious illness or injury can be identified, intervention provided, and transport initiated without delay.

Once the patient's most serious conditions have been managed (or if none can be determined), the continued assessment is performed. The continued assessment is a more detailed examination and always includes continued reevaluation of the patient while in the paramedic's care. With serious conditions, the continued assessment is usually performed en route to the hospital.

SUGGESTED READINGS

1. **Ali J, et al:** Advanced Trauma Life Support Course for Physicians. American College of Surgeons, 1989.

2. **Bledsoe B:** *Paramedic Emergency Care,* ed 3. Englewood Cliffs, NJ, 1997: Prentice-Hall, Inc.

3. **Campbell J E, ed:** Basic Trauma Life Support for Paramedics and Advanced EMS Providers, ed 3, Englewood Cliffs, NJ, 1995, Prentice-Hall, Inc.

4. **Caroline N:** Emergency Care in the Streets, ed 5, Boston, 1995, Little, Brown and Company.

5. **Dunham M C, Adams C R:** Initial Evaluation and Management of the Trauma Patient. Shock Trauma/Critical Care Manual. Maryland Institute for Emergency Medical Services Systems, 1991.

6. **Dunham M C, Adams C R:** Systems Injury. Shock Trauma/Critical Care Manual. Maryland Institute for Emergency Medical Services Systems, 1991.

7. **Dunham M C, Adams C R:** Systems Failure. Shock Trauma/Critical Care Manual. Maryland Institute for Emergency Medical Services Systems, 1991.

8. **Leslie D J:** Patient Assessment: History Taking and Physical Examination. Neurologic Problems. *Nurse Review.* 1986.

9. **Leslie D J:** Evaluation. Neurologic Problems. *Nurse Review.* 1986.

10. **Nicholas B S:** Pain: Transmission and Theories. Special Neurologic Problems. *Nurse Review.* 1986.

11. **Paris P M, Stewart R D:** Pain Management in Emergency Medicine. 1988.

12. **Potter P A, Perry A G:** Fundamentals of Nursing: Concepts, Process, and Practice. St. Louis, 1993, Mosby–Year Book, Inc.

13. **Seidel H M, et al:** Mosby's Guide to Physical Examination. St. Louis, 1995, Mosby–Year Book, Inc.

Larry Mellick, MD, FAAP, FACEP

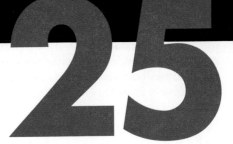

Chapter 25

Pediatric Assessment

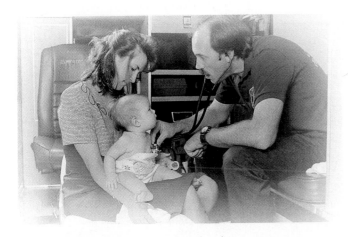

A paramedic should be able to:

1. Describe the unique physiological, anatomical, and psychological characteristics of the pediatric patient.

2. Describe appropriate interaction with the pediatric patient's parents or guardian.

3. Identify ways to become better prepared to deal with pediatric patients.

4. Describe how the assessment process and management of the pediatric patient should be altered based on the child's developmental level.

5. Describe the essential components of the history and physical exam of a pediatric patient.

6. Identify priorities of care for a pediatric patient based on assessment findings.

The subject of managing patients with pediatric emergencies often leads to one central question: Are children medically similar to adults, or are there enough specific differences to require a modified approach?

This chapter assumes that much of the anatomic, physiologic, and assessment knowledge acquired for use in the care for adults is applicable to the care of pediatric patients. Infants and children certainly have differences that go beyond physical size, but these differences are best learned in the context of a thorough grounding in general patient care skills.

As such, this chapter focuses on special differences in young patients, avoiding duplication of general material and emphasizing additional knowledge that paramedics will need to care for infants and children. The assessment and management of critical pediatric patients are explained in Chapter 22.

Psychosocial Aspects of Pediatric Care

Developmental Stages

Pediatric patients are commonly grouped in age ranges to help the paramedic understand the similarities among, and differences between, the many stages of the patients' mental and emotional development from birth to adulthood. The following descriptions summarize actions and responses that paramedics can expect, based on patient age.

Of course, the following are general categories; not all patients will fit these descriptions perfectly. Infants, in particular, could easily be divided into several additional groups because of the rapid changes in the first year of life. Also, some pediatric patients may regress to earlier behavior patterns under the stress of situations that lead to ambulance calls. Still, the characteristics of these stages are an important starting point for the assessment of children.

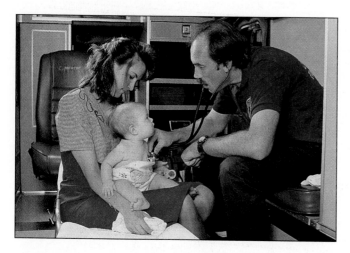

Infants (Birth to 12 Months of Age)

Infants are completely dependent on their environment (primarily their parents), for all physical and emotional needs. This dependence leads to a natural "separation anxiety" in the older infant that makes it important to keep the child in phys-

ical contact with a parent in assessment situations. Because these children are also likely to be frightened by the sudden appearance of strangers, a calm and unthreatening entry by paramedics is important.

As with other pediatric patients, the paramedic should ensure that examining hands and equipment are warm, to help avoid unnecessary surprises that may startle the patient. Reassuring parents is another key. Because the child takes many emotional cues from the parents, the parent's comfort, or agitation, has a direct impact on the patient-paramedic interaction. Giving the patient a pacifier to suck on may also provide a comforting familiarity that helps an infant tolerate a physical examination by a stranger.

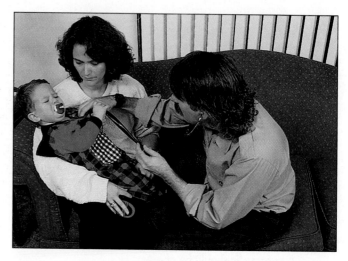

From Stoy WA: Center for Emergency Medicine: Mosby's EMT-Basic Textbook, St. Louis, 1996, Mosby Lifeline.

Toddlers (1 to 3 Years of Age)

Toddlers are in the beginning stages of experiencing life directly, rather than through parents. Separation anxiety and fear of strangers continue in this age group, and these situations often make it difficult for the paramedic to maintain a cooperative attitude. Toddlers must be left in a parent's lap when possible, and may be comforted by allowing them to hold a favorite toy or other possession during the examination. The examination should be gentle, quick, and limited only to the pertinent essentials.

Offering the patient some choices is important for the patient in this age group, and will continue on throughout the older patient groups. The choices and their true relevance to the medical situation vary according to what the child can understand. However, the importance of granting respect and some self-control to the individual does not vary.

Pain becomes a more distinct concept for toddlers; paramedics must choose their approach with an understanding of the patient's acute awareness and fear of pain. Language development is very basic, so explanations must be kept simple. Much of the patient history must come from the parent.

The patient's mind wanders quickly and easily at this age. Responders must be inventive, and sometimes playful, to keep the patient's attention focused where it is needed. The patient's high activity level also means that toddlers will be upset about restraint of any kind; immobilization requires both the paramedic's psychological and physical skill, and is best accomplished with parental cooperation.

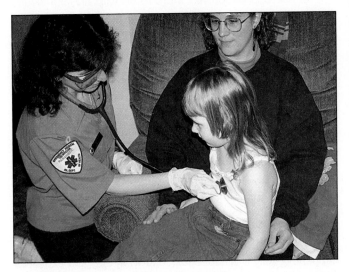

From Stoy WA: Center for Emergency Medicine: Mosby's EMT-Basic Textbook, St. Louis, 1996, Mosby Lifeline.

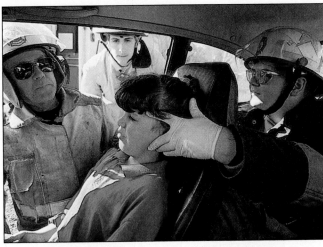

From Stoy WA: Center for Emergency Medicine: Mosby's EMT-Basic Textbook, St. Louis, 1996, Mosby Lifeline.

Preschool-Aged Children (4 to 5 Years of Age)

Many preschooler age children are more self-confident than toddlers, increasing their potential cooperation with responders. Their language skills may permit them to help with their history, and their ability to understand often goes beyond what they can express.

Toddlers' fears about their bodies can be simplistic, and they may interpret paramedics' statements literally. This is the youngest group of pediatric patients that may become upset at careless, although seemingly innocent, statements. A paramedic's reference to a broken bone may suggest a catastrophe, for instance, because the child knows that broken toys are often thrown away. The paramedic instead should use thoughtfully chosen words, and keep an emphasis on recovery and positive outcomes.

Fears that often arise in the patient of this age group include abandonment, darkness, loss of control, and unknown and unfamiliar situations. Body fears are often vivid, including anxieties about blood and mutilation or disfigurement. An explanation by the rescuer that the body is intact can be reassuring to the patient, and covering injuries from the patient's view is important. Offering the patient a chance to hold or examine equipment and help with some part of the examination can spark the child's natural curiosity and cooperation.

School-Aged Children (6 to 11 Years of Age)

School-aged children are often able to cooperate with the examination and are capable of providing most of the needed history. This is a modest age group; the paramedic should be sensitive to the patient's concerns of privacy and body exposure. The modesty may arise partly from the value placed on what the children's peers think.

Language skills make natural interaction with responders easier than it is with children at earlier ages. School-aged children appreciate honest communication, emphasized with positive outcomes, explanations of the reasons for procedures. With this age group, there is a strong need to please adults. These children often benefit from reassurance and praise about their courage and self-control. The paramedic's language skills can also mask confusion; school children may appear to understand more than they do. It is a good idea for to paramedic to ask an occasional question to check the patient's level of understanding.

Fears about mutilation and loss of control continue in patients at this age, along with a new-found awareness and fear of death. Paramedics must expect questions about the long-term results of injury or illness and may reduce anxiety by answering them before asked. It is often helpful to explain that the child has done nothing wrong and is not in trouble.

Adolescents (12 to 18 Years of Age)

Adolescents often approach adult levels of communication and cognition, and must be treated with adult respect. Concern about image among peers is intense and may matter more to the patient than what their parents think. Peer pressure adds to the patient's need for privacy, a need further compounded by the patient's growing awareness of sexual identity.

Although quite independent, adolescents often tend to overreact emotionally to stress and pain. They are acutely aware of possible body disfigurement and other changes in physical image, and fear of death can be strong. These patients need reassurance that is tempered with honest talk about long-term consequences and outcomes.

Both peer pressure and emotional alienation from parents can make history and examination procedures very sensitive. Cooperation is unlikely without a clear commitment to privacy and this situation may require promises of confidentiality that can create legal and ethical problems. Paramedics must understand local law and practice in advance to ensure that they know how much confidentiality they can promise (also see Chapter 5).

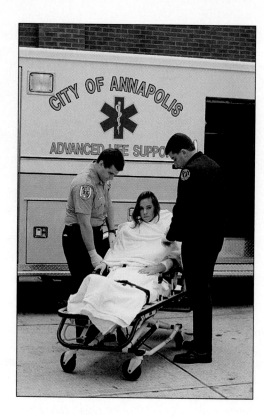

As near-adults, adolescents dislike feeling dependent, and so must be included in their treatment decisions. The paramedic should offer choices wherever possible and, in difficult situations such as confidentiality problems, be clear and candid about why information is needed and what the possible medical consequences are of withholding it. It may enhance the patient history to interview the patient privately, before talking to parents.

Approach to the Patient

From the age-range characteristics previously discussed, the paramedic can draw many of the factors that are important in approaching the pediatric patient. Most of these factors are also appropriate for adults but require special focus with young patients.

Confidence and Calmness

Both parents and children tend to be anxious when a child is ill or injured. The paramedic's behavior can either lessen or aggravate the problem for both parties. Direct communication with both parties is important, as is a manner that indicates competent professionalism. This interaction involves a balance between being gentle and taking firm control. It is a balance based on observations of the specific situation, as well as the moods and personalities involved. There is no one-size-fits-all approach.

Paramedic anxiety, which is common during pediatric responses, can be a major obstacle to overcome when calming other parties involved. The confidence that helps parents and children to relax and trust the responder grows out of the responder's own strength and ability to handle the problem.

Paramedics who find themselves routinely or intensely uncomfortable with pediatric situations can address this problem in two ways. The first option is further study of pediatric care, which is a specialty in itself that requires ongoing education throughout the paramedic's career.

The second option has more to do with life experience than with training. Paramedics who do not have children or who have not spent much time around young people may simply need more direct contact with this age group. Extra training in pediatric units or simply volunteering in a day care setting can be valuable for developing communication skills and comfort levels around children.

Honesty

Although it may be tempting at times to shade the truth for children or their parents, it must be done with care. Anything that could be construed later as deliberate deception can compromise trust in paramedics and other caregivers and could affect care in a way that hurts the patient.

This does not mean that brutal honesty is necessarily appropriate, but those involved do need explanations of what is happening, why it is happening, and what they can expect as the situation progresses. This includes fair warning about procedures that may hurt or be frightening to the patient. It also includes some caution about promises made; optimism can be very reassuring ("No more shots now"), but optimism must also be balanced with the range of possibilities to come (another IV at the hospital). "I don't know" is a better answer than a false-positive answer, especially when accompanied by an offer to find out information or to pass along the concern to future caregivers.

A good approach for the paramedic to use is to give a general explanation of the need for a transport or procedure, and then focus on the necessities for a positive outcome. Depending on the ages and emotions of patients and others involved, two explanations may work well: a simple explanation for the patient, and a more detailed one for the parent, delivered out of the patient's earshot.

Consistency

The stress and uncertainty of emergencies can often be reduced by designating one caregiver to develop rapport immediately and remain with the patient until transfer of care. Most children will naturally include this "primary responder" as part of their emotional support system. The primary responder then makes introductions (of new responders and receiving staff) and explanations to the patient to reduce stranger anxiety and fears about unknown situations and events.

Consistency also applies to "honesty." If the answer to a previous question has changed or a promise must be broken, it is best done with an admission of the mistake made by the paramedic and an apology that acknowledges the distress the change may cause.

Respect for Patient Dignity

At every age, respect for an individual's dignity is a central factor in maintaining trust in the care setting. Even though infants are too young to express this need directly, the parents will feel it strongly on their behalf. Several related factors contribute to the patient's sense of being respected.

- *Physical approach.* Smaller children, in particular, are intimidated by strangers who approach and touch them too quickly. When time permits, the paramedic should take a moment to talk with parents and begin verbal and eye contact that will let the child accept his or her approach more gradually. This also gives the paramedic an initial chance to observe the child's general condition (e.g., skin, breathing, mood, guarded body areas). Behavioral changes triggered by direct stranger contact may be easier to sort out from symptoms of the underlying problem. Another way to reduce the intimidation factor is for the paramedic to be positioned at face level with the patient, rather than towering above, which can often be intimidating.
- *Self-determination.* People have a need to feel in control of their bodies, feelings, and decisions. One key is to offer as many choices to the patient as possible and many opportunities to participate in the care process (more critical conditions lessen the opportunities, of course). However, the paramedic must be sure the choice exists before offering it. Asking, "Do you want to go for a ride in the ambulance?" is a mistake with a child who requires transport, but "Do you want to go in Mom's lap or ride on the stretcher?" grants the patient some control.
- *Privacy.* Being unclothed in front of others is sometimes more sensitive for children than for adults. Simple precautions can help preserve patient modesty and help convince patients and parents that responders have their best interests in mind. In smaller children, modesty regarding strangers is often quite intense. Outside of trauma settings (when shielded stripping may be necessary), having a child identify parts on a doll can help in history taking. Adolescents present added concerns about image among their peers. Anxiety about privacy of information also increases with age, reaching a stage in adolescence at which it may shape the entire patient encounter.
- *Expression of feelings.* Giving the patient permission to cry or otherwise express pain or fear can be reassuring for those who are stressed by illness or other crises. It helps to prepare the patient for painful procedures such as IV insertion, and demonstrates that the responder wants to help. Venting emotion can also be remarkably calming for the adults involved, if responders listen and acknowledge the feelings, rather than react to them as threats or challenges. Paramedics should praise the patient's courage and thank the child for cooperating with difficult procedures; these actions will validate the patient's feelings and dignity.
- *Parental involvement.* Parental dignity is also part of the pediatric care scenario. Paramedics should avoid questions and comments that carry a critical or judgmental tone. Parents must be validated for seeking help, included in choices and explanations, and offered the opportunity to accompany the child during transport (parents often feel guilty for a child's illness or injury, even when they have done nothing wrong).

Medical Assessment

Although children are born with all of the anatomical and physiological systems of adults, many of these systems are incompletely developed and incapable of full function. Some structures are also positioned differently from adult anatomy, particularly in the respiratory system.

When discussing differences between children and adults, it is important for the paramedic to realize that there is no "magic age" or dividing line between the two groups. CPR guidelines define any patient over 8 years of age as an adult. In terms of disease processes and response to trauma, the paramedic might well consider all patients under 15 years of age to fall into a separate category or several special categories. In legal and psychosocial terms, some experts argue that full adulthood is not achieved until a patient reaches 18 to 21 years of age.

It may be simplest to view changes in the pediatric population as a gradual spectrum from birth until the mid-to-late teenage years. By far the most dramatic differences are seen in the neonatal period (generally defined as the first month of life) and during infancy (the remainder of the first year). Reference charts for vital signs (Table 25-1) and for equipment use

TABLE 25-1	Weight and Vital Signs by Age Group			
Age	Weight, kg (lb)	Respirations	Pulse	Systolic Blood Pressure
Newborn	3–4 kg (6–9 lb)	30–50	120–160	60–80
6 mo–1 yr	8–10 kg (16–22 lb)	30–40	120–140	70–80
2–4 yr	12–16 kg (24–34 lb)	20–30	100–110	80–95
5–8 yr	18–26 kg (36–55 lb)	14–20	90–100	90–100
8–12 yr	26–50 kg (55–110 lb)	12–20	80–100	100–110
> 12 yr	>50 kg (110 lb)	12–16	60–90	100–120

TABLE 25-2   Suggested Pediatric Equipment and Medications

Medication	Standard supply	Minimum quantity
Albuterol sulfate 0.5%	20 ml bottle	1
Atropine sulfate	0.1 mg/ml in 10 ml prefilled syringe	2
Dextrose 25%	12.5 gm in 10 ml prefilled syringe	2
Dextrose 50%	25 gm in 50 ml prefilled syringe	2
Diazepam	5.0 mg/ml in 2.0 ml vial	1
Diphenhydramine HCL	50 mg/ml in 1.0 ml vial	1
Epinephrine 1:1,000	1.0 mg/ml in 1.0 ml ampule	2
Epinephrine 1:10,000	0.1 mg/ml in 10 ml prefilled syringe	3
Glucagon	1.0 mg in vials (mixing required)	1
Lidocaine HCL	10 mg/ml in 10 ml prefilled syringe	2
Metapreterenol sulfate 5%	10 ml or 30 ml bottle	1
Naloxone HCL	1.0 mg/ml in 2.0 ml ampule	2
Normal saline	500 or 1000 ml bag	3
Sodium bicarbonate 8.4%	1.0 mEq/ml in 50 ml prefilled syringe	1
Sodium chloride injection 0.9%	10 ml vial	4

Airway

Laryngoscope handle	Penlite size	1
Miller blades	#0, #1, #2, #3	1 each
Macintosh blades	#2, #3	1 each
Stylet	6F and 14F	1 each
Oropharyngeal airways	00-5	1 each
Nasopharyngeal airways	5.5, 6.0, 7.0, 8.0	1 each
Endotracheal tubes (uncuffed)	2.5, 3.0, 3.5, 4.0, 4.5, 5.0, 5.5	2 each
Endotracheal tubes (cuffed)	6.0, 7.0, 8.0	2 each
Nasogastric tubes	5F, 8F, 10F and 14F	1 each
Suction catheters	6F, 7F, 10F, 12F, and 14F	1 each
Magill forceps	Pediatric size	1
Magill forceps	Adult size	1
Oxygen supply tubing		1
High concentration mask	Pediatric size	1
Nebulizer		1
Bag-valve-mask resuscitator	Child and infant size	1 each
Transparent ventilation masks	Premature, newborn, infant, child, and small adult sizes	1 each

Adapted from Eichelberger: Pediatric Trauma, 1993, St. Louis, Mosby-Year Book.

(Table 25-2) typically divide pediatric patients into several age ranges. These charts are useful, although the paramedic must remember to allow some variation for individual rates of development, especially when the patient borders between two age groups.

Attempting to memorize normal vital signs for the various patient age ranges is discouraged, particularly in the paramedic's early learning stages. Instead, the paramedic should focus on general concepts and ensure that quick reference guides are available in the field, as they must be for equipment selection and medication dosages.

History

Information required in a pediatric patient history is generally similar to that needed for adults. Differences for specific conditions are covered as those conditions are addressed within this textbook. What more often differs is the patient's ability to communicate pertinent data; the paramedic's related communications skills and accompanying strategies are fundamental. Parents or other caretakers should always be considered potential sources of background information. In general, the younger the patient, the more critical adult input will be for completion of the historical picture.

TABLE 25-2 Suggested Pediatric Equipment and Medications (Continued)	
Medication	**Minimum quantity**
Bulb syringe	1
Syringes	
1 cc	3
3 cc	3
5 cc	5
10 cc	5
Intraosseous needle	
Jamshidi/Kormed disposable bone marrow needle (sternal/ileac aspiration needle), 15 gauge	2
Intravenous catheters	
24 gauge	2
22 gauge	2
20 gauge	2
18 gauge	2
16 gauge	2
14 gauge	2
Miscellaneous	
Pediatric defibrillator paddles	1 set
Child size sphygmomanometer	1
Baby No Neck, pediatric, and short cervical spine extrication collars	1 each
Stockinette cap	1
Pediatric monitoring electrodes	6
Minidrip administration set	2
Maxidrip administration set	2
Intravenous extension set	2
Alcohol prep pads	
Band Aids	
Tape, 1 in and 1/2 in	
Arm boards	
Topical antiseptic ointment (single use)	
Isolation masks	
Venous constricting bands (Penrose drain, elastic band)	
Spare AA batteries	
Spare laryngoscope bulb	

Physical Examination

The following section discusses the differences in the major body systems of young patients in comparison with those of adults, and the ways in which assessment must be focused to locate the needed information.

Respiratory System

The most important medical aspect of pediatric care is the critical priority that patient respiratory status receives in assessment and management. Infants and children seldom experience cardiac arrest as the result of a primary cardiac condition; cardiac arrest more often follows a decline in ventilation and oxygenation. Unfortunately, the successful resuscitation of children in cardiac arrest is poor, even in sophisticated medical centers.

This poor success rate, coupled with the fact that most pediatric cardiac arrests can be prevented by early detection of respiratory decline and aggressive interventions in early stages, combine to place a primary emphasis on respiratory matters in this patient group. The paramedic who reaches a pediatric patient before severe respiratory failure occurs and who takes the necessary steps to support ventilation and oxygenation, can usually contribute to a positive patient outcome.

A number of special aspects of pediatric respiratory care arise from the way in which children, especially neonates, infants, and toddlers, differ anatomically from adults (Fig. 25-1):

- The larynx is more cephalad (closer to the head).
- The tongue is larger in relation to the rest of the upper airway.

- The less rigid ribs and intercostal cartilages lend less support to the chest wall.
- Poorly developed intercostal muscles are less able to assist the diaphragm in the breathing process.
- The softer lower airways are less able to retain their shape, and therefore more likely to collapse in the presence of mild-to-moderate pressure changes.
- The cricoid ring is the smallest in diameter of the structures between the pharynx and the bronchi (in the adult, the larynx is smallest).
- Everything is smaller, particularly the sizes of the structures in the larynx and trachea, and the distances between them.

From this list, the rescuer can draw many conclusions regarding special pediatric respiratory assessment and care:

- Increased pressures in the airways, such as those caused by added breathing effort in the presence of airway obstruction, can easily lead to collapse of small airways and sometimes of the bronchi or trachea.
- Pressure changes, in combination with weak support from soft tissues in the chest wall, also cause some of the telltale signs of pediatric respiratory distress: sternal and intercostal retractions upon inspiration.
- The patient's attempt to develop increased pressures to compensate for some type of obstruction, lead to another group of classic respiratory distress signs: grunting, nasal flaring, head bobbing with each breath, and inspiratory abdominal distention (i.e., exaggerated diaphragmatic effort).
- Relatively minor swelling, foreign body presence, or change in airway position can lead to partial or even full airway obstruction.
- Soft tissue weakness leads to lowered lung compliance, which makes mechanical ventilation easy but also creates a need for caution to avoid overinflation and lung damage. (Neonates are the exception; lung compliance is quite high, especially immediately after birth and requires more ventilatory effort than in infants.)
- Endotracheal intubation can be more challenging. Visualizing the cords is sometimes difficult because of the large tongue and the sharper angle between the mouth and glottis. The small size of the cricoid ring also poses the potential of inserting a tube that will fit through the glottis but then be stopped by the cricoid just below it.
- Small sizes and distances mean that tracheal tubes can be displaced with less movement, leading to bronchial or esophageal intubations.

Respiratory Assessment. Physical assessment of pediatric respiratory status can be divided into five major categories: rate, mechanics, skin color, breath sounds, and arterial oxygen sat-

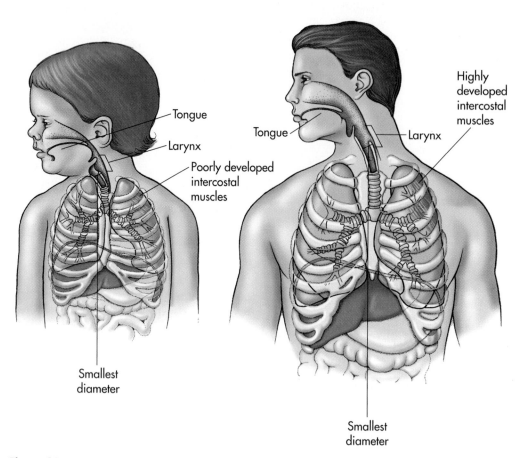

Figure 25-1

Anatomical changes occur as a child develops into an adult. These differences in the respiratory system have a significant impact on assessment and management.

uration. Mentation and level of responsiveness will also be discussed here.

Rate Pediatric respiratory rates are normally faster than those of adults (Table 25-1). The pediatric rate should be even higher in the presence of pain, anxiety, fever, or any specific cause of cardiac compromise or respiratory distress, such as shock.

Paramedics must be particularly attentive to patients who present with any of these conditions and whose respiratory rates are normal or slow. As with adults, tachypnea is a compensatory response. When fatigue and advancing hypoxia begin to weaken the compensation, breathing will slow and eventually stop.

There may be periods during the lapse into respiratory failure when respiratory status appears normal, especially if rate is the only sign assessed; it is critical for the rescuer to recognize the possibility of impending failure and intervene early in the process. The patient who looks somewhat normal just before collapsing emphasizes the value of a big-picture assessment; the other factors discussed in following paragraphs will help differentiate the healthy child from the distressed child.

Pediatric respiratory rates are often variable or cyclic, particularly in neonates and infants. Accurate respiratory rate determination requires a minimum 30-second observation; a 1-minute assessment is preferable in the youngest patients.

Mechanics Assessment of respiratory mechanics includes the general observation of visible chest movement and specific check for the physical signs of pressure changes in respiratory distress: grunting, nasal flaring, head bobbing, and suprasternal, intercostal, and subcostal inspiratory retractions. Prolonged expiration, usually caused by obstruction or disease in the lower airways, is another mechanical sign of ventilatory difficulty.

One specific abnormal sign sometimes indicates fatigue after a period of respiratory distress. "Seesaw," or paradoxical, respirations feature abdominal distention with each breath. Tiring of the chest wall muscles, which are somewhat weak to begin with, also leads to a reduction in chest expansion or to chest contraction during inspiration. This is another indication that respiratory failure is near unless rapid action is taken.

The younger the patient, the more important it is for the rescuer to note these signs. As described here, auscultation of pediatric lungs can be challenging; mechanics and other indications are often required to complete the picture and enable the paramedic to recognize respiratory failure early in its course.

Skin Color Skin color changes do not automatically indicate respiratory problems. Color changes also occur as a result of circulatory trouble, and in some cases, these changes occur as a normal part of less-threatening conditions. Color changes may also be absent in a young patient whose condition has already deteriorated considerably.

As nonspecific as they may be, skin signs remain important in the total picture. No single clinical sign can be reliable to indicate compromised respiratory function. In combination with other signs skin color can be an important warning signal of the need for immediate intervention.

Although they may be caused by circulatory insufficiency, skin changes such as mottling, duskiness, and cyanosis should be assumed to indicate respiratory decline and hypoxia until proven otherwise. Because shock and other circulatory emergencies often accompany or result from a respiratory deterioration, this assumption is a logical starting point.

In neonates and young infants, central cyanosis is a late and dire sign when present. However, it does not appear consistently, so its absence cannot be trusted as a sign of adequate tissue oxygenation.

When the patient's color is inconsistent from one body area to another, several pointers will help guide the paramedic's assessment:

- The paramedic should check the mucous membranes inside the patient's eyelids and lips; pink membranes indicate that the central blood supply is well oxygenated, and that peripheral color changes are more likely related to circulatory factors.
- Circulatory signs should be evaluated in more depth to help broaden the overall health picture.
- If available, a pulse oximeter should be used to measure arterial oxygen saturation directly.

Breath Sounds As in adults, noisy breathing of any kind is abnormal in children. Abnormal respiratory sounds audible without a stethoscope deserve immediate attention as possible signs of serious respiratory insufficiency. These sounds can include wheezing (lower airway obstruction), stridor (upper airway obstruction), and grunting (extreme effort added to normal respiratory mechanics to increase pressures and move air past some kind of obstruction). As usual, the absence of these signs does not rule out trouble.

Auscultating lung sounds, especially in infants and small children, can be more difficult than in adults. Figure 25-2 shows the auscultation locations. The thin chest wall and relatively short distance between different lung areas in children mean that a sound heard at any spot could easily have originated in another part of the chest (or even in the upper airways) and been conducted to the point of auscultation. To solve this problem, the paramedic should concentrate more on differences between lung areas than on absolutes (presence or absence of particular sounds) and use other aspects of the examination to confirm suspicions.

As an example, a child with a rapid respiratory rate, good skin and membrane color, normal mechanics, and consistent lung sounds would not appear to be in immediate danger. The same child with prolonged expirations, intercostal retractions, and dusky membranes would obviously require a more aggressive response, even if lung sounds appeared normal. A wheeze heard upon expiration would further heighten concern, and so on.

Arterial Oxygen Saturation The use of a pulse oximeter for measurement of arterial oxygen saturation is discussed in detail in Chapter 18. Its use and shortcomings in children are very similar to those described for adults, with the exception of methods for proper sensor attachment to children's small fingers and earlobes.

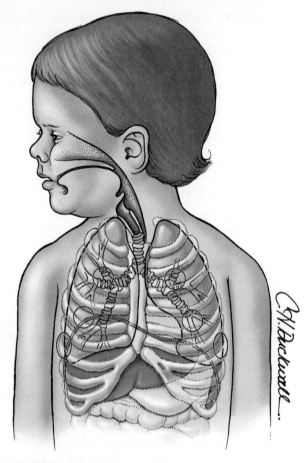

Figure 25-2

Sites for auscultation of lung sounds in a child.

The use of pulse oximetry is valuable in focusing the clinical assessment and evaluating the patient's response to oxygen therapy, especially when considering the occassional difficulty encountered in pediatric respiratory status assessment.

Mentation and Level of Responsiveness Among patients too young to provide adequate medical history, mentation and level of responsiveness is an important indicator of the patient's general perfusion status. Parental advice is sometimes necessary to confirm variations from normal behavior, especially in infants, for factors such as pain response and alertness to parents and environment.

Mentation is another nonspecific sign. Mentation changes can point to circulatory deficiency and other problems but should also be considered possible signs of respiratory compromise. Central nervous system assessment is described in more detail in a following section.

Cardiovascular System

Because primary cardiac problems are rare in children, cardiovascular assessment is emphasized by identification of two broad categories of problems: 1) secondary results of respiratory insufficiency, as described above; and 2) perfusion failure caused by any of the mechanisms that can lead to shock. Hemorrhage, dehydration, burns, anaphylaxis, and sepsis are among the most common of these mechanisms.

Children lack one important compensatory mechanism for volume loss that adults have: increased cardiac contractility. Because contractility is relatively fixed, heart rate and systemic vascular resistance bear a greater burden for maintaining perfusion in the face of volume loss. This, in turn, puts greater emphasis on evaluations of heart rate and skin signs. It also helps explain why a bradycardic child is viewed as being in grave danger: the child's primary compensatory mechanism may already be exhausted.

Cardiovascular Assessment Cardiac monitoring of children can be useful, but primary cardiovascular assessment can usually be accomplished without it. The basic categories of cardiovascular assessment are heart rate, peripheral perfusion signs, blood pressure, and mentation and level of responsiveness.

Heart Rate As with respirations, pediatric heart rate is faster than the normal rate of adults (Table 25-1) and should rise further in the face of physiological stressors such as fever, trauma, pain, fear, and hypoxia. Sinus tachycardia is a normal compensatory response which bears more of the responsibility for reinforcing perfusion in shock situations than is true for adults.

Also in keeping with the significance of respiratory rate, the patient should be assumed to be in critical condition by the time heart rate drops. Generally, bradycardia is a late and very serious sign, often immediately followed by cardiac arrest unless treatment is quick and intensive.

Peripheral Perfusion Signs

- *Pulse characteristics.* In most forms of shock, peripheral pulses will gradually weaken and disappear as systemic vascular resistance increases to compensate for perfusion compromise. Septic shock is sometimes an exception; peripheral pulses may actually strengthen. In addition to common adult pulse sites, the brachial artery in the upper arm is a common site to try in children, and the apical pulse can often be palpated in neonates and infants (Fig. 25-3).
- *Skin signs.* Skin perfusion is another indicator of the extent to which the cardiovascular system is using changes in vascular resistance to compensate for circulatory problems.

Signs of concern include both color and temperature changes. Mottling and pallor indicate selective and total capillary shutdown, respectively, as the system shunts blood to the core. Cyanosis can fall in this category, although it may have respiratory as well as circulatory causes.

It is important to remember that skin exposed to a cold environment may exhibit some of these signs in a patient who is otherwise in normal condition. In a warm environment, however, cold skin has a special importance. As part of the compensatory peripheral shutdown, fingers and toes will start to cool, followed by the hands and feet, then gradually the arms and legs. This can be a subtle sign if not carefully sought out, but it is another useful hint that the patient is in the early stages of compensated shock.

Two factors predispose pediatric patients, especially preschool-aged children, to larger and faster swings in

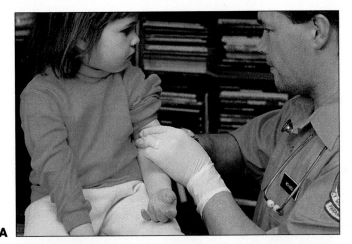

A

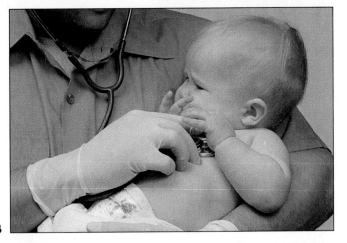

B

Figure 25-3

A) The brachial artery in the upper arm is a common site to assess pulse in children, and B) the apical pulse can often be palpated in neonates and infants.

body temperature than are usually seen in adults. Thermoregulatory controls are not completely developed, and the child has more body surface (skin) area relative to body mass. The latter can be an advantage in the febrile patient who requires cooling, but this condition also subjects children to quicker development of hypothermia when wet or in cool environments.

- *Capillary refill.* The patient's nail beds are good places to check capillary refill. A normal response after the nail is squeezed to "blanch" the color out of it is the return of color in 2 seconds or less. The hand or foot to be checked should be placed at or slightly above the level of the patient's heart; if the extremity is placed lower, the capillary refill may appear normal as a result of gravity (venous backflow) rather than true arterial perfusion.

  Capillary refill is not an absolute sign, but it can be useful in conjunction with other signs in early-to-moderate shock stages and is considered more reliable than blood pressure. As with color changes, capillary refill assessment may be less reliable if the extremity is cold.

- *Fontanelles.* The "soft spots" between cranial plates in infants, called *fontanelles*, provide another way to assess for volume loss. When observed with the child placed in a

sitting position, fontanelles sunken visibly below skull level suggest dehydration (Fig. 25-4A). Fontanelles that appear tight or that bulge slightly may also be a sign of increased intracranial pressure caused by infection or trauma (Fig. 25-4B).

Blood Pressure Falling blood pressure is a late and unreliable sign of shock. When present, it confirms a grave situation, but the paramedic must hope for earlier opportunities to recognize and treat the problem. When other signs make perfusion compromise obvious, blood pressure measurement may have to be prioritized to follow more urgent assessment and management interventions.

Blood pressure may also be difficult to measure in children whose peripheral circulation is already reduced by the compensatory increase in vascular resistance. Proper measurement requires a cuff whose width is approximately two-thirds the length of the patient's upper arm (*see* Table 25-1 for normal blood pressures by age).

Mentation and Level of Responsiveness Mentation and level of responsiveness changes often point to perfusion difficulties, although a number of other causes are possible. In a child with other signs of cardiovascular inadequacy, signs such as lethargy, irritability, combativeness, and confusion are significant.

Toddlers and younger patients will show mental changes more in response to the environment: pain response, eye contact, awareness of surroundings, response to parents, and so on. This younger patient group may also show advanced signs of central nervous system hypoxia, such as loss of muscle tone.

Central Nervous System

Young patients' nervous systems differ in a few basic ways from more fully developed systems of adults. Structurally, incomplete fusion of cranial bones renders neonates and infants more vulnerable to serious brain injury with mild-to-moderate mechanisms of injury.

Physiologically, temperature control is less predictable. The higher ratio of body surface area (skin) to body volume means that heat loss takes place more quickly. Underdeveloped compensatory mechanisms, such as shivering, can also affect the patient's response to heat loss.

The child's age and state of social, mental, and verbal development also have a major impact on the approach to assessment. Infants and toddlers require more careful observation of objective signs and more detailed communications with parents than do older children who can interact effectively with paramedics.

CNS Assessment. Mentation and Level of Responsiveness

In older children, mentation and level of responsiveness can be assessed in much the same manner as for adults. Younger patients will often show a predictable, observable decline that begins with irritability and continues on to lethargy and eventually unresponsiveness. At the lethargy stage, the situation is already serious.

Response to the environment is especially useful in infants and young children. Eyes are a central point to observe. Any

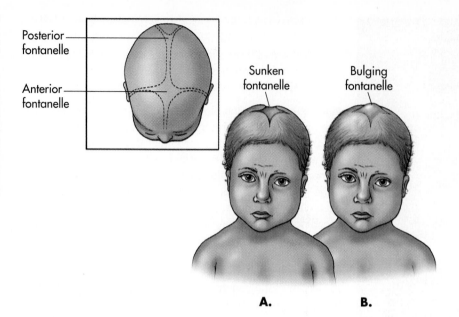

Figure 25-4

The appearance of the fontanelles in infants should be assessed. A, Sunken fontanelles can be indicative of dehydration. B, Bulging" or firm fontanelles may indicate increased intracranial pressure in the pediatric patient.

child more than 1 month of age should be able to track a moving object, such as a responder's hand, near his or her face, and many will make eye contact in a way that indicates awareness of another person's presence. Response to noises and touch may also be useful. However, all of these responses are somewhat subjective in the youngest patients. Parental input about variation from normal response levels helps confirm the paramedic's observations.

Level of responsiveness can be documented objectively using the AVPU scale to describe the patient's best response level to stimulus. This assessment avoids the inconsistency of using poorly defined adjectives (stuporous, obtunded) to describe unresponsive states. Another method is use of a version of the Glasgow Coma Scale (GCS) modified for pediatric use (*see* Chapter 21). This method is particularly useful for establishing a baseline that can be used for comparison in later, serial observations.

In addition to level of responsiveness, there are several areas in which parents can provide important perspective about how the presenting picture differs from the patient's normal state. Signs to evaluate, as well as observe directly are the patient's mood, activity level, attention span, and willingness and ability to cooperate.

Other than fixed and dilated pupils, progressive loss of responsiveness may be the only major sign of increasing intracranial pressure in these patients. Children do not always show Cushing's reflex (bradycardia and hypertension) and when they do, it may be very late in the process.

Motor Function Motor function can be observed generally in the coordination of the patient's movements, ability to stand and change position, and so on. Motor tests used in adults, such as hand-grip strength and leg strength, can also be used in older children who will cooperate.

Sensory Function In lethargic or unresponsive children, response to pain stimulus (e.g., pinch, pin prick) can be used, although it is important for the paramedic to consider the need and possible results before proceeding with this test. The child who becomes further distressed or uncooperative as a result of this evaluation technique will be more difficult to manage and could be harmed as a result. As with motor response, more typical adult methods ("Can you feel my hand on your toes?") are preferable when they will work.

Trauma Assessment

Only a few aspects of trauma assessment differ between adults and children; most aspects are the same: the priority of ABCs in the initial assessment, the need to expedite scene times in critical patients, the emphasis on airway management and spinal immobilization, and the importance of multiple, serial examinations, including vital signs, during transport to identify developing crises. The latter is even more important in pediatric patients, in whom relatively small amounts of bleeding can lead quickly to shock.

Many of the notable differences between large and small patients have been discussed above. A number of anatomical differences in the airway predispose infants and small children to airway obstruction. Incomplete closure of fontanelles in neonates and infants creates a higher chance of brain injury with what would be considered in adults to be only minor or moderate blows to the head. Observation of fontanelles as an indicator of dehydration or increased intracranial pressure, as well as the use of a modified Glasgow Coma Scale to supplement the more basic AVPU scale in assessing and reassessing level of responsiveness, are important in pediatric trauma assessment.

Anatomical differences account for a higher incidence of certain chest and abdominal injuries in children. The softer chest walls and larger internal organs of children make pulmonary contusion and injuries to both liver and spleen more likely in blunt trauma. Deceleration, particularly in vehicle accidents when the patient is unrestrained or ejected, is a common mechanism that leads to these injuries and the respiratory distress or shock that can follow.

SUMMARY

Providing effective emergency care for pediatric patients requires an understanding of the ways in which these patients are medically similar to adults, as well as the ways in which they differ. Despite areas of contrast, most knowledge about adult care is at least generally applicable to children.

Psychosocially, young patients fall into several general age ranges. The paramedic who communicates with an awareness of the common traits and fears in these age groups will create a cooperative atmosphere that makes it easier to deliver needed care. Some aspects of the responder's approach to the child and parents remain important regardless of the patient's age. These include confidence, calmness, honesty and respect for individual dignity.

The medical changes that occur throughout childhod span a spectrum that is not well suited to rote memorization or absolute statements of what is normal for a given age. Paramedics will need to focus on basic clinical observations, and have quick-reference materials readily available in the field, to evaluate and care for the broad scope of possibilities in this patient group.

Even more than in adults, airway and ventilatory concerns deserve top priority in young patients. Most other aspects of emergency pediatric care arise from, or can be closely related to, a thorough understanding of this area.

REFERENCES

1. **Altieri M, Bellet J, Scott H:** Preparedness for pediatric emergencies encountered in the practitioner's office. *Pediatrics* 85:710–714, 1990.

2. **American College of Emergency Physicians Policy Statement:** Pediatric Equipment Guidelines, April, 1994.

3. **American College of Emergency Physicians Police Statement:** Equipment for Ambulances, September, 1994

4. **American Heart Association and American Academy of Pediatrics, Chameides L, Hazinski MF (eds):** Pediatric Advanced Life Support.

5. **Fuchs S, Jaffe DM, Cristoffel KK:** Pediatric emergencies in office practices: prevalence and office preparedness. *Pediatrics* 83:931–939, 1989.

6. **Kissoon N, Walia MS:** The critically ill child in the pediatric emergency department. *Ann Emerg Med* 18(1):30–33, 1989.

7. **Kissoon N, Frewen TC, Kronick JB, Mohammed A:** The child requiring transport: lessons and implications for the pediatric emergency physician. *Pediatr Emerg Care* 4:1–4, 1988.

8. **Krauss BS, Karaka T, Flesicher GR:** The spectrum and frequency of illness presenting to a pediatric emergency department. *Pediatr Emerg Care* 7:67–71, 1991.

9. **Maze A, Bloch E:** Stridor in pediatric patients. *Anesthesiol* 50:132–145, 1979.

10. **McCarthy PL, Sharpe RM, Spiesel SZ, et al:** Observation scales to identify serious illness in febrile children. *Pediatrics* 70:802–809, 1982.

11. **Mellick LB, Guy JR:** Approaching the infant and child in the prehospital arena. *JEMS* 17:126–136, 1992.

12. **Rivara FP, Kamitsuka MD, Quan L:** Injuries to children younger than 1 year of age. *Pediatrics* 81:93–97, 1988.

13. **Sager M:** Scoring systems in emergency pediatrics: one cannot see the forest for the trees. *Pediatr Emerg Care* 5:142–144, 1989.

14. **Seidel JS, Henderson DP, Lewis JB:** Emergency medical services and the pediatric patient III: resources of ambulatory care centers. *Pediatrics* 88:230–235, 1991.

15. **Seidel JS, Henderson DP, Ward P, Wayland BW, Ness B:** Pediatric prehospital care in urban and rural areas. *Pediatrics* 88:681–690, 1991.

16. **Tsai A, Kallsen G, et al:** Epidemiology of pediatric prehospital care. *Ann Emerg Med* 16:284–92, 1987.

17. **Wood DW, Downes JJ, Lecks HJ:** A clinical scoring system for diagnosis of respiratory failure. *Am J Dis Child* 123:227–228, 1972.

Daniel L. Storer, MD, FACEP

Chapter 26

Geriatric Assessment

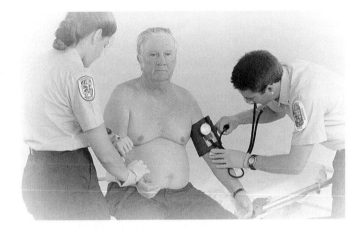

KEY TERMS

1. **Alzheimer's disease**—a disease marked by progressive loss of mental capacity (e.g., impaired memory, thinking, and behavior) resulting from degeneration of the brain cells.

2. **Elder abuse**—a syndrome in which an elderly person has sustained serious physical or psychological injury from another person (e.g., psychological injury from his or her children or other care providers).

3. **Geriatrics**—the study and treatment of diseases of the aged.

The paramedic should be able to:

OBJECTIVES

1. Identify changes in anatomy and physiology that occur with aging.

2. Describe the special problems associated with assessment of the elderly and techniques to overcome them.

3. Describe the incidence and unique features of selected medical and trauma related problems in the elderly patient.

4. Describe the special problems that exist regarding management of various illnesses and injuries in the elderly patient.

5. Identify the special problems associated with medication use by the elderly.

6. Identify factors associated with elder abuse and neglect.

Scene Survey

Initial Assessment

Focused History
and Physical Exam

Continued Assessment

Following the initial assessment and management of life-threatening emergencies, the focused history and physical examination of the elderly patient should follow the same sequence as that in other patients. However, the findings may be different because of the aging process. Because elderly people are living longer, the birth rate is declining, and no major wars or catastrophes have occurred, the percentage of people over 65 years of age grows each year. According to data from the Bureau of the Census, in 1993 there were approximately 32.8 million persons in the United States who were 65 years of age or older. Experts predict that by the year 2000, there will be 35.3 million people 65 years of age or older, and 70.2 million by the year 2030.[13]

Evaluation and treatment of the elderly is sometimes more complex than treatment provided for other age groups. Older patients often have at least one chronic condition, and many may have multiple conditions, such as arthritis, hypertension, hearing impairments, and heart problems. The leading causes of death among the elderly are coronary artery disease, cancer, and stroke.[3]

Aging and the Human Body

To better understand some of the changes in symptoms and physical signs among elderly patients, it is necessary to discuss the changes that occur in anatomy and physiology during aging (Fig 26-1).

Endocrine, Gastrointestinal, and Metabolic Systems

In general, aging results in a decrease in the amount of total body water and total body fat. There is no clear evidence of a decline in metabolic activity, but the total number of body cells decreases. Many elderly patients have gastrointestinal complaints. These patients may experience a decrease in the amount of saliva and a decrease in gastric secretions. The elderly patient has fewer taste buds, which may contribute to loss of appetite and poor nutrition. Esophageal activity decreases, and decreased gastric motility may cause digestion difficulties and increased risk of aspiration.

Skin

Changes in the skin associated with aging make us keenly aware of the aging process. The skin gradually becomes dry, transparent, and wrinkled. There is an uneven discoloration and loss of elasticity. Dryness of the mucous membranes in the mouth and skin may cause the paramedic to mistakenly believe that the patient is dehydrated. Contributing to this misconception, the patient's skin may have poor elasticity even without dehydration. These changes contribute to the increase in skin wrinkling and may also delay wound healing abilities. Aging skin may have a thinner outer layer (epidermis), and

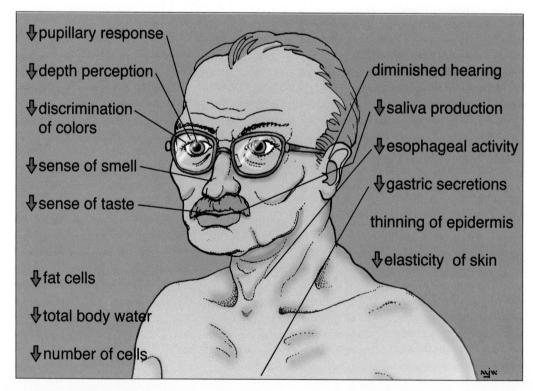

Figure 26-1

Physiologic changes seen with the aging process.

capillaries can be fragile and easily bruised. Considering these changes, the paramedic should handle the elderly patient with care to avoid additional epidermal bruising and tearing.

Senses

There are significant changes in the eyes, ears, nose, and throat of the elderly patient. With increasing age, the pupils show decreased ability to accommodate to varying levels of light. As a result, the older patient requires more time to adjust to lighting changes in order to ambulate safely. There is greater sensitivity of the aging eye to glare and bright lights. There is an increase in cataract formation, which interferes with the passage of light rays to the retina and results in diminished vision and further increased sensitivity to bright lights (Fig. 26-2). The presence of cataracts may also contribute to the decreased ability to discriminate between colors of similar intensities such as blue and green, which can affect the elderly patient's ability to distinguish between medications. Depth perception also may be diminished, interfering with the elderly patient's ability to use grab bars or hand rails, especially when they are similar in color to the surrounding walls.

Diminished hearing, especially of high-pitched sounds, is common among the elderly. In the 75- to 84-year-old age group, approximately 70% of people have hearing impairments.[11] Elderly men are more frequently affected by hearing impairment. Speaking loudly, which actually distorts sounds, does not solve the communications problem; rather, speaking slowly in a normal tone and at the patient's level gives the patient a chance to hear without distortion and to read lips. Elderly patients may also experience decreased senses of smell and taste, which can affect appetite and result in malnutrition and dehydration.

Respiratory System

From 30 to 80 years of age, there are changes in the respiratory system (Fig. 26-3). Lung function decreases, resulting in a

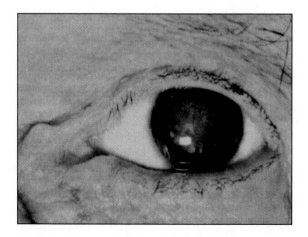

Figure 26-2

Example of cataract. *From Bedford, MA: Color Atlas of Ophthalmologic Diagnosis, ed. 2, 1986, Wolfe Medical Publishing.*

decrease in oxygen uptake. The cough reflex is diminished and the ability to clear secretions is lessened.

Cardiovascular System

As age increases, cardiac output drops and the heart rate slows, decreasing compensatory ability. The conduction system degenerates, and the left ventricle thickens and becomes more rigid. There is also an increase in coronary artery occlusion and a rise in both systolic and diastolic blood pressures.

Renal System

In the renal system of the elderly patient, there is a decline in kidney function. There is a decrease in blood flow to the kidneys and a decrease in responsiveness to hormones that regulate fluid and electrolyte balance.[9] These changes may contribute to fluid and electrolyte disturbances.

Central Nervous System

The central nervous system of the elderly patient experiences a 45% loss of cells in certain areas of the brain. There is also decreased blood flow to the brain, with increased resistance in the cerebral blood vessels. Oxygen consumption drops, and a 15% reduction in nerve conduction velocity occurs. As a result of these changes, the patient may experience slowed reflexes and decreased pain perception, sense of equilibrium, and perception of touch and temperature. Many of these changes contribute to the increased incidence of falls and injury in the elderly.

Musculoskeletal System

Muscles and bones undergo a change with aging (Fig. 26-4). There may be a decrease in an individual's height of 2 to 3 inches, which is caused by narrowing of the spinal disc spaces. Posture changes often occur as a slight flexion develops at the knees and hips and the spine deteriorates. There is a decrease in total skeletal muscle weight and a decreased density of some bones (osteoporosis). Hip injuries are more frequent in this population than in any other age group.

Scene Survey

Initial Assessment

Focused History and Physical Exam

Continued Assessment

Assessing the Elderly Patient

Several common problems may be encountered during the assessment of an elderly patient. Paramedics and other health care providers sometimes focus too closely on the presenting problem without identifying possible underlying conditions, both medical and social, that may have contributed to the

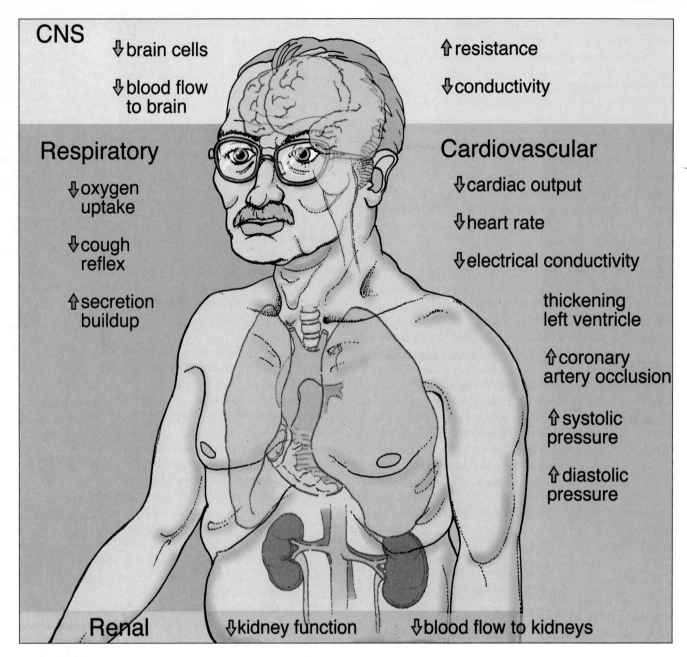

CNS
⇩brain cells
⇩blood flow to brain
⇧resistance
⇩conductivity

Respiratory
⇩oxygen uptake
⇩cough reflex
⇧secretion buildup

Cardiovascular
⇩cardiac output
⇩heart rate
⇩electrical conductivity
thickening left ventricle
⇧coronary artery occlusion
⇧systolic pressure
⇧diastolic pressure

Renal   ⇩kidney function   ⇩blood flow to kidneys

Figure 26-3

Respiratory, cardiovascular, renal, and CNS changes seen with the aging process.

patient's condition. The chief complaint can be trivial, with the patient failing to report important symptoms, possibly because the elderly patient is threatened by the thought of hospitalization and the resulting loss of independence.

Elderly patients are likely to suffer from more than one disease at a time, either chronic or acute. Chronic problems make assessment of acute problems more difficult because the symptoms can intermix.

As an example, an acute fall may be mistakenly evaluated and treated only as a minor injury problem when a serious medical or social problem may have caused the fall. Falls are a major source of suffering and death among the elderly. The fall may have resulted from a correctable medical problem, such as one of many causes of syncope. Falls can also be caused by correctable environmental problems such as poor lighting, hazardous rugs, or bulky clothing.

To further complicate assessment, the individual's response to illness or injury may be different than expected. Because pain sensation can be diminished or absent, the patient and the paramedic can easily underestimate the severity of the condition. Temperature regulation mechanisms may be depressed, so fever can be minimal or absent even when the patient has severe infection. Elderly patients are also more likely to be affected by environmental temperature extremes, making them more vulnerable to both hypothermia and hyperthermia. Social and emotional factors also have a greater impact on health in the elderly than in any other age group.

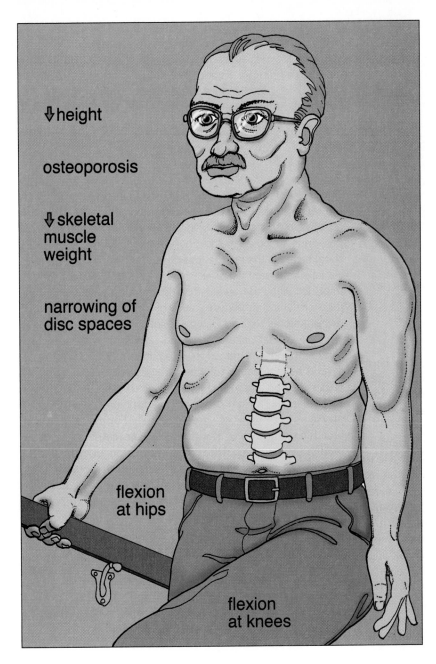

Figure 26-4

Musculoskeletal system changes seen with the aging process.

Within the figure:

↓height

osteoporosis

↓skeletal muscle weight

narrowing of disc spaces

flexion at hips

flexion at knees

History

Several of the complaints common to geriatric patients are nonspecific and require further investigation. These include fatigue, weakness, dizziness, falls, headache, inability to sleep, difficulty swallowing, loss of appetite, and problems with urination, constipation, or diarrhea. The patient's chief complaint may not reflect the total problem. When taking a history, the paramedic should search for other significant symptoms rather than assuming that this type of complaint is insignificant. The geriatric patient may not volunteer significant information until asked and may attribute symptoms to advanced age.

The paramedic may face communication problems while taking the patient history. Problems that may interfere with clear communication are depression and diminished sight, hearing, and mental status. Diminished sight fosters increased anxiety, as the inability to see surroundings clearly contributes

to a feeling of loss of control. Many elderly patients wear glasses; the paramedic should assist the patient in finding his or her glasses when attempting to obtain information. It also helps to speak clearly and be positioned in good light and at eye level so that the patient can watch (lip-read) and listen to the questions (Fig. 26-5).

Diminished hearing and deafness can make obtaining a history difficult or even impossible. If the patient appears unable to hear the questions, ask others whether the patient has hearing difficulty rather than assuming hearing loss. Speak in a normal tone and avoid shouting. Many elderly patients wear hearing aids, which can contribute to sound distortion if other than normal speaking tones are used. Shouting is also not helpful for patients who are totally deaf. Writing notes may be necessary. Speaking slowly and directly toward the patient will help those who can lip read. Whenever possible, the paramedic should verify the patient history with relatives or others

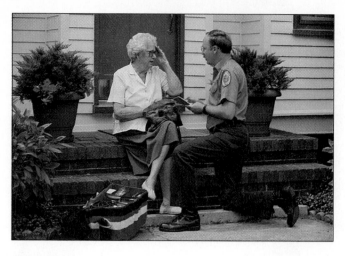

Figure 26-5

Paramedics should position themselves at eye level in a well-lit area to assess the geriatric patient.

who are knowledgeable about the patient's condition. These relatives or friends may also be able to help with communication. When attempting to get a history, the paramedic should eliminate noises, such as radios, ECG alarms, strange voices, and other sounds that could distract the patient.

A patient's diminished mental status also complicates the history, because the patient may be confused and unable to remember details. The diminished mental status may be chronic, as in Alzheimer's disease, or acute and the paramedic should attempt to differentiate between the two. They may present similarly. The paramedic should attempt to determine from people at the scene if the patient's mental status represents a significant change from normal. A paramedic must never assume that a confused, disoriented patient is "just senile;" he or she should probe for underlying problems. A possible contributing factor to confusion and change in mental status is the presence of alcohol or other drugs. Alcoholism is more common among the elderly than generally realized.

Depression among the elderly is also more common than suspected. Depression may mimic senility or organic brain syndrome; it also may be the cause of a patient's lack of cooperation. The depressed patient may be malnourished, dehydrated, overdosed on medication, contemplating suicide, or simply imagining physical ailments for attention. Ask questions regarding drug ingestion and suicidal thoughts. Suicide is a significant cause of death among the elderly in the United States.

When obtaining a past medical history, the paramedic should try to determine what is significant. The history may be complicated. Medication history is important; any drugs or medication containers found at the scene should be brought to the hospital with the patient. Elderly patients usually take multiple drugs, and medication errors and noncompliance are common. If possible, current and old medications should be identified, including nonprescription drugs.

The paramedic should try to verify history with reliable family or friends. To avoid offending the patient, questions can be repeated out of the patient's earshot.

The surrounding scene may help clarify the origins of the patient's condition. The paramedic should observe the environment for indications of inadequate self-care, and look for evidence of drug or alcohol ingestion. The patient should be checked for "Medic Alert" tags, "vial of life" programs, or other indicators. Paramedics must also be alert for signs of violence or elderly abuse.

Physical Examination

The physical examination of the geriatric patient should follow the same general sequence as those for patients in other age groups, but should involve additional considerations. In preparing to perform the physical examination, paramedics should explain the process clearly before beginning. This is especially important when examining an elderly patient with diminished sight. Be aware that the elderly patient may minimize or deny symptoms because of a fear of being bedridden or institutionalized and losing self sufficiency.

The elderly patient may wear excessive clothing, which can hamper the examination. The patient can also fatigue easily and have difficulty tolerating the examination. Peripheral pulses may be diminished and difficult to evaluate, and it can be challenging for the paramedic to distinguish signs of acute problems from those of chronic disease. For example, mouth breathing and loss of skin elasticity can cause dry mucous membranes that give the false impression of dehydration. Chronic nonpathologic rales are common without the presence of congestive heart failure or pneumonia. Likewise, edema in the lower extremities can be secondary to poor circulation and inactivity, rather than congestive heart failure.

Trauma, Medical, and Psychiatric Disorders

Several considerations related to trauma, medical diseases, and psychiatric illnesses deserve special attention.

Trauma

Studies show that the death rate among elderly trauma patients is higher than in any other age group. Falls, motor vehicle accidents and burns account for more than 80% of the injuries.[13] The elderly are also at high risk for assault. They tend to suffer more serious injury and to recover more slowly than younger patients. The elderly victim may have slower reflexes, failing eye sight and hearing, arthritis, fragile tissues and bones, and inelastic blood vessels. Falls are the single largest cause of accidental death in the elderly and account for one half of all deaths.[1]

The elderly are also more prone to serious head injury, even from relatively minor trauma. Shrinkage of brain tissue with aging allows more free space inside the skull. The brain can then move more freely with sudden blows to the head, leading to increased blood vessel tearing and likelihood of cerebral bleeds such as subdural hematomas. Signs of brain compression may develop more slowly, sometimes over days or weeks, because of the increased space available for swelling. The patient may even have forgotten the injury by the time symptoms develop.

Spine injuries result more frequently with trauma in elderly patients because of chronic bone changes that cause stiffening of the spine, and bone spurs pressing against the spinal cord can result in significant spinal cord injury with relatively minor trauma. The spinal stiffness increases the likelihood of fracture. Assessment of the spine is limited by the potential for reduced pain sensation, so the paramedic should have an increased level of suspicion.

Changes in bone associated with aging similarly affect the ability of the chest to tolerate blunt trauma; minor injuries in the elderly patient can often break ribs. With less protection from the chest wall, the lungs, heart, and aorta are more susceptible to injuries, such as lung and cardiac contusions and aortic tears. Among elderly trauma patients, the leading cause of death in the first 24 hours after injury is adult respiratory distress syndrome.[1]

Trauma management in elderly patients demands special consideration to proper immobilization techniques because of fragile bones and an increased tendency for fracture. Positioning and immobilization may have to be modified to accommodate physical deformities resulting from arthritis, spinal abnormalities, or frozen limbs (Fig. 26-6).

The elderly patient is more likely to have dentures that will have to be removed to facilitate proper airway management. Oxygen therapy is important because of the potential for increased vascular disease. Past myocardial infarctions contribute to the risk of dysrhythmias and congestive heart failure. The trauma may even have been the result of an accident that occurred when the patient suffered an acute myocardial infarction.

The paramedic should keep the patient warm following a traumatic incident. Elderly patients are particularly susceptible to temperature loss because of diminished subcutaneous fat reserves. Hypothermia further raises the risk of cardiac dysrhythmias in elderly patients. Cardiac monitoring should be standard procedure in these cases.

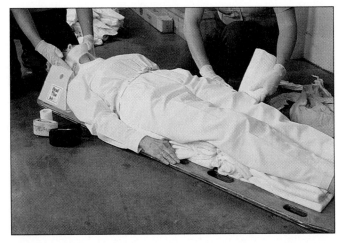

Figure 26-6

Immobilization techniques may require modification when involving geriatric patients.

Elderly patients may require a higher than normal blood pressure to maintain perfusion of vital organs, because of increased peripheral resistance. At the same time, there is a decreased ability to respond to blood loss; an elderly patient may not have the ability to increase heart rate in response to blood loss, because of medications or pre-existing cardiovascular disease. The paramedic, therefore, must pay special attention to early signs of shock. IV fluid administration is indicated but should be given with care, because of decreased myocardial reserve and the increased likelihood of congestive heart failure.

As with trauma injuries in other age groups, the elderly patient should be transported as quickly as possible to the nearest appropriate facility. Field stabilization should be brief, concentrating on the initial assessment, life-threatening situations, and the focused history and physical examination prior to transport. Continued assessment, IV therapy, and secondary immobilization other than the cervical spine, should occur during transport.

Respiratory Disorders

The changes in pulmonary physiology that occur with increased age increase the danger of acute pulmonary disorders in the elderly. Several respiratory disorders affect elderly patients more than patients of other age groups, including:

- COPD (including chronic bronchitis and asthma)
- Pneumonia
- Pulmonary embolism
- Lung cancer

COPD is one of the major health problems in the United States. It is the fourth leading cause of death (following heart diseases, malignant cancer, and cerebrovascular disease) in patients 60 to 79 years of age.[11] Most elderly patients with COPD fall into the category of asthma, chronic bronchitis or emphysema. Many elderly patients will present with an overlap of these conditions. For example, chronic bronchitis can be worsened by an acute asthma attack. The typical cause of deterioration in the elderly patient with COPD is acute airway infection. Respiratory infections cause edema of the involved mucosa, increased bronchial smooth muscle irritability leading to spasm, and increased mucous secretion. Air flow is limited, and breathing becomes more difficult.

Management of wheezing in the elderly patient is the same as management for other age groups, except for subcutaneous epinephrine therapy, which is commonly reserved for younger patients. In patients over 40 years of age, there is an increased likelihood of adverse cardiac effects with the use of epinephrine, and subcutaneous absorption rates vary. Paramedics should give the patient a hand-held, aerosolized bronchodilator agent when authorized by medical direction (Fig. 26-7). These agents work quickly and are effective in relieving bronchial spasms without significant cardiovascular side effects.

Pneumonia is the leading infectious cause of death in the geriatric age group and the fourth leading cause of death in patients over 75 years of age.[3] Symptoms commonly include shortness of breath, cough, and fever. Although the classic

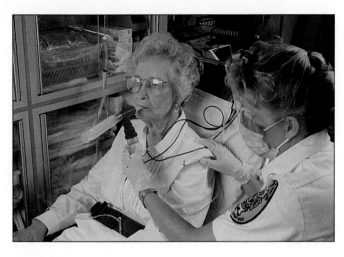

Figure 26-7

Bronchodilator therapy can improve breathing and causes few side effects.

signs and symptoms may not be present early in the infection, physical examination typically reveals audible rales over the affected area. Bilateral pneumonia may sound similar to pulmonary edema, with bilateral rales. Differentiation between pneumonia and pulmonary edema is difficult in the absence of other associated signs such as fever or history of infection, but the differentiation is important to make because of the differences in eventual treatment. Field management of the elderly patient with pneumonia includes standard airway management, including supplemental oxygen.

Pulmonary embolism must be considered in the elderly patient with shortness of breath. It is a life-threatening problem that is frequently missed during early patient assessment. In most patients, the blood clot originates in the veins of the pelvis or thigh. Elderly patients considered at high risk for pulmonary embolus are those with immobility, recent surgery, recent hip or long bone fracture, congestive heart failure, venous disease, obesity, malignancy, or any other state that increases blood clot formation. Symptoms of pulmonary embolus in the elderly patient are similar to those symptoms seen in other age groups. Treatment is the same, including appropriate airway management and supplemental oxygen.

Cardiovascular Disorders

Because of the probability of advanced atherosclerotic disease, the elderly patient is more likely to have acute cardiac disease, stroke, syncope, and ruptured aneurysm.

Acute myocardial infarction (AMI) is a leading cause of death among the elderly. Assessment of AMI presents a considerable challenge, because the elderly patient may not present with the classic symptoms; chest pain, in particular, is not common. The most frequent symptoms of AMI are shortness of breath, fatigue, and abdominal or epigastric discomfort. AMI should be considered a possibility in any elderly patient with an acute change in medical condition or behavior.

Congestive heart failure will present, as it does in other age groups, with shortness of breath and orthopnea. Management of elderly patients is similar to management of younger

patients. Aortic dissection, aortic aneurysm, and peripheral vascular disease are all more common in geriatric patients and are also treated much the same as in other age groups.

Gastrointestinal Disorders

Elderly patients frequently complain of problems related to the gastrointestinal (GI) system. Bowel habits are often mentioned. Bleeding is the most common of the more serious GI disorders. Major causes of upper GI bleeding include peptic ulcer disease, gastritis, esophageal varices, and esophageal tears from excessive vomiting. Lower GI bleeding is less common; major causes include tumors, ischemic bowel, arteriovenous (AV) malformations, and diverticula of the large bowel. Because of increased vascular compromise secondary to atherosclerotic changes, ischemic bowel should always be considered when an elderly patient complains of abdominal discomfort or lower GI bleeding.

"Coffee-ground" or bloody vomitus, black stools (melena), bloody stool, orthostatic hypotension, tachycardia, and confusion are common presenting signs and symptoms of GI bleeding. However, the paramedic should watch for increasing confusion or shortness of breath or a worsening or new onset of angina, as blood flow to the brain and heart drops. Any condition that lowers cardiac output may worsen conditions caused by atherosclerosis, especially in the brain and heart. In addition, the ability to react to changes in blood flow by peripheral vasoconstriction and increasing heart rate may be compromised.

Another GI emergency worth noting in the elderly patient is the acute abdomen. Elderly patients often fail to exhibit the usual signs and symptoms of guarding, rigidity, and localized pain. However, the paramedic must have a high index of suspicion, because of the possible absence of classic signs.

Neurological Disorders

Cerebrovascular accidents (CVA), transient ischemic attacks (TIA), and syncope are found more commonly in the elderly population, because advanced atherosclerotic disease limits blood flow to the brain. Occlusive stroke, in which the artery is blocked, is statistically more common than the hemorrhagic type.[5] TIAs are often preliminary to strokes. Once TIAs have begun, approximately 25% of patients will have a major, permanent stroke within 3 years, and 10% to 15% of patients will have a stroke within 1 year.[2]

When seizures occur for the first time in an elderly individual, this is evidence of some underlying neurologic disease. Cerebrovascular disease and brain tumors are the two most common causes. A seizure can also be the presenting symptom of a stroke or may occur as a later complication. Seizures following a stroke can begin months or even years after the stroke and after a full recovery. Focal seizures may present at the beginning of a cerebral infarction. Chronic seizure disorder, recent or past head trauma, mass lesion such as a tumor or expanding blood clot, alcohol withdrawal, and diabetic hypoglycemia are other possible seizure causes the paramedic should consider.

Syncope in the elderly patient represents a major challenge (see Chapter 29). Syncope is a patient's generalized weakness of muscles, inability to stand, and transient loss of consciousness. This condition is the result of temporarily inadequate blood flow to the brain that causes brain ischemia and a sudden halt in brain metabolism. Presyncope, or faintness, contrasts with syncope in that there is no loss of consciousness, but the sensation of impending loss of consciousness. The causes of syncope in the elderly patient are multiple; many represent conditions that can lead to disability or death.

Approximately 75% of the total blood volume is contained in the venous bed. Any interference with venous return to the heart may lead to a decrease in cardiac output. Cerebral perfusion is maintained if resulting arterial vasoconstriction occurs. However, if this adjustment fails, as is likely with the elderly patient, significant hypotension and cerebral hypoperfusion will occur.

There are multiple types of syncope, each having a list of causes. There is a higher incidence of both cardiac and cerebral causes of stroke in the geriatric population. In managing the elderly syncope patient, the paramedic must give special attention to obtaining a history. This information may be crucial to the physician's subsequent diagnosis of the cause of syncope.

Determining the cause of dizziness, like syncope, presents a major assessment challenge for the paramedic (see Chapter 34). There are many major and minor causes of dizziness, including impairment of any of the systems that orient the body to its environment such as vision, the inner ear, peripheral sensation, and the central nervous system. Alcohol and other drugs also are a common cause of dizziness among the elderly.

Vertigo is a specific sensation of motion perceived by the patient as spinning or whirling, as opposed to simple dizziness. Vertigo is commonly accompanied by sweating, pallor, nausea, and vomiting. It can be difficult to differentiate between dizziness, vertigo, presyncope, and syncope.

Altered mental status is a common presenting complaint in the elderly (see Chapter 30). Determining the cause is more difficult because relevant acute changes must be sorted from chronic conditions (see Box 26-1). The paramedic and all subsequent emergency care providers must collect information to determine if the patient's condition represents a substantial change from his or her previous level of function. If the change is significant, paramedics must also learn whether the mental disturbance indicates the presence of an acute neurologic disorder or a decompensation of a chronic mental status change caused by non-neurologic factors such as psychological illness, medical conditions, or social influences. An acute mental status change that is sudden in onset is called delirium and is often reversible. Dementia is a chronic mental status change with a gradual onset.

As aging progresses, it is normal for mental processes to undergo change. Memory capacity begins to decline as early as the teenage years. Loss of functioning brain cells begins slowly in the 40s and 50s, and continues at a progressive rate into the later decades. However, it is incorrect to assume that senility is a normal process in the elderly. Many people in their 70s, 80s, and 90s continue to be productive and enjoy the use of their intellects. Severe mental impairment resulting in loss of independence indicates the presence of disease and is abnormal at any age.

Acute mental status changes are important to identify because they may be reversible. Reversible causes can be related to general medical illness, medications, or specific neurologic diseases. Some of the most common general medical illnesses that cause changes in elderly patient mental status are metabolic disorders and nutritional deficiencies. An underactive thyroid (hypothyroid) and low blood sugar (hypoglycemia) are examples of metabolic disorders that can cause a change in mental status. Vitamin B_{12} deficiency (pernicious anemia) and thiamine deficiency are nutritional examples.

Cardiopulmonary diseases in the elderly that compromise cardiac output and lung function may lead to diffuse cerebral hypoxia, which can result in a decline in mental function. Electrolyte abnormalities also cause acute mental status changes.

Subdural hematoma and other mass lesions, such as tumors, may produce subtle, slowly progressive changes in mental status. Generalized cerebrovascular disease, such as atherosclerosis, multiple small strokes, and chronic infection of the spinal fluid or brain tissue, can produce slowly progressive deterioration of mental status.

The possibility of excessive medication doses, drug interactions, or alcohol intoxication should not be overlooked as possible causes of change in mental status. Elderly patients often take a large number of medications with complicated dosing schedules. All important information about the patient including medications should be obtained by the paramedic to determine the possibility of acute, reversible changes.

Alzheimer's disease is the most common of the chronic degenerative disorders producing progressive deterioration of mental status. Alzheimer's is a degenerative disorder of unknown cause in which nerve cells of the cerebral cortex die. The cerebral cortex becomes shrunken or atrophic. Although these changes do not directly cause death, patients ultimately stop eating and become malnourished and immobilized, making them prone to infections.

BOX 26-1	Causes of Altered Mental Status in the Elderly
Acute (Delirium)	**Chronic (Dementia)**
Medication error	Multi-infarct dementia (small strokes)
Hypoglycemia	Stroke
Hypothyroid	Alzheimer's disease
Pernicious anemia	Brain tumor
Thiamine deficiency	
Electrolyte disturbances	
Hypoxia	
Alcohol intoxication	
Depression	
Pneumonia	
Meningitis	

Psychiatric Illness

Progressive deterioration of mental status is a disease process almost entirely limited to older age groups. A change in mental status often presents as a psychiatric illness and is often listed as a psychiatric illness. This classification increases the possibility that important reversible medical causes may be overlooked.

Depression is common in the elderly. Symptoms vary from mild to severe and from mildly bothersome to totally incapacitating. Depression may be difficult to identify, because it can accompany other psychiatric or medical illnesses. The symptoms may mimic common conditions such as Alzheimer's disease. Apathy, loss of motivation, lack of energy, social withdrawal, difficulties with memory, and the inability to perform tasks are common to both conditions.

It has been estimated that more than 25% of suicides occur in the population group over 65 years of age. The real figure may be two to three times that number because of under-recognition of suicide and under-reporting of suicide cases.[1] Alcoholism also is common among the elderly; it is the second most frequent reason for the admission of elderly patients to psychiatric facilities. Schizophrenia is also present, but appears less prominently than in other age groups.

The Use of Pharmacological Agents

Elderly patients are at increased risk for adverse drug reactions because of age-related alterations in body composition, and in drug distribution, metabolism, and excretion. In addition, elderly patients are often prescribed multiple medications. To complicate recognition of adverse drug reactions, the elderly patient's symptoms may be mistakenly attributed to multiple medical problems or to the aging process in general.

Because of the changes in drug absorption, distribution, metabolism, and excretion, the effects of drugs may be exaggerated. Accidental overdosing can be caused by poor vision, confusion, poor memory, or self-selection of drugs. Overdosing may also be intentional because of the belief that, "if one tablet is good, two tablets might be better," or as a response to depression with suicidal thoughts. Underdosing is also a major source of medication errors in the elderly. Forgetfulness and limited income are frequent contributing factors to this problem.

Studies report that 3% to 8% of hospital admissions are a consequence of adverse drug reactions, and this percentage increases with patient age.[6] Drugs that commonly cause toxicity in elderly patients include diuretics, digitalis (the leading cause), and other heart medications and medications for high blood pressure, diabetes, blood thinning, nerves, and pain.

Because of the complexities of multiple medications and the physiologic changes that occur with aging, the paramedic should make every attempt to get an accurate drug history and to transport all drug containers with the patient.

Environmental Emergencies

Constant high and low temperatures are poorly tolerated by elderly patients, because of the decreasing efficiency of compensatory mechanisms. Predisposing factors for hypothermia include neurologic disorders such as stroke, endocrine disorders (diabetes, hypothyroid), chronic illness with debilitation, drug therapy that interferes with heat production, accidental exposure, and a low or fixed income that limits the ability of the patient to maintain a protective environment.

Predisposing factors for hyperthermia include decreased function of the temperature regulation center in the brain, commonly prescribed drugs that interfere with perspiration, and a low or fixed income.

Elderly Abuse and Neglect

According to the United States House of Representatives Select Committee on Aging, approximately 4% of the nation's elderly population are victims of abuse or neglect. The Committee reported, "...elderly abuse is far from an isolated or localized problem involving a few frail elderly and their pathologic offspring. The problem is a full-scale national problem which exists with a frequency that few have dared to imagine. In fact, abuse of the elderly by their loved ones and care takers exists with a frequency and rate only slightly less than child abuse."[14] There has been a general problem in identifying the abused elder patient because of a lack of agreement in definition and ambiguity in state reporting laws.

Of the different types of geriatric abuse, physical abuse and physical neglect will be encountered most by the paramedic (see Box 26-2 and Chapter 56).

BOX 26-2		Types of Geriatric Abuse	
Physical Abuse	**Physical Neglect**	**Psychological Abuse**	**Material Abuse**
Assault	Dehydration	Verbal or emotional abuse	Withholding finances
Rough handling	Malnutrition	Threats	Misuse of funds
Burns	Poor hygiene	Isolation or confinement	Theft
Sexual abuse	Inappropriate or soiled clothing		Withholding means of daily
Unreasonable physical	Medications given improperly		living
confinement	Lack of medical care		

Elderly abuse knows no socioeconomic bounds. The situation usually occurs when the older person is unable to be totally independent, and the family has difficulty upholding the commitment to care for the older family member.

The potential geriatric abuser is often stressed (loss of job, illness or marital discord), over 50 years of age, a family member, dependent on the victim for financial support, an alcohol or drug user, ill prepared or reluctant to provide, poor at impulse control, and has a history of domestic violence (e.g., spouse or child abuse).

Common characteristics of the abused victim include age more than 75 years (average age of 80), severe mental impairment, multiple chronic medical problems, problematic behavior (e.g., incontinence), shouting (especially at night), paranoia, dependence on the caregiver for most daily care needs, social isolation, and multiple psychosomatic complaints.

Unexplained trauma is the primary finding. The paramedic should try to obtain a complete patient and family history, as previously above in the appropriate method for obtaining patient history. To help identify elderly abuse, the paramedic should note and report all inconsistencies to the health care team who receives the patient at the hospital. Because of increased awareness of elder abuse, most states now have legislation providing a system of protective services for the elderly patient. The paramedic can play an important role in helping to identify elder abuse cases.

SUMMARY

The assessment and management of the elderly patient should follow the same procedure as that of other patients. However, the findings may be different because of consequences of the aging process. Emergency medical service providers will see an increasing proportion of elderly patients as a result of increased survival and declining birth rates.

Evaluation and treatment of the elderly is more complicated than in other age groups. Older patients may have an acute illness or injury complicated by one or more chronic conditions, such as arthritis, hypertension, hearing impairments, and heart disease.

To better understand some of the changes in physical signs and symptoms among the elderly, the paramedic should have an understanding of the physiologic and psychologic changes that occur as a result of aging. It is important for the paramedic not to focus too closely on the presenting problem without identifying possible underlying conditions, both medical and social, that may have contributed to the problem at hand.

REFERENCES

1. **Bosker G, et al:** Geriatric emergency medicine. St. Louis, 1990, Mosby–Year Book.

2. **Easton JD, Hart RG, Sherman DG, et al:** Diagnosis and management of ischemia. Stroke: Part 1. Threatened stroke and its management. In Harvey WP (ed): Current problems in cardiology, VIII. Chicago, 1983, Yearbook Medical Publishers.

3. **Gaylord S: Demography of aging, Geriatrics Review Syllabus:** A Core Curriculum in Geriatric Medicine, American Geriatrics Society, New York, 1991–1992.

4. **Gerson LW, Schelble DT, Wilson JE:** Using paramedics to identify at risk elderly. Ann Emerg Med, 21:688–691, 1992.

5. **The National Institute of Neurological Disorders and Stroke, rt-PA Stroke Study Group:** Tissue Plasminogen Activator for Acute Ischemic Stroke, N Engl J Med, 333(24):1581–1587, 1996.

6. **Nolan L, O'Malley K:** Sensitivity of the elderly to adverse drug reactions; prescribing for the elderly, Part I. Am Geriatr Soc, 36:142–149, 1988.

7. **Olsky M, Murray J:** Dizziness and Fainting in the Elderly, Emerg Med Clin North Am, 8(2):295–307, 1990.

8. **Rubens AJ:** Geriatric Emergencies, Emergency Medical Services. J Emerg Care Trans, 20(7), 1991.

9. **Sanders A:** Emergency care of the elder person, Geriatric Emergency Medicine. Society for Academic Emergency Medicine, St. Louis, 1996, Beverly Cracom Publications.

10. **Stewart CP:** Elder Abuse, Emergency Medical Services. J Emerg Care Trans, 20(7), 1991.

11. **United States Department of Health and Human Services, Public Health Service, Centers for Disease Control, National Center for Health Statistics:** Health Data on Older Americans: United States. Hyattsville, 1993.

12. **United States Department of Transportation, Geriatrics/Gerontology, Emergency Medical Technician-Paramedic:** National Standard Curriculum, Washington, 1985.

13. **United States Department of Health and Human Services:** A profile of older americans: Washington, 1994, American Association of Retired Persons and the Administration of Aging.

14. **United States House of Representatives Select Committee on Aging:** Elder Abuse: An Examination of a Hidden Problem, 1981, publication 97-277, 97th Congress, Washington, United States Government Printing Office.

Section

Patient Presentations—Medical

4A

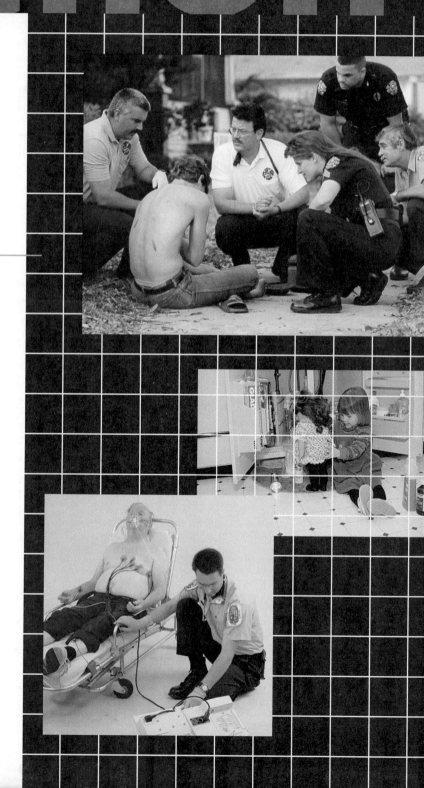

Included In This Section:

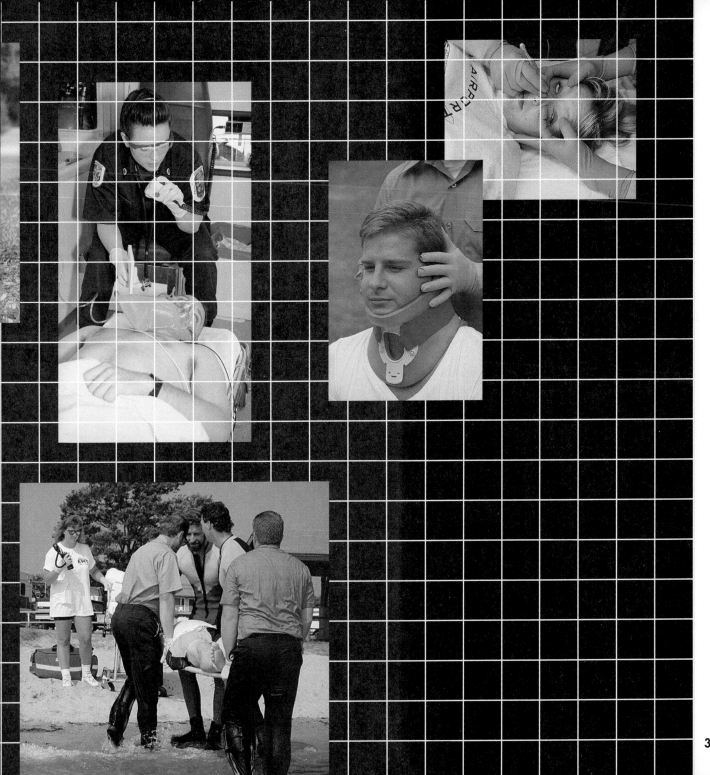

369

Howard A. Werman, MD, FACEP

Chapter 27
Dyspnea

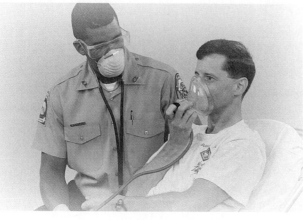

A paramedic should be able to:

1. Describe the normal physiology of breathing.
2. Define dyspnea.
3. Describe the history and assessment of the patient complaining of dyspnea.
4. Define and list signs and symptoms of respiratory failure.
5. Describe and differentiate among various causes of dyspnea in the prehospital setting.
6. In an examination of a patient with dyspnea, explain the significance of a silent chest, abnormal breath sounds, vital signs, and cardiac rhythm.
7. Describe general prehospital management of the patient with dyspnea.
8. Describe the different management approaches to various patient conditions that present with dyspnea.
9. List indications, actions, side effects, and precautions of various medications used to treat specific causes of dyspnea.

1. **Cyanosis**—a bluish discoloration of the skin and mucous membranes caused by reduced hemoglobin in the blood.
2. **Dyspnea**—an unpleasant or uncomfortable sensation of breathing, or an inappropriate awareness of breathing that is accompanied by obvious signs of difficulty or discomfort breathing.
3. **Hemoptysis**—coughing up blood from the respiratory tract.
4. **Hypoxia**—inadequate delivery of oxygen to the tissues of the body.
5. **Tachypnea**—greater than normal respiratory rate.

yspnea is an unpleasant or uncomfortable breathing sensation or an inappropriate awareness of breathing with obvious signs of difficulty or discomfort. Dyspnea is a symptom common in many illnesses and injuries seen in the prehospital setting. This chapter will discuss nontraumatic causes of dyspnea.

Pathophysiology

Under normal circumstances, the respiratory muscles receive input from both the cortex of the brain and the lower brain stem (Fig. 27-1). Breathing is usually an involuntary activity. The most important stimulus for breathing is the blood level of carbon dioxide. The accumulation of carbon dioxide in the blood causes the respiratory centers of the brain to increase the rate and depth of ventilation to return the amount of CO_2 to normal levels.

Low blood oxygen levels (hypoxia) and low blood pH (acidosis) also play a role in stimulating respiratory effort but to a lesser extent. Conditions that cause dyspnea are those in which the patient cannot adequately eliminate carbon dioxide or oxygenate the blood.

The exact mechanisms that result in dyspnea are not well understood. Dyspnea is noted when the work of breathing is excessive or resistance to airflow increases. An increase in both in the activity of the brain centers that control respiration and the activity of the respiratory muscles themselves appear to be necessary for the patient to experience dyspnea.

There is not always a direct relationship between hypoxia and the amount of dyspnea described by the patient. As a result, some hypoxic patients do not complain of breathlessness. This is particularly true of patients with chronic obstructive pulmonary disease (COPD), who usually have some degree of hypoxia from underlying lung damage. Conversely, dyspnea may also occasionally be described by patients with normal blood oxygen levels, such as patients with asthma having a mild attack. This results from the constriction of bronchioles which makes it more difficult for the patient to exhale. Factors that can produce bronchoconstriction include infections, exercise, food, allergens, environmental irritants such as dust, and in many patients, unknown precipitants.

Dyspnea is a frequent field complaint, because most conditions that affect a patient's upper airway, lower airway, lung, or heart, can cause dyspnea. Edema, constriction, or foreign body or substance in the upper airway can cause the sensation of shortness of breath. An allergic reaction, a chemical or thermal injury, or laryngeal infection can all cause upper airway compromise and dyspnea.

Pathology that affects the lower airway and the lungs includes inflammation, irritation, increased secretions, alveoli destruction, bronchiole spasm, or blood or fluid in the pleural space. COPD is the result of alveolar wall destruction and collapse along with an irritated, narrowed bronchial tree and

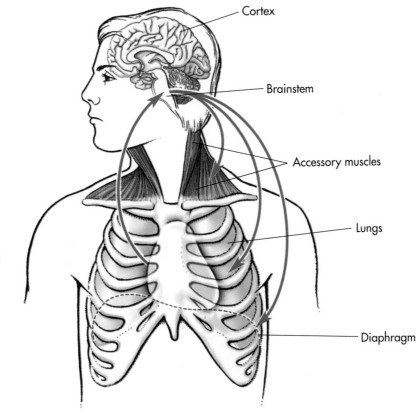

↑ Rate of respiration

↑ Depth of respiration

Cortex

Brainstem

Accessory muscles

Lungs

Diaphragm

Figure 27-1

In a healthy patient, the amount of carbon dioxide present in the blood is the primary trigger for respirations.

excessive mucous production. Figures 27-2 and 27-3 show the pathology from **chronic bronchitis** and **emphysema.** Asthma is another commonly encountered condition affecting the lower airway (Fig. 27-4). Edema, secretions, inflammation, and bronchospasm characterize asthma, which causes dyspnea. **Pulmonary edema** results from a back-up of blood into the pulmonary system and alveoli, usually caused by **heart failure,** but also a possible result of **toxic inhalation.**

Cardiac pathology causes dyspnea, most commonly with a **myocardial infarction** and heart failure (Fig. 27-5).

Patient Assessment

The patient's environment should be quickly evaluated. Toxic inhalation exposure from fire, carbon monoxide, corrosive acids or alkalis, or cyanide may be observed or smelled. Pill bottles and cigarettes may be helpful environmental clues as to the cause of the patient's condition.

History

A carefully focused patient history can often provide useful clues to the paramedic in directing patient management. Although in most cases, a complete evaluation can be performed, a patient with signs of impending respiratory failure (Box 27-1) requires immediate intervention without the benefit of a careful history or physical examination.

The paramedic should not attribute dyspnea to a known medical condition before a thorough patient evaluation can be performed. It is common for other causes of dyspnea to occur in patients with a previously diagnosed condition. For example, it could be disastrous to assume that respiratory complaints in the patient with heart disease are only a result of underlying lung disease.

With that in mind, there are several important questions the paramedic should ask to determine a possible underlying cause for dyspnea.

- *Over what period of time did the patient become dyspneic?* Often, the acuteness of onset will provide some clue about the underlying cause of dyspnea. Patients with pulmonary embolism or spontaneous **pneumothorax** will report the sudden onset of dyspnea, and patients with COPD, asthma, or pneumonia may note a more gradual worsening of symptoms.
- *How limiting is the patient's dyspnea?* In attempting to determine the degree of severity of dyspnea, it is best for the paramedic to ask the patient to relate the shortness of

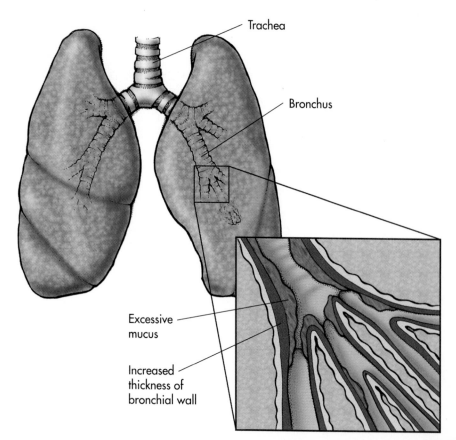

Trachea

Bronchus

Excessive mucus

Increased thickness of bronchial wall

Figure 27-2

Chronic infections result in the formation of scar tissue. In the presence of mucus during an episode of bronchitis, breathing is impaired.

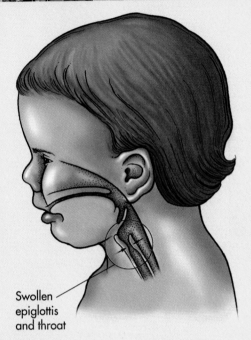

Swollen
epiglottis
and throat

- Dyspnea, as it relates to children, is perhaps better defined as respiratory distress or an increased work of breathing.
- Dyspnea in children, with the exception of foreign body obstruction and trauma, is rarely acute in nature. It usually has a gradual presentation and if not recognized early and treated appropriately, it has the potential to become life threatening. It is usually the result of abnormalities in the pulmonary, cardsiovascular, or metabolic systems. CNS disturbances should also be a consideration.
- Infants and children have small airways, an underdeveloped musculoskeletal system, and increased metabolic requirements that make them more susceptible to decompensation from respiratory emergencies. Anatomically, a newborn's trachea and bronchi are significantly smaller in diameter than an adolescent and/or adult. There is also a lesser elastic recoil of the alveoli in newborns as well. The tongue is relatively large and can obstruct the airway.
- In infants, the diaphragm and abdominal muscles are primarily used for breathing. In older children, the intercostal muscles are primarily used.
- Some physiological factors which affect respiration in infants and children include skeletal defects, abdominal distention (ascites, peritonitis), and tumor.
- Healthy children usually make little visible effort in breathing; therefore, several signs of dyspnea can

be recognized from a distance. These signs include supraclavicular, intercostal, and substernal retractions, nasal flaring, and use of the child's accessory muscles. Other signs include an unequal respiratory ratio (inspiratory/expiratory). A normal I/E ratio should be 1:1. The child may also display mental status changes, become irritable or lethargic, have skin color changes, and progress to complete loss of consciousness.

- Some causes of respiratory distress in children include infectious diseases such as croup, epiglottis, bronchiolitis, and pneumonia.
- Infants and children with congenital heart disease, especially of the cyanotic type, may present with dyspnea. This is due to an increase in the right-to-left shunting of blood and the bodies increased demand for oxygen. Most episodes follow feeding, crying, and even when defacating. An acute episode can occur as well.
- Other cardiovascular causes of dyspnea include CHF, pulmonary edema, pulmonary hypertension, pulmonary embolism and carditis.
- Cyanotic breath-holding spells are quite common in young children following excessive crying due to fear, anger, or frustration. Respiration will cease shortly thereafter and cyanosis will occur. Flaccidity and complete loss of consciousness may also follow, as can seizure-like movements. Spontaneous breathing will resume fairly rapidly. The child will usually sleep following the spell and have no effects.
- Cystic fibrosis is also a chronic lung infection that leads to a progressive loss of pulmonary function.
- Intubation requires an understanding of the unique anatomy of the infant and child, including more anterior cords and the relatively larger tongue. The trachea is shorter, making ETT placement in the right mainstem bronchus easier.

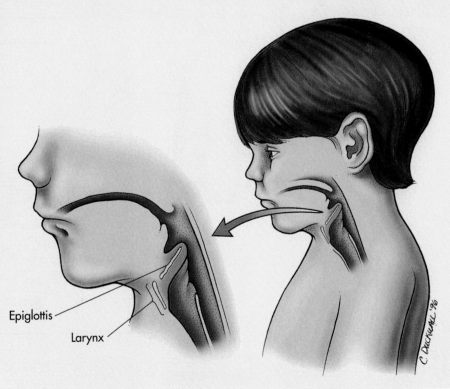

Epiglottis

Larynx

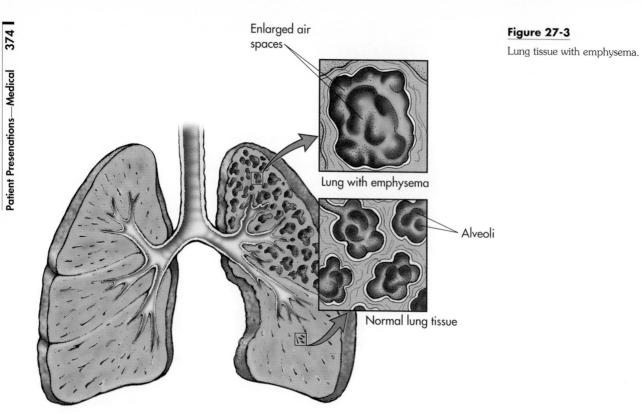

Enlarged air spaces

Figure 27-3

Lung tissue with emphysema.

Lung with emphysema

Alveoli

Normal lung tissue

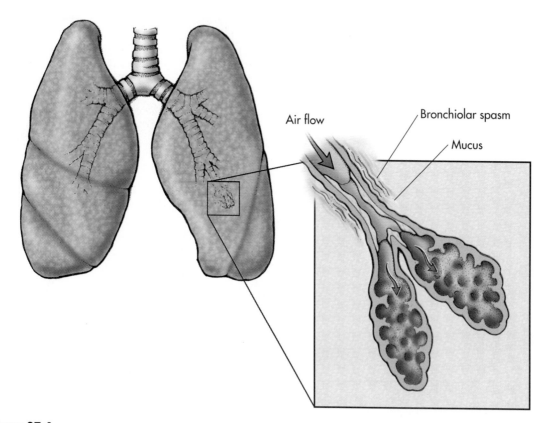

Air flow

Bronchiolar spasm

Mucus

Figure 27-4

Bronchiolar spasm and mucous plugging during an asthma attack result in severe dyspnea.

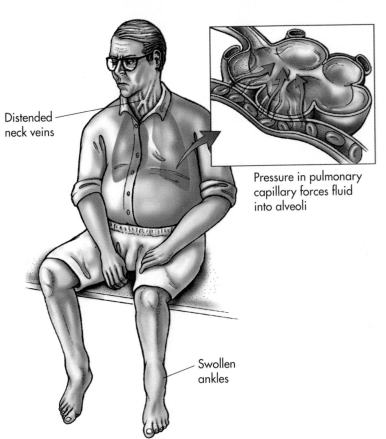

Distended
neck veins

Pressure in pulmonary
capillary forces fluid
into alveoli

Swollen
ankles

Figure 27-5

Dyspnea results from pulmonary hypertension, causing fluids
from the circulatory system to be driven into the alveoli. This
fluid widens the gap between the alveoli/capillary membrane,
making diffusion of oxygen and carbon dioxide less efficient.

breath to a specific activity that he or she might normally
perform. Walking around the block and climbing a flight
of stairs are examples of activities that may produce
symptoms.

- *What was the patient doing when the dypsnea occurred? Does the dyspnea occur at rest?* Dyspnea that
  occurs when the patient is at rest is particularly worrisome
  because it implies that the patient is unable to meet respiratory demands, even in the resting state. Cardiac causes
  are often precipitated by exertion associated with increased heart rate. Some patients with asthma have attacks which are caused by exercise. Patients with chronic
  lung diseases, such as emphysema or bronchitis, often
  become dyspneic with only mild exertion.
- *Are there any associated symptoms?* Patients who are
  experiencing breathlessness from infectious processes often report other symptoms such as fever, chills, pleuritic
  chest pain, headache, and muscle aches. On the other
  hand, dyspnea associated with chest heaviness, chest
  tightness, or heartburn may suggest a cardiac cause of
  dyspnea.

Tightness in the throat, flushing, itching, and hoarseness
may accompany an allergic reaction with airway compromise
progressing to complete **airway obstruction** (Fig. 27-6).
Lower leg pain or swelling may indicate **thrombophlebitis**
that has led to pulmonary embolism. Such a condition would
likely be accompanied by hemoptysis. Sputum production is a
classic symptom of patients with chronic bronchitis. Ankle
edema may be the paramedic's clue that heart failure exists,
possibly a result of COPD.

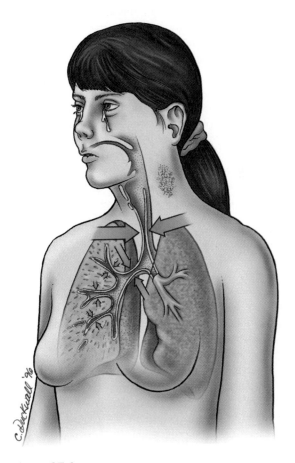

Figure 27-6

Suspect anaphylaxis as the cause of an acute airway emergency presenting with flushed skin, itching, and hoarseness.

Numbness and tingling around the mouth, hands, and feet or spasm of the fingers (carpopedal spasm) may indicate **hyperventilation syndrome.**

- *What factors worsen or improve the patient's dyspnea?* Such factors may be helpful in determining the cause for the patient's symptoms. In patients with heart problems, dyspnea may be relieved by moving the patient into an upright position. Patients with chronic lung problems may report improvement in their breathing after a deep cough. Specific questions about the patient's response to medication used and the patient's compliance with prescribed drugs should be included.

- *What is the patient's past medical history?* Many underlying medical conditions that result in dyspnea, such as asthma, COPD, or congestive heart failure (CHF), tend to occur repeatedly. In addition, the patient should be asked how the current episode compares in severity with previous ones. A recent history of prolonged immobilization or a surgical procedure may lead to a suspicion of deep vein thrombosis with pulmonary embolism. A patient with **HIV** will be more susceptible to pneumonia.

- *What therapies have worked in the past?* Evaluation of effective therapies often provides clues to both the underlying medical condition and the initial management of the patient. A patient with asthma who is unresponsive to therapies that have been previously successful is in jeopardy of respiratory arrest. A previous episode requiring intubation or mechanical ventilation is an ominous finding.

- *Is the patient taking any medications?* Often medical conditions contributing to dyspnea can be identified by the medications that the patient is currently taking. Patients taking theophylline, corticosteroids, inhalers such as beclomethasone, or beta-agonist inhalers such as albuterol are more likely to have dyspnea caused by worsening of asthma or COPD. However, if a patient is taking digoxin, furosemide, or nitroglycerin, a primary cardiac problem is more likely the cause. See Table 27-1 for patient medications related to dyspnea.

- *Does the patient have any allergies?* Both asthma and **anaphylaxis** may indicate dyspnea caused by allergic reaction.

Physical Examination

The physical assessment also helps evaluate the extent of respiratory distress and guides initial patient therapy. In assessing and re-evaluating the dyspneic patient, paramedics must be alert for signs suggestive of impending respiration failure. Patients with these signs require immediate intervention.

Some observations can be made prior to physical examination of the patient. The patient should be examined for pale, mottled, or cyanotic skin and facial color. Patients with emphysema tend to have a pink skin color caused by an excess of red blood cells (polycythemia). Patients with chronic bronchitis may have some chronic cyanosis. The position in which the patient is found should also be noted. Does the patient assume an upright position? Is the patient pursing the lips or showing muscle retractions (Fig. 27-7). Inspection is performed primarily to determine the patient's effort used in breathing.

One simple method that can be used to quantitate the severity of the dyspnea is to observe how many words the patient can speak before requiring a breath. A patient able to speak in full sentences when relating a medical history is in less serious condition than the patient who must stop for breath after only a few words.

Particular attention should be focused on the patient's use of the accessory muscles for respiration—intercostal muscles and sternocleidomastoid muscles of the neck. When the accessory muscles are used to assist respiration, the patient is most likely experiencing severe respiratory distress.

The patient's vital signs should be assessed next. The rate and quality of respirations should be determined. Adults typically take 12–20 breaths per minute. An early sign of a respiratory problem is a rise in the respiratory rate. Any adult patient breathing more than 24 times per minute is considered tachypneic and should be monitored closely. Ventilatory assistance with a bag-valve-mask is often required in these patients.

Irregularities in the pulse rhythm may indicate cardiac **dysrhythmias,** which are commonly found in the patient with dyspnea. Tachycardia is usually seen in patients with dyspnea, particularly those using bronchodilators. A slowing of an adult's pulse to a rate of 80 to 100 beats per minute with therapy suggests an adequate response to treatment.

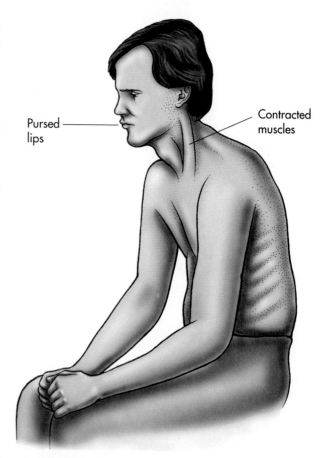

Pursed lips — — — — — —

Contracted muscles

Figure 27-7

Pursed lip breathing, retractions, and accessory muscle use during respiration signal dyspnea.

TABLE 27-1 Dyspnea-Related Patient Medications

Classification	Specific Drug	Indication	Therapeutic Action	Side Effects and Precautions
BRONCHODILATORS Oral	Aminophylline Theodur Somophylline Elixophylline Brethine	Asthma COPD	Dilates the bronchi	Cardiac dysrhythmias Tachydysrhythmias Nervousness N/V
Inhalants	Proventil Ventolin Alupent Albuterol			
ANTICOAGULANTS	Coumadin Heparin Persantine	Pulmonary embolism DVT Thrombophlebitis AMI	Increased clotting time	Hemorrhage
ANTI-INFLAMMATORY Steroid	Medrol Prednisone	Arthritis Asthma Allergies Inflammation	Reduces inflammation from severe disease	Masks symptoms of other diseases Mood swings Weight gain
ANTIHYPERTENSIVE Diuretics	Lasix (Furosemide) Esidrex (Hydrochlorothiazide) Hydrodiuril Diuril Oretic Aldactone	HTN Congestive heart failure	Increases urinary output Decreases circulating volume	Dehydration Electrolyte imbalances Hypotension Hypokalemia
CARDIOTONICS	Digitalis (Digoxin) Lanoxin	CHF A-fib/A-flutter/PSVT	Increases force of contraction Slows conduction through the AV node—decreases heart rate	Bradycardia Digitalis toxicity

Although tachycardia can be seen in patients with primary cardiac problems and associated dyspnea, it is more commonly seen in patients with hypoxia and impending respiratory failure. The dyspneic patient commonly demonstrates a normal or elevated blood pressure. Blood pressure and pulse elevations are the result of increased circulating catecholamines, such as epinephrine, which are released when the patient experiences breathlessness.

Bradycardia is a critical finding in a patient with dyspnea. It is usually caused by prolonged hypoxia and indicates imminent respiratory failure.

A complete lung assessment should be performed to determine a pulmonary cause of symptoms. This examination should include inspection and palpation of the patient's chest wall and auscultation of lung sounds. Palpation is helpful in identifying any asymmetry of chest wall movement or crepitus caused by subcutaneous air from a pneumothorax. A barrel chest with an increased anterior/posterior chest diameter may be observed and indicates emphysema as an underlying condition.

The lungs are then auscultated. First, the paramedic gains a sense of the ease of air movement through the lungs. Clearly audible breath sounds throughout a full inspiration indicates good air flow.

Markedly decreased air movement is a worrisome finding that suggests a worsening of the patient's ventilatory status.

The paramedic must be prepared to support the patient's ventilations and provide oxygen supplementation.

There are several abnormal lung findings that may be identified in the dyspneic patient. Snoring respirations indicate obstruction of the upper airway. Gurgling noises are associated with fluid collections in the patient's airway. Stridor, heard best over the trachea, is a continuous crowing or musical, high-pitched sound heard primarily during inspiration. It usually indicates a partial upper airway obstruction.

Wheezing is also a continuous, high-pitched lung sound that is heard best in the lung peripheries and is more pronounced during expiration. Wheezing indicates narrowing of the bronchioles, usually by bronchospams as seen in asthma and COPD. Crackles, or rales, are generally recognized as fine, high-pitched sounds heard during inspiration when there is fluid in the alveoli such as that which occurs in CHF or pneumonia. Rhonchi are lower-pitched, harsh sounds usually heard on expiration and related to mucus or foreign matter in the bronchi, such as occurs in bronchitis or pneumonia. Rhonchi often clear after coughing.

Noisy breathing that becomes quiet does not always indicate an improvement in the patient's condition. Sounds of partial obstruction become quiet when the patient develops a *complete* obstruction. Similarly, a decrease in wheezing a patient with asthma may indicate a decrease in air movement. Patients in these situations require aggressive ventilatory support and airway management.

The equality of the breath sounds should also be evaluated. Decreased or absent breath sounds on one side suggest the possibility of a pneumothorax.

When possible, a more complete physical assessment of the patient should be performed to reveal other possible supportive findings. Examination of the neck may reveal jugular venous distention (JVD) caused by obstruction of venous return to the heart indicating possible heart failure. The skin and mucous membranes may show cyanosis, suggesting hypoxia, or pallor and mottling resulting from **hypoperfusion** or **anemia.** Finally, the extremities may demonstrate swelling as fluid builds up because of worsening CHF.

Key Conditions and Findings

- *Upper airway obstruction.* Obstruction can be caused by a foreign body, throat trauma, or swelling of the oropharynx. Such swelling can be seen with allergic reactions (e.g., anaphylaxis, angioedema) or infections (e.g., epiglottitis, croup, **peritonsillar abscesses**).
- *Pulmonary pathologies.* These diseases include: asthma, COPD, infections (pneumonia, **tuberculosis**), pulmonary embolism, and pneumothorax.
- *Cardiac problems.* Dyspnea can be related to left ventricular failure that causes hypoperfusion or myocardial ischemia (e.g., myocardial infarction, dysrhythmias) or pulmonary edema (e.g., congestive heart failure).
- *Miscellaneous causes.* Another concern is anemia, which results in dyspnea because of the reduced oxygen-carrying capacity of blood. Inhalation of toxins (e.g., cyanide, pesticides, chlorine gas, hydrocarbons) can result in damage to lung tissue. Shock or sepsis from any source may also be a consideration.

Management

Initially, all dyspneic patients should be placed in a position of comfort. Next, the paramedic must determine if an upper airway obstruction is present. Patients with airway obstruction are identified by complaints of foreign body sensation, hoarseness, difficulty speaking, drooling, grunting respirations, coughing, or stridor. Observation and management to prevent complete airway obstruction is imperative (*see* Chapter 18).

The initial intervention for all dyspneic patients is administration of oxygen. In many cases, the oxygen alone will significantly relieve dyspnea. Supplemental oxygen should be given at near 100% concentration with a nonrebreather mask.

The paramedic should be prepared to assist ventilations if indicated.

Although it is true that some patients with COPD depend on low blood oxygen levels to stimulate their respiratory drive, these patients only lose respiratory stimulus after receiving oxygen for a period longer than the majority of transport times. Therefore, high concentrations of oxygen should not be withheld from any patient whose clinical condition requires it.

The prehospital management indicated for a patient who is wheezing includes inhalation of a selective beta-2 agonist such as albuterol or metaproteranol. Such agents may provide significant improvement in patients with asthma or COPD and may provide symptomatic relief in patients with wheezing from other causes. Subcutaneously injected epinephrine may be useful in some resistant cases of wheezing caused by asthma or allergic reactions, particularly in younger patients.

If crackles or rales are heard, it is important for the paramedic to determine if the symptoms are a result of CHF. Patients in these siutations usually demonstrate other signs suggestive of heart failure, including JVD and swelling of the feet and ankles (pedal edema). A prior history of heart problems or episodes of CHF and medications including diuretics, digoxin, and nitrates, support this suspicion.

Other conditions can cause rales or crackles, including pneumonia, pulmonary embolism, COPD, and toxic inhalation. Only those patients with a history strongly suggestive of CHF should receive vasodilators, which are medications effective at reducing venous return (preload). Such medications include nitroglycerin and morphine sulfate; furosemide may also be considered.

Patients with suspected myocardial infarction or ischemia should be treated accordingly (*see* Chapter 31). Some patients with underlying cardiac disease will present with only a complaint of dyspnea, not chest pain or discomfort. This is particularly true of elderly patients.

Patients with unilaterally absent breath sounds should be suspected of having a spontaneous pneumothorax. Should a patient develop tension pneumothorax, JVD, hypotension, subcutaneous emphysema, and severe respiratory distress are likely. The management of a tension pneumothorax requires needle decompression of the involved side (*see* Skill #36 in the Skills Section).

As respiratory failure approaches, the patient's mental status changes from anxious to agitated and confused, and finally to tired and lethargic just prior to respiratory arrest. If these findings are noted, the patient's ventilation should be supported and preparation should be made for endotracheal intubation.

Other supportive measures should be initiated for every patient with a chief complaint of dyspnea. IV access should be established so that drug therapy can be initiated if necessary; crystalloid at a keep open rate is appropriate in this setting. Cardiac monitoring should also be instituted, because hypoxia can lead to PVCs and other cardiac rhythm disturbances. Also, myocardial ischemia and cardiac rhythm disturbances can present as dyspnea. Finally, where available, pulse oximetry is a rapid, noninvasive method use to determine the oxygen saturation of the blood. This technology is not only useful in evaluating the severity of the patient's initial condition but also in monitoring the patient's response to therapies.

SUMMARY

Dyspnea is a patient complaint that is commonly encountered by prehospital personnel. A directed patient assessment is necessary to determine the severity of respiratory distress experienced by the patient and the type of intervention required. The patient should be closely observed for signs of impending respiratory failure. Initial management includes supplemental oxygen, IV access, and electrocardiographic monitoring, as well as general supportive measures. More specific therapy depends on the ability to identify the underlying cause, which may involve systems other than the pulmonary system.

SUGGESTED READINGS

1. **Barrett S:** Dyspnea and shortness of breath. In *Emergency Medicine: concepts and clinical practice,* ed 3, St. Louis, 1992, CV Mosby.

2. **Daily RH:** Difficulty in breathing. In *Principles and Practice of Emergency Medicine,* ed 2, Philadelphia, 1992, WB Saunders.

3. **McEwen JI:** Pleural Disease. in *Emergency Medicine: concepts and clinical practice,* ed 3, St. Louis, 1992, CV Mosby.

4. **Murphy C:** Acute dyspnea. in *Current Practice of Emergency Medicine,* ed 2, Philadelphia, 1991, BC Decker.

5. **Sternbach G:** Dyspnea. in *Current Therapy in Emergency Medicine,* Philadelphia, 1991, JB Lippincott.

6. **Wright SW:** Acute dyspnea. In *Emergency Medicine: An approach to clinical problem-solving,* Philadelphia, 1991, WB Saunders.

Francis Mencl, MD

Chapter 28

Nontraumatic Bleeding

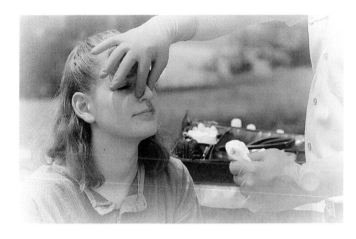

A paramedic should be able to:

1. Define homeostasis, and discuss how it is accomplished in the body.
2. List diseases or conditions that may be associated with inadequate clotting ability.
3. Define the following terms.
   a. Epistaxis   d. Hemoptysis
   b. Hematemesis   e. Melena
   c. Hematuria
4. Discuss assessment procedures to perform on a patient who has non-traumatic bleeding and key assessment findings.
5. Identify causes, potential sites, signs and symptoms and field treatment for patients who present with:
   a. Epistaxis   d. Hemoptysis
   b. Hematemesis   e. Melena
   c. Hematuria

1. **Epistaxis**—bleeding from the nose.
2. **Hematemesis**—vomiting of blood.
3. **Hematuria**—a dark-colored urine caused by the presence of hemoglobin.
4. **Hemoptysis**—coughing up blood from the respiratory tract.
5. **Hemostasis**—the termination of bleeding by mechanical or chemical means or by the complex coagulation process of the body, consisting of vasoconstriction, platelet aggregation, and thrombin or fibrin synthesis.
6. **Melena**—abnormal, black, tarry stool containing digested blood.

Acute nontraumatic bleeding nearly always provokes fear in the patient and anxiety in the prehospital care provider and indeed may represent a true life-threatening process. The sudden onset of rapid bleeding can cause syncope or light-headedness in the patient because of hypovolemia. It may strain a heart already weakened by cardiac disease. Severe bleeding from the nose or into the airway may cause acute respiratory distress. At times, the source, extent, and rate of nontraumatic bleeding are not readily apparent.

Pathophysiology

One process of clotting (hemostasis) is complex and is accomplished by several different mechanisms. The first mechanism is vascular spasm, or the instantaneous contraction of the vessel wall. This process reduces the flow of blood from the injured vessel and causes a reflex that, in turn, causes vessel spasm for the area surrounding the injury. The intensity of this vascular spasm can be so significant that lacerated large arteries do not result in serious blood loss.

The second mechanism that is activated in hemostasis is an attempt made by the platelets to plug the torn vessel. Platelets in this case become sticky, and layers upon layers adhere to each other to fill the hole.

The third mechanism in hemostasis is blood clot formation. Blood clot formation can begin within 20 seconds of severe injury and is activated by substances from the traumatized vessel wall and from the platelets that have gathered at the injury.

This clotting process depends upon the interaction of numerous clotting factors but has three primary steps (Fig. 28-1): 1) the prothrombin activator is formed as a result of the vessel injury; 2) the prothrombin activator breaks down the prothrombin into thrombin; and 3) the thrombin converts fibrinogen into fibrin threads that allow the red blood cells and plasma to form the clot.

There can be a deficiency or dysfunction in any of these or other involved factors. For example, people with hemophilia lack factor VIII and bleed easily with minimal or no trauma. Many of the clotting factors are produced in the liver. Not surprisingly, individuals with severe liver disease, such as cirrhosis and hepatitis, have problems with blood clotting. Patients with certain cancers, especially leukemias, are also prone to bleeding complications. Some medications, such as blood thinners (coumadin) and aspirin, can interfere with the clotting process and cause the patient to bleed heavily or chronically.

Epistaxis, or nasal bleeding, is a common complaint affecting approximately 15% of the adult population each year.[1] Most cases can be resolved quickly without treatment. Those that result in an EMS call tend to have been prolonged, severe, or recurrent. Epistaxis is commonly associated with hypertension, which is not considered a cause, but may complicate control of the hemorrhage. Epistaxis can also occur spontaneously without special underlying causes, especially at higher altitudes or dry climates.

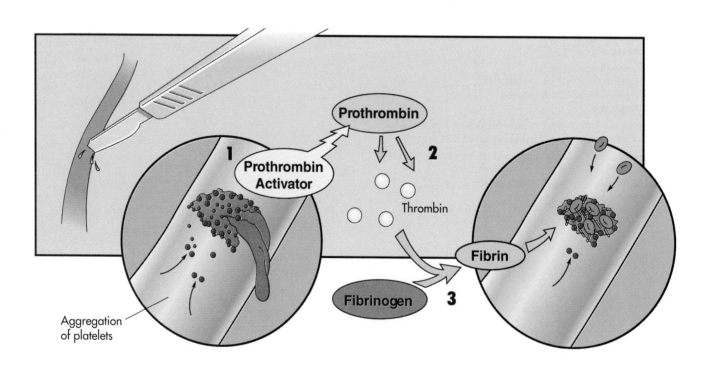

Figure 28-1

The three primary steps of the clotting process.

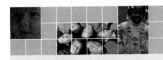

PEDIATRIC PERSPECTIVE

- Nosebleeds, or epistaxis, in children can cause great fear and alarm for children and parents as they may tend to overestimate the episode and the amount of blood loss. Through the nose is a common site of minor trauma, from clumsiness to picking, it contains minimal support for the small blood vessels that supply it, making it more prone to bleeding from other non-traumatic causes.

- Another common cause of alarm to parents is the presence of blood in the child's emesis and/or stool. Most children who present with some sort of GI bleeding are hemodynamically stable. Non GI sources such as a recent epistaxis, possible ingestion of red Kool-Aid or Jell-O, etc. should be sought. It should be noted that 80–85% of GI bleeding in children will stop before or early in the hospital course of treatment or stay, whatever the source. Also, severe lower GI bleeding leading to respiratory, cardiovascular or hemodynamic instability which requires transfusion is rare in children.

- Hematologic diseases, such as hemophilia A and B, leukemia, and hepatic disorders cause non-traumatic bleeding in children as well. Children with hemophilia have abnormalities in normal coagulation and may pre-sent with numerous locations of bleeding such as at the joints, muscles, and oral cavity. These children will complain of pain to the affected area and possibly a decrease in their normal range of motion. Bruising may also be found. Prehospital treatment for these children is primarily supportive as they need a more disease specific therapy, such as Factor VIII replacement, cryoprecipitate, and fresh frozen plasma.

- Non-traumatic bleeding within the lungs is potentially life threatening to the child with **cystic fibrosis.** These children already have diminished lung function and capacity due to their disease. The first presentation of this may be hemoptysis. It can also be noticed by the presence of a cough which can sometimes produce a "wet" sound upon auscultation. If undetected, pulmonary hemorrhage can be life threatening and may require emergent airway maintenance with attempts made to suction the increased bloody secretions from the lungs via the endotrachael tube. Poor compliance will be noted when assisting ventilations in these children. Rapid transport with optimal airway maintenance is imperative.

Patients coughing up blood (hemoptysis) is a problem that has multiple causes. Although most patients who have an episode of hemoptysis have relatively benign disorders (such as **bronchitis**), there can also be serious underlying illness; **pneumonia, lung abscess, tuberculosis,** tumors, and **pulmonary emboli** are examples. Hemoptysis can also arise from severe left heart failure and valvular heart disease (mitral stenosis).

Bleeding from the gastrointestinal (GI) tract is classified according to location (Fig. 28-2). Upper **GI bleeding** originates from the esophagus, stomach, or proximal duodenum. Lower GI bleeding can originate in the small intestine, colon, or rectal regions.

Patients with upper GI bleeding frequently present with hematemesis (vomiting of blood). When combined with stomach

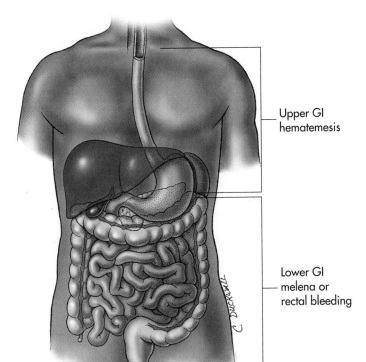

Upper GI
hematemesis

Lower GI
melena or
rectal bleeding

Figure 28-2

Upper GI bleeding results in hematemesis (bloody vomit), whereas lower GI bleeding results in dark, tarry appearing stools (melena) or bright red rectal bleeding.

acid, blood forms an iron compound that is very irritating to the stomach and usually causes vomiting. Bright red blood in the emesis indicates a recent or vigorous bleed. However, when the stomach accumulates blood that becomes partially digested, the emesis may resemble "coffee grounds." Forceful and repeated vomiting may also cause hematemesis by tearing the small blood vessels that line the stomach and esophagus.

The color of blood in the stool is determined by the site of the bleeding and the amount of time the blood has spent in the GI tract. Slow bleeding from upper GI sources results in digested blood that gives the stool a black, tarry appearance (melena). Blood coming from the lower colon or rectal area usually appears bright red and may be on the surface of the stool or streaked into it. A considerable amount of blood may remain "hidden" in the stomach or intestines, so that the amount of blood found in the stool or emesis does not accurately indicate the total amount of blood loss.

Vaginal bleeding, one of the most common gynecologic symptoms, usually is sudden in onset, dramatic, and frightening to the patient. Vaginal bleeding can be the first sign of a pregnancy-related problem, pelvic cancer, or bleeding disorder; it can also simply be heavy menstrual bleeding.

Blood noted in the urine (hematuria) is a relatively common complaint. Common nontraumatic causes of hematuria include **urinary tract infections, kidney stones,** and tumors.

Patient Assessment

History

Assuming there is no hemodynamic instability, pertinent historical facts will be very useful in directing patient management.

- *What is the source of the bleeding?* Determining the source of bleeding can be a challenge. Patients often find it difficult to differentiate between hematemesis and hemoptysis. A patient suffering from epistaxis may swallow a great deal of blood and then vomit.

CRITICAL ISSUE

Hematemesis and hemoptysis are easily confused. Blood from a nasal source may be swallowed by a patient and then vomited. Careful questioning and observation by the paramedic can help to differentiate the bleeding site.

- *What are the characteristics of the bleeding and when did the bleeding begin?* In most cases, bright red or arterial bleeding is of the most concern because hemodynamic compromise is apt to follow. The time factor may be critical in alerting the EMS provider that an aggressive approach is required; the patient's estimates of blood loss are often inaccurate, and in most cases, there is substantial blood volume in hidden, internal sites.
- *Does the patient have epistaxis?* If so, many patients have a prior history of nosebleeds or are on medication

for hypertension. Epistaxis may also be related to sinus infections or surgeries.
- *Is hemoptysis noted?* The most frequent presentation of hemoptysis is coughing up small amounts of blood that appear as small dark blood clots or blood-streaked sputum. This is usually from a small, slow bleed in the mucosa of the bronchial tree. Bright red blood with minimal sputum indicates rapid bleeding, carries the risk of airway compromise, and may be immediately life threatening. Foamy, pink-tinged sputum, indicating small amounts of blood which has not clotted prior to being coughed up, is seen in acute pulmonary edema.
- *Are any respiratory symptoms noted?* The presence of chest pain, cough, shortness of breath or wheezing are useful in directing management plans. The paramedic should note if the patient has been treated for any significant respiratory diseases in the past.
- *Is GI bleeding present?* The presence of frank hematemesis or "coffee ground emesis" can indicate an upper GI bleed. The paramedic should inquire about the presence of dark, tarry appearing stools and a history of peptic ulcer disease or alcohol abuse.
- *If vaginal bleeding is present, what is the patient's menstrual history?* The patient may state that the character of this menstrual period is heavier or lighter than usual periods. The paramedic should inquire about possible results available from a recent pregnancy test. Any patient who is in the early stages of pregnancy or having menstrual irregularities should be assumed to have an **ectopic (tubal) pregnancy.** These women are at risk for life-threatening hemorrhage and aggressive management is mandatory.
- *What medications does the patient take?* Certain medications, such as aspirin and coumadin, interfere with the blood clotting process. Patients taking these medications may note a tendency to bruise easily and bleed spontaneously from any source. Anti-inflammatory agents, such as aspirin or ibuprofen, cause irritation of the mucosal lining of the stomach and have been associated with formation of upper GI bleeding. Patients treated for **ulcer disease** commonly take histamine blockers, such as cimetidine, to prevent excess stomach acid production.

Physical Examination

Hypovolemia caused by uncontrolled hemorrhage usually presents telltale signs. Initial efforts at physical examination should revolve around detecting any evidence of **shock.**

CRITICAL ISSUE

Shock and hypoperfusion may be seen in all types of hemorrhage, regardless of site.

Many of these patients manifest changes in their vital signs and mental status. Patients who slowly lose blood over a period of time will compensate for a longer period of time, and vital sign changes will occur more slowly. The earliest sign of hypoperfusion is seen in a patient who presents with anxiety, combativeness, or other mentation changes. Tachycardia and tachypnea are likely to be the first shifts seen in vital signs. As blood loss continues, the body loses the ability to compensate, and frank hypotension ensues.

Skin signs are very helpful in evaluating the bleeding patient. The skin may be cool, pale, and moist as a result of sympathetic stimulation. Patients with significant blood loss often show pallor of the conjunctiva and mucous membranes. If the patient is in respiratory distress, cyanosis may appear early at the fingernail beds and later progress to the lips.

Severe respiratory distress may develop in patients with hemoptysis. Auscultate the lungs for the presence of crackles or wheezing, and determine the adequacy of air movement in all lung fields. The presence of neck vein distention or peripheral edema points toward cardiac failure.

When inspecting the abdomen, visible swelling or distention of superficial veins, particularly around the umbilicus (belly button), suggests liver disease. Tenderness on palpation may be absent and does not correlate with the severity of bleeding. Liver disorders are often discovered by checking for a firm, enlarged liver in the right upper quadrant, as well as visible jaundice. Because blood acts as an irritant to the lining of the intestine, auscultation of the abdomen can reveal hyperactive bowel sounds if the bleeding is significant.

The healthy pregnant patient has a lower blood pressure and faster heart rate than normal. Blood volume is increased, so the patient can lose a large quantity of blood before typical hypovolemic changes in blood pressure and heart rate begin to take place.

CRITICAL ISSUE

Because they may not show early signs of hypoperfusion, pregnant patients with possible bleeding must be treated aggressively and watched carefully. All pregnant patients, regardless of apparent hemodynamic stability, should be transported for further evaluation.

Key Conditions and Findings

- *Epistaxis.* Bleeding from the nose may occur directly from the anterior or posterior nasopharynx, where there are rich vascular networks. Epistaxis may also be associated with sinus disorders and hypertension.
- *Hemoptysis.* Most commonly, bleeding from the respiratory tract is caused by pulmonary infections, such as bronchitis or pneumonia. Bleeding can also be present with more serious infections, such as tuberculosis and lung abscesses. Hemoptysis and weight loss are the first signs of many lung tumors. Pulmonary embolus, heart failure, and valvular heart disease account for a smaller percentage of patients.
- *Hematemesis.* Vomited blood generally originates in the upper GI tract. Bleeding from esophageal varices can be seen when pressure backs up in the vessels surrounding the esophagus because of liver disease. Irritation of

the lining of the esophagus or stomach can cause erosion into the capillary beds of these organs, a condition known as esophagitis or gastritis. When this process becomes more extensive, ulcers form in the stomach or duodenum.

- *Rectal Bleeding.* Rectal bleeding usually presents as melena from upper GI sources or with bright red blood emerging locally from lower GI sources. Causes of lower GI hemorrhage include inflammatory bowel diseases, tumors, hemorrhoids, and anal fissures.
- *Vaginal Bleeding.* Early in pregnancy, most cases are secondary to ectopic pregnancy, or spontaneous and threatened abortions (see Chapter 37). In contrast, third-trimester bleeding may be caused by imminent delivery, or more importantly by placenta previa or abruptio placenta, where both the mother and fetus may be at risk. In nonpregnant patients, hemorrhage may be associated with tumors, infections, and hormonal irregularities.
- *Hematuria.* Occasionally, paramedics are called to evaluate someone with blood in his or her urine. Most often in young patients, this is caused by infection, kidney stones, or blunt trauma. Hematuria in older patients may signify a urinary tract cancer.
- *Clotting Disorders (coagulopathies).* Patients with clotting problems may have inherited disorders (hemophilia) or be taking medications which interfere with the clotting process (coumadin or aspirin). Severe medical conditions, such as liver and renal failure, can also cause coagulopathies. The important fact about this group of patients is that they may bleed spontaneously and extensively from any site.

Management

Many patients with uncontrolled bleeding are at risk for airway compromise and pulmonary aspiration. Most often, this occurs in patients suffering from severe hematemesis or hemoptysis, but it also may be seen in a few epistaxis patients. If an individual shows a decreasing level of mentation and an inability to control these secretions, airway management becomes a priority. Adequate suction must be available. Endotracheal intubation is performed orally under direct visualization. Nasotracheal intubation is relatively contraindicated because many of these patients will have coagulation problems. Trauma to the nares or oropharynx during the blind attempt could worsen an already serious situation.

Because of the lowered concentration of hemoglobin, all patients should receive 100% oxygen at a high-flow rate, which maximizes oxygen delivery and minimizes tissue hypoxia. Pulse oximetry can be used to monitor respiratory status if available, but it can be very misleading in patients with severe anemia, who can be hypoxic even when fully saturated.

Intravenous access with a normal saline or Ringer's lactate solution should be obtained with a large-bore catheter. For patients with signs of hemodynamic compromise, fluid boluses should be administered according to local protocols. Because hypotension is caused by hypovolemia in these cases, pressor agents such as dopamine are not indicated.

A cardiac monitor is useful for monitoring hemodynamic status and demonstrating evidence of myocardial ischemia in those patients who may be unusually sensitive to hypovolemia.

Epistaxis may be controlled by pinching the nose after allowing the patient to first blow out all blood and clots. The patient is usually kept in an upright position. Suctioning should be available and used as needed (*see* Chapter 39).

Managing patients with massive hemoptysis is a different problem. The patient should be placed in a slight head-down position (Trendelenburg position). This position will facilitate drainage of blood from the lungs and airway. If it is known which lung is involved, position the patient with that side down; this position prevents drainage of blood into the airway and the unaffected lung. All other patients should be transported in the position of comfort, or a position that logically minimizes the risk of aspiration from the bleeding site.

Because of the risk of acquiring an infection, it is important to take respiratory precautions by wearing a mask, and placing one on the patient, if tolerated, for all patients presenting with hemoptysis.

Transport of patients with evidence of hemodynamic compromise should be to a facility capable of providing a prompt surgical response, often a trauma center.

SUMMARY

The severity of nontraumatic bleeding can vary from minimal to life threatening. Although minimal hemorrhage may only require assessment and reassurance, life-threatening bleeding must be recognized and swiftly managed. Immediate life threats center around airway obstruction and hypoperfusion from uncontrolled hemorrhage.

REFERENCES

1. **Hamilton G, et al (ed):** Emergency medicine: an approach to clinical problem solving, Philadelphia, 1991, WB Saunders, p. 537.

Chapter 29

Syncope

William Roush, MD

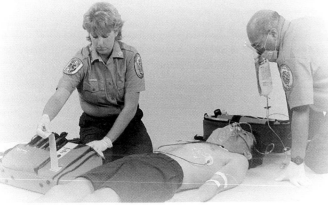

KEY TERMS

1. **Orthostatic hypotension**—abnormally low blood pressure occurring when an individual assumes the standing posture.

2. **Syncope**—a transient loss of responsiveness (a few seconds to several minutes) in which the patient regains mentation when placed in a supine position.

3. **Vasovagal response**—increased parasympathetic tone which results in slowing the heart rate.

A paramedic should be able to:

OBJECTIVES

1. Define syncope and discuss its pathophysiology.

2. Identify the possible causes of syncope.

3. Discuss the following conditions in terms of pathophysiology, clinical significance, and prehospital management:
   a. Vasovagal response
   b. Orthostatic hypotension

4. Identify key historical questions to ask a patient who has experienced syncope.

5. Describe aspects of the physical examination that are indicated for a patient experiencing syncope.

6. Discuss the clinical significance of orthostatic vital signs (tilt test) as related to syncope.

7. Discuss the significance and probable cause of syncope in a patient who has no warning signs.

8. Describe the prehospital management of a patient with syncope.

Syncope, or fainting, is a common presenting complaint for patients entering the EMS system. Syncope is a transient loss of responsiveness (lasting a few seconds to several minutes), in which the patient regains mentation when placed in a supine position.

By far the most frequent cause of syncope is decreased blood flow to the brain. Normal brain function and a responsive state depend on a constant supply of oxygen and glucose to the brain. Because the brain is unable to store these nutrients, an interruption of cerebral blood flow for 5 to 10 seconds will result in unresponsiveness.[1]

Pathophysiology

Syncope occurs frequently in otherwise healthy individuals and is usually referred to as fainting. Fainting is often associated with experiencing or anticipating an unpleasant situation (e.g., feeling afraid, seeing blood, feeling pain). In response to these situations, the individual has a temporary sympathetic response followed by a reflex vagal reaction that causes decreased heart rate and dilation of blood vessels. This "vasovagal" response can cause major, transient decreases in blood pressure and cerebral blood flow.

A temporary decrease in the amount of blood returned to the heart occurs whenever the patient holds his or her breath and bears down, strains to urinate or defecate, or has prolonged bouts of coughing. These maneuvers not only decrease blood return to the heart because of increased intrathoracic pressure, but may also cause a vagal response that slows the heart. A similar response can occur following pressure on the carotid sinus in the neck. Some individuals have carotid sinus hypersensitivity; minimal stimulation can result in significant cardiac slowing, decreased blood pressure, and syncope in these patients.

Orthostatic hypotension frequently results in syncope. Under normal circumstances, when an individual stands, the sympathetic nervous system causes peripheral blood vessel constriction and an increase in heart rate in order to maintain cardiac output and blood flow to the brain (Fig. 29-1). If these reflex changes do not occur, blood return to the heart decreases because of blood pooling in the abdomen and lower extremities. The result is a drop in blood pressure that may be severe enough to cause syncope.

Older individuals are especially susceptible to positional changes in blood pressure, particularly after long periods of inactivity. Such changes may be reflected by the increase in pulse rate or decrease in blood pressure seen when orthostatic vital signs (tilt test) are performed.

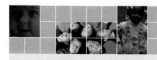

PEDIATRIC PERSPECTIVE

- Close attention should be paid to the child with syncope because it is usually secondary to a current illness or serious underlying medical condition. Therefore, any child with syncope should be transported to an ED and have a thorough examination performed.
- Simple fainting can occur when a child is provoked or overcome with fear or apprehension, such as when exposed to certain medical procedures or domestic disturbances. In simple fainting, the physical assessment will be unremarkable and transport would consist only of supportive care.
- While orthostatic hypotension in children can be normal, it can also be caused by dehydration and hypovolemia secondary to GI losses (vomiting and diarrhea), sepsis, and malnutrition. Orthostatic vital signs ("tilt-test") should be obtained. Management includes IV fluid boluses of normal saline or Ringer's lactate at 20 mL/kg.
- Diagnosed or undiagnosed cardiovascular disease and congenital heart anomalies can also cause syncope in children. If the syncope is cardiac related, the episode usually will occur following exercise or exertion. The most common cardiac causes of syncope in children are dysrhythmias and obstructive structural disorders of the heart (aortic stenosis). These cardia causes have the potential to become lethal. The child who experiences syncope secondary to bradycardia, tachycardia, or frequent ventricular aberrancy also has decreased cardiac output, which should be recognized and treated aggressively. Treatment of pediatric

cardiac-related syncope should be geared toward correcting the underlying cause(s).
- The child with syncope should be closely observed, because the episode is usually secondary to a current illness or serious underlying medical condition. Therefore, any child with syncope should be transported to an ED for a thorough examination.
- The two most common metabolic causes of syncope in children are hypoglycemia and anemia. Hypoglycemia is usually preceded by a gradual change in the child's normal status, diaphoresis, and weakness.
- Hyperventilation syndrome can cause a syncopal episode in children as well. This syndrome occurs because of the decrease in cerebral perfusion secondary to a reduction of CO_2 from the tachypnea. The child may also complain of numbness and tingling of the hands. This may be more common in school-aged children and adolescents. Episodes of purposeful breath holding can also cause syncope.
- Numerous drugs, both prescription and nonprescription, can cause syncope in children. This condition is mainly caused by the medication's effect on the blood pressure. Examples of such medications are antihypertensives (HCTZ, diazide) and diuretics (Lasix, Bumex). It is important to remember that children on these medications have an underlying medical condition that may be causing the syncope.

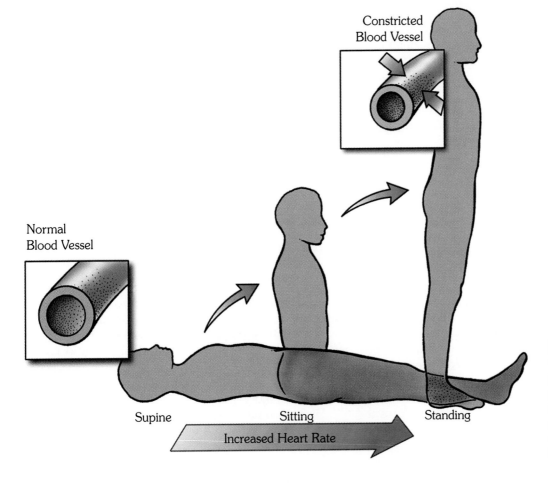

Normal
Blood Vessel

Constricted
Blood Vessel

Supine   Sitting   Standing

Increased Heart Rate

Figure 29-1

To maintain blood flow to the brain during postural changes, the sympathetic nervous system must increase peripheral vascular resistance (through vasoconstriction) and increase heart rate.

The potential for orthostatic problems increases with medical conditions (diabetes mellitus) or medications (especially for blood pressure or tranquilizers) that interfere with the ability of the blood vessels to respond quickly to position changes.

Orthostatic syncope can also be the result of diminished blood volume caused by dehydration (vomiting, diarrhea, heat) or blood loss. Syncope may be the first indication of unrecognized bleeding, such as GI bleeding, leaking aortic aneurysm, or ruptured ectopic pregnancy.

Syncope is sometimes the only symptom of a dysrhythmia and may occur without associated chest pain or other symptoms suggestive of myocardial ischemia. Patients with valvular heart disease (particularly aortic stenosis) that causes blockage of blood flow through the heart may not be able to respond with increased cardiac output during periods of increased demand, such as exercise. The result is decreased blood flow to the brain and near-syncope or syncope.

Patient Assessment

History

The prehospital provider must carefully assess each patient for altered mental status. During the initial assessment, any awake patient who is not alert and aware is probably not experiencing simple syncope. The patient who demonstrates any abnormalities in the ability to understand questions or respond appropriately must be evaluated for other causes of the altered mental status.

- *What was the history of the event?* Ask about the patient's position and level of activity prior to the episode.
- *Were there any symptoms before the event?* Ask the patient about any warning symptoms. Patients about to "pass out" usually realize they are having a problem when they experience weakness, light-headedness, sweating or dizziness, or progressive narrowing of the visual field. The presence of other symptoms, such as chest pains or palpitations, prior to or following the event may be significant.

CRITICAL ISSUE

Any patient developing syncope without warning symptoms or while in the supine position must be assumed to have a cardiac cause for syncope and treated accordingly.

If the patient recognizes impending syncope and lowers his or her head quickly enough to improve blood flow to the brain, unresponsiveness may be averted (called near-syncope). Many times, the patient can prevent syncope by siting or lying down. Patients who experience near-syncope can have serious medical problems and should be evaluated as thoroughly as patients who have a complete syncopal event.

- *Does the patient complain of palpitations?* Acute dysrhythmias, especially those associated with very slow or very rapid heart rates (< 40 min or > 150/min) may cause a marked decrease in cardiac output and cerebral blood flow. Syncope caused by dysrhythmias can occur with the patient in any position.

- *Could the patient be pregnant?* A similar problem of hypotension and syncope can occur during pregnancy when the enlarged uterus compresses the inferior vena cava and decreases blood return to the heart (supine hypotensive syndrome). To relieve the pressure on the vena cava, a pregnant patient should be positioned on her left side (left lateral recumbent position) rather than the supine position.

- *Were any other observers present?* Other individuals at the scene should be questioned in an effort to identify a significant medical history and determine the sequence of events. The duration of patient unresponsiveness as estimated by observers, the occurrence of any involuntary movements, and the duration of any confusion or disorientation after awakening must all be investigated.

- *Is there any evidence of trauma?* The patient or bystanders should be questioned regarding the possibility of falls or other trauma sustained. Patients who are alert can usually give an adequate history of pain and possible injuries. An examination to identify trauma should focus attention to the head, neck, and spine.

- *What is the patient's past medical history?* Are there medications? Low blood sugar causes progressive confusion and a decreased level of mentation. If the condition remains untreated, unresponsiveness results. Diabetic patients who take insulin can usually be identified by history provided by the patient or family or by a Medic Alert® tag.

Seizures, particularly grand mal seizures, can cause temporary unresponsiveness. However, unlike syncope, the patient may not be aware of the surroundings upon awakening and may not be able to give a meaningful medical history. Additional findings of urinary incontinence, bitten tongue, a Medic Alert® tag signifying a seizure disorder, or bottles of antiseizure medication can also be helpful.

The patient should be specifically questioned regarding any medication he or she is currently taking and previous episodes of syncope experienced.

Physical Examination

When a patient's vital signs are assessed, pulse irregularities can indicate a dysrhythmia as the cause of the syncope. Abnormalities in patient pulse rate, especially those that are very rapid (>150) or very slow (<40) must be recognized early and treated appropriately. Extremely fast or slow pulse rates can result in insufficient cardiac output, hypoperfusion, and increased cardiac workload, causing unconsciousness when the patient attemps to stand. If the paramedic recognizes significant bradycardia causing hypoperfusion, this condition must be given the highest treatment priority. Pulse rates above 150/min may be associated with a marked decrease in cardiac output as well as increased cardiac work and may not be tolerated for extended periods of time, especially in the elderly patient.

Pulse rates greater than 100 but not critically fast (<150) may indicate that the patient is attempting to compensate for hypovolemia and this situation should prompt a search for a hidden source of bleeding.

A normal blood pressure in a supine patient does not necessarily indicate a normal pressure when sitting or standing. It may be necessary for the paramedic to obtain orthostatic vital signs from the patient to determine the true status of the patient's volume. Orthostatic vital signs should not be performed if tachycardia or outright hypotension is present.

CRITICAL ISSUE

Positive orthostatic vital sign changes in a patient are a strong indication of decreased circulating blood volume.

To obtain orthostatic vital signs, the patient should be moved from a supine position to sitting or standing position for 30 seconds. A drop in systolic pressure of 20 mm Hg or a pulse increase of 20/min is considered significant. A patient who becomes dizzy or develops near-syncope or syncope when sitting or standing indicates a positive test result; no further attempts should be made to raise the patient.

High blood pressure and a negative tilt-test result in a patient who has experienced temporary loss of consciousness should cause the provider to suspect causes other than simple syncope.

Mild elevation of the patient's respiratory rate can be expected if the patient is anxious about the medical problem, but this elevation should be temporary. Persistent tachypnea may indicate a cardiopulmonary cause for syncope that requires its own evaluation (*see* Chapter 27).

Evaluation of the patient's skin may demonstrate cool, moist, and pale skin. These findings are the result of an attempt by the sympathetic nervous system to re-establish blood flow to the brain. The symptoms should resolve once the patient is in a supine position and the blood pressure is restored. Persistent cool, clammy skin indicates that the patient is experiencing hypoperfusion caused by hypovolemia or a primary cardiac problem.

Hot or warm, dry skin may indicate a fever that has resulted in dehydration and hypovolemia. Further confirmation can be obtained by checking the patient for dry oral mucous membranes and a decrease in the normal elasticity of the skin.

All patients experiencing syncope must have a complete prehospital neurologic evaluation to establish a baseline, and level of consciousness must be specifically documented. If the patient's level of consciousness is not completely normal, he or she must be evaluated for a more serious cause of altered level of consciousness. The patient's pupil size and reaction also should be confirmed. Equally dilated pupils may be the result of a sympathetic response from anxiety or fear. Constricted pupils may indicate opiate intoxication.

The patient should also be checked for muscle or facial weakness on one side of the body. Any localized abnormalities should be investigated for the possibility of a cerebrovascular accident or other central nervous system problem.

Key Conditions and Findings

- *Vasovagal Reaction.* A vasovagal reaction is a common cause of syncope. However, the EMS provider must suspect and determine any other causes.
- *Inadequate Sympathetic Response to a Position Change.* This can be a cause of syncope, particularly in the elderly patient or in the patient who is taking blood pressure medication or sedatives.
- *Hypovolemia.* Hypovolemia is a cause of syncope that often occurs secondary to unrecognized bleeding from the GI tract or an ectopic pregnancy. Dehydration can also be a source of hypovolemia and consequently syncope.
- *Cardiovascular Conditions.* An acute **myocardial infarction** (AMI) can present with an episode of syncope or near-syncope, as can a **cerebrovascular accident** (stroke) and **pulmonary embolus.**
- *Dysrhythmia.* Syncope may be the first manifestation of an acute dysrhythmia such as bradycardia, tachycardia, or ventricular ectopy. This condition is a more common cause of syncope in the elderly.

Management

Many patients who experience no trauma with the syncopal episode will feel well and deny the need for further medical evaluation or treatment. The prehospital provider should make every attempt to convince the patient of the need for appropriate evaluation.

The patient should be transported in a position of comfort; if orthostatic signs are positive, a supine position is appropriate. As a minimum for patients who demonstrate no history or physical findings suggestive of a life-threatening problem, high-flow oxygen should be administered and an IV initiated at a keep open rate. Cardiac monitoring is indicated for all patients unless an obvious noncardiac etiology of syncope is identified.

Oral or IV glucose should be given if there is a clinical suspicion of **hypoglycemia,** preferably after blood glucose levels have been determined (when available).

If conditions such as dysrhythmia, hypovolemia, or cardiovascular or central nervous system problems are noted, the patient should receive treatment appropriate to the specific problem.

Because the loss of responsiveness during syncope is only temporary, the patient probably will have regained normal mentation and feel better by the time the EMS provider arrives on the scene. An awake patient may feel embarrassed by the apparent weakness and temporary loss of control and may frequently deny a problem and refuse treatment. Prehospital providers may have to use his or her best bedside manner to convince the patient that evaluation is necessary.

SUMMARY

Syncope can be the result of either benign or life-threatening conditions. Although the patient may be awake and denying a medical problem at the time of EMS arrival, it is the paramedic's responsibility to evaluate the patient completely and be aware that acute problems can develop at any time. Treatment depends upon the patient's history, general health, and associated signs and symptoms. Any treatment decisions should be made according to local protocols and in consultation with medical direction.

REFERENCE

1. **Hunt M:** Syncope. In Rosen P, Barkin RM, Braen R, et al (eds): Emergency Medicine: Concepts and Clinical Practice, ed 3, St. Louis, 1992, CV Mosby.

William R. Roush, MD

Chapter 30

Altered Mental Status

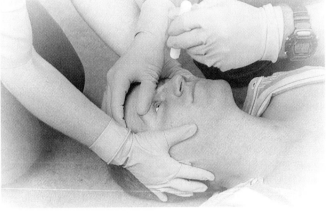

OBJECTIVES

A paramedic should be able to:

1. Explain the pathophysiology related to altered mental status.

2. Describe the pathophysiology and identify subjective and objective findings of the following potentially life-threatening causes of altered mental status:
   a. Cerebrovascular accident
   b. Hypoglycemia
   c. Hypoperfusion
   d. Hypoxia
   e. Meningitis
   f. Seizures
   g. Toxins
   h. Tumors

3. Identify the key historical features in the assessment of a patient with altered mental status.

4. Outline the components of a rapid, directed physical examination in evaluating patients with altered status.

5. Given any of the following descriptive mental status terms, identify the corresponding patient behavior: lethargic, awake, oriented, alert, confusion, agitation, aware.

6. Describe the prehospital management of patients with altered mental status.

KEY TERMS

1. **Aphasia**—an abnormal neurologic condition in which language function is defective or absent because of an injury to certain areas of the cerebral cortex.

2. **Cerebrovascular attack (CVA)**—an abnormal condition of the blood vessels of the brain characterized by occlusion by an embolus, thrombus, or cerebrovascular hemorrhage resulting in ischemia of the brain tissues normally perfused by the damaged vessels.

3. **Disorientation**—a state of mental confusion characterized by inadequate or incorrect perceptions of place, time, or identity.

4. **Encephalitis**—an inflammatory condition of the brain, usually caused by an infection transmitted by the bite of an infected mosquito. This condition may also result from lead or other poisoning, or from hemorrhage.

5. **Hyperthermia**—significantly elevated core body temperature.

6. **Hypoglycemia**—a condition in which the glucose level in the blood is abnormally low.

7. **Hypoperfusion**—inadequate circulation; insufficient delivery of oxygen and nutrients necessary for normal tissue and cellular function.

8. **Hypothermia**—an abnormally low core body temperature.

9. **Hypoxia**—inadequate delivery of oxygen to the body.

10. **Intracranial pressure (ICP)**—pressure that occurs within the cranium.

11. **Level of consciousness**—a degree of cognitive function involving arousal mechanisms of the reticular formation of the brain.

12. **Meningitis**—any inflammation of the membranes covering the brain and spinal cord.

13. **Mental status**—the degree of competence shown by a person in intellectual, emotional, psychologic, and personality functionings as measured by psychologic testing with reference to a statistical norm.

14. **Postictal**—after a convulsion.

15. **Seizure**—a hyperexcitation of neurons in the brain leading to a sudden, violent, involuntary series of contractions of a group of muscles that may be paroxysmal and episodic, as in a seizure disorder, or transient and acute, as after a head concussion.

16. **Status epilepticus**—continuous seizure activity or repeated seizures without the patient regaining consciousness.

17. **Subarachnoid hemorrhage**—an acute, often spontaneous, bleed in the brain usually caused by cerebral artery aneurysm or an arteriovenous malformation.

393

Altered mental status is a challenging condition in the prehospital setting. Mental status refers to a variety of components of mental function. Level or depth of consciousness is one mental status component that is assessed in every patient by determining their level of responsiveness to various stimuli. Other components of mental status may include cognitive functions, such as orientation to person, place, time and event, recent and remote memory, mood, speech characteristics, and the thought process. Sometimes the terms mental status and level of responsiveness are used interchangeably; however, the meaning of these terms is not the same. Altered mental status in a patient may be reported to EMS as fainting, disorientation, strange behavior, seizure activity, or unresponsiveness. There are variations of altered mental status, and a patient's mental status may change during the course of prehospital care.

For the paramedic, obtaining a reliable patient history is often difficult in this situation, but a thorough, focused assessment is crucial to detect life threats and manage reversible causes of the patient's condition.

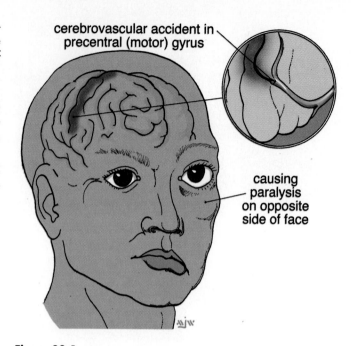

Figure 30-1

The face of cerebrovascular accident.

Pathophysiology

Normal brain function requires an intact brain anatomy and a continuous supply of glucose and oxygen. A number of intracranial structural abnormalities, as well as toxic and metabolic problems, can interfere with brain activity and result in abnormal mental status.

Sudden patient unresponsiveness, that occurs within a few seconds of the onset of symptoms, is associated with complete recovery shortly after the patient assumes a supine position, and causes no residual neurological problems, is usually the result of a temporary interruption of blood supply to the brain (*see* Chapter 29).

Cerebrovascular accident (CVA) can cause the sudden onset of localizing neurologic signs that are not necessarily associated with unresponsivenes (Fig. 30-1). Localizing neurologic signs are those that involve a specific portion of the brain. For example, weakness or paralysis of the right arm and leg usually result from an injury or lesion involving the left cerebral hemisphere. Some examples of possible CVA origins are: acute intracranial hemorrhage and blockage of blood vessels in the neck or head by an embolism or a thrombosis.

Generalized seizures involving sudden loss of responsiveness and characteristic stiffening and jerking movements of extremities are not difficult to recognize if the onset of the seizure is witnessed. Generalized seizures are typically associated with a period of confusion and disorientation after awakening (postictal state) that can last from a few minutes to several hours. If there are no witnesses and the patient is confused, it may be difficult for EMS providers to identify seizure as the cause of the altered mental status.

Seizure activity that persists, or several generalized seizures that occur without a period of responsiveness between awakening is termed status epilepticus—a potentially life-threatening event that requires immediate treatment and transport. Patients with status epilepticus use tremendous

amounts of body energy and can develop aspiration, hypoxia, hyperthermia, and hypoglycemia.

Cellular brain dysfunction resulting from metabolic, toxic, or infectious causes can lead to the gradual onset of altered mental status (Fig. 30-2). Confusion, disorientation, agitation, or lethargy (usually without other localizing neurologic signs), may worsen over hours or days and end in patient unresponsiveness. Patients with slowly increasing intracranial pressure from infections, tumors, or hypertension can also present in this fashion.

Patient Assessment

History

Obtaining a history in patients with altered mental status can be problematic. In many cases, the patient cannot provide accurate information, and the paramedic is forced to rely on data gathered from bystanders on the scene.

If the patient who is awake and alert at the time of EMS arrival denies the presence of a problem, additional history must be obtained from bystanders. If the patient remains confused, disoriented, agitated, responds only to pain, or continues to have seizures, a rapid assessment must be made to determine if there is an immediate threat to life.

- *How quickly did the patient's mental status change?* Determining the progression of symptoms from onset to the patient's current status is essential and may provide insight into the cause of the altered mental status. If the patient is unable to provide a coherent history, an attempt should be made to obtain this information from family or bystanders. Observers may also be able to offer a description of the patient's baseline mental status.

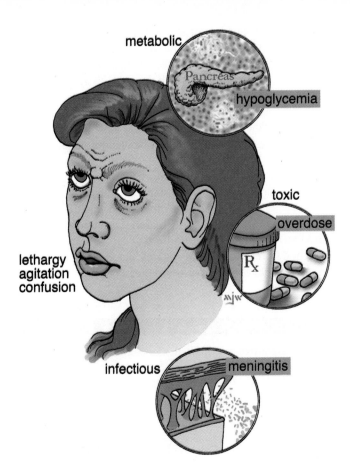

metabolic

Pancreas

hypoglycemia

toxic

overdose

R_x

lethargy
agitation
confusion

infectious   meningitis

Figure 30-2

Cellular brain dysfunction can have many causes.

- *Is there evidence of a seizure?* Findings in a patient of a bitten tongue, urinary incontinence, a "Medic Alert" tag signifying a seizure disorder, or bottles of antiseizure medication near the scene may suggest seizure as the cause of the patient's confusion and disorientation.

- *What do the surroundings show?* The paramedic must be sure to check the scene for pill bottles, syringes, or other items that may be helpful in discovering a cause for the change in the patient's mental status. Any odors in the house that might indicate a toxicologic problem should be noted. Articles of significance should be brought to the emergency department with the patient.

Physical Examination

The physical examination begins with an assessment of the patient's mental status (also *see* Chapter 45 regarding the mental status exam). The thorough documentation of these findings can be of critical importance. There are some commonly used descriptive terms (*see* Box 30-1), but when these terms are used, they should be accompanied by a more specific description of what was observed. For example, the notation of "alert and oriented times two" or "A&O × 2" warrants further explanation: "The patient gave name, age, and location, but did not know the current date or year."

The AVPU scale is a simple way to evaluate and record the level of patient responsiveness (*see* Chapter 17). This assessment of mental status should be performed initially as a baseline and repeated at short intervals during patient assessment and care.

Awake and Alert responsiveness is measured by the patient's orientation to person, place, time, and ability to relate to surroundings. Occasionally, EMS providers will be unable to

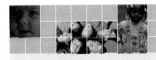

PEDIATRIC PERSPECTIVE

- A wide variety of conditions can cause altered mental status in infants and children. The most common causes are hypoxia, head trauma, seizures, infection, hypoglycemia, and drug or alcohol intoxication.
- Mental status in infants and small children is best determined by assessment of the child's alertness, eye contact, recognition of parents, spontaneous movement of extremities, reach for objects, strength of cry, and withdrawing to pain. Parents may note that their child is "not acting right."
- A sudden change in the child's level of responsiveness is unusual and may indicate an infection, a seizure, or hypoglycemia.
- Infants have inadequate glycogen stores, that predispose them to hypoglycemia when stressed. Hypoglycemia is a serum glucose level less than 60 mg in a child or less than 40 mg in a newborn. $D_{25}W$ is administered to the hypoglycemic child, and $D_{10}W$ for the newborn and to the child 1 year of

age. It is important to note that a secure IV line is essential when administering D_{10} or D_{25}. Hypertonic glucose solutions can cause severe damage to tissues if the IV infiltrates.
- Seizures are a common pediatric medical emergency. In childhood, seizures are most commonly caused by fever. Other causes include hypoxia, brain hemorrhage, meningitis, encephalitis, and intoxication.
- Status epilepticus may occur as the child's first seizure. Status epilepticus is a serious emergency requiring immediate treatment to decrease the likelihood of brain injury. Status epilepticus in children less than 3 years of age is typically caused by hypoxia or toxins.
- Rectally administered diazepam (Valium®) is a practical and relatively safe form of seizure management if the child is seizing when paramedics arrive. The rectal dosage is higher than the normal pediatric IV dosage. Observation for respiratory depression is necessary.

BOX 30-1 Mental Status Descriptive Terms

Awake The patient is obviously awake or sleeping patient can be easily awakened.

Alert The patient is awake and responds to surroundings. The patient may be acting appropriately or inappropriately according to accepted norms.

Aware The patient understands present circumstances: "I was in an auto accident. I was with two friends." Other questions to determine awareness include questions such as the name of the current president. Aware patients should be able to give a meaningful history.

Oriented The patient is able to identify in order from most difficult to the least difficult, the date, day of week, month, year, place (where they are now, i.e., home?, hospital? city? state?), and person (who he or she is).

Lethargic The patient can be awakened but returns to sleep when external stimulation ends.

Agitated The patient is restless, unable to remain still, and unable to control behavior.

Confused The patient demonstrates a slowed thinking process and is unable to think clearly.

Unresponsiveness indicates no observable response in the patient to either verbal or painful stimuli. When a patient is unresponsive, the extremities should be checked to determine if there is muscle tone or if the limb drops lifelessly.

Very slow or very rapid pulse rates (< 40 or > 160) may cause generalized hypoperfusion that reduces cerebral blood flow sufficiently enough to alter a patient's mental status. Life-threatening dysrhythmias also must be recognized and treated rapidly.

Markedly elevated blood pressure may directly cause cerebral edema and altered mental status in patients with uncontrolled **hypertension.** On the other hand, high blood pressure also can result from increased intracranial pressure caused by cerebral edema or an **intracranial hemorrhage,** as the body's reflexes elevate systemic blood pressure in an effort to maintain cerebral perfusion pressure.

CRITICAL ISSUE

Unresponsive patients with markedly elevated blood pressure are usually suffering from intracranial bleeding or swelling.

determine whether abnormal findings are either acute or representational of the patient's usual mental status, as the result of previous medical or psychiatric problems.

Verbal responsiveness indicates an appropriate response to verbal stimuli, such as a patient who is not awake but can be aroused and follows commands.

Pain responsiveness is used as a stimulus to elicit a response from a patient who does not respond to verbal stimuli. Painful stimuli can include rubbing the sternum or applying nail bed pressure. The patient's response to pain varies, from trying to remove the offending stimulus (localizing response), to poorly directed random movements. In more serious conditions, posturing is present—a reflex response that indicates severe impairment of higher brain functions.

Decorticate posturing generally indicates loss of cerebral cortex (outermost portion of the brain) function. Without input from this level, the reflex response to external stimuli is arm flexion at the elbows and wrists, leg extension, and pointing of the toes.

Decerebrate posturing usually indicates injury to areas of the brain below the cerebral cortex. External stimulation results in extension of the elbows with the wrist flexed and leg extension with the toes pointed. Decorticate and decerebrate posturing are discussed in Chapter 47.

CRITICAL ISSUE

Any patient who demonstrates a decreasing level of responsiveness from a higher level of function to a lower one (i.e., who is initially awake and later responds only to pain) has an acute medical emergency that is possibly life threatening, and must be transported rapidly to the nearest appropriate medical facility.

The patient's breathing pattern should be observed. Certain respiratory abnormalities may provide clues to the cause of the patient's altered mental status (see Chapter 23). Acute hypoxia, with labored or inadequate ventilation resulting from pulmonary or cardiac causes, may lead to confusion, restlessness, agitation, or unresponsiveness. Hyperventilation with continuous, rapid, deep inspirations may be caused by **metabolic acidosis** or hypoxia but can also result from brain injury caused by stroke, bleeding, or swelling (central neurogenic hyperventilation).

Cheyne-Stokes respirations involve rhythmic changes in rate and depth of respirations. The patient appears to be hyperventilating and suddenly shows a period of apnea. Cheyne-Stokes respirations may be caused by **congestive heart failure,** metabolic abnormalities, or intracranial lesions.

The patient's skin condition should be checked. Hot, dry skin could indicate a fever from infection or heat exposure. A generalized rash may indicate an infectious or allergic problem. Also, the paramedic should note any evidence of extensive bruising (possibly in various stages of healing), which suggests that the patient has been falling frequently. Bruising could also point to a clotting or bleeding disorder.

The paramedic should evaluate the patient for facial paralysis. Weakness of one side of the face (e.g., one eye that does not close completely when the patient blinks, or the inability to retract one corner of the mouth when smiling) in association with altered mental status is an indication of a CVA.

When the patient's eyes are examined (under room light), a light shone in one eye should result in contraction of both pupils. A normal reaction indicates an intact reflex at the midbrain level. However, the test is difficult to interpret if the patient's pupils are quite small—in the case of a narcotic overdose, for instance.

The awake patient should have a systematic evaluation of muscle strength. The strength of the right side should be compared with that of the left side, and strength in the lower extremities compared with that of the upper extremities. Weakness limited to the arm and leg on one side is usually caused by a CVA involving the opposite side of the brain. Unresponsive patients with CVA may demonstrate muscle tone detected by movement of extremities on one side of the body, while the affected side remains flaccid, offering no resistance to passive motion.

Key Conditions and Findings

The causes of altered mental status are many, but with a systematic approach a reasonable management plan can be developed. The origins of altered mental status include:

- *Trauma.* Closed head injury usually presents with a history of trauma that has caused either brief or sustained unresponsiveness. Bleeding within or around brain tissue can cause hematoma formation. The expanding hematoma, in turn, can create an increase in intracranial pressure that disturbs or damages brain structures. Alcoholics are at particular risk for hematoma formation following even minor trauma, because they commonly have liver disease, which compromises clotting functions.
- *Bleeding.* Bleeding may occur spontaneously in or around the brain in conditions such as subarachnoid hemorrhage secondary to a ruptured aneurysm. In these cases, profound alteration of mental status usually follows the onset of a sudden, severe headache, often described as the "worst the patient has ever experienced." Spontaneous intracerebral bleeding may also result from prolonged hypertension. Whether or not a cerebral bleed will cause altered mental status depends upon the portion of the brain that is affected.
- *Tumors.* Tumors involving the central nervous system (CNS) often become symptomatic over a long period of time and the patient presents with vague behavioral complaints such as memory difficulties or personality changes. A recurring headache may also be part of the clinical presentation. Altered mental status is a late finding, suggesting that the tumor has grown enough to cause an increase in intracranial pressure.
- *Infections.* Meningitis, an infection involving the meninges surrounding the brain, is the more common CNS infection. It can result from bloodborne infection spread or travel from nearby sites, such as the middle ear. It sometimes occurs in adults, but is more frequently a concern in the pediatric age group. The classic signs of headache, fever, and neck stiffness precede the onset of altered mental status. Encephalitis is another common, usually viral, brain infection that causes behavioral changes or a chronic, generalized headache before more severe mentation changes appear.
- *Ischemia.* Cerebral blood flow may be compromised by blood clot formation and atherosclerotic narrowing in an artery. Clots, which sometimes travel from proximal sites to smaller distal arteries, can occlude blood flow to tissue beyond the obstruction. As with intracerebral bleeding, the presence of altered mental status depends upon the area of the brain that is affected.
- *Toxins.* This category accounts for most sources of altered mental status. Examining the environment and gathering historical data, such as the patient's medications and past medical history, can provide critical clues to the exact substance involved. Toxins and high drug concentrations cause dysfunction at the cellular level, often disturbing cellular metabolism. Alcohol is the most widely used toxin, but any medication, whether prescription or over-the-counter, can cause altered mental status when taken in overdose amounts. Among chemical exposures, carbon monoxide inhalation is seen most frequently in winter months, when household furnaces often malfunction. Headache often precedes behavioral changes, as the blood level of carbon dioxide rises.
- *Metabolic disruptions.* Cellular malfunctions can occur secondary to other metabolic abnormalities. Hypoglycemia is the most common metabolic problem that can lead to altered mental status. Glucose is the energy source needed for most cellular reactions, and the brain is the organ most dependent on glucose availability. Electrolyte abnormalities, particularly hyponatremia (sodium deficiency), also disrupt cellular metabolism. Hypoxia, renal failure, and disorders of temperature regulation (e.g., hyperthermia and hypothermia) are other common causes of metabolic disruption.
- *Seizure.* If a massive discharge of excitable neurons spreads to involve major portions of the central brain, a generalized seizure results. Seizures consume the brain's metabolic energy resources and can produce temporary cerebral hypoxia and acidosis. There is a variable time period during which the patient's mental status remains altered as the body works to correct these metabolic problems. In most cases, the patient's mental status improves gradually. Presentations vary from minor mentation deficits that resolve quickly to unresponsiveness or paralysis.

Management

Management for the patient with an altered mental status depends upon the specific findings of each particular patient. A paramedic's attention to the important basics of airway, breathing, and circulation may adequately sustain the patient until hospital intervention is available. Unfortunately, neither prehospital personnel nor in-hospital physicians may be able to significantly impact the outcome of some patients with altered mental status.

Reversible causes of altered mental status that will likely benefit from immediate treatment in the prehospital setting include hypoxia, hypoperfusion, hypoglycemia, and status epilepticus. All patients with altered mental status should receive high-concentration oxygen, with assisted ventilation and airway control if needed. Controlled airway management and hyperventilation (20 to 24/min) may be beneficial for patients who are suspected of having altered mental status because of increased intracranial pressure and brain swelling. If evidence or suspicion of history of trauma is present, spinal stabilization should occur.

CRITICAL ISSUE

Paramedics should be particularly attentive to the airway of a patient with altered mental status. Difficulty with secretions, vomiting, and inadequate tidal volume are common and significant problems.

All patients should have cardiac monitoring, and IV access should be established. If there is evidence of hypoperfusion, 200 mL of normal saline or Ringer's lactate should be administered rapidly as a bolus. Following the fluid bolus, the rate of IV administration is determined by the patient's clinical response.

Although controversial (see Sidebar), some EMS experts recommend that 50% dextrose must be administered IV to all adult patients with altered mental status unless blood glucose can be determined. Naloxone should be administered IV to patients with suspected narcotic overdose. Diazepam is the appropriate medication to be administered IV to any patient presenting with status epilepticus.

If trauma is not suspected, patients should be transported in the lateral recumbent position to minimize the risk of aspiration.

Any patient who cannot stay awake for questioning or does not understand current circumstances and recognize the surroundings probably cannot give a reliable history and must be considered incapable of making informed decisions regarding his or her treatment or refusal of treatment.

D50—SUGARY SUCCESS OR SICKENINGLY SWEET?

By Jedd Roe, M.D., FACEP

Hypoglycemia has been reported in 8.5% of patients with the complaint of altered mental status. However, controversy exists regarding the empiric administration of hypertonic glucose solutions (50% glucose or D50) to these patients.

Some clinicians have expressed concern for those patients with a normal or elevated blood sugar, noting that additional glucose may be harmful in this setting. Other clinicians have shown that one dose of D50 does not alter the patient's serum glucose level or osmolarity to a clinically significant degree. A number of human and animal studies also have demonstrated that in cerebral ischemia, an elevated blood glucose is associated with an increase in infarct size and mortality. The counterpoint to this argument is that the animal studies used glucose doses much larger than the usual field dose, and one large, long-term human study showed no effect on long-term survival or functional ability.

Further complicating the issue is the ability to diagnose hypoglycemia. Combining the classic signs of hypoglycemia with a history of diabetes may misdiagnose as many as 25% of hypoglycemic patients. Rapid reagent tests for blood glucose fail to diagnose hypoglycemia in 6% to 8% of cases, when this test is used in the prehospital setting. Strict quality control programs have been advocated to enhance accuracy of the reagent strips, but these programs have encountered logistical difficulties being implemented into EMS systems.

There is some danger in relying solely on numbers (most

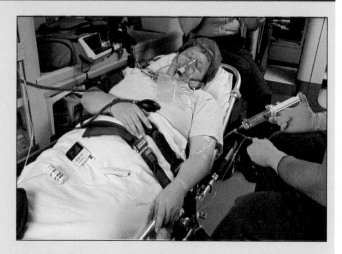

EMS providers follow the indication of a serum glucose less than 60 mg/dL) to determine hypoglycemia. Some poorly controlled diabetics showed clinical evidence of hypoglycemia with an average serum glucose level of 77 mg/dL.

Certainly there is no debate that glucose should be administered when blood glucose determination is impossible. When the patient continues to manifest an altered mental status, the provider is left to balance the benefit of a potential cause of permanent brain damage against the potential risks described above.[1]

SUMMARY

The prehospital provider must take a systematic approach to the evaluation of a patient with altered mental status. Alterations in mentation may vary from confusion, to loss of awareness of surroundings, to complete unresponsiveness without reaction to painful stimuli. Paramedic evaluation must identify life threats and give priority to recognition and management of correctable problems such as airway and ventilation problems, hypoperfusion, and hypoglycemia. Any patient demonstrating a decreasing level of response to stimuli must receive rapid transport to the nearest appropriate facility.

REFERENCES

1. **Hoffman RS, Goldfrank LR:** The poisoned patient with altered consciousness in one use of a "coma cocktail." *JAMA*, 274(7):562–569, 1995.

William R. Roush, MD

Chapter 31

Chest Pain

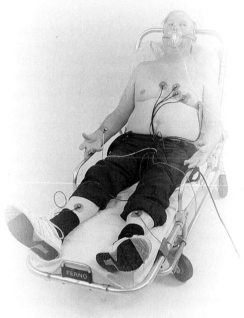

A paramedic should be able to:

OBJECTIVES

1. Explain the pathophysiology of the various types of chest pain.
2. Identify the key historical features in the assessment of chest pain.
3. Describe a rapid, directed physical examination when evaluating patients with chest pain.
4. Identify the subjective and objective findings associated with potentially life-threatening processes in patients with chest pain.
5. Describe the prehospital management of patients with chest pain.

KEY TERMS

1. **Acute aortic dissection**—a sudden tear in the inner lining of the aorta that allows blood to enter the space between the inner and outer layers.
2. **Angina**—the pattern of cardiac chest pain that occurs with exertion and is relieved by rest or vasodilators such as nitroglycerin.
3. **Atherosclerosis**—thickening, hardening and loss of elasticity of arterial walls.
4. **Bronchitis**—an acute or chronic inflammation of the mucous membranes of the tracheobronchial tree.
5. **Dysrhythmias**—variation from a normal rhythm.
6. **Ischemia**—a decreased supply of oxygenated blood to a body organ or part, often marked by pain and organ dysfunction.
7. **Myocardial infarction**—necrosis of a portion of cardiac muscle caused by obstruction in a coronary artery from either atherosclerosis or an embolis. Also called "heart attack."
8. **Nitroglycerin**—a potent smooth muscle relaxant and vasodilator; often prescribed for the relief of heart symptoms.
9. **Pericarditis**—inflammation of the pericardium (the membrane that surrounds the heart).
11. **Pneumothorax**—a collection of air or gas in the pleural space; collapse of a lung.
10. **Pneumonia**—infection of the lung tissue.
12. **Pulmonary embolism**—the blockage of a pulmonary artery by foreign matter such as fat, air, tumor tissue, or a thrombus that usually arises from a peripheral vein.

hest pain is one of the most frequent medical complaints prompting a call to EMS. This patient presentation may be difficult to evaluate because of the varied medical problems involving the organs located in the chest and upper abdomen.

Some patients with acute chest pain present with signs and symptoms that indicate they are in danger of developing a life-threatening process; others have atypical pain that is difficult to evaluate. Although the patient may not present in a typical fashion, the prehospital provider should always consider chest pain as representing a significant problem.

Pathophysiology

Cardiac chest pain most frequently originates from ischemia, or deficiency of blood supply, of the cardiac muscle, and usually results from coronary artery disease (CAD). CAD is the development of plaques (atherosclerosis) in the arteries that may narrow them enough to cause a significant decrease in blood flow to the heart muscle (Fig. 31-1). As the vessel narrows, it becomes much easier for a blood clot to form and completely occlude the artery. Once the supply of blood and oxygen is cut off, the heart muscle begins to die (myocardial infarction). Until the coronary artery is completely blocked, the narrowing of the vessel in combination with episodes of coronary artery spasm can produce episodes of pain which are usually induced by exertion and relieved with rest. These attacks of pain result from an inadequate supply of oxygen which does not meet the demand, but because the supply of oxygen is not completely cut off, the cardiac muscle does not die. These episodes are referred to as angina attacks or "angina pectoris." When deprived of oxygen, the heart muscle also becomes irritable and can develop dysrhythmias. These dysrhythmias can lead to inadequate cardiac output, hypoperfusion, or cardiac arrest (see Chapter 32). Dysrhythmias are the most common specific cause of sudden death caused by heart disease.

Ischemia, causing chest pain, can also result in a significant decrease in the heart's ability to contract effectively. If the dysfunction is severe and the heart muscle is not strong enough to pump adequate amounts of blood, the patient will accumulate fluid in the lungs (pulmonary edema). As ventricular failure proceeds, cardiac output falls and signs of hypoperfusion appear. Immediate life threats associated with chest pain are summarized in Box 31-1.

Severe chest pain may occur with acute aortic dissection, a sudden tear in the inner lining of the aorta that allows blood to enter the space between the inner and outer layers. The pain is often described by the patient as "tearing" in nature and frequently is referred to the back or between the shoulder blades.

Chest pain secondary to pulmonary conditions usually occurs when the pleural lining becomes inflamed and the two irritated layers of pleura rub against each other. The patient typically reports a sharp pain that worsens with deep inspiration or coughing (pleuritic pain). This description helps to identify noncardiac chest pain; pleuritic pain is usually not cardiac in origin. Common causes of pleuritic pain include pneumonia, bronchitis, pneumothorax, and pulmonary embolism. Pericarditis (inflammation of the pericardium) causes similar, pleuritic pain that is classically relieved by the patient sitting up and leaning forward.

Pain originating from the esophagus may be virtually indistinguishable from pain of cardiac etiology, possibly because both structures share a common nerve supply (Fig. 31-2). Esophageal pain usually arises in the presence of acid (ingested or from the stomach) or from severe spasms of esophageal muscles. The patient may describe characteristics similar to cardiac pain, such as retrosternal pressure with radiation, and that is not necessarily relieved by antacids. To further complicate the issue, nitroglycerin, which is taken to re-

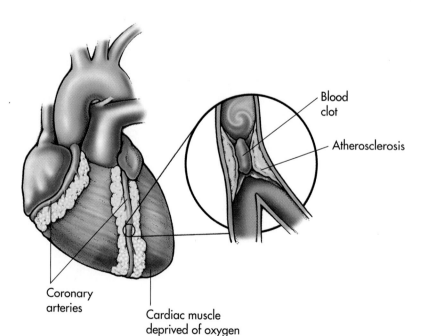

Coronary arteries

Cardiac muscle deprived of oxygen

Blood clot

Atherosclerosis

Figure 31-1

The combination of coronary artery disease and a thrombus can occlude blood flow to tissues distal to the site of the clot, resulting in ischemia and myocardial infarction.

- Chest pain is unusual in the pediatric patient. Cardiac causes of chest pain in the infant and child include acute dysrhythmias, congenital heart defects or diseases, such as carditis (viral and bacterial).
- Thoracic causes of chest pain in the pediatric patient include pleuritis, costrochondritis, and chest trauma.
- Respiratory causes of pediatric chest pain include viral or bacterial infections and illnesses including cough, bronchitis, pneumonia, and asthma. Pneumothorax, pleural infusion, hyperventilation and muscle fatigue are other possible causes.

- Gastrointestinal disorders can cause chest pain in the pediatric patient. Types of these disorders include gastritis, esophagitis, ulcers, hiatal hernia, and severe vomiting. Substance abuse and ingestion can be causes as well.
- Children with sickle cell anemia can develop a condition known as "acute chest syndrome." This condition can be the result of pulmonary infections or pulmonary infarctions caused by the disease.

lieve cardiac ischemia pain, often relieves esophageal symptoms. All of these patients should be treated as if they have cardiac disease, because historical features will not separate esophageal from cardiac processes.

Lastly, many abdominal disease processes can produce irritation and inflammation of the underside of the diaphragm. However, this process may be "felt" as chest pain because of the overlapping nerve innervation and the patient's inability to differentiate exactly where the problem is located.

Patient Assessment

History

In the absence of an immediate life threat to the patient, the first step in assessment is for the paramedic to obtain a history. A detailed, accurate patient history is important to distinguish among the various causes of chest pain. The most important element of the patient history is an accurate characterization of the type of pain the patient is experiencing, because that is also the most important determinant of future management.

- *What is the location and character of the pain?* Critical findings that suggest cardiac chest pain and acute myocardial infarction include: 1) pain that is centered in the chest, but is diffuse or poorly localized; 2) pain that is described by the patient as severe, aching, crushing, squeez-

ing, or heavy ("like a weight on my chest"); and 3) pain that lasts more than 5 minutes. In an effort to describe the pain, the patient may make a fist and place it over the center of the chest. (Fig. 31-3)

The patient may have an atypical presentation of cardiac pain and interpret the discomfort as originating from indigestion ("heart burn") or muscular pain, especially if the patient has been involved in physical activity. These less typical presentations can cause the patient to delay seeking medical attention and make it difficult for the EMS provider to determine whether the complaint is significant and potentially dangerous.

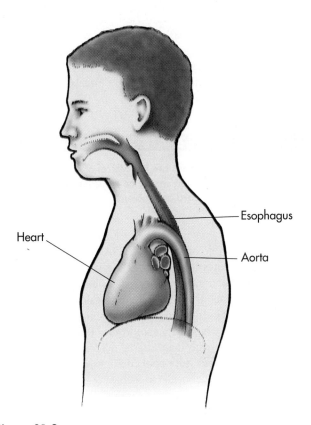

Esophagus

Heart

Aorta

Figure 31-2

Because of the close proximity of the aorta and esophagus, it is difficult to distinguish the origin of pain from these sites.

BOX 31-1	Immediate Life Threats Associated with Chest Pain

- **Dysrhythmias**—Recognition of initial dysrhythmias may alert the provider to impending, lethal cardiac rhythms causing cardiac arrest.
- **Hypoperfusion**—This may develop rapidly from heart muscle weakness, dysrhythmias, ruptured aneurysm or pulmonary embolus.
- **Hypoventilation**—This is associated with acute respiratory failure and congestive heart failure.

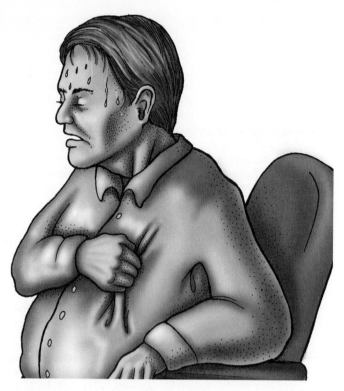

Figure 31-3

A sick-looking patient and a patient with a clenched fist are common presentations of acute myocardial infarction.

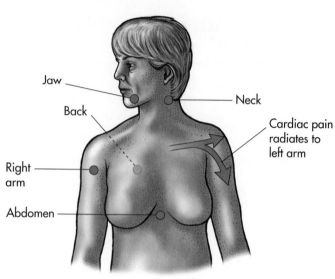

Figure 31-4

Pain and discomfort associated with an acute myocardial infarction can radiate to numerous sites.

Even when the symptoms are not typical of cardiac pain, all adult patients with chest pain should be considered to have a cardiac problem; this potentially serious cause cannot be ruled out until further evaluation is performed at a hospital. Pain that is characterized by the patient as sharp and exacerbated by breathing suggests a potential pulmonary cause.

CRITICAL ISSUE

Even when the symptoms are not typical of cardiac pain, all adults with chest pain should be considered to have a cardiac problem.

- *Does the pain go anywhere else?* Although classical cardiac pain radiates to the patient's left arm, it can be "referred" to the right arm, neck, jaw, back, or upper abdomen as well (Fig. 31-4). Patients sometimes also describe numbness or tingling in these areas.
- *Are there any associated symptoms?* Patients with chest pain associated with diaphoresis, dyspnea, transient loss of responsiveness (syncope), dizziness, or nausea and vomiting must be considered as having an acute myocardial infarction. They require careful observation for sudden deterioration. Cough, sputum production, hemoptysis, or fever and chills point toward a pulmonary source as the cause of the chest pain. Pain in either of the patient's shoulders may represent cardiac or pulmonary problems but should also raise the paramedic's suspicion of an abdominal process which is causing diaphragmatic irritation.
- *What are the patient's past medical history and medications?* Of particular interest is a patient history of problems related to the heart, lungs, and GI tract. Many patients have previously diagnosed problems and will be able to relate such problems to the paramedic. A history of **diabetes** is particularly important, because many diabetics who develop an acute myocardial infarction often present with minimal or atypical symptoms (chest pain is a relatively minor component). Medications the patient is taking will provide information about underlying diseases. In particular, the use of nitroglycerin indicates prior cardiac disease (*see* Table 31-1 for related patient medications).
- *Are there any aggravating or relieving factors?* Identifying associated factors that intensify or relieve the patient's chest pain may help to determine its significance. Pain that develops during or after physical exertion (especially if the patient describes as squeezing or heavy in nature) and does not subside immediately with rest is highly suggestive of cardiac pain. However, angina refers to the pattern of cardiac chest pain that occurs with exertion and is relieved by rest or by vasodilators, such as nitroglycerin. Thus, it is important for the paramedic to ask if the patient has nitroglycerin, if a dose was taken, and what effect it had on the pain.

However, activity is not necessary for the development of cardiac ischemia. Some patients experience cardiac chest pain at rest or after a large meal. The pain may be dismissed as "in-

TABLE 31-1 Chest Pain—Related Patient Medications

Classification	Specific Drug	Indication	Therapeutic Action	Side Effects and Precautions
CORONARY VASODILATORS	Nitroglycerin Isordil Nitrobid Nitropaste	Angina—pain relief Coronary artery disease	Dilates vascular smooth muscles Decreases myocardial O_2 demand Decreases cardiac workload in patients with AMI or CHF	Orthostatic hypotension Check potency—Headache, bitter taste Store away from light
ANTIDYSRHYTHMICS	Pronestyl (Procainamide) Procan SR Norpace Quinidine (Quinidex, Quinora) Tonocard (Tocainide) Procardia Verapamil	Preventing reoccurence of V-Tach after conversion Preventing PVCs Ventricular dysrhythmias	Decreases ventricular irritability Slows conduction of impulses through AV node	Hypotension ($\downarrow$HR = $\downarrow$CO = $\downarrow$BP) Bradycardia Contraindicated in complete heart block (can cause progressive widening of QRS and prolonged PR interval). GI disturbances.
CARDIOTONICS	Digitalis (Digoxin) Lanoxin	CHF A-fib/A-flutter/PSVT	Increases force of contraction Slows conduction through the AV node-decrease heart rate	Bradycardia Digitalis Toxicity: Cardiac: PVCs, V-Tach GI: anorexia, nausea, vomiting, diarrhea, abdominal pain CNS: visual disturbances (green/yellow halos around lights), confusion, headache, LOC changes, lethargy There is a very narrow range between toxic and therapeutic doses.

digestion" and the patient may take antacids or other home remedies prior to seeking professional help. The patient should also be asked if movement or body position influences the pain. Pain that is worse with deep inspiration or coughing is also more suggestive of a pulmonary cause.

Physical Examination

A pulse that is very rapid (>150/min), or very slow (<40/min) or irregular should alert the paramedic to the possibility of a cardiac dysrhythmia. Any pulse abnormalities should be evaluated by ECG. Absent or unequal peripheral pulses may indicate a serious vascular problem.

Blood pressure outside the accepted normal range for the patient's age should be considered a potential problem. Low blood pressure (<90 systolic) is a cause for concern as it may indicate cardiogenic shock. Markedly elevated blood pressures (systolic >200 or diastolic >120), may be contributing to the chest pain and could result in other medical emergencies such as aortic dissection, cerebrovascular accident (CVA) or congestive heart failure (CHF). If aortic dissection is a possibility, blood pressure measurement in both arms may reveal a difference, and a reading greater than 10 mm Hg difference is highly suggestive of dissection.

Respirations should be evaluated for rate and respiratory effort. Observations that suggest respiratory compromise are the patient's use of accessory muscles of respiration and the presence of retractions.

A patient with diaphoresis and cool skin may indicate a sympathetic response to maintain blood circulation to the vital organs. Flushed, warm skin in a patient may indicate a temperature elevation, indicating an infectious process, such as pericarditis or pneumonia. Cyanosis, especially involving the patient's lips and nail beds, indicates hypoxia and a life-threatening condition.

Jugular venous distention (JVD) is recognized by distention of the neck veins above the clavicle with the patient sitting at a 45° angle (Fig. 31-5). Any distention of the neck veins that occurs when the patient is sitting upright is abnormal. Neck veins that remain distended during the respiratory cycle

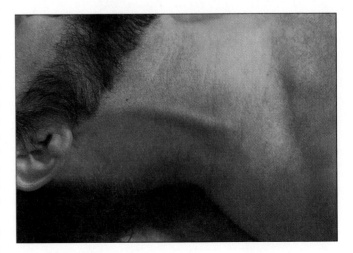

Figure 31-5

Distention of the jugular veins (JVD). From NAEMT: PHTLS: Basic and Advanced Prehospital Trauma Life Support, ed 3, St. Louis, 1994, Mosby-Year Book.

indicate increased pressure in the venous system and is usually caused by right heart failure.

Palpation of the chest wall in a nontrauma patient with chest pain may not be helpful, although palpation of the abdomen may identify possible abdominal sources for chest pain, such as gall bladder, liver, or pancreatic disease. Also, the patient's feet and ankles may demonstrate swelling or edema as CHF worsens.

Auscultating the patient's heart sounds may help to determine rate and rhythm when the pulse is weak and difficult to evaluate (Fig. 31-6). Auscultation of the lungs is necessary to determine potentially serious problems. Absent breath sounds on one side of the patient's chest may indicate a pneumothorax or accumulation of fluid in the chest cavity. Crackles, or rales, heard near the periphery of the lungs indicate fluid in the alveoli; those sounds localized to one area and associated with fever suggest pneumonia. When crackles are heard over both sides of the patient's chest, especially the lower lung fields, he or she may be experiencing pulmonary edema caused by left heart failure. If wheezing is present, it usually indicates the presence of bronchospastic disease, but in a minority of patients, wheezing can also be present with CHF.

CRITICAL ISSUE

Suspicion of acute MI is based on history. Do not be reassured by a normal interpretation of a Lead II monitor strip or by normal vital signs.

Key Conditions and Findings

- *Myocardial Ischemia/Acute Myocardial Infarction.* Patients with significant coronary artery disease frequently experience cardiac chest pain when cardiac muscle has more demand for oxygen than the blood flow through the coronary arteries can supply. Short-lasting episodes (less than 5 to 10 minutes) of chest pain which resolve with rest and reveal no signs of permanent muscle damage are called angina attacks. If the pain lasts longer and later reveals evidence, from ECG or blood work, of cardiac muscle damage, the episode is called an acute myocardial infarction, or more commonly, a heart attack.
- *Esophageal Spasm.* Esophageal spasm can be quite severe in some patients, and indistinguishable from the pain of angina or an acute myocardial infarction. Strong, prolonged contraction of the esophageal smooth muscle can be triggered by direct irritation (stomach acid or food that is too cold) or distention by a large bolus of food.
- *Pleuritic Chest Pain.* Conditions that inflame the pleura cause pain that is well localized to the chest wall; the patient can usually identify a specific area. The pain typically intensifies by breathing or by movement, but may not be aggravated by direct palpation. Pleuritic pain may represent pulmonary embolus, pneumonia or pneumothorax, and bronchitis.
- *Aortic Dissection.* A tear in the lining of the thoracic aorta presents an immediate threat to life (Fig. 31-7). A hypertensive patient may present with the complaint of

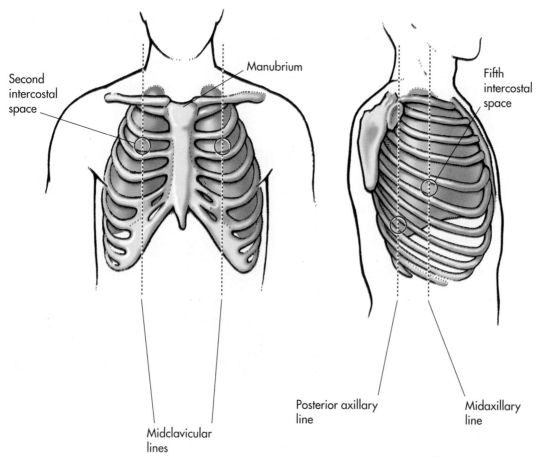

Second intercostal space

Manubrium

Fifth intercostal space

Midclavicular lines

Posterior axillary line

Midaxillary line

Figure 31-6

Some common auscultatory sites for lung assessment. These sites allow every lobe of the lung to be assessed.

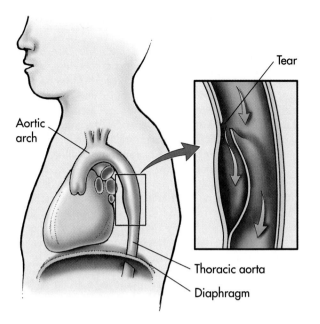

Figure 31-7

Aortic dissection occurs when a tear in the internal lining of the aorta allows blood to enter and gather within the walls of the vessel.

sudden, severe, deep, tearing pain centered in the upper back or anterior chest.

- *Pericarditis.* Pericarditis may occur in patients, such as younger individuals, who are not usually considered to be at high risk for AMI. The pain is classically worsened by deep inspiration, by the patient lying in a supine position, or by the patient turning onto his or her side; however, the pain may be dramatically relieved if the patient sits or leans forward. Pericarditis is commonly associated with both bacterial and viral infections, inflammatory diseases such as lupus, chronic renal failure, and tumors. Thus, many other symptoms may also be present.
- *Gall Bladder Disease.* Gall bladder disease (or cholecystitis), presenting as spasm in the presence of gallstones (biliary colic) or infection, may refer pain to the right side of the back and upper chest.
- *Intra-abdominal Disorders.* Irritation of the diaphragm can be caused by ectopic pregnancy, perforation of hollow organs such as the stomach and bowel, or rupture of solid organs such as the kidney and spleen. The pain is described as dull and aching and may be aggravated by breathing.

Management

Early management of patients with chest pain and possible AMI is outlined in Figure 31-8.

Patients with chest pain should receive oxygen at a high-flow rate, and attention must be paid to the possible development of hypoventilation or respiratory arrest. If the patient's respirations are inadequate, the paramedic should establish an airway and assist ventilations.

Continuous cardiac rhythm monitoring is important to establish in all patients with chest pain. The paramedic should observe the patient carefully for rhythm disturbances that require prompt treatment.

CRITICAL ISSUE

Constant monitoring of the patient with chest pain is essential. Many patients with AMI who develop ventricular fibrillation have no warning dysrhythmias.

Intravenous access should be established in all patients with acute chest pain. This access is necessary, in case the patient's condition suddenly deteriorates, necessitating fluid or medications. Usually, the IV is D_5W administered at a keep open rate, although some medical directors prefer normal saline or Ringer's lactate be used. The important point is the keep open rate, because the patient who may be experiencing AMI could develop pulmonary edema caused by the presence of extra fluid.

CRITICAL ISSUE

Monitor IV fluids carefully. It is easy to inadvertently fluid-overload these patients and put them into pulmonary edema.

If myocardial ischemia is suspected as the cause of acute chest pain, sublingual nitroglycerin may be appropriate. Because myocardial ischemia causes systemic vasodilation that can lead to significant hypotension, nitroglycerin should be used with caution; this medication cannot be used as a diagnostic tool. However, nitroglycerin may also relieve many noncardiac etiologies of pain, such as esophageal spasm and biliary colic.

Morphine sulfate is effective in both relieving acute chest pain and reducing anxiety. Anxiety may lead to agitation and increased catecholamine release, which then adds to the stress on the injured heart muscle. Morphine is usually an option considered in conjunction with, or after failure of, nitroglycerin. Aspirin is also included in the prehospital management of patients who may be experiencing an AMI. One tablet is taken orally, either chewed or swallowed with a small amount of water. Aspirin decreases platelet clumping and may assist in breaking up the clot.

The paramedic must continue to assess the patient frequently for a worsening in cardiac function, indicated by hypotension or signs of pulmonary edema.

Transport must be initiated with the intent to transfer the AMI patient quickly to the nearest facility capable of offering thrombolytic therapy. Thrombolytic agents are medications that dissolve blood clots which obstruct coronary blood flow. The sooner these agents are administered, the sooner blood flow can be restored to the myocardium, thus reducing the amount of muscle damage and necrosis. Reduction of future complications of AMI, such as left ventricular failure, is directly

by Rob Carter, EMT-P

The care of a patient with an acute myocardial infarction (AMI) has changed dramatically over the past 10 to 12 years. "Clot-busters" (thrombolytic agents) and emergency angioplasty have provided an opportunity to save myocardium and minimize damage and disability caused by an infarct.

A clot in a coronary artery is the primary cause of an AMI. The clot occludes blood flow through an already narrowed coronary artery, causing an acute lack of oxygen to the myocardium, subsequently resulting in infarction. Ninety percent of patients have a clot in the affected coronary artery during the first 4 hours of their AMI. By reperfusing the vessel and increasing the amount of oxygen delivered to ischemic cardiac muscle, myocardium can be salvaged. Breakdown (lysis) of the clot to allow reperfusion can be achieved by the IV administration of drugs known as thrombolytics (e.g., streptokinase, urokinase, or tissue plasminogen activator [T-PA]).

Because 50% of deaths from AMI occur within 3 to 4 hours of the onset of symptoms, thrombolytic therapy has proven most effective when initiated early, especially within the first hour of the onset of symptoms. Research has shown that patients, given a thrombolytic drug within 60 to 90 minutes after onset of chest pain, benefit the most and often have minimal cardiac damage. The time from onset of chest pain to initiation of thrombolytic therapy is vital ("Time is muscle").

Patients who receive thrombolytic therapy must meet certain criteria and be free from contraindications. Therapy is generally safe and effective, but there are side effects including bleeding, hypotension, tachycardia and other dysrhythmias and, in severe cases, stroke.

This change in management of AMI patients has important implications for EMS providers. Lessening drug administration time allows EMS providers to identify patients with AMI and those patients who may be candidates for thrombolytics. A prehospital 12-lead ECG (when available) and notification of the receiving hospital and telemetry station can decrease the "door-to-drug" time.[2,5]

Although few EMS services currently have 12-lead ECG capabilities, this equipment is becoming more popular in the prehospital setting. Because of recent advances in computerized technology, 12-lead ECGs can be easily performed in the prehospital setting and transmitted to emergency department telemetry stations with little or no distortion. EMS providers also can be trained to correctly obtain a standard 12-lead ECG and, with more training, to interpret the results. Most computerized 12-lead ECG monitors are equipped with interpretation capabilities.

Along with the use of prehospital 12-lead ECGs, chest pain checklists may be used in the field to evaluate potential candidates for thrombolytic therapy. The prehospital checklist consists of specific questions and guidelines aimed at indications and contraindications of therapy, vital sign criteria, as well as other evaluation tools. The information is then transmitted to the emergency department via radio or telephone. The emergency department team will then evaluate all information and determine whether thrombolytic therapy is indicated and beneficial for the patient.[1,3]

So what about the administration of thrombolytics in the prehospital setting? Theoretically, patients suffering from chest pain who have a suspected AMI could receive thrombolytic therapy earlier in the management if EMS units carried the drug. However, there are several additional aspects to consider. First, most EMS departments have limited budgets; the cost for providing an entire fleet with thrombolytic therapy capabilities is significant. The equipment necessary for this endeavor includes cardiac monitors equipped with 12-lead ECG capabilities and telemetry equipment, as well as EMS provider training. Additionally, studies report that initiation of thrombolytic therapy in the prehospital setting has actually shown no significant change in the morbidity and mortality of patients suffering from an AMI compared with minimizing the time to drug administration in the emergency department.[1,3]

For years, the American Heart Association (AHA) has provided both medical personnel and the public with information and recommendations concerning detection and recognition of heart disease and the treatment and prevention of AMI. The AHA and the National Heart Attack Alert Program recommend that the primary goal of treatment and management of patient with an AMI is the initiation of thrombolytic (reperfusion) therapy within 1 hour of the onset of initial signs and symptoms. This should also be the goal of EMS and emergency department personnel.

By initiating and following these recommendations, there will hopefully be a decreased morbidity and mortality rate for AMI patients. This method of patient management will help salvage heart muscle and improve patients' chances of survival.

REFERENCES

1. The European Myocardial Infarction Group: Prehospital thrombolytic therapy in patients with suspected acute myocardial infarction. *N Engl J Med* 329(6):383–389, 1993.

2. National Heart, Lung, and Blood Institute: Staffing and equipping emergency medical services systems; rapid identification and treatment of acute myocardial infarction, Bethesda, United States Department of Health and Human Services, Public Health Service, National Institutes of Health.

3. Weaver TD, et al: Prehospital-initiated vs. Hospital-initiated thrombolytic therapy: the myocardial infarction triage and intervention trail. *JAMA* 270(10):1211–1216, 1993.

4. MacCallum, et al: Reduction in hospital time to thrombolytic therapy by audit of policy guidelines. *Eur Heart J* 11(Suppl F):48–52, 1990.

5. National Heart, Lung, and Blood Institute: Emergency department: rapid identification and treatment of patients with acute myocardial infarction, Bethesda, United States Department of Health and Human Services, Public Health Service, National Institute of Health.

6. National Heart, Lung, and Blood Institute: National Heart Attack Alert Program Coordination Committee 60 Minutes to Treatment Working Group, United States Department of Health and Human Services, Public Health Service, National Institutes of Health.

7. Olin, et al (ed): Facts and Comparisons, St. Louis.

Acute Myocardial Infarction Algorithm

Early Management of Patients with Chest Pain and Possible Acute Myocardial Infarction (AMI) in Three Management Settings

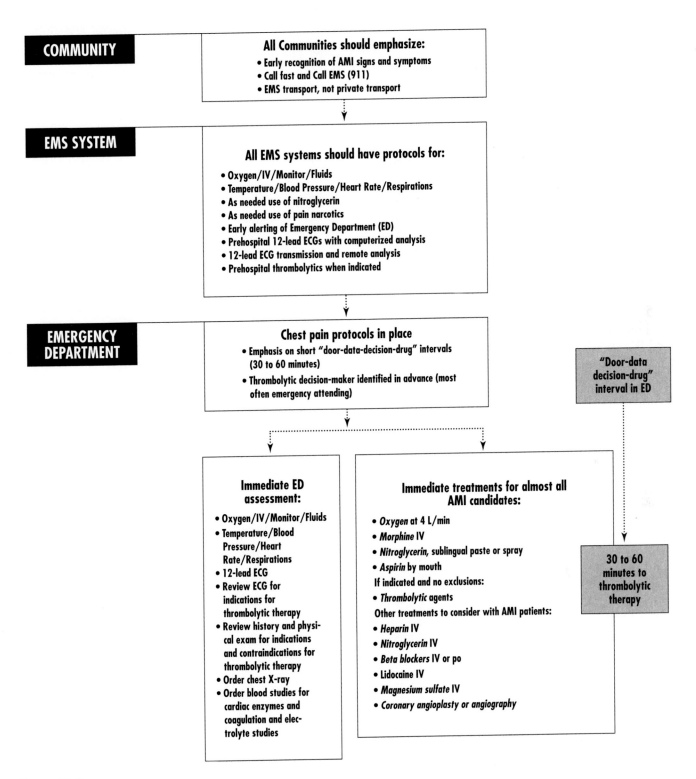

COMMUNITY

All Communities should emphasize:
- Early recognition of AMI signs and symptoms
- Call fast and Call EMS (911)
- EMS transport, not private transport

EMS SYSTEM

All EMS systems should have protocols for:
- Oxygen/IV/Monitor/Fluids
- Temperature/Blood Pressure/Heart Rate/Respirations
- As needed use of nitroglycerin
- As needed use of pain narcotics
- Early alerting of Emergency Department (ED)
- Prehospital 12-lead ECGs with computerized analysis
- 12-lead ECG transmission and remote analysis
- Prehospital thrombolytics when indicated

EMERGENCY DEPARTMENT

Chest pain protocols in place
- Emphasis on short "door-data-decision-drug" intervals (30 to 60 minutes)
- Thrombolytic decision-maker identified in advance (most often emergency attending)

"Door-data decision-drug" interval in ED

Immediate ED assessment:
- Oxygen/IV/Monitor/Fluids
- Temperature/Blood Pressure/Heart Rate/Respirations
- 12-lead ECG
- Review ECG for indications for thrombolytic therapy
- Review history and physical exam for indications and contraindications for thrombolytic therapy
- Order chest X-ray
- Order blood studies for cardiac enzymes and coagulation and electrolyte studies

Immediate treatments for almost all AMI candidates:
- *Oxygen* at 4 L/min
- *Morphine* IV
- *Nitroglycerin*, sublingual paste or spray
- *Aspirin* by mouth
If indicated and no exclusions:
- *Thrombolytic* agents
Other treatments to consider with AMI patients:
- *Heparin* IV
- *Nitroglycerin* IV
- *Beta blockers* IV or po
- *Lidocaine* IV
- *Magnesium sulfate* IV
- *Coronary angioplasty or angiography*

30 to 60 minutes to thrombolytic therapy

Figure 31-8

The algorithm for acute myocardial infarction. Adapted from Cummins: ACLS Scenarios: Core Concepts for Case-Based Learning, St. Louis, 1996, Mosby-Year Book. Adapted with permission, Journal of the American Medical Association: Guidelines for Cardiopulmonary Resuscitation and Emergency Cardiac Care, vol 268, ©1992, American Medical Association.

related to the speed with which thrombolytic agents are administered. Recent studies have not shown improvement in patient outcome with the prehospital administration of thrombolytics, perhaps because of the quick arrival time to most urban emergency departments. However, obtaining 12-lead electrocardiograms in the field may be an effective strategy to reduce the time to thrombolytic administration, because this procedure can be time consuming in the emergency department (see Sidebar).

All patients should be transported in a position of comfort. Patients who develop signs of hypoperfusion should be transported in a supine position to facilitate blood flow to the heart and brain.

CRITICAL ISSUE

Transport with lights and siren only for patients in cardiogenic shock or with uncontrollable dysrhythmias. In others, the catecholamine surge from this stress may be harmful.

SUMMARY

Chest pain can be caused by many conditions, some of which may be immediately life threatening to the patient. Because the most common of these conditions are associated with cardiac disease, prehospital providers should assess each patient for a cardiac source of pain. Even when the patient is stable and in no acute distress, the complaint of chest pain must be considered a potentially serious problem until thoroughly evaluated. The paramedic must be prepared for sudden deterioration of the patient's condition; rapid intervention may improve patient outcome.

William Roush, MD
Phil Fontanarosa, MD, FACEP

Chapter 32

Palpitations and Dysrhythmias

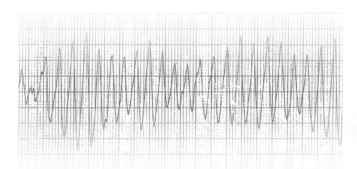

A paramedic should be able to:

OBJECTIVES

1. Describe the significance and common causes of palpitations.

2. Identify the key historical findings in the assessment of a patient with palpitations/dysrhythmias.

3. Identify 4 classifications of patient medications commonly used to treat palpitations/dysrhythmias

4. Describe the rapid, directed physical examination of patients with palpitation and dysrhythmias.

5. Identify the subjective and objective assessment findings that indicate the need for prehospital intervention in patients with palpitation and dysrhythmias.

6. Describe the specific causes, signs and symptoms, potential problems and prehospital treatment for the following:
   a. Bradycardias (sinus, junctional)
   b. AV heart block
   c. Narrow complex tachycardia
   d. Wide complex tachycardia
   e. Atrial fibrillation
   f. Premature ventricular contractions.

KEY TERMS

1. **Artificial pacemaker**—electronic device used to stimulate the heartbeat when the electrical conduction system of the heart malfunctions.

2. **Bradycardia**—dysrhythmia with rate of less than 60 beats per minute.

3. **Cardiovert**—delivery of energy to correct a potentially lethal dysrhythmia.

4. **Defibrillation**—delivery of an unsynchronized pulsation of energy to correct a life-threatening dysrhythmia.

5. **Dysrhythmia**—a rhythm other than a normal sinus rhythm. Also sometimes called *arrhythmia*.

6. **Palpitation**—a sensation of fluttering or slipped beats caused by a dysrhythmia.

7. **Synchronized cardioversion**—delivery of an electrical pulsation that is timed so it does not fall during the relative refactory period.

8. **Tachycardia**—considered to be three or more beats occurring at a rate greater than 100 beats per minute.

9. **Tachydysrhythmia**—heart rate greater than 100 beats per minute.

10. **Transcutaneous pacing**—the delivery of electrical impulses through the skin.

ardiac rhythm disturbances, or *dysrhythmias*, are a common problem encountered by paramedics. The presentation can range from an incidental finding upon patient assessment, to a patient complaint of palpitations, to signs of life-threatening dysrhythmias. The proper assessment and management of patients with cardiac dysrhythmias is one of the most important responsibilities of prehospital emergency care providers.

Pathophysiology

Many dysrhythmias are perceived by the patient as palpitations. Palpitations are an awareness of forceful heart beating, usually with an increased rate, and either with or without rhythm irregularity. Patients use various terms to describe palpitations, including skipping beats, flipping, fluttering, pounding, running away, going too fast or too slow, and stopping.

However, not all dysrhythmias are perceived by the patient as palpitations; one of the most serious dysrhythmias, ventricular tachycardia, frequently does not cause this sensation.

Palpitations that occur during or after strenuous exercise may be normal, but those related to mild exertion suggest underlying poor physical conditioning, dysrhythmias, heart failure, or anemia. Other common triggering factors that contribute to palpitations include smoking, stress or fatigue, alcohol ingestion, caffeine-containing beverages, and certain medications, such as stimulant drugs.

Many dysrhythmias reduce cardiac output and produce symptoms related to decreased blood flow and perfusion (Fig. 32-1). For example, there may be reduced cerebral blood flow and symptoms related to decreased delivery of oxygen and

glucose to the brain. Cerebral blood flow reduction can be further aggravated by atherosclerosis found in cerebral vessels.

Light-headedness, confusion, or syncope in a patient may result from an extremely rapid heart rate or from profound bradycardia. If the dysrhythmias is temporary, the symptoms often resolve when the patient is supine, because the horizontal position improves cardiac output and blood flow to the brain.

In addition, decreased cardiac output may compromise coronary artery perfusion and thus present as ischemic chest pain, such as that seen with angina pectoris (*see* Chapter 31). Another common complication is shortness of breath related to congestive heart failure or pulmonary edema.

Bradycardia, which is defined as a heart rate less than 60 beats per minute, can result from slowing of the natural pacemaker function of the heart. Parasympathetic stimulation of the vagus nerve decreases depolarization frequency in the SA node, which then slows the heart rate (Fig. 32-2). Vagal slowing of the heart can result from a number of sources, including severe pain of any origin, urination, defecation, vomiting, and acute emotional distress. Slowing also occurs when ischemia affects the heart's electrical conduction system, particularly in the setting of inferior myocardial infarction.

Tachycardia is defined as a heart rate greater than 100 beats per minute. Under circumstances of increased demand, such as exercise, this results from a sympathetic response to increase cardiac output. However, with advancing age, the maximum achievable and tolerable heart rate decreases. The average 80-year-old patient generally cannot sustain a heart rate greater than 150 beats per minute for a significant length of time without developing symptoms of myocardial ischemia, such as chest pain or shortness of breath.

Many pathologic conditions, such as ischemic heart disease, hypoxia, and drug toxicity, can also produce a variety of tachydysrhythmias that require field treatment. These conditions include paroxysmal supraventricular tachycardia

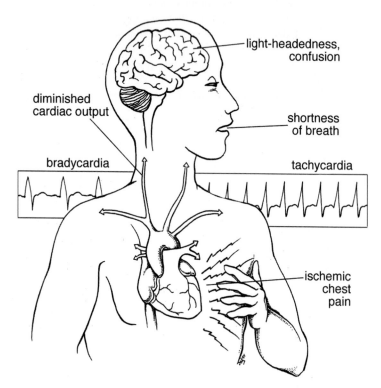

Figure 32-1

Dysrhythmias which cause reduced cardiac output and decreased blood pressure.

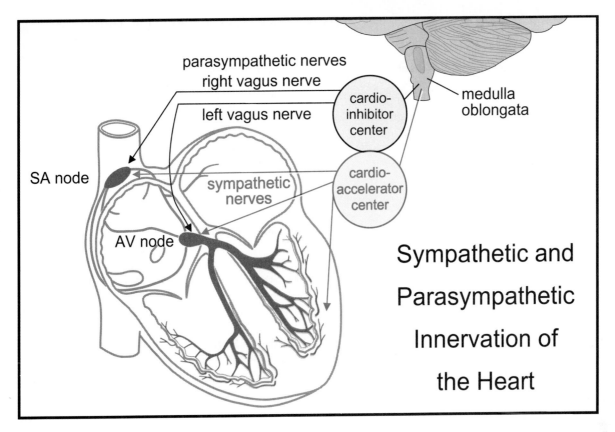

parasympathetic nerves
right vagus nerve

left vagus nerve

cardio-inhibitor center

medulla oblongata

cardio-accelerator center

SA node

sympathetic nerves

AV node

Sympathetic and Parasympathetic Innervation of the Heart

Figure 32-2

Effects from the vagus nerve (cranial nerve X). *From Huszar: Basic dysrhythmias, second edition, 1994, Mosby Lifeline.*

and ventricular tachycardia and are usually associated with ischemic cardiac disease.

Patient Assessment

History

Historical information about the patient can be helpful in differentiating serious dysrhythmias from more benign presentations of palpitations.

- *Does the patient complain of palpitations?* Palpitations are perhaps the most common symptom in patients with cardiac rhythm disturbances. Even though the cause is often benign, most patients consider palpitations to be serious and frequently are concerned that the symptom signals the presence of heart disease.
- *Does the patient note chest pain or shortness of breath?* Some patients with dysrhythmias have symptoms, such as chest pain or dyspnea, and others experience syncope. The dangers of any dysrhythmia and the need for immediate treatment are based largely on the severity of the associated symptoms. Significant symptoms caused by cardiac rhythm disturbances generally result from insufficient cerebral blood flow or inadequate myocardial perfusion. For example, chest pain associated with a rapid heart rate suggests myocardial ischemia re-

sulting from increased cardiac muscle oxygen demands. Inadequate cardiac output can be the cause of chest pain in very slow heart rates.
- *Does the patient note any light-headedness or dizziness?* Dysrhythmias producing mild-to-moderate decreases in cerebral blood flow may cause dizziness, a sensation of light-headedness, dimming or narrowing of vision. These symptoms typically worsen when the patient tries to stand.
- *What is the patient's past medical history?* Many patients will have experienced dysrhythmias in the past or have a history of other cardiac disease or cardiac surgery. If a patient has had an artificial pacemaker implanted, a mechanical malfunction may be responsible for the current symptoms. Thyroid disease can cause **atrial fibrillation**. The rescuer should note the patient's use of any medications, particularly those for cardiac diseases as listed in Table 32-1. Substance abuse, especially cocaine or other stimulants, is often a precipitating factor. Drug overdoses also cause dysrhythmias, particularly cardiac drugs, tricyclic antidepressants, and stimulants. Organophosphate poisoning causes a bradycardia.

Physical Examination

Physical examination begins with determination of vital signs, which should be directed at evaluating the patient for evidence

TABLE 32-1 Medications Related to Palpitations and Dysrhythmias

Classification	Drug Name	Indication	Therapeutic Action	Side Effects and Precautions
Calcium channel blocker	Calan (verapamil)	Rapid atrial dysrhythmias	Slows heart rate	Bradycardia
	Isoptin (verapamil)			Hypotension
	Cardizem (diltiazem)			
Antidysrhythmics	Pronestyl (procainamide)	Prevents reoccurrence of VT after conversion	Decreases ventricular irritability	Hypotension
	Norpace			Bradycardia
	Quinidine (Quinidex)	PVCs		GI disturbances
	Tonocard (tocainide)	Ventricular dysrhythmias	Slows conduction through AV node	
Beta blocker	Tenormin	Supraventricular tachycardia	Slows conduction through AV node	Hypotension
	Lopresor			Bradycardia
			Slows sinus node	Increases AV block Bronchospasms in asthma patients
Cardiotonic	Digitalis (digoxin)	Atrial fibrillation	Increases force of contraction	Bradycardia
	Lanoxin	Atrial flutter		Digitalis toxicity: PVCs, V-tach, nausea, vomiting, visual disturbances, confusion, lethargy. There is a narrow range between therapeutic and toxic dosages
		PSVT	Slows conduction through AV node; decreases heart rate	

of hypoperfusion. The patient should always be examined first for evidence of airway compromise and respiratory distress or tachypnea. Hypoxia may be a manifestation of, or caused by, a dysrhythmia.

The presence of a dysrhythmia may be suspected by noting abnormalities in the patient's pulse (e.g., is it rapid, slow or irregular?). Hypoperfusion is indicated by a weak, thready pulse, and cool, moist (clammy) skin. Hypotension will be present if hypoperfusion is severe and compensatory mechanisms are failing. The patient's mental status should be evaluated. Poor cerebral blood flow is initially demonstrated by confusion or syncope and may progress to seizures or unresponsiveness if cardiac output remains inadequate.

The neck should be examined for jugular vein distention. The patient's use of accessory muscles during respiration should also be noted . The paramedic should auscultate the patient's chest for the presence of crackles (rales). These findings frequently suggest left ventricular failure.

The rescuer should palpate the extremities for pulses and compare the quality and character. If pitting, dependant peripheral edema is noted, it usually represents chronic heart failure and is not a result of the acute event.

A cardiac monitor is essential for any patient complaining of palpitations. Most common dysrhythmias can be recognized on the monitor screen. However, detailed analysis and systematic interpretation of rhythm strips are required to assure accurate identification of dysrhythmias (*see* Chapter 12). Although dysrhythmia interpretation is essential, findings must be correlated with the patient's presenting complaint and medical condition.

CRITICAL ISSUE

Documentation of prehospital dysrhythmias with the tracing is extremely important. The prehospital information may be the only guidance for long-term management.

Management

All patients with dysrhythmias and cardiac symptoms should be considered unstable with a potentially life-threatening problem. The provider should be prepared for immediate intervention to stabilize the condition.

CRITICAL ISSUE

Paramedics must remember to treat the patient not the dysrhythmia. Signs of adequate perfusion mean the patient may not require emergent treatment in the field.

After considering the need for airway management, the rescuer should apply high-concentration oxygen to the patient. Pulse oximetry should be used if available. The patient should be placed in a position of comfort, and intravenous access should be initiated with normal saline or lactated Ringer's. Unless shock is present, the IV should be run at a keep open rate.

The need for field intervention for a dysrhythmia can be determined by answering the following questions:

1. Is the patient stable or unstable?
2. Is the heart rate fast or slow?
3. Are the QRS complexes wide or narrow?
4. Is the rhythm regular or irregular?
5. Are the P waves (atrial activity) associated with QRS complexes (ventricular activity)?

The answers to these questions generally lead to an appropriate management strategy. Dysrhythmia management is generally presented as algorithms which outline in a stepwise fashion recommended guidelines for treating specific abnormal rhythms.

Stable vs Unstable

The first step in management is to determine if there is evidence of compromised cardiac output. The patient should be evaluated to be stable or unstable. This evaluation is indicated by complaints of chest pain or dyspnea, unresponsiveness, or signs of hypoperfusion. If the patient is stable, a more thorough evaluation can be undertaken. If, the patient is unstable, rapid evaluation and therapy are required.

Fast or Slow

Dysrhythmias that significantly decrease cardiac output typically involve abnormalities in heart rate. Simplistically, if the heart rate is slow, it must be increased; if the heart rate is fast, it must be decreased. The method by which this is done depends on the rhythm identified. The presence of a slow rate does not automatically indicate a significant cardiac problem. Many well-conditioned athletes have a normal resting pulse rate of less than 60 per minute.

> ### CRITICAL ISSUE
>
> Paramedics must remember to treat the patient not the dysrhythmia. Signs of adequate perfusion mean the patient may not require emergent treatment in the field.

If, on the other hand, the patient is bradycardic and shows signs of hypoperfusion, treatment generally includes transcutaneous pacing and/or atropine. (*See* Bradycardia Algorithm in Chapter 20.) Pacing should not be delayed if there is any difficulty in obtaining IV access. Analgesia or sedation is often helpful if the patient is experiencing any pain caused by transcutaneous pacing.

Occasionally, the hypoperfusing bradycardia patient will develop **premature ventricular complexes** (PVCs) caused by hypoxia or as escape beats. After administering oxygen, the rate should be treated and then, if necessary, the PVCs. Increasing the rate will hopefully improve perfusion and oxygenation of the myocardium, thus eliminating the PVCs.

Mobitz Type II **second-degree AV block** prevents atrial impulses from reaching the ventricle, and represents a potentially dangerous situation for the patient (*see* Chapter 12). This type of block frequently progresses to complete, or **third-**

degree block, and is associated with a high mortality rate. In the setting of these advanced-degree blocks, a transcutaneous pacer should be applied early, in case the patient's condition deteriorates.

The use of atropine with Mobitz II and third-degree blocks may be associated with some increased risk. In this setting, atropine may increase the atrial rate and worsen the AV block. Paradoxically, the ventricular rate can fall and diminish the hemodynamic status further. This is a concern that should be addressed in local protocol. In any case, if atropine is used in this setting, transcutaneous pacing must be immediately available.[1]

Any patient with a tachydysrhythmia and myocardial dysfunction is considered unstable, regardless of the QRS width. (*See* Tachycardia Algorithm in Chapter 20.) After evaluation of blood pressure, mental status and chief complaints, the caregivers may decide to prepare for synchronized cardioversion. (*See* Electrical Cardioversion Algorithm in Chapter 20.) Synchronized cardioversion is the administration of a timed pulsation of electrical current through the patient's heart to depolarize cells. This method is performed during the down slope of the R wave or during the S wave, to avoid causing **ventricular fibrillation** (*see* Skill #16 in Skill Section). When possible, the patient should be sedated in advance with an agent such as diazepam. Suction should be available in the event the sedated patient vomits.

QRS Wide or Narrow?

If the patient with a fast rhythm appears stable, treatment will be guided by the interpretation of the rhythm. The first step will be to determine if the QRS complex is narrow, indicating a supraventricular origin, or wide, suggesting a ventricular cause.

Sinus tachycardia is a normal response to the demand for an increased heart rate. The demand can arise from exercise, anxiety, and compensation for certain medical problems, such as blood loss, fever, and hypoxia. Sinus tachycardia can be an expected physiologic response, particularly when the heart rate is less than 160 beats per minute. In these cases, it requires no specific treatment beyond addressing the underlying cause.

Narrow-complex tachycardias (heart rate > 160) can usually be terminated by medications that temporarily slow or interrupt AV conduction, such as adenosine and verapamil. Adenosine, with its short half-life, is most commonly used and should be considered for long transport times or awake patients with signs of mild hypoperfusion. Verapamil is also effective, but because it commonly causes significant hypotension, adenosine is the first choice for field use.

Wide-complex tachycardias are initially treated with IV lidocaine. If it is not effective, repeat doses of lidocaine, bretylium, or adenosine (for possible supraventricular etiologies) may be considered to attempt to produce a more effective rhythm. Medications that require large doses which must be administered slowly over prolonged periods of time, such as procainamide, are often not utilized in the prehospital setting.

Ventricular fibrillation and pulseless wide-complex tachycardia (ventricular tachycardia) are treated identically, with CPR, defibrillation, and medications such as epinephrine and lidocaine (*see* Ventricular Fibrillation and Pulseless Ventricular Tachycardia Algorithm in Chapter 19).

Magnesium sulfate is the drug of choice for torsades de pointes (Fig. 32-3). Torsades de pointes is a version of ventricular tachycardia whereby the QRSs are constantly changing. The dysrhythmia is usually secondary to drug toxicity which produces a prolonged Q—T interval and predisposes to ventricular tachycardia.

CRITICAL   ISSUE

The single most important management consideration for the patient in ventricular fibrillation is rapid defibrillation.

• *Is the rhythm regular or irregular and are there P waves associated with each QRS complex?* The presence of atrial fibrillation may be chronic or acute. Rapid ventricular rates in response to atrial fibrillation can be problematic for older patients and those with heart disease. The lack of a coordinated atrial contraction compromises the efficiency of ventricular filling and decreases cardiac output. Microemboli (tiny blood clots) can be caused by sluggish blood in the atria due to atrial fibrillation and can lead to cerebrovascular accidents.

If tachycardia is determined to be the result of atrial fibrillation or **atrial flutter**, a number of medications are acceptable to slow or regulate the rate. These include diltiazem, certain betablockers, verapamil, and digoxin.[1] These medications are usually given in the emergency department setting. Because atrial fibrillation can be very difficult to cardiovert, this treatment is not used routinely.

Atrial fibrillation present in patients with a history of abnormalities may be an incidental finding during physical assessment. If the patient does not have a specific cardiac complaint and the pulse rate is in the normal range, additional prehospital treatment is not required for the dysrhythmia.

PVCs indicate irritability of the cardiac muscle usually from hypoxia and should be evaluated carefully to determine if they require advanced treatment. They commonly occur in the setting of acute cardiac ischemia and myocardial infarction. On the other hand, some individuals chronically experience PVCs without developing other significant cardiac symptoms. PVCs in patients who are not experiencing cardiac problems

---

CRITICAL   ISSUE

The first treatment of any PVC activity is to apply high-concentration oxygen.

---

do not necessitate treatment. Further evaluation of the clinical status of the patient leads to the proper decision.

In the situation of chest pain that is secondary to cardiac ischemia, PVC activity may warn of impending ventricular tachycardia or fibrillation. Specifically, PVCs that are in excess of 6 per minute, occur on the T wave (R on T phenomenon) of the preceding beat, are multifocal, in couplets (groups of 2), runs (2 or more), or bigeminy (every other complex is a PVC), suggest that treatment is warranted (Fig. 32-4). Following contact with medical direction, or based on standing orders, these PVCs are treated with IV lidocaine bolus that may be repeated as necessary to a total dose of 3 mg/kg.[1] PVCs in the setting of atrial fibrillation or in the presence of bradycardia should not be treated prior to consultation with medical direction.

Asystole is the complete lack of cardiac electrical activity. The presence should be confirmed in at least two leads. (*See* Asystole Treatment Algorithm in Chapter 19.) A patient presenting in **asystole** is unlikely to respond to medications or pacing. However, should the patient progress to asystole from another rhythm, pacing is initiated as soon as possible.

Pulseless electrical activity (PEA, formerly called *electromechanical dissociation*) is the presence of cardiac electrical activity without apparent mechanical activity or a pulse. It is generally managed by giving epinephrine, atropine, fluid boluses, and considering possible underlying causes. (*See* Pulseless Electrical Activity Algorithm in Chapter 19.)

Although prompt transport is indicated for any symptomatic dysrhythmia, treatment for cardiac arrest and life-threatening dysrhythmias should be initiated in the field. The patient receives better care when the duration of hypoperfusion is minimized.

On occasion, the paramedic will discover an abnormal cardiac rhythm during evaluation of a noncardiac complaint. The dysrhythmia may be unrelated to the chief complaint and may be identified when assessing vital signs or during routine cardiac monitoring. Although the paramedic should be suspicious of an underlying cardiac disorder, it is not necessary to treat every patient with a benign incidental dysrhythmia.

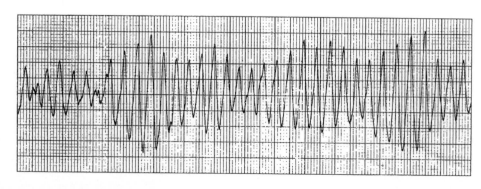

Figure 32-3

Torsades de Pointes. *From Aehlert: ACLS quick review study guide, 1994, Mosby Lifeline.*

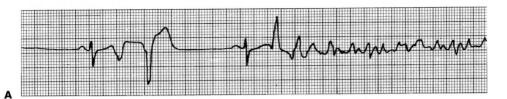

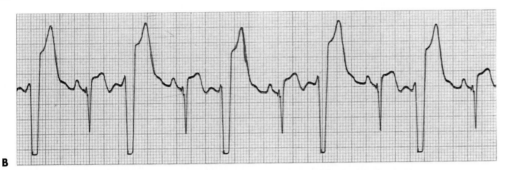

A

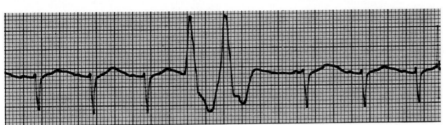

B

C

Figure 32-4

A) V fib as a result of R on T in a heart with ischemic disease. B) Ventricular bigeminy. C) Couplets of PVCs. *From Conover: Understanding electrocardiography, Seventh edition, 1996, St. Louis, Mosby-Year Book.*

SUMMARY

Rapid, accurate analysis of the cardiac rhythm on a monitor or rhythm strip is one of the most important responsibilities of the paramedic. Not all dysrhythmias require prehospital intervention, but precise patient assessment will identify those situations in which prompt management is indicated to improve patient outcome.

REFERENCE

1. Guidelines for Cardiopulmonary Resuscitation and Emergency Cardiac Care. *JAMA* 268:2171–2298, 1992.

Chapter 33

Headache

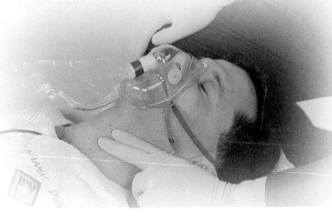

KEY TERMS

1. **Meningitis**—an infection of the membranes covering the brain and spinal cord, usually caused by bacteria, virus or fungus.

2. **Subarachnoid hemorrhage**—an acute spontaneous bleed in the brain, usually caused by cerebral artery aneurysm or an arteriovenous malformation.

3. **Hypertensive encephalopathy**—a set of symptoms, including headache, convulsions, and coma, associated with glomerulonephritis.

A paramedic should be able to:

OBJECTIVES

1. Describe the pathophysiology of headache disorders.

2. Describe the general assessment of a patient with a headache and explain the significance of specific findings.

3. Describe the specific neurological patient evaluation and explain the significance of specific findings.

4. Given a description of several patients complaining of headache with different clinical findings, identify a patient who potentially has: a subarachnoid or other intracranial hemorrhage; meningitis; hypertensive encephalopathy; preeclampsia; carbon monoxide poisoning; tension headache; sinusitis; migraine; glaucoma; and hemophilia.

5. List potential complications for patients who present with a headache disorder.

6. Describe the general management of patients with the following specific headache disorders:
   a. Subarachnoid (or other intracranial) hemorrhage
   b. Meningitis
   c. Hypertensive encephalopathy
   d. Preeclampsia (toxemia of pregnancy)
   e. Carbon monoxide poisoning and other toxins
   f. Tension headache
   g. Sinusitis and dental disease
   h. Migraine
   i. Glaucoma
   j. Hemophilia

Headache is a common, usually benign condition experienced by virtually everyone at some time in their lives. Occasionally, headache is the presenting symptom of an acute, life-threatening emergency requiring immediate intervention.

The paramedic can distinguish life-threatening causes from those that are non-life threatening by determining the characteristics, associated signs and symptoms, and the patient's past medical history. A brief physical assessment of the patient should follow, with emphasis on the neurologic examination.

In general, patients with a headache severe enough to warrant a call to 9-1-1 should be transported for physician evaluation. If a life-threatening cause of headache is recognized, rapid stabilization and transport is crucial.

Pathophysiology

There are many pain-sensitive structures in the head and neck. These include all of the extracranial structures, such as the skin, blood vessels, nerves, and muscles. However, in the intracranial structures, only the meninges and a small portion of intracranial vasculature are pain sensitive.

The most common cause of pain in headache patients is tension or traction on anatomic structures (Fig. 33-1). Tension can cause spasm in scalp and neck muscles and result in a tension headache. If an intracranial mass or bleeding is present, the lesion activates sensory fibers to send impulses that are interpreted by the body as pain.

Vascular headaches, such as migraines, are caused by dilation and distention of blood vessels. Patients usually describe these headaches as "throbbing." Hypertension and certain toxic substances can also trigger headaches through the contraction or enlarging of blood vessels.

Lastly, inflammatory processes such as infection and hemorrhage can irritate peripheral nerves in the head and neck. Headache caused by meningitis occurs in a similar way. For instance, when the meninges at the base of the brain become inflamed, the patient will describe pain at the base of the skull.

Patient Assessment

History

Because only a minority of patients are found to have neurologic findings during physical examination, medical history questions take on added significance and provide clues to the underlying cause of headache in a majority of circumstances.

- *When did the headache start, and how severe is it?* Headache that begins suddenly (within seconds), rather than gradually (minutes to hours), usually indicates a more serious problem. "Sudden onset of the worst headache of my life" is a classic description of subarachnoid hemorrhage, which is a life-threatening emergency. In contrast, a tension headache, which is the most common type of headache, usually begins gradually over a period of 30 to 60 minutes.
- *Where is the pain located?* In a tension headache, pain is usually bilateral and involves the occipital and frontal areas of the head.

  Localized pain, particularly over one side of the face or forehead, may indicate sinusitis. Sinusitis occurs when the large air cells, or sinuses, underlying the face and forehead become congested or infected (Fig. 33-2).
- *Are there any associated symptoms?* Classic examples of headache may include fever, visual changes (e.g., blurred vision, double vision, vision loss, flashes of light), localized weakness or numbness (arm, leg, face), and vomiting. Associated symptoms such as these often indicate a more serious cause of headache.

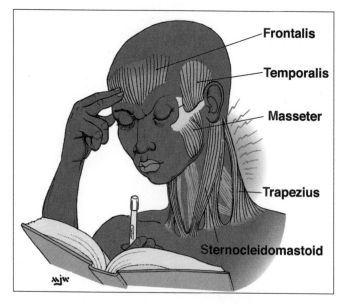

Figure 33-1

Tension headaches are usually caused by spasms of muscles in the head or neck.

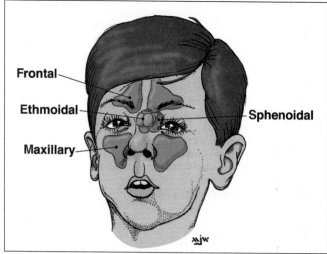

Figure 33-2

Expect localized pain when sinusitis (due to congestion or infection) is present.

- *Has there been a toxic exposure?* The possibility of patient exposure to toxic fumes should be explored, particularly in late fall or early winter when faulty heating systems may emit carbon monoxide and cause **carbon monoxide poisoning.** Patients who have been exposed to fumes and who complain of headache require immediate intervention. Carbon monoxide is the most likely inhaled toxic substance to cause headache. It may be present as either a component gas of fumes, such as in smoke or exhaust emission, or as a product of internal metabolism of certain body chemicals, such as methylene chloride, a common chemical in paint strippers.

- *What is the patient's past medical history?* The paramedic should ask whether the patient has experienced similar headaches in the past. Previous headaches of this type often indicate conditions such as tension or migraine headaches. Migraine sufferers often experience a neurologic prodrome (a symptom that precedes the onset of headache) such as flashes of light, half-loss of vision, and rarely, unilateral weakness or numbness.

- *Does the patient have a history of bleeding abnormalities or use of blood thinners?* Patients complaining of headache who have underlying bleeding abnormalities often have intracranial hemorrhage. An obvious example of such an abnormality is **hemophilia;** other examples include patients taking blood-thinning drugs (such as Coumadin) and patients with severe liver disease (e.g., alcoholic **cirrhosis and cancer**). Patients with bleeding abnormalities can have blood flow into the brain either spontaneously or following a minor injury.

CRITICAL ISSUE

A patient with an underlying bleeding abnormality (hemophilia) or a patient who is taking blood-thinning drugs who presents with severe headache is at extreme risk for an intracerebral hemorrhage.

- *Is the patient pregnant?* Women in the third trimester of pregnancy, in labor, or in the early postpartum period who complain of headache and who have elevated blood pressure should be considered to have **preeclampsia** (toxemia of pregnancy). Even a seemingly mild blood pressure elevation (a reading of 140/90 or greater) should be considered serious if it occurs during pregnancy.

Physical Examination

The physical examination should begin with a determination of the patient's mental status according to the AVPU scale (*see* Chapter 17). The patient's vital signs are also important. Hypertension, particularly when the diastolic pressure is above 120 mm Hg, can also cause headache. Severe hypertension that causes headache can suggest hypertensive crisis. Hypertensive **encephalopathy** may develop if appropriate treatment is not initiated.

Fever may be suggested by warm, flushed skin. Symptoms such as these in a patient with headache and stiff neck should raise the concern for the presence of meningitis.

CRITICAL ISSUE

Headache associated with fever and neck stiffness should be regarded as possible meningitis until proven otherwise.

The paramedic should examine the patient's pupils for size and reactivity, and look for gross abnormalities, such as redness or a cloudy cornea, which could indicate the presence of **glaucoma.**

Upon examination, the patient may either move the neck freely or hold it stiff and rigid. This stiffness, called *nuchal rigidity,* is seen with conditions of meningitis and subarachnoid hemorrhage.

Finally, a neurologic examination of the patient should be performed, including tests for motor strength in all extremities. The patient's face should be examined for signs of weakness, such as a unilateral facial droop. Is there any seizure activity on one or both sides of the patient's body? Patients experiencing subarachnoid hemorrhage may display a wide range of physical findings, from normal behavior to an altered mental status, pupil abnormalities, localized weakness, or seizures.

CRITICAL ISSUE

The patient who complains of headache and displays any neurologic abnormality should be considered to have a potentially life-threatening condition.

The paramedic must carefully note and document all neurologic findings on the prehospital care report. Periodic reexamination and documentation of changes in the patient's neurologic status during transport are also important.

With the exception of rare migraine episodes, most headaches do not result in neurologic abnormalities. However, the prehospital provider should regard the headache patient as having a potentially serious condition, even when neurologic findings are normal.

Key Conditions and Findings

- *Subarachnoid (or other **intracranial) hemorrhage.*** Subarachnoid hemorrhage is an acute spontaneous bleed in the brain, usually caused by a cerebral artery **aneurysm** or an arteriovenous malformation (Fig. 33-3). These patients often experience a sudden onset of a severe headache, vomiting, photophobia, neck stiffness, and great discomfort.

- *Meningitis.* Meningitis is an infection of the membranes covering the brain and spinal cord, usually caused by

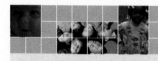
- Though headaches are usually mild and short lasting in children, they may, as in adults, be the only sign or symptom of a serious underlying medical condition or illness. The most common types of headaches in children are 1) inflammation or infection headaches, 2) vascular headaches, 3) trauma induced headaches and 4) other various causes.

- The two most serious causes of headaches due to an inflammation or infection are meningitis and encephalitis. Headaches are common with these conditions due to the inflammation of pain-sensitive structures or swelling and an increase in intracranial pressure. Fever, an altered level of consciousness for the child's age, lethargy,

pain in the neck, and increased irritability are other findings.

- Tumors, abscesses, eye strain, migraine, and epilepsy can also cause headaches in children. These causes are usually accompanied by other specific signs and symptoms related to the specific cause. Most common signs and symptoms include ataxia, lethargy, nausea, vomiting, as well as others. Headaches secondary to trauma are common and will be discussed in a separate chapter.

- Sinus infections and dental infections can also cause headaches in children. These are usually accompanied by pain to a specific area (jaw, eyes).

bacteria, virus, or fungus. In addition to headache, fever and neck stiffness, patients often complain of photophobia, nausea, vomiting, and chills.

- *Hypertensive encephalopathy.* Hypertensive encephalopathy is a diffuse (scattered) brain injury resulting from severe, uncontrolled hypertension. If, in addition to headache and hypertension, the patient experiences blurred vision, altered mental status, confusion, neck stiffness, or seizures, then hypertensive encephalopathy should be suspected.

- *Preeclampsia (toxemia of pregnancy).* Toxemia of pregnancy is characterized by elevated blood pressure, proteinuria, and edema and usually occurs in the last trimester. If not treated promptly, preeclampsia can result in death of both the mother and fetus.

- *Carbon monoxide and other toxic poisoning.* Patients exposed to carbon monoxide or other toxic gases may

present with headache, nausea, vomiting, chest pain, confusion, seizures, or unresponsiveness.

- *Tension headache.* This throbbing headache often can be stress-related. It begins bilaterally in front of the head and often radiates to the occipital region.

- *Sinusitis and dental disease.* Patients with sinusitis often complain of nasal congestion, tenderness over the cheeks or forehead, and pain that intensifies when he or she lowers the head. Dental pain can also frequently cause headache on the same side as the dental problem.

- *Migraine.* This headache is severe and throbbing in nature and may be unilateral or bilateral in origin. Nausea and vomiting are common symptoms.

- *Glaucoma.* Localized pain, redness, visual loss, a cloudy cornea, and pupillary abnormalities involving one eye usually indicate the presence of acute glaucoma in a patient.

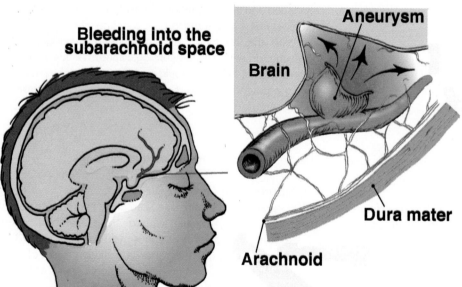

Figure 33-3

A subarachnoid hemorrhage is a life-threatening condition and can occur anywhere within the arachnoid space. It is often caused by an aneurysm or AV malformation.

- *Hemophilia.* This includes a number of disorders, usually hereditary, that prevent the blood from clotting normally after injury. Hemophiliac patients are prone to internal bleeding, often following minor trauma.

Management

Most patients with headaches can be managed supportively and should be transported in a position of comfort.

Intravenous access, 100% oxygen, and cardiac monitoring are indicated when any potentially life-threatening condition is recognized in a patient. The IV is established in case the patient develops seizures, dysrhythmias, or severe hypertension or hypotension. Generally, the IV should be maintained at a keep-open rate, unless hypotension requires fluid boluses. High-concentration oxygen is particularly important for patients who suffer from possible carbon-monoxide exposure. Severe hypertension (systolic greater than 200 mm Hg, diastolic greater than 120 mm Hg) is generally treated using standard protocols in consultation with medical direction. An effective antihypertensive medication often used in the prehospital setting is nitroglycerin, administered sublingually or orally in spray form. Medical direction should be consulted prior to treating hypertension, particularly in the pregnant patient.

Finally, the patient should be transported rapidly to the nearest appropriate facility. Patients with suspected intracranial hemorrhage should be transported *immediately* to a hospital with neurosurgical capabilities. Pregnant women with headache and hypertension should be transported to a facility with emergency obstetric capabilities. Although not a life-threatening condition, glaucoma can cause permanent blindness; it is important for these patients to receive prompt evaluation by an ophthalmologist. Finally, patients with suspected carbon monoxide poisoning should be transported to a hospital with a hyperbaric oxygen chamber.

Because certain forms of meningitis are contagious, prehospital providers should protect themselves by wearing masks, gowns, and gloves when meningitis is suspected.

SUMMARY

Life-threatening causes of headache can be recognized during the initial patient assessment. Characteristics of such headache include sudden onset in pain, fever and neck stiffness, history of bleeding abnormalities, severe hypertension, pregnancy, exposure to fumes, and abnormal neurologic examination results. Once a life-threatening condition is recognized, treatment must be quick and decisive. Airway control, oxygen administration, IV initiation, and treatment of associated dysrhythmias, seizures, and severe blood pressure elevations are all crucial. Finally, the patient should be transported rapidly to the nearest appropriate facility.

REFERENCES

1. **Henry GL: Headache.** In Rosen P (ed): *Emergency Medicine, Concepts and Clinical Practice,* ed 2, St. Louis, 1988, CV Mosby.

2. **Hoffman GL: Headache.** In Tintinalli (ed): *Emergency Medicine, A Comprehensive Study Guide,* ed 3, New York, 1992, McGraw-Hill.

Richard N. Nelson, MD, FACEP

Chapter 34

Weak, Dizzy, and Malaise

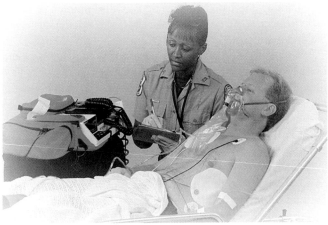

A paramedic should be able to:

OBJECTIVES

1. Describe the pathophysiology, common causes, and signs and symptoms for the following chief complaints:
   a. Weakness
   b. Dizziness/lightheadedness
   c. Malaise
2. Identify the structures that control the functions of equilibrium and spatial orientation.
3. Identify the historical and physical examination data to obtain for patients with these complaints.
4. Describe the significance and potential life-threatening conditions that can be associated with these complaints.
5. Discuss general field management for patients with these complaints and specific management of life-threatening conditions.

KEY TERMS

1. **Anemia**—a disorder characterized by a decrease in hemoglobin in the blood to levels below the normal range, caused by decreased red cell production, or increased red cell destruction, or blood loss.
2. **Vertigo**—a sensation of movement: as if the external world were revolving around the person, or the body itself were spinning.
3. **Hyperkalemia**—a condition in which the potassium in the blood is abnormally high.
4. **Hypoglycemia**—a condition in which the glucose in the blood is abnormally low.
5. **Infection**—the growth of an organism in a suitable host, with or without detectable signs of illness.
6. **Malaise**—a vague feeling of bodily discomfort.
7. **Shock**—a condition in which body tissues are not receiving adequate blood and oxygen; often related to a drop in blood pressure or cardiac output.

O ccasionally, paramedics will encounter a patient whose symptoms are vague and nonspecific. "I feel weak," "I'm dizzy," and "I ache all over" are complaints dreaded by emergency care workers because of the number of conditions they may represent. Although many of these patients will not have true emergencies, some patients do have life-threatening conditions. The EMS provider who is skilled in patient assessment will recognize patients who require rapid intervention and transport.

Pathophysiology

Generalized weakness implies a condition affecting the patient's entire body, and localized weakness implies a cause affecting only the brain (e.g., a stroke) or a specific nerve.

Electrolyte disorders are common causes of generalized weakness; usually an abnormally high or low potassium level is involved. Potassium is essential for transmission of electrical impulses through nerves and muscles, including the heart. Severe elevation or depression of potassium levels (hyper- or hypokalemia, respectively) slows these impulses, causing the patient to feel extremely weak. The most common cause of hyperkalemia is renal failure, because nonfunctioning kidneys cannot excrete potassium. Patients with renal failure who have missed their dialysis sessions or have eaten foods high in potassium are at special risk. The most common cause of hypokalemia is diuretic use, especially among patients being treated for hypertension or congestive heart failure.

Anemia is defined as a deficiency of hemoglobin in the blood (Fig. 34-1). Because hemoglobin carries oxygen to the tissues, low hemoglobin levels result in less oxygen delivered throughout the body. Consequently, the anemic patient feels weak, tired and sometimes short of breath. The most common causes of anemia are related to chronic blood loss.

Sickle cell anemia is a hereditary form of anemia occurring primarily in black patients. Because the hemoglobin is abnormal, the red blood cells develop a "sickle" shape and are more prone to hemolysis (bursting) as the blood becomes more acidotic.

Severe infections are often associated with weakness or malaise (a vague feeling of bodily discomfort). Sepsis is a life-threatening infection, usually caused by bacteria in the bloodstream. The condition usually starts as a local infection (e.g., pneumonia, cellulitis, urinary tract infection) before spreading to the bloodstream. Signs and symptoms of sepsis include fever, hypothermia (especially in the elderly), tachycardia and hypotension.

An example of localized weakness is seen when pressure on the spinal cord produces cord dysfunction. Causes include tumor, blood clot, infection (abscess formation) and herniated disc. Patients with cord compression in the neck develop weakness and numbness of the arms and legs. Patients with cord compression in the lower back develop weakness and numbness in the legs only.

Dizziness is a very imprecise term which patients may use to describe vertigo or a general feeling of light-headedness or faintness. Vertigo is often described as feeling that the environment around the patient is spinning, and usually is caused by an abnormality in the structures controlling the functions of equilibrium and spatial orientation. These structures include

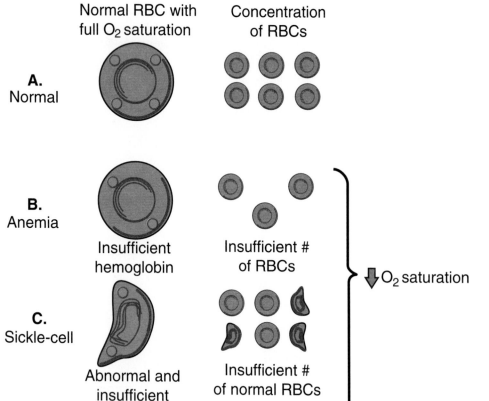

A.
Normal

Normal RBC with full O₂ saturation

Concentration of RBCs

B.
Anemia

Insufficient hemoglobin

Insufficient # of RBCs

C.
Sickle-cell

Abnormal and insufficient hemoglobin

Insufficient # of normal RBCs

↓O₂ saturation

Figure 34-1

Normal concentration of RBCs with complete saturation of oxygen (A) contrasted with anemia conditions in which there is an insufficient amount of hemoglobin or an insufficient number of normal RBCs (B and C).

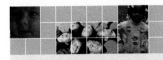

PEDIATRIC PERSPECTIVE

- Weakness, dizziness, and malaise alone do not alert the paramedic to one specific pediatric illness or emergency. They are, however, signs and symptoms of other illnesses which include diabetic emergencies, GI disorders, sepsis, dehydration, and others. These signs and symptoms can also be the result of drug ingestions, overdoses or intoxications, and trauma.

the middle and inner ear, brainstem, cerebellum, and cerebral cortex.

Light-headedness is a common complaint that may be associated with any disease process that results in an alteration of mental status or a decrease in cerebral blood flow. Among the many mechanisms that may result in this symptom is any cause of decreased cardiac output, such as hypovolemia or a dysrhythmia. The central nervous system can be affected by hypoxia, medications (sedatives, antihistamines), and psychogenic causes (such as hyperventilation syndrome), producing this symptom as well.

Patient Assessment

When evaluating the patient who complains of weakness, dizziness, or malaise, the paramedic must attempt to define the complaints further.

History

- *Is the weakness generalized or localized?* With generalized weakness, all movements and extremities are equally affected. Localized weakness involves a specific region of the body, such as the left side of the body or the right arm.
- *Does the patient feel dizzy or lightheaded?* The word *dizzy* means different things to different people. To some, dizziness means a spinning sensation as if the room is moving in circles. This is called *vertigo* and is often associated with nausea and vomiting. Vertigo usually involves an abnormality of the balance center located in the inner ear, but may also be caused by a central nervous system disease. To others, dizziness means light-headedness, such as the sensation a patient experiences prior to passing out. Light-headedness implies temporary hypoperfusion and may have numerous causes, the most serious of which are related to diminished cerebral perfusion pressure from shock or dysrhythmias. Generally, the paramedic should attempt to identify a patient as suffering from vertigo or light-headedness.

- *Does the patient complain of malaise? Malaise* is defined as a vague feeling of bodily discomfort. The most common causes of malaise are related to illness from bacteria or viruses, often leading to fever and generalized discomfort. If nausea, vomiting, diarrhea, and poor oral intake are part of the patient's illness, dehydration can occur, furthering the feeling of malaise.
- *Is there any history of bleeding?* The presence of black, tarry stools indicates blood loss in the GI tract. There may be a history of congenital blood disorders, such as sickle cell anemia, which can result in similar complaints. Excessively heavy or prolonged menstrual periods can result in anemia and the complaint of weakness or light-headedness.
- *Are there any aggravating or relieving factors?* Light-headedness can worsen when the patient moves from a lying to a sitting or standing position, possibly indicating hypovolemia.

CRITICAL ISSUE

Sudden, nonpositional light-headedness associated with syncope often occurs secondary to a cardiac dysrhythmia.

- *Are there any associated symptoms?* Fever often potentiates the feeling of weakness and malaise. Associated pain, particularly in the head, neck, or back, may be associated with certain types of stroke or spinal cord compression. Nausea and vomiting often occur with disorders causing vertigo, and patients may also exhibit uncoordination (ataxia) or an unsteady gait. The complaint of palpitations can be seen in the presence of a cardiac dysrhythmia and may be accompanied by a syncopal event.
- *What is the patient's past medical history?* Past medical history is crucial when evaluating the weak and dizzy patient. Such patients may have experienced similar episodes in the past. In many cases, underlying medical conditions, such as diabetes, renal failure, cancer, hypertension, and cardiac disease, are contributing factors.

CRITICAL ISSUE

Although many of these complaints are frustratingly nonspecific, they should not be attributed to a benign, psychogenic cause in the prehospital setting. Patient management strategies should be chosen based on the possible presence of life-threatening conditions.

CRITICAL ISSUE

Severe, generalized weakness in a renal dialysis patient is frequently the result of hyperkalemia.

- *Is the patient taking medication?* Diuretics are commonly prescribed and have been repeatedly associated with electrolyte abnormalities such as hypokalemia. Sedatives are also used frequently and can cause weakness, either individually or in combination with other medications.

Physical Examination

The physical examination begins with an accurate set of vital signs, including a tilt–test evaluation (*see* Chapter 29, Syncope). Tachycardic patients or patients with positive orthostatic signs may be suffering from hypovolemia secondary to blood loss or dehydration.

The skin may show evidence of hypoperfusion by being cool, moist, or pale. Other signs of anemia may include pallor of the conjunctivae or the oral mucous membranes. Capillary refill of the extremities may also be delayed longer than 2 seconds.

Respiratory examination is performed next. The patient may appear to be in respiratory distress and using accessory muscles of respiration. Tidal volume may also be diminished as a result of inadequate respiratory excursion caused by muscular fatigue. In such cases, the patient's breath sounds will be decreased in all fields. It is important to rule out primary respiratory disease, as well as the potential cause of respiratory distress.

Finally, a neurologic examination should be performed. Disorientation is often the initial sign of a toxic or metabolic problem (e.g., drugs, carbon monoxide poisoning, hypoglycemia) or a cerebral perfusion problem (e.g., shock or cardiac dysrhythmia). The patient's pupils should be checked for reactivity and it should be noted if the patient is able to move the eyes in all four directions. As eye movement is tested, the patient may exhibit rapid, alternating movements of the eye known as nystagmus. Nystagmus is usually present with vertigo and often is caused by inner ear dysfunction but may also be related to drug toxicity or cerebellar dysfunction. The patient should be examined for abnormal motor or sensory findings. Any deficits, particularly if they are localized, should be noted.

Key Conditions and Findings

Generalized Weakness

Weakness presenting as a generalized symptom may indicate:

- *Anemia.* The most common causes of anemia are chronic blood loss and congenital abnormalities, usually in the form of abnormal hemoglobin.
- *Electrolyte Abnormalities.* Abnormal levels of potassium frequently result in weakness from muscular dysfunction. In many cases, patients will have a history of renal failure or diuretic use.
- *Cardiac Ischemia.* In elderly or diabetic patients, cardiac ischemia may present without the typical complaints and only be demonstrated by lethargy or weakness.

Localized Weakness

Localized weakness may be seen with:

- *Cerebrovascular Accident.* Usually, weakness or paralysis involves one or both extremities on the same side of the patient's body.
- *Nerve Compression.* Pressure can be placed on nerves from a variety of sources. A common cause of spinal nerve root compression is a herniated disc, which usually occurs at lumbar levels.

Dizziness

Dizziness is generally classified into two groups of causes. Those presenting with vertigo include:

- *Inner Ear Disorders.* These disorders can result from viral infections or trauma; and can also be positional in nature.
- *Central Nervous System Disorders.* In most cases, the area of the brain that is involved is the cerebellum. Tumors, hemorrhage, and ischemia all can initiate cerebellar dysfunction. Because the cerebellum controls coordination, ataxia is often present.

Causes presenting as light-headedness include:

- *Hypoperfusion.* Shock or decreased blood flow causing light-headedness is most concerning when caused by hypovolemia and when cardiac dysfunction arises from a dysrhythmia.
- *Toxicologic and Metabolic Conditions.* Many drugs, particularly antihypertensives and antidepressants, can result in orthostatic hypotension. Hypoglycemia and inhaled toxins, such as carbon monoxide, are also sources of concern.

Malaise

Malaise is often present with:

- *Infections.* Whether bacterial, viral or fungal, infections frequently cause malaise. The more systemic an infection has become, the more probable it is that a patient will show signs of malaise.
- *Dehydration.* Dehydration accompanies many of the disorders already mentioned and worsens many metabolic abnormalities already present.

Management

When a potentially life-threatening cause of weakness, dizziness, or malaise is recognized, the EMS provider must act quickly. If the patient is unable to protect the airway or shows evidence of respiratory compromise, the patient should be intubated and ventilated with 100% oxygen. Other patients may be placed on oxygen at lower flow rates.

Intravenous access with a large-bore catheter is then established. Patients with signs of hypoperfusion should receive

A. MILD-MODERATE

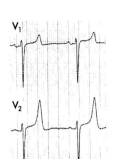

B. MODERATE-SEVERE

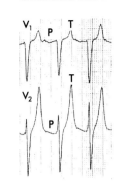

C. VERY SEVERE

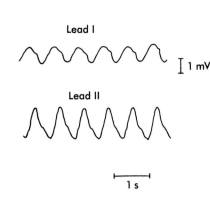

Lead I

Lead II

1 mV

1 s

Figure 34-2

ECG changes seen with hyperkalemia include tall, peaked T-waves, widened QRS, and a loss of P-waves. From Goldberger: Clinical electrocardiography, ed 5, 1994, Mosby-Year Book, Inc.

normal saline or Ringer's lactate fluid boluses to support blood pressure and improve tissue perfusion.

Patients with an altered level of responsiveness require rapid blood glucose determination when available, and may be given 50% IV dextrose. Patients with pinpoint pupils or other evidence of opiate overdose should receive IV naloxone.

Cardiac monitoring is important in patients complaining of weakness or dizziness, especially those in whom cardiac disease, hypoperfusion, or metabolic abnormalities are suspected. Hyperkalemia causes characteristic ECG changes which include tall, peaked T-waves and loss of P-waves (Fig. 34-2). At higher blood potassium levels, the QRS complex widens. If hyperkalemia is suspected, medical direction should be contacted to consider the IV administration of sodium bicarbonate or calcium chloride. Other therapies used in the emergency department include IV dextrose, insulin, and oral potassium-binding resins. Definitive management is achieved with hemodialysis.

The remainder of prehospital management is supportive. Generally, patient transport should be to the nearest appropriate hospital in a position of comfort. Patients who are reluctant to be transported must be informed of a possible recurrence or worsening of the problem. Patients should also be made aware that symptoms may recur during routine activities, such as driving a car, operating machinery, or climbing stairs.

SUMMARY

Patients complaining of weakness, dizziness, and malaise present a challenge to even the most experienced EMS providers. Historical data concerning the patient's symptoms (e.g., vertigo, light-headedness, generalized weakness, localized weakness) are the most useful in directing management. Life-threatening causes, such as hypovolemia, sepsis, arrhythmias, hypoglycemia, hyperkalemia, stroke, and myocardial ischemia, should be recognized early and treated accordingly.

SUGGESTED READINGS

1. **Davis E:** Emergency department approach to vertigo. *Emerg Med Clin North Am* 5(2):1987.

2. **Kohn MS:** Weakness. In Rosen P (ed): Emergency Medicine, Concepts and Clinical Practice, ed 2, St. Louis, 1988, CV Mosby.

3. **Little N:** Vertigo and dizziness. In Tintinalli (ed): Emergency Medicine. A Comprehensive Study Guide, ed 3, New York, 1992, McGraw-Hill.

4. **Schultz KE:** Vertigo and syncope. In Rosen P (ed): Emergency Medicine Concepts and Clinical Practice, ed 2, St. Louis, 1988, CV Mosby.

Michelle Blanda, MD, FACEP
Paul Clancy, MD

Chapter 35

Diabetic Emergencies

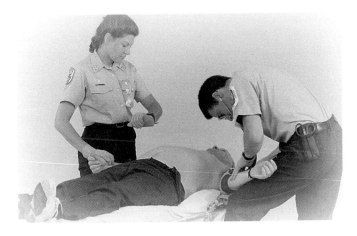

A paramedic should be able to:

iabetes mellitus (DM) is the most common endocrine disorder, affecting many organs and leading to multiple complications. Diabetes mellitus occurs in an estimated 3% of the American population.[12] Insulin-dependent diabetes mellitus comprises 7% to 10% of these cases. Because the EMS system is used frequently by patients with diabetes, it is important for the paramedic to be aware of the problems associated with the disease and its complications.

Pathophysiology

Insulin is produced in the pancreas and released into the blood stream in response to elevations in blood sugar. Insulin assists glucose uptake by the cells, allows excess glucose to be stored in the liver and muscle, and aids in fat synthesis (Fig. 35-1).

Other cells in the pancreas make different hormones that are also important in glucose metabolism. One of these is glucagon. When glucose is not reaching cells, either because of inadequate food intake or lack of insulin, the body perceives

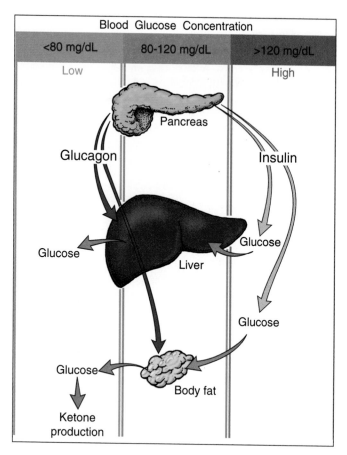

Figure 35-1

The interaction of the hormones insulin and glucagon with the body. Glucose can enter cells because of the presence of the hormone insulin. When glucagon is present, glucose is released from its stored form in the liver and is available for the body's cells.

a fasting state and releases glucagon to elevate blood sugar. Glucagon causes the breakdown of stored sugars in the liver and stored fat in the body. Fat metabolism results in ketone production as a breakdown product. Ketones are acidic and lead to a lowered blood pH (acidosis). It is this process of ketone and acid formation (ketoacidosis) that can lead to one of the acute diabetic complications called diabetic ketoacidosis.

Diabetes Mellitus

Diabetes mellitus is a disorder of carbohydrate metabolism caused by inadequate amounts of insulin. The hallmark of the disease is elevated blood sugar (hyperglycemia). Diabetes can be separated into disease presentations. Type I, also known as insulin-dependent diabetes mellitus (IDDM) or "juvenile onset diabetes mellitus," usually develops prior to early adulthood. Insulin dependent diabetes mellitus in the United States is estimated to develop in approximately 120,000 individuals aged 19 years and under.[10] Patients with Type I DM produce almost no insulin and consequently may develop markedly elevated glucose levels. Ketoacidosis can develop when metabolic acids accumulate in the blood secondary to the breakdown of stored body fat. Patients with IDDM are dependent on insulin therapy for survival.

Type II, or noninsulin-dependent diabetes mellitus (NIDDM), usually appears in patients over 40 years of age. Patients with NIDDM are able to produce insulin, but only in decreased amounts. These patients require diet control, oral medication, or additional insulin to control blood sugar levels. Ketoacidosis rarely occurs in Type II diabetics because some insulin is produced. Differences between the two types of diabetes are listed in Table 35-1.

Hypoglycemia

The most common diabetes-related emergencies that lead to EMS calls relate to either too little or too much sugar in the blood. Normal blood sugar levels are between 80 to 120 mg/dL. Abnormally low blood sugar, referred to as hypoglycemia, may result from a decrease in food intake with regular insulin administration, an error in insulin administration, or a combination of the two. Patients who follow a strict insulin protocol to keep blood sugar tightly controlled are prone to more frequent and more severe hypoglycemic episodes. Patients taking certain oral hypoglycemic agents are also at risk for hypoglycemia for up to 36 hours after administration of these medications.

Unrecognized hypoglycemia will lead to death. The cells of the body, especially the brain, are dependent on glucose to function. Without glucose, the cells may find other sources of energy, but their breakdown products will be toxic and eventually lethal if the process is not reversed. Permanent brain damage may occur in patients who survive hypoglycemic events because the cells of the brain do not have the ability to store or use other sources of energy, as does the rest of the body.[1,7,10]

- Type I diabetes, or insulin-dependent diabetes, is the most common type of diabetes encountered in children and adolescents. Type II diabetes (noninsulin dependent) is less common in children under 18 years of age, but can occur in teenagers who are either overweight or obese.
- In the child and the adolescent, it is often difficult to regulate food intake and insulin dosage because of growth and physical activity.
- The clinical presentations of hyperglycemia and hypoglycemia are subtle and variable in children. Rapid glucose determination is recommended prior to treatment.
- Infants are more prone to hypoglycemia when stressed, because their bodies inadequately store glycogen. A symptomatic newborn with a glucose level of less than 40 mg should be treated with 10% Dextrose. This solution is prepared by diluting 1 part $D_{50}W$ into 4 parts of sterile water or normal saline. A 3- to 4-mL/kg bolus is administered in the infant. It is important to note that a secure IV line is essential when administering D_{10} or D_{25}. Hypertonic glucose solutions can cause severe damage to tissues if the IV infiltrates.
- Infants with prematurity, infants with sepsis, infants of diabetic mothers, infants with hypothermia, and infants experiencing a prolonged or stressful delivery are at risk for hypoglycemia.
- Signs and symptoms of hypoglycemia in the neonate include apnea, respiratory distress, decreased muscle tone, jitteriness or seizures, or lethargy.
- A child is considered hypoglycemic with a blood sugar level of less than 60 mg and should be treated with 25% Dextrose. This solution is prepared by diluting 1 part $D_{50}W$ into 1 part sterile water or normal saline. A 2-mL/kg dose is administered IV.

Diabetic Ketoacidosis

Diabetic ketoacidosis (DKA) is a dangerous complication of diabetes. This condition occurs approximately 10 times more often in patients less than 15 years of age.[5] The overall mortality rate is 9% to 14% per episode.[6] It generally occurs in patients who are insulin-dependent, but 20% to 30% of all cases of DKA are the first manifestation of undiagnosed diabetes mellitus.[4] Precipitating causes are found in 70% to 80% of patients, with infection and medication noncompliance being the most common factors.

DKA is caused by an insufficient amount of insulin. In the liver, stored glucose is released into the blood and hyperglycemia results. Once these stores are depleted, body fats containing fatty acids are broken down to form glucose. The byproducts of fatty acid breakdown are ketone bodies, which acidify the blood. As glucose levels rise, the kidney's ability to retain glucose is overwhelmed, and glucose is lost into the urine (Fig. 35-2). This glucose loss also draws water and electrolytes out of the blood and into the urine. Urination increases, resulting in volume loss and dehydration. Volume loss in adult DKA patients ranges from 4 to 10 liters.[2,8]

Ketones are excreted poorly by the kidneys, and then only when combined with sodium. As sodium is excreted, it is replaced by hydrogen ions; this substitution further elevates the acidosis.

Hyperglycemia

Hyperglycemia can occur in some patients without the development of DKA. Many diabetics routinely have elevated blood sugars with essentially normal acid-base status. Insulin deficiency, other glucose regulating hormones, and dehydration can all contribute to hyperglycemia. It is not known why some patients develop acidosis and others do not.

Hyperosmolar Coma

Nonketotic hyperosmolar coma (NKHC), also called hyperosmolar hyperglycemic nonketotic coma (HHNC), is characterized by central nervous system dysfunction associated with severe hyperglycemia, dehydration and hyperosmolarity. It is similar to DKA, but there is no ketosis. The reason for the

TABLE 35-1	Comparison of Type I and Type II Diabetes	
	Type I (IDDM)	**Type II (NIDDM)**
Name	Insulin-dependent diabetes mellitus	NonInsulin-dependent diabetes mellitus
Pathology	No insulin production	Decreased insulin production
Age of Onset	Childhood peak age 10–14	Adulthood > age 40
Required Treatment	Insulin	Diet control, oral agents, insulin
Tendency for Ketoacidosis	Strong	Weak

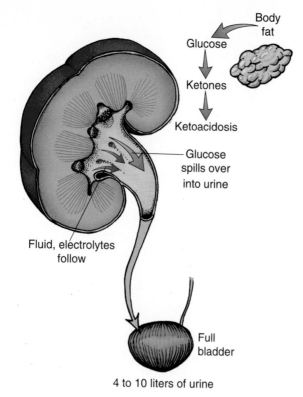

Glucose

Body
fat

Ketones

Ketoacidosis

Glucose
spills over
into urine

Fluid, electrolytes
follow

Full
bladder

4 to 10 liters of urine

Figure 35-2

Diabetic ketoacidosis (DKA) affects the kidney and results in an increase in urination.

---

lack of ketosis is not well understood. It is more common in patients over 60 years of age who have NIDDM. Caucasians, women, and institutionalized or mentally impaired individuals are also found to be at risk for NIDDM. Precipitating factors include dehydration, medications such as steroids and thiazides, acute illness, cerebral vacular disease, advanced age, and rarely new diagnosis of diabetes.[11] This occurrence may be because these patients have abnormal thirst mechanisms that lead to dehydration. Mortality may be as high as 50% in this patient group.

The predominant presentation is that of abnormal mental status, which may vary from lethargy to coma. Unlike DKA, focal neurologic deficits, such as seizures or hemiplegia, can occur and may resolve with treatment of the hyperosmolar state.

Chronic Diabetic Problems

Longstanding diabetes can lead to multisystem problems that may require EMS intervention. There is evidence that diabetics with well-controlled blood sugars will likely have fewer complications from the disease.[3] Diabetic neuropathy is damage to nerves that results in numbness, tingling, and decreased sensation. It accounts for the lack of pain in some diabetics who have heart attacks, impotence, orthostatic hypotension, and an inability to urinate.

It is likely that all blood vessels in a diabetic patient are abnormal. Small-vessel disease (microangiopathy) is caused by thickening of the lining of the vessels. The small vessels of the

eyes and kidneys are commonly affected, and the condition can progress to renal failure or blindness.

Large vessels of the heart, brain, and lower extremities develop atherosclerosis plaque formation more often in diabetic patients than in nondiabetic. This is why heart disease and cerebrovascular disease are major contributors to the decreased life expectancy in diabetics.

Foot problems are also common. Ulcers form and do not heal well because of poor blood supply, impaired wound healing, and decreased nerve function. Infections commonly develop, and may become chronic. When the bones become infected (osteomyelitis), amputation is inevitable.

Patient Assessment

When assessing diabetic patients, the paramedic must be aware of potential conditions that can cause rapid deterioration and death. These conditions are frequently identified by history, physical findings, and rapid blood glucose determination or administration (Table 35-2).

The signs and symptoms of hypoglycemia are rapidly reversible. Its diagnosis and management are based on obtaining a history of diabetes dependent on insulin or medication and on observing altered mental status. Because of the easily reversible nature of this disease, management may precede a complete patient assessment.

History

- *Is there any complaint or report of altered mental status?* A common reason for EMS system activation for a diabetic is an altered level of responsiveness. The mental status change may range from "not feeling right" to confusion or unresponsiveness. Complaints of being weak, dizzy, and lightheaded are frequent because of poor oral intake, vomiting, or increased urination, all of which lead to dehydration in the patient. Hypoglycemia causes central nervous system dysfunction that may also present as irritability, headache, seizures, or loss of coordination. Bizarre behavior and inappropriate anger can also be caused by hypoglycemia.
- *How quickly did the patient's mental status change?* A rapid onset of altered mentation suggests hypoglycemia, whereas gradual onset more likely indicates hyperglycemia (either DKA or hyperosmolar coma).
- *Does the patient complain of thirst or frequent urination?* Polydipsia (excessive thirst), polyuria (frequent urination), and polyphagia (excessive eating) are common presenting symptoms of new-onset or worsening diabetes and are characteristics of the hyperosmolar state and dehydration seen with elevated blood sugar levels.

    Other associated symptoms include abdominal complaints (nausea, vomiting, and abdominal pain), fatigue, and visual disturbances.
- *What is the patient's medication history and diet?* Patients and their families should be questioned specifically

TABLE 35-2	Assessment Findings of Diabetic Emergencies		
Findings	Hyperglycemia with Diabetic Ketoacidosis	Hyperosmolar Hyperglycemic Nonketotic Coma	Hypoglycemia
History			
Onset of episode	Gradual, over several days	Gradual, over several days	Usually rapid, over a period of hours or minutes
Precipitating event	Infection, illness, medication noncompliance	Stroke, infection	Not eating and taking insulin, excessive exercise
Hunger	No appetite	Normal to decreased	Intense
Thirst	Intense	Intense	Absent
Insulin history	Insufficient or absent	Insufficient or absent	Regular or excessive
Food/sugar intake	Normal or excessive	Normal or excessive	Insufficient
Urination	Increased frequency	Increased frequency	Unchanged, possible incontinence
General	Weak, dehydrated	Weak, usually elderly	Weak
Physical Examination			
LOC	Decreased LOC, restless to unresponsive	Lethargy to unresponsive	Altered—irritable, abnormally aggressive, bizarre behavior, to unresponsive
CNS	Headache, visual disturbances	Seizures, hemiplegia	Headache, dizziness, tremors, seizures
Respiratory Early Late	Slight increase in rate Kussmaul's breathing— deep and rapid breathing	Normal to increased rate	Slowed or normal rate
Cardiovascular	Weak, rapid pulse, normal or low blood pressure; dysrhythmias may occur secondary to electrolyte imbalance	Weak, rapid pulse, decreasing blood pressure	Normal or rapid and full pulse, normal blood pressure
Gastrointestinal Nausea/vomiting Abdominal pain	Present nonspecific pain, tenderness, distention	Rare Absent	Rare Absent
Odor (Ketone) on breath	Present	Absent	Absent unless fasting has occurred over several days and muscle tissue is breaking down into ketones
Skin	Dry, warm, possible tenting	Possible tenting	Pale, cool, clammy

about similar episodes, because many are familiar with the signs and symptoms of high and low blood sugar. A decrease in the usual amount of food intake is a common precipitating factor for hypoglycemia. Malnutrition secondary to chronic diseases or alcoholism may also predispose to hypoglycemia. The paramedic should inquire as to any recent changes in the type or dose of insulin or oral hypoglycemic agents being used (see Table 35-3 for related patient medications). A patient may have an insulin pump implanted that can malfunction or administer an excessive dose of medication.

Physical Examination

The physical examination begins with assessment of patient airway and respiratory status, mental status, skin color, and temperature. Many diabetic patients wear Medic Alert[R] tags that can provide diagnostic clues in patients who are unresponsive.

The patient's rate and rhythm of respirations should be assessed. A slight increase in respiratory rate is seen early in DKA. Kussmaul respirations (deep, rapid and intense respirations) may develop later. Hypoglycemic patients may have slowed or normal respiratory rates.

Tachycardia is commonly seen in hypoglycemic patients and those in DKA. Irregular or bradycardic rates may represent underlying cardiac disease or a serious dysrhythmia caused by electrolyte imbalance. Blood pressure may be decreased secondary to dehydration or underlying cardiac disease. Orthostatic vital signs can be less reliable in a diabetic because of diabetic neuropathy.

The patient's skin should also be assessed for tenting or loss of elasticity, both conditions suggesting dehydration. Cool, clammy skin with diaphoresis often accompanies hypoglycemia because of sympathetic nervous system activation. Hypothermia is a common presentation.

Facial features suggestive of dehydration include sunken eyes, a furrowed tongue, and dry mucous membranes.

TABLE 35-3 Medications Related to Diabetes

Classification	Specific Drug		Indication	Therapeutic Action	Side Effects And Precautions
DIABETIC MEDICATIONS					
Oral Hypoglycemics	Orinase Dymelor Tolinase	Micronase Diabinese Diabeta	Diabetes mellitus (adult onset, Type II)	Stimulates body's production of insulin	Hypoglycemia Brain death caused by hypoglycemia
Insulin	Regular NPH Lente		Diabetes mellitus (Juvenile onset, Type I)	Replaces body's insulin Transports glucose across cell membranes	

Abdominal examination may show nonspecific pain, tenderness, or distention which occur in DKA. Focal findings such as right lower quadrant tenderness may also be present. The paramedic should remember that infection and pregnancy are common causes of DKA and should be considered.

Neurologic evaluation is important and should focus on determination of the patient's mental status. Seizures may occur secondary to hypoglycemia, and usually resolve with administration of glucose. Hypoglycemic patients may be psychotic, violent, or hyperactive, although DKA patients can appear apathetic.

CRITICAL ISSUE

Neurologic deficits may be seen in patients with high or low blood sugar levels.

Management

Establishment of an adequate airway is always a first priority, and diabetes is no exception. Airway should be assessed while patient history is obtained. Any patient with respiratory distress requires airway stabilization and administration of high-flow oxygen by mask. Cardiac monitoring and pulse oximetry should be used if available.

A rapid blood sugar determination is ideal for all known diabetic patients and all patients with altered mental status, preferably prior to any glucose administration. Any diabetic adult who is not awake and oriented, or a patient with a blood glucose reading of 70 or less, should receive 50 mL of IV 50% dextrose (D50). A red- or gray-top tube of blood should be drawn so that a more precise blood sugar evaluation can be performed at the hospital. Symptomatic children with a blood glucose level of 50 or less should receive 2 to 4 mL/kg of 25% dextrose (D25). Symptomatic infants should receive 10% dextrose when blood sugar levels are below 40 mg %.

CRITICAL ISSUE

Glucose should be administered to all diabetic patients with a severely altered mental status, unless a blood glucose reading in the high range is obtained. This procedure may be life saving in a hypoglycemic patient and will do no harm to a patient with hyperglycemia.

Intravenous glucose should also be administered to unresponsive patients with an unknown blood glucose level. This administration will not harm hyperglycemic patients as long as definitive therapy is initiated promptly. $D_{50}W$ is extremely irritating to the peripheral veins and should be administered slowly over 3 to 5 minutes, with a maintenance IV continuing to run open. Most patients should be functioning at their normal, baseline mentation within 5 to 10 minutes. Some patients who have had a prolonged hypoglycemic period may have a longer recovery time. Rarely, patients who are hypoglycemic for extended amounts of time sustain irreversible brain injury. If IV access is unobtainable, glucagon can be administered IM. If the patient is alert and refusing treatment or transport, sugar can be administered orally and then recommend complex carbohydrates. A quick boost of simple sugar (glucose) without a more prolonged carbohydrate load will lead to repeat hypoglycemia in the patient.

If there is a possibility that the patient is alcoholic, D50 administration should be preceded or closely followed by IV thiamine, if available. Alcoholics generally have depleted most of their stored thiamine, and some evidence suggests that Wernicke's encephalopathy can be precipitated by a large load of glucose that rapidly exhausts the small remaining thiamine reserve.

Awake patients with glucose levels less than 70 can be given juice or other similar forms of glucose by mouth, as long as they are competent to administer the liquid themselves without assistance.

Hypotensive patients and patients with signs of dehydration or hypoperfusion should be administered isotonic IV fluids, such as normal saline (NS) or lactated Ringer's solution, to replace fluid volume.

If the patient is hyperglycemic, especially with a blood sugar level greater than 350 to 400 mg/dL, the patient is considered to be dehydrated. Children should be given 20 mL/kg of NS or LR as an initial fluid bolus, repeated once if vital signs do not respond. Adults can be given boluses of 500 cc of NS or LR repeated as needed to a total volume of 2 liters. Fluid replacement is the mainstay of therapy for DKA and NKHC, and should be undertaken aggressively because of the huge volume of fluid already lost. Ultimately, these patients will require insulin in addition to continuous volume replacement. Although the patient may be acidotic, bicarbonate should not be given; the acidosis will correct with fluid and electrolyte replacement and insulin. The patient's ECG should also be monitored, because decreased potassium levels can lead to serious dysrhythmias.

Should complications of diabetes, such as foot ulcers or skin infections be identified, supportive care, such as cleaning wounds and applying sterile dressings, should be given.

Once therapy has been initiated, the patient should be transported to the closest emergency department in accordance with local protocols. Further definitive therapy will include continuing fluid replacement and electrolyte monitoring, and insulin administration for patients with DKA or NKHC.

SUMMARY

Evaluation and management of diabetic patients is a challenging problem for paramedics. The key to appropriate management is thorough patient assessment and rapid blood sugar level measurement. Knowledge of diabetic complications and their predisposing factors is important for the paramedic to accurately identify and manage diabetic problems.

REFERENCES

1. **Auer RN et al:** Neuropathologic findings in three cases of profound hypoglycemia, *Clin Neuropathol* 8:63, 1989.

2. **Bergenstal RM:** Diabetic ketoacidosis: How to treat and, when possible, prevent, *Postgrad Med* 77:151, 1985.

3. **The Diabetes Control and Complications Trial Research Group:** The effect of intensive treatment of diabetes on the development and progression of long term complications in insulin-treated diabetes mellitus. *N Engl. J Med* 329:977-986, 1993.

4. **Faich GA, Fishbein HA, Ellis SE:** The epidemiology of diabetic acidosis: A population-based study, *Am J Epidemiol* 117-551, 1983.

5. **Fishbein H, Palumbo PJ:** Acute Metabolic Complications in Diabetes. In *Diabetes in America,* ed 2, National Institute of Health, 1995, NIH Publication #95-1468.

6. **Harris M:** Summary. In *Diabetes in America,* ed 2, National Institute of Health, 1995, NIH Publication #95-1468.

7. **Iwai A, et al:** Computed tomographic imaging of the brain in after hypoglycemia coma, *Neuroradiology* 29:398, 1987.

8. **Keller U:** Diabetic ketoacidosis: Current views on pathogenesis and treatment, *Diabetologia* 29:71, 1986.

9. **Klatt EC, Beatie C, Noguchi TT:** Evaluation of death from hypoglycemia, *Am J Forensic Med Pathol* 9:122, 1988.

10. **LaPorte DE, Matsushima M, Chang YF:** Prevalence and Incidence of Insulin-Dependent Diabetes. In *Diabetes in America,* ed 2, National Institute of Health, 1995, NIH Publication #95-1468.

11. **National Center for Health Statistics, United States National Hospital Discharge Survey:** Average annual number of hospital discharge listing hyperosmolar nonketotic coma (ICD 250.2), United States, 1989-1991, *United States National Hospital Discharge Survey, National Center for Health Statistics.*

12. **United States Department of Health and Human Services, Public Health Services:** Diabetes Statistics, National Institutes of Health, 1995, NIH Publication *96-3926.

SUGGESTED READINGS

1. **Green DA:** Diabetic Ketoacidosis. *Top Emerg Med* 5(4): 17-31, 1984.

2. **Finegold DN:** Hypoglycemia. *Top Emerg Med* (Jan):57-63, 1984.

3. **Feingold KR, Gavin LA, Schambelan M, et al:** Hypoglycemia. In Andreoli TE, Carpenter C, Plum F, et al (eds): *Cecil Essentials of Medicine,* Philadelphia, 1990, WB Saunders.

4. **Kolodzik JM, Dobbert D:** Complications of Diabetes. In Hamilton G: *Emergency Medicine: An approach to clinical problem solving,* Philadelphia, 1991, WB Saunders.

chapter 36

Abdominal, Genitourinary, and Back Pain

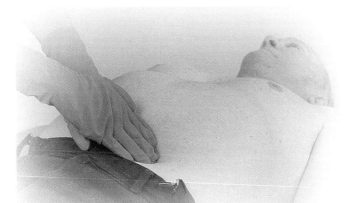

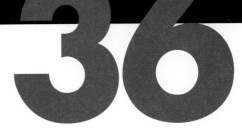

Acute abdominal pain is a frequent complaint encountered by prehospital providers and accounts for 5% to 10% of all emergency department visits. Between 15% and 30% of patients presenting with acute abdominal pain eventually require surgical intervention.

Because the potential causes of acute abdominal pain include a wide variety of conditions that range from minor to life threatening, the evaluation and management of patients with this common complaint create special challenges for prehospital care providers, emergency physicians, and surgeons. Although it is not necessary to establish the precise cause of abdominal pain in the prehospital setting, the paramedic must be able to recognize the basic signs of serious conditions to provide necessary intervention and begin rapid transport.

Pathophysiology

To evaluate acute abdominal pain, a working knowledge of the types of pain and of the mechanisms responsible for its production and perception is essential. Because of the abdomen's complex innervation, abdominal pain is usually not as well localized as pain in other regions, such as the extremities. However, the majority of patients with acute abdominal pain generally manifest one of three pain patterns: visceral, somatic (parietal) or referred, or some combination of these patterns.

Visceral Pain

Visceral pain fibers are located in the walls of hollow organs and the capsules of solid organs. Mechanisms that stimulate these fibers and produce visceral pain include increased wall tension from distention of hollow organs (such as the intestine or gallbladder), stretch of the capsule of solid organs (kidney or liver), vascular impairment with inadequate perfusion of abdominal organs, and chemical irritation caused by leakage of bowel contents or blood.

Visceral pain is often the earliest sign of an acute intra-abdominal process. A patient feels pain that is usually intermittent, worsens with time, and may be described as dull, cramping, or even gaseous. Because visceral pain impulses are carried by nerve fibers that return to the spinal cord at several levels (Fig. 36-1), the pain is typically perceived by the patient as being poorly localized and ill-defined. Because sensory fibers return to the spinal cord from both sides of the body, visceral pain is usually felt in the midline of the abdomen.

Although there may be a difference between the site the pain is felt and the precise location of the underlying disease process, involvement of certain intra-abdominal structures is suggested by the general location of visceral pain (Fig. 36-2). Visceral pain perceived in the upper abdomen (epigastric region) may originate from the esophagus, stomach, gallbladder, or liver. Pain originating in the small intestine, appendix, and right colon is typically felt in the midabdominal or periumbilical area. Pain in the lower midabdomen between the umbilicus and the pubic bone (hypogastric region) generally originates in

Even though the abdominal examination may fail to reveal localized abdominal tenderness, many patients with visceral pain appear in moderate distress. They may be unable to find a comfortable position and often appear restless and moving. In addition, visceral pain is frequently accompanied by systemic symptoms, such as nausea, vomiting, palpitations, and weakness.

Somatic Pain

In contrast to visceral pain, somatic, or parietal, pain impulses arise from the parietal peritoneum, abdominal wall, or diaphragm. These structures are innervated by sensory nerve fibers that return to the spinal cord along specific nerve pathways located on the same side as the site of pain (Fig. 36-3). Consequently, somatic pain is more localized than visceral pain to the site of the underlying disease process.

Somatic pain frequently is characterized as sharp or knife-like, constant, and aggravated by movement or coughing. Most patients can localize somatic pain to a specific area of the abdomen, such as the epigastric region or one of the four abdominal quadrants.

Somatic pain may be caused by bacterial or chemical inflammation of the peritoneum and occurs following visceral pain in many disease processes. Once parietal peritoneal irritation occurs, the abdominal examination will reveal localized tenderness that corresponds to the specific inflamed area. As more of the peritoneum becomes involved, local abdominal tenderness is accompanied by guarding (an increase in ab-

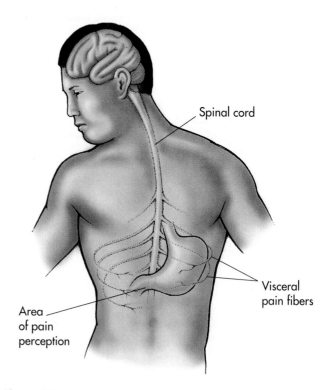

Figure 36-1

Visceral pain is often difficult to localize because the nerves pass through many parts of the abdomen before joining with the spinal cord.

dominal wall muscle tone when palpated) and muscle rigidity over the involved structure. If peritoneal involvement is extensive, as may occur with leakage of blood, gastric juice, or intestinal contents, somatic pain progresses from well-localized to a generalized pain involving the entire abdomen. This produces the "boardlike" muscle rigidity characteristic of an acute abdomen.

Referred Pain

Referred pain is experienced by the patient at a location distant from the affected site; pain originating in the abdomen can be noticed at an extra-abdominal location (Fig. 36-4). This results from overlapping nerve segments that provide sensation to both areas.

Referred pain is usually intense and most commonly occurs in association with an inflammatory condition. Several abdominal disorders commonly produce referred pain, and the pattern of radiation is helpful in determining the source of the pain. One of the best-known patterns occurs when intra-abdominal blood or fluid causes irritation of the abdominal surface of the diaphragm, usually on the left side. This produces pain that is perceived along the left side of the neck and over the top of the shoulder.

Patient Assessment

History

In the absence of recognizable life threat, evaluation of the patient with acute abdominal pain should be logical, systematic, and efficient. Historical data is extremely valuable in distin-

guishing between the various causes of abdominal pain. Because of the importance of the history, the paramedic should avoid asking leading questions ("does the pain feel sharp?").

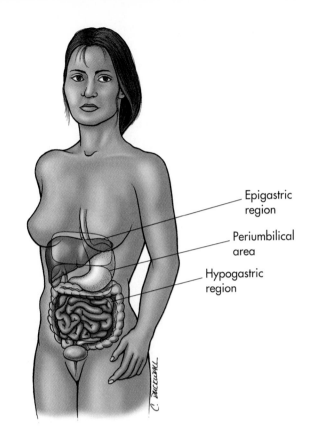

Figure 36-2
Pain resulting from diseased or injured organs within the abdomen frequently manifests itself in predictable locations such as the epigastric, periumbilical and hypogastric regions.

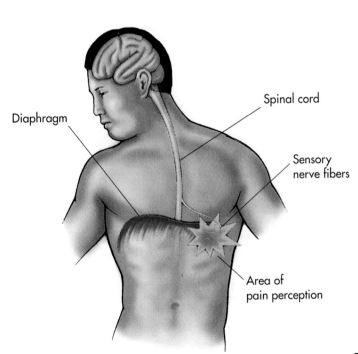

Figure 36-3
Somatic pain is isolated to the nerve pathway of the origin of the pain.

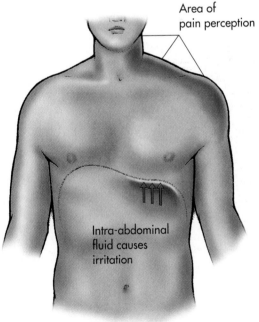

Figure 36-4
Referred pain results from overlapping nerve fibers that transmit sensation to areas other than where the injury or disease occurs.

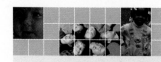

- Younger children cannot accurately localize the pain as can adults, making an accurate diagnosis often difficult.
- Common causes of abdominal pain in children include constipation, diarrhea, increased frequency of stools, vomiting, colic, torsion of the testicle, as well as associated gastrointestinal illnesses of childhood. Other causes include appendicitis, Meckel's diverticulum, pelvic inflammatory disease, hernias (intra-abdominal or inguinal), gastroenteritis, ulcers, hepatitis, and pancreatitis.
- Less common presenting conditions in infants and children include intussusception, intestinal malrotation, volvulus, renal calculus, inflammatory bowel disease, and Hirschprung's disease, a disorder affecting the peristalsis of the large bowel.
- Other medical emergencies can cause abdominal pain, such as pneumonia, diabetic ketoacidosis, and Reye's syndrome. Trauma can be a cause as well.
- A sudden onset of abdominal pain can be suggestive of intussusception, abdominal perforations, etc. A more gradual onset of abdominal pain can be suggestive of constipation, pancreatitis, or cholecystitis. A chronic abdominal pain can be due to inflammatory bowel diseases or tumor.

The use of open-ended questions ("Can you describe how your pain feels?") will not bias the patient during later assessment in the emergency department. For the prehospital provider, the primary objectives of the history are to characterize the pain episode and identify factors suggestive of a potentially dangerous condition (Box 36-1).

- *When did the pain begin?* The rapidity of onset of acute abdominal pain generally reflects the severity of the underlying process. Pain that is abrupt and explosive in onset and reaches a peak within minutes usually signifies a serious intra-abdominal process or vascular emergency, such as a perforated intestine or ruptured abdominal aortic aneurysm. Conditions, such as intestinal bowel obstruction, or appendicitis, have a less dramatic clinical picture, with steadily progressive pain that localizes over several hours.

- *What is the character of the pain?* Although the quality and intensity of abdominal pain are the most subjective aspects of the history, some intra-abdominal disease processes are associated with a characteristic quality of pain. For example, pain caused by an abdominal aortic aneurysm may be described as "tearing" in nature while pain from gastritis or peptic ulcer disease is often characterized as "burning." It is important for the paramedic to note that visceral types of pain are classically described as cramping that "comes and goes," while somatic pain is sharp and localized.

The severity of acute abdominal pain is often difficult to determine and is of limited value in providing clues to the underlying cause. Although agonizing pain generally denotes significant disease, milder nonspecific pain may be present with serious intra-abdominal processes, particularly in elderly patients and diabetics. Asking patients to compare the current episode of abdominal pain with previous pain from a known cause (such as childbirth) may help gauge severity.

- *Where is the pain and does it move to another site?* Somatic pain originating from some abdominal structures provides reasonably good clues to identifying the organ involved. The sudden onset of well-localized abdominal pain that rapidly becomes generalized throughout the abdomen may indicate perforation of an abdominal structure with leakage of irritating fluid into the peritoneal cavity.

Acute abdominal pain may follow specific referral patterns that are highly suggestive of a certain problem. For instance, sudden midabdominal pain that radiates directly to the back or the flank in an elderly patient suggests a ruptured or leaking aneurysm, and gradually worsening epigastric pain that radiates through to the back is associated with pancreatitis (inflammation of the pancreas) or peptic ulcer disease. Kidney stone pain often radiates to the lower abdomen, genitalia, or inner aspect of the thigh.

- *Are there associated gastrointestinal symptoms?* Nausea, vomiting, and diarrhea frequently accompany acute abdominal pain. Vomiting is a prominent symptom in upper GI tract diseases and, if this symptom continues for an extended period of time, may lead to dehydration. The presence of bright red or dark brown "coffee ground" emesis indicates acute upper GI bleeding.

BOX 36-1	Historical Data of Acute Abdominal Pain

- Sudden, unheralded, severe abdominal pain suggests an intra-abdominal catastrophe.
- Abdominal pain precedes the onset of associated symptoms, such as nausea and vomiting, in most cases of acute abdominal pain that require surgery.
- Pain that awakens the patient from sleep usually indicates significant disease.
- Acute, severe abdominal pain that occurs in a previously healthy patient and lasts longer than 6 hours usually requires surgical intervention.

CRITICAL ISSUE

Prehospital providers should consider the possibility of GI hemorrhage in any patient with acute abdominal pain, especially if syncope has occurred or evidence of blood loss is present.

Severe pain that precedes the onset of vomiting and is longer than 6 hours in duration is likely to be caused by a surgically correctable illness.

Changes in bowel habits, such as diarrhea or constipation, also occur frequently with acute abdominal disorders but are nonspecific symptoms. The absence of both stool and intestinal gas passage is a common finding with bowel obstruction. Grossly bloody stools or foul-smelling black stools that look like tar (melena) also signify GI bleeding as either the primary cause for abdominal pain or an associated complication.

- *Are there urinary symptoms?* Burning with urination, urinary frequency, or bloody urine suggests the urinary tract as a potential source of abdominal pain. Flank pain similar to pain experienced during prior episodes of kidney stones may indicate recurrent stone disease.
- *When was the patient's last menstrual period?* A history of missed, abnormal or irregular menstrual periods in women of child-bearing age with abdominal pain may suggest a complication of pregnancy such as an ectopic pregnancy. Cramping and intermittent abdominal pain associated with vaginal bleeding in a woman in the first trimester of pregnancy may signify a threatened abortion (possible miscarriage). A history of significant vaginal discharge, recent abortion, or chronic pelvic pain also points to a gynecologic source for acute abdominal pain, frequently due to infection.

All women of childbearing age with acute lower abdominal pain must be considered to have an ectopic pregnancy until proven otherwise.

- *Is there a significant past medical history?* The paramedic should ask the patient about underlying medical conditions, including cardiac disease, pulmonary disorders, diabetes, and kidney disease. Pulmonary diseases such as pneumonia, and cardiac problems including myocardial infarction, may present with complaints of abdominal discomfort or pain, again because of overlapping nerve supplies. Previous surgeries not only indicate a prior disease process, but can also point to an individual at risk for development of an intestinal obstruction secondary to scar formation in the peritoneal cavity.

Pertinent medications should be identified. For example, anticoagulants may inadvertently cause bleeding complications. Antibiotics may blunt the patient's pain response to an intra-abdominal infection. Corticosteroid medications can cause GI tract perforation and, more no-tably, mask the signs of serious intra-abdominal processes, even in cases of advanced peritoneal inflammation (see Table 36-1 for related patient medications).

Physical Examination

A skillful, directed, and rapid physical assessment is necessary to identify patients with acute abdominal pain caused by potentially dangerous disorders (see Boxes 36-2 and 36-3). If evidence of a life-threatening condition is discovered or suspected, resuscitation, stabilization, and transport procedures must be instituted immediately, even before a complete assessment is performed.

The assessment begins with a rapid overview, focusing attention on the airway, breathing, and circulation. During evaluation of circulation, the provider should pay close attention to the patient's skin temperature, color, state of hydration, and evidence of discoloration or bruising. The presence of diaphoresis, pallor, and cool, wet skin generally signifies shock and serious illness. Circulatory evaluation should also include assessment of capillary refill and palpation of carotid, radial, and femoral pulses. Decreased femoral pulses may be present in patients with a leaking or ruptured aortic aneurysm.

The initial overview requires a rapid assessment of the patient's level of responsiveness, because this influences the reliability of the abdominal examination. Most patients with abdominal pain are alert, and although they may be markedly uncomfortable, generally remain calm.

At this point, the patient can be placed in a position of most comfort. Patients with severe visceral pain (such as pain from kidney stones) may be doubled over in pain with their knees drawn toward their chest, or writhing about in search of a comfortable position. In contrast, patients with peritoneal inflammation usually remain motionless, because even the slightest movement can cause the pain to intensify.

Vital signs, with a tilt test, provide critical information regarding the immediate danger associated with acute abdominal pain. Mild tachycardia, mild blood pressure elevation, and minor increases in respiratory rate are common findings in patients with acute abdominal pain. However, a positive tilt test or other evidence of hypoperfusion such as a rapid, weak pulse, hypotension, rapid respirations, and decreased mental status indicates a serious, rapidly progressive disorder. Aggressive resuscitation and prompt transport are critical in these patients, and surgical intervention will usually be required.

The goal of the abdominal evaluation is to determine the extent and location of the underlying process, while taking care to avoid producing unnecessary discomfort for the patient. Establishing rapport and providing explanations during assessment increase the patient's understanding and cooperation and greatly enhance the yield of information.

Assessment begins with inspection of the abdomen for distention, scars from prior surgeries or trauma, discoloration such as jaundice, and obvious masses. The absence of abdominal wall movement during respiration may indicate peritoneal irritation.

TABLE 36-1		Medications Related to Abdominal, Genitourinary, and Back Pain		
Classification	**Specific Drug**	**Indication**	**Therapeutic Action**	**Side Effects and Precautions**
Antiemetics	Antivert Phenergan Dramamine Compazine Torcan	Nausea/vomiting Vertigo	Inhibits vomiting/vertigo	Drowsiness Dystonic reaction
Antibiotics	Penicillin Keflex Ceclor Flagyl Doxycycline Bactrim	Infection	Destroys bacteria	Diarrhea Yeast infections Allergic reaction
Antidiarrheals	Paragoric Lomotil Donnatol	Diarrhea	Inhibits GI motility	CNS depression Constipation
Anti–Inflammatories Steroid	Medrol Prednisone	Arthritis Asthma Allergies Inflammation	Reduces inflammation	Masks symptoms of other diseases Mood swings Weight gain
Nonsteroid	Tolectin Motrin Ibuprofen Indocin Clinoril Naprosyn	Pain Arthritis	Unknown mechanism	GI disturbances Allergic reaction
Antisecretory Gastrointestinal Drugs	Tagamet (Cimetidine) Pepcid Carafate Zantac Axid	Duodenal ulcers Prevention of stress Ulceration	Inhibits gastric acid secretion	GI disturbances
Acid-Neutralizing Drugs	Maalox Mylanta Riopan Di-Gel	Gastric ulcers Duodenal ulcers Gastritis	Neutralize acid	Diarrhea Constipation

Palpation follows inspection and is the most important element of the abdominal examination. Prehospital providers must be aware that the information obtained from palpation is directly proportional to the gentleness of the examination. Before beginning, the paramedic should ask the patient to indicate the location of pain. Patients with diffuse or nonlocalized abdominal disorders may be unable to identify a specific area of pain, whereas those with well-localized disease processes frequently can point to the exact site with a finger.

The examiner should begin palpating the abdomen in the quadrant farthest from the site indicated by the patient, and should use gentle fingertip pressure (Fig. 36-5). After determining the general "feel" of the abdomen, noting whether it is soft, firm or rigid, the provider should palpate each abdominal quadrant to assess for masses, pulsations, enlarged organs, tenderness, and muscle guarding.

Abdominal tenderness may be localized, generalized, or absent. Localized tenderness often provides a valuable clue to

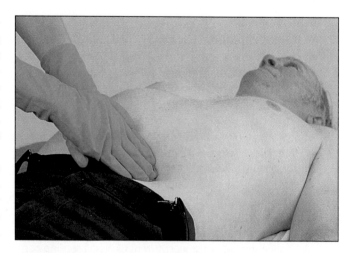

Figure 36-5

Palpation of the abdomen should begin by placing the hands on the part farthest away from the reported area of pain.

Factors Suggesting Serious Disease in Patients with Acute Abdominal Pain

- Abrupt onset of pain
- Cardiac symptoms (chest pain)
- Syncope or profound weakness
- Excruciating abdominal pain or severe distress
- Altered level of responsiveness
- Skin pallor and diaphoresis
- Evidence of dehydration
- Sustained tachycardia (> 120 beats/min)
- Hypotension
- Respiratory distress
- Evidence of sepsis (fever, chills, decreased alertness)
- Marked abdominal tenderness
- Abdominal muscle guarding with "boardlike" rigidity
- Evidence of gastrointestinal hemorrhage
- Elderly patient
- Immune compromise (malignancy, diabetes, HIV infection)
- Chronic steroid therapy

Potentially Life-Threatening Processes in Acute Abdominal Pain

Hemorrhage
  Ruptured abdominal aortic aneurysm
  Ruptured ectopic pregnancy
  Acute gastrointestinal hemorrhage
  Ruptured ovarian cyst with bleeding
  Spontaneous splenic rupture (rare)
Hypovolemia
  Peritonitis
  Pancreatitis
  Perforated viscus (internal organ)
  Intestinal obstruction
  Mesenteric ischemia
    Contributing factors for dehydration
      Protracted vomiting
      Severe diarrhea
      Poor oral intake
      Fluid losses from fever and rapid respirations
Sepsis
  Underlying origins
    Intestinal perforation
    Perforated appendicitis
    Perforated diverticulitis
    Gallbladder perforation
    Pyelonephritis
Acute cardiac decompression
  Aggravation of underlying cardiac disease
    Myocardial ischemia
    Cardiac dysrhythmias
    Acute pulmonary edema
  Atypical presentation of acute myocardial infarction (more common in elderly patients)
    Inferior wall myocardial infarction
    Abdominal pain associated with dyspnea and diaphoresis

the site of the underlying disease process. The presence of guarding, that causes resistance to palpation, should also be noted.

Rebound tenderness, a sharp increase in abdominal pain following sudden release of the examiner's palpating hand, indicates irritation of the peritoneum. However, testing for rebound tenderness should not be assessed in the prehospital setting. Doing so increases the patient's pain unnecessarily, serves to make the patient more guarded and less cooperative for the next examiner, and does not provide any information that will alter the prehospital management.

Indirect evidence of peritoneal irritation can be determined by noting increased abdominal pain that occurs when the patient coughs, when the patient is moved onto the stretcher, or when the patient is jarred while the transporting vehicle hits bumps in the road.

Given the time constraints and noisy environment of the prehospital setting, auscultation of the abdomen has no place in the prehospital evaluation of patients with abdominal pain. Even if performed, auscultation would not change the plan for patient management.

Evaluation of patients with acute abdominal pain should include pulmonary and cardiovascular examinations. Severe abdominal pain frequently causes an increased respiratory rate, although marked respiratory distress is unusual. The chest should be examined for evidence of an intra-thoracic process causing or contributing to abdominal pain, as may occur with pneumonia. Carotid, radial, and femoral pulses should be palpated bilaterally, noting their quality, regularity and symmetry.

Key Conditions and Findings

Life-threatening disorders in patients with nontraumatic acute abdominal pain generally are the result of either hypoperfu-

sion or acute cardiac decompensation, or both. However, at times, these dangerous complications may manifest initially with only minor alterations in vital signs and without significant abdominal findings, particularly among elderly patients. Nevertheless, the prehospital provider must keep life-threatening processes uppermost in mind when evaluating patients with acute abdominal pain (Table 36-2).

- *Abdominal aortic aneurysm (AAA).* AAA is one of the most rapidly lethal conditions that can present with acute abdominal pain. Aortic aneurysms are caused by localized weakening and dilation of the wall of the aorta and usually result from atherosclerosis (Fig. 36-6). An estimated 2% to 7% of the adult population have AAAs, with an 11% incidence in men older than 65 years of age. Mortality from ruptured AAA is nearly 80% in patients who present with shock.

    The characteristic clinical presentation of a ruptured or leaking AAA is sudden onset of severe, constant pain in the abdomen or back. The pain may be confined to the middle of the back or abdomen, or may radiate to the lower back, flank, or pelvis. Femoral pulses may be de-

TABLE 36-2 Characteristics of Common Causes of Acute Abdominal Pain

Disorder By Location	Pain Quality	Pain Pattern and Radiation	Abdominal Findings	Associated Findings
EPIGASTRIC				
Perforated viscus	Abrupt, severe	Rapidly becomes generalized	Guarding; "boardlike" rigidity	Tachycardia, shock, fever
Acute pancreatitis	Steady, boring	Both upper quadrants; radiates to midback	Epigastric tenderness; guarding	Vomiting; dehydration; history of alcoholism
RIGHT UPPER QUADRANT				
Cholecystitis	Cramping, colicky	Localizes to RUQ; radiates to right scapula	Tender RUQ with guarding	Vomiting; fever; possibly jaundice
PERIUMBILICAL				
Appendicitis	Steady, achy	Diffuse, then localizes to RLQ	RLQ tenderness with guarding	Fever, vomiting, loss of appetite
Intestinal obstruction	Crampy, diffuse	Becomes generalized	Distension; diffuse tenderness	Vomiting; fever; dehydration
Aortic aneurysm (ruptured or leaking)	Abrupt, severe	Rapidly becomes generalized	Diffuse tenderness; pulsatile mass	Shock, pallor, decreased femoral pulses
Gastroenteritis	Mild, crampy	Nonlocalized	Generalized mild tenderness	vomiting, watery diarrhea
Intestinal ischemia	Aching, diffuse	Progressive, severe	Initial examination relatively normal; later, guarding and rebound tenderness	Hypotension, tachycardia, bloody stool
LOWER QUADRANT				
Ectopic pregnancy (ruptured)	Sudden, severe	Initially local in LQ; may become diffuse	Lower quadrant tenderness with guarding	Shock, pallor, possibly vaginal bleeding
Diverticulitis	Steady, aching	Usually LLQ; may radiate to back or groin	LLQ tenderness; guarding; possible mass	Fever, possibly bloody stools
Kidney stone	Abrupt, colicky, excruciating pain	Begins in flank or lower back; radiates to groin	Flank tenderness; abdomen nontender	Vomiting; writhing in bed; blood in urine

RUQ—right upper quadrant; RLQ—right lower quadrant; LLQ—left lower quadrant; LQ—lower quadrant.

creased. Patients often have syncopal episodes caused by loss of blood if they attempt to stand and may present in frank shock from hemorrhage into the abdominal cavity. A pulsatile abdominal mass may be detected in some patients and is an ominous finding, signaling impending rupture, if rupture has not already occurred.

CRITICAL ISSUE

Patients with a palpable, pulsating mass should be immediately transported to the closest hospital that has in-hospital surgeons and anesthesia. These patients require immediate surgical intervention.

- *Ectopic pregnancy.* Ectopic pregnancy occurs when the fertilized ovum implants outside of the uterus, usually in the fallopian tube. An estimated 70,000 ectopic pregnancies occur annually in the United States, and the incidence appears to be increasing. Ruptured ectopic pregnancy is the leading cause of death during the first trimester of pregnancy, with mortality primarily resulting from acute hemorrhage. If the ectopic pregnancy ruptures, the patient usually experiences sudden, severe abdominal pain originating on one side of the lower abdomen.

   Abdominal findings include marked tenderness with guarding and evidence of peritoneal irritation. On occasion, vital signs may be deceptively normal while the pa-

tient is in a supine position, even with moderate bleeding. However, when these patients are upright, weakness, dizziness, and syncope may occur.

- *Acute gastrointestinal (GI) bleeding.* Although patients with acute GI bleeding may experience mild abdominal pain, evidence of hypoperfusion, and clinical signs of bleeding generally overshadow the degree of pain. On occasion, patients with GI bleeding fail to demonstrate the obvious signs of bleeding.

- *Dehydration.* Several other intra-abdominal processes associated with acute abdominal pain can produce hypoperfusion and even cardiovascular collapse because of volume loss. A number of abdominal diseases, including processes that are inflammatory (such as pancreatitis), infectious (gastroenteritis), obstructive, and ischemic (mesenteric artery thrombosis) can cause rapid shifts of large volumes of intravascular fluid into the peritoneal cavity or the intestine. Fluid deficits are compounded by other problems that accompany intra-abdominal conditions, including lack of oral intake, vomiting, diarrhea, and fluid loss from fever and increased respiratory rate.

- *Sepsis.* Sepsis is a potential cause of hypoperfusion and hemodynamic compromise in patients with acute abdominal pain. Serious intra-abdominal infections can lead to bacterial invasion of the bloodstream, particularly among elderly patients and patients with impaired immune function caused by **cancer,** malignancy, diabetes mellitus, or **human immunodeficiency virus** (HIV) infection. Find-

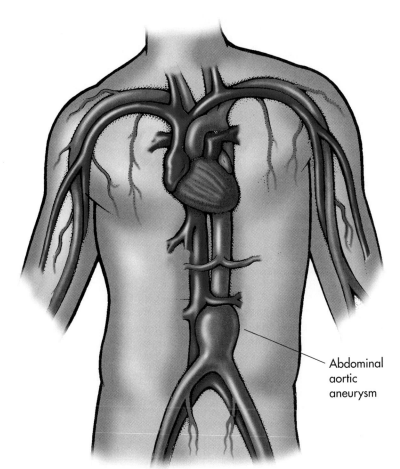

Abdominal aortic aneurysm

Figure 36-6

A common site for an abdominal aortic aneurysm.

ings suggestive of **sepsis** from an intra-abdominal source include abdominal pain and tenderness associated with chills, fever, tachycardia, rapid respirations, decreased alertness, and possibly hypotension.

- *Myocardial ischemia.* Some patients with acute cardiac disorders may complain primarily of acute abdominal pain. Patients with acute myocardial infarction (AMI) may present with abdominal pain, not associated with chest pain, as the only manifestation of decreased blood flow to the heart muscle. This atypical presentation of AMI is most common among elderly patients, diabetic patients, and patients with myocardial infarction involving the posterior wall or inferior wall of the heart.

  Abdominal pain caused by cardiac problems may occur suddenly or be gradual in onset. The pain usually is a dull ache, typically located in the epigastric region and upper quadrants of the abdomen, and may mimic other common abdominal disorders, such as an ulcer or **gallbladder disease.** Significant abdominal examination findings are usually absent.

  Acute abdominal pain may result from numerous, relatively common disease processes. These include acute disorders requiring emergency surgery, as well as chronic, recurrent conditions and benign, self-limited illnesses. Some of these conditions are:

- *Appendicitis.* Caused by obstruction and infection of the appendix, its clinical features include loss of appetite, nausea, vomiting, diffuse abdominal pain that begins in the mid-abdomen and localizes to the right lower abdomen, and right lower quadrant tenderness with guarding.

- *Cholecystitis.* This obstruction and infection of the gallbladder, usually caused by gallstones, is characterized by upper abdominal pain, nausea and vomiting after meals, and with right upper quadrant tenderness and guarding.

- *Bowel obstruction.* Blockage of the normal passage of intestinal contents is usually associated with cramping abdominal pain, vomiting, abdominal distension, diffuse abdominal tenderness, and decreased or no passage of stool and flatus. It occurs most often in patients who have had prior surgery.

- *Gastroenteritis.* This inflammation of the intestinal tract is caused by infection or an ingested toxic substance and is characterized by vomiting, diarrhea, abdominal cramping, and mild diffuse abdominal tenderness.

- *Pelvic inflammatory disease.* Pelvic inflammatory disease (PID) is a sexually transmitted infection involving the uterus, fallopian tubes, and ovaries. It is usually associated with fever, vaginal discharge, and lower abdominal pain and tenderness.

- *Pancreatitis.* Pain from pancreatic inflammation varies from mild to very severe and is usually located in the epigastric area or right upper quadrant. Nausea and vomiting also occur, as well as a low-grade fever.

- *Diverticulitis.* Pain from inflammation of diverticula, which are little out-pouchings located in the wall of the large bowel. The discomfort is usually noted in the left lower quadrant and may be associated with episodes of rectal bleeding.

- *Urinary tract disease.* Infections or stones involving the kidneys or ureters are perceived as pain in the flank or low back, which may radiate to the lower abdomen or the genitalia.

Lastly, **diabetic ketoacidosis** (DKA) may develop rapidly or over several days. It can be precipitated by the patient's failure to take prescribed insulin or by acute stress from infection, myocardial infarction, pregnancy, or trauma. Nausea, vomiting, abdominal pain, and tenderness are common presenting features in DKA, and the symptoms are accompanied by dehydration, rapid respirations, acetone (fruity) breath, tachycardia, and occasionally hypotension.

Acute abdominal pain can also be caused by nonabdominal processes or metabolic disorders. Cardiac and pulmonary problems should always be considered as a possible cause of acute abdominal pain, especially when pain is located in the patient's upper abdomen or when pain radiates to the chest. In addition to myocardial infarction, patients with other disorders of the chest including pneumonia, **pulmonary embolus,** and esophageal problems may present with acute abdominal pain. **Sickle cell disease** can present as a "crisis" with acute abdominal pain; lead poisoning, renal failure, and **thyroid disease** are other possible causes.

The paramedic should bear in mind that the most common diagnosis assigned to patients presenting to the emergency department with abdominal pain is "abdominal pain of unknown etiology." It is usually difficult to come up with a specific diagnosis in the prehospital setting, and determining a diagnosis often would not contribute to patient management.

Management

After completion of the initial assessment, the patient should be placed in a position of comfort. Unless contraindicated, patients who are vomiting or pregnant should be transported in the left lateral decubitus position. Given the possibility of disease that will require surgery, patients with abdominal pain should be given nothing orally.

If evidence of hypoperfusion or signs of significant dehydration are present, aggressive management is warranted. Paramedics should ensure airway patency, provide supplemental high-flow oxygen, establish large-bore IV access, and institute rapid fluid resuscitation with normal saline or lactated Ringer's. Cardiac monitoring and pulse oximetry determination, if available, are also indicated.

Although controversial, the prehospital use of narcotic analgesics for patients with abdominal pain is not recommended. Administering narcotics can mask ongoing symptoms and impair the evaluation of the patient by the emergency physician or surgeon after arrival at the hospital.

Management priorities for patients with acute abdominal pain and no evidence of life-threatening complications are di-

rected toward the specific problems encountered and generally involve only supportive care. The majority of patients with acute abdominal pain should have an IV line established en route to the hospital, provided transport is not delayed. Careful monitoring is essential and should include repeat vital signs and gentle, repeat abdominal examination during transport.

In terms of transport, the most urgent patients are those who demonstrate the possibility of catastrophic internal bleeding. Many of these patients will present with shock. In these cases, the paramedic should consider transporting the patient to a trauma center where prompt surgical consultation and resources are readily available.

SUMMARY

Evaluation and management of patients with acute abdominal pain is a common problem that represents a significant challenge for all emergency care personnel. Acute abdominal pain can be the manifestation of an intra-abdominal emergency, or it may represent a progressive disease process that, if unrecognized and untreated, is potentially catastrophic. The cornerstones of prehospital care include performance of a rapid, orderly and accurate assessment, prompt recognition of life-threatening processes, institution of appropriate stabilization measures, and transport to the nearest appropriate medical facility.

SUGGESTED READINGS

1. **Davidson SJ, McNamara RM:** Surgical causes of acute abdominal pain. In Harwood-Nuss A, Linden CH, Luten RC, et al (eds): *Clinical Practice of Emergency Medicine*, Philadelphia, 1991, JB Lippincott.

2. **Davidson SJ, Wagner DK:** Approach to Acute Abdominal Pain. In Callaham ML (ed): *Current Therapy in Emergency Medicine*, Toronto, 1987, BC Decker.

3. **Fontanarosa PB:** Approach to acute abdominal pain. *Emerg Care Quart* 5:1–11, 1989.

4. **Fontanarosa PB:** Acute abdominal pain. *Emerg Med Serv* 14:9(11):28–41, 1989.

5. **Hickey MS, Keirnan GJ, Weaver KE:** Evaluation of Abdominal Pain, *Emerg Med Clin North Am* 7:437–452, 1989.

6. **Hirsch E, Birkett D:** Challenges of the Acute Abdomen. In Noble J (ed): *General Medicine and Primary Care*, 1987, Little, Brown, and Co.

7. **Hockberger RS:** Ectopic pregnancy, *Emerg Med Clin North Am* 5:481–493, 1987.

8. **Hockberger RS, Henneman PL, Boniface K:** Disorders of the small intestine. In Rosen P, Barkin RM, Braen GR, et al (eds): *Emergency Medicine: Concepts and Clinical Practice*, ed 3, St. Louis, 1992, CV Mosby.

9. **Hoekstra JW:** Acute abdominal pain. In Hamilton G: *Emergency Medicine: An Approach to clinical problem solving*, Philadelphia, 1991, WB Saunders.

10. **Marston WA, Alquist R, Johnson G, et al:** Misdiagnosis of ruptured abdominal aortic aneurysms. *J Vasc Surg* 16:17–22, 1992.

11. **Overton DT:** Abdominal Pain. In Tintinalli J, Krome R, Ruiz E (eds): *Emergency Medicine: A Comprehensive Study Guide*, ed 3, New York, 1992, McGraw-Hill.

12. **Trott AT, Greenberg R:** Acute abdominal pain. In Rosen P, Barkin RM, Braen GR, et al (eds): *Emergency Medicine—Concepts and Clinical Practice*, ed 3, St. Louis, 1992, CV Mosby.

13. **Young GP:** Abdominal Catastrophes. *Emerg Med Clin North Am* 7:699–720, 1989.

Greg Mears, MD

Chapter 37
Pregnancy and Childbirth

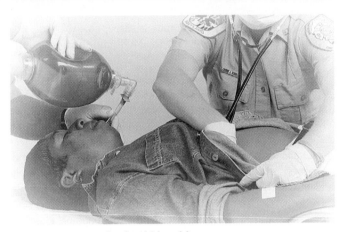

A paramedic should be able to:

1. Define the following terms:
   - a. Ovary
   - b. Vagina
   - c. Uterus
   - d. Fallopian tubes
   - e. Amniotic fluid
   - f. Placenta
   - g. Umbilical cord
   - h. Supine hypotensive syndrome
2. Describe physiological changes that occur during pregnancy.
3. Describe the effects of decreased maternal circulation on the fetus.
4. Describe the pathophysiology, risk factors, signs and symptoms, complications and management for:
   - a. Spontaneous abortion
   - b. Threatened abortion
   - c. Ectopic pregnancy
   - d. Hyperemesis gravidum
   - e. Premature labor
   - f. Toxemia of pregnancy (preeclampsia and eclampsia)
   - g. Abruptio placenta
   - h. Placenta previa
   - i. Multiple pregnancies
5. Describe the pathophysiology and management for the following labor and delivery complications:
   - a. Prolapsed cord
   - b. Breech presentation
   - c. Limb presentation
   - d. Postpartum hemorrhage/ infection
   - e. Meconium stained amniotic fluid
6. Identify the signs and symptoms and management of a patient in normal labor.
7. Describe the appropriate assessment of the pregnant patient.
8. Describe three phases of labor and delivery.
9. Describe the actions and uses of drugs used for labor and delivery complications.
10. Identify the signs and symptoms of imminent delivery.
11. Identify the appropriate equipment and steps that are necessary to manage an uncomplicated prehospital delivery.
12. Describe the appropriate steps involved in newborn care, including resuscitation.

1. **Amniotic fluid**—the fluid contained in the gestational sac which surrounds the fetus.
2. **APGAR score**—a postpartum numeric score based on infant heart rate, respiratory effort, muscle tone, color, and response to stimuli.
3. **Cervix**—the lower part of the uterus.
4. **Delivery**—the actual passing of the products of conception, including the placenta.
5. **Eclampsia**—the occurrence of a seizure in the presence of preeclampsia.
6. **Fallopian tubes**—two trumpet-shaped muscular tubes that extend from the ovaries to the base of the uterus.
7. **Fetus**—a general term for an unborn infant.
8. **Gestation**—the period from the fertilization of the ovum until birth.
9. **Gravidity**—the total number of pregnancies a woman has had, including abortions and miscarriages.
10. **Labor**—the coordinated sequence of involuntary uterine contractions producing effacement and dilatation of the cervix, and leading to delivery.
11. **Ovulation**—release of an ovum from the vesicular follicle.
12. **Parity**—the total number of live deliveries a patient has experienced.
13. **Placenta**—the vascular structure in the uterus that connects to the maternal circulation and exchange nutrients and wastes for the fetus.
14. **Postpartum**—the time period after delivery.
15. **Preeclampsia**—the presence of hypertension, proteinuria, and edema associated with pregnancy, generally occurring in the later half of pregnancy.
16. **Trimester**—pregnancy is divided into 3 equal intervals, each approximately three months in length, referred to as first, second, and third trimesters.
17. **Umbilical cord**—the cord containing the blood vessels that connect the fetus and the placenta, transporting nutrients and wastes.
18. **Uterus**—the pear-shaped muscular organ that houses the fetus in pregnancy, also often called the womb.

The management of labor and delivery outside of the hospital is a stressful situation regardless of the individual circumstances. But it can also be one of the most rewarding and memorable experiences of a paramedic's career. It is important for paramedics to be prepared for imminent delivery and to appropriately manage any complication that might occur, giving both the mother and infant the best chances for a positive outcome.

Anatomy and Physiology of Pregnancy

The internal female reproductive anatomy includes the vagina, the uterus, the fallopian tubes, and the ovaries (Fig. 37-1). The vagina is the passageway from the uterus to the outside of the body that allows for menstrual flow and childbirth. The ovaries are located in the pelvis on either side of the uterus. The two primary functions of the ovaries are to develop and expel the ova (eggs), and to secrete hormones. At birth, each ovary contains the total number of ova that will be stored and released during the woman's life.

The uterus is a hollow, thick-walled, muscular organ with two important functions: it is the organ of menstruation, and it receives and nourishes the fertilized ovum during pregnancy, expelling the fetus during labor. The fallopian tubes are two trumpet-shaped muscular tubes that extend from the ovaries to the base of the uterus. The fallopian tubes each have two openings, one into the uterine cavity and the other into the abdominal cavity. The fallopian tube provides a temporary environment for the ovum and the sperm, where fertilization can occur. The fertilized ovum then passes through the tube to the uterus.

In women who have reached the age of menstruation, ovulation occurs monthly with considerable regularity. This release of a mature egg is stimulated by estrogen, which also stimulates the formation of a special lining of cells and blood in the uterus that will nourish the egg after fertilization. If the egg is not fertilized, the uterus sheds this lining, and menstruation occurs.

The ovum in the fallopian tube is susceptible to successful fertilization by a sperm for 12 to 24 hours after ovulation. Sperm can survive for 48 to 72 hours in the female reproductive tract. Over the 7 days following fertilization, the ovum normally continues through the fallopian tube and implants in the specially prepared uterine lining. Implantation allows the newly created embryo to obtain nourishment from the blood and tissues of the endometrium.

Once the embryo is implanted in the endometrium and nourished, the amniotic cavity develops around the embryo. It is filled with fluid that originates from the fetal urine and other secretions. The amniotic fluid (or the "bag of waters") has several important functions. It cushions the fetus against possible

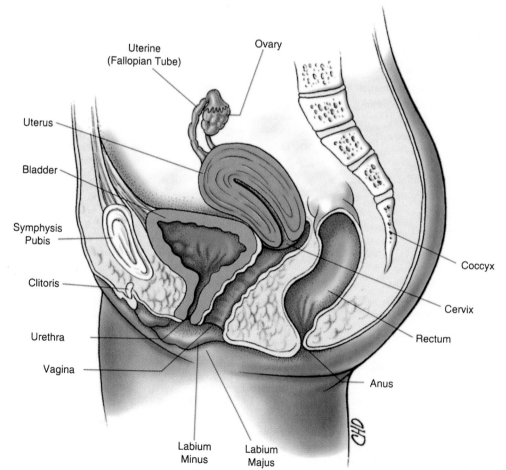

Uterine
(Fallopian Tube)

Ovary

Uterus

Bladder

Symphysis
Pubis

Clitoris

Urethra

Vagina

Coccyx

Cervix

Rectum

Anus

Labium
Minus

Labium
Majus

Figure 37-1

The female reproductive system. From McSwain et al: Instructor's Resource Kit to Accompany The Basic EMT: Comprehensive Prehospital Patient Care, St. Louis, 1996, Mosby Lifeline.

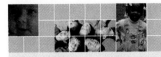

- The onset of menses generally occurs from age 12 to 16 years. Initial periods are anovulatory and irregular. Teenage pregnancy has become a major problem in the United States.

- Low birth weight and prematurity often occur with adolescent pregnancy. Prenatal care and nutritional counseling are especially important for the adolescent ob patient.

injury, maintains the fetus at a consistent temperature, and provides an environment in which the fetus can be mobile. At full term, the amount of amniotic fluid present in the sac is 500 to 1000 mL.

By the third month after fertilization, the placenta has formed. This is a disk-shaped organ that is approximately 20 cm in diameter and 2 cm thick in late pregnancy. At term, it weighs approximately 500 g. The placenta is a very versatile organ that functions in place of lungs, kidneys, GI tract, skin, endocrine glands and even the liver, to a degree. The placenta transfers gasses, excretes waste, transports nutrients, transfers heat, produces hormones, and acts as a barrier against some harmful substances.

The umbilical cord is the organ that connects the fetus to the placenta. It is approximately 45 cm long and 1.5 cm in diameter. The umbilical cord contains two arteries that carry deoxygenated blood from the fetus to the placenta, and a large vein returning oxygenated blood to the fetus. The umbilical

cord typically leaves the placenta near its center and enters the fetal abdominal wall just below the middle of the median line. The fetal blood remains in its own closed system, separate from the mother's circulation. Figure 37-2 illustrates the anatomic structures of pregnancy.

Pathophysiology

Pregnancy is generally divided into three separate 3-month periods, called *trimesters*. The first trimester (months 1 to 3) is the general time period in which the egg is fertilized, implants into the endometrium of the uterus, and the critical development of the fetus occurs.

During the second trimester (months 4 to 6), the majority of fetal development is completed and the growth phase begins. During this time, pregnancy is made more noticeable by the physical enlargement of the uterus and abdomen.

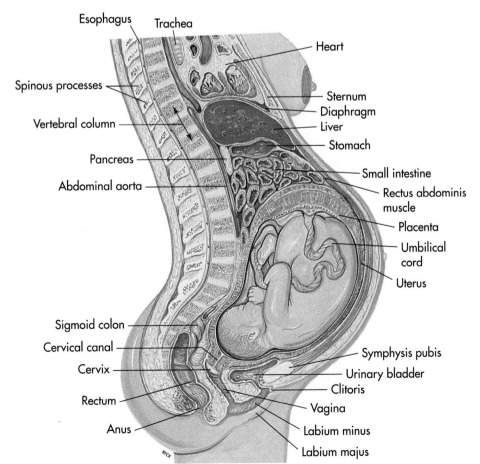

Figure 37-2

Anatomic structures of full-term pregnancy. From Thibodeau GA: Anatomy and Physiology, ed 2, St. Louis, 1993, Mosby–Year Book.

The third trimester (months 7 to 9) begins with the seventh month and progresses to labor and delivery at the end of the ninth month (approximately 40 weeks). This final trimester is a rapid growth period for the fetus; during this period the fetus is capable of surviving on its own should labor and delivery occur. Box 37-1 summarizes embryonic, fetal, and placental milestones.

Nearly every organ system in the mother's body is affected by pregnancy. These changes are most noticeable beginning in the second trimester, and they progress until delivery. A paramedic must have an understanding of these changes to anticipate problems and adequately evaluate and manage any illness or injury.

As the fetus grows within the uterus, a large amount of the mother's resources, such as blood, nutrients, and energy, are required for a healthy pregnancy. By the third trimester,

---

BOX 37-1 — Embryonic, Fetal, and Placental Milestones

3 minutes to 48 hours
Fertilization
7 to 8 Days
Implantation occurs
18 to 21 Days
Heart begins to twitch
Primitive eyes, ears exist
Placenta covers approximately one fifteenth of uterus, begins to function
4 weeks (1 month)
Heart begins asynchronous pulsations; blood pumped
Brain differentiates into forebrain, midbrain, hindbrain
   head large in proportion to body
Outlines of eyes seen above primitive mouth cavity
   lung buds appear
Gastrointestinal tract, liver, thyroid gland, pancreas, gallbladder can be identified
8 weeks (2 months)
Hands, feet well formed
Eyes move to front of face; eyelids fuse
Heart has four chambers, beats 40 to 80 times per minute
Major blood vessels form; circulation through umbilical cord occurs
Thyroid, adrenal glands, taste buds well formed
External genitalia can be distinguished as male or female
Placenta covers one third of uterine lining
Crown-rump (C-R) length is 3 cm; weight is 2 g
12 weeks (3 months)
Lungs take shape; respiratory motion seen
Thumb, forefinger oppose
Swallowing reflex present
Liver begins production of red blood cells
C-R length is 9 cm; weight is 45 g
Second Trimester
16 weeks (4 months)
Fingerprints develop
Arms, legs move frequently
Lips form; facial contours fill out
Skin still loose, wrinkled, pink
Brain forms ridges, cerebrum grows rapidly
Bladder fully formed
Fetus sensitive to light
Meconium (dead cells, mucus, gland secretions) forms, will make up newborn's first stool
C-R length is 14 cm; weight is 180 to 200 g
200 mL of amniotic fluid present
20 weeks (5 months)
Eyelashes, eyebrows, hair on head more abundant
Vernix caseosa (grayish-white, cheeselike substance), lanugo (soft hair) cover, protect fetus

Fetus sucks, swallows, hears sounds
Circadian rhythm begins
Respiratory movements occur, become more regular
C-R length is 19 cm; weight is 430 to 480 g
Placenta covers half of uterine lining, weighs 120 g
400 mL amniotic fluid present
24 weeks (6 months)
Eyes complete; eyelids open, close
Alveolar ducts, sacs present
Bone ossification begins
Thick vernix covers fetus; head hair very long
Skin layers on hands, feet thicken
Many reflexes appear
C-R length is 23 to 24 cm; weight is 700 to 800 g
Third Trimester
28 weeks (7 months)
Respiratory, circulatory systems function
Respiratory movements *in utero* seen by ultrasound
Testes begin to descend
Skin very thin, red, wrinkled, with prominent capillaries underneath
Eyebrows, eyelashes prominent; nails appear; lanugo begins to disappear
C-R length is 28 cm; weight is 1000 to 12000 g
32 weeks (8 months)
Subcutaneous fat deposits form to insulate fetus from temperature changes at birth
Skin becomes less wrinkled, red
Fingernails, toenails complete
More reflexes present
C-R length is 29 to 32 cm; weight is 1300 to 1200 g
36 weeks
Sleep-wake cycle more definite
Maternal antibodies transfer to fetus and last for approximately 6 months
C-R length is 32 to 35 cm; weight is 2500 to 2800 g
Approximately 1000 mL of amniotic fluid present
38 weeks (term)
Fetus less active due to limited space
Meconium accumulates in intestines
Nails have grown to tips of toes, fingers; creases prominent on soles of feet
Fetus may be able to lift head
Fetal circulation developed
C-R length is 35 to 37 cm; crown-heel (C-H) length is 46 to 52 cm; weight is 3000 to 3600 g
800 mL of amniotic fluid present

Adapted from Dickason, et al: Maternal and Infant Nursing, ed. 2, 1994, St. Louis, Mosby–Year Book.

BOX 37-2 — Maternal Changes During Pregnancy

- Cardiovascular
    - Increased blood volume 30%–50%
    - Increased heart rate 15–20 bpm
    - Decreased blood pressure systolic 5–15 mm Hg; diastolic 10–15 mm Hg
    - Increased cardiac output 30%–50%
    - Increased total body water
    - Increased RBC mass 10%–15%
    - Increased plasma and blood volume
- Respiratory
    - Increased oxygen consumption 20%–30% due to cardiac work, renal performance, breast, uterine and placenta demand
    - Increased tidal volume and depth of respiration
    - Increased perception of dyspnea
- Renal
    - Increase in size and weight of kidney
    - Increase in blood flow through kidney
    - Increased frequency and urgency
    - Increased urine production, especially at night
- Gastrointestinal
    - Gums become more sensitive and bleed easily
    - Increased gastric secretions causing heartburn in the third trimester
    - Nausea and vomiting in the first trimester
    - Increased incidence of constipation
    - Increased incidence of hemorrhoids
- Skin
    - Stretchmarks occur on breasts, lower abdomen, or thighs
    - Increased sweating
    - Increased pigment of skin, especially on nipples, umbilicus, and perineum
    - Increased nail and hair growth
- Musculoskeletal
    - Increased backache caused by forward curvature of the spine and increased uterus weight
    - Relaxation of pelvic and hip joints causing pelvic discomfort
    - Increased muscle cramping, especially in third trimester and at night

---

the mother's blood volume increases by as much as 50%, her resting heart rate increases as much as 15 to 20 beats per minute, and blood pressure, both systolic and diastolic, normally falls by 5 to 15 mm Hg. All of these circulation changes are the result of increased requirements of the fetus. Box 37-2 summaries maternal changes during pregnancy.

In addition, potential circulatory problems are created by the weight of the enlarging uterus. A pregnant woman placed in a supine position can become hypotensive as the weight of the uterus compresses the inferior vena cava, reducing both venous return to the heart and cardiac output **supine hypotensive syndrome.** This may also be referred to as *vena cava syndrome.*

The respiratory rate is usually not increased during pregnancy, but as the uterus enlarges in the abdomen, the diaphragm is pushed up, increasing ventilatory work.

The hormones of pregnancy also have an effect on the GI tract by relaxing the smooth muscle in the intestines, decreas-

ing the rate of food passage. This places the patient at risk for vomiting and aspiration. Morning sickness and nausea occur in some women, typically in the first trimester.

The blood pressure on the fetal side of the placenta is very low compared with the maternal circulation, in the range of 10 to 30 mm Hg. If the maternal circulation has a decreased cardiac output, such as in trauma or shock, the fetal circulation is also quickly affected. It is possible for the mother to withstand a great deal of blood loss and not show evidence of shock, when the fetus may be dying of hypoxia.

Evidence of a circulation problem or lack of oxygen to the fetus is most easily monitored by the fetal heart rate. With significant stress, the fetal heart rate will drop below its normal rate of 120 to 160 beats per minute. Unfortunately, monitoring the fetal heart rate either by Doppler or Fetascope is extremely difficult in a moving, noisy ambulance. When a Doppler or Fetascope is available in the prehospital environment, fetal heart tones (FHTs) or sounds can be auscultated after approximately the sixteenth week of pregnancy.

The doppler microphone or fetascope bell is firmly placed on the mother's abdomen, close to the mother's umbilicus. The instrument should be moved around the area until a fetal heart tone can be discerned.

The fetal heart rate should be counted as any other heart rate. Normal FHTs are in the 120 to 160 beats per minute range, with higher or lower rates signifying some type of early fetal distress. Contractions (or tensing of the uterine muscles) of labor will often cause a short period of acceleration, although a rise of more than 20 beats per minute may indicate fetal or maternal problems. This information, if available, should be promptly reported to medical direction and the receiving hospital.

Complications of Pregnancy

A wide variety of complications can occur during the course of a pregnancy. Some relate directly to the pregnancy itself, and others relate to the effect of the pregnancy on the mother.

Vaginal bleeding can occur at any time during a pregnancy. The conditions that cause bleeding vary, depending on whether the event occurs early in the pregnancy (before the fifth month) or later.

Some fertilized ova that implant in the wall of the uterus are imperfect or develop abnormally, and sometimes the environment in the uterus is not exactly right to allow for continued development. When this occurs, the body may rid itself of the imperfect embryo by expelling it. This is known as a **spontaneous abortion.** This may also occur with an apparently normal embryo. In a spontaneous abortion, the uterine muscles contract to expel the contents, causing cramping abdominal pain. Vaginal bleeding is noted as the process progresses. This most commonly occurs early in the pregnancy (6 to 20 weeks).

A **threatened abortion** is the occurrence of vaginal bleeding in the first half of pregnancy, possibly accompanied by abdominal cramping, in which the fetus remains viable. Twenty percent of threatened abortions progress to fetal demise and abortion, and more than 50% of these fetuses exhibit chromosomal abnormalities not compatible with life.[1]

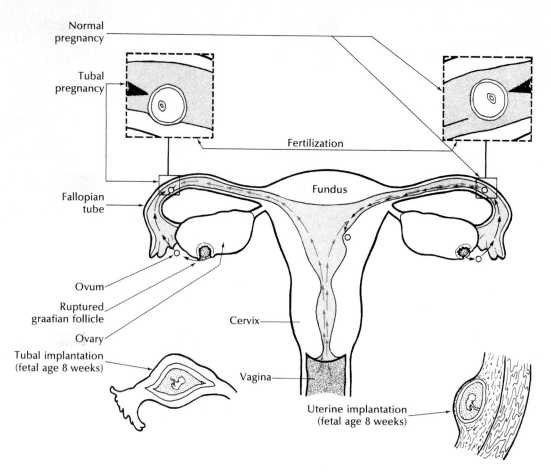

Normal
pregnancy

Tubal
pregnancy

Fertilization

Fundus

Fallopian
tube

Ovum

Ruptured
graafian follicle

Ovary

Tubal implantation
(fetal age 8 weeks)

Cervix

Vagina

Uterine implantation
(fetal age 8 weeks)

Figure 37-3

During a normal pregnancy, the fertilized ovum implants within the uterine wall. During an ectopic
pregnancy, the fertilized ovum implants at a different site, frequently within the fallopian tube. From
Jensen MD, Bobak IM: Maternity and Gynecoloigic Care, ed 3, St. Louis, 1985, CV Mosby.

Sometimes the fertilized ovum cannot progress normally through the fallopian tube to implant in the uterus. Instead it implants in the wall of the tube. This is called an **ectopic pregnancy** (Fig. 37-3). This implanted embryo can continue to grow there until it erodes through the wall or becomes large enough to rupture it, causing sudden abdominal pain and bleeding, usually intra-abdominally, that may lead to shock. Rupture usually occurs at 8 to 12 weeks gestation.

Risk factors for ectopic pregnancy involve those processes that can distort fallopian tube structure, including **pelvic inflammatory disease,** previous ectopic pregnancy, tubal ligation, prior pelvic surgery, and intrauterine device (IUD) use. Ectopic pregnancies also occasionally implant in the abdominal cavity when the fertilized ovum exits the tube through the wrong opening.

Another complication is when labor begins before the expected timeframe. Premature, or preterm, labor has been identified as the largest problem in obstetrics because of the high infant morbidity and mortality rates.[2] Premature labor is defined as regular uterine contractions with dilation of the cervix after the twentieth week and before the thirty-seventh week of gestation. This condition may be caused by or associated with rupture of the membranes and leaking amniotic fluid. Once membrane rupture has occurred, the baby is exposed to the potential of infection.

Preeclampsia (also known as toxemia of pregnancy) is defined as the presence of hypertension (systolic of 140 or >; diastolic 90 or >), protein in the urine, and edema during pregnancy. The edema associated with preeclampsia is generally caused by abnormal retention of sodium and water. It usually occurs in the third trimester, but can appear at any time in the latter half of pregnancy.

Eclampsia is the occurrence of a seizure in the presence of preeclampsia. Symptoms suggesting the development of preeclampsia in the patient include the presence of headache, visual disturbances, and other complaints related to the increased blood pressure. All of these conditions are considered life threatening to mother and baby.

Abruptio placenta is the premature separation of the placenta from the uterus prior to delivery of the fetus (Fig. 37-4). This condition occurs most commonly in the third trimester. The abruption produces some bleeding, loss of oxygen, and nutrient exchange in the area of separation, with potential risk to the fetus. If the separation occurs along the edge of the placenta, blood can escape through the cervical os (opening), and produce vaginal bleeding. If the separation occurs in the central area of the placenta, no bleeding will be noted and a hematoma will form inside the uterus. Once the placenta separates, the muscles of the uterus usually go into spasm, causing the pain typical of this condition.

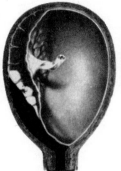
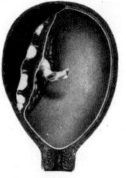
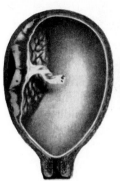

Partial separation (concealed hemorrhage)

Partial separation (apparent hemorrhage)

Complete separation (concealed hemorrhage)

Figure 37-4

Abruptio placenta: Degrees of separation of the placenta from the uterine wall. From Dickason EJ, Silverman BL, Schult MO: Maternal-Infant Nursing Care, ed 2, St. Louis, 1994, Mosby–Year Book. Used with permission of Ross Products Division, Abbott Laboratories, Columbus, Ohio.

In some cases, the fertilized ovum implants in the lower part of the uterus and the developing placenta grows over the opening of the cervix, either partially or completely. The location of the placenta over the cervical os, known as **placenta previa,** can result in uncontrollable hemorrhage directly from the placenta (Fig. 37-5). In this situation, unlike abruption, the bleeding is usually painless. The bleeding can be profuse and life threatening, but as in abruption, little or no blood may escape vaginally. Placenta previa is noted in 1 in 200 births, and is much more common in multiparous women.[2] Table 37-1 compares placenta previa with abruptio placentae.

Multiple pregnancies also present challenges. Twin pregnancies occur in approximately 1 out of 83 conceptions, and triplets occur once in 8000.[2] Multiple pregnancy is associated with much greater maternal risk, and infant mortality rate approximately three to four times higher than normal.[2] These increased problems are primarily caused by prematurity and complications of pregnancy, labor, and delivery.

Although many women experience nausea during the first trimester of pregnancy, a small percentage of women experience persistent and severe vomiting and subsequent dehydration. Hyperemesis gravidarum can compromise nutritional and hydration status of the mother.

Complications of Labor and Delivery

Labor is defined as the coordinated sequence of involuntary uterine contractions producing effacement (thinning) and dilation of the cervix leading to delivery. *Delivery* is the actual passing of the products of conception, including the placenta. A number of complications may occur during this process.

Sometimes during delivery, the umbilical cord presents itself first through the cervix and vagina, rather than the baby's head. This is called *prolapse of the umbilical cord* (Fig. 37-6). With uterine contractions, the head or presenting part of the baby compresses the cord against the birth canal, obstructing blood flow through the cord. This can result in fetal hypoxia, anoxic brain injury, and death.

The position of the baby inside the uterus is a very important factor in the difficulty of the labor and delivery process. *Fetal presentation* is the term used to describe the part of the baby that lies over the cervix. In 95% of pregnancies, a vertex, or head down, presentation is noted (Fig. 37-7). Frank breech, or buttock down, presentation occurs in 4% to 5% of deliveries. In this presentation, the lower extremities are flexed at the hips and extended at the knees, thus presenting the buttocks instead of the head. A footling breech is one or both feet at the opening.

The postpartum period is the period after labor and delivery when the body changes from its pregnant state back to normal. Most complications associated with this process occur in the first week following delivery; **postpartum hemorrhage** and infection account for the most serious problems.

Patient Assessment

History

Diagnosis of any abdominal abnormality in a pregnant woman is made more difficult by the changes associated with pregnancy. The enlarging uterus displaces abdominal organs and

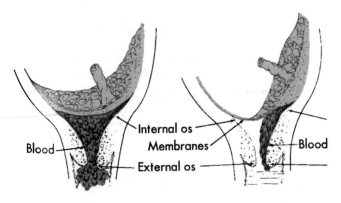
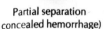

Blood — Internal os — Membranes — External os — Blood

Figure 37-5

Placenta previa occurs when the placenta grows over the internal os, causing hemorrhage. From Jensen MD, Bobak IM: Maternity and Gynecologic Care, ed 3, St. Louis, 1985, CV Mosby.

TABLE 37-1	Comparison of Placenta Previa and Abruptio Placentae	
Placenta Previa	**Abruptio Placentae**	
No underlying chronic disease	Associated with hypertension, diabetes, and kidney diseases	
Warning sign of spotting hemorrhage always externally visible	Usually no warning signs; hemorrhage may be internal or externally visible	
No pain	Pain may be present in varying degrees	
Placenta in lower uterine segment	Placental attachment in normal locations	
Soft uterus	Uterus tender to rigid	

Adapted from Dickason, et al: Maternal and Infant Nursing Care, ed 2, St. Louis, 1994, Mosby–Year Book.

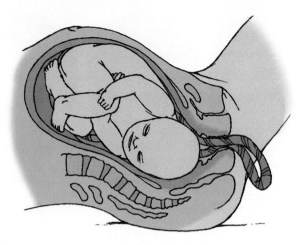

Figure 37-6

In the condition of a prolapsed cord, the umbilical cord can be compressed between the baby's head and the wall of the vaginal canal. From Stoy WA, Center for Emergency Medicine: Mosby's EMT–Basic Textbook, St. Louis, 1996, Mosby Lifeline.

can produce pain from nonpregnancy related abdominal processes that is perceived in sites distant from their "classical" locations. In addition, conditions can occur within the uterus that produce true emergencies for the mother and fetus.

- *Is the patient pregnant?* This is often difficult to verify early in the pregnancy when symptoms are often subtle and some women do not yet realize they are pregnant. Even as the pregnancy progresses, some assign their physical changes to weight gain rather than pregnancy. Thus, it is always important for prehospital providers to consider the possibility of pregnancy, even if the patient does not mention it. Over-the-counter pregnancy tests have made it much easier for women to have an accurate determination of pregnancy very early after a missed menstrual period.
- *How far along is the pregnancy?* The determination of which trimester the pregnancy is in will help the patient assessment. In women who know they are pregnant, this can be estimated by asking the date of her last menstrual period and determining the elapsed time less 2 weeks. If the pregnancy has progressed beyond 12 weeks, the uterus can be palpated in the abdomen. Spontaneous abortion and ectopic pregnancy generally occur in the first trimester. Abruption placenta, placenta previa, preeclampsia, and eclampsia generally occur in the third trimester.
- *Is abdominal pain present?* Constant abdominal pain of sudden onset may be related to abruptio placenta or ectopic pregnancy. Many of the conditions that occur in nonpregnant individuals, such as appendicitis, can also be present during pregnancy. If the pain is cramping in nature and is felt in the lower back or abdomen, premature or full-term labor should be considered. Preeclampsia may be accompanied by epigastric pain.
- *Does the patient note vaginal bleeding?* If the patient is in the first trimester of pregnancy, vaginal bleeding may indicate a threatened or complete abortion, or less commonly, an ectopic pregnancy. In the third trimester, vaginal bleeding with abdominal pain suggests abruptio placenta; depending on the size of the separation and the degree of circulatory loss, fetal distress may also develop.

CRITICAL ISSUE

Vaginal bleeding, abdominal pain, or shock presenting in a women in the first trimester of pregnancy must be considered to be an ectopic pregnancy, and preparations for aggressive resuscitation should be instituted until proven otherwise.

Placenta previa usually causes painless vaginal bleeding that may be profuse and life threatening. Fetal distress can occur if **hypovolemia** and maternal hypoperfusion develop. Placenta previa must be considered as a source of vaginal bleeding in any pregnant woman. The amount of bleeding can be approximated by quantifying the number of pads used in a period of time and how soaked with blood they are at each pad change. The difficulty of blood loss estimation is compounded, however, by the possibility of further bleeding concealed by the placenta.

CRITICAL ISSUE

Vaginal bleeding in the third trimester is a serious condition. There can be a large amount of bleeding or severe fetal distress that is not evident in maternal vital signs.

- *Are contractions occurring?* It is important to note the time between contractions and the duration of each. Determine when the contractions began, and if the patient's membranes have ruptured. The longer the contractions have been going on, the longer the duration of each contraction and the shorter the intervals between them, the closer the patient is to delivery.
- *Has the patient been pregnant before?* Patients are often described based on their gravidity and parity. *Gravidity* is the total number of pregnancies a woman has had including abortions or miscarriages, while *parity* describes the number of previous live births. As a very general rule,

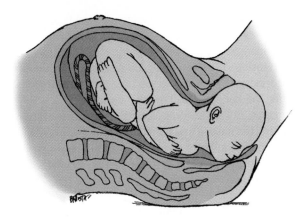

Figure 37-7

Cephalic delivery position. From Stoy WA, Center for Emergency Medicine: Mosby's EMT–Basic Textbook, St. Louis, 1996, Mosby Lifeline.

the time between the onset of labor and delivery of the baby is greater in the first pregnancy than in later ones. Preeclampsia is also more common during the first pregnancy.

CRITICAL ISSUE

If the patient has had a prior delivery, she can usually tell if delivery is imminent.

- *Is this a multiple pregnancy?* Some patients may be aware that their pregnancy consists of multiple fetuses. Multiple pregnancy results in increased abdominal distention, backache, nausea, anemia, fetal activity, and nearly every other symptom of pregnancy.
- *Has the patient had any prenatal care?* Women who have not had prenatal care are not likely to have had complications or problems treated, and thus are at higher risk for complicated labor and delivery. Prenatal care is regular preventive medical care of the mother and fetus during the pregnancy. Care is aimed at improving the health of the fetus and mother with nutritional counseling, information about normal body changes, emotional support, and hazard warnings such as smoking, alcohol, and illicit and prescribed drugs. Maternal chronic diseases such as **diabetes, hypertension,** and cardiovascular disease are managed to prevent complications for the mother and baby.
- *Has the patient had a cesarean section previously?* Women in labor who have had previous cesarean sections (surgical delivery of the baby through the abdomen) are at increased risk of **rupture of the uterus** along the scar. Additionally a cesarean may be indicated again for subsequent pregnancies depending on why it was done in the first place.

Physical Examination

The prehospital physical examination of the pregnant patient begins with evaluation of vital signs. Remember that the pulse may be elevated by as much as 20 beats per minute during a normal pregnancy.

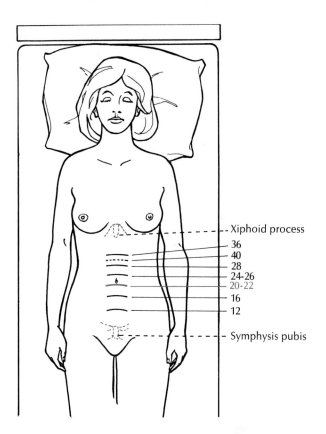

Xiphoid process
36
40
28
24-26
20-22
16
12
Symphysis pubis

Figure 37-8

Height of fundus by weeks of gestation. These measurements refer to the normally growing single conceptus within the uterus. The paramedic must remember that fundal height measurements are offset by numerous factors, for example: molar preganancy, multiple pregnancy, or growth-retarded fetus (large for gestational age {LGS}). From Jensen MD, Bobak IM: Maternity and Gynecologic Care, 3d 3, St. Louis, 1985, CV Mosby.

Hypertension in a pregnant women is considered to be a systolic pressure of 140 mm Hg or greater, or a rise of 30 mm Hg from the patient's nonpregnant systolic level, if known. A diastolic pressure of 90 mm Hg or greater, or a rise of 15 mm Hg above the patient's nonpregnant reading, is also considered hypertensive.

The abdominal examination can provide information about the stage of pregnancy duration. The abdomen can be observed for evidence of distention, and in many cases the fundus (top of the uterus) is palpable. Beginning with the twelfth week of pregnancy, the uterus can be felt above the pelvic rim (Fig. 37-8). By the twentieth week of pregnancy, the top of the uterus can be felt at the level of the umbilicus. In the third trimester, the fundal height is generally palpated between the xiphoid and the umbilicus. Contractions can also be felt as the patient begins labor.

As a general rule, internal vaginal examinations should not be performed in a prehospital setting. The perineum should be visually assessed with as much privacy as can be accomplished for the patient. Visual inspection is necessary to evaluate for any crowning—presentation of a body part or the umbilical cord at the opening of the vagina during a contraction (Fig. 37-9).

If vaginal bleeding is present, the color of the blood and the presence of clots or tissue should be noted. When the

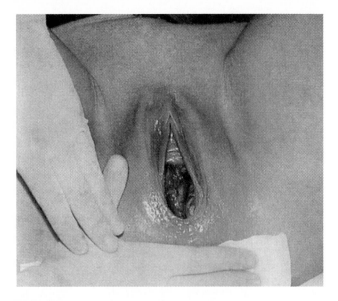

Figure 37-9

Crowning refers to the presence of a fetal body part or umbilical cord during uterine contraction. From Al-Azzawi: Color Atlas of Childbirth and Obstetric Techniques, St. Louis, 1990, Mosby–Year Book.

mother's membranes rupture, amniotic fluid is released. If this fluid is visible, the paramedic should examine for the presence of meconium, which is fecal material produced *in utero*. The presence of meconium indicates possible fetal asphyxia and the need for special airway care at birth.

Key Conditions and Findings

- *Threatened or Spontaneous Abortion.* This condition occurs before 20 weeks of gestation, usually at 6 to 12 weeks and is associated with vaginal bleeding and cramping abdominal pain. If the fetus remains viable, it is a threatened abortion; if fetal tissue is expelled, it is a spontaneous abortion.
- *Ectopic Pregnancy.* This condition usually occurs between 6 and 12 weeks of gestation. The patient presents with the sudden onset of abdominal pain and lightheadedness, and syncope or shock from intra-abdominal hemorrhage. Vaginal bleeding may or may not be noted.
- *Abruptio Placenta.* Abruptio placenta is associated with hypertension, diabetes, preeclampsia, eclampsia, chronic renal disease, and even minor trauma. Abruption is more common in multiparous women and in women who have had an abruption during a previous pregnancy.
- *Placenta Previa.* Several conditions increase the likelihood of placenta previa, including previous cesarean section, a large placenta, and poor uterine vascular supply.
- *Premature Labor.* Patients at risk for premature labor are those with trauma, previous preterm deliveries, urinary tract infections, twins or multiple pregnancies, and anatomic abnormalities of the uterus.
- *Preeclampsia.* Preeclampsia is most common in very young (less than 17 years of age) and older (more than 35

years of age) pregnant patients. Approximately 65% of the cases occur during the first pregnancy.[2] The incidence also increases with multiple pregnancies. A history of hypertension, diabetes, vascular disease, or renal disease also increases the risk of occurence. Once a seizure occurs, the patient is said to have eclampsia.

- **Hyperemesis Gravidarum.** Some women will develop protracted nausea and vomiting during the pregnancy, resulting in significant **dehydration** and requiring IV fluid replacement. In some cases, antiemetic medications may be prescribed to aid the patient in recovery.
- *Prolapse of the Umbilical Cord.* Risk factors for the development of a prolapsed cord include breech or abnormal presentations, multiple pregnancies such as twins, premature rupture of membranes, low implantation of the placenta, abnormally long cord, and a small pelvis. Prolapse of the umbilical cord occurs in approximately 1 in 200 births.[2] When the water bag breaks and fluid rushes out the vagina, the cord can be pulled with it through the vaginal opening.
- *Uterine Rupture.* The rupture of the uterus during pregnancy is a rare but major cause of maternal and fetal death, occurring in approximately 1 in 1500 deliveries.[2] This condition usually occurs during labor but can also be associated with trauma to the gravid uterus. Assessment reveals severe lower abdominal pain, a distended abdomen, and presence of hypovolemic shock.
- *Postpartum Hemorrhage.* A common complication in the postpartum period is hemorrhage. The uterus, which has been much larger as it enclosed the placenta and fetus, is now empty and must contract to control bleeding. The most common cause of bleeding is the inability of the uterus to contract adequately. Other causes include coagulation defects and retained products of conception.
- *Postpartum Infection.* Postpartum infection typically occurs within the first few days after delivery. The majority of patients with infection have **endometritis,** an infection of the lining of the uterus. This is associated with abdominal or uterine tenderness, fever, and a foul-smelling vaginal discharge or bleeding. The infection may spread rapidly and progress to systemic **sepsis.** Other potential sources of infection include the genital tract, urinary tract, and the breasts.

Management

Prehospital evaluation and treatment of any complaint of abdominal pain or vaginal bleeding is based on an assumption that the problem is potentially life threatening. This begins with assessing the need for airway management and placing the patient on 100% oxygen at a high-flow rate. The paramedic must remember that normal maternal vital signs do not necessarily reflect the absence of fetal distress, and that supplemental oxygen provides the best environment for the fetal circulation.

Intravenous access should be established in all pregnant patients using a large—bore catheter (16g or larger). If there

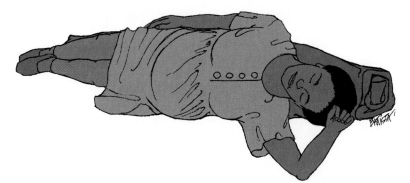

Figure 37-10

Transporting the mother on her left side will reduce the pressure that the fetus places on her circulatory system. From Stoy WA, Center for Emergency Medicine: Mosby's EMT–Basic Textbook, St. Louis, 1996, Mosby Lifeline.

is evidence of hypoperfusion, normal saline or Ringer's lactate fluid boluses should be administered and a second IV established.

All patients in the third trimester should be placed on their left side (in left lateral decubitus position), conditions permitting, to shift the uterus off of the vena cava and aorta, and improve blood return to the heart (Fig. 37-10). If the patient is immobilized on a long backboard, the entire board can be tilted to the left by placing a blanket or padding under the right side.

The patient with suspected preeclampsia must be aggressively treated and is considered a high-risk pregnancy. Consultation with medical direction for IV magnesium sulfate may be necessary if available if severe hypertension is noted. If seizure activity is present, IV magnesium or diazepam will likely be necessary (see Box 37-3).

In a patient in premature labor or with any other high-risk pregnancy, transport should be rapid and to a facility capable of handling a complicated obstetrical condition. Contact with the hospital must be made early to allow for prompt notification of obstetricians and neonatologists.

Most standard ACLS procedures can and should be used as they would for a nonpregnant patient. Events that may produce cardiac arrest in the pregnant patient include ventricular dysrhythmias, congestive heart failure, myocardial infarction, and complications of preeclampsia or eclampsia.

Labor and Delivery

The process of labor is usually divided into three stages (Fig. 37-11). The first stage consists of regular uterine contractions that gradually become more frequent and forceful and longer in duration. The uterine contents are pushed against the cervix, and effacement and dilation of the cervix occur. During this period, the mucous plug that fills the cervical os is expelled usually with some associated bleeding. This is commonly referred to as a "bloody show." This process also involves some amount of cramping pain, generally in the lower abdomen and back.

As the cervix dilates and the presenting part (normally the head) moves down toward the pelvis, more perineal pain is noted. The average duration of the first stage is 8 to 12 hours for the first pregnancy and 6 to 8 hours in subsequent ones. Uterine contractions gradually increase in intensity and frequency during this stage, occurring every 2 to 3 minutes and

lasting 30 to 45 seconds. Contractions may be felt and timed by feeling the uterine wall become hard during the contractions, and relaxing and becoming soft between them.

Rupture of the membranes that contain the amniotic fluid and enclose the baby can occur prior to the onset of labor or at any time during the first stage. Once the membranes have ruptured, 90% of women will go into labor within 24 hours.[2]

The second stage of labor is the period from complete cervical dilation to delivery of the baby. This period does not usually last longer than 2 hours. The fetal head enters the birth canal, and contractions occur more frequently and strongly. The mother may have the urge to bear down or push, as the fetal head presses against the rectum.

The third stage of labor begins at birth and ends with delivery of the placenta. The placenta generally separates from the uterus within 5 minutes after delivery of the infant and delivers within 20 to 30 minutes.

The management of labor and delivery outside the hospital is a stressful situation regardless of the circumstance. Every effort should be made by the paramedic to reassure the mother and provide emotional support for her. The spouse or a neighbor may be enlisted to help with the mother's emotional needs. It is important for EMS providers to be prepared in the event that a patient's labor has progressed and delivery is imminent. The mother should be moved into a left lateral decubitus position during labor and then placed supine for delivery.

BOX 37-3	Magnesium Sulfate

- Therapeutic Action
  Stops convulsive seizures associated with toxemia of pregnancy
  Central nervous system depressant
- Indications
  Seizures associated with eclampsia
  Torsades de Pointes (a rare variation of ventricular tachycardia)
  Refractory ventricular tachycardia and fibrillation
- Contraindications
  Kidney failure
  Heart block
  Respiratory depression
- Adverse Reactions
  Hypotension
  Respiratory depression or arrest

Emergency vehicles should carry an obstetrical kit, which is a sterile setup containing the items found in Box 37-4.

If a prolapsed cord is noted, the prehospital provider should place a hand in the vagina and push up on the fetal head to decrease cord compression until management can be assumed by a physician in the emergency department (Fig. 37-12). "Knee chest" position will also add gravitational assistance, although it can be difficult to maintain during transport.

Delivery is imminent when the patient is straining as if to have a bowel movement, the vagina is bulging and the fetal head is visible at the vaginal opening. The mother should be placed on her back with her knees widely separated. The buttocks can be elevated with pillows to allow for access to the perineal area. A sterile field should be made around the vaginal opening with sterile towels or paper barriers. Once the head is visible, no attempts should be made to delay or prevent delivery.

BOX 37-4   **The Delivery Kit**

Births can be very spontaneous. Prepackaged equipment is essential for a successful and organized delivery. The delivery kit should include the following components:

- Surgical scissors—used for cutting the cord
- Hemostats or cord clamp—used for clamping the cord
- Umbilical tape or sterilized cord—used for tying off the placenta side of the umbilical cord
- Bulb syringe—used for suctioning the mouth and nose of the infant
- Towels—used for drying and stimulating the infant
- 2 times 10 gauze sponges—used to clear secretions from the infant's mouth and to pat the ends of the cut umbilical cord
- Sterile gloves—used for body substance isolation
- One baby blanket—used to keep the baby warm
- Sanitary napkins—used to absorb the drainage of blood from the vagina
- Plastic bag—used as a receptacle for transporting the placenta

Ideally, the kit should be packaged in a moisture-resistant receptacle with a date of expiration to prevent deterioration of the contents.

From McSwain, et al: The Basic EMT, St. Louis, 1996, Mosby Lifeline.

C R I T I C A L   I S S U E

If a prolapsed cord is noted, the prehospital provider should place a hand in the vagina and push up on the fetal head to decrease cord compression until management can be assumed by a physician in the emergency department.

The paramedic places the palm of one hand over the advancing head of the fetus (Fig. 37-13). The head should be slightly flexed to make delivery easier and at the same time held to prevent it from popping out too quickly. As the head emerges, the mother should be encouraged not to push so

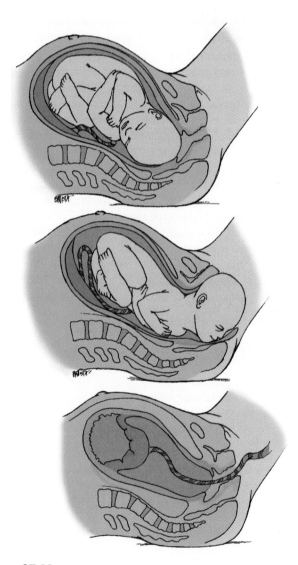

Figure 37-11

The three stages of labor: A, contraction and dilation. B, The baby moves through the birth canal and is born. C, Delivery of the placenta. From Stoy WA, Center for Emergency Medicine: Mosby's EMT–Basic Textbook, St. Louis, 1996, Mosby Lifeline.

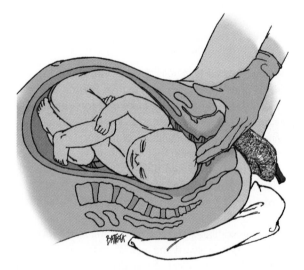

Figure 37-12

Pressure on the fetal head may decrease cord compression. From Stoy WA, Center for Emergency Medicine: Mosby's EMT–Basic Textbook, St. Louis, 1996, Mosby Lifeline.

that the delivery can continue slowly and with minimal trauma to the perineal area. Having the mother take slow deep breaths through her mouth will help to overcome the strong urge to push.

Once the head is delivered, the baby's mouth and nasal passages should be cleared of secretions by suctioning the nose first with a bulb syringe (Fig. 37-14). If the umbilical cord is wrapped around the infant's neck, it can usually be slipped down over the shoulder. If the cord is too tightly wrapped around the neck, it can be clamped and cut (Fig. 37-15).

One shoulder is then delivered with the next contraction. The anterior (upper) shoulder should usually passes first with gentle downward pressure on the head during the contraction. The posterior (lower) shoulder can then be delivered with gentle upward pressure on the head. Once the shoulders are free, the remainder of the infant's body normally delivers easily.

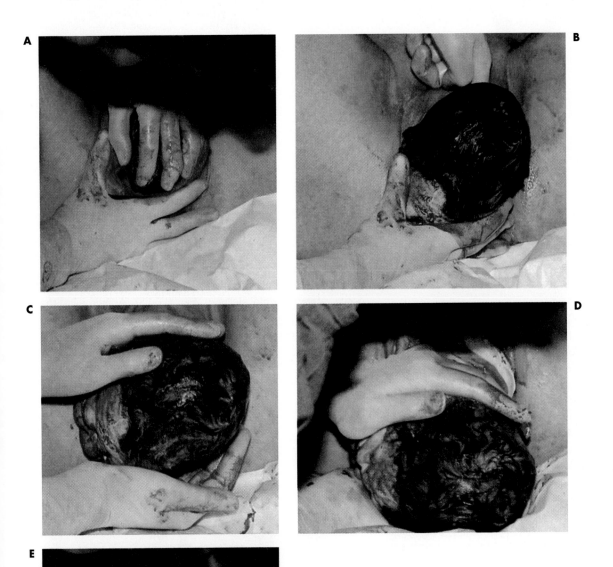

Figure 37-13

The delivery process: A, Crowning. B, the baby's neck should be checked for the presence of the umbilical cord. C, The baby's head is supported as it rotates. D, The baby's head is guided downward to deliver the shoulder. E, The baby's other shoulder is delivered. From Al-Azzawi: Color Atlas of Childbirth and Obstetric Techniques, St. Louis, 1990, Mosby–Year Book.

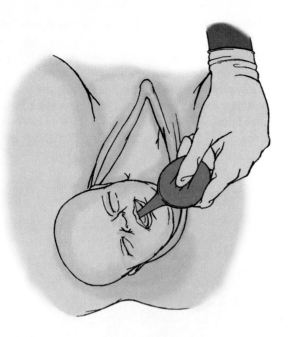

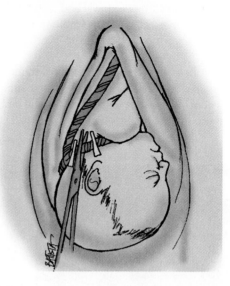

Figure 37-15

If the umbilical cord is wrapped around the baby's neck and cannot be removed, the cord should be clamped in two places and cut between the clamps. From Stoy WA, Center for Emergency Medicine: Mosby's EMT–Basic Textbook, St. Louis, 1996, Mosby Lifeline.

Figure 37-14

After the infant's head is born, the head should be supported and the baby's mouth and nose wiped. The baby's nose and mouth should then be suctioned with a bulb syringe. From Stoy WA, Center for Emergency Medicine: Mosby's EMT–Basic Textbook, St. Louis, 1996, Mosby Lifeline.

Postpartum bleeding can sometimes be controlled by external uterine massage, encouraging the uterus to clamp down, after placental delivery (Fig. 37-18). Additionally, the mother should be encouraged to breast feed, as stimulation of the nipples may promote uterine contraction. Some EMS systems use the drug oxytocin to contract uterine smooth muscle and decrease bleeding (Box 37-5). Vaginal lacerations may occur as the result of delivery and may be limited or extend into

Once delivered, the infant should be held at the level of the vagina or below until the cord can be clamped with two clamps, then cut in between (Fig. 37-16). The cord should be clamped permanently with an umbilical clamp or cord about 6 cm from the infant's abdomen.

Complicated deliveries such as breech presentations, brow, or face presentations, the head or shoulders not moving further down the birth canal, and multiple births should not be delivered in the field if at all possible.

Although it can be done, field delivery of a frank breech presentation requires specific training and is best left to hospital personnel when possible. If a paramedic must deliver a frank breech, he or she should allow the fetus to deliver spontaneously to the level of the umbilicus. Next, the paramedic should palpate the fetal shoulder and rotate the arm across the chest and over the posterior vagina. The fetal head usually delivers spontaneously; if not, the trunk of the infant should be supported with the paramedic's forearm, and the paramedic should place his or her fingers on the infant's maxilla and exert mild downward traction (Fig. 37-17). Traction should not be exerted by using fingers in the infant's mouth. Breech presentations of an isolated extremity require a caesarean section for delivery and cannot be delivered in the prehospital environment.

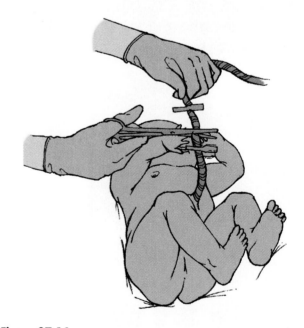

Figure 37-16

The umbilical cord can be cut between the two clamps approximately 6 cm from the baby. From Stoy WA, Center for Emergency Medicine: Mosby's EMT–Basic Textbook, St. Louis, 1996, Mosby Lifeline.

C R I T I C A L   I S S U E

Rapid transport to a hospital is indicated for any breech presentation or other condition causing prolonged labor.

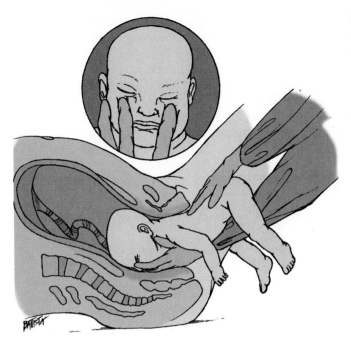

Figure 37-17

The technique for management of a breech birth with an undelivered head. From Stoy WA, Center for Emergency Medicine: Mosby's EMT–Basic Textbook, St. Louis, 1996, Mosby Lifeline.

the rectum. Prehospital management should be directed at applying direct pressure to control hemorrhage.

Transport of the patient to the hospital should occur immediately. Delivery of the placenta may occur spontaneously, but unless significant bleeding is noted, it may be postponed until arrival at the receiving hospital. Destination policies should reflect a desire to transport the patient to a facility that optimizes the outcome for both mother and fetus. High-risk pregnancies (e.g., breech presentations, multiple births, preterm labor) should be transported to a facility where spe-

cialized care is available for both patients, when possible. Otherwise, patients in active labor should generally be transported to the closest emergency department.

Newborn Care

The essentials of newborn care include drying and heat conservation, airway clearing, proper positioning to maintain the airway and encourage fluid drainage, and physical stimulation to promote breathing.

Newborns have difficulty maintaining their body temperature because of the children's large surface area-to-core ratio and the presence of amniotic fluid. Heat loss can be prevented by using an infant warmer if available. If not, warm towels may be used and the infant can be placed against the mother. Head covering is also important to maintain warmth and can be done with a blanket if a cap is not available. The infant should be dried as soon as possible, and positioned in a slight head-down (Trendelenburg) position on the baby's side to help nasal and airway secretions drain. Stimulation of the infant is important and can improve the respiratory effort. This can be performed by rubbing or drying the infant with a towel.

C R I T I C A L   I S S U E

The primary enemy of newborns is hypothermia, which can occur within minutes because of evaporative heat loss.

If meconium-stained amniotic fluid has been noted, it is necessary to examine the infant's pharynx for evidence of meconium, because this material does not usually pass below the vocal cords until after birth. In this setting, the paramedic should perform laryngoscopy and suction any visible meconium. Aggressive respiratory support may be required. Neonatal resuscitation is described in Chapter 22.

Any resuscitation required after the aforementioned items have been completed usually involves the use of high-flow oxygen. It may be necessary to use a bag-valve-mask or to intubate the infant. In the majority of cases, however, a proper airway and oxygenation are the only corrective measures required.

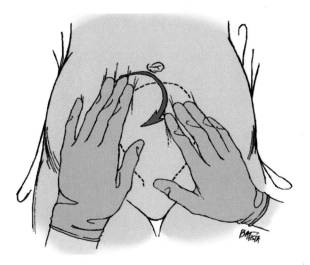

Figure 37-18

Uterine massage helps to control bleeding after delivery. From Stoy WA, Center for Emergency Medicine: Mosby's EMT–Basic Textbook, St. Louis, 1996, Mosby Lifeline.

BOX 37-5   **Oxytocin**

- Therapeutic Action
  Stimulates contraction of uterine smooth muscle to decrease bleeding from uterine vessels
- Indications
  Postpartum hemorrhage
- Contraindications
  Do not use prior to delivery of the baby or placenta; multiple gestations
- Adverse Reactions
  Cardiac dysrhythmia, uterine rupture, anaphylaxis, nausea, and vomiting

TABLE 37-2	The APGAR Scoring System		
Sign	**0**	**1**	**2**
Appearance (skin color)	Blue, pale	Body pink, blue extremities	Completely pink
Pulse Rate (heart rate)	Absent	< 100/minute	> 100/minute
Grimace (irritability)	No response	Grimace	Cough, sneeze, cry
Activity (muscle tone)	Limp	Some flexion	Active motion
Respirations (respiratory effort)	Absent	Slow, irregular	Good, crying

From Aehlert: Pediatric Advanced Life Support Study Guide, St. Louis, 1994, Mosby Lifeline.

An APGAR score should be determined at intervals of 1 and 5 minutes after delivery. The score is based on the assessment of the infant's heart rate, respiratory effort, muscle tone, color, and response to stimulation (Table 37-2). Infants with APGAR scores of less than 7 are more likely to require aggressive resuscitation and should be monitored closely and frequently.

SUMMARY

The evaluation and treatment of the woman of childbearing age requires a knowledge of the changes and conditions associated with pregnancy. The presentation of the pregnant woman generally involves the presence of abdominal pain or vaginal bleeding.

It is important for the paramedic to note the differences in blood volume, heart rate, and blood pressure in the initial assessment of the pregnant patient, and to remember that changes affecting the baby may be occurring without obvious effect on the mother.

REFERENCES

1. **Apgar BS, Churgay CA.** Spontaneous abortion. Prim Care 1993; 20:621–7

2. **Benson RC.** Current obstetric and gynecologic diagnosis and treatment. Los Altos, CA, Lange Medical Publications, 1992.

SUGGESTED READINGS

1. **American College of Surgeons.** Advanced Trauma Life Support Course. Chicago, 1993.

2. **American Heart Association.** Textbook of advanced cardiac life support. Dallas, TX, 1990.

3. **Campbell JE.** Basic trauma life support: advanced prehospital care. Englewood Cliffs, NJ, Brady, 1988.

4. **Chameides L.** Textbook of pediatric advanced life support. American Heart Association and American Academy of Pediatrics, 1990.

Carol Goodykoontz, RN, MS, EMT-P

Chapter 38

Fever

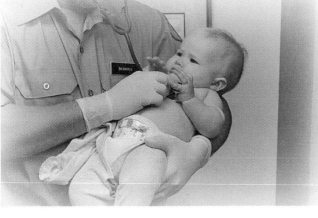

A paramedic should be able to:

KEY TERMS

1. **Febrile seizure**—a seizure associated with a febrile illness.
2. **Hypothalamus**—a portion of the diencephalon of the brain that activates, controls, and integrates the peripheral autonomic nervous system, endocrine processes, and many somatic functions, such as body temperature, sleep, and appetite.
3. **Pyrogens**—any agent or substance that tends to cause a rise in body temperature, such as some bacterial toxins.
4. **Sepsis**—infection or contamination.
5. **Septic shock**—a form of shock that most often results from a serious systemic bacterial infection.

ever is a classic and reliable sign of illness or disease, and in some cases may indicate a life-threatening condition. A basic understanding of body temperature regulation and the common causes of fever will assist the EMS provider in evaluating and managing patients with fever. This chapter focuses on the recognition of life-threatening febrile illnesses.

TABLE 38-1	Normal Body Temperature by Location
Oral	98.6°F (37° C)
Rectal	99.6°F (37.6° C)
Axillary	97.6°F (36.4°C)

Pathophysiology

Temperature Regulation

Body temperature is maintained by balancing heat loss and heat production. Heat production takes place during the transformation of food into energy (metabolism) and during physical exercise. Most heat loss occurs through the skin, primarily by radiation from exposed areas and evaporation of sweat (Fig. 38-1). Under other circumstances, heat loss may be accelerated by convection (wind blowing across exposed skin) or conduction (the direct transfer of heat to another substance, such as water).

The brain's primary control of body temperature and heat regulation takes place in the hypothalamus. The hypothalamus receives body temperature messages directly from circulating blood and from peripheral skin receptors. It acts as a thermostat, maintaining body temperature very near 98.6° F (37° C). Body temperature is higher near the center, or core, of the body. Under average conditions, body temperature is maintained within a narrow range, although it can vary 1° above and 2° below 98.6° F and still be considered normal (Fig. 38-2).

Table 38-1 lists normal body temperature measurements for the oral, rectal, and axillary locations. Table 38-2 shows the comparison of Fahrenheit and Celsius readings and gives conversion formulas.

TABLE 38-2	Comparison of Fahrenheit and Celsius Readings	
Fahrenheit	**Celsius**	
96.8°	36°	
98.6°	37°	
100.4°	38°	
102.2°	39°	
104°	40°	

Conversion Formulas
Fahrenheit to Celsius: (Fahrenheit reading − 32) × 5 / 9
Celsius to Fahrenheit: (Celsius reading × 9 / 5) + 32

The Mechanism of Fever

Fever is defined simply as an elevation of body temperature, which can occur for a variety of reasons. The most common cause of fever is infection by virus, bacteria, or fungus.

This condition differs from other factors that can affect temperature control, such as high environmental temperature and humidity, or factors that directly affect the hypothalamus (e.g., stroke, tumors, or central nervous system [CNS] stimulants).

Infectious agents cause the release of stored protein substances known as pyrogens. These proteins promote an

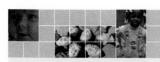

PEDIATRIC PERSPECTIVE

- Fever is a common medical presentation in the pediatric population. Although it is usually benign and self-limiting, a fever can signal a potentially serious or even fatal illness, such as meningitis.
- Pediatric patients, particularly preschool-aged children, are predisposed to larger and faster ranges in body temperature than are usually seen in adults. The reasons for this occurence are that thermoregulatory controls are not completely developed, and the child has more body surface (skin) area relative to body mass.
- The increased body surface area relative to body mass in an infant and child allows for effective cooling of a febrile patient but also subjects these patients to quicker development of hypothermia, either when wet or when exposed to cool environments.

- Dehydration is a concern with febrile infants and children. Signs of volume depletion include tachycardia, dry mucous membranes, delayed capillary refill, altered mental status, and an absence of tears when the child cries. In an infant, the number of wet diapers can give an indication of hydration status.
- Febrile seizures are a particular risk in children (commonly between 6 months and 3 years of age) with fever. A rapid rise in temperature, rather than a high temperature itself, usually triggers the seizure.
- Management of the infant or child with fever includes removal of heavy clothing, administration of acetaminophen, and keeping the child in a cool environment. Transport to a physician is also important.

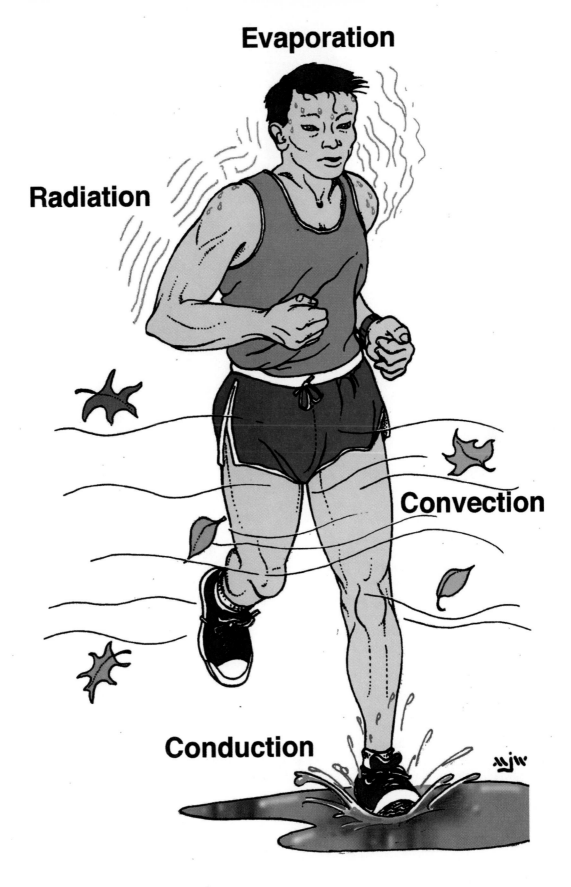

Figure 38-1

Types of heat loss.

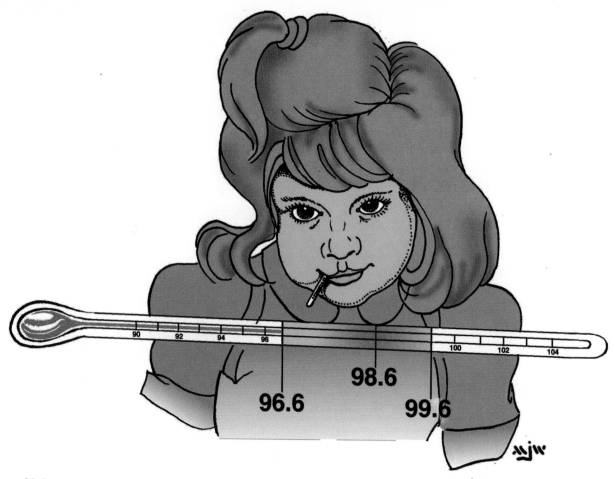

Figure 38-2

The range of normal body temperature.

increased production of chemical agents called prostaglandins, which raise the thermostatic "set point" of the hypothalamus (usually 98.6° F or 37° C) to a higher level. Because bacteria and viruses reproduce more slowly at temperatures higher than the normal core temperature, fever serves as a defense mechanism against intruding organisms. Pyrogens are also released when tissue is destroyed, which explains why temperature elevation sometimes occurs in patients with myocardial infarction or severe injuries.

Chills may occur as the body attempts to maintain temperature at the higher set point through shivering (heat production) and peripheral vasoconstriction (heat conservation). When the pyrogen release ends following antibiotic or other treatment methods, or simply because the disease has run its course, the hypothalamus will reset to a lower point, and the fever "breaks." Peripheral vasodilation allows the excess heat to be eliminated by the body through evaporation of sweat, and body temperature returns to normal.

Patient Assessment

History

If the initial patient assessment does not reveal immediate life threats, the history should focus on key questions related to the fever.

- *When did the fever begin, and how high is it?* Determining the time of onset of a fever can provide some indication about the duration of the disease process. Although the degree of temperature elevation may not be representative of the severity of illness, in general, the higher the fever, the greater the concern should be about the presence of serious illness.
- *What is the pattern of fever?* The pattern of fever may be sustained, intermittent, or remittent (Table 38-3). A sustained fever is most commonly found in severe cases of pneumonia or meningitis.
- *Are there any associated symptoms?* Often a fever is accompanied by chills, headache, and malaise. Other patient complaints that may signify an infection include ear

TABLE 38-3	Patterns of Fever	
Sustained	**Intermittent**	**Remittent**
Fever remains consistently elevated with minimal variation during the day.	Fever rises to a peak in the late afternoon then returns to normal.	Fever is present each day although the degree fluctuates. Temperature does not return to normal (most common type).

Adapted from Luckman J, Sorensen K: Medical-Surgical Nursing, A Psychophysiologic Approach, ed 3, Philadelphia, 1987, WB Saunders.

pain, sore throat, cough, flank pain, and painful or frequent urination.

- *In infants, what are the associated complaints?* In addition to fever, signs and symptoms of infection in infants are lethargy, poor feeding habits, irritability, bulging fontanels, rash, and a stiff neck. Neck stiffness is a significant sign but difficult to evaluate in young children.

- *Is this patient at special risk from a fever?* Certain individuals should be considered to have a serious problem any time they present with body temperature elevation. These include patients with impaired immunity, such as those with diabetes, alcoholics, and AIDS patients, and patients on an immunosuppression regimen, such as transplant recipients.

Children with fever account for a significant proportion of pediatric EMS calls. The risk of a child contracting a serious infection, such as meningitis, is greater than the risk in an adult patient because children lack a fully developed immune system. Childhood illnesses are frequently accompanied by fever.

In elderly patients, the hypothalamus temperature regulation is often compromised. Because baseline temperature is usually lower than normal (temperature is typically in the range of 96° F [35.6° C] to 98° F [36.7° C] oral) in the elderly, a life-threatening infection can be present without significant temperature elevation. The lack of effective temperature control can also cause elderly patients to develop dangerously high temperatures in response to elevated environmental temperatures.

- *Does the patient admit to any recreational drug use?* Sympathetic stimulants, such as cocaine and amphetamines, can produce a hyperactive, hypermetabolic state that is associated with the production of fever and can pose a life threat.

Physical Examination

The physical examination is directed by information obtained in the patient history. The most important initial observation is the patient's tolerance of the fever. If toxicity is readily apparent, a more aggressive management plan will be necessary. Altered mental status in a patient may often be the only sign of severe sepsis, particularly in the elderly.

A complete set of vital signs is imperative. The patient's pulse can be expected to increase 10 beats per minute for each 1.3° F (0.6° C) rise in temperature. Fever may also be associated with an elevated respiratory rate, especially when respiratory infections are present.

Although some EMS systems do not record patient temperatures in the prehospital environment, the technology exists to do so quickly and accurately if desired.

Audiothermy, or temperature measurement in the ear, and temperature strips placed on the forehead are used by some services rather than traditional thermometers. It must be noted that these techniques can be misleading because they can be inaccurate. The temperature reading is helpful when elevated but may be unhelpful when reading normal.

If thermometers are used, axillary temperatures are somewhat unreliable and may take 5 to 7 minutes to obtain a reading. These thermometers are therefore not recommended for the prehospital setting. Oral temperatures are taken in most situations, although the reading can be altered by recent eating or drinking. Rectal temperatures should be assessed on any patient who has an altered level of responsiveness or confusion; a patient under the age of 5; or a patient with a history of seizures. The rectal temperature reading is the most accurate reflection of body core temperature.

Body temperature can also be estimated clinically by the appearance of the patient's skin, which may be flushed and warm to the touch but usually dry. In the later stages of a serious infectious process, there may be a pale, cool, moist appearance indicating hypoperfusion.

A purple or maroon rash on the skin that does not blanch under pressure is called purpura and may indicate the presence of meningitis. Other rashes may indicate drug reactions, other systemic infections, or a localized skin infection.

Nuchal rigidity, or neck stiffness, can signify meningitis but is difficult to assess; a patient may complain of pain or flex the knees in response to flexion of the neck.

Assessment of lung sounds is important if there is a cough or other respiratory complaint. Localized crackles or decreased breath sounds may indicate the presence of pneumonia.

Palpation of the abdomen for signs of tenderness or guarding should be performed if the patient has any associated GI symptoms.

Key Conditions and Findings

- *Sepsis.* Sepsis is a life-threatening condition that may present with fever. It occurs when an infection, such as cellulitis, pneumonia, or a kidney infection, spreads to the general circulation.

When bacteria invades the bloodstream, shock is an imminent concern. The circulating bacteria release toxins, which then cause blood vessels to dilate. As a result of peripheral blood pooling, venous return to the heart decreases, and shock can result.

A number of conditions can be associated with sepsis. Patients with meningitis, pneumonia, diabetes, AIDS, abdominal or genitourinary surgery, indwelling urinary catheters, and IV lines are more likely to develop sepsis. Infants and the elderly are also at higher risk to develop sepsis.

Field management of these patients includes blood pressure support with fluids and administration of vasopressors, such as dopamine, if blood pressure does not respond to volume replacement. Immediate transportation to an emergency department is necessary to start the patient on antibiotics.

CRITICAL ISSUE

The paramedic must have a high index of suspicion to identify the septic shock patient and rapidly transport to a hospital to reverse the life-threatening condition.

- *Febrile children.* Fever in a child younger than 3 months of age is abnormal and always cause for concern. The possibility of meningitis should be considered in any child with a fever.

- *Febrile seizures.* Febrile seizure is a particular risk in children with fever. These seizures occur most commonly between 6 months and 3 years of age, and are characterized by a rapid rise in body temperature. Acute management is aimed at lowering the core temperature until the cause of the fever can be identified at the hospital. Any child with a fever should be observed closely for a seizure.
- *Heat stroke.* Heat stroke is an immediate life threat that occurs following exposure to elevated environmental temperatures. Hypothalamic regulation fails when temperatures reach 106° F (41.1° C), resulting in continued body temperature elevation. Patients with heat stroke usually have temperature measurements of 106° F (41.1° C) rectally and present with CNS signs including confusion, unresponsiveness, or seizures. The skin is usually flushed and dry, because sweating ceases following shutdown of the temperature regulating system (*see* Chapter 43). Rapid cooling with cold packs is essential for the heat stroke patient.

- *Drug reactions.* Toxic ingestion or overdoses of certain medications, such as aspirin, anticholinergics, and CNS stimulants, may produce fever. In addition, a fever may be seen as a complication of administration of multiple prescription medications.
- *Central nervous system lesions.* Cerebrovascular accidents or tumors may directly influence hypothalamic temperature control.
- *Malignant tumors.* Patients with lymphomas or leukemia may present with fever as the initial manifestation of disease. Because of immune system depression, these patients are at special risk for developing infections.

Management

Airway management should be undertaken as indicated during the initial patient assessment.

All tachycardic patients or those in respiratory distress require 100% oxygen administered at a high-flow rate via a nonrebreather mask. If a pulse oximeter is available, the respiratory status of the patient can be monitored continuously. If any respiratory signs or symptoms are present, a mask should be worn by EMS providers to avoid transmission of infection.

Intravenous access and infusion of normal saline or Ringer's lactate can be established with a large-bore catheter. If signs of hypoperfusion are present, resuscitation can begin with fluid boluses in accordance with local protocols. A cardiac monitor is appropriate for detecting possible dysrhythmias.

Efforts to lower core temperature should be instituted before arrival at the hospital for those patients with temperatures in excess of 104° F (40° C) or patients who have had a febrile seizure. If possible, place the patient in a cool environment and remove clothing. When fever is in excess of 104° F (40° C) and the patient is conscious, acetaminophen (Tylenol) is effective in lowering the temperature elevation by blocking the production of prostaglandins. Because most EMS providers do not usually carry acetaminophen, contact medical direction to consider administration of acetaminophen found on the scene, if the patient has not already taken the medication. Aspirin is no longer considered appropriate treatment for children with a fever because of the chance of provoking Reye's syndrome.

Sponging the patient with tepid, lukewarm water (100° to 105° F, 37.8° to 40.6° C) is an effective cooling method if transport time is extended. Ice and cold water baths should be avoided, because they cause shivering and constriction of skin blood vessels, which then increases the core temperature. Alcohol baths are also discouraged because the alcohol can be absorbed through the skin.

All patients should be transported to the nearest appropriate facility based upon their clinical status. Upon arrival, consult with emergency department personnel regarding the paramedic's need for prophylactic treatment of an infectious disease exposure. EMS providers are most commonly given treatment when exposed to potential cases of meningitis, but other types of infections may require therapy as well (*see* Chapter 10).

SUMMARY

Evaluation of the patient with fever requires a thorough patient history and close assessment for life-threatening illnesses. Care should be exercised to complete a relevant physical examination and begin appropriate treatment.

SUGGESTED READINGS

1. **Bates B:** A Guide to Physical Examination and History Taking, ed 4, Philadelphia, 1987, JB Lippincott.
2. **Bledsoe BE, et al:** Paramedic Emergency Care, ed 2, Englewood Cliffs, 1994, Prentice Hall.
3. **Caroline N:** Emergency Care in the Streets, ed 4, Boston, 1991, Little, Brown, and Co.
4. **Dierking BH, Everidge JM, Ramenofsky ML:** Initial Prehospital Assessment of the Pediatric Patient. *J Emerg Med Serv,* 13(4):59, 1988.

5. **Jones S, et al:** Advanced Emergency Care for Paramedic Practice, ed 1, Philadelphia, 1992, JB Lippincott.

6. **Kravis TC, Warner CG, et al:** Emergency Medicine: A Comprehensive Review, ed 2, Rockville, 1987, Aspen.

7. **Luckman J, Sorensen K:** Medical-Surgical Nursing, A Psychophysiologic Approach, ed 3, Philadelphia, 1987, WB Saunders.

8. **Rosen P (ed):** Emergency Medicine, Concepts and Clinical Practice, vol 2, St. Louis, 1992, Mosby–Year Book.

Mark Hauswald, MD, FACEP

Chapter 39

Eye, Ear, Nose, and Throat Complaints—Medical

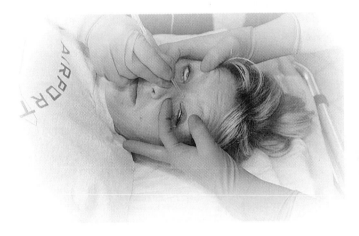

A paramedic should be able to:

OBJECTIVES

1. Describe the basic anatomy and function of the following eye structures:
   a. Sclera
   b. Conjunctiva
   c. Cornea
   d. Retina

2. Describe the following eye conditions including the management of them:
   a. Corneal abrasions
   b. Conjunctivitis
   c. Cataract
   d. Foreign Body

3. Identify two assessment findings of the eye that constitute an emergency situation.

4. Discuss the basic pathophysiology, signs, symptoms, and complications of acute glaucoma.

5. Describe four conditions that may result in loss of vision or blindness.

6. Identify two functions of the ear.

7. Define and discuss the following terms/conditions:
   a. Pharyngitis
   b. Otitis
   c. Vertigo

8. Identify potential causes, complications, and management of patients with epistaxis.

9. Discuss the clinical significance and management of a:
   a. Peritonsillar abscess
   b. Dystonis reaction
   c. Partial airway obstruction

10. Describe the appropriate assessment and significant findings for patients with complaints involving the eye, ear, nose, or throat.

KEY TERMS

1. **Acute glaucoma**—rapid increase of pressure within the eye.

2. **Cataract**—an abnormal, progressive condition of the lens of the eye, characterized by loss of transparency.

3. **Conjunctivitis**—inflammation of the mucous membrane covering the anterior surface of the eyeball and lining of the eyelids; caused by bacterial or viral infection, allergy, or environmental factors.

4. **Corneal abrasion**—scrape of the convex, transparent, anterior part of the eye.

5. **Croup**—an acute viral infection of the upper and lower respiratory tract that occurs primarily in infants and young children.

6. **Dystonic reaction**—muscle stiffness.

7. **Epiglottitis**—inflammation of the lidlike cartilage overhanging the entrance to the larynx.

8. **Epistaxis**—bleeding from the nose.

9. **Otitis**—inflammation or infection of the ear.

10. **Retinal artery occlusion**—decreases blood supply to the retina caused by a clot or embolus in the retinal artery.

11. **Vertigo**—the sensation that the world is spinning. True vertigo is caused by an abnormality of the inner ear balance organs, or rarely, the brain.

475

The face contains the primary sense organs: the eyes for vision, the ears for hearing, the nose for smell, and the throat for taste. The face also includes the upper airway, upper gastrointestinal tract, and many muscles. Unlike the rest of the body, nerves serving this area travel through small holes in the skull between the face and the brain, rather than through the spinal cord.

This chapter focuses on nontrauma related problems affecting these organs. Trauma to the head and the face is presented in Chapter 47.

To simplify the presentation, each of the facial organs is discussed individually.

Eye

Anatomy and Physiology

The function of the eye is to translate light into nervous impulses for interpretation in the brain's occipital cortex. Its most superficial anatomical structures are the eyelids, which provide a protective covering and secrete lubricant and tears to keep the front of the eye moisturized and adequately oxygenated (Fig. 39-1). The white portion of the eye, called the sclera, is a relatively dense, opaque, fibrous tissue. The conjunctiva is a transparent membrane covering the anterior sclera that forms sacs under each eyelid. Its function is to secrete mucus and hold the lubricants secreted by the tear ducts.

The cornea, a thin but extremely tough transparent membrane, allows light to pass through the front of the eyeball (the anterior chamber). The light then passes through the lens and posterior chamber to the retina. The retina contains blood vessels and the actual light receptors (rod and cone cells). The rods and cones respond to light by sending nervous impulses through the optic nerve to the brain.

Patient Assessment

A few questions will help to direct the patient assessment and management:

- *Is there eye pain?* The cornea is extremely sensitive. Most patients with eye pain, even patients who do not remember injuring the eye, have scratched or burned the cornea. **Corneal abrasions** (scrapes) may be caused by foreign objects caught under the lid or by damaged contact lenses. Burns may be caused by ultraviolet light from sunlight ("snow blindness") or welding. Eyes burned by ultraviolet rays usually begin to hurt several hours after exposure.

C R I T I C A L   I S S U E

The patient with a red, painful eye is considered to have an ophthalmologic emergency, and prompt patient transport is indicated.

Few medical problems cause severe eye pain. The most serious is rapid increase in pressure within the eye, **acute glaucoma**. This problem may occur in patients at any age, but it is more frequent in the elderly. Unilateral eye pain may spread to the rest of the head and cause nausea and vomiting. The patient may appear quite ill and often complains of decreased vision and seeing "haloes" around lights.

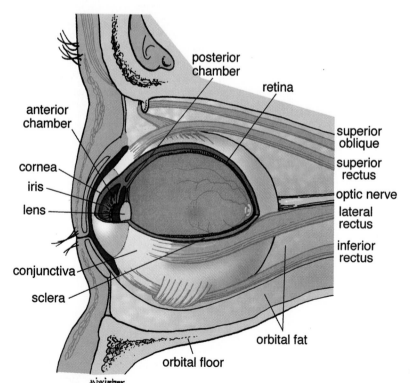

posterior chamber
retina
anterior chamber
cornea
iris
lens
conjunctiva
sclera
superior oblique
superior rectus
optic nerve
lateral rectus
inferior rectus
orbital fat
orbital floor

Figure 39-1

Structures of the eye.

- *Does the patient complain of loss of vision?* Rapid loss of vision is always an emergency. Anything that makes the anterior chamber, lens, or posterior chamber unable to transmit light, especially infection and bleeding, can cause blindness. Detachment of the retina, which commonly occurs after a direct blow, also prevents conversion of light into nervous impulses and subsequently results in loss of sight. Decreased blood supply to the retina caused by a clot or embolus in the retinal artery (retinal artery occlusion) may result in partial blindness, either temporary or permanent. Temporary blindness, often limited to part of the visual field, may also result from a cerebrovascular accident.

CRITICAL ISSUE

The patient with sudden onset of decreased vision is considered to have an ophthalmologic emergency, and prompt transport is indicated.

- *Does the patient wear contact lenses?* There are three basic kinds of contact lenses: hard, soft, and extended-wear. All three types can cause abrasions by trapping foreign bodies against the eye, and all three increase the risk of infection or conjunctivitis. Hard lenses and some soft lenses prevent air from reaching the cornea. Because the cornea's only source of oxygen is contact with air, hard lenses cause hypoxia and lead to pain if left in place for longer than approximately 12 hours.
- *Is there any history of surgery to the eye?* If the lens of the eye has been removed because of a cataract, an artificial lens is often substituted. These intraocular lenses may be displaced and cause acute pressure increases, and they may become infected. Any pain or vision change in an eye with an intraocular lens is a true emergency.
- *Is there a history of trauma?* Trauma includes direct blows to the face, penetrating injuries, and foreign bodies. Although a complete examination of the eye requires sophisticated instruments, a surprising amount of information can be gained using only inspection and a penlight.

First, the patient's vision is checked. Is the patient able to see the paramedic, count fingers at 3-foot distance, and read normally? Of course, a person who wears glasses or contacts (if they are in place) should have vision tested with these in place. However, if contacts are not already in place, they should not be inserted in order to check the vision. Next, the paramedic should inspect the sclera. Is it irritated and reddened? This finding may indicate infection, allergy, or minor trauma. If pus is present or crusting of the eyelids is noted, the presence of conjunctivitis is likely. The paramedic should be sure to use gloves in this setting, because it is easy to transmit infection to oneself or others. Subconjunctival bleeding can be dramatic. The entire white area of the eye may be stained blood-red, but the hemorrhage itself is not serious.

A penlight can be used to examine the cornea while looking for a contact lens or scratches. Are the cornea and anterior chamber clear? If the cornea is cloudy, glaucoma may be present. Is the pupil round or is it irregular from surgery or prior trauma?

The paramedic should evaluate the patient's pupillary function by shining a light directly into the eye (Fig. 39-2). If the pupil reacts, this proves that the light has traveled through the eye to the retina, the retina has reacted, the optic nerve has transmitted the information to the brain and the brain has told the iris muscle to constrict. If the pupil does not react, something in this pathway is not working properly. A fixed and dilated pupil may indicate trauma (local or intracranial) or glaucoma. Pupils may be different sizes or irregular, either normally or after surgery.

Artificial eyes made from glass or plastic are created to look identical to the natural eye. These eyes are not attached to the eye muscles, so they don't move normally. They may be scratched inadvertently, but if examined carefully are clearly not real eyes. Paramedics must be certain that the fixed, unreactive pupil is not an artificial one.

Management

If a foreign body is in the eye, gentle irrigation may be helpful (Fig. 39-3). The paramedic or patient must hold both eyes open during the procedure because it is nearly impossible to keep the irritated eye open if the other is clenched shut. Body-temperature normal saline is easier to tolerate than cold water, but either will do. Irrigation is also the treatment of choice for chemical exposures to eyes.

Contact lenses should be removed from painful eyes. The patient who wears contact lenses is usually quite adept at removing them and should be allowed to do so as a first choice. Irritated eyes are best kept shut during patient transport. This will minimize pain and further injury. In most cases, the eyes can be patched.

Topical ophthalmic anesthetic agent, such as proparacaine, may be used for pain control in patients who present with eye pain and a foreign-body sensation. Topical anesthetics are contraindicated in patients with rupture or laceration of the globe. Also, these medications should only be administered after a patient has consented to be transported to the emergency department to prevent an inappropriate refusal of care after relief of pain. Consultation with on-line medical direction may be necessary prior to administration of topical anesthetics.

This is no specific prehospital treatment for acute glaucoma, but medications (pilocarpine) to decrease intraocular pressure must be initiated promptly in the emergency department or the patient can become blind within hours.

Ear

Anatomy and Physiology

The ear actually has two functions: it converts sound waves into nerve impulses which allow us to hear and also provides information to the brain to maintain balance. Anatomically, the ear is divided into three parts: the outer ear, including the

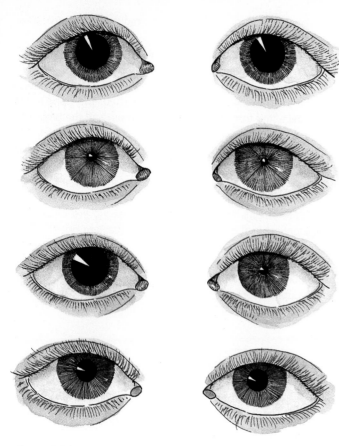

Figure 39-2

A, Pupil dilation. B, Pupil constriction. C, Unequal pupils. D, Normal pupils. *From McSwain et al: The Basic EMT: Comprehensive Prehospital Patient Care, St. Louis, 1996, Mosby Lifeline.*

external canal and the ear drum; the middle ear, containing small bones that amplify the motion of the eardrum and therefore sound waves; and the inner ear, which contains the balance organs and the auditory nerve that send sound and balance information to the brain (Fig. 39-4).

Patient Assessment

- *Does the patient complain of ear pain?* The most common cause of ear pain in adults and older children is infection of the external canal (otitis externa) or the middle ear (otitis media). While painful, neither is particularly dangerous unless the infection spreads through the skull to the brain. Direct spread of infection to the brain is rare except in infants, the elderly, and **immunosuppressed patients.**
- *Could a foreign body be present?* Insects occasionally crawl into ears, and their scratching against the eardrum can be agonizing. If still alive when paramedics arrive, the insect can be drowned using room-temperature mineral oil. Children place a wide variety of objects into their ears that can become lodged inside and sometimes infected.
- *Is vertigo present?* The sensation that the world is spinning (vertigo) is usually caused by damage to the balance portion of the inner ear, the auditory nerve, or the corre-

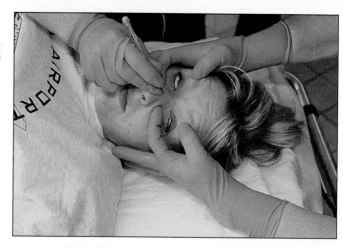

Figure 39-3

Irrigation of the eye may help to remove a foreign body.

sponding part of the brain. This condition may be the result of an infection or trauma. Patients often describe the spinning sensation as "dizziness." If severe, inner-ear problems will cause vomiting, and the patient may need sedation or rehydration with IV fluids.

- *Does the patient note hearing loss?* Deafness alone, whether partial or total, rarely results in an EMS call. The condition can be caused by foreign bodies (usually wax) in the ear canal or damage to the inner ear, nerve, or brain. Injuries to the inner ear or nerve may occur when a **skull fracture** cuts through them. This causes sudden, complete deafness in the patient's affected ear and may be accompanied by severe vertigo.

  Examining the ear is simple because only the external ear is visible. The paramedic can look for discharge (pus or bleeding) and signs of infection in the external ear canal (redness or warmth and swelling in and behind the ear). The patients' hearing can be tested by gently rubbing fingers together near each ear.

Management

Most patients with ear complaints require no active intervention and can be transported in a position of comfort. Any patient with vertigo and a neurologic deficit should have attention to the airway and high-flow oxygen administration. In these cases, IV access and cardiac monitoring should be established.

CRITICAL ISSUE

Ear pain in the presence of any mental status change is a true emergency.

Nose

Pathophysiology

The nose is designed to warm and humidify air before it reaches the lungs. The inside of the nose is lined with a thin, moist mucosal layer (Fig. 39-5). Blood flows through the mu-

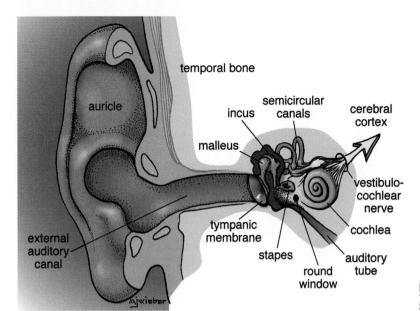

Figure 39-4

Structures of the ear.

cosa and warms the air. The paranasal sinuses drain into the back part of the nasal cavity.

Bleeding from the nose, or **epistaxis,** is a common complaint in adults. In acute epistaxis, most bleeding episodes originate from small blood vessels located on the nasal septum in the anterior portion of the nose. Anterior epistaxis is usually unilateral and can be compressed by local pressure to the nares (Fig. 39-6).

Posterior epistaxis is more serious, because the passage of blood and blood clots is posterior into the nasopharynx. The location of these blood vessels makes them inaccessible to direct pressure. Posterior epistaxis is most common in elderly patients, but can also occur in patients with bleeding disorders or patients taking anticoagulant medications, such as coumadin.

Patient Assessment

- *Does the patient note epistaxis?* The most common causes of epistaxis are local trauma, low atmospheric humidity (particularly during winter months), upper respiratory infections, and allergies. Overuse of nasal spray or cocaine and medications that increase bleeding (e.g., aspirin and coumadin), also increase the risk of anterior nosebleeds. Clotting disorders, such as **hemophilia,** may be considered in patients with epistaxis but are uncommon without a prior history or other signs of a bleeding disorder, such as bruising. **Hypertension** is not believed to be a direct cause of spontaneous nasal bleeding, although significant blood pressure elevation may make control of epistaxis difficult.

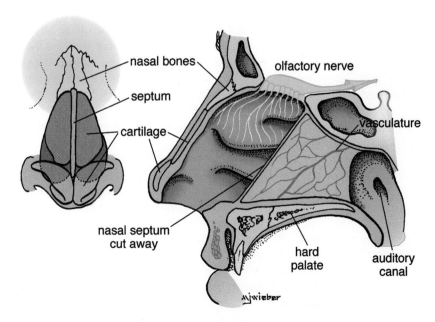

Figure 39-5

Bones, cartilage, and nerves of the nose.

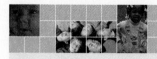

- The most common pediatric eye, ear, nose, and throat complaints are earache, sore throat, epistaxis, foreign body placement, and breathing difficulty.
- Epistaxis in children is commonly caused by trauma, but can also be caused by exposure to dry air, medical problems such as idiopathic thrombocytopenia, leukemia, and other bleeding disorders.
- Foreign bodies in the nose and ears are commonly encountered and usually a result of self-insertion, but have the potential to become true emergencies.
- Respiratory distress, difficulty swallowing, and throat pain can be associated with two common infectious abscesses: peritonsillar and retropharyngeal abscesses. A peritonsillar abscess (most often seen in the teen-age years) is usually the result of tonsillitis and is the most common pediatric infection of the head and neck. A retropharyngeal abscess, a bacterial infection, is most often seen in children under 2 years of age. This has the potential to become a true emergency because of both potential airway compromise and sepsis if left untreated.
- Drooling, sore throat, and voice impairment are usually indicative of an infectious process, such as the abscesses mentioned earlier. It can also accompany epiglottitis, allergic reactions, and ingestions.
- Ear pain with associated discharge from one or both ears is usually caused by an otitis media or externa. It can, however, represent a foreign body in the ear or a basilar skull fracture.
- Otitis media and externa are common conditions in children and are easily treatable by the physician. The child will usually complain of ear pain, sometimes severe, and itching or may tug at the ear lobe.
- Allergic reactions and infections can cause abnormal nasal discharge as well. Be alert for potential nasal obstruction secondary to this discharge.

- *How long has epistaxis been present?* Most episodes of epistaxis resolve quickly and spontaneously, and relatively few patients with nasal bleeding actually need medical assistance. However, patients with epistaxis who have been unable to stop the bleeding or patients who have recurrent bleeding may call for EMS assistance. Patients with active nosebleeds usually are anxious and apprehensive. These patients also are commonly nauseated or have vomited because of the irritating effect of swallowed blood on the GI tract. If bleeding is severe, rapid, or prolonged, the patient may develop signs and symptoms of hypovolemia.
- *Is there a nasal discharge?* As a general rule, three things cause nasal discharge: allergies, viral infections, and foreign bodies. Children put an amazing variety of objects into their noses. If these objects are left in place for a few days, infection results. The paramedic is almost never justified in trying to remove foreign bodies from the patient's nose. These objects are usually very difficult to remove, and pushing them deeper into the nose may cause more damage or may push the objects into the trachea.

Examination of the nose is limited to what can be accomplished by inspection. The source of any discharge may be localizable, and the patient's hemodynamic status should be assessed with vital signs.

Management

The patient who experiences epistaxis should be positioned upright and, after the patient blows his or her nose into a towel, the nares should be pinched firmly for 10 to 15 minutes without releasing pressure. Many patients will release the pressure frequently to determine whether bleeding has stopped. If the patient will not perform the procedure as instructed, the paramedic should apply direct pressure by firmly pinching the patient's nostrils closed for the prescribed duration of time. In most cases of anterior epistaxis, direct pressure will control the bleeding.

In some patients with significant anterior epistaxis, and patients with posterior epistaxis, pinching the nose will be ineffective in controlling hemorrhage, and active bleeding may continue. Blood and blood clots pass into the throat, causing patients to experience a sensation of choking, develop gagging and coughing, and swallow moderate amounts of blood. These patients should be positioned leaning forward to permit blood to flow from the nostrils rather than into the throat, and the patient should be encouraged to spit and have suction provided as needed.

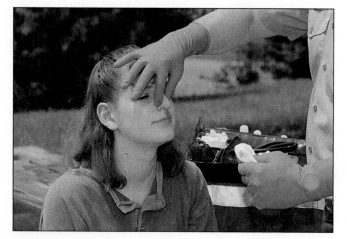

Figure 39-6

Local pressure is used to control anterior epistaxis.

In cases of uncontrollable epistaxis, patient transport must be expedited. These patients are often elderly and chronically ill, and establishment of IV access and cardiac monitoring is required in these cases. Fluid boluses with normal saline or Ringer's lactate can be administered if the patient's hemodynamic status warrants.

Throat

Pathophysiology

The mouth and the throat are not covered with skin, but by a thin, moist, mucosal membrane. The mucosa is bathed in saliva which contains antibodies and white blood cells that prevent infection. The tongue is a muscle covered by thin musoca and studded with sensory (taste and pain) cells. At the base of the tongue is the epiglottis, and beyond that lie the vocal chords and the trachea. The tonsils are two masses of tissue that are part of the immune system and are located on the lateral aspects of the posterior pharynx (Fig. 39-7).

The pharyngeal mucosa is fragile and has minimal supporting structures. As a result, infection of the throat is common and can penetrate deeply to form abscesses in the deep spaces of the neck. These infections are always serious and may threaten airway patency.

Some patients have a hole through the front of the trachea (tracheostomy) that bypasses the upper airway. A tracheostomy may be performed for patients with mouth cancer or severe lung disease or because long-term endotracheal intubation is required. A short tube is placed through the tracheostomy hole to maintain the airway. Some special tracheostomy tubes are designed so that, by plugging the external hold, air can be diverted through the vocal chords, allowing the patient to speak. However, most tubes make speech impossible.

Patient Assessment

If evidence of respiratory distress is detected upon the initial patient assessment, management will take precedence over further assessment. Assuming this is not the case, the following historical questions may provide useful information.

- *Does the patient complain of throat pain?* The mucosa of the throat, particularly the tongue and the epiglottis, are extremely sensitive. Pain without other symptoms is rare and usually has an obvious cause, such as airway burn or obstruction by foreign body. Pain and fever indicate infection, such as pharyngitis and tonsillitis. Infection causes swelling, which can be fatal in the narrow air passages of the throat. Such patients usually complain of pain when swallowing.
- *Does the patient complain of hoarseness or recent voice change?* An acute charge in the vocal character may indicate a throat infection or the presence of a foreign body and can also accompany neck trauma. Changes developing over a long period of time can be seen with tumors of the larynx or abscesses of the deep spaces of the neck.

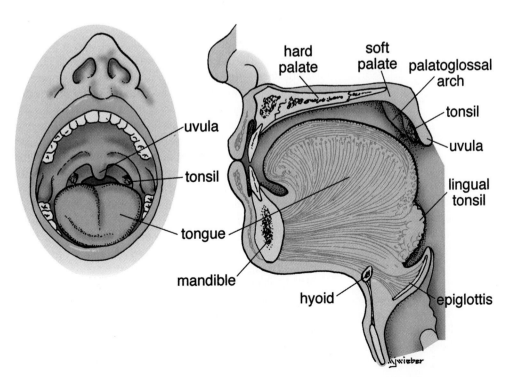

Figure 39-7

Structures that form the mouth and pharynx.

- *Is there a history of recent surgery?* As is true after any surgery, operations involving the face and neck may result in bleeding or infection. These problems are the same as when they appear for any other reason. For example, operations for tonsil removal may be associated with delayed bleeding. Clots break down several days after the operation; *any* bleeding is potentially serious since the carotid artery is located immediately beneath the tonsils.

- *Does the patient take any medications?* Most of the major tranquilizers (e.g., haloperidol, droperidol, etc.) used to treat psychoses and, in lower doses, vomiting, can cause muscle stiffness and difficulty swallowing (dystonic reaction) even if taken in normal doses. A certain class of antihypertensive agents, angiotensin-converting enzyme (ACE) inhibitors such as enalapril, are associated with life-threatening swelling of mucous membranes of the tongue and oropharynx (angioedema).

When the neck and throat are examined, the airway should be the focus. Any obvious signs of airway obstruction should be noted. If obstruction is present, treatment must begin and the remainder of the examination postponed until the patient's condition is stabilized.

High-pitched sounds heard upon inspiration (stridor) indicate the presence of upper airway obstruction. This symptom can be seen in young children presenting with viral illnesses such as **croup** or in patients of all ages with **epiglottitis.** There may be other evidence of respiratory distress present in the patient, such as the use of the accessory muscles of respiration or retractions in the supraclavicular area. If drooling occurs because the patient cannot swallow saliva, it usually indicates significant upper airway swelling and potentially impending obstruction.

The patient's lips should be observed for swelling that may be present with an **allergic reaction.** The teeth, tongue, and back of the throat can be assessed for evidence of swelling, redness, or pus. A tongue blade should not be used; a partial airway obstruction may be made complete by such stimulation. The epiglottis is not usually visible. If the epiglottis is visible and is swollen, the patient may have epiglottitis that can progress to include the entire diameter of the airway.

Lastly, the neck is examined for evidence of swelling or palpable masses. Swelling could be caused by infection deep in the patient's neck muscles.

Management

For the patient who has complete airway obstruction or who is unresponsive, the reader can refer to Chapter 18. If the patient with upper airway problems is awake and breathing, it is necessary for the paramedic to work quickly, decisively, and with a plan.

First, the patient should be administered high-flow oxygen. Oxygen will not relieve an obstruction, and its effect on the work of breathing is only psychological. However, if the patient stops breathing, oxygenation will be maximal and there will be several minutes to correct the problem before brain damage occurs in the patient.

If possible, the oxygen should be humidified. Cool mist is particularly helpful in patients with croup but may also help other types of throat swelling. It is possible, but difficult, to assist a responsive patient with a bag-valve-mask. If the patient can cooperate by holding the mask and the patient does not fight the effort, the paramedic can carefully time the respiratory assistance to the patient's inhalations. This greatly relieves the work of breathing. A few assisted ventilations with the bag-valve-mask may be all that is required to stabilize a patient's respiratory status. The paramedic must always be prepared to increase the level of airway management as necessary.

If time permits, two or three means of airway management should be prepared at once. If the patient can not be ventilated with a bag-valve-mask device, the paramedic should be prepared for endotracheal intubation or, if local protocol permits and the worst case develops, a needle or formal cricothyroidotomy.

Upper airway obstruction must be treated somewhat differently than airway management in other situations. The paramedic should use an endotracheal tube one size smaller than usual and only intubate the patient as a last resort. Procedures involving intubation are likely to make the airway obstruction worse, and the obstruction will make intubation more difficult. Placing the patient in the supine position allows the tongue to fall back onto the airway. Inserting the laryngoscope blade will stimulate the gag reflex and narrow the airway. The blade itself will fill most of the narrowed airway passage. If the tube fails to pass on the first attempt, the patient's vocal chords may swell shut.

CRITICAL ISSUE

Patients with partial airway obstruction should be transported in a position of comfort. Intubation should be considered only as a last resort.

The other airway adjuncts—nasal, oral, and pharyngeal airways (including the Pharyngo-Tracheal Lumen [PTL] and similar devices)—are relatively contraindicated in upper airway problems because they are likely to make the obstruction worse.

In the case of a **foreign body causing complete airway obstruction,** removal may be attempted using a laryngoscope and Magill forceps. In rare circumstances, a small foreign body may need to be pushed below the level of the carina with an endotracheal tube to allow ventilation of at least one lung. Other patients who are ventilating adequately with a partial airway obstruction should be transported with administration of high-flow oxygen and respiratory assistance, if tolerated, for definitive removal of the foreign body in the more controlled emergency department setting.

When allergic reactions jeopardize the airway, aggressive pharmacologic therapy is indicated. Epinephrine is the drug of choice to initiate recovery from such conditions, and is usually administered subcutaneously. Epinephrine or racemic epinephrine can also be given by oral inhalation with a nebulizer. These medications promote local vasoconstriction to reduce swelling of the upper airway. Diphenhydramine (Benadryl) provides a useful effect in countering the histamine effects of an allergic reaction but does not have as rapid an onset as epinephrine, and is therefore most useful when long transport times are anticipated.

In severe dystonic reactions, the patient may appear rigid, sitting forward with tongue out, drooling and eyes rolled back but with a normal level of responsiveness. Some patients will hold the tongue because they feel they are going to swallow it. Although these reactions are emotionally disturbing, they are rarely life-threatening. The paramedic should consult with medical direction to consider IV diphenhydramine, which rapidly reverses this effect.

Tracheostomy tubes may become clogged with mucus, but they can be cleared with suction just as an endotracheal tube can. A bag-valve-mask can be attached to the opening or a small pediatric mask fitted over it. If the patient coughs the tube out of position, it is usually easy to slide a small cuffed endotracheal tube gently through the hole into the trachea. Forceful insertion of a tube, particularly in the first weeks after surgery, may result in the creation of a false passage outside the trachea and a total airway obstruction.

For a respiratory complaint or sign of upper airway obstruction, rapid transport to the closest hospital is indicated.

SUMMARY

The discussion of the face and neck was separated into four parts to simplify discussion in this chapter. These organs are packed tightly together in a small area and may share the same blood supply and innervation. Also, problems with the brain may affect the face, and infection in the face may drain back into the brain. For these reasons, paramedics should be careful to examine all of the adjacent structures if one part of the patient's face is affected.

Robert Suter, DO, MHA, FACEP

Chapter 40

Nontraumatic Extremity Complaints

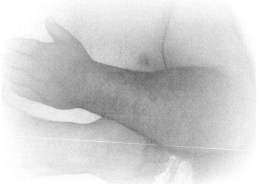

KEY TERMS

1. **Arthritis**—a disease of inflammation and destruction of joints which is accompanied by pain and leads to loss of function in affected joints.

2. **Compartment syndrome**—a pathologic condition caused by the progressive development of arterial compression and reduced blood supply.

3. **Deep vein thrombosis**—a disorder involving a thrombus in one of the deep veins of the body; symptoms include tenderness, pain, swelling, warmth, and discoloration of skin.

4. **Occlusion**—the state of being closed or stopped up.

5. **Sickle cell crisis**—an acute, episodic condition that occurs in children with sickle cell anemia.

A paramedic should be able to:

OBJECTIVES

1. Identify potential life threats associated with nontraumatic extremity complaints.

2. Describe the causes, pathophysiology, signs and symptoms, and potential complications of the following:
   a. Deep vein thrombosis
   b. Arterial occlusion
   c. Arthritis
   d. Compartment syndrome
   e. Sickle cell crises
   f. Hemarthrosis

3. Explain why a patient with a nontraumatic extremity complaint could possibly have a life-threatening or serious condition requiring physician care.

4. Given a patient with a nontraumatic extremity complaint, discuss the appropriate history and physical exam necessary for proper assessment.

With the increasing use of the 9-1-1 system as access to health care, patients with nontraumatic extremity complaints often receive their initial care from paramedics.

It can be dangerous to minimize the significance of nontraumatic extremity complaints. Although many of these patients have minor injuries, some patients with extremity complaints have life- or limb-threatening conditions that require immediate intervention. Therefore, paramedics must approach these patients with knowledge, skill, and appropriate concern.

Most EMS patients with complaints of this type will have suffered extremity injuries. The approach to patients who volunteer a history of trauma occurring immediately before the onset of symptoms is covered in Chapter 48.

Pathophysiology

The approach to patients with extremity complaints unrelated to an injury is challenging. Most life or limb threats related to extremity injuries are atypical presentations of problems involving major organ systems.

One type of vascular problem, arterial occlusion, is the most urgent extremity-specific condition causing generalized extremity pain (Fig. 40-1). Arterial occlusion may be caused by prolonged compression, thrombosis or embolus. Symptoms of occlusion can occur suddenly or begin gradually as a result of arterial insufficiency resulting from arteriosclerosis. Arterial emboli usually originate with thrombus formation in the heart. Clots can form in the left ventricle at the site of myocardial infarctions or in the atrium as a result of valvular stenosis or atrial fibrillation. The size of the clot determines how far it will travel through the blood vessels. The smaller the clot, the further it will travel until it finally becomes lodged. Embolized clots can obstruct any artery, but most frequently involve those in the lower extremities (Fig. 40-2).

Compartment syndrome results from tissue swelling and pressure increases in a tissue compartment confined by fascia (Fig. 40-3). Although compartment syndrome is often trauma-related, the patient may not initially connect the complaint to trauma. In the absence of trauma, compartment syndrome is often seen in patients who are "down" after a prolonged period of time, sometimes caused by alcohol intoxication, drug overdose, or stroke. High blood pressures are possible because of the lack of flexibility of surrounding fascia or external compression by a constricting cast or bandage. Pressure-induced muscle, nerve, and blood vessel damage accounts for the associated sensory loss, diminished pulses, and pain with passive extension.

Patients with hematologic disorders often have extremity complaints. Patients with sickle cell disease can have periods of "crisis" during which they experience intense pain. Sickle cell crisis occurs when the abnormal red blood cells (sickle cells) block smaller blood vessels and prevent blood flow (Fig. 40-4). The blockage and hypoxia further aggravate the sickling problem. Tissue damage as a result of sickle cell crisis can involve almost any organ. The crisis is associated with severe, aching pain most often occurring in the abdomen, chest, back, and extremities. Patients with hemophilia may suddenly bleed into a joint and present because of pain and swelling.

Deep venous thrombosis (DVT) is the development of blood clots in the large veins, typically in the pelvis and legs. The thrombus slows blood return from the extremity and may cause swelling (Fig. 40-5). DVT is not usually considered a limb threat, but it can threaten the patient's life if a thrombus breaks away, passes through the vascular system, and becomes a pulmonary embolus.

Infection involving the soft tissue of an extremity or a joint is a common problem. As the infection spreads, the tissues react by becoming red, swollen, and tender. Localized warmth is also noted when palpated. Joint infection can result in complete destruction of the cartilage and joint, rendering the joint immobile and useless.

Patient Assessment

If a life- or limb-threatening emergency is not immediately suspected, the assessment should continue prior to initiating treatment.

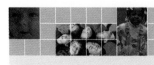

PEDIATRIC PERSPECTIVE

- Most often, the first sign or symptom of an extremity problem in a child is the child's refusal to stand, walk, or use the extremities.
- After viral illnesses in infants and children, a syndrome known as Guillain-Barre syndrome can develop.[1] It is characterized by a slow, ascending weakness which affects both sides of the body equally. This syndrome has also been seen after scheduled immunizations.

- If extremity weakness is the only complaint in a child, weakness usually implies a nerve disorder, whereas proximal weakness usually implies some type of myopathy.
- Children with a seizure disorder may present with one-sided weakness or paralysis (Todd's paralysis) which may resolve in minutes or last longer.
- Vasoocclusive crisis, such as in sickle cell anemia and leukemia, can be the cause of extremity pain.

Figure 40-1

A, Arterial insufficiency is caused by a partially occluded vessel, resulting in an inadequate flow of
blood distal to the occlusion. B, Arterial occlusion
results when the vessel is totally blocked due to the
presence of a spasm or compression, thrombus, or
embolus.

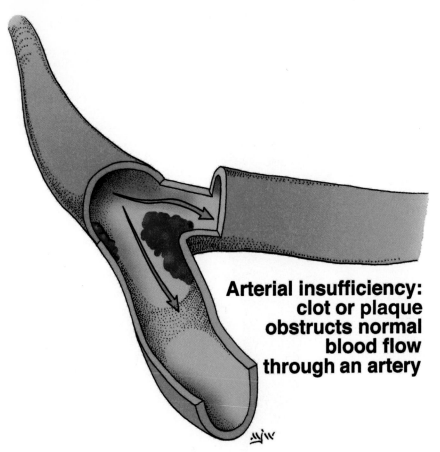

**Arterial insufficiency:
clot or plaque
obstructs normal
blood flow
through an artery**

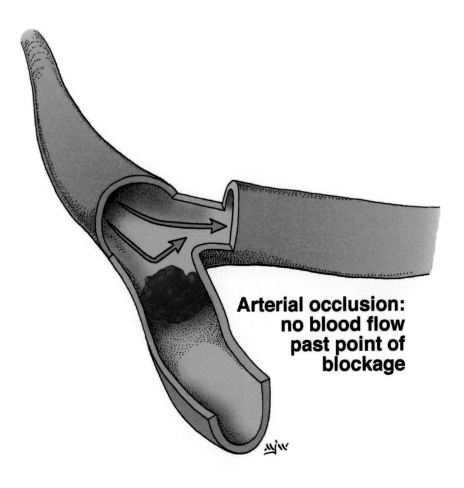

**Arterial occlusion:
no blood flow
past point of
blockage**

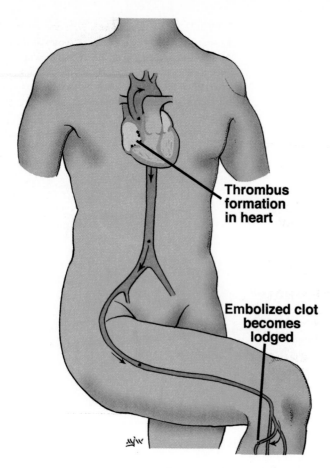

Figure 40-2

Often small arterial thrombi will lodge in a lower extremity.

History

Extremity complaints can be divided into two broad categories: pain and weakness. Pain assessment is described in Table 40-1.

What is the character of the pain? Sensations can be described as burning, cramping, numbness, tingling, and hot or cold. Whether the pain is of gradual or sudden onset is another useful discriminating characteristic. A generalized, unpleasant, single-extremity sensation of sudden or rapid onset that is constant and dull, aching, throbbing, or cold suggests vascular origin.

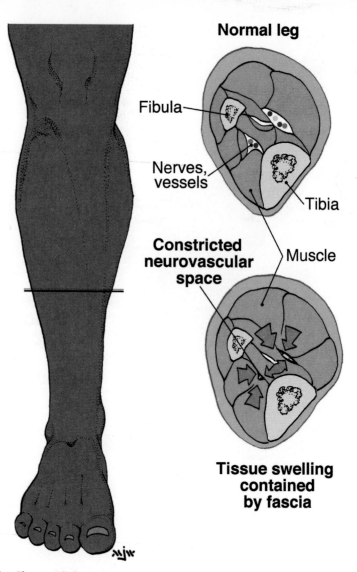

Figure 40-3

The protective covering surrounding muscles, called fascia, is tough and inelastic. Swelling of tissues within the intact fascia results in compartment syndrome. If the pressure is not relieved, ischemic tissues can necrose and die.

How severe is the pain? Pain intensity is difficult to evaluate because of differences in individual thresholds to pain and underlying conditions that may diminish pain, such as diabetes or advanced age. Pain of decreasing intensity can be caused by an inadequate blood supply to the nerves or by compensatory responses to pain. Therefore, even patients whose pain is completely resolved should be transported for physician evaluation.

Where is the pain located? It is important to determine if the pain is generalized to the entire extremity or localized to a specific area. The paramedic should identify the origin of the discomfort and note any radiation. Isolated upper extremity pain, particularly on the left side, can be the sole indicator of cardiac ischemia.

TABLE 40-1	Pain Assessment
Pain Assessment	**Description**
Character	Burning, cramping, tearing, numbness, tingling, hot or cold sensations, sharp, dull
Intensity	Increasing, decreasing, continuous, severity on a 1-to-10 scale
Location	Generalized, localized
Onset	Sudden, gradual, recent, chronic
Radiation	Location and direction, constant, shooting

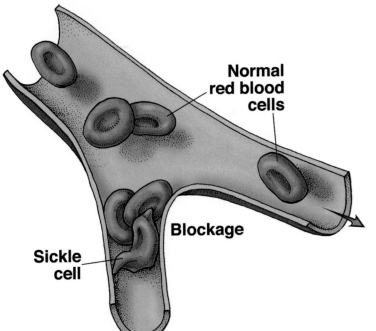

Normal red blood cells

Blockage

Sickle cell

Figure 40-4
For patients with sickle cell anemia, abnormally shaped RBCs can block capillary beds, resulting in the formation of clots and severe pain. Prehospital care includes oxygenation and pain management.

CRITICAL ISSUE

Symptoms in the arms caused by stress or activity, not involving the affected extremity and not relieved by rest, are likely to represent cardiac ischemia.

Does the extremity feel cold? Painful sensations perceived as cold are usually secondary to decreased or blocked circulation. Extremity complaints associated with acute thrombosis or arterial emboli will be rapid or sudden in onset. The classic syndrome is recognized by the "Five Ps:" Pain, Paresthesia (numbness or tingling), Pallor, Pulselessness, and Paralysis.[1] The patient may also have cyanotic color, loss of warmth, loss of strength, or any combination of these symptoms. Time of onset is crucial, as in many cases it will determine treatment op-

tions. If there have been periods of improvement, the potential for saving the extremity is increased.

What was the patient doing when the pain began, and are there any aggravating or relieving factors? Pain caused by arterial insufficiency may at first occur only after exercise and later progress to a constant complaint. **Claudication** is an ischemic type of pain resulting from an inability to increase arterial blood flow to a muscle during exercise because of partial occlusion. It rarely occurs in patients less than 40 years of age and classically involves the calf muscles of the lower legs during and immediately after walking or exercise. Claudication can also occur in other muscle groups if there is a significant decrease in blood flow (Fig. 40-6). Relief quickly follows the cessation of physical activity.

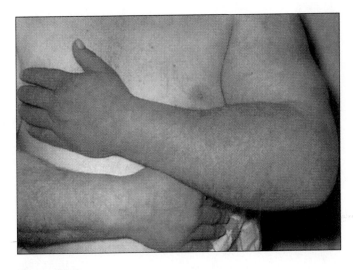

Figure 40-5
Venous thrombosis—swelling of the arm. *From Walker: Color Atlas of Peripheral Vascular Disease, 1980, Wolfe Medical Publications Ltd.*

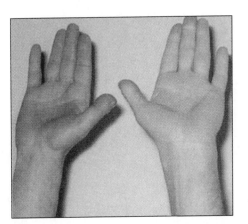

Figure 40-6
Claudication of forearm. *From Walker: Color Atlas of Peripheral Vascular Disease, 1980, Wolfe Medical Publications Ltd.*

Are there any risk factors for deep vein thrombosis? DVT normally occurs in older patients with underlying medical problems, but may also be found in younger persons with risk factors for DVT. One of the most common of these factors is immobilization of the extremity. This can occur when the patient is confined to bed for medical reasons, wears a cast, or takes a long trip with few opportunities to stretch. Other risk factors include obesity, recent surgery, some types of birth control pills, and either recent or remote trauma to the extremity.

Does the patient complain of weakness in the involved extremity? Weakness localized to an extremity may suggest nerve compression (Fig. 40-7) or be a manifestation of central nervous system disease, such as a cerebrovascular accident, or compression of the spinal cord from tumor, abscess, or ruptured disc. In some cases, increasing pressure in a muscular compartment will also be present with weakness.

What is the patient's past medical history? The hemophilia patient is usually aware of the condition and able to supply an adequate history. The presence of bruises in various stages of healing may help identify those at risk for bleeding into a joint or hemarthrosis (Fig. 40-8).

Physical Examination

The first step in physical examination is to evaluate the patient's vital signs. The paramedic should take pulses in all extremities and determine if they are bilaterally equal in strength. The patient's radial pulse (in the arm) and the dorsalis pedis pulse (in the foot) should both be assessed. If the radial pulse is absent or decreased, the brachial pulse can be checked. Should the dorsalis pedis pulse be diminished, the popliteal and femoral pulses can be used for comparison. Capillary refill can also be compared bilaterally; it should be less than 2 seconds.

> **CRITICAL ISSUE**
>
> If the weakness is in one arm and the leg on the same side, a cerebrovascular event may be in progress. The patient's airway, mental status, and blood pressure and ECG should be monitored carefully, and oxygen therapy is important.

> **CRITICAL ISSUE**
>
> If the initial approach reveals a patient who appears pale, cool, clammy, or cyanotic or has an extremity with any of these characteristics, the paramedic should assume a life- or limb-threatening emergency and transport the patient rapidly to an emergency department.

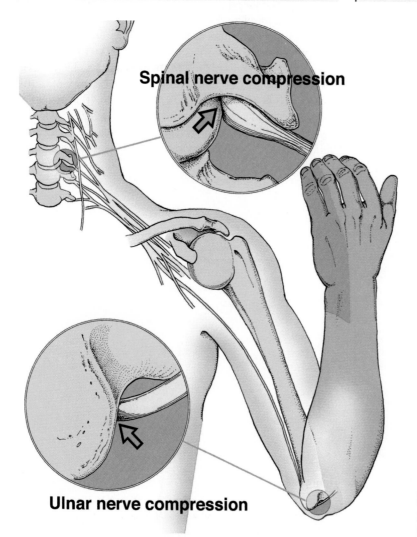

Spinal nerve compression

Ulnar nerve compression

Figure 40-7

Nerve compression can result in pain or changes in the level of sensation of an isolated area of the body.

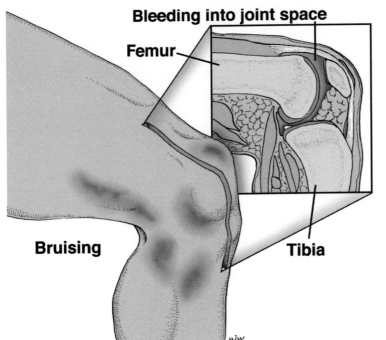

Bleeding into joint space

Femur

Bruising

Tibia

Figure 40-8

Look for bruising, joint stiffness or immovability, and soft-tissue swelling as an indication of hemarthrosis.

The patient's blood pressure should be assessed in both the affected and unaffected extremities if possible. For complaints involving the legs, this may be more difficult and depends on the availability of a large-size sphygmomanometer.

A detailed examination of the involved extremities should be performed; asymptomatic extremities can be used for comparison. The color of the skin and nailbeds may be pale when hypoperfused or demonstrate cyanosis in the hypoxic patient. Note bruises or other evidence of trauma.

Obvious swelling and asymmetry when compared with the other extremity can be a sign of venous obstruction. The patient with DVT will usually complain of pain and swelling in the region of the thrombus. The extremity is also usually tender to touch, with localized tenderness over the site of obstruction and swelling of the surrounding tissue. In some cases, there is a palpable "cord" that reveals the thrombosed vein (Fig. 40-9). The skin overlying the area of pain may be warm and red.

Palpation for abnormal temperature may identify a cold extremity, which promptly identifies the patient at risk from vascular compromise. With arterial occlusion, the most common physical finding is a pale, cold, pulseless extremity. Compression or squeezing the affected location of an extremity with DVT or compartment will elicit pain.

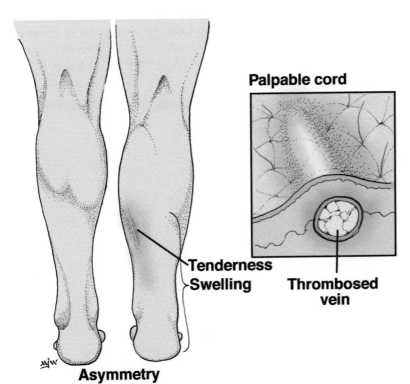

Palpable cord

Tenderness
Swelling

Thrombosed vein

Asymmetry

Figure 40-9

DVT is recognizable when a palpable cord is present in the area of pain and swelling.

Range of motion of the affected extremity should be assessed. In cases of compartment syndrome, attempts at passive extension (examiner moving the extremity) can cause severe pain, and movement may not be possible. The absence of pulses is classic, but this is a late sign. In addition, movement which places a vein with a thrombosis under tension or stretch (such as dorsiflexion of the foot [Homans' sign] in a patient with a DVT in the calf) may elicit pain (Fig. 40-10).

In patients complaining of joint pain without a history of trauma or other associated extremity complaints, a major concern is septic arthritis, or infection of the joint space. The skin over the joint will be hot, red, and swollen, and the pain will usually intensify with motion. Strength may be decreased because of pain. Despite these findings, distal skin color and pulses are normally not affected.

Pain of musculoskeletal origin may limit muscular effort and give the patient a false sense of weakness. Determining whether extremity weakness is really a result of decreased strength is critical to assessment of the patient. This requires comparison of one side of the body with the other. The paramedic should test motor strength in each extremity and check sensation to further evaluate nerve function. The latter is performed by lightly touching the tip of a finger to the extremity and evaluating the patient's response.

Key Conditions and Findings

Findings that suggest serious conditions in patients with extremity complaints are summarized in Box 40-1.

- *Arterial occlusion.* Blockages of the arterial supply can be caused by several mechanisms. Arterial thrombosis is the occlusion of an artery by clot formation at the site of atherosclerotic plaques. Claudication occurs when plaque growth significantly impedes vascular flow and is often associated with other vascular disease such as myocardial infarction or CVA. A thrombus may break loose from a central or proximal site such as the heart or aorta and cause occlusion peripherally as an embolus.

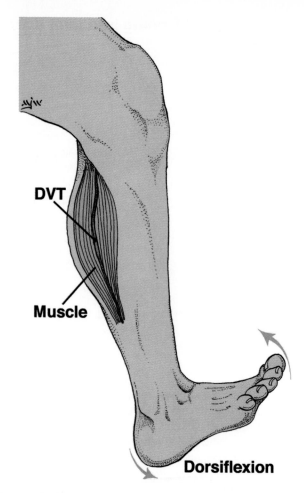

Figure 40-10

A positive finding of Homan's sign indicates DVT, and is present when dorsiflexion of the foot results in a stretching and pain of the thrombosed vein.

- *Deep vein thrombosis.* Deep vein thrombosis is defined as blood clots that form in the larger veins of the legs, pelvis, or arms usually present with swelling of the involved extremity and pain and tenderness in the area overlying the clot. Although there is no direct limb threat, this condition could be life-threatening to the patient if

BOX 40-1	Findings Suggestive of Serious Conditions in Patients with Nontraumatic Extremity Complaints

- Patient appears pale, cool, clammy, or cyanotic
- Extremity appears pale, cold, or cyanotic
- Associated chest pain, shortness of breath, or severe headache
- Patient over 40 years of age (especially men)
- Medical history of diabetes, heart disease, arteriosclerosis, or high blood pressure
- Symptoms occurring in a **dermatomal** distribution
- Sudden onset
- Recent onset (minutes, hours, days)
- Pain originating from the chest, abdomen, or spine
- Symptoms caused by stress or activity which did not involve the symptomatic extremity and is not relieved by rest
- Abnormal vital signs (systolic blood pressure > 160 or < 100; heart rate > 100; or respiratory rate > 20)
- Abnormal ECG
- Obvious hypoperfusion or respiratory distress
- Abnormal lung sounds
- Obvious difference in pulses, sensation, or strength between extremities

part of the thrombus broke free and travelled through the vascular system, passing through the patient's heart and lodging in the lung (forming a pulmonary embolus).

- *Compartment syndrome.* Generalized single-extremity pain with diminished pulses and sensation can be caused by an elevation of pressure within the fascial compartments of the extremity. Because the fascia cannot expand, pressure increases result in compression of blood vessels, nerves, and other structures. Check for patient history of recent trauma, especially crushing blunt injury or prolonged direct pressure that occurs in unresponsive patients. A cast or constricting bandage that cuts off circulation can also cause compartment syndrome.
- *Septic arthritis.* This limb-threatening emergency is an infection of the joint space. Septic arthritis usually only involves one joint, and most frequently occurs in the lower extremities.
- *Noninfectious arthritis.* Joint pain in a patient with no history of trauma or swelling is usually caused by less alarming musculoskeletal conditions, such as types of noninfectious or inflammatory arthritis (Fig. 40-11). This is differentiated from septic arthritis by the absence of both fever and localized redness or warmth at the pain site. In addition, the pain from inflammatory arthritis tends to be more gradual in onset and follows a prolonged, chronic course.
- *Sickle cell crisis.* Extremity pain in the patient with a history of sickle cell disease may be caused by the condition sickle cell crisis. Patients will usually complain of severe, aching pain, although the physical examination may be normal.
- *Hemarthrosis.* Individuals with bleeding disorders may develop bleeding into a joint space, or hemarthrosis, with minimal or no apparent trauma. The potential for bleeding problems occurs in patients who have inherited diseases such as hemophilia, patients taking anticoagulant drugs, or patients with poor liver function, such as alcoholics.
- *Skin infections.* Reddened, warm skin associated with swelling and tenderness from infection is called cellulitis (Fig. 40-12). Abscesses are well-localized infections. The abscess will be palpated as a lump under the warm, reddened skin that may feel soft and fluid filled.

- *Muscle cramps.* Uncontrolled spasms of musculature are a common extremity complaint. Simple muscle cramps are frequently a result of overuse of the affected muscle. This may be through either repetition or excessive stress on the muscle. If overuse did not occur, electrolyte abnormalities should be considered.
- *Extremity weakness.* Extremity pain or weakness associated with neck or back pain can be caused by conditions affecting the spine or spinal cord (Fig. 40-13). Compression of the spinal canal or nerve roots may be the result of spinal arthritis, tumor, or trauma.
- *Cardiac ischemia.* Extremity pain associated with exertion, chest pain, nausea, lightheadedness, or shortness of breath may be cardiovascular in origin. This aching discomfort or numbness will usually affect the patient in one or both arms, more commonly the left side. Rarely, the extremity may be the only source of complaint for patients with cardiac ischemia.

Management

The patient with generalized, single-extremity pain and any evidence of abnormal vital signs or decreased color, warmth, or pulses should be viewed as a vascular emergency. Rapid identification and treatment of vascular occlusion or insufficiency is crucial if the extremity is to be saved. If the clot or obstruction is not removed within 6 hours, the extremity may have to be amputated.

After management of any conditions identified upon initial assessment, patients suspected of vascular or cardiac disease should receive 100% oxygen administered at a high-flow rate. The patient should also be placed on a cardiac monitor. The presence of atrial fibrillation suggests the possibility of an arterial embolus.

Intravenous access should be established using a large-bore catheter; the use of fluid boluses depends on local protocols and detection of systemic hypoperfusion. The IV access site should be an unaffected extremity.

Patients should be transported in a position of comfort, ensuring minimized motion of affected extremities and protection from further injury and extreme temperatures.

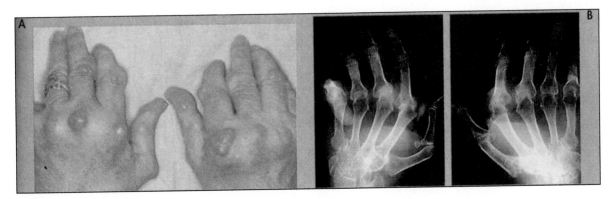

Figure 40-11

Rheumatoid arthritis. *From Seeley: Essentials of Anatomy and Physiology, ed 2, 1996, Mosby-Year Book.*

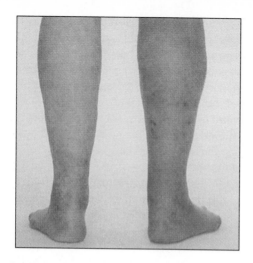

Patient assessment should continue during transport. When arterial occlusion is strongly suspected, the destination is ideally a facility capable of performing immediate vascular surgery. Such capabilities are usually found at Level I or II trauma centers.

Patients with suspected sickle cell crisis require rapid transport with 100% oxygen administration, IV fluids, and pain medication as determined by local protocols or medical direction.

Figure 40-12

Cellulitis. *From Seeley: Essentials of Anatomy and Physiology, ed 2, 1996, Mosby-Year Book.*

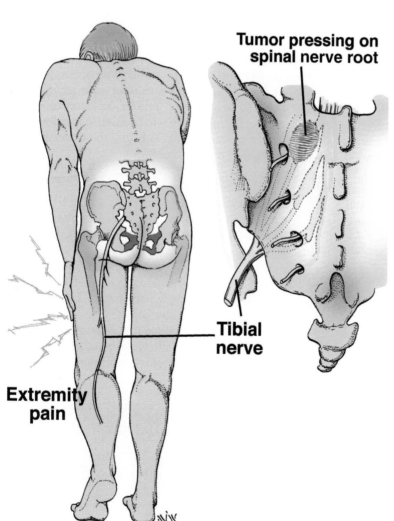

Tumor pressing on spinal nerve root

Tibial nerve

Extremity pain

Figure 40-13

A tumor pressing on a spinal nerve near the cord can result in distal pain or weakness in an extremity.

SUMMARY

The patient with any nontraumatic extremity complaint has a potential life- or limb-threatening emergency requiring immediate treatment. The paramedic should maintain a high level of suspicion for serious causes and provide appropriate assessment and management.

REFERENCE

1. **Magnusson AR:** Humerus and Elbow. In Rosen P (ed): Emergency Medicine, ed 3, St. Louis, 1992, Mosby–Year Book.

SUGGESTED READINGS

1. **Barkin RM (ed):** Pediatric emergency medicine: concepts and clinical practice, St. Louis, 1992, Mosby–Year Book.

2. **Hamilton GC (ed):** Presenting signs and symptoms in the emergency department, Baltimore, 1992, Williams & Wilkins.

3. **May HL, et al:** Emergency medicine, ed 2, Boston, 1992, Little, Brown, and Company.

4. **Rosen P (ed):** Emergency Medicine: concepts and clinical practice, ed 3, St. Louis, 1992, Mosby–Year Book.

5. **Schwartz GR (ed):** Principles and practice of emergency medicine, ed 3, Baltimore, 1992, Williams & Wilkins.

Kathleen Delaney, MD

Chapter 41

Poisoning and Overdose

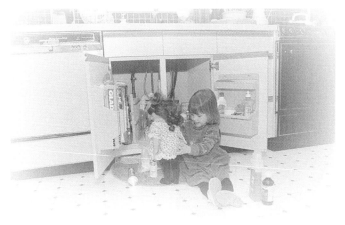

A paramedic should be able to:

1. Describe the various entry routes by which toxic substances enter the body.
2. Identify characteristic findings of an opiate, adrenergic, and anticholinergic toxidrome.
3. Describe the general principles for assessing and managing patients who have overdosed or been poisoned.
4. Given a group of patients who have overdosed or been poisoned, describe the specific management for each.
5. Describe the action and indication for specific antidotes.

1. **Adrenergic**—of or pertaining to sympathetic nerve fibers of the autonomic nervous system that use epinephrine or epinephrinelike substances as neurotransmitters.
2. **Anticholinergic**—of or pertaining to a blockade of acetylcholine receptors that results in the inhibition of the transmission of parasympathetic nerve impulses
3. **Antidote**—a drug or other substance that opposes the action of a poison. An antidote may coat the stomach and prevent absorption, make the toxin inert, or oppose the action of the poison.
4. **Opioid**—pertaining to natural and synthetic chemicals that have opium-like effects, although they are not derived from opium.
5. **Poisoning**—the act of administering a toxic substance; the condition or physical state produced by ingestion, injection, inhalation, or exposure to a poisonous substance.
6. **Toxidrome**—a group of characteristic findings on physical examination that may be useful in determining which drug the patient had ingested.

his chapter presents an overview of poisoning and overdose through a general approach to patient presentation and management. The term *poisoning* is used to refer to a harmful effect on the body caused by any drug or nonpharmaceutical chemical. Poisoned patients can be exposed through ingestion, inhalation, injection, or skin contact (Fig. 41-1). This chapter's emphasis is on ingested poisons. The term *overdose* refers to poisoning caused by an excess of a pharmaceutical agent, whether prescribed as a medication or used illicitly. A toxin is a nonpharmaceutical chemical poison, such as cyanide, kerosene, or an insecticide.

Pathophysiology and Etiology

Serious poisonings occur in many ways, both accidental and intentional. Accidental poisonings are most common in children. For example, in the absence of child-proof latches, the exploring toddler may sample substances stored under the sink or in the medicine chest (Fig. 41-2). When a child who is too young to explore is poisoned, the possibility of error, child abuse, or administration by an older sibling must be considered. Bad taste does not appear to be a significant deterrent to the ingestion of poisonous substances by small children. Sometimes the resemblance of medications to familiar candies prompts the ingestion of large quantities (Fig. 41-3).

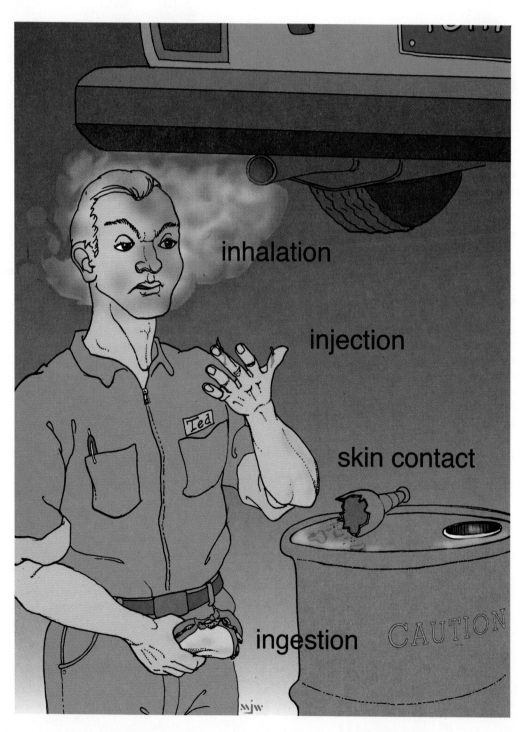

Figure 41-1

Routes of exposure.

Figure 41-2

A unsecured cabinet can easily lead to a poisoned child.

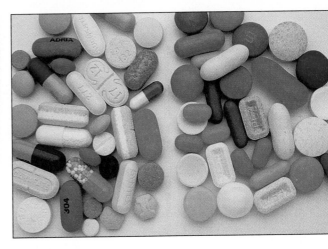

Figure 41-3

Picture how these items appear to a toddler. Could you tell the difference?

Although more common in small children, accidental poisonings also occur in adults and adolescents. Attempts to get "high" or "down" by using drugs stolen, purchased on the street, or supplied by acquaintances often result in unintended overdose. Occasionally, attempts at self-medication may result in poisoning by herbs, vitamin preparations, or less traditional medicines. Accidental ingestions may also involve medication errors caused by forgetfulness or failing eyesight in the elderly.

Group poisonings may result from errors by a chef, such as the misidentification of mushrooms, berries, or a salad ingredient or the serving of food that has not been properly preserved or prepared. Such occurrences also present in work settings where toxic agents are used and at the scenes of accidental leaks or spills of chemicals.

Intentional ingestions occur most often in the adolescent and the adult. Suicidal ingestions may involve very large amounts of a single substance or several substances with different toxic effects.

Although life-threatening, some common ingestants result in delayed or minimal symptoms on initial presentation (Box 41-1). Both the rescuer's failure to recognize the significance of ingestion of these substances and misidentification of the ingestant have resulted in unnecessary deaths. Other agents have a rapid onset of symptoms (Box 41-2).

A toxidrome is a group of characteristic findings discovered upon physical examination of the patient which may be useful in determining which drug was ingested, especially if no patient history is available.

The opioid toxidrome, resulting from overdosage of narcotics, includes the following signs of toxicity: pinpoint pupils, decreased respirations, hypotension, bradycardia, hypothermia, and sedation. Hypoventilation and a mental status decreasing to unresponsiveness are the hallmarks of opioid overdose in a patient.

Some substances result in signs of adrenergic excess such as dilated pupils, sweating, tachycardia and hyperthermia. Common medications that can cause adrenergic hyperactivity are cocaine, theophylline, caffeine, and pseudoephedrine. These patients are at risk for hyperthermia and seizures.

The anticholinergic toxidrome shows evidence of atropinelike effects including dilated pupils, flushed and dry skin, delirium or sedation, hyperthermia, and tachycardia. Among

---

BOX 41-1	Common Ingestants with Delayed Onset of Symptoms

- Acetaminophen (Tylenol, Paracetamol)
- Acetonitrile
- Clonidine (in children)
- Colchicine (a common medication for treatment of gout)
- Hydrofluoric acid
- Lithium
- Lomotil (diphenoxylate-atropine)
- Long-acting calcium channel blockers (Procardia-SL, Calan-SR, Cardizem-CD)
- Long-acting theophylline preparations (Slo-Bid, Theodur, Unasyn, etc.)
- Monoamine oxidase inhibitors (Phenylzine, Nardil, etc.)
- Podophyllin (a common topical therapy for warts)
- Salicylates (aspirin, oil of wintergreen)

BOX 41-2	Common Ingestants with Rapid Onset of Symptoms (Within 1 Hour)

- Camphor
- Chloroquine (a widely available antimalarial agent)
- Cocaine
- Cyanide
- Hydrocarbons
- Isoniazid (INH, a tuberculosis medication)
- Most cardiac and blood pressure medications
- Most opioids
- Most sedatives
- Most antidepressants and antipsychotic drugs

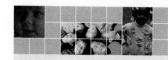

- Poisoning is the fourth leading cause of death in pediatric patients. More than three fourths of all pediatric poisonings are accidents, and occur in children less than 5 years of age.[2] Adolescent poisonings are usually intentional and may include several different substances and mixtures.[1]
- Acetaminophen overdoses are quite common in children, possibly because of the over-the-counter availability of the drug and its presence as a common household medication. A dose of > 140 mg/kg is considered toxic in older children.[1] The child may be initially asymptomatic after ingestion or may present with nausea, vomiting, and GI problems. If untreated, liver damage may occur approximately 72 hours after ingestion and possibly develop into complete liver failure.[1,2]
- Alcohol ingestions are also quite common in older children. They can occur in young children as well ("Sunday Morning Syndrome").

- Syrup of Ipecac administration is not recommended for children less than 1 year of age or for children with altered mental status, children who are comatose, and children with respiratory depression.[1,2]
- Local guidelines and protocols should be followed for dosage of activated charcoal. The recommended dose for children less than 6 years of age is 25 to 50 g; for older children, the dosage is 50 to 100 g. A total dose of 1 g/kg of body weight is also a recommendation.[1,2]

REFERENCES

1. **Barkin R, et al:** *Pediatric emergency medicine. Concepts and clinical practice.* St. Louis, 1992, Mosby–Year Book.

2. **Nichols E, et al:** *Golden hour: the handbook of advanced pediatric life support,* ed 2, St. Louis, 1996, Mosby–Year Book.

the atropinelike substances that present in this manner are tricyclic antidepressants, antihistamines such as diphenhydramine and belladonna alkaloids found in eye drops, and certain plant extracts.

Other chemicals can cause signs of cholinergic or parasympathetic stimulation: pinpoint pupils, sweating, hypothermia, bradycardia, vomiting, diarrhea, increased salivation, and bronchial secretions. Toxins that cause these effects are most commonly found among organophosphate and carbamate insecticides.

Carbon monoxide, an odorless, colorless gas, binds to normal hemoglobin to form carboxyhemoglobin, which cannot carry oxygen. Carbon monoxide is formed during the partial combustion of organic fuels, such as gasoline, natural gas, and wood. Carbon monoxide poisoning should be considered in any person who develops a headache, nausea and vomiting, or loses responsiveness in a closed space or near a stove, furnace, fire, or combustion engine.

Patient Assessment

History

Patients often have a rapid onset of symptoms in the absence of poisoning history, posing a significant challenge to responders. Cardiac dysrhythmias, hypoperfusion, seizures, hyperthermia, altered mental status, and respiratory failure are life-threatening manifestations of serious poisonings.

At scenes where presence of an environmental toxin is suspected, paramedics should determine the risk to themselves and the need for special protective equipment before attempting rescue or patient assessment. For example, EMS providers may be poisoned by contact with a patient suffering from a toxic organophosphate (insecticide) exposure, because this chemical can be absorbed through skin contact.

CRITICAL ISSUE

Inhalation poisoning is particularly dangerous to rescuers. The paramedic should be able to recognize a hazardous environment and know not to enter without adequate protection.

Historical data and patient information from the prehospital scene are crucial to the emergency department management of the poisoned patient.

- *What agent is suspected in the poisoning?* Because clinical signs of serious poisoning may be delayed for many hours, identification of the toxic agent is important so that therapy can be planned and possible patient deterioration anticipated. Identification of the poison or drug is crucial because an antidote may be available for a specific substance.

CRITICAL ISSUE

Acids should not be neutralized with alkalis, or the reverse. This method can cause heat-releasing chemical reactions that further injure the gastrointestinal tract.

- *What was the approximate time of the exposure?* Acute ingestions may be managed differently in the emergency department than would chronic exposures. The time from the patient's ingestion of the toxin is critical when considering antidote administration and gastric emptying.
- *What medications are available in the home?* The paramedic should bring all the medications found in the home to the emergency department with the patient. This helps narrow the possibilities in an unknown ingestion, and may offer evidence of a mixed overdose.

Pill bottles or the container of suspected poison should always be transported to the hospital with the patient.

- *Can the family identify illnesses for which they have received medicines?* Family members may be able to give a history of the patient's conditions such as hypertension, heart disease, diabetes, or seizures that gives clues about the type of medication ingested.
- *Were any seizures noted?* The paramedic should ask bystanders or family members to describe the characteristics of the seizure; seizures are more prevalent with exposure to certain chemicals and medications. Drugs that commonly cause seizures are listed in Box 41-3.
- *Are there any chemicals in the household?* The rescuer should ask about special hobbies and the presence of chemicals related to those activities (e.g., mercury used for gold extraction, cyanide to clean jewelry, or selenium compounds for gun cleaning).
- *Did this exposure take place at work?* In occupational accidents, the paramedic should ask the work supervisor what job the employee performs and what chemicals could be involved.
- *Is there any history of psychiatric problems or recent emotional stressors?* Many poisonings are intentional. The suicidal patient will often relate that an overdose has been taken; family and friends may have witnessed the ingestion or know of the patient's desire to die.

All patients with intentional ingestions must be transported; psychiatric evaluation of suicidal intent is mandatory.

With intentional ingestions, the patient history cannot be relied upon to exclude a serious medical condition.

However, the paramedic must not assume drug overdose in a patient with a history of psychiatric problems. It is always important to look for clues that may reveal the cause of the patient's condition.

Physical Examination

The physical examination begins with assessment of the patient's mental status and vital signs. These physical findings are usually the most helpful data when it comes to differentiating between types of poisonings.

First, the paramedic should assess the need for airway management. Poisoned patients often hypoventilate and are at risk for aspiration. Opioids and barbiturates are very strong respiratory depressants, but antidepressant drugs and benzodiazepines are milder. Patients poisoned with these substances may be cyanotic and have a decreased rate of respirations. Hypoxia and hypoventilation also occur when caustic ingestants, such as acids and alkalis, cause swelling of the throat and obstruct the airway.

Several factors can assist in assessing hemodynamic status. Cool, pale, and moist skin suggests the presence of hypoperfusion. Very slow heart rates occur commonly with overdoses of cardiac and antihypertensive drugs such as digoxin, beta blockers, and calcium channel blockers. Wide-complex tachycardias (wide QRS complex) occur commonly with ingestions of medications that affect cardiac electrical conduction. Narrow complex tachycardias (narrow QRS complex) occur commonly with overdoses of stimulants and drugs with anticholinergic effects.

The paramedic should evaluate the patient's mental status and be prepared to describe the condition accurately to medical direction. Unresponsiveness commonly follows exposure to sedating agents such as barbiturates and opioids. Most stimulant drugs cause agitated behavior when taken in overdose. However, agitation can also be caused by hypoglycemia, hypoxia, hypoperfusion, or a recent seizure.

The patient's temperature can be estimated by inspecting the skin for flushing, palpating for warmth, and taking core temperature, when appropriate.

Many drugs decrease the body's ability to maintain a normal body temperature. Drugs that cause agitated behavior or seizures increase heat production by increasing muscle activity. Life-threatening elevation of body temperature can occur in poisoned patients.

The paramedic should study the patient for evidence of respiratory distress. The patient's skin may be cyanotic and the patient tachypneic, using the accessory muscles of respiration. The rescuer should auscultate the patient's chest for the presence of rales. Noncardiogenic pulmonary edema can occur with any overdose that has led to apnea. It is also common following the patient's inhalation exposure to toxic gases, such as nitrogen dioxide, chlorine, phosgene, or mustard gases, and after aspiration of chemicals such as kerosene and gasoline.

Organophosphate insecticides cause a dramatic increase in pulmonary secretions, literally suffocating the patient with fluid. Certain ingested drugs, such as salicylates (aspirin, oil of wintergreen), are directly toxic to the lung tissue.

BOX 41-3	Drugs and Chemicals That Commonly Cause Seizures

- Aminophylline (Theodur, Slobid, asthma medications)
- Antidepressants
- Beta-blockers
- Camphor (a mothball usually eaten by a child)
- Certain insecticides (organophosphates, carbamates)
- Cocaine
- Insulin and oral diabetic drugs (seizure caused by low blood sugar)
- Isoniazid (INH, an antituberculosis medication)

by Robert Carter, NREMT-P

Poison control centers exist throughout the United States to aid in the management of poisonings. They are used by health care providers and the general public and offer a wide variety of resources and responsibility including information and treatment suggestions.

Poison control centers have many resources of information and references to legal and illegal drugs and medications, as well as toxic agents, such as chemicals and hazardous materials. These centers also have information regarding animal bites (e.g., insect, snake, fish), plants, cosmetics, and a host of other "poisons."

Most poison control centers are located at major medical centers or large teaching hospitals and are staffed by physicians, pharmacists, and specially trained job-related professionals, including specially trained paramedics.

Poison control centers can be accessed 24 hours a day by telephone, medical dispatch centers, or portable EMS radios, depending on local guidelines and resources.

Information required by the poison control center to provide appropriate advice includes: 1) specific agent(s) involved; 2) route of exposure (inhalation, ingestion, absorption, etc.); 3) amount of agent(s) ingested; 4) time (duration) of exposure; 5) patient demographics (age, weight, etc.); 6) medical condition of the patient (assessment, vital signs, etc.); 7) any treatment already rendered by either EMS or family; and 8) any additional information.

The amount and type of assistance provided by each facility varies from center to center. In addition to offering advice to the caller, poison centers may notify the receiving facility, provide information related to the incident, and offer treatment suggestions. These facilities may also assist in transporting medical attention to the exposed or poisoned individuals if needed.

After a request has been made to the poison control center, each incident is followed up to determine the outcome and to gather epidemiological information concerning the incident.

Respiratory failure occurs with poisons, such as cyanide or carbon monoxide, that prevent cells from using oxygen. Patients poisoned with these agents are not cyanotic. Respiratory failure also occurs with poisons that alter hemoglobin so that it cannot carry oxygen (e.g., carbon monoxide, nitrites, nitroglycerine).

Respiratory distress and tachypnea occur with poisons that cause metabolic acidosis. The rapid, deep respirations decrease the amount of acid in the blood and may prevent fatal acidosis from developing. Toxins that cause metabolic acidosis are salicylates, toxic alcohols (e.g., methanol, ethylene glycol), iron, cyanide, and carbon monoxide.

After mental status evaluation, pupillary findings are the most helpful data obtained by neurologic examination of the patient. Pinpoint pupils may provide evidence of opioid toxicity or cholinergic excess. Dilated pupils are more likely seen with ingestions of adrenergic stimulators or as part of an anticholinergic toxidrome.

Oxygen delivered at high concentrations by nonrebreather mask is critical for victims of carbon monoxide exposure. High concentrations of oxygen help displace carbon monoxide from the hemoglobin molecule, freeing it for oxygen transport. Those patients exposed to carbon monoxide who exhibit an altered mental status, syncope, or seizures ideally require transport to a facility capable of delivering hyperbaric oxygen therapy.

Hypoglycemia is a common cause of agitated behavior or unresponsiveness and should be diagnosed by rapid glucose determination if possible. However, necessary treatment can be given on the basis of history and more general examination by administering 50% dextrose IV.

Naloxone (Narcan) is an antidote that specifically reverses the effects of opioids. It has no effect on any other sedating drugs such as ethanol, barbiturates, or benzodiazepines. An IV bolus is indicated in patients who have altered mental status or respiratory depression in the presence of signs of opioid toxic-

Management

During the initial evaluation, the paramedic should detect and treat the patient for the immediate life threats from poisoning (Box 41-4). While life threats are assessed, the patient should be evaluated for airway management, given oxygen, placed on a cardiac monitor, and started on an IV. Blood tubes can be drawn when initiating the IV and saved for later laboratory analysis.

BOX 41-4	Immediate Life Threats from Poisoning

- Altered mental status
- Cardiac dysrhythmias
- Hyperthermia
- Hypoperfusion
- Respiratory failure
- Seizures

ity. Naloxone rapidly reverses both lowered mental status and respiratory depression in these patients. It may precipitate vomiting in patients who are addicted to opioids, necessitating airway protection and appropriate positioning. Opioid-addicted patients may also awaken with combative behavior, and EMS personnel should take appropriate precautions. Narcan lasts approximately 30 minutes and may need to be repeated if transport time is extended.

Some drugs and toxins have a specific antidote to counteract poisonous effects. For example, cyanide poisoning is managed with a Cyanide Antidote Kit which contains amyl nitrite ampules, sodium nitrite, and sodium thiosulfate solution. These drugs counteract the poisonous effects of cyanide. Contact with a Poison Control Center can assist EMS personnel or medical direction with the appropriate antidote as well as other information about the toxin. Other specific antidotes are listed in Table 41-1.

Unless the patient is in pulmonary edema, the initial approach to the poisoned patient with hypoperfusion should involve the administration of IV boluses of normal saline or lactated Ringer's. If volume administration is not effective or the patient is in pulmonary edema, administration of a pressor agent, such as dopamine, may be appropriate.

Patients with dysrhythmias following overdose require rapid transport to an emergency department for specialized care.

Routine ACLS measures may need to be modified, depending on the agent ingested by the patient. For instance, sodium bicarbonate is the preferred treatment for wide complex tachycardia caused by tricyclic antidepressant toxicity.

CRITICAL ISSUE

Drug-related wide complex tachycardia may not respond to standard ACLS treatment. Patient management requires rapid transport and consultation with medical direction to consider alternative strategies.

TABLE 41-1	Toxins and Specific Antidotes
Toxin	**Antidote**
Acetaminophen	N-acetyl-cysteine
Anticholinergics	Physostigmine
Benzodiazepines	Flumazenil
Beta blockers	Glycagon
Calcium channel blockers	Calcium, glucagon
Digoxin	Digibind (antibodies to digoxin)
Isoniazid	Vitamin B_6
Methanol, ethylene glycol	Ethanol
Opioids	Naloxone
Organophosphates	Atropine, praladoxime
Tricyclic antidepressants	Sodium bicarbonate

There are two methods that may be used outside of the hospital to "decontaminate" the stomach:

1. Activated charcoal, an agent which absorbs toxins in the stomach
2. Syrup of Ipecac, an oral medication which induces vomiting

Activated charcoal effectively absorbs many toxic agents and is as effective or more effective than methods which involve gastric emptying, such as administration of syrup of Ipecac or gastric lavage. It is mixed with water or sorbitol (a cathartic) and is ideally administered orally. Limitations of its use in the prehospital setting are primarily caused by its lack of palatability, which limits compliance. Contraindications to its administration include a caustic ingestion and mental state of depression that would increase the possibility of aspiration. Activated charcoal does not bind alcohols, hydrocarbons, or metals, such as lithium and iron.

Syrup of Ipecac should only be used in consultation with on-line medical direction or poison control. The administration of ipecac may be indicated for a patient following very recent ingestions of large amounts of aspirin, acetaminophen, iron, lithium, or aminophylline preparations. In general, ipecac is not given following the ingestion of hydrocarbons, such as gasoline or kerosene, unless they are mixed with very serious poisons, such as arsenic or insecticides. The administration of ipecac is contraindicated following ingestions of caustics, drugs with rapid onset of seizures, and sedatives with rapid onset of mental status depression.

The administration of ipecac is contraindicated if the patient:

- has a decreased level of responsiveness
- has already seized
- shows signs of hypoperfusion
- has respiratory insufficiency
- is already vomiting

Ipecac should be given with a minimum of 8 ounces of water. Complications of Syrup of Ipecac include continued and uncontrolled vomiting, inability to retain more useful antidotes, GI hemorrhage, and aspiration. In the hospital, gastric lavage may be used to remove poisons from the GI tract.

If a patient is actively seizing, the paramedic should ensure adequate respirations and administer oxygen, because hypoxia may be the cause. If the patient is not hypoxic or continues to seize, diazepam IV may be administered based on local protocol and medical direction consulted for the possible use of other medications (such as sodium bicarbonate in the setting of tricyclic antidepressant overdose).

Severe agitation can lead to injury to the patient or the paramedic. Use of physical restraints should be directed by local protocols. With long transport time, IV sedation may be indicated, but such therapy should only be initiated after contact with medical direction.

If the patient is hyperthermic, cooling is a high priority. The paramedic should remove clothing and constricting materials, apply lukewarm water, and fan the patient to increase evaporative cooling.

Management Considerations for Common Drugs

Because every drug and poison is different, it is difficult to make treatment generalities. The following section offers a brief discussion regarding individual agents that the paramedic will likely encounter.

Salicylates

There are many different forms of salicylates, the most common of which include aspirin and topical pain relieving compounds, such as oil of wintergreen. Oil of wintergreen is highly concentrated and has been associated with many cases of fatal salicylate toxicity.

Signs and Symptoms

Following ingestion, patients note ringing in their ears followed by the slow onset of hyperventilation and confusion. Death has been associated with severe metabolic acidosis, seizures, and hypoperfusion.

Management

Ipecac is safe to administer if the patient has very recently ingested the drug. The drug is well bound by activated charcoal. Alkalinization of the urine with sodium bicarbonate increases elimination. Hemodialysis is used in severe cases.

Acetaminophen (Tylenol[R])

This is a common drug involved in suicidal and sometimes accidental poisonings.

Signs and Symptoms

Initially, there may be only mild nausea or no symptoms at all. Over several days, vomiting, abdominal pain, and jaundice occur, caused by potentially fatal injury to the liver.

Management

Ipecac is safe for very early ingestions. The drug is well bound by activated charcoal. The specific antidote N-Acetyl Cysteine (NAC, or "Mucomyst") is highly effective and must be administered within 8 hours of the ingestion.

Carbon Monoxide

Carbon monoxide is an odorless, colorless gas which binds to normal hemoglobin causing the formation of "carboxyhemoglobin" which cannot carry oxygen. It is formed during the partial combustion of organic fuels such as gasoline, natural gas, or wood. The diagnosis should be considered in any person who develops a headache, nausea, and vomiting, or loses responsiveness in a closed space or near a stove, furnace, or fire.

Signs and Symptoms

Initially, headache and nausea may be the only signs of poisoning, slowly followed by confusion, seizures, unresponsiveness, and hypoperfusion. Children and pets are more susceptible to the effects of carbon monoxide and may have more serious signs of poisoning. Most poisoned patients have normal skin color. The famous "cherry red" skin coloring is seen only in the most severe cases (usually, by the coroner or medical examiner). Pulse oximetry will be inaccurate in the patient with possible carbon monoxide poisoning.

Management

High concentrations of oxygen help to displace CO from hemoglobin. Seriously poisoned patients are treated with hyperbaric oxygen at 3 atmospheres of pressure.

Cyanide

Cyanide is a highly toxic chemical which occurs in the form of a gas, such as in industrial accidents or fires in which plastics are burning, or a salt which usually appears with suicide attempts and occasionally accidental ingestion.

Signs and Symptoms

The patient initially experiences panic and shortness of breath, followed by unresponsiveness, seizures, bradycardia, and respiratory arrest. Severe metabolic acidosis occurs early. Patients with mild symptoms from gas exposure recover quickly when the exposure is stopped. Rescue personnel may be poisoned by the same environment which injured the victim, or by exposure to oral secretions during mouth-to-mouth resuscitation.

Management

The most important treatment involves airway management, assisted ventilation, and administration of oxygen, followed by the IV administration of sodium nitrite and sodium thiosulfate (Lilly Cyanide Kit[R]). When the diagnosis is suspected but not certain, only the soduim thiosulfate is given, especially if carbon monoxide may also be present.

Hydrocarbons

Hydrocarbons are familiar products of oil distillation, including gasoline, kerosene, and other solvents. In a pure form, they are not seriously toxic unless aspiration occurs. Most serious poisonings are caused by aspiration or by poisons dissolved in the solvent, such as insecticides or arsenic.

Signs and Symptoms

Coughing and respiratory distress as a result of noncardiogenic pulmonary edema.

Management

Oxygen should be administered and the patient intubated if indicated. If the solvent contained a large amount of a life-threatening toxin, ipecac is sometimes used to empty the stomach. Studies suggest that alert patients are less likely to aspirate when ipecac is used than when gastric lavage is used.[1] A poison specialist should always be consulted prior to the administration of ipecac to a patient with a hydrocarbon ingestion.

Caustics

Strong acids and strong alkalis cause injury to the mouth, throat, esophagus, and stomach. These substances may be found in many homes and many work places. Lye, dishwasher detergent, and battery acid are examples of common caustics.

Signs and Symptoms

Serious injury may occur without any evidence of injury to the mouth or throat. Patients complain of difficulty swallowing, difficulty breathing, and severe pain.

Management

Water or milk may be given to the patient to drink. Ipecac should not be given. The rescuer should intubate early if there is stridor or respiratory distress.

Iron Pills

Large ingestions of iron-containing vitamins may be very toxic to small children and sometimes to adults. Some formulations of iron pills appear identical to familiar candies.

Signs and Symptoms

Iron is very irritating to the stomach so that early vomiting and diarrhea, occasionally with evidence of **GI bleeding,** are common. Unresponsiveness, shock, and severe acidosis are consequences of severe poisoning. In survivors, severe scarring and obstruction of the GI tract may develop.

Management

Iron is not bound to activated charcoal. With documented large ingestions, administration of ipecac is indicated, unless the patient is vomiting already. If the amount ingested is believed to be small, ipecac should not be given, because the development of spontaneous vomiting will be an indication of a more significant ingestion than initially suspected. When there is uncertainty as to whether the amount of iron ingested by a child might be toxic, a poison control center should always be consulted. In the hospital, x-rays will demonstrate the amount of tablets in the stomach. IV chelation therapy with desferoxamine is used to treat severely poisoned patients.

Theophylline Preparations

Long-acting theophylline preparations are used in the treatment of **asthma.** Intentional ingestion by adults is common and may be fatal. Chronic toxicity also occurs, usually accidentally, with serious consequences in older patients.

Signs and Symptoms

Rapid heart rate, tremor, diaphoresis, and vomiting are common, and may be followed by seizures.

Management

This drug is very well bound by activated charcoal, which is the best therapy to administer in the field. This drug may be removed by hemodialysis in the hospital.

Cocaine

This is a commonly abused drug which is "sniffed" or injected in the form of a salt or smoked in the alkaloid form called "crack" or "freebase" (*also see* Chapter 42).

Signs and Symptoms

Agitated behavior, hyperthermia, **hypertension,** tachycardia, seizures, **myocardial infarction,** and **strokes** are possible symptoms in overdose patients.

Management

Treatment is symptomatic. IV benzodiazepines are very useful for agitation and seizures and also will lower the blood pressure. Severe cardiac chest pain should be treated with oxygen and nitroglycerin. Activated charcoal or ipecac are not indicated. If an ingestion is suspected, advice from a poison center or specialist should be obtained prior to treatment (*see* Chapter 42).

Tricyclic Antidepressants

These drugs are commonly used to treat depression and are frequently involved in suicide attempts by adults and accidental ingestions by children.

Signs and Symptoms

Rapid development of unresponsiveness, seizures, and hypotension occur in serious overdoses. Wide-complex tachycardia is common. Anticholinergic signs such as dilated pupils, flushed dry skin, dry mouth, and decreased bowel sounds are often present.

Management

Ipecac is absolutely contraindicated. Activated charcoal is useful and should be administered early. Seizures respond to IV benzodiazepines. Wide-complex tachycardia responds to the administration of sodium bicarbonate. Hypotension is treated with IV fluids, followed by norepinephrine infusion if needed.

Drugs and Toxins with Delayed Effects

Certain poisons have few initial side effects but may cause life-threatening problems hours following the ingestion. All patients with significant ingested amounts of these agents require evaluation and observation in a hospital. The most common of these agents are:

- *Lomotil.* A common opioid agent for treatment of diarrhea, this drug has been the cause of delayed deaths in small children. Death is caused by respiratory failure and is preventable. The respiratory depression is reversed with naloxone.
- *Clonidine.* A drug used to treat high blood pressure, clonidine has caused delayed respiratory arrest in small children. Death is caused by respiratory failure and is preventable.
- *Acetonitrile.* This agent, which is a solvent in nail polish removers, is metabolized to cyanide and has led to delayed death in small children. Effective antidotes are available. In these cases, careful identification of the ingestant and consultation with a poison control center will prevent error.
- *Monoamine oxidase inhibitors or MAOIs.* These substances are used to treat certain forms of depression but may cause death after an initial asymptomatic period lasting as long as 12 hours.
- *Hydrofluoric acid.* This material is used to clean bricks and remove rust from metals and has caused delayed death following an initial asymptomatic period after ingestion. Oral administration of magnesium or calcium solutions may bind the toxic fluoride ion.
- *Tylenol (acetaminophen).* Death occurs from liver failure 2 to 3 days after ingestion. A very effective antidote is available (Mucomyst or N-acetyl cysteine) which must be administered within 8 hours of ingestion. Acetaminophen is effectively bound to activated charcoal.
- *Aspirin.* Death may occur many hours later with status epilepticus, pulmonary edema, shock, or severe metabolic acidosis after an initial asymptomatic period. Hemodialysis is effective in preventing death if used early.
- *Toxic alcohols (methanol and ethylene glycol).* Death associated with severe metabolic acidosis occurs many hours after ingestion. Initially, the patient may appear only slightly intoxicated. Effective treatment is available if used early.

SUMMARY

Because of the wide availability of toxins in our environment, the EMS provider will frequently encounter poisoned or potentially poisoned patients. The role of the paramedic is to identify life-threatening complications and institute appropriate management strategies. For more stable patients, attempts to identify the toxin using clues at the scene can provide invaluable information.

REFERENCE

1. **Ng RC, Darwish H, Stewart DA:** Emergency treatment of petroleum distillate and turpentine ingestion. *Can Med Assoc J* 111:537, 1974.

Mahesh Shrestha, MD, FACEP and Lena Day Williams, BS, RN

Chapter 42

Drugs of Abuse

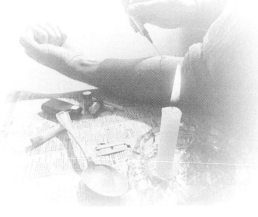

A paramedic should be able to:

1. Identify major life threats that need to be identified in the drug abuse patient.

2. Describe the physiological effects of cocaine.

3. List potential complications associated with cocaine use.

4. Describe the general effects of alcohol when combined with other drugs.

5. Identify the signs, symptoms and complications associated with acute alcohol intoxication and alcohol withdrawal syndrome.

6. Given a description of several patients with different clinical findings, identify patients suffering from acute alcohol intoxication and alcohol withdrawal, and describe the appropriate patient treatment for both conditions.

7. Identify commonly abused drugs, including their street names, and classify them according to category.

8. Given a description of several patients with different clinical findings, identify the drug of abuse and describe the appropriate patient treatment.

1. **Amphetamines**—a group of central nervous system stimulants that are subject to abuse because of their ability to produce feelings of euphoria.

2. **Barbiturate**—a derivative of barbituric acid that acts as a sedative or hypnotic.

3. **Benzodiazepines**—general term used to describe a group of tranquilizing drugs with similar chemical structures.

4. **Cocaine**—a white crystalline powder used as a local anesthetic.

5. **Endorphin**—any one of the neuropeptides composed of many amino acids, elaborated by the pituitary gland and acting on the central and the peripheral nervous systems to reduce pain.

6. **Inhalant**—substance drawn in of breath vapor or gas into the lungs.

7. **Marijuana**—a psychoactive herb derived from the flowering tops of hemp plants.

8. **Methaqualones**—a sedative-hypnotic.

9. **Narcotics**—a class of drugs that affect the nervous system. Legally used to relieve pain; illicit use to produce an intense state of relaxation.

10. **Phencyclidine**—a piperidine derivative administered parenterally to achieve neuroleptic anesthesia. Also called "angel dust."

Substance abuse is prevalent in American society and plays a significant role in the types of situations in which the paramedic may be called. Thirty-three percent of all Americans have tried marijuana; 5% to 6% of people over 12 years of age are marijuana users, 1.5% of Americans are current cocaine users.[6] Alcohol was a factor in approximately 50% of the 46,386 motor vehicle fatalities that occurred in 1987.[25]

A wide range of illnesses and injuries result from drug abuse. Examples of these injuries and illnesses range from a higher incidence of falls,[9] fires,[25] drownings,[16] and suicides[17] in alcoholic patients, to fatal respiratory depression caused by sedatives such as narcotic and barbiturate drugs, to fatal hyperthermia and hypertension caused by central nervous system (CNS) affecting drugs, such as amphetamines and cocaine. Knowledge of the manner in which these drugs present is important, so that treatment can begin in the field. For example, in the case of a young, agitated patient with track marks caused by IV drug abuse on the veins (Fig. 42-1), the most likely cause is stimulant (cocaine or amphetamine) abuse. The drug which should be administered in the field in this case is a benzodiazepine. Administration of naloxone (Narcan) would at best be a waste of time and could make the situation worse if the patient had also taken a narcotic.

The paramedic must not discount a patient's call for help because the patient is a drug abuser. A patient who appears to be drunk could actually have a subdural hematoma. The patient who is belligerent, instead of simply high on cocaine, may also be suffering from malignant hypertension and hyperthermia.

This chapter briefly reviews various drugs of abuse, the physiology, methods of administration, signs and symptoms, and management of intoxication, overdose, and withdrawal (see Table 42-1).

Cocaine

Cocaine has become one of the most popular street drugs today (Fig. 42-2). The drug is known by street names such as coke, snow, flake, blow, and many others; these names may be specific to regions of the country. Crack is a special preparation of cocaine that can be smoked. The term "speedball" refers to a combination of cocaine and heroin, and "liquid lady" refers to a combination of cocaine and alcohol. The purity of cocaine varies considerably. Substances from common foodstuffs, such as cornstarch and glucose, and drugs such as benzocaine, phencyclidine and strychnine, have been used to "cut," or dilute, cocaine.

Physiology

Cocaine is a CNS stimulant. Through its action on pleasure centers of the brain, the patient may initially become euphoric, self-confident, and hyperactive.[8] Actions in other areas can lead to tremors, hyperreflexia, and seizures. Unlike amphetamines, cocaine is rapidly metabolized. As the levels drop, irritability, anxiety, restlessness, and depression develop. These "lows" can be decreased by the concurrent use of alcohol or narcotics, accounting for the popularity of these combinations. The effects can be reversed by using more cocaine, leading to "binges" that may last for days. These combinations can leave the cocaine abuser listless and sleepy. One characteristic the paramedic must watch for in the cocaine user is paranoia, which is experienced by more than two thirds of patients.[20] Erratic, violent behavior may be seen when paranoia is combined with the increased energy and self-confidence also caused by cocaine.

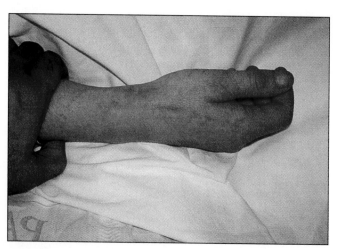

Figure 42-1

Track marks are visible from repeated punctures from nonsterile needles on unclean skin.

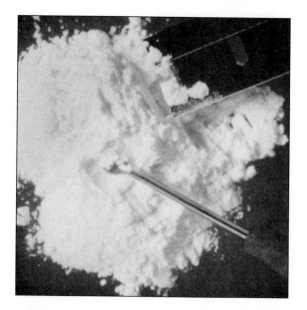

Figure 42-2

Cocaine in powdered form can be inhaled or mixed with other drugs and injected. From Ray/Ksir: *Drugs, Society, and Human Behavior,* ed 7, St. Louis, 1996, Mosby–Year Book. (Courtesy Drugs of Abuse, US Department of Justice, Drug Enforcement Administration.)

TABLE 42-1 Commonly Abused Drugs

Drug	Street Names	Route of Administration	Pharmacokinetics	Effect	Overdose	Withdrawal
NARCOTICS						
Morphine	Big M, Birdie powder, Dreamer, Dust, Gunk, Happy medicine, Morph, M.S., Piece, Red cross, Sweet Morpheus, Witch	Oral IM IV SQ	Oral: Effect within half hour, lasting around 4 hours. IM: Effect within minutes IV: Near immediate effects	Euphoria, drowsiness, constricted pupils, nausea, weight loss, respiratory depression	Slow and shallow breathing (even apnea), decreased heart rate and blood pressure, chest wall rigidity, clammy skin, pulmonary edema, convulsions, coma, death	Tremulousness, agitation, restlessness, anxiety, nausea, stomach cramps, diarrhea, cold sweats, insomnia, runny nose, watery eyes, yawning, pain, muscle cramps
Heroin	Anti-freeze, Big Harry, Caca, China White, Hombre, Horse, Caballo, Mojo, Poison, Smack, Texas Tea	Oral SQ IM IV (most common)	Effects seen nearly immediately after IV injection. Blood half-life is less than 20 minutes.			
Codeine	Schoolboy					
Meperidine (Demerol)				MPTP (methyl-phenyltetra hydropyridine) was a contaminant in MPPP which caused Parkinson's syndrome (muscular tremor and rigidity)		
Methylphenylpropion-oxypiperidine (MPPP)						
Hydromorphone (Dilaudid)	Lords					
Pentazocine (Talwin)	T's (T's and Blues refers to a combination of pentazocine and tripelennamine [Pyribenzamine], an antihistamine)	Oral T's and blues: IV				
Oxycodone (in Percodan)		Oral				
Methadone	Dollies, Dolls, Amidone	Oral				
Fentanyl	Tango and Cash, China white, synthetic heroin	Oral, SC, IM	Effects within 30 min of oral dose. Half-life 15 hours			
BENZODIAZEPINES			Oral absorption is good. Peak plasma levels occur in 1–3 hours. IV effects with diazepam is nearly immediate. IM absorption is erratic Half-life of drugs:	Slurred speech, disorientations, drunken behavior (without odor of alcohol). Paradoxical excitement can be seen in the very young or the very old.	Shallow respirations (even apnea), clammy skin, may have dilated pupils, weak and rapid pulse, sleepy, coma, possible death	Anxiety, headache, insomnia, tension, sweating, difficulty concentrating, tremor, fear, fatigue, agitation, seizures
Diazepam (Valium)	Downs	Oral IV	20–50 hours			
Chlodiazepoxide (Librium)		Oral	5–30 hours			
Alprazolam (Xanax)		Oral	11–14 hours			
Lorazepam (Ativan)		Oral	10–20 hours			

TABLE 42-1   Commonly Abused Drugs (Continued)

Drug	Street Names	Route of Administration	Pharmacokinetics	Effect	Overdose	Withdrawal
BARBITURATES			All are rapidly absorbed through the GI tract. Their half-lives vary:		Lethargic, shallow respirations (even apnea), may have dilated pupils, weak and rapid pulse, coma, possibly death	Anxiety, hallucinations, tremor, nausea, vomiting, abdominal cramps, insomnia, agitation, convulsions
Phenobarbital	Barbs, Blue birds, Blues, Candy, Crosses, Downs, Downers, Drowsy high, Phennies, Purple hearts, yellow jackets	Oral IM	48–144 hours	Sleepy, slurred speech, drunken behavior (without odor of alcohol).		
Butalbital (in Fiorinal, Esgic and Buff-A Comp.)		Oral	34–42 hours			
Secobarbital (Seconal)		Oral	22–29 hours			
AMPHETAMINES						
Amphetamine	"A", Bennies, Black Beauties, Black Mollies, Crosses, Jelly beans, Lid poppers, Uppers	Oral IM	Half-life: 8 hours	Euphoria, increased alertness, insomnia, excitation, grinding of jaw, increased pulse and blood pressure, perspiration, loss of appetite, Lethargy, depression is seen after a "speed run" (days of taking amphetamines)	Restlessness, dizziness, tremor, agitation, irritibility, weakness, nausea, dilated pupils, hyperthermia, chest pain, arrhythmias, combative, hallucinations, convulsions, possibly death	Listless, lack of energy, hypersomnia
Methylenedioxy-methamphetamine (MDMA)	Ecstasy, Adam, X, XTC, hug drug, clarity	Oral IM				
Methylenedioxy-ethylamphetamine (MDEA)	Eve	Oral IM	Oral onset of action is 30 minutes			
Methamphetamine	Crank, crystal meth, meth, speed	IV (most common) Oral Snorted	Effect within minutes if smoked or IV Half-life: 12 hours Duration of effects is 4–6 hours			
Ice (pure (+) methamphetamine)	Crystal, glass	Smoked (only amphetamine that is pure enough to be inhaled) Oral IM				
COCAINE						
Cocaine powder	Bernie's, Blow, Cadillac, Candy, Coke, Coconut, Dream, Flake, Girl, Happy dust, Leaf, Nose candy, Snow, Toot, White horse, White powder	Snort SQ (skin popping) IV	Snorting: peak effect in one half hour Plasma half-life approximately 12 minutes.	Euphoria, Feeling all powerful, able to do anything, excitation, increased blood pressure, loss of appetite. Chronic users appear thin. Chronic nasal drainage, red/raw nostrils (even perforated nasal septum) in snorters.	Agitation, belligerence, dilated pupils, hyperthermia, severely increased blood pressure, convulsions. Some may have lethargy, slurred speech, coma, especially after a long binge. Death.	Psychological depression, listlessness, lack of initiative, lethargy.
Crack cocaine (Freebase)	Crack, Rock	Smoke	IV and smoking: peak effect within minutes, (IV slightly slower than smoking). Effects last only a few minutes.			
PHENCYCLIDINE (PCP)	Angle dust, crystal, Dead on arrival (DOA), Embalming, Hog, Killer weed, Loveboat, Peace pill, Pop, Supergrass	Smoked Oral IM IV snorted	Effects nearly immediate if smoked or IV. Oral may take 30 minutes Half-life is on the order of 24 hours.	Illusions and hallucinations, poor perception of time	Severe agitation and belligerence, paranoia, nystagmus, hyperthermia, increased blood pressure, convulsions, possibly death	Psychological depression

TABLE 42-1 Commonly Abused Drugs (Continued)

Drug	Street Names	Route of Administration	Pharmacokinetics	Effect	Overdose	Withdrawal
LYSERGIC ACID DIETHYLAMINE (LSD)	Acid, Beast, Haze, Lucy in the sky with diamonds, Mind detergent, Peace, Strawberry fields, Sunshine, Zen	Smoked Snorting Oral	Peak serum levels in 1–2 hours. Half-life is approximately 3 hours. "Trips" may last several minutes or hours	Illusions and hallucinations, emotional swings, unpredictable behavior, altered perceptions, psychosis, dilated pupils. Violent/bizarre behavior can result in murder and suicide.	Same as effects but more severe	Psychological depression
CANNABIS Marijuana/Hashish	Acapulco gold, Baby, Flowers, Ganja, Goof butts, Happy cigarette, Indian boy, Jane, Juan Valdez, Lobo, Mary Jane, M.J., Poke, Pot, Reefer, Salt and pepper, Sinsemilla, Smoke, Tea, Weed, Yerba	Smoke Oral	Effects in 7–8 minutes, effects lasting 20–30 minutes Effects in 40 minutes, lasting 4–6 hours	Euphoria, relaxed inhibitions, disoriented behavior	Fatigue, paranoia, possibly psychosis	Psychological depression
METHAQUALONE (Quaalude, Sopor)	Lude, quay, quad, sopor, soaps, soapers, 714's, luding out (combined with wine)	Oral IV (much less common)	Peak levels achieved 1–2 hours after ingestion, half life of 2–6 hours.	Used to be prescribed for pain relief and sleep induction. Drowsiness, euphoria ("luding out"), sense of indestructibility.	Hallucinations, anxiety, numbness, tingling, tremors, altered sleep patterns, hypotension and respiratory depression (even death)	Headache, coma, loss of appetite, nausea, sleep disturbances, hallucinations, hypertension, convulsions.
INHALANTS Vapors of paints, glues, fuels, cleaning and beauty agents (toluene and other hydrocarbons)	spray	sniff	Effect almost immediate	Stimulation of mood, decreased inhibitions, euphoria. Often followed by nausea, drowsiness and headaches. Red and watery eyes	Muscle weakness and loss of control, confusion, "sudden sniffing death", loss of consciousness. Suffocation more likely if breathes into paper bag.	Psychological depression

It is believed that cocaine acts through sympathetic stimulation in the peripheral nervous system,[24] causing dilated pupils, sweating, hypertension, cardiac tachyarrhythmias and, if overdose is severe, hyperthermia. If the intoxication is mild, the tachycardia may be a sinus tachycardia, but supraventricular tachycardia is also frequent. In extreme overdose, ventricular tachycardia may be seen.

The sympathetic activation is also believed to be responsible for the vasoconstriction that occurs in numerous organs with cocaine overdose. In the coronary blood vessels, vasoconstriction can take place even with the ingestion of a very small amount of cocaine.[11] On occasion, a patient without a history of heart disease, such as an adolescent, will sustain a myocardial infarction (MI) as a result of cocaine overdose.[2] The incidence of chest pain in cocaine users is so common that the paramedic should consider cocaine use in patients who would otherwise be unlikely to have angina.[21]

Because of heightened metabolic activity from the sympathetic activation, the patient may exert himself or herself sufficiently enough to cause damage to skeletal muscle (rhabdomyolysis).[14] The breakdown product of skeletal muscle in this process is toxic to the kidneys and can result in renal failure. This process is often seen in the cocaine-intoxicated patient attempting to flee from or struggle with police. The cause of sudden deaths reported in such struggles is most likely MI. The cocaine has already caused coronary vasoconstriction and a heightened metabolic rate. When excessive physical activity is added, the demands on the heart may be more than the organ can withstand.

Crack is the alkali base of cocaine. It can be made from cocaine with simple extraction kits that are available on the street. Creation of the drug involves the use of solvents, such as ether. The use of materials such as these sometimes results in explosions if contact with a flame occurs. The resulting crystals, also called "rocks," are heat stable and can be smoked in a pipe.

Methods of Administration

- *Sniffing or "snorting."* Cocaine crystals are chopped into a fine powder and inhaled into the nostril through a straw or rolled up piece of paper, usually a dollar bill. Maximal euphoric sensations occur after 10 to 15 minutes.
- *Smoking or "free basing."* Because crack is rapidly absorbed by the lungs, the feeling of euphoria occurs almost immediately. However, it usually lasts less than 30 minutes, and is followed by more of a psychological "low" than with other methods of administration. The strong desire to smoke more often results in binges.
- *Intravenous use.* Effects of this method are similar to smoking, only slightly delayed. The use of the IV route causes medical problems of its own, such as bacterial endocarditis, local abscess formation, thrombosis of the injected vessel, and possible loss of limb if injected into an artery.

Signs and Symptoms

Mildly intoxicated patients may appear euphoric and talkative or irritable, tremulous, and hallucinatory. The paramedic may observe twitching of small muscles or grinding of the teeth. As the intoxication becomes worse, patients may seize, become hyperthermic (body temperature as high as 114°F have been recorded[19]), hypertensive, and lethargic. Finally, the patient can pass into coma and then die from seizures, respiratory arrest, intracranial hemorrhage, dysrhythmias, MI, or other causes.

Withdrawal from cocaine is mainly psychological. Patients usually display some degree of paranoia, insomnia, depression, nausea and vomiting. Abusers of crack cocaine appear to experience more of these symptoms, perhaps because of the more rapid drop in blood levels after use. Withdrawal does not lead to death, but the addict will do nearly anything to avoid the withdrawal process.

Management of Intoxication and Overdose

Management in general is supportive. The patient is in a CNS–excited state with possible paranoia, and paramedics must avoid sudden movement or other actions that the patient may find threatening. If the patient is struggling, excessive physical force in restraint is not recommended, because this action increases the stress on the patient's already stressed cardiovascular and muscular systems. Instead, benzodiazepines should be given in sufficient doses to calm the patient. Diazepam (Valium) should only be given IV; Lorazepam (Ativan) may be given IM if an IV line is not yet established. Benzodiazepines are also useful in controlling seizures, hyperthermia, hypertension, and tachycardia in the patient.

If chest pain is present and believed to be caused by coronary vasoconstriction, nitroglycerin administration may be of benefit.[5] Cardiac dysrhythmias are treated in the usual fashion. The paramedic should not be surprised, however, if supraventricular tachycardia returns after initial cardioversion or fails to convert.

Propranolol and other beta-blockers should not be given in the field, because these drugs could have adverse effects on the patient's condition. Naloxone (Narcan) should not be used in the patient without a decreased level of responsiveness; the presence of a narcotic counteracts some effects of the cocaine, a desirable action that would be abolished by naloxone. By the same token, the benzodiazepine antagonist flumazenil (Mazecon) should not be used, even if the patient has a decreased level of responsiveness, because this would abolish any therapeutic use of benzodiazepines.

Amphetamines

Colloquially called "uppers" or "speed," amphetamines produce excitement, euphoria and a sense of energy (Fig. 42-3). Some of the synthetic amphetamines, commonly known as MDA and PMA have hallucinogenic properties and are referred to as "love" drugs. The names of some common examples are Adam, Eve, and Ecstasy.

"Ice" is a very pure formulation of methamphetamine that can be smoked. It thus has an exaggerated effect when compared with less pure compounds. "Crank," which should not be confused with crack cocaine, is methamphetamine sulfate which can be orally ingested, injected IV, or snorted. The use of amphetamines has declined because of the popularity of cocaine and the rising medical awareness of prescription drug abuse.

Physiology

The symptoms of intoxication are those of increased CNS and sympathetic nervous system activity, similar to symptoms seen with cocaine but longer lasting. The psychological dependance is somewhat less, and amphetamines have not been implicated to the same degree in coronary vasospasm and MI. With oral usage, symptoms appear within 30 to 60 minutes and persist for 4 to 6 hours.

Methods of Administration

Different compounds can be administered in different ways. The most popular mode of administration is oral ingestion. IV injection gives a more intense "rush" or "flash." Increasing tolerance can lead to "speed runs" of repeated injections for up to 24 hours. Ice can also be snorted. Because the amphetamine inhalers for asthma (Benzadrine and Benedrex) were banned, the Vicks inhaler, which contains only a small amount of amphetamine, is the only inhalation formula available.[7]

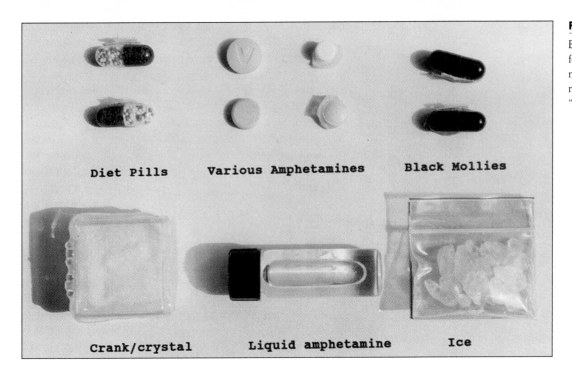

Figure 42-3

Examples of various forms of amphetamines, which increase metabolism and "speed" up the body.

Signs and Symptoms

The symptoms cover a range from mild restlessness, talkativity, flushing, diaphoresis, dry mucous membranes, dilated pupils, and nausea to moderate effects such as confusion, hypertension, tachypnea, tachycardia, premature ventricular contractions, chest pain, elevated temperature, repetitive behaviors and hallucinations, and finally to severe results that include delirium, marked hypertension, hyperthermia, seizures, coma, and serious cardiac dysrhythmias. Death can occur from those symptoms or dysrhythmias or from acute congestive heart failure, hyperthermia, malignant hypertension and even intracranial hemorrhage in the seriously overdosed patient.

Abrupt discontinuation does not produce life-threatening consequences, although chronic users may experience depression and lethargy.

Management of Intoxication and Overdose

There is no antidote for acute intoxication. Treatment is supportive, similar to the treatment of cocaine overdose, including normal treatment of dysrhythmias, hypertension, hyperthermia, and seizure activity. As with cocaine management, benzodiazepines are also useful.

Narcotics

Narcotics have been abused since ancient times. Today, the naturally occurring narcotics (i.e., opium, morphine and codeine) are joined by various semisynthetic derivatives such as heroin, hydrocodone (with acetaminophen in Loretab), oxycodone (with aspirin in Percodan, and acetaminophen in Percocet), hydromorphone (Dilaudid), and fully synthetic compounds such as meperidine (Demerol), propoxyphene (Darvon), methadone (Dolophine), pentazocine (Talwin), and fentanyl (Sublimaze), which has 200 times the potency of morphine. With the exception of heroin, these drugs can all be legally prescribed by physicians for patients with severe pain.

Physiology

Narcotics are CNS depressants. They act by binding to and stimulating receptors in the CNS that release endorphins and enkephalins, substances that produce euphoria, a sense of well being and increased pain tolerance. Severe overdose depresses the respiratory control center in the brain, decreasing the rate of breathing, sometimes to point of total apnea. In less-extreme overdoses, the patient may have various degrees of decreased responsiveness. Through their effects on the cardiovascular system, narcotics can cause hypotension, which can not always be reversed with naloxone (Narcan).

Methods of Administration

Oral, IV, IM, rectal, and even intranasal forms of delivery are available. In general, the IV form is the most reliable and quickest acting (Fig. 42-4). This method of administration exposes the abuser to all of the medical complications of IV drug use.

Signs and Symptoms

Constricted pupils (miosis) and decreased level of responsiveness are the important signs and symptoms the paramedic should look for in the patient. The presence of either should

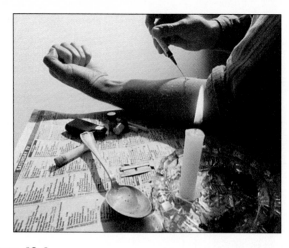

Figure 42-4

Intravenous heroin. From Ray/Ksir: *Drugs, Society, and Human Behavior,* ed 7, St. Louis, 1996, Mosby–Year Book.

make the paramedic suspicious of a narcotic overdose. Constricted pupils are not always seen, especially with meperidine (Demerol) overdoses. Needle track marks, empty bottles, and other hints may also point toward narcotic abuse.

Management of Intoxication, Overdose and Withdrawal

The availability of a very safe antidote, naloxone (Narcan), makes the identification of narcotic overdose especially important. It reverses both unresponsiveness and respiratory depression. Naloxone can be administered IV, endotracheally, IM, subcutaneously, or intralingually, although intralingual injection should be the last resort.[12] The usual dosage is 0.4 to 2.0 mg IV. The higher dose is recommended in the patient with respiratory compromise. If there is no response, naloxone may be repeated to a maximum of 10 mg. Propoxyphene and pentazocine overdoses are particularly likely to require multiple doses. Some degree of caution must be exercised in treating the narcotic-addicted patient. Smaller doses should be used, because the paramedic can precipitate withdrawal, making the patient much more difficult to manage and transport.

If the analgesic effect of the narcotic is desired without the toxic effects, the paramedic can administer small amounts of naloxone (0.04 mg) at 2-minute intervals until the desired response is achieved.[28] In long transports, the paramedic must remember that the duration of naloxone effects varies between 40 and 90 minutes. Some narcotic effects last longer, so that the patient may again become toxic and require further doses. The concept of duration of drug action is also important in the patient who has used a speedball (cocaine and heroin). Initially, the patient may be agitated, at which time naloxone may not be necessary and may even make transport of the patient more difficult. Because cocaine has a shorter duration of action than heroin, the patient may develop respiratory compromise after the cocaine wears off; administration of naloxone may be life saving.

Narcotic withdrawal begins 6 to 8 hours after the last dose taken, peaks at 2 days, and can last for 5 to 10 days. Withdrawal is not fatal but can cause the patient serious discomfort.

Early withdrawal symptoms include yawning, insomnia and restlessness. This progresses to abdominal pain, pupillary dilation and muscle spasm. Late symptoms include nausea and vomiting, tachypnea, tachycardia, hypertension, and diaphoresis. These symptoms can sometimes be avoided by decreasing the dosage by approximately 20% each day.

Methadone is a long-acting narcotic given at addiction treatment centers to selected addicts who are unable to come off narcotics totally. Clonidine (Catapres) is an antihypertensive medication which appears to decrease the symptoms of withdrawal.

Barbiturates

Barbiturates, often called "downers," were a leading cause of drug-induced death until the early 1970s. Recognition of the addictive potential and dangerous effects in overdose led to the development of the safer benzodiazepines, which are now much more commonly used (Fig. 42-5). Barbiturates are still used in anesthesia, for seizure control and in certain combinations for pain control. On the street, phenobarbital is the most commonly abused type of barbiturate.

Physiology

Barbiturates are CNS depressants. These agents are believed to work through the same mechanism in the CNS as that used by the benzodiazepines.[18] Low doses cause drowsiness, and toxic doses lead to total unresponsiveness. Patients with barbiturate intoxication can appear dead. When overdose is fatal, death results from respiratory depression. High doses also depress skeletal, smooth, and cardiac muscle, leading to weakness, vasodilation, reduced gastrointestinal motility, congestive heart failure, and hypotension. One of the reasons the

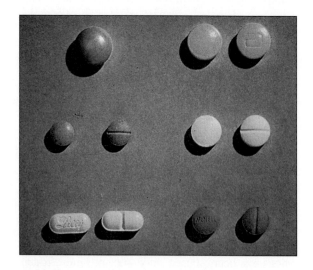

Figure 42-5

Barbiturates are taken to calm the nerves or to help bring on sleep. From Ray/Ksir: *Drugs, Society, and Human Behavior,* ed 7, St. Louis, 1996, Mosby–Year Book.

barbiturates have caused so many medical problems is the small difference between therapeutic and toxic doses: the average toxic dose is only five times the therapeutic dose.

The different forms of barbiturates differ in their duration of action. Pentobarbital (Nembutal) and secobarbital (Seconal) are short acting, lasting approximately 3 hours. Amobarbital (Amytal) and butalbital (contained in many combination preparations, such as Esgic, Fiorinal, and Buff-A. Comp) are intermediate acting, lasting approximately 3 to 6 hours. Phenobarbital (Luminal) is long acting, lasting approximately 6 to 12 hours.

Methods of Administration

These are taken either orally, IV, or as an IM injection.

Signs and Symptoms

The observable effects of barbiturates in usual and toxic doses are those expected from a CNS depressant. Thus, in low and moderate doses, the patient has slurred speech, disorientation, and drunken behavior. In toxic doses, there are shallow respirations, clammy skin, weak and rapid pulse, and dilated pupils (early in the overdose these are actually constricted) and eventually lack of reflexes, total unresponsiveness, apnea, and death.

Withdrawal from barbiturates can be severe, resulting in symptoms that can range from minor (e.g., anxiety, agitation, sleep disturbance, nausea, vomiting, anorexia and tremor) to severe (e.g., bizarre, jerky movement of the extremities, and seizures) to ominous (e.g., hallucinosis, hyperthermia and death). Symptoms of withdrawal can last for up to 14 days.[10]

Management of Intoxication, Overdose, and Withdrawal

In the mildly intoxicated patient, no treatment other than observation is needed. In overdose, treatment is supportive. If there is a decrease in ventilatory effect, intubation and assisted ventilation may be necessary. Blood pressure support with fluids and possible dopamine may also be needed. If the ingestion was oral, activated charcoal should be given to bind the patient's stomach contents.[4]

Methaqualone

Methaqualone was introduced in 1965 in the United States as a substitute for barbiturates. "Quaaludes" quickly gained popularity as a street aphrodisiac. Although they were once believed to be nonaddictive, reports of physical and psychological dependence surfaced quickly. Legal production of methaqualone has ceased in the United States.

Physiology

Methaqualone is a CNS depressant. Paradoxically, high doses result in increased motor tone and reflexes, sometimes requir-

ing paralysis for control.[1] The other effects are similar to those of barbiturates and alcohol.

Signs and Symptoms

Like barbiturates, with methaqualone use the patient appears drunk but does not have the odor of alcohol. The unique symptom seen frequently in severe overdoses (55% to 75% of the time) is increased muscle tension. There is also a high rate of pulmonary edema. Withdrawal may occur, with symptoms similar to barbiturate withdrawal.

Management of Intoxication, Overdose, and Withdrawal

Management is similar to that of barbiturate overdose. Activated charcoal should be administered if the patient is able to swallow. Withdrawal can be treated by reinstituting the medication and gradually decreasing the dose.

Benzodiazepines

This class of medication is among the most widely prescribed, especially Diazepam (Valium) and alprazolam (Xanax) (Fig. 42-6).

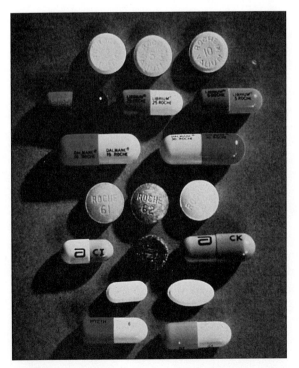

Figure 42-6

Benzodiazepines are psychotropic drugs which include many tranquilizers. The prehospital drug diazepam (Valium) is in this class as well. From Ray/Ksir: *Drugs, Society, and Human Behavior,* ed 7, St. Louis, 1996, Mosby–Year Book. (Courtesy Drugs of Abuse, US Department of Justice, Drug Enforcement Administration.)

Physiology

Benzodiazepines are CNS depressants and are prescribed for anxiety and sleeplessness. They are occasionally used as muscle relaxants and as anticonvulsants in patients with status epilepticus. If death occurs, it usually results from respiratory depression, which is more likely if other drugs with depressive effects are taken at same time, such as barbiturate, narcotics, or alcohol. The difference between the various preparations of benzodiazepines is the half-life. Diazepam (Valium) and chlordiazepoxide (Librium) are long acting but are often prescribed at more frequent doses to keep blood levels from dropping. Alprazolam (Xanax) and lorazepam (Ativan) are shorter acting forms (10 to 24 hours). The ultrashort (< 10 hours) acting agents, triazolam (Halcion), and temazepam (Restoril) are used mainly for sleep induction.

Withdrawal symptoms rarely appear, unless large doses of benzodiazepines are used chronically. If signs appear, they do so 1 to 11 days after discontinuation, depending on whether the particular benzodiazepine was long or short acting. The most common symptoms are insomnia, anxiety, headache, muscle spasm, involuntary movements, appetite loss, nausea, vomiting, tremor, ringing in the ears, and weakness. Seizures may develop but rarely. These symptoms are similar to, but much less common, dramatic, and serious than those seen with barbiturate, alcohol, or narcotic withdrawal. In fact, benzodiazepines are the mainstay of alcohol withdrawal treatment.

Methods of Administration

These include oral, IV, IM, endotracheal, rectal and intranasal, depending on the availability of the formulation. Most abusers use the IV and oral routes.

Signs and Symptoms

Sedation, drowsiness, slurred speech, double vision, difficulty walking, and difficulty concentrating are the most common effects. Symptoms are mild, even in the overdose situation, distinguishing benzodiazepine overdose from other CNS–depressant drugs, such as barbiturates and alcohol. It would be unusual for a healthy young patient to stop breathing as a result of benzodiazepine overdose unless other drugs were involved. Older patients and patients with chronic diseases, such as chronic obstructive pulmonary disease (COPD), may become apneic with benzodiazepine overdose.

Management of Intoxication, Overdose, and Withdrawal

Flumazenil (Mazicon) is a recently approved medication that reverses the effects of benzodiazepines. However, unlike naloxone, it is not recommended for routine prehospital use. There have been cases of intractable seizures and death from its use, especially in patients who also overdosed on a medication that could cause seizures, such as tricyclic antidepressants or cocaine.[13] The medication is not necessary in the prehospital setting; assisted ventilation is sufficient to stabilize patients during transport.

The treatment is supportive for patients with benzodiazepine overdose. The patient is observed for signs of respiratory compromise and prohibited from engaging in potentially dangerous activity requiring judgement or coordination. Withdrawal generally does not require treatment, if it occurs at all.

Alcohol

Ethanol, the ingestible form of alcohol, is the most commonly abused drug in the United States (Fig. 42-7). An estimated

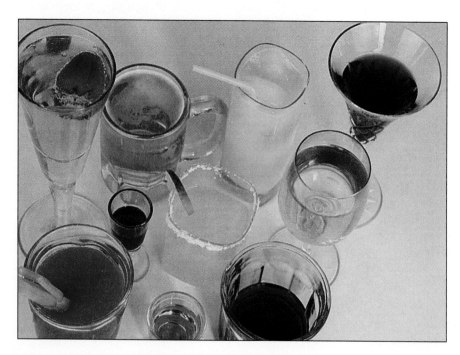

Figure 42-7

Alcohol is one of the most abused readily available drugs. From Ray/Ksir: *Drugs, Society, and Human Behavior,* ed 7, St. Louis, 1996, Mosby–Year Book.

6.2% of all deaths in California were related to alcohol, making this cause one of the top ten causes of death in the state.[23]

Physiology

In large, acute ingestions, alcohol is a CNS depressant. In smaller doses, alcohol can appear to stimulate the patient because of its effects on the patient's psychological inhibitions and judgement. A patient's degree of tolerance, genetic ability to metabolize alcohol, underlying nutritional status, amount of alcohol ingested, rising blood level rate, and coingestion of other drugs are determinants of the effect alcohol will have. The effects of alcohol are additive in the presence of other CNS depressants, such as benzodiazepines and barbiturates. Only very rarely does alcohol itself cause fatal respiratory depression.

Malnutrition is associated with alcohol abuse because foods, which contain vitamins and protein, are replaced with alcohol. Deficiency of thiamine (vitamin B^3) can lead to circulatory and neurological problems that include congestive heart failure and peripheral neuropathy with decreased sensation in the distal arms and legs. As thiamine deficiency continues, the patient may develop Wernicke's syndrome (mental status changes, ataxia and abnormalities in eye movement) and Korsakoff's psychosis (characterized by the mental habit of making things up). Treatment with thiamine injections is effective only in the early stages. The symptoms of thiamine deficiency, particularly congestive heart failure, can be precipitated by the administration of dextrose, which increases metabolic rate and thiamine demand. Thus, thiamine, usually 100 mg IM or IV, should be administered before, with, or within a short period of time after dextrose.

Methods of Administration

Alcohol is limited to the oral route. Occasionally, IV ethanol will be given therapeutically in ethylene glycol overdoses. Aside from the usual sources of alcohol, such as beer, wine and hard liquor, alcohol is also present in many cold remedies and hygiene products, such as mouthwash, that are easily available over-the-counter. Some of these products can contain as much as 25% alcohol. Alcohol-dependent patients may also resort to drinking substances such as methanol (wood alcohol), isopropyl alcohol (rubbing alcohol), and ethylene glycol (found in antifreeze). These substances are much more toxic than ethanol and mandate transport to an emergency department.

Signs and Symptoms

Signs of mild intoxication in a patient range from euphoria to loss of temper. With progressive intoxication, slurred speech, ataxia (poor physical coordination), nystagmus (abnormal eye movements), tachycardia, and distortion of sensory perceptions occur. With severe intoxication, the patient becomes less and less responsive. Breathing can slow or even stop. The patient's blood pressure and body temperature may also drop to fatal levels.

Death usually does not occur as a direct result of alcohol ingestion. More often, the alcohol-intoxicated person engages in an activity, such as driving a car, in which lack of judgement or coordination can be fatal. Children become dangerously intoxicated at smaller doses. Fatalities are also more likely if the patient is taking another CNS depressant.

Alcohol withdrawal has many manifestations. The first stage is usually shakiness which, for alcoholics, can begin after 8 hours of sleep. Approximately 1 day after the patient's last drink, seizures and hallucinations can occur. The seizures are the generalized tonic-clonic type. A common hallucination is the feeling of ants crawling over the body. The life-threatening withdrawal syndrome is called **delirium tremens** (DTs). Patients often mistakenly refer to simple tremors as DTs. Delirium is a changing level of responsiveness or orientation. The patient may be alert but not know where he is, then be lethargic or think he is someone else. Tremens refers to an excessive output of the sympathetic nervous system. The patient's pupils will be dilated, skin will be wet with perspiration, and blood pressure, heart rate, and temperature will be elevated. The patient startles very easily and appears to threaten or retreat from anyone close by.

Management of Intoxication, Overdose, and Withdrawal

Simple alcohol overdose generally requires no treatment other than observation until the ingested ethanol is sufficiently metabolized. Respiratory depression, either from a very large ingestion or a concurrent depressant overdose, is treated supportively by assisting ventilation. In the unresponsive patient, Narcan and D$_{50}$ should be used. Thiamine should also be given soon after arrival at the emergency department, if not in the field. Evidence for other mechanisms of injury, such as head trauma, should also be sought.

Treatment for withdrawal includes benzodiazepines, such as diazepam (Valium) or chlordiazepam (Librium). If the withdrawal involves serious problems, such as repeated seizures or DTs, a longer hospital stay is required. Patients suffering from Wernicke's encephalopathy (also called Wernicke's syndrome) or Korsakoff's psychosis will need hospitalization for thiamine administration.

Phencyclidine

Phencyclidine (PCP) was originally developed in the 1920s as an anesthetic. Because of its hallucinogenic and seizure promoting properties, its manufacturer voluntarily discontinued production in 1963. Illicit PCP use peaked in the 1970s when clandestine laboratories found it inexpensive to produce.

Physiology

PCP most likely works through its effects in areas of the brain important to emotion, behavior, and motor control. The drug is slowly metabolized; its effects last 4 to 6 hours, much longer than cocaine. Similar to cocaine and amphetamines, PCP also increases the sympathetic nervous system's activity and thus can lead to hypertension and tachycardia.

Methods of Administration

The most popular form of use is smoking PCP sprinkled on parsley or marijuana leaves (Fig. 42-8). Cigarettes can be dipped into liquid PCP and smoked. More rarely, PCP is snorted or ingested. IV use is very common. Because it can be administered through all of these routes, PCP is a common adulterant in other illicit drugs.

Signs and Symptoms

Signs and symptoms can be separated into major and minor patterns. Symptoms of major intoxication include total unresponsiveness, bizarre or repetitive posturing, repetition of nonsense, and violent behavior with hallucinations. These patients will require hospitalization. Minor patterns include lethargy, euphoria, and somewhat violent behavior without hallucinations. Nystagmus is common. Heart rate and blood pressure are generally elevated unless the overdose is very large. Agitation and violent behavior may last from a few hours to a few days.

Withdrawal may last only 1 day and consists of goose bumps and increased sensory sensitivity. Most first-time abusers have a pleasurable experience. However, with repeated use, the unpleasurable effects predominate.

Management of Intoxication and Overdose

There is no specific treatment for patient with PCP intoxication. It is nearly impossible to "talk down" an agitated, paranoid patient on PCP. Initially, the use of physical force and restraints may be necessary to gain control of the patient, but this method can result in serious injury. When the stress of a physical struggle is added to the major physiological stress the PCP-intoxicated patient is already experiencing, significant injury can result to the patient's muscle and internal organs, such as the heart and liver. These injuries can be severe enough to cause death. It is best for "chemical restraints" to be

used, such as a diazepam (Valium), lorazepam (Ativan), or haloperidol (Haldol), as soon as possible. Withdrawal requires no treatment.

Lysergic Acid Diethylamide (LSD)

Use of lysergic acid diethylamide (LSD) peaked in the 1960s and then gradually waned, although its use may have increased recently. LSD is also called "acid" and other street names.

Physiology

LSD probably has its effects through certain chemicals in key parts of the brain. Effects generally develop within 40 to 90 minutes after ingestion and begin to abate after approximately 4 hours. Tolerance develops with continued use but physical withdrawal symptoms do not occur.

Routes of Administration

LSD is nearly always taken orally (Fig. 42-9). It can be taken IV or nasally, but these routes are seldom employed.

Signs and Symptoms

Pupillary dilation is the most frequent physical sign. Mild increases in heart rate, body temperature, and respirations are also common. Blood pressure is usually normal. There may be some parasympathetic signs such as salivation, tearing, nausea, and vomiting, and some neuromuscular effects, such as weakness, tremor, and ataxia.

The most notable psychological experience is that of sensory distortion. Visual afterimages are prolonged, flat surfaces may show depth, and objects with depth may appear flat. There may be amplification of background noise. Time appears to slow. The patient's thought process is altered, and behavior patterns are difficult to predict. Other side effects include acute panic attacks, memory flashbacks, acute psychotic reactions, mania, behavior-induced trauma, seizures, and coma. Life-threatening reactions are rare.

Management

There is no specific treatment.

Marijuana

Marijuana is derived from the dried leaf of the Indian hemp plant, Cannabis sativa (Fig. 42-10A). Its street names include pot, Mary Jane, weed, and grass. Hashish is the concentrated, dried resin collected from the flower tops of the hemp plant (Fig. 42-10B). This form is commonly produced in the Middle East and North Africa.

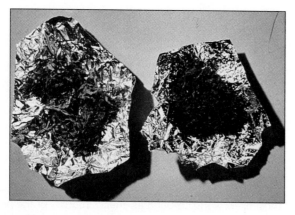

Figure 42-8

PCP, an animal tranquilizer, is found naturally occurring on plants. From Ray/Ksir: *Drugs, Society, and Human Behavior,* ed 7, St. Louis, 1996, Mosby–Year Book. (Courtesy Drugs of Abuse, US Department of Justice, Drug Enforcement Administration.)

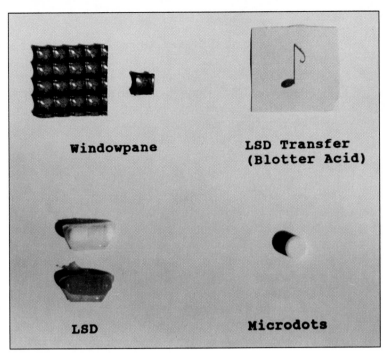

Figure 42-9
LSD was a popular drug during the 1960s, and its use is again on the rise.

Physiology

The exact mechanism of marijuana's effects is not understood.

Methods of Administration

The most popular route of administration is smoking (Fig. 42-10C). Maximal psychological effects occur within 20 to 30 minutes and decrease over the following minutes. Approximately 3 times more marijuana is required for the same effect if taken orally. The effect is slower, with peak effects 2 to 3 hours after ingestion, but longer lasting. There have been only a handful of reports of IV use.

Signs and Symptoms

The effects are mainly psychological. In addition to its desired effect of relaxation and euphoria, acute ingestion may cause anxiety, fear, disorientation, paranoia, confusion, and hallucinations. The more severe effects are more common with larger ingestion doses. The patient develops tolerance with repeated use and there is a mild withdrawal reaction which consists of restlessness, insomnia, irritability, and decreased appetite.

Recently, marijuana has been proposed to be used legally in the treatment of patients with terminal cancer or HIV-related disease, mainly for its antivomiting and pain-reducing effects.

Management

Treatment of acute marijuana intoxication is supportive.

Inhalants

Many household compounds are inhaled by patients for recreational purposes, including model airplane glue, rubber cement, spray paint, aerosol propellants, lighter fluid, gasoline, nail-polish removers, and substances easily available in some workplaces such as nitrous oxide (laughing gas) and industrial solvents (Fig. 42-11). Typically, the abuser is a boy less than 14 years of age; occasionally, the patient is as young as 7 to 8 years of age.[15]

Physiology

These volatile substances contain hydrocarbons that are rapidly absorbed into the bloodstream and enter the CNS almost immediately. Many abused substances contain a combination of different volatile chemicals. The "high" that is achieved is characterized by euphoria, lightheadedness, excitement, occasional hallucinations, and depression, similar to the effects of alcohol. In general, tolerance and dependence (with a minor withdrawal syndrome) do develop.

Some of the toxic effects are specific to certain agents. Toluene (found in many glues, paints and industrial solvents) can cause nerve damage with pain, tingling, weakness, tremors, and ataxia. With chronic use, this substance can cause a very severe hypokalemia through loss of potassium in the urine, leading to an acute paralysis. Gasoline causes pulmonary symptoms by irritating the respiratory tract and causing possible visual hallucinations. Most of these substances increase the chances of serious ventricular arrhythmias if the patient is startled.

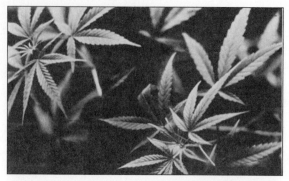

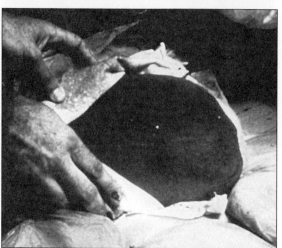

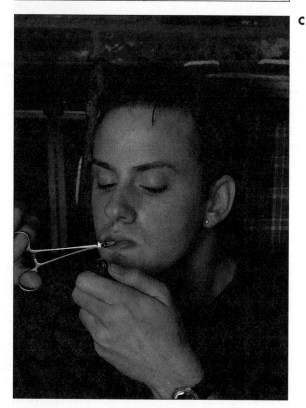

Methods of Administration

The wide availability of these substances and ease of administration have made them popular. Abusers generally start by "sniffing." As the abuse progresses they may move to "huffing," which is inhaling from a cloth soaked in the solvent. More experienced abusers may also breath in and out of a paper or plastic bag containing the chemical ("bagging").

Signs and Symptoms

Many of the effects are similar to those seen with alcohol intoxication. Euphoria, blurred or double vision, slurred speech, ataxia, nausea and vomiting can all be seen with inhalant abuse. Visual hallucinations and disorientation to time and place are more common symptoms than with alcohol intoxication. It is important that the paramedic monitor the patient for cardiac dysrhythmias.

The smell of the abused substance on the patient or at the scene is an important clue which must be reported. Various paraphernalia such as rags, containers, and bags should be recovered if present.

Management

Treatment is supportive. In patients with mental status changes, the paramedic should make every effort to disturb the patient as little as possible to avoid causing cardiac dysrhythmias. Usual care, such as 100% oxygen, establishment of an IV line, and cardiac monitoring are necessary for transport. Patient withdrawal generally does not require special treatment.

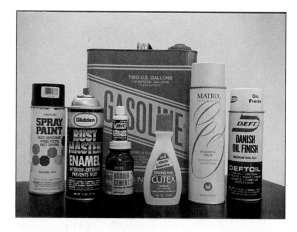

Figure 42-10

A, The cannabis plant, from which marijuana is derived. B, Hashish is a concentrated form of marijuana that is frequently mixed with other drugs. C, The most common way to consume marijuana is by smoking it. From Ray/Ksir: *Drugs, Society, and Human Behavior,* ed 7, St. Louis, 1996, Mosby–Year Book. (A & B courtesy of Drugs of Abuse, US Department of Justice, Drug Enforcement Administration.)

Figure 42-11

The use of inhalants is on the rise, seen commonly with teenagers and preteens. Volatile chemicals that are readily available, such as gasoline, lacquer thinner, spray paint, and other household chemicals make this potentially deadly drug use very popular. From Ray/Ksir: *Drugs, Society, and Human Behavior,* ed 7, St. Louis, 1996, Mosby–Year Book.

SUMMARY

The dramatic increase in drug abuse in the United States and the violence that often accompanies it, often places the prehospital provider in dangerous situations. Familiarity with the drugs of abuse, their common street names, and how to recognize and manage drug-related calls is essential to providing appropriate prehospital care.

REFERENCES

1. **Abboud PT, Freedman, MT, Rogers RM, et al:** Methaqualone poisoning with muscular hyperactivity necessitating the use of curare. *Chest* 65:204–205, 1974.

2. **Ascher EK, Stauffer JC, Gaasch W:** Coronary artery spasm, cardiac arrest, transient electrocardiographic Q waves and stunned myocardium in cocaine associated myocardial infarction. *Am J Cardiol* 61:939–1941, 1988.

3. Barbiturate coma and blisters (editorial). *Lancet* 1:733, 1972.

4. **Berg MJ, Berlinger WG, Goldberg MJ, et al:** Acceleration of the body clearance of phenobarbital by oral activated charcoal. *N Engl J Med* 307:642–644, 1982.

5. **Brogan WC, Lange RA, Kim AS, et al:** Alleviation of cocaine induced vasoconstriction by nitroglycerin. *J Am Coll Cardiol* 17:174A (abstract), 1991.

6. **Coleman P:** Overview of substance abuse. *Primary Care* 20(1):5–6, 1993.

7. **Gal J:** Amphetamines in nasal inhalers. *J Toxicol Clin Toxicol* 19:577–578, 1982.

8. **Hammer P:** Cocaine alters opiate receptor binding in critical brain reward regions. *Synapse* 3:55–60, 1989.

9. **Honkanen R, Ertama L, Kuosmanen P, et al:** The role of alcohol in accidental falls. *J Stud Alcohol* 44:231–245, 1983.

10. **Khantzian EJ, McKenna GJ:** Acute toxic and withdrawal reactions associated with drug and abuse. *Ann Intern Med* 90:364, 1979.

11. **Lange RA, Cigarroa RG, Yancy CW, et al:** Cocaine induced coronary artery vasoconstriction. *N Engl J Med* 321:1557–1572, 1989.

12. **Maio RF, Gaukel B, Freeman B:** Intralingual naloxone injection for naloxone-induced respiratory depression. *Ann Emerg Med* 16:572, 1987.

13. **Marchant B, Wray R, Leach A, Nama M:** Flumazenil causing convulsions and ventricular tachycardia (letter). *Brit Med J* 299:860, 1989.

14. **Merigan KS, Roberts JR:** Cocaine intoxication: hyperpyrexia, rhabdomyolysis and acute renal failure. *J Toxicol Clin Toxicol* 25:135–148, 1987.

15. **Miller NS, Gold MS:** Organic solvent and aerosol abuse. *Am Fam Phys* 44:183–189, 1991.

16. **Mooney A:** Alcohol and drug abuse. American Academy of Family Practice Monologue 107, 1988.

17. **National Institute on Alcohol Abuse and Alcoholism:** 7th Special Report to Congress on Alcohol and Health, Washington, 1990, United States Government Printing Office.

18. **Olsen RW, Yang J, King RG, et al:** Barbiturate and benzodiazepine modulation of GABA receptor binding and function. *Life Sci* 39:1969, 1986.

19. **Roberts JR, Quattrocchi E, Howland MA:** Severe hyperthermia secondary to intravenous drug abuse. *Am J Emerg Med* 2:373, 1984.

20. **Satel SL, Southwick SM, Gawin FH:** Clinical features of cocaine induced paranoia. *Am Psych* 148:495–498, 1991.

21. **Schwarts RH:** Chest pain in adolescent: think of cocaine. *Pediatrics* 83:639–640, 1989.

22. **Stabenau JR:** Is risk for substance abuse unitary. *J Nerv Mental Dis* 180:583–588, 1992.

23. **Sutockey JW, Shultz JM, Kizer KW:** Alcohol related mortality in California, 1980–1989. *Am J Pub Health* 83:817–823, 1993.

24. **Van Dyke C, Byck R:** Cocaine. *Sci Am* 246:139, 1982.

25. **United States Department of Health and Human Services, Centers for Disease Control:** Update: alcohol-related traffic fatalities—United States 1982–1993. *Morb Mort Wkly Rep* 43(47):861–867, 1994.

26. **Waller JA:** Nonhighway injury fatalities—the roles of alcohol and problem drinking, drugs, and medical impairment. *J Chron Dis* 25:33–45, 1972.

27. **West LJ, Maxwell DS, Noble EP, et al:** Alcoholism. *Ann Intern Med* 100:405–416, 1984.

28. **Wright DJM, Phillips M, Weller MPI:** Naloxone in shock. *Lancet* i, ii:1261, 1980.

Michael D. Mackan, MD, FACEP
and Jedd Roe, MD, FACEP

Chapter 43

Environmental Emergencies

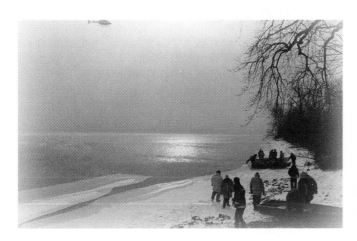

A paramedic should be able to:

1. Describe the pathophysiology, assessment, and prehospital management of patients who have been stung or bitten by an insect, reptile, or animal.

2. Describe the basic mechanism for body temperature regulation.

3. Identify individuals who are at high risk for developing heat and cold related illnesses.

4. Describe the pathophysiology, assessment, and management of patients who have heat related illness.

5. Describe the pathophysiology, assessment, and management of patients who have been struck by lightning.

6. Describe the pathophysiology, assessment, and management of patients who have cold related illness or injury.

7. Describe the pathophysiology, assessment, and management of patients who have high altitude illness.

1. **Allergic reaction**—a hypersensitive response to an allergen to which an organism has previously been exposed and to which the organism has developed antibodies.

2. **Anaphylaxis**—acute, severe immune response resulting in a life-threatening emergency reaction.

3. **Antivenin**—a suspension of venom-neutralizing antibodies prepared from the serum of immunized horses; confers passive immunity and is given as a part of emergency first aid for various snake and insect bites. Also called *antivenom*.

4. **Core temperature**—the temperature of deep structures of the body, such as the liver, as compared with temperatures of peripheral tissues.

5. **Envenomation**—a poisoning caused by a bite or a sting.

6. **Frostbite**—injury to the skin caused by prolonged exposure to cold. The liquid content of the skin freezes and ruptures the cell membranes; may be superficial (frostnip) or deep.

7. **Heat cramps**—the first and mildest form of heat exposure; muscle cramping caused by excessive loss of body fluids and salts.

8. **Heat exhaustion**—a form of heat exposure that occurs when the body's circulation system fails to maintain its normal function due to excessive loss of body fluids and salts; patients present with shocklike symptoms.

9. **Heat stroke**—a severe, potentially fatal condition that results from failure of the body's temperature-regulating capacity; primarily caused by prolonged exposure to the sun or to high temperatures.

10. **High-altitude cerebral edema (HACE)**—the most severe form of acute high-altitude illness; characterized by a progression of global cerebral signs in the presence of acute mountain sickness that are probably related to increased intracranial pressure.

11. **High-altitude pulmonary edema (HAPE)**—A noncardiac pulmonary edema believed to be related, at least in part, to increased pulmonary artery pressure that develops in response to hypoxia; results in increased pulmonary arteriolar permeability and in leakage of fluid into extravascular locations.

12. **Histamine**—an amine released by mast cells and basophils that promotes inflammation.

13. **Hyperthermia**—significantly elevated core body temperature.

14. **Hypothermia**—an abnormally low core body temperature.

15. **Metabolism**—the aggregate of all biochemical reactions that take place in living organisms, resulting in growth, generation of energy, elimination of wastes, and other bodily functions.

nvironmental emergencies arise from a wide variety of etiologies and sources. These emergencies include such disparate entities as lightning strike, heat illness, and bites and stings. In this chapter, each environmental emergency is discussed in a separate section.

SECTION I

Envenomations—Bites and Stings

Thousands of people each year are affected by the bites and stings of various animals. Most commonly, bites are inflicted by domestic dogs and cats, but they can also involve species of mammals, reptiles, and insects that are capable of injecting venom. This section of the chapter discusses some of the more common effects of bites and stings and how these injuries should be managed.

Pathophysiology

One of the most problematic effects of an insect bite is **anaphylaxis** or an **allergic reaction**. The *hymenoptera* group of insects accounts for the greatest number of life-threatening stings in the United States. Members of the group include the honey bee, wasp, hornet, yellow jacket, and fire ant. Approximately 100 people die from insect stings annually.[15] Although it is estimated that it takes 300 to 500 stings to kill a person on a poisoning basis, it only takes one in a patient who is allergic to the venom.

On initial exposure to venom, an individual usually develops a local inflammatory reaction at the sting site, and the immune system responds by producing immunoglobulins (IgE)

specific to that venom. If the patient is stung a second time, an allergic reaction occurs; the venom and IgE combine to form a complex that attaches itself to cells in the bloodstream or becomes fixed to target organs. As a result, numerous substances are released that affect blood vessels and other organs. One of these is histamine, the effects of which include vasodilatation, capillary membrane leakage, bronchoconstriction, smooth muscle spasm, cardiac irritability and depression, and itching. These effects combine to produce the signs and symptoms of an allergic reaction (Fig. 43-1).

Spider bites typically cause a reaction by the toxic venom. There are two principal species of spiders that are of major concern—the black widow and the brown recluse (Fig. 43-2). The black widow is black with a red hourglass-shaped marking on its abdomen; this species is found in most areas of the United States. Its bite is usually immediately painful, as its venom causes the release of acetylcholine and norepinephrine from nerve endings. This results in muscle spasm, abdominal pain, diaphoresis, tachycardia, and hypertension. Two small "fang" marks may be present as well as a papule (red raised area on the skin).

The brown recluse, a light- to dark-brown colored spider with a yellow violin-shaped marking on its back, is usually seen in the midwest and southwest areas of the United States. The venom has a high concentration of enzymes that can produce extensive local tissue destruction (ulcers) although the initial bite may go unnoticed. Within a few hours, redness and pain will be present at the site of the bite. Within 24 to 48 hours, a blister will develop surrounded by redness. This is called the "bullseye sign." Necrosis may involve the surrounding tissue with severe **cellulitis**. Some patients, especially children, will also exhibit the systemic responses of malaise, weakness, nausea, and pain in muscles and joints.

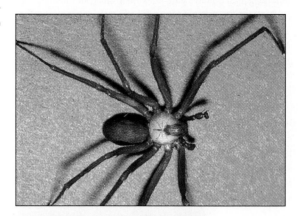

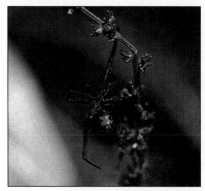

Figure 43-1

Signs and symptoms of an allergic reaction. *From Lewis, et al: Medical Surgical Nursing, ed. 4, St. Louis, 1996, Mosby-Year Book.*

Figure 43-2

A) Brown recluse spider B) North American black widow spider. *From Auerbach, PS: Wilderness Medicine: Management of Wilderness and Environmental Emergencies, ed. 3, St. Louis, 1995, Mosby-Year Book.*

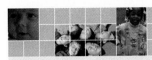

- Bites (human and animal) and stings are common in childhood. Children are susceptible to such injuries due in part to their curiosity with animals and interesting environmental objects such as nests or spider webs.
- Tick bites are also a common occurrence in childhood. The rescuer should avoid squeezing the site where the tick is embedded, because of the possibility of releasing more blood into the child's system. Health concerns associated with tick bites include lyme disease and rocky mountain spotted fever.
- Snake bites in children, as compared to adults, produce an increased risk of significant injury and even death and thus require more antivenin. Rapid transport to an appropriate emergency department is imperative in these situations.
- Infants and neonates are the most susceptible to heat loss because of their inability to shiver, the minimal amount of subcutaneous tissue, the large body surface area in relation to weight, and their inability to cover or shield themselves from the elements.
- Cystic fibrosis impairs heat dissipation as a result of ineffective sweat glands.
- Most children suffering from high-altitude illness experience no more than mild headaches and fatigue. However, some patients progress to pulmonary edema.

Poisonous snakes exist in most of the United States and account for approximately 8000 bites annually.[7] Most of the bites are caused by pit vipers, such as rattlesnakes and cottonmouths, which inject venom through fangs (Fig. 43-3). Although some snakebites do not result in envenomation, most result in exposure to venom and a combination of local and systemic effects. The digestive enzymes contained in the venom cause local tissue destruction; systemically, they can destroy blood cells and disrupt nervous control of the muscles (Table 43-1).

Most animal bites seen by emergency personnel are inflicted by dogs and cats. There are two major problems seen with animal bites: local trauma and subsequent infection. Trauma from animal bites, while usually limited to extremities, can be severe and cause damage to major nerves and blood vessels.

Dog bites are similar to crush injuries that destroy tissue by tearing it. Because the wounds are usually superficial and accessible for care, the infection rate is relatively low.

Because of the shape of their teeth, cats tend to inflict puncture wounds that deposit saliva in deep tissue areas, and the infection rate is substantially higher than that seen in dog bites.

Rabies is a disease caused by a virus passed to the human host in the saliva of a biting animal. Since the development of a veterinary rabies vaccine, the presence of the virus in domestic animals has dropped sharply. Wild animals, mostly bats, skunks, and raccoons, are the source of the rabies virus in the majority of cases. It may take weeks or months for a human to begin showing symptoms of rabies. The virus usually invades the central nervous system and can be fatal.

Patient Assessment

History

The paramedic must assess the patient for signs and symptoms of life-threatening, systemic complications of a sting or bite. This discussion assumes that responders have removed

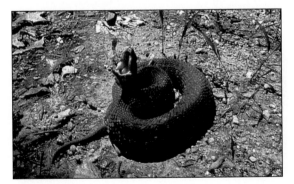

Figure 43-3

Cottonmouth. (Courtesy Sherman Minton, M.D.) *From Auerbach, PS: Wilderness Medicine, ed. 3, St. Louis, 1995, Mosby-Year Book.*

TABLE 43-1	Characteristics of Snake Envenomations	
Type of Snake	**Characteristics**	**Signs of Envenomation**
Pit Viper (ratttlesnake, water moccasin, copperhead)	• Triangular head distinct from body • Depressed pit in maxillary bone (heat-sensing mechanism) • Vertical, elliptical eyes • Hollow fang on each side of the head • Strikes typically defensive	• Scratch marks; one or more fang marks • Local swelling, edema, pain, may extend beyond site • Bruising around bite area • Bite may cause weakness, nausea, vomiting, or shock
Coral Snake	• "Red on yellow, kill a fellow; red on black, venom lack" • Round pupils • Bullet-shaped head • Small fangs near front of the maxilla • Envenomation occurs only with "chewing"	• Semicircular marking on the skin from teeth • Little or no pain • Bite may cause confusion, dilated pupils, difficulty swallowing, seizures, and respiratory and cardiac failure

any risk to themselves of being exposed to the offending insect, reptile, or animal.

- *When did the patient suffer the sting or bite?* Symptoms of envenomation or allergy which occur soon after the bite or sting and progress rapidly are indicative of severe response that will require prompt and aggressive management.
- *If the patient has suffered an insect sting, are there symptoms of allergy?* Usually, patients with allergic reactions will first note localized pain, itching, or urticaria (hives) about the area of the sting (Fig. 43-4). In more severe cases, there will also be complaints of shortness of breath, wheezing, difficulty swallowing, weakness, dizziness, or other signs of circulatory collapse.

CRITICAL ISSUE

The possibility of severe allergic reaction (anaphylaxis) secondary to a bee sting should be considered in a patient with shock of unknown etiology.

- *Has the patient been exposed to a sting or bite previously?* With previous exposure, there is a higher risk of a more severe response to the venom. The paramedic should inquire carefully about the type of symptoms the patient experienced beforehand and what therapy was required.
- *Was the patient bitten by a spider?* If the spider is dead or safely contained, bring it in to the emergency department for evaluation. Most often, the spider is never seen. In many cases, patients may only be able to report being in environments frequented by spiders (e.g., garages, basements, outdoors).

Patients with black widow spider bites often present with severe pain from muscle cramping; if the bite is on the chest or abdomen, it may be difficult to distinguish from other causes of acute chest or abdominal pain.

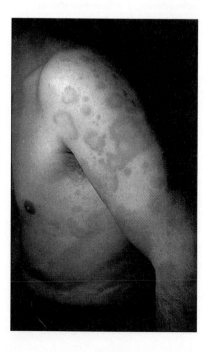

Figure 43-4

Victim of delayed reaction to a wasp sting. *From Auerbach, PS: Wilderness Medicine, ed. 3, St. Louis, 1995, Mosby-Year Book.*

- *Was the patient bitten by a snake?* Usually, patients will be aware of and recall an encounter with the snake and can provide a description. In some instances, bystanders or friends may have begun first aid. Inquiry into the nature of this assistance is often valuable. Remember that a dead snake can still bite by reflex if handled.
- *Was the patient bitten by another type of animal?* The paramedic should try to determine the type of animal involved and the elapsed time since the bite. If infection is occurring, the patient may complain of pain and localized swelling or rash. Systemically, there may be fever, chills, aches in muscles and joints, weakness, or malaise. If a domestic animal is involved, ask the owner about the status of the pet's rabies vaccination.

Physical Examination

Assessment of vital signs may show tachypnea, tachycardia, or hypotension in the setting of anaphylactic shock, although a snake-bite victim may become hypertensive. The patient's airway should be evaluated for evidence of stridor, increased secretions, and swelling of the tongue or oropharynx. If any of these signs are evident, rapid institution of therapy for allergic reactions is required. The patient should be observed for respiratory distress and use of accessory muscles for respiration. Wheezing is possible in severe allergic reactions and also demands an aggressive approach.

In the case of insect sting such as bees, there will be erythema (redness), swelling, and local tenderness at the site (Fig. 43-5). The paramedic should note the presence or absence of a stinger and venom sac. Spider bites may show themselves as two small puncture wounds, but usually there is no significant swelling noted. Occasionally, a "halo" lesion may be seen, described as an area of pallor immediately about the bite surrounded by a ring of erythema. Ulcers that form hours to weeks after a bite are typical of a brown recluse spider.

CRITICAL ISSUE

The initial appearance of the bite does not reflect the severity or likelihood of envenomation, because symptoms and signs of toxicity may develop over time.

Bites of a pit viper are seen as puncture wounds corresponding to the location of the snake's fangs. Typically, there is surrounding swelling and erythema with bloody drainage

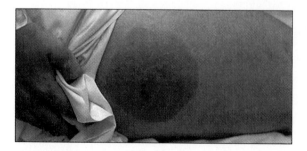

Figure 43-5

Brown recluse spider bite after 48 hours. *From Auerbach, PS: Wilderness Medicine, ed. 3, St. Louis, 1995, Mosby-Year Book.*

from the wound. It is not possible to determine by examination of the wound whether or not envenomation has occurred. Snakes without fangs may leave an imprint of their jaw on the victim's skin.

Animal bites commonly cause soft tissue injury, hemorrhage, and rarely fractures. On occasion, life-threatening injury can be produced by injury to major blood vessels, the trachea, or the head.

Management

The first priority is safety. The paramedic should not attempt to catch live animals or reptiles. If an insect is contained, it should be brought into the emergency department with the patient for evaluation. If local statute makes notification an EMS responsibility, the paramedic must be sure local animal control agencies are notified about an animal causing a bite and remove the patient from the environment to reduce the possibility of further exposure.

Patients should be transported in a position of comfort. High-concentration oxygen should be administered to any patient showing evidence of a systemic reaction. In cases of suspected envenomation, IV access should be established and a cardiac monitor applied.

In the case of bee stings, if there is a stinger and venom sac present, it should be removed; envenomation can occur for up to 20 minutes after the sting. The paramedic should be careful not to squeeze the venom sac. Rather, the stinger should be removed with forceps or by scraping the skin with a straight-edge blade. This is called the "flicking technique."

Although a cold pack may be applied locally to decrease pain, it is important to institute therapy for allergic reactions quickly. Some patients will have their own bee-sting kits that contain autoinjectable epinephrine and an oral antihistamine. Most EMS systems will allow patients to use such kits without contacting medical direction.

If there is any evidence of airway involvement or respiratory distress, epinephrine (1:1000, SQ) should be administered promptly. The patient can also receive IV diphenhydramine for this type of allergic reaction or for the treatment of itching or hives. Hypotensive patients require aggressive fluid resuscitation with normal saline or Ringer's lactate. Transportation is indicated for all patients with respiratory or systemic symptoms or previous history of systemic involvement. Consider intravenous epinephrine 1:10,000 when patients are in severe shock.

Care for victims of spider bites focuses initially on supportive care for systemic symptoms. When the problem is clear (i.e., the spider and its bite are seen), the patient's pain should be treated either by relieving muscle spasm with diazepam or administering an analgesic, such as morphine sulfate. Analgesia may also be indicated for victims of brown recluse spider bites. Local wound care, in the form of elevation, irrigation with sterile saline, and application of sterile dressings, is also important. In both cases, the short-term application of ice may also reduce pain.

For snake-bite victims, efforts are directed at keeping the patient calm and the extremity immobilized at the level of the heart, which helps to minimize venom absorption. Rings, watches, or other bands that may cause vascular compromise as swelling increases should be removed. Although tourniquets are not recommended, if one has been applied by a bystander, it should be left in place until IV access is established. When an IV is in place, the tourniquet can be removed slowly while the patient's status is closely monitored. Ice should not be used because it may cause local tissue destruction. The paramedic should evaluate the injured area for swelling (mark the edge of the swelling with a pen and note the time) and transport the patient to a facility capable of providing antivenin. Antivenin is a medication used to neutralize the venom and prevent or reverse the poisonous effects.

Most animal bites only require local wound care with elevation, irrigation with sterile saline, and use of sterile dressings. Immobilization is useful to reduce bleeding and further damage.

Transport to an emergency department should be encouraged, and the paramedic should explain to the patient that early definitive wound care (i.e., irrigation, debridement, antibiotic therapy) lowers the risk of subsequent infection. Tetanus immunization is also required for all victims of bites or stings whose status is not current.

Section I Summary

This section addresses the pathophysiology and clinical presentation of common bites and stings. The importance of scene safety, aggressive support and treatment of envenomations, and prompt transport for definitive administration of antivenin is emphasized.

Section II

Heat Illness

Approximately 4000 people die from heat-related illness in the United States every year.[1] Although more than 50% of these victims are over 50 years of age, heat stroke is also the second leading cause of death (behind trauma) in amateur athletes.[4] Environmental factors are important; heat-related illness is more prevalent in areas where heat and humidity are commonly elevated (temperature > 95° F; humidity > 60 %). The higher concentration of streets and buildings in urban areas creates an environment that is hotter and dissipates heat more slowly than rural settings. Saunas, hot tubs, and work environments can also provide the warm, enclosed areas that can lead to heat-related illness.

Temperature Regulation in the Body

The human body is continuously producing heat through the normal chemical reactions known as *metabolism*. An increased metabolic rate (up to 10 times normal) is required when people work, exercise, experience stress, or must meet other special demands. Extra heat is produced during this increased metabolism; unless the body dissipates this heat, normal chemical reactions and cellular functions begin to fail. Failure to meet increased cellular demands for oxygen and nutrition contributes further to cellular dysfunction and necrosis.

In cool environments, the body dissipates heat primarily by transferring it to the environment through vasodilated vessels in the skin by radiation and convection. Radiation directly transfers heat by emitting it into a cooler environment, and is responsible for the majority of heat loss. Convection, which requires water or air movement over the skin to carry the heat away from the body, varies with the velocity of air movement and accounts for only a small fraction of total heat loss. However, when the outside temperature rises above 92° F (33.3° C), these methods fail. A small amount of heat may be lost by physical contact and conduction into objects of lower temperature, but this method is of little help in a practical sense.

One of the most important methods of heat dissipation in warm environments is evaporation of sweat. Evaporation of sweat is important because it is the only method of dissipating heat when the environmental temperature is high. During exertion, fluid losses may approach 2 liters per hour. This represents a significant volume loss that can also be accompanied by major electrolyte losses. It is dangerous for a person to lose more than 7% of the body weight through fluid losses of any kind. Unfortunately, evaporation of sweat becomes ineffective as humidity rises, particularly above 50% (Box 43-1).

The cardiovascular and nervous systems are involved in adaptive mechanisms. The hypothalamus and spinal cord regulate body temperature. When cooling is required, peripheral vasodilation is promoted, which allows greater blood flow to the skin and more effective radiation of excess heat. The cardiovascular system responds by increasing myocardial contractility and rate to maintain an adequate blood pressure in the face of this decreased peripheral vascular resistance. All of these activities require an increased amount of energy. Metabolic rates may increase by 100% over normal. Nutritional reserves must be able to supply the demands of the various systems or they will begin to fail.

Factors Associated with Heat Illness

The many factors associated with heat-related illness can be considered in three major categories. First, there is the risk of heat gain from outside the body. This condition is especially prevalent when environmental temperature is above 95° F (35° C), and humidity is above 50% for more than 2 days.[18] These conditions reduce the body's ability to shed heat.

Second, increased production of heat is an additional concern, particularly during work or exercise in a hot environment. Military recruits, construction workers, athletes wearing heavy uniforms, foundry and laundry workers, and firefighters are at special risk. When engaging in extraordinary sustained physical exertion, these individuals can produce more heat than the body can dissipate. Pathologic conditions in patients with fever, infections, seizures, and conditions that increase the metabolic rate, such as hyperthyroidism, can also lead to excess heat production. Drugs, including LSD, PCP, speed, and cocaine can act in a similar fashion.

Although alcohol is commonly associated with hypothermia, alcohol consumption can also increase the likelihood of a heat illness. Alcohol may be consumed in place of water or other liquid. Alcohol can cause dehydration by acting as a diuretic, increasing urine production. This is a result of alcohol's inhibition of antidiuretic hormone (ADH).

Certain conditions impair the body's ability to dissipate heat. Examples include obesity, heavy clothing, and skin abnormalities such as in sweat gland function or structure (large burns or scars, or the sweat gland malfunction seen in cystic fibrosis). Drugs that interfere with sweat production are also a concern, including anticholinergics, antihistamines, antispasmodics, phenothiazines, antidepressants, lithium, MAO inhibitors, and diuretics.

High-Risk Groups

Very young and very old patients are at the greatest risk for heat illness, because these groups have either not yet developed a tolerant, adaptable metabolic system or are losing it through aging, underlying diseases, or medication use. Chronic diseases of the cardiovascular, neurologic, hepatic, and renal systems impair a patient's ability to regulate temperature. Conditions that reduce the nutritional support available to combat heat stress, such as diabetes, thyroid disease, malnutrition, and alcoholism also pose a threat to the patient.

Acclimatization

The body adapts to heat in a process called *acclimatization*. Although full acclimatization takes up to 8 weeks, exposure to heat stress for approximately 10 to 20 days will result in a significant level of acclimatization. With acclimatization, the body sweats more effectively, with less sodium loss and an increase in cellular metabolic efficiency.

Pathophysiology

Debate continues regarding the origin of heat-related illness involving either a failure of central heat regulation in the hypothalamus and brain stem or a peripheral sweat gland dysfunction. In either case, multiple body systems are affected when normal regulatory mechanisms cannot cope with heat stress.

Heat-related illness is a broad spectrum of disease ranging from mild dehydration that causes muscle cramping, to complex multisystem involvement with direct cellular thermal in-

BOX 43-1	Normal Temperature Regulation

Heat Production → Must Equal → Heat Loss

Heat Production	Heat Loss
Metabolism	Conduction (if cool environment)
Muscle contractions:	Radiation (if cool environment)
Exercise	
Shivering	Evaporation of sweat (as long as humidity is low)
Conduction (if hot environment)	
Radiation (if hot environment)	
Convection (if hot environment)	

jury, protein destruction, and inability to keep up with increased metabolic demands. Heat-related illness has been categorized broadly into three classes based upon the severity of the signs and symptoms present. These are heat cramps (mild), heat exhaustion, and heat stroke (severe). Heat stroke is usually divided into two types: the classic heat stroke, in which the hypothalamus fails, and exertional heat stroke, whereby sustained, high exertion causes more heat production than the body can dissipate (*see* Table 43-2).

When temperature regulation fails, as in the classic heat stroke, sensitive CNS structures are often affected first by hypoxia and direct heat injury to cellular proteins. Altered mental status is usually the initial presentation; syncope occurs in most heat stroke victims. Headache, disorientation, ataxia, seizures, and coma are also seen.

The cardiovascular system faces tremendous stresses as it attempts to maintain cardiac output in the face of maximum vasodilation, falling peripheral resistance, hypoxia, and acidosis from low cellular blood flow. Direct myocardial damage may also occur, causing dysrhythmias, ischemia, and infarction.

Blood Chemistry

Abnormalities result as coagulation factors (proteins) produced by the liver are altered by the heat stress. This can lead to abnormal bleeding (disseminated intravascular coagulopathy [DIC]) from sites of IV access, the GI tract, and other areas. Red blood cells may burst (lyse), releasing hemoglobin, and causing anemia. As degeneration and necrosis of liver tissue continues, jaundice may be seen.

Heat and hypoxia may lead to muscle cell damage and muscle necrosis, known as rhabdomyolysis. Weakness, pain, and decreased muscle function occur. Myoglobin, a muscle protein, is released as cells are destroyed and—in combination with hypoxia and decreased renal blood flow—induces acute renal failure in a significant number of heat stroke victims.

Patient Assessment

Critical observations that require immediate intervention for victims of heat illness include altered mental status, seizures, hypotension, cardiac dysrhythmias, a rectal temperature of 105° F or higher, and the need for airway management.

History

- *What are the environmental factors?* While noting the ambient temperature and humidity, the paramedic should consult with the patient or bystanders regarding the duration of heat exposure and exertion. The paramedic should also determine if the patient was protected from sunlight or if he or she is wearing constrictive or excessive clothing.

  Apartments or homes without air conditioning contribute to the heat illness problem during prolonged heat spells. In lower socioeconomic neighborhoods, fear pro-

TABLE 43-2	**Heat Emergencies**		
	Heat Cramps (Localized)	**Heat Exhaustion (Systemic)**	**Heat Stroke (Systemic)**
Cause	Salt from heavily exercised muscles, without serious volume loss. Patients typically replace fluid loss, but not salt loss	Systemic salt and/or water loss with peripheral blood pooling and hypovolemia	Damage to the hypothalamus and heat regulatory center caused by prolonged exposure to heat *Classic Type:* Develops over days as a result of exposure to high heat and humidity. Usually seen in patients with no mechanical means for cooling and/or poor fluid intake (especially the elderly) *Exertional Type:* Prolonged exertion produces more heat than the body can expel
High-Risk Groups	Unconditioned, nonacclimatized workers/athletes; patients who have ingested alcohol; patients with chronic diseases	Same as Heat Cramps, with the addition of elderly and very young patients	Same as Heat Exhaustion
Signs and Symptoms	Localized muscle cramps in extremities, occasionally in abdomen. Patients are awake and alert. Vital signs usually normal with some tachycardia. Body temperature normal. Skin cool or slightly warm	Patients are awake or have slightly decreased level of responsiveness (dizziness, light-headedness, headache, or irritability). Normal or decreased BP and tilt; tachycardia, increased respirations; body temperature normal or slightly elevated. Skin pale with excessive sweating	*Early:* Dizziness, headache, followed quickly by bizarre or unusual behavior, seizures, and coma. Vital signs reveal normal or decreased BP, tachycardia with a bounding pulse, increase in respirations. Temperature highly elevated rectally. Skin usually hot, red, and dry. Condition caused by exercise (exertional type), skin hot, red, and wet; patient may be volume depleted
Management	Move patient to a cool environment and transport	Move patient to a cool environment, administer O_2, normal saline, or lactated Ringer's, possible D_5W, and transport	ABCs— intubate if necessary. Administer O_2, rapidly cool patient with cold packs around head, axilla and groin. Avoid alcohol rubs. Initiate IV of normal saline or lactated Ringer's, monitor ECG, transport rapidly

Used with permission from UT Southwestern Emergency Medicine Education paramedic course syllabus.

hibits many from opening windows at night to allow cooling of their homes.

- *Are there patient-specific factors?* Examples of these factors include the patient's age and acclimatization to the warm environment. The patient's past medical history should be obtained and the paramedic should consider whether there are conditions or medications that might augment heat production or impair dissipation.
- *Does the patient complain of muscle cramping?* Cramping of extremity and abdominal muscle groups is common with physical exertion in a warm climate. Although often associated with dehydration and seen during exercise, heat cramps can occur up to several hours after physical exertion. These cramps are believed to be secondary to the significant salt losses from sweating.
- *Is the patient weak or fatigued?* In patients with heat exhaustion, often the bodies have not acclimatized to the environment, and these patients may present initially with vague complaints such as weakness, malaise, nausea, and light-headedness. As fluid and salt losses continue, headache, muscle cramping, gait difficulties, and confusion can occur.

Physical Examination

Patients with heat-related illness present with a variety of physical signs that range from mild to severe. Minor heat illness is associated with profuse sweating and results from salt and water depletion. The clinical syndrome is characterized by severe muscle cramping.

If the patient has progressed in the spectrum of heat illness and becomes volume depleted, symptoms will include tachycardia and tachypnea. A severely dehydrated patient is frankly hypotensive or has positive orthostatic vital signs. As the severity of the heat illness progresses, the patient may become disoriented, anxious, combative, or unresponsive.

Body temperature is reported to be normal in patients with heat exhaustion and markedly elevated in heat stroke. Although thermometers are more accurate, skin signs can aid the paramedic in forming an initial impression about the severity of the condition. Patients with heat exhaustion have skin described as cool and moist, and classic heat stroke presents with hot, dry skin. This differentiation may not always hold true, because sweating can be seen with hot skin in exertional heat stroke patients. Other features of these conditions are described in Table 43-3.

CRITICAL ISSUE

Altered mental status and a rectal temperature of 105° F (40.6° C) or higher are the most important distinguishing features of a heat stroke in a patient.

The EMS provider may arrive at a scene with a number of victims with heat-related illness. This is especially true at sporting events and other mass gatherings. In such situations, the paramedic will be faced with the additional task of triaging those patients at greatest risk of developing heat stroke.

The patient with heat exhaustion sweats profusely, losing volume and electrolytes, and becomes **hypovolemic** with a narrow pulse pressure. The heat stroke victim often does not lose large volumes of fluid, but instead suffers cardiovascular collapse with a widened pulse pressure.

Heat stroke patients have rectal temperatures of 105° F (40.6° C) or higher, unless they are already undergoing cooling. Heat exhaustion is typified by normal or slightly elevated temperatures, usually in the range of normal to 101° F (38.3° C). It should be noted that these are core temperatures, which are most reliably assessed with a rectal thermometer.

Management

Heat Cramps and Heat Exhaustion. Heat cramps are managed first by removing the individual from the hot environment. Because heat cramps typically occur several hours after heat exposure, the patient may already be out of the hot environment. The patient should have oral replacement of salt losses, typically with a commercially available electrolyte solution or "sport drink." Individuals who are prone to heat cramps can typically prevent them by continuously replacing sweat losses with an electrolyte solution instead of water alone. Salt tablets should be avoided.

The patient with heat exhaustion should also be removed from the hot environment, with any excessive clothing removed. Moving the victim to a fan or air-conditioned environment is all the cooling that is usually necessary, because ice or cold packs may cause shivering and consequently increase heat production. Oral fluid replacement with an electrolyte solution is appropriate if the patient is awake and alert and not nauseated or vomiting. In the case of an unresponsive patient, an IV solution of normal saline or Ringer's lactate should be administered slowly. Some patients with heat exhaustion suffer primarily from water (not salt) loss, and these patients can be rehydrated with D_5W.

TABLE 43-3	Characteristics of Heat Stroke and Heat Exhaustion		
	Classic Heat Stroke	**Exertional Heat Stroke**	**Heat Exhaustion**
Skin	Hot, "drier," mottled; inappropriate lack of sweating	Hot, red, wet (sweaty)	"Cooler," clammy, pale; appropriate sweating
Central Nervous System	Syncope, coma; seizures, disoriented, combative	Syncope, coma; seizures, disoriented, combative	"Exhausted," dizzy, fatigue; weak, headache; irritable
Core Temperature	105° F (40.6° C) or higher	105° F (40.6° C) or higher	Normal or slightly elevated < 105° F (40.6° C)
Blood Pressure	Widened pulse pressure; normal or low, usually < 90 systolic	Widened pulse pressure; normal or low, usually < 90 systolic	Narrowed pulse pressure; usually > 90 systolic, often positive orthostatic upon tilt test

Heat Stroke. Heat stroke is often a fatal event in the untreated patient.

The airway should be intubated if the patient is unresponsive, and an IV of normal saline or Ringer's lactate should be initiated. The fluid should be cautiously administered, because vigorous administration especially in the elderly or those with decreased cardiac function, can result in fluid overload and pulmonary edema. Hypotension is usually the result of fluid shift to the dilated superficial vessels in the skin, and cooling will result in the return of blood to the central circulation. If cooling does not restore the patient's blood pressure, a 250- to 500-mL bolus of fluid can be administered. Reassess pulmonary status for rales between repeat boluses.

Cooling is achieved by cold packs, particularly in the neck, axilla, groin, and chest over large vessels. Air conditioning or a fan can enhance cooling by convection and evaporation. Rectal temperature should be monitored, and cooling measures should be stopped when this temperature reaches 102° F (38.9° C). This return can be achieved with cold packs within approximately 1 hour or less. The patient may experience seizures or shivering, and these conditions can be managed with diazepam.

Some evidence exists that rapid body cooling can be accomplished with 59° to 61° F (15° to 16° C) water baths, which will avoid problems with vasoconstriction, seizures, and shivering. However, this method is difficult and ineffective in the ambulance.

Section II Summary

This section reviews the predisposing factors of heat-related illnesses and pathophysiologic mechanisms that lead to typical patient presentations. Priorities in management center around prompt institution of cooling measures, fluid resuscitation, and timely transport to an emergency department for additional evaluation and therapy.

Section III

Lightning Injuries

Lightning strikes, although uncommon, cause more deaths in the United States than other natural disasters including hurricanes, tornadoes, volcanoes, and floods. Precise statistics on the number of persons killed by lightning strikes in this country are difficult to obtain, but estimates place the number of deaths between 100 and 600 per year.[1] Fatal strikes are more common in summer and fall, tend to happen in early after-

noon and evening, and are more likely to occur in rural than urban environments.[1] Lightning strikes cause serious injuries in an estimated 1000 to 1500 patients annually, and 74% of survivors have significant permanent complications.[3]

Pathophysiology

Lightning is produced by differences in electrical potential that exist among the water droplets in a cloud. Layers of positive and negative charges exist, the lowest layer being negatively charged. When the potential difference between the ground and the cloud's lowest layer becomes great enough, lightning strikes move back and forth between the earth and cloud. A lightning strike can be thought of as a massive electrical spark of direct current with an energy level of 2000 to 2 billion volts and a short duration (less than 1 millisecond).

Lightning may strike a victim directly or, more commonly, may strike nearby and jump through the air to "flashover" or "splash" the victim. Direct strikes have the greatest mortality. The effect of a direct strike is to act as a massive countershock that causes depolarization of the entire myocardium and usually results in asystole. Although the inherent automaticity of the heart usually reestablishes an organized rhythm, respiratory arrest may persist as brain stem respiratory control centers continue to be affected. Victims of direct strikes may also demonstrate evidence of myocardial dysfunction or dysrhythmias. With "splashes" of lightning, there is usually not enough current applied to internal organs to cause interference with cardiac and respiratory function.

Neurologic results of lightning strikes are seen in the form of amnesia, coma, seizures, paralysis, intracranial hemorrhage, and brain injury. Blunt trauma, such as fractures, dislocations, and contusions, can also result from sudden, extreme muscle contractions or being thrown by shock wave impact.

As the victim is struck, a shock wave is created by expanding hot air that ruptures tympanic membranes in approximately 50% of these patients. Lightning, particularly in exposure to side splashes, can also cause skin burns, sometimes in a fern or featherlike pattern.

Autonomic dysfunction may manifest itself in the form of intense vasospasm. As a result, the extremities can appear cold, mottled, and pulseless. The transient malfunction of autonomic nerves also presents with fixed, dilated pupils.

Patient Assessment

History

Most information regarding the circumstances of the lightning strike is gathered from bystanders; in most serious cases, the patient will be unresponsive or have an altered mental status.

- *When did the lightning strike?* This will provide information about how long the patient was down after the strike.
- *Was the patient knocked to the ground or found unresponsive?* This information will help determine the severity of the patient's injury. Patients who were knocked down should undergo a complete physical examination for blunt injury, such as fractures, and chest, abdominal, or head trauma. Unresponsive patients may have sustained respiratory or cardiac arrest and could have an associated hypoxic brain injury.
- *Was the patient standing near or holding a metal object?* If so, the object's conductivity may have caused a more concentrated direct strike of energy than would be otherwise suspected.

Physical Examination

Given the likelihood of cardiac or respiratory arrest, the initial assessment takes on additional significance. Most patients will become unresponsive at the time of the strike and will begin to regain cognitive functions as long as cardiac and pulmonary function has been maintained. Commonly, patients will be unable to remember events before and after the strike.

The patient's pupils should be examined for dilation and the ears examined for bleeding or decreased hearing suggestive of tympanic membrane rupture. Pulses in the extremities may not only be abnormal in the presence of dysrhythmias, but also may be absent in extreme vasospasm. In the latter case, the patient's extremity will also be cold and ashen. The skin should be examined for evidence of burns (Fig. 43-6). Al-

though ferning and superficial burns may be seen with lightning splashes, energy may pass from the ground and enter the patient through the leg or foot. In this instance, the entrance wound may resemble a high-voltage entrance burn.

Management

Rescuers must first assess scene safety and obtain access to the patient. If the patient is in cardiac or respiratory arrest, standard treatment measures should be initiated.

If there are multiple patients, a different triage strategy than usual should be followed. In most mass-casualty situations, patients found in respiratory or cardiac arrest are considered dead, and treatment priorities are aimed at the living. After a lightning strike, patients with asystole promptly convert to a viable rhythm, but the primary respiratory arrest continues. Further cardiac deterioration can be avoided by the early correction of hypoxia. Because these individuals with respirations and a pulse typically survive, victims in cardiac or respiratory arrest as a result of a lightning strike are the first priority.

CRITICAL ISSUE

Patients with cardiac or respiratory arrest are the first priority in the setting of a mass-casualty incident involving lightning strikes.

Standard advanced life support methods are provided as indicated, including intubation and administration of appropriate medication. When working with the airway, the patient's cervical spine should be protected, because these patients are considered victims of major trauma. Full spinal immobilization is appropriate.

A cardiac monitor should be applied and IV access obtained using normal saline or Ringer's lactate solution. Fluid administration rates depend on the setting. Without the presence of hypotension, which would suggest serious blunt trauma injuries, extensive volume resuscitation is seldom nec-

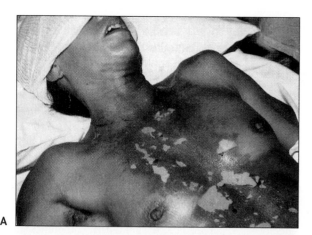

A

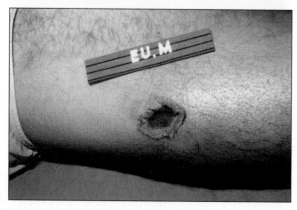

B

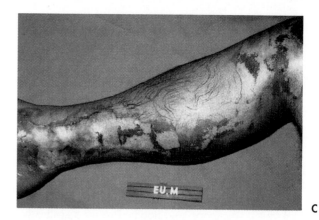

C

Figure 43-6

A) Thoracic lesions caused by a melted gold chain B) Entry point of lightning on the thigh C) Exit point on the leg. *From Vallotton J. and Dubas F. (eds): Color Atlas of Mountain Medicine, 1991, London, Wolfe Publishing Co.*

essary. In addition, cerebral edema and other intracranial injuries may become worse if uncontrolled fluid resuscitation is initiated. The patient should be rapidly transported to an appropriate receiving hospital and monitored en route.

Common-sense tactics can be life saving during a lightning storm. Activity planners, outdoor workers, sports teams, marching bands, and outdoor recreationists should always be aware of weather conditions and changes. When lightning is present, it is best to seek shelter or remain inside a building or vehicle. Care should be taken to avoid metal objects such as bicycles, golf clubs, fences, and grandstands. Open fields, golf courses, high terrain, and bodies of water are high-risk areas, as are ungrounded structures, including most tents, sheds, and cabanas.

If caught in an open area, a person should quickly seek a low spot and lie down. It is also best to avoid use of phones and showers during a thunderstorm, because these may provide a path for a lightning strike.[14] One myth that may prove deadly is that lightning never strikes the same place twice. Conditions that created the first lightning strike may rapidly develop again, and another strike can occur quickly.

Section III Summary

This section reviews the origin of a lightning strike and the mechanisms of cardiac, respiratory, and neurologic dysfunction as a result. In this setting, patients must be carefully assessed for evidence of trauma and monitored for dysrhythmias and respiratory failure. Appropriate prioritization and aggressive management of cardiac or respiratory arrest is required.

Section IV

Hypothermia and Frostbite

Classically, a person visualizes accidental hypothermia involving winter outdoor enthusiasts but in reality, the condition can involve any season or location. In the United States, urban settings account for the majority of cases of accidental hypothermia; homeless, the alcoholic, and elderly patients are common victims of these situations.[5]

Pathophysiology

Systemically, the symptoms of hypothermia appear when the patient's core body temperature falls below 95° F (35° C). At this point, heat losses from the body exceed the ability to produce heat and maintain a constant body temperature.

Heat Production and Loss

Body temperature is controlled by the hypothalamus, the area of the brain that maintains a balance between the production and loss of heat. Heat is produced by cellular metabolism, muscular activity, and shivering.[10] Shivering can begin shortly after the victim is exposed to cold; the involuntary muscle activity increases heat production by increasing the metabolic rate to several times its normal level.

Heat loss takes place through four physical mechanisms. First, *radiant heat* losses from uncovered surfaces can account for more than 50% of total heat loss. For instance, a patient's exposed head can result in the loss of 50% of internal heat production. Heat can also be lost by direct contact with cooler substances or objects. Known as *conduction*, this type of heat loss in particularly important during immersion in water, which dissipates heat 25 times faster than air.

Convection occurs when air moves across exposed skin surfaces, replacing air and water vapor already heated by the body. Finally, heat is lost by *evaporation* from the skin and the lungs. Evaporative losses increase with lower humidity and heavier perspiration.

Systemic Hypothermia

Hypothermia can be mild, moderate, or severe and can be classified as either primary or secondary (Table 43-4). Primary hypothermia occurs when an individual is exposed to environmental extremes of cold and is usually acute in onset. Secondary hypothermia arises more gradually under the influence of other clinical conditions, such as shock, overwhelming infection, intoxication, or the extremes of age.

Physiologic Response. A lowering of body temperature is initially detected by sensory receptors. The receptors transmit this information to the hypothalamus, which stimulates direct nervous reflexes and the release of catecholamines and thyroid hormone. As a result, the initial physiologic response generates shivering and vasoconstriction. Shivering augments heat production metabolically, and vasoconstriction reduces heat loss by shunting blood to the core. Other physiologic compensations include an initial tachycardia and increased respiratory rate.

At a core body temperature of 95° F (35° C), heat production by shivering is at its maximum. At this mild stage of hypothermia, the central nervous system is affected by a gradual decrease in cerebral metabolism. This appears first in the patient as trouble with thought processes such as memory, speech, and judgment. Later, patients show lethargy and difficulty with gait (ataxia).

At body temperatures below 90° F (32° C), other body functions slow and dysrhythmias are commonly seen. Atrial fibrillation may be the earliest dysrhythmia seen. Bradycardia begins and progresses; at temperatures below 82° F (28° C), the likelihood of ventricular fibrillation is greatly increased. Because hypoventilation decreases the amount of oxygen delivered to the tissues, hypothermia increases the affinity of hemoglobin for oxygen, and less oxygen is available for cellular metabolism. A progression of altered mental status is noted, and voluntary motion decreases.

When hypothermia becomes severe, all body systems are affected, including the liver and kidneys. Acidosis develops and nitrogenous wastes from the body are unable to be cleared. Systemic blood flow drops as cardiac output falls to half the normal level, hypoperfused organs malfunction, the acidosis intensifies, and reflexes are absent. At body temperatures of 72° F (22° C), the risk of ventricular fibrillation is highest, and

TABLE 43-4	Characteristics of the Three Zones of Hypothermia		
Stage	**Core Temperature** °C	°F	**Characteristics**
Mild	37.6	99.6±1	Normal rectal temperature
	37.0	98.6±1	Normal rectal temperature
	36.0	96.8	Increase in metabolic rate, blood pressure, and preshivering muscle tone
	35.0	95.0	Urine temperature 34.8° C; maximum shivering for generating heat
	34.0	93.2	Amnesia, dysarthria, and poor judgment develop; maladaptive behavior; normal blood pressure; maximum respiratory stimulation; tachycardia, then progressive bradycardia
	33.0	91.4	Ataxia and apathy develop; depression of cerebral metabolism; tachypnea, then progressive decrease in respiratory minute volume
Moderate	32.0	89.6	Stupor; 25% decrease in oxygen consumption
	31.0	87.8	Shivering; heat generation ceases
	30.0	86.0	Atrial fibrillation, other arrhythmias develop; pupils; cardiac output two thirds of normal; insulin ineffective
	29.0	85.2	Progressive decrease in level of responsiveness, pulse, and respirations, pupils dilated; paradoxical undressing
	28.0	82.4	Decreased ventricular fibrillation threshold; 50% decrease in oxygen consumption and pulse; hypoventilation
	27.0	80.6	Loss of reflexes and voluntary motion
	26.0	78.8	Major acid-base disturbances; no reflexes or response to pain
	25.0	77.0	Cerebral blood flow one third of normal; loss of cerebrovascular autoregulation; cardiac output 45% of normal; pulmonary edema may develop
	24.0	75.2	Significant hypotension and bradycardia
	23.0	73.4	No corneal or oculocephalic reflexes; areflexia
	22.0	71.6	Maximum risk of ventricular fibrillation; 75% decrease in oxygen consumption
	20.0	68.0	Lowest resumption of cardiac electromechanical activity; pulse 20% of normal
	19.0	66.2	Electroencephalographic silencing
	18.0	64.6	Asystole
	10.0	50.0	95% decrease in oxygen consumption

From Auerbach PS: Wilderness Medicine, ed 3, St. Louis, 1995, Mosby–Year Book.

at 64° F (18° C), asystole ensues. The lowest recorded temperature that an adult patient has survived in accidental hypothermia is 61° F (16° C).[5]

Predisposing Factors. Many factors predispose an individual to hypothermia. Some do so by increasing heat loss, others by decreasing heat production. A final group may impair thermoregulation. The factor seen most frequently in the United States is the abuse of alcohol.[2]

Alcohol counteracts many of the normal physiologic responses to cold by promoting vasodilation and impairing the heat-generating mechanism of shivering. By clouding thought processes, alcohol abuse can also lead to a decreased perception and appreciation of environmental risk or ability to seek shelter from the environment.

Malnutrition, seen particularly in the elderly, also decreases the resources available for heat production. Many drugs interfere with the central mechanism of temperature control. Examples include benzodiazepines, phenothiazines, barbiturates, and opiates. Up to 25% of overdose patients present to the emergency department in a hypothermic state.[5]

Localized Hypothermia

Frostbite is the localized freezing of body tissue to the extent that cellular damage occurs. The condition may or may not be seen together with hypothermia.

Frostbite has traditionally been classified by the extent of tissue damage. Frostnip, which is the presence of superficial ice crystals on the skin with underlying cellular damage, is a reversible injury. Varying degrees of frostbite are clinical descriptions of mild through complete tissue loss (Fig. 43-7). The extremities account for 60% of frostbite cases in patients, and the majority of the remaining cases involve the face, particularly the ears and nose.[19]

One of the first physiologic responses to cold is vasoconstriction of peripheral blood vessels. As this occurs, peripheral tissue temperature begins to drop. Below 59° F (15° C), cellular ischemia begins as a result of immobile blood, coagulation in the capillaries, and the shunting of blood to the core. Because of the underlying heat radiated from the body's core, ice crystals do not begin to form until tissue temperature reaches 25° F (−4° C). As ice forms, the cells become dehydrated, resulting in cellular shrinkage, abnormally high electrolyte concentrations, and destruction of cellular proteins. Most cases of frostbite involve a chronic time course (hours); as a result, ice forms principally in extracellular spaces and the cells may survive. When frostbite occurs acutely (minutes or less), intracellular ice is more likely, and the prognosis for cellular survival is bleak.[7] There is an immediate risk for frostbite at −25°F. Wind chill factor contributes as a risk.

Chief among the predisposing factors for the development of frostbite is a previous history of frostbite. The reasons for this condition are not entirely clear, but frostbite may induce permanent vascular instability in the tissue, making it more sensitive to colder environments. Any disease process that causes narrowing of peripheral blood vessels, such as diabetes or atherosclerosis, or a patient who smokes cigarettes, results in an increased susceptibility to frostbite because of the decreased tissue blood flow. Alcohol abuse is present in nearly all cases of urban frostbite and is a direct contributor in 50% of all cases.[19]

Patient Assessment

History

After the initial assessment, continued patient assessment should be performed not only on the patient, but also the environment.

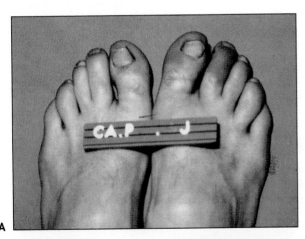

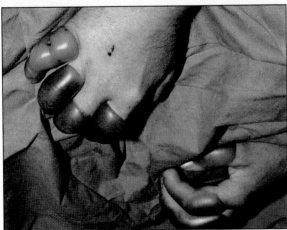

- *What environmental factors were present?* The air temperature, humidity, and duration of time in which the patient was exposed to these conditions are of particular importance. Exposure to or immersion in water may enhance heat loss; knowledge of water temperature is helpful. The presence of wind adds to heat loss by convection. If the patient's clothing is wet, the paramedic should determine the lengh of time of the patient's exposure. Although commonly believed to be effective insulation, the temperature beneath deep snow may be as much as 50° F (10° C) below that of the surface. These same factors are important in determining the extent of tissue damage in the patient.

- *Is there any potential for trauma?* Many outdoor activities have the potential for both hypothermia and trauma. In some cases this will be obvious, as in an avalanche, and some instances of falls or auto–pedestrian accidents may be more difficult to realize when discovered after the fact.

- *Is there any significant past medical history or evidence of drug abuse?* Alcohol and drugs have already been identified as significant predisposing factors for hypothermia, and a thorough assessment should be made for evidence of substance abuse. Other medical conditions, such as diabetes mellitus, systemic infections, and intracranial hemorrhage may be associated with hypothermia.

CRITICAL ISSUE

The paramedic should search diligently for secondary causes of hypothermia in the patient, and treat the patient's altered mental status accordingly.

- *Does the patient complain of numbness in the extremities?* Often the patient will report that the involved extremity feels numb and cold in the early stages of frostbite. Subsequently, feeling is absent in the involved tissue, and movement of the extremities become clumsy or uncoordinated.

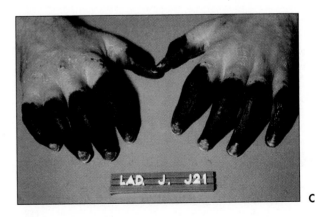

Figure 43-7

A) First degree frostbite B) Second superficial degree frostbite C) Third degree frostbite. *From Vallotton J. and Dubas F. (eds.): Color Atlas of Mountain Medicine, 1991, London, Wolfe Publishing Co.*

• *What kind of clothing was the patient wearing?* Inadequate protective clothing may contribute greatly to heat loss. Wet clothing conducts more heat from the body, and tight-fitting or constrictive clothing may further reduce blood supply to the periphery. Tight gloves and boots also increase the risk of frostbite to digits. Layered, dry clothing helps prevent frostbite.

Physical Examination

After the initial assessment, the rescuer should evaluate the patient's mental status. The first signs of hypothermia can include apathy, confusion, lethargy, and difficulty with speech and gait. With severe hypothermia, patients become disoriented, more lethargic and finally, completely unresponsive.

In mild hypothermia, respirations and pulse rate are initially elevated. As the body's core temperature drops, so do cardiac and respiratory functions. Because bradycardia and hypoventilation are common in severe hypothermia, the paramedic must be sure to evaluate the patient for pulse and respirations for at least 1 to 2 minutes. Atrial fibrillation is suggested by the presence of an irregular pulse.

Body temperature can be estimated by noting cool, pale skin. In early hypothermia, expect to see shivering (occurring at a core temperature of 88° to 95° F, or 31° to 35° C). As core temperature drops, muscles stiffen and may mimic rigor mortis, reflexes are lost, and pupils dilate.

Frostbitten skin appears white or mottled blue in color and is firm or solid when palpated. Sensation in this skin is decreased or absent. If the involved tissue has undergone any rewarming prior to paramedic arrival, the skin may appear pink, warm, and tender. With more severe forms of frostbite (second and third degree), vesicles and bullae (similar to the blisters of a partial-thickness burn) appear that are indicative of deeper dermal involvement. In the most severe cases (fourth degree), subcutaneous structures including muscle, tendon, and bone are involved. Absence of a peripheral pulse usually indicates significant involvement of deeper structures. The paramedic should keep in mind that such classifications are usually determined after rewarming; initial impressions often underestimate the extent of injury.[5]

Management

Although the cold, stiff, and blue hypothermic patient often appears dead, the paramedic's ability to predict patient viability is not accurate until a patient has been rewarmed. Thus, the adage for paramedics remains, "No one is dead until warm and dead."

CRITICAL ISSUE

Patients who appear dead in the setting of exposure to cold should not be pronounced as such until rewarmed.

After removing the patient from the environment, he or she should be protected from further cooling. If possible, the patient should be moved promptly to a warm environment, such as a heated ambulance, and any wet clothing should be replaced with warm blankets. Heat packs should be placed around the head, neck, axilla, and groin. Do not massage the patient.

Airway management in hypothermic patients is controversial. Ventricular fibrillation has been induced by CPR, endotracheal intubation, and even roughly moving a patient. Therefore, it is recommended that all patients with spontaneous respirations receive 100% oxygen with assistance from a bag-valve-mask device if necessary. Warmed (113° F; 45° C), humidified oxygen is the first line of active rewarming when available because it takes advantage of the large alveolar surface area. Definitive airway management by endotracheal intubation should be reserved for apneic patients or in patients where the airway cannot be protected by other means. Because aggressive suctioning can also trigger ventricular fibrillation, this method should be avoided whenever possible.

All hypothermic patients require cardiac monitoring. Although any dysrhythmia may be seen with a core body temperature less than 90° F (32° C), atrial fibrillation is common early on in the condition, deteriorating to bradycardic rhythms as hypothermia progresses. The J wave (Osborn wave or hypothermic hump) is frequently seen in lead II, and is described as a "hump" or elevation of the ST segment at the junction of the QRS complex and the ST segment (Fig. 43-8). The size of the wave increases as the patient's core body temperature drops.

In contrast to normothermic patients, pharmacologic or electric treatment of dysrhythmias at core body temperatures less than 82° F (28° C) is usually ineffective. Bradycardic rhythms will not benefit from pacing or atropine, and these methods should not be attempted. In the case of ventricular fibrillation, it may be reasonable to attempt one series of three countershocks; medications, if used, may not be effective until rewarming is achieved.

CRITICAL ISSUE

In severe hypothermia, ACLS drugs and electrical therapy should be used rarely, if at all, because these therapeutic measures are generally ineffective and may cause harm to the patient.

With hypothermia, the percentage of a drug that is protein bound increases. Thus, if several rounds of a medication are given, the patient may receive a toxic dose during the rewarming process. Some animal studies have suggested that bretylium tosylate decreases the core temperature at which defibrillation is possible.[4] Further investigation will be required before this practice can be routinely recommended. Vasopressors will have minimal effect on the already vasoconstricted vascular bed. These drugs may induce dysrhythmias and will offer no benefit to the patient.

All patients require IV access with normal saline or Ringer's lactate (warmed if possible) through a large-bore catheter; this procedure can wait until the patient is loaded

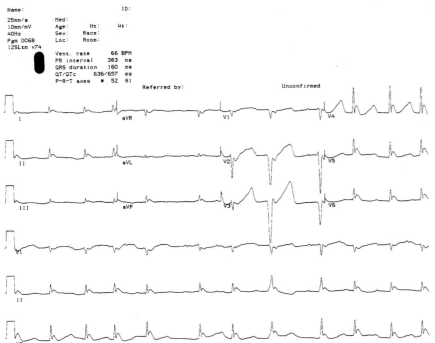

Figure 43-8

The J or Osborn wave of hypothermia. *From Auerbach, PS: Wilderness Medicine, ed. 3, St. Louis 1995, Mosby-Year Book.*

into the warm ambulance. Most hypothermic patients are dehydrated and will also require volume expansion.

Many patients with hypothermia present with altered mental status, and those patients with hypoglycemia or heroin overdose may present in a hypothermic state. Hypothermic patients should therefore be tested for blood sugar level, examined for signs of opiate overdose, and treated appropriately. Hyperglycemia may be found in non-diabetics due to the inactivation of insulin below 90° F (30° C). Do not administer or help in the administration of insulin after rewarming since hypoglycemia may occur.

Rapid rewarming is the definitive care for frostbite, and is best carried out in the emergency department. If a frostbitten area is allowed to thaw and refreeze, greater tissue destruction results than if the tissue remains frozen until arrival at the hospital. Attempting to rewarm the area using a fire, stove, or heater may not only initiate the thaw–refreeze cycle, but can also result in thermal injury to the numb skin.

All wet, constricting clothing should be removed (if not frozen to the skin), and core body temperature can be maintained with warm blankets. Ideally, an affected extremity is best transported in a supported, elevated position. Frostbitten skin can be covered gently with dry, sterile dressings, taking care to keep any blisters or bullae intact. Manipulation or rubbing of the frostbitten tissue also increases the potential for tissue damage.[7]

CRITICAL ISSUE

Rewarming of frostbitten tissue is best performed in the controlled setting of the emergency department. The paramedic should avoid the potential damage done by the "thaw-refreeze" cycle and not rub or manipulate frozen tissue.

Except for very mild cases of hypothermia, all patients with hypothermia or frostbite require physician evaluation. If a patient is severely hypothermic, the best destination choice is a facility with ready access to cardiopulmonary bypass, because this is the ideal technology to control the active rewarming process in unstable, severely hypothermic (90° F/30° C) patients not responding to usual rewarming techniques.

Section IV Summary

Hypothermia can occur in a variety of settings and at any time during the year. Particular care should be directed to identifying predisposing factors and elements suggesting secondary hypothermia. Prehospital care centers around removing the patient promptly from the cold environment, passive external rewarming (with blankets), initiating IV fluid replacement, active internal rewarming (with warmed oxygen) when available, supportive care, and close monitoring designed to avoid precipitating a worse dysrhythmia than is already present. Patient transport should be to a definitive care center capable of providing controlled, active rewarming. Patients with areas of frostbite must be transported promptly to an emergency department for active thawing of the affected area. Care should be taken to avoid further tissue damage and refreezing of frostbitten tissue.

Section V

High-Altitude Illness

With the ease of modern air and automobile travel, many more people not only arrive at high-altitude environments, but get there more rapidly than ever before. In Colorado alone, millions of people ski at elevations of more than 8000 feet.[13] Hiking, mountain climbing, camping, and other tourist activities have grown in popularity and commonly occur at high altitudes. High-altitude illness is a spectrum of disease reflecting the physiologic responses in an unacclimatized individual to the hypoxia encountered when the partial pressure of oxygen falls at altitude. It can range from insomnia and headache to respiratory failure and coma.[14] Symptoms may be seen in 20% to 50% of individuals and depends on both the altitude achieved and rate of ascent.[9]

Pathophysiology

When one ascends to high altitude, atmospheric (barometric) pressure falls. Although the percentage of atmospheric oxygen remains the same (21%), this pressure drop affects the partial pressure of inspired oxygen and commonly causes hypoxia in healthy individuals at altitudes above 8000 feet (2438) meters). Over time, through an individual's physiologic responses to hypoxia, acclimatization to high altitude occurs. The first of these is an increase in ventilation. As the oxygen content of blood falls, the brain stem respiratory center acts to stimulate respirations. Catecholamine release results in mild rises in pulse and blood pressure, increasing delivery of oxygen to the tissues. Finally, as a result of hormonal influences, the bone marrow is stimulated to produce more oxygen-carrying red blood cells, although this process may take 4 to 5 days.[8]

Hypoxia is the primary physiologic event leading to high-altitude illness, but the exact mechanism by which this occurs is unclear. It has been proposed that some individuals have a decreased respiratory response to hypoxia. Subsequent pulmonary vasoconstriction may lead to pulmonary hypertension and a noncardiogenic pulmonary edema known as *high-altitude pulmonary edema (HAPE)*. There may be an element of alveolar leakage in the development of HAPE, as well.

It has also been suggested that the body's fluid regulation mechanisms are abnormal, resulting in fluid retention and a shift of fluid to the intracellular spaces. One consequence is that plasma volume drops by 20%; with exertion, dehydration is more likely. With hypoxia, cerebral blood vessels dilate and elevated pressure may lead to breakdown of the blood-brain barrier. A combination of these two factors is believed to cause high-altitude cerebral edema (HACE). As intracranial pressure increases, HACE formation may act centrally to cause a neurogenic pulmonary edema and further aggravate HAPE.[18]

Several factors predispose an individual to development of high-altitude illness. Travel to over 2500 to 3000 meters and a rapid ascent may be the most common factors. Prior episodes of high-altitude illness make an individual more prone to future attacks. The use of alcohol or medications that are respiratory depressants (e.g., benzodiazepines and opiates) inhibits the normal ventilatory physiologic response necessary for adaptation and may hasten the onset of symptoms.

Patient Assessment

History

Because high-altitude illness can be subtle and present with

nonspecific symptoms, historical data are of particular significance to patient assessment.

- *Does the patient have a history of travel?* The most critical factors related to the onset of high-altitude illness are a rapid ascent, usually from altitiudes below 3000 feet to those above 8000 feet and the duration of time spent at high altitudes. Most commonly, symptoms develop 8 to 24 hours after arrival at the sleeping altitude. During some airline flights, the cabin may be pressurized to the equivalent of an altitude of 8000 feet or more, which can result in symptoms in some patients.[15]
- *Is there a complaint of malaise?* The mild, early symptoms of high-altitude illness often include complaints of nausea, malaise, fatigue, and headache. The headache is throbbing, and bilateral in nature and is often worsened by exercise. Patients may note difficulty sleeping because of variations in respiratory patterns commonly seen secondary to hypoxia. As illness progresses, vomiting ensues and the headache is unrelieved by common pain medication.[8] Mild disease generally resolves with acclimatization in 3 to 7 days.
- *Are there any respiratory symptoms?* Any complaint of shortness of breath (especially at rest), cough, or hemoptysis should be considered secondary to HAPE until proven otherwise. HAPE can be seen in up to 15% of people who ascend rapidly to high altitudes.[14]
- *Does the patient appear confused or exhibit poor judgment?* These symptoms, along with complaints suggestive of increased intracranial pressure, such as headache, vomiting, seizures, or difficulty with gait, can indicate the onset of HACE. HACE usually occurs at altitudes over 12,000 feet but has been reported at altitudes under 9000 feet.[18]

C R I T I C A L   I S S U E

The paramedic should remember to consider other causes of altered mental status, such as hypoglycemia or CVA, in patients with possible HACE.

- *What is the patient's past medical history?* Patients with previous cardiac or respiratory disease will experience enhanced effects of altitude and hypoxia, as will patients with sickle cell disease who are more prone to vasoocclusive crisis when artrial oxygen levels fall. The paramedic should inquire about any previous episodes of high-altitude illness, alcohol use, smoking, or the use of medications that may lead to altitude-related complaints.

Physical Examination

Mild high-altitude illness is particularly lacking in specific physical signs. Blood pressure, pulse, and respiratory rate may all be mildly elevated as a result of early physiologic compensation. The rescuer should check the patient for a lowered body temperature; hypothermia and high-altitude illness often appear together. Skin signs can include pallor or cyanosis in the setting of hypoxia.

CRITICAL ISSUE

Even mild, nonspecific symptoms should be considered high-altitude illness until proven otherwise.

Upon auscultation of the patient's chest, the paramedic may note the presence of crackles (rales), seen in many patients at altitudes over 14,000 feet. The presence of this symptom indicates that acclimatization is necessary prior to further ascent. Other signs of respiratory distress (retractions and use of accessory muscles for respiration) can herald the onset of HAPE.[8] With severe cases, peripheral or facial edema can be noted.

A thorough examination of the patient's mental status is crucial. Confusion, lethargy, and poor judgment (declining food or water intake, poor appreciation of surroundings) indicate a progression of disease, possibly leading to HAPE or HACE. An initial clumsiness or lack of dexterity, proceeding to an ataxic gait, is believed to be one of the most accurate warnings of a deterioration of the patient's status.[18] Mental status worsens with severity of disease to demonstrate hallucinations, stupor, and coma, and less frequently reported symptoms such as seizures and focal neurologic findings.

Management

After patient assessment, management of high-altitude illness principally involves rest, descent, and administration of oxygen. Mild cases of high-altitude illness may be managed without descent in young, healthy patients as long as further ascent is curtailed until acclimatization occurs. Increasing fluid intake, limiting physical exercise, avoiding alcohol, and reducing salt consumption are other measures that may be helpful in preventing the progression of symptoms.

Absolute rest alone may reduce symptoms by reducing internal oxygen demands. Oxygen should be administered at high concentration by mask to all patients with moderate to severe high-altitude illness (including HAPE and HACE). The paramedic must recognize that, although patients may improve with oxygen administration, this therapy is not a replacement for descent. Respirations should be assisted with endotracheal intubation, if necessary, for those patients with signs of respiratory distress, cyanosis, or altered mental status.

The most effective therapy for high-altitude illness is descent. Dramatic improvement may be seen with a descent of as little as 1000 feet. A Gamon bag may be used to increase the atmospheric pressure around the patient, thus stimulating a partial descent and buying some time while arranging the evacuation of the patient to a lower altitude.

CRITICAL ISSUE

Descent is the cornerstone of therapy for all but the mildest forms of high-altitude illness.

Intravenous access with normal saline or Ringer's lactate should be established in all patients undergoing descent. The paramedic must take care to avoid fluid overload, because patients are at risk for the pulmonary hypertension and leaky alveoli that lead to HAPE. Fluid boluses should therefore be limited to those necessary to maintain vital signs.

Cardiac monitoring can be used as indicated by patient status or previous history of cardiac or respiratory disease. Diuretics, such as furosemide, are not useful in the acute phase of treatment of HAPE, but may not be ordered for HACE.

All patients with moderate to severe high-altitude illness, HAPE, and HACE, require evacuation, descent, and transfer to an emergency department at an appropriate altitude for further evaluation, observation, and possible hospital admission.

Section V Summary

The most important aspect of managing high-altitude illness is recognizing the symptom complex when the patient first presents. Careful initial assessment is particularly important because the major complications, HAPE and HACE, can be avoided with prompt oxygen therapy and descent. Individuals can prevent high-altitude illness by remaining well hydrated, ascending slowly enough to allow acclimatization, and avoiding physical overexertion.

SUMMARY

Environmental emergencies represent a microcosm of the challenges a paramedic must face daily, from the management of traumatic injury caused by a significant animal bite to the assessment and treatment of the hypo- or hyperthermic patient. The etiologies for these emergencies vary widely; however, the prehospital interventions are crucial components for successful recovery.

REFERENCES

1. Browne BJ, Gaasch WR. Electrical injuries and lightning. **Emerg Med Clin North Am** 1992; 10:211–29.

2. Center for Disease Control. Hypothemia-related deaths—Cook County, Illinois, November 1992–March 1993. MMWR 1993; 42:917–919.

3. Cooper MA. Lightning injuries: prognostic signs for death. **Ann Emerg Med** 1980; 9:134–8.

4. Danzl DF, Hedges JR, et al. Hypothermia outcome score: development and implications. **Crit Care Med** 1989; 17:227–231.

5. Danzl DF, Pozos RS, et al. Accidental hypothermia. In Auerbach PS, Geehr EC (eds). Management of wilderness and environmental emergencies, ed 2, St. Louis, Mosby–Year Book, Inc. 1995.

6. Dart RC, Sullivan JB, Jr. Crotalid snake envenomations. In The clinical practice of emergency medicine, ed 2, Harwood-Nuss AL (eds), Lippincott-Raven, Philadelphia, 1996: 1450–53.

7. Gonzalez F, Majidan AM. Cold-induced tissue injuries. In Harwood-Nuss A, Linden C, et al (eds). The clinical practice of emergency medicine, Philadelphia, Lippincott–Raven, 1996.

8. Hackett PH, Roach RC, et al. High altitude medicine. In Auerbach PS, Geehr EC (eds). Management of wilderness and environmental emergencies, ed 2, St. Louis, Mosby–Year Book, Inc. 1995.

9. Honigman B, Theis MK, Koziol-McLain J, et al. Acute mountain sickness in a general tourist population at moderate altitudes. **Ann Intern Med** 1993: 118:587–592.

10. Klainer PH, Mongillo B. Hypothermia. In Harwood-Nuss A, Linden C, et al (eds). The clinical practice of emergency medicine, Philadelphia, Lippincott–Raven, 1996.

11. Knochel JP. Dog days and siriasis: how to kill a football player. **JAMA** 1975; 233(6):513.

12. Patten BM. Lightning and electrical injuries. **Neurol Clin** 1992, 10:1047–59.

13. Reisman RE. Stinging insect allergy. **Med Clin North Am** 1992; 76:883–94.

14. Richardson DM. High altitude illness. In Harwood-Nuss A, Linden C, et al (eds). The clinical practice of emergency medicine, Philadelphia, Lippincott–Raven, 1996.

15. Stafford CT. Life-threatening allergic reactions: anticipating and preparing are the best defenses. **Postgrad Med** 86:235, 1989.

16. Stewart CE. Preventing progression of heat injury. **Emerg Med Rep** 1987; 8:121–8.

17. Tek D, Olshaker JS. Heat illness. **Emerg Med Clin North Am** 1992; 10:299–310.

18. Tso E. High altitude illness. **Emerg Med Clin Nor Am** 1992; 10:231–247.

19. Urschel JD. Frostbite: predisposing factors and predictors of poor outcome. **J Trauma** 1990; 30:340–342.

Richard N. Nelson, MD, FACEP

Chapter 44

Aquatic Emergencies

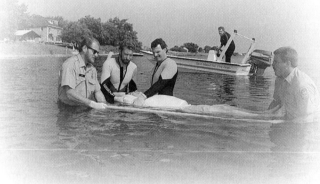

The aquatic environment is an important source of recreation for millions. When an accident occurs, it usually involves a young, previously healthy and potentially productive person. The EMS provider may be the first person to render treatment at the scene of an aquatic emergency, and this initial management frequently determines whether the victim goes on to recovery or suffers permanent disability or death.

Scuba (Self-Contained Underwater Breathing Apparatus) diving and snorkeling have become popular sports in recent years. Diving accidents are seen not only in coastal areas, but also in inland communities; dive accidents occur in rivers, lakes, and abandoned quarries. Victims may present hours after leaving a dive site. Thus, EMS providers everywhere should be familiar with the prehospital management of underwater diving emergencies.

Pathophysiology

Drowning and Near-Drowning

Drowning is a major cause of death and disability. Of the 140,000 annual deaths due to drowning worldwide, approximately 8000 of these incidents occur in the United States.[4] Many more patients are injured and permanently disabled from the neurologic complications of near-drowning.

Drowning is defined as death by submersion in a liquid medium, usually water. Near-drowning involves a submersion accident in which the patient survives for at least 24 hours after submersion.

Wet drowning occurs when water or other liquid is aspirated into the lungs, usually after the victim has lost protective airway reflexes and is unable to suppress respirations. When freshwater is aspirated, it is absorbed quickly through the alveoli into the circulation by osmosis. This dilutes the more concentrated plasma and disrupts the surfactant lining of the alveoli, resulting in decreased lung compliance, atelectasis, capillary leakage, and **pulmonary edema.** These conditions ultimately lead to poor ventilation and severe hypoxia (Fig. 44-1).

Saltwater is more concentrated than plasma; aspiration of saltwater results in fluid from the circulation passing into the lungs, again drawn by osmosis. Victims who have aspirated saltwater are more likely to have fluid in their lungs at the time of initial resuscitation. Aspiration of polluted water can result in bacterial contamination, infection, or chemical inflammation of the lungs, depending on the pollutants in the water. Both saltwater and polluted water also cause surfactant washout and capillary leakage, resulting in effects similar to freshwater aspiration.

Approximately 10% of drownings occur without aspiration.[3] Laryngospasm during the initial struggle prevents water from entering the lungs, leading to death by airway occlusion and asphyxiation rather than aspiration. Although these victims theoretically stand a better chance of successful resuscitation owing to less severely damaged lungs, "dry drowning" cannot be differentiated from "wet drowning" in the prehospital setting.

Respiratory compromise occurs immediately in most submersion victims, but some patients are stable after initial rescue only to develop respiratory distress later (Table 44-1). Respiratory distress after an initial period of recovery is called postimmersion syndrome, or "secondary drowning." This syndrome usually occurs within 12 hours of rescue, but can be delayed for as long as 72 hours. Its existence emphasizes the importance of hospital evaluation after any submersion accident.

Sudden death that occurs as a result of contact with water, usually cold water, is called immersion syndrome. This poorly defined syndrome is probably the result of severe bradycardia or cardiac arrest with subsequent loss of responsiveness and aspiration. Alcohol ingestion by the patient is considered an important predisposing factor.

Often the submersion incident results from exhaustion, muscle cramps, or the victim's inability to swim. In many cases, there is a precipitating event or associated condition that, when recognized, significantly alters prehospital management.

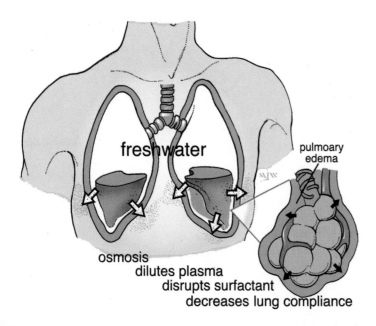

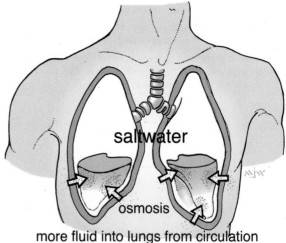

Figure 44-1

The effects of freshwater and saltwater on the lungs.

- Drowning and near-drowning episodes are becoming a leading cause of accidental death in children less than 5 years of age.[1] However, these occurrences are frequently preventable, because they often result from lack of parental or guardian supervision or poor barriers allowing easier access to hazards. Environmental hazards include beaches, lakes, rivers, swimming pools, hot tubs, and bathtubs. Medical conditions such as epilepsy, drug overdoses, and head trauma contribute as well.

- Children lose body heat (temperature) more rapidly than do adults, particularly when they are wet. This occurrence is caused by the larger surface area as compared to body weight, a larger head in relation to body size, and minimal subcutaneous tissue.

- After a near-drowning event, the child's neurologic status often improves within 72 hours, if there is to be a favorable outcome.[2] On the other hand, a prolonged period of time may be required to properly evaluate the child's complete neurologic status and outcome.[2]

- The "diving" reflex (bradycardia and shunting the circulating blood volume to the heart and brain) is believed to be an important factor in the sometimes favorable outcome of a child suffering from a near-drowning event.[1,2]

- Physical assessment and clinical findings directly reflect the mechanism of the aquatic emergency and the length of the event. Water temperature and cleanliness, as well as preexisting medical conditions of the child, are factors.

- Any child suffering from an aquatic emergency should receive prompt prehospital pediatric advanced cardiac life support and treatment even if the child is found pulseless and apneic with profound hypothermia.

REFERENCE

1. Barkin R, et al: Pediatric emergency medicine. Concepts and clinical practice. St. Louis, 1992, Mosby–Year Book.

2. Nichols D, et al: Golden hour: the handbook of advanced pediatric life support, ed 2, St. Louis, 1996, Mosby–Year Book.

A common scenario is that of a young person drowning after a head-first dive into shallow water or an accident in a swimming pool causing either a head injury and loss of responsiveness or a cervical spine fracture with subsequent paralysis (Fig. 44-2). Cervical spine injuries associated with drownings also occur in surfing, water skiing, and boating accidents.

Many submersion victims are later found to have high blood levels of drugs or alcohol. Intoxicants impair the patient's judgment and lead to inappropriate and dangerous actions. They also predispose the individual to unresponsiveness, exhaustion, hypothermia, and hypoglycemia, all of which make aspiration and drowning more likely.

Hypothermia is very common in submersion victims and is possible both in summer and winter. Hypothermia is not necessarily a bad sign, as it greatly reduces cerebral oxygen

TABLE 44-1	Medical Conditions Caused by Near Drowning	
Condition	**Other Name(s)**	**Description (Partial)**
Acute respiratory distress syndrome (ARDS)	Shock lung Wet lung	Shortness of breath, rapid breathing. **Cause:** damaged lung tissue; hemorrhage; fluid buildup in lungs.
Acute renal failure	Acute kidney failure	Inability of kidneys to excrete wastes. **Cause:** hemorrhage; toxic injury. May cause heart failure.
Hemolysis	Hemolytic anemia	Breakdown of red blood cells. **Cause:** dilution of blood by excessive amounts of hypotonic solutions.
Diffuse intravascular coagulation	Internal Clotting	Clotting in blood vessels and organs throughout the body **Cause:** breakdown and dilution of blood cells, followed by massive internal bleeding.

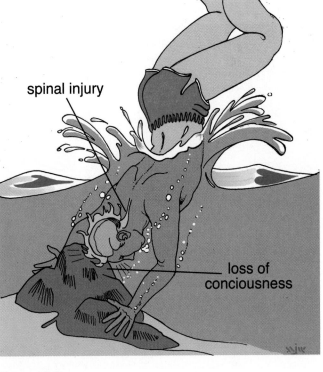

spinal injury

loss of conciousness

Figure 44-2

Drowning occurs during diving accidents because of spinal injuries or loss of responsiveness.

requirements and thus increases the time the brain can withstand anoxia. Hypothermic near-drowning victims, particularly children, have sustained submersion times of more than 40 minutes with complete neurologic recovery.

Underlying medical conditions, such as seizures and cardiac dysrhythmias, can be catastrophic if they occur while the victim is in the water. The unresponsiveness and loss of protective reflexes that follow can lead to aspiration and drowning even in shallow water.

Suicides, homicides, and child abuse may present as submersion events. Bathtub or toilet drownings and other suspicious findings should alert the EMS provider to the possibility of child or adult abuse (see Chapter 56).

Patients with submersion times less than 5 minutes who regain spontaneous circulation with less than 10 minutes of resuscitative efforts generally have good outcomes.[2] Factors associated with poor outcomes include prolonged submersion, delay in CPR, severe acidosis, fixed and dilated pupils, a Glasgow Coma Score of less than five, and asystole upon arrival at the hospital. Still, submersion victims with all of these findings have gone on to complete recovery, particularly if these patients are hypothermic.

Pressure-Related Diving Accidents

Decompression Sickness

When the body travels from higher to lower atmospheric pressure environments, inert gas dissolved in the blood and tissues (most commonly nitrogen) comes out of solution (Fig. 44-3). Usually, this excess gas is exhaled harmlessly through the

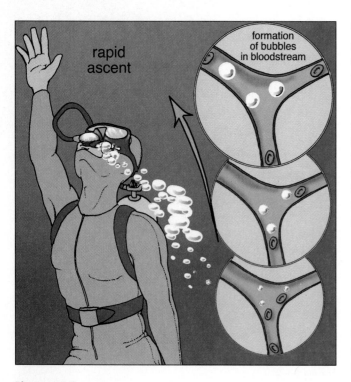

Figure 44-3

Rapid changes in atmospheric pressure result in decompression sickness.

lungs. However, if the change in pressure occurs too quickly, bubbles form in the blood vessels and body tissues. The resulting signs and symptoms are known as decompression sickness (DCS), "the bends," or "caisson disease." Although scuba divers most often develop DCS, anyone exposed to compressed air is at risk; underwater tunnel workers are another group affected.

Most patients with DCS notice symptoms within 4 hours of surfacing, but some patients may be asymptomatic for 12 hours or more. DCS is usually not a risk unless the patient has been exposed to depths of at least 33 feet. Because DCS is caused by nitrogen bubbles in the vasculature and tissues, the actual symptoms correlate to the sites of bubble formation.

Also known as "pain-only bends," Type I DCS usually manifests as a deep pain or throbbing in the large joints, usually shoulders and elbows, made worse with movement. Bubbles forming in the brain, spinal cord, heart, lungs, or inner ear produce potentially life-threatening effects known as Type II DCS. Manifestations of Type II DCS can include paralysis, dyspnea, hemoptysis, numbness and tingling, headache, auditory disturbances, dizziness, or loss of responsiveness.

Barotrauma

Barotrauma occurs when air contained in certain body cavities is unable to equilibrate with atmospheric pressure as the body moves from one pressure level to another. The pressure gradient that occurs between the body cavity and the atmosphere makes the cavity either collapse or expand, and often causes injury (Fig. 44-4). Common areas affected are the external, inner, and middle ear, the sinuses, and the lungs. In addition to affecting scuba divers, barotrauma is a common affliction among snorkelers, platform divers, tram riders, and aircraft passengers.

Air Embolism

Air embolism is the second most common cause of death among scuba divers, after drowning.[1] This condition occurs when the diver either surfaces too quickly or breath-holds during ascent. Expansion of air in the lung during ascent forces air through the alveoli into the pulmonary circulation, from which it can obstruct any of numerous vessels. Although the signs and symptoms of air embolism vary depending on which vessels are occluded, the brain is most commonly affected. Although less often involved, the coronary circulation can manifest involvement as acute myocardial infarction and cardiac arrest. Unlike decompression sickness, air embolism can occur after ascent from a dive as shallow as 4 feet underwater.

Patient Assessment

In aquatic emergencies, patient assessment begins with a survey of the scene and initial assessment. After ABC's are taken care of, patient assessment continues with historical questions and interviews of bystanders.

- *Is the scene safe?* One possible hazard is malfunctioning electrical equipment near home swimming pools. Electric-

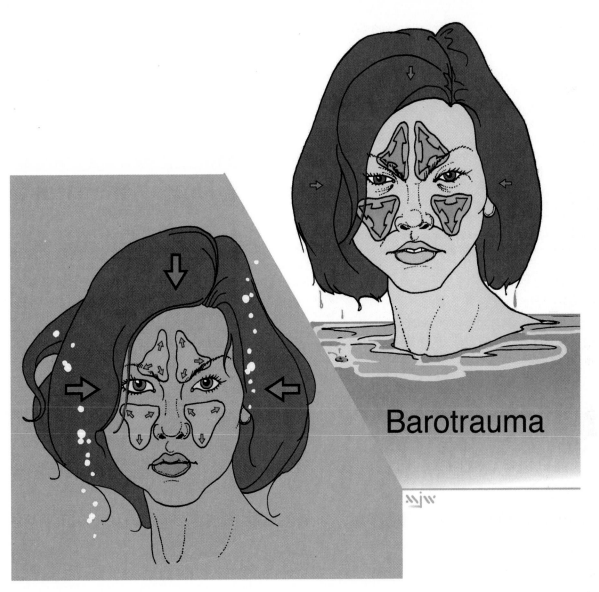

Figure 44-4

Body cavities that contain air, such as the sinuses, are susceptible to barotrauma caused by pressure changes.

ity transmitted through the water may not only have caused the drowning, but also could be a potential hazard to the rescuer. Other potential hazards include currents or undertows which might pose a danger to the rescuers.

- *Is the victim still in the water?* If the victim is still in the water, extrication may be dangerous. Ice water rescues are particularly treacherous; many would-be rescuers themselves fall through the ice during extrication attempts each year. The temperature of the water and the patient's time of submersion must be noted.

History

- *Is there a history of scuba diving?* If time allows, the paramedic should obtain as much history of the dive as possible. Important information includes the type of equipment used; the number and depth of all dives in the past 48 hours; the amount of in-water decompression if any; the site of the dive; the approximate water temperature; and the time of onset of symptoms.

- *Do the patient's complaints suggest barotrauma?* Ear pain accompanies barotrauma involving any portion of the ear, and occasionally the tympanic membrane (eardrum) actually ruptures. The patient's hearing is diminished as the air of the middle ear is replaced with fluid. Inner-ear barotrauma is characterized by tinnitus (ringing in the ears) and dizziness. Symptoms of sinus involvement include headache, cheek pain, upper tooth pain, or nosebleed.

- *Does the patient complain of chest pain, dyspnea, or hemoptysis?* If a scuba diver does not exhale sufficiently during ascent, the air in the lungs will expand, sometimes resulting in **pulmonary overpressurization syndrome** (POPS) or "burst lung." Air can leak through the lungs into the surrounding tissue and cause **pneumothorax,** pneumopericardium, or pneumomediastinum.

- *Is air embolism a possibility?* Air embolism typically manifests itself within seconds after a diver surfaces. If symptoms occur more than 10 minutes after surfacing, the symptoms are probably not the result of air embolism. Because the bubbles tend to float to the cerebral circulation, neurologic findings are most common in patients and resemble those seen in an acute stroke. Common symptoms are altered mental status, seizures, weakness, visual disturbances, difficulty speaking, dizziness, headache, dyspnea, and hemoptysis.

CRITICAL ISSUE

A patient's sudden loss of responsiveness immediately upon surfacing from a dive is usually a sign of air embolism.

Physical Examination

The physical examination begins with determination of vital signs and mental status. Many patients will be tachypneic; if a pulse is present, the rate and strength should be determined, and capillary refill assessed.

The paramedic should evaluate the patency of the patient's airway and listen carefully to breath sounds. Wheezing and crackles are common findings following aspiration and can indicate the presence of pulmonary edema. Unequal breath sounds and subcutaneous emphysema, particularly about the patient's chest and neck, may follow pulmonary injuries from diving accidents.

CRITICAL ISSUE

The Heimlich maneuver should be used only if a foreign body or mechanical airway obstruction is suspected. In all other cases of near-drowning, the technique is not indicated.

Submersion victims may appear entirely normal, or they may appear dead with no movement or pupillary response. Between these two extremes are confusion, combativeness, and decorticate or decerebrate posturing. Perform a careful neurologic assessment, paying particular attention to level of responsiveness, pupillary response, and motor and sensory function. If possible, the paramedic should determine a Glasgow Coma Score and document this information on the patient care report.

Management

Managing submersion victims requires consideration of trauma to the patient's head and spine. Any patient found unresponsive with an unknown etiology must be suspected of having a head or spine injury until proven otherwise. For this reason, any patient rescued from a submersion accident requires airway management in conjunction with precautions to protect the cervical spine. This is even true of victims who have been rescued from the water by lifeguards or bystanders prior to the arrival of EMS personnel. If the accident was not witnessed, the paramedic cannot rule out head or spine injury. In situations in which the mechanism of injury clearly suggests the potential for head and spine injury (e.g., a person injured when diving in shallow water), it is even more important to appropriately manage the airway and spine.

CRITICAL ISSUE

If the accident was not witnessed, the paramedic cannot rule out head or spine injury.

Most protocols addressing the management of submersion victims identify the need for spinal immobilization, unless it is determined that the victim did not sustain a head or spine injury. If a near-drowning victim is found in cardiac arrest, CPR must be performed on a firm surface. In this case, a backboard can be used thus to provide partial immobilization. The use of in-line stabilization techniques protects against additional injury.

In most cases, the near-drowning victim will already have been removed from the water before EMS personnel arrive. In a few instances, however, EMS personnel will be on the scene, participating in a search and rescue effort. Once located, the victim must be removed from the water to be properly managed.

Removing the victim from the water is a team effort. Because the victim is often found face down in the water, the rescuer should begin by positioning the victim face up, while supporting the head and spine. There are several methods that can be used to accomplish this task. One of the simplest methods is to place the victim's arms against his or her ears and hold the head in-line with the body (Fig. 44-5). The victim is rotated toward the rescuer, until he or she is face up in the water (Fig. 44-6). Another rescuer submerges a backboard and raises it under the victim (Fig. 44-7). A third rescuer takes over control of the victim's head, while the other two rescuers now support the board and move it to safety (Fig. 44-8).

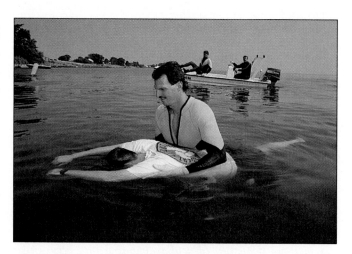

Figure 44-5

The victim's arms should be placed against his or her ears, and the head should be held in line with the body.

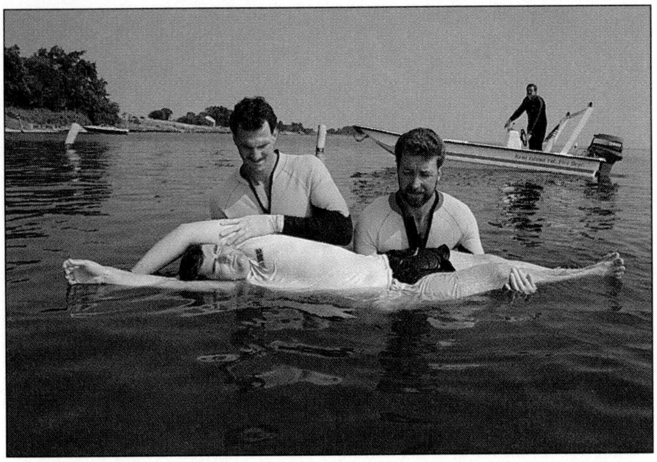

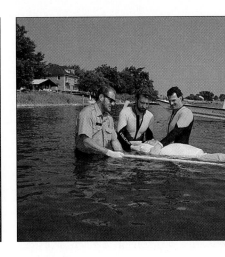

Figure 44-6

The victim is rotated toward the rescuer until he or she is face up in the water.

Figure 44-7

Another rescuer submerges a backboard and raises it under the victim.

If the victim's airway is clear and he or she is breathing adequately, rescuers may apply a cervical collar and complete the immobilization procedures (apply and secure the straps) while the patient is in the water. Depending on the conditions, this maneuver may require additional assistance. If the victim is experiencing respiratory distress, is apneic, or is unresponsive, appropriate care is best accomplished on land. If adequate personnel are available to assist, the rescuer must remove the patient from the water immediately and begin care. The key to proper management is to ensure a patent airway and avoid hypothermia. This generally means that rescuers should not take time to secure the straps for patient removal unless absolutely necessary. As long as in-line stabilization can be maintained, the patient should be removed from the water. Once removed, endotracheal intubation is indicated if the victim is apneic, unresponsive, or if respirations are inadequate.

For years, rescuers have been instructed to begin mouth-to-mouth breathing in the water, as soon as a victim is brought to the surface. Other techniques have included attempting to use a pocket mask or bag-valve-mask. These techniques are impractical, because 1) these techniques are difficult to perform without significant practice; 2) these techniques require the use of antiquated methods (i.e., mouth-to-mouth) that are inconsistent with body substance isolation precautions; and 3) these techniques require many sets of free hands working in the water.

For this reason, even lifeguards are currently being instructed to remove victims rapidly from the water and begin care on land. The only time that resuscitation efforts should be performed in the water is when circumstances prevent removal, such as patient entrapment in a partially submerged vehicle. Even so, CPR cannot be performed effectively in the water.

All submersion victims should receive 100% oxygen. A nonrebreather mask is adequate in the awake patient. The paramedic must always assume the presence of hypoxic brain injury in the unresponsive submersion victim and hyperventilate with 100% oxygen. Suction may aid ventilation, particularly in saltwater aspiration. If available, pulse oximetry can be used to monitor oxygenation.

The paramedic should begin CPR immediately if no pulse is present. In general, patients who have been submerged for less than 1 hour should undergo aggressive resuscitative efforts in the field and be transported to the hospital.

CRITICAL ISSUE

Resuscitation efforts for the near-drowning patient should be aggressive, even following prolonged submersion times.

Intravenous access should be established on all patients using normal saline or lactated Ringer's, with an initial rate sufficient to keep the vein open. Fluids must be carefully monitored, because overhydration may worsen pulmonary or cerebral edema.

Cardiac dysrhythmias are common in submersion victims, especially if the patient is hypothermic, so cardiac monitoring is mandatory. Dysrhythmias are treated according to Advanced

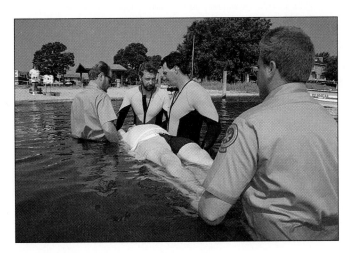

Figure 44-8

A third rescuer takes over control of the victim's head, while the other two rescuers support the board and move it to safety.

Life Support guidelines, with the exception that only one course of ACLS drugs should be administered until the patient is warmed to 92° F.

CRITICAL ISSUE

If the patient is hypothermic, defibrillation and other ACLS strategies are likely to be unsuccessful until the patient is rewarmed. Prolonged CPR may be required.

The paramedic should remove the patient's wet clothing, dry the patient, and apply blankets to reduce further heat loss and hypothermia.

As soon as air embolism is suspected, the patient should be placed in Trendelenburg's position on the left side (Fig. 44-9). This position keeps air bubbles away from the brain and coronary arteries. After 30 to 60 minutes, the patient should be placed in a neutral flat position; over time, the original head-down positioning may worsen cerebral edema.

If ear or sinus barotrauma is suspected, further medical evaluation is warranted to determine if the patient has a surgically correctable problem. All POPS patients should receive 100% oxygen and respiratory support as indicated, with the warning that positive pressure ventilation must be accompanied by careful observation for development of tension pneumothorax.

All submersion victims should be transported to the hospital for evaluation and observation because of the possibility of postimmersion syndrome. The submersion victim who is hypothermic and in cardiac arrest should be transported rapidly to the nearest appropriate facility, with advanced rewarming capabilities, such as cardiopulmonary bypass, if available.

Recompression is the mainstay of therapy for patients with DCS or air embolus. Because recompression is provided in a hyperbaric oxygen chamber, all patients with suspected DCS should be transported as quickly as possible to the closest hyperbaric facility.

If a patient must be flown to the hospital, either a helicopter or a fixed-wing aircraft is acceptable if it can be safely flown at altitudes under 1000 feet. If this is not possible, an aircraft capable of maintaining a cabin pressure of less than 1000 feet is needed; exposure to lower atmospheric pressures, such as those found in most commercial aircraft at high altitude, can precipitate or worsen DCS.

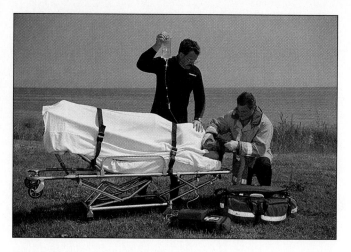

Figure 44-9

As soon as an air embolism is suspected, the patient should be placed in the Trendelenburg position on the left side.

SUMMARY

The aquatic environment is popular for work and play but is also a common source of injury. EMS personnel are often the first to respond to aquatic emergencies involving near-drowning patients, and patients with decompression sickness, barotrauma, and air embolism. This initial response can be the main factor in determining whether the patient survives neurologically intact or suffers permanent disability or death.

REFERENCES

1. **Bennett PB, Elliot DH (eds):** The physiology and medicine of diving, ed 4, London, 1993, WB Saunders.

2. **Jain KK:** Textbook of hyperbaric medicine, Toronto, 1990, Hogrefe and Huber Publishers.

3. **Nelson RN:** Drowning and near-drowning. In Nelson RN, Rund DA, Keller MD (eds): *Environmental Emergencies,* Philadelphia, 1985, WB Saunders.

4. **Olshanker JS:** Near drowning. *Emerg Med Clin North Am* 10(2):339–350, 1992.

Jeffrey T. Mitchell, PhD

Chapter 45

Behavioral Emergencies

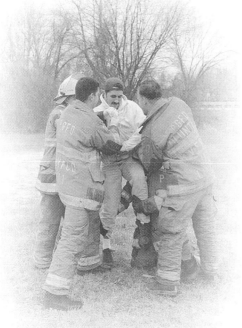

A paramedic should be able to:

1. Define the following behavioral terms and describe the characteristics and appropriate management of each:
   a. Situational crisis
   b. Maturation crisis
   c. Anxiety
   d. Psychosis
   e. Depression
   f. Manic behavior
   g. Bipolar disorder

2. Identify two conditions that are considered transient personality disorders.

3. Describe the appropriate interpersonal and intervention skills that should be utilized when assessing and managing a patient with a behavioral emergency.

4. Describe the five steps in a mental status evaluation.

5. Identify suicide risk factors using the SAD PERSONS mnemonic and describe the management of the suicidal patient.

6. Define crisis intervention and describe its four goals.

7. Discuss the impact of drug/alcohol abuse on behavioral emergencies.

8. Discuss the significance of the psychological component of illness and injury.

9. Describe the legal obligations that apply to behavioral emergencies.

1. **Affective disorders**—a class of disorders characterized by feelings, emotions, moods, and dispositions.

2. **Anxiety**—a vague, uneasy feeling, the source of which is often nonspecific and unknown to the individual.

3. **Crisis intervention**—a set of helpful techniques designed to achieve rapid intervention in a crisis with the goals of stabilizing the situation, mobilizing the resources to resolve the crisis, and restoring the person to function as quickly as possible.

4. **Delusions**—irrational beliefs contrary to reality and despite evidence and common sense.

5. **Hallucinations**—hearing, seeing, smelling, tasting, or feeling things which do not exist in reality. Hallucinations come from within a person's mind.

6. **Mental status examination**—a short assessment tool used to determine the current mental condition of a patient. It includes an assessment of the person's speech patterns, emotions, appearance, awareness (orientation), actions, or behaviors.

7. **Phobia**—a persistent irrational fear of some stimulus or of humiliation or embarrassment (as in social phobia). Exposure to the stimulus almost always provides an immediate anxiety response.

8. **Psychosis**—a mental disorder which interferes seriously with the usual functions of life.

9. **Schizophrenia**—a group of psychotic reactions characterized by fundamental disturbances in reality and concept formations and behavioral, affect and intellectual disturbances in varying degrees.

10. **Situational crisis**—an event that produces emotional distress.

It would be difficult to imagine an emergency call in which human emotions and behaviors did not play a role. They are an integral component of all human experience. The primary victims of an incident, their loved ones, bystanders, and even paramedics all are affected during emergencies. Knowledge of normal and abnormal behaviors is therefore essential for paramedics to perform optimally.

This chapter emphasizes a practical approach to understanding and managing the behaviors that paramedics are likely to encounter in the daily performance of their duties. The goals of management include facilitating control of patients exhibiting abnormal behavior, achieving an appropriate resolution, and managing any life-threatening conditions.

Pathophysiology

Human experience covers a broad scope of thoughts, feelings, and behaviors that range from normal to abnormal or psychopathological. "Normal" implies thoughts, feelings, and behaviors that promote health, happiness, and the achievement of a balanced and productive life. "Psychopathological" refers to a psychological disturbance that produces thoughts, feelings, and behaviors that are destructive to oneself or another. Box 45-1 provides an overview of the commonly encountered behavioral disorders.

Disorders

Another word that is commonly used in the psychological field is *disorder,* a broad term applied to a wide range of mental and behavioral disturbances. A disorder is best described as an emotionally painful state that causes suffering.

Anxiety

An anxiety state is one of the most common types of mental disorders. There are many anxiety states and all are characterized by high levels of worry and fear. Other symptoms include

anger, loss of self-confidence, poor self-esteem, guilt, and disturbances in interpersonal relationships. The symptoms range from mild to severe. When an anxiety state is severe, it can appear as a generalized anxiety disorder, panic attacks, a hysterical reaction, or a conversion disorder, in which a body part does not work or sensation is lost but there is no physiological cause.

CRITICAL ISSUE

Some patients with serious medical problems, such as pulmonary embolus or myocardial infarction, may present with anxiety as a manifestation of their disease.

Psychosis

The most serious psychological disturbances are called psychoses. Psychoses are less common than anxiety states and may be produced by organic (genetic or physiological) conditions, by developmental (childhood) mechanisms, or by stress. Toxicity, head trauma, and metabolic disturbances can cause or contribute to psychoses as well.

A person with psychosis typically has at least three of the following severe symptom patterns, all of which involve an impaired or distorted perception of reality. The patient may experience hallucinations, which are false perceptions that exist only in the person's mind. Hallucinations are usually auditory (e.g., hearing voices), but rarely may also be visual, olfactory, or tactile.

Psychotic people frequently experience delusions, which are false beliefs that have no foundation in fact. Examples of common delusion include the belief that one is being persecuted (paranoia) or that one is very important (grandeur).

Lastly, a significant symptom of psychosis is behavioral change. Psychotic patients exhibit unusual and bizarre behaviors that do not fit with stimuli present in the environment.

CRITICAL ISSUE

Psychotic patients have a dramatically increased potential for violence and suicide.

Psychosis may be represented in serious thought disorders, such as schizophrenia. Although there are several types of schizophrenia, all types will typically manifest the symptoms described previously to some degree. A detailed psychiatric evaluation is required to diagnose a specific subtype of schizophrenia.

Affective disorders are those that cause disturbances in a person's emotions. A frequently encountered example is psychotic depression. The patient is severely depressed and has little energy for self-care. Depressed patients are rarely dangerous to others, but they may be a threat to themselves because they cannot take proper care of themselves and become suicidal.

Manic psychosis is characterized by intense agitation, constant movement, restlessness, uncontrollable thinking,

---

BOX 45-1	Behavioral Disorders

Psychopathological Disorders
    Anxiety state
    Psychoses
        Schizophrenia
            Paranoid
            Catatonic
            Undifferentiated
        Affective
            Depressive
            Manic
Transient Personality Disorders
    Crisis
        Maturational
        Situational

rapid speech, and emotional outbursts. Angry outbursts may present a danger for paramedics; caution and slow, gentle intervention are recommended in the management of these patients.

Psychotic patients may jump back and forth between manic and depressed states. It is a common feature of the condition for the affected patient to swing from one extreme mood to the other. It generally takes several hours to several days for a patient to complete the mood swing. A patient who moves from a normal state to either a manic or a depressed state, but who only goes in one direction, is considered "unipolar." When the patient swings from normal to manic states, or from normal to depressed states, the condition is considered "bipolar."

Transient Personality Disorders

Even healthy people occasionally experience situations that negatively affect their thoughts, feelings, or behaviors. The result is an emotional crisis or transient personality disorder, which is defined as any temporary mental disturbance that occurs as a direct result of severe stress or exposure to a crisis situation. This is the most common type of mental disturbance encountered by paramedics, as every EMS call involves emotional reactions that are considered crisis events to the people experiencing them. Anyone can have a transient personality disorder at any time in life.

The onset of the crisis situation that causes a transient personality disorder is sudden. A key characteristic of people in a transient personality disorder or crisis reaction is that their reactions have a distinct starting point. They do not have any significant degree of the emotional crisis symptoms until a specific event begins. Another characteristic is that their reactions are rational given the context in which they occur; in the same situation, most people would have similar reactions.

In the majority of cases, people's reactions to crisis events are normal and are not extreme or bizarre enough as to be considered psychotic. Under the worst circumstances, an anxiety state or psychotic symptom may appear in a patient, but these usually disappear quickly once the crisis has been resolved. Recovery is expected in nearly all cases.

There are two types of crises: maturational and situational. Maturational crises include such life situations as entering puberty or reaching retirement age. Situational crises include illnesses, injuries, disasters (such as fires or floods), and exposure to grotesque experiences, such as viewing death or dismemberment. Situation crises are events outside the range of ordinary experience.

Both types of crises can produce a state of emotional disturbance or turmoil, which generally is time limited and resolves within a period of hours or days. In unusual cases, a crisis may last a few weeks. An emotional crisis can lead a person to greater growth or, if it is not managed quickly and appropriately, to permanent damage. Deterioration of the crisis state can lead to moods, thoughts, or behaviors so disordered or disturbed that patients can harm themselves or others. Posttraumatic stress disorder is example of a situation disorder that can affect paramedics (see Chapter 58).

Patients exhibit suicidal thinking or attempt suicide when they have lost hope in themselves and the future. They are in pain because of illness, the loss of a loved one by death or divorce, the breakup of a close relationship, economic hardships, failure, retirement, imprisonment, or some other painful emotional event.

Suicide remains a leading cause of death, and there has been an increasing incidence in the young and in patients with Acquired Immune Deficiency Syndrome (AIDS). Patients who have previously attempted suicide, are depressed, or are under the influence of drugs or alcohol also have a greater potential to attempt suicide. The paramedic should keep in mind that patients frequently present with a variety of nonspecific medical complaints prior to committing suicide.

Patient Assessment

People experiencing behavioral emergencies may be a danger to themselves or to others. Rapid intervention is required to lessen the danger to all involved. Thus, assessment is first directed at determining if there is a risk to the patient or others, or if the patient is disabled to the point of being unable to function independently. Examples include suicidal thoughts, severe psychosis, violent behavior, severe depression, and mental derangement so extreme that a person is incapable of self-care.

Some cases may dictate a less aggressive approach. For instance, panic attacks, intoxicated patients, situational crises, a lone person (often homeless or elderly) in need of emotional support, or mild, general anxiety, may only require reassurance and referral to friends, family or other professionals.

Initial Approach

Some of the most important work involved in managing a mental disturbance, crisis, or behavioral emergency takes place in the initial approach to the patient. The first contact is crucial and sets the tone for the remainder of the interaction with paramedics and other caregivers. First, the paramedic must be certain the surrounding scene is safe. Many patients have the potential for violence to themselves or others. The paramedic should also be aware of potential weapons, and if the patient is acting in a suspicious manner, the paramedic should wait for police assistance.

The paramedic should think first and plan out the core elements of the intervention with the patient. Teamwork makes for safety; one paramedic can survey the scene and the patient while the attending paramedic conducts the patient interview.

The patient intervention should not be rushed. The paramedic should gather as much information directly from the patient as possible. Confrontation inhibits communication and makes the patient more resistant to help, so the paramedic should avoid argumentative statements or questioning. A better approach is to acknowledge the patient's statements without agreeing with irrational thoughts. After hearing the patient out, a paramedic can sort out the details and make better sense of the situation. An interviewer is most effective when appearing to be calm, understanding, and nonjudgmental.

When communicating with a disturbed or distressed person, it is important that the paramedic use simple, concise terms to explain what is happening and what is being done to help. Comments should be explained fully and important concepts repeated as often as necessary to be sure the patient understands. The paramedic should ask open-ended questions rather than questions that require a "yes" or "no" answer. The aim is to establish rapport and get the person talking. Open-ended questions elicit a better assessment of the nature of the patient's disorder or crisis than narrow questions do.

The assessment of the emotionally distressed or disturbed patient is often further complicated by an impaired ability to cooperate in the assessment. Emotional distress may cause the patient to be upset and agitated and to disregard or misinterpret questions. For example, distressed people are often so distracted and disorganized that they are unable to give complete or accurate information about their physical condition. Assessing the person in a state of emotional crisis or mental disturbance is a significant challenge for the paramedic.

Mental Status Examination

The mental status examination is a useful interview techinique that provides insights into the nature of human thoughts and feelings. The brief examination presented here was designed for quick gathering of information about a person's emotions, thought processes, and behaviors. This examination assumes the patient's level or depth of responsiveness is awake and alert. The process is quite simple and can be employed easily by paramedics under field conditions. The five steps are: 1) observations on approach to the patient; 2) characteristics of the patient's speech; 3) characteristics of the patient's mood; 4) evaluation of the patient's thoughts; and 5) determination of the patient's orientation (Box 45-2).

BOX 45-2	Five-Step Mental Status Examination

1. Observations upon Approach
   General appearance
   Surroundings
   Posture/hand position
   Facial expressions
2. Speech Characteristics
   Rate, clarity, pitch, volume, inflection
   Rational/coherence
3. Mood
   Direct/indirect response
   Words
   Perception
4. Thought Processes
   Hallucinations
   Illusions/misinterpretations/delusions
   Suicidal ideation
   Phobias
5. Orientation
   Person, place, time, event
   Concentration
   Attentiveness
   Cooperation

- *What does the paramedic observe upon approaching the patient?* The mental status examination begins with the observations a paramedic makes upon approaching the patient. The paramedic should note the patient's general appearance: Is the patient groomed and clean or dirty with disheveled clothing? The more disordered a patient's appearance and surroundings are, the more likely it is that the patient is experiencing a behavioral emergency. The paramedic must remember to accept these observations within the general context of the overall situation.

  The patient's posture should be observed, because this often reflects the patient's emotional state. Depressed patients appear overwhelmed. Their shoulders may droop or they may move slowly and sit in a slumped position. Agitated patients may pace back and forth, wring their hands, and make hand gestures that suggest intense rage or irritability.

  Facial grimaces and violent actions may indicate a patient who is unable to control psychotic impulses. People also display emotions with facial expressions. Psychotic patients tend to manifest a "flat affect," or the inappropriate absence of emotion in facial features.
- *What are the characteristics of the patient's speech?* The manner and content of a patient's speech can be very revealing. Calm, spontaneous, controlled speech that answers questions rationally is suggestive of a healthy mind. Pressured, rapid, excessively loud speech may indicate an anxious, agitated, or even psychotic patient. Slowed, excessively soft, or slurred speech is seen with patients who have a low self-image or who are depressed. Speech that is unintelligible, made up of nonsense words, or garbled by disordered sentence structure can indicate psychosis. A psychotic patient may also display speech that conveys a rapid shifting of ideas without any association between them.
- *What is the patient's mood?* Mood is defined as a person's predominant emotional state at a specific time. Patients will often describe the mood or emotions they are experiencing and often answer questions about their mood directly. These patients may portray feelings of anger, frustration, or sadness. Indirect or evasive answers are seen in a depressed state. Important mood cues are often nonverbal; words may say one thing, but other perceptions can indicate an entirely different emotional condition. Euphoria, guilt, fear, and anger are other examples of moods.
- *What are the patient's thought processes?* Thoughts are evaluated during the mental status examination by listening carefully to determine if the thought processes are normal or abnormal. Abnormal mental states, particularly psychoses, exist when a patient has hallucinations. That means that the person sees, hears, smells, tastes, or feels things that do not exist in reality.

  Other indications of psychosis are illusions, or misinterpretations of actual stimuli in the environment, and delusions, false beliefs held despite contradictory facts. Hallucinations, delusions, and illusions are indicative of a serious disruption in a patient's thought process.

Many people are not psychotic, yet have disturbing thoughts that can cause great suffering. Suicidal thinking is one such thought process, and a phobia, a persistent fear that is excessive or unreasonable, is another.

- *What is the patient's orientation?* The fifth and final step in the mental status examination is orientation. A person oriented to person, place, time, and event is usually able to pay attention, concentrate, and cooperate with the patient care a paramedic is providing. He or she should be able to describe the individuals involved, the occurrences, the symptoms, and their intensity. Patients with obvious psychiatric illness usually are oriented, even in the face of significant hallucinations or delusions. On the other hand, patients with medical illness as a source of their hallucinations are usually not oriented. The paramedic should note if there are other mitigating factors, such as the use of alcohol. Other important considerations of the mental examination include the risk of suicide, the patient's past medical history, alcohol or drug abuse, and input from family or bystanders.

- *Are there any risk factors for suicide?* The most important facet in prehospital management of a suicidal threat is recognition. This can be difficult because patients may deny or hide their suicidal thoughts. There are high-risk factors, which can be remembered and assessed with the SAD PERSONS mnemonic. These factors have assigned point values, and are generally useful even without the scoring (Table 45-1). The number of risk factors has been found to correlate with the risk of suicide. Generally, less than six total points is considered low risk, and more than eight points indicates a patient at high risk. There is no risk in questioning suicidal thoughts, because the questions will not provoke the thought. Many patients will acknowledge that they were thinking about killing themselves, and some find it a relief to be able to talk about it.

- *What is the patient's past medical history?* Find out the characteristics of previous episodes, the frequency of occurrence, the symptoms that developed, and the patient's actions to resolve the problem. Inquiry also includes family information, history of psychiatric problems, suicides within the family, and the use of alcohol or other substances of abuse. The exact medication prescribed to a patient may hint at the specific disorder being treated and will be important in treating medication overdoses. For example, medications such as thorazine, stelazine and haloperidol are often prescribed for patients with psychosis, amitriptylene and prozac are used for depression, and lithium is given to patients with bipolar disease.

- *Is there evidence of alcohol or substance abuse?* When assessing an alcohol or substance abuse situation, it is necessary for the paramedic to know the type of substance, its dosage, and the time of injection or ingestion. Mental attitudes and motivation will often influence how a drug affects the victim. Other factors include personality, maturity level, psychological state, and history of drug use. Tolerance levels (i.e., how much of the drug it takes to get the same effect after repeated use) and the presence of contaminants may also affect the behavioral response. Alcohol tends to decrease inhibitions, possibly making intoxicated patients more likely to harm themselves or others. Once the patient is sober, the destructive behavior may disappear (*also see* Chapter 42).

- *Are bystanders or family members present?* If it is difficult for the paramedic to communicate with the patient directly, family, friends, neighbors, coworkers, or bystanders may be able to supply helpful information. Police officers and clergy personnel who may have been called to the scene prior to paramedic arrival can be consulted. Paramedics may also find other sources of patient information, including notes written by the patient.

The paramedic must remember that many medical conditions can present with altered mentation. A physical examination should be directed toward these problems (*see* Chapter 30).

CRITICAL ISSUE

Many life-threatening physical complaints can present with abnormal behavior.

Management

A patient's reaction to a crisis situation during the first 3 hours of the incident is usually characterized by a high level of anxiety, denial, and anger. Distressed people must express themselves and should be encouraged to do so as often as necessary.

The emergency team has to balance support for the person's emotions with efforts to contain and resolve the problem. The rescuer should move slowly to avoid frightening a distressed patient and establish eye contact or touch the patient to help gain rapport. Later, remorse, grief, relief, and feeling resigned to the experience are the predominant emotional reactions. People are usually calmer and easier to manage in the later phases of the crisis.

Numerous techniques can be used to manage people in crises. Reducing outside stimulus is one of the first steps. This

TABLE 45-1	Suicide Risk Factors Using the "SAD PERSONS" Mnemonic
Risk Factor	**Point Value**
S—Sex Male	1 point
A—Age < 19 or > 45	1 point
D—Depression	2 points
P—Previous suicide attempts	1 point
E—Excessive alcohol or drug use	1 point
R—Rational thinking loss (organic disease or psychosis)	2 points
S—Separated, divorced or widowed	1 point
O—Organized suicide plan, or actual life-threatening attempt	2 points
N—No social support	1 point
S—Stated future intent to repeat attempt	2 points

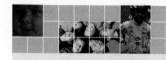

- Behavioral problems in children are usually related to pre-existing psychosocial or developmental disorders such as learning disabilities, substance abuse, emotional or sexual abuse, underachievement, depression, and attention deficit disorder.
- Temper tantrums are common in young children and are characterized by excessive screaming, kicking, or rolling around on the floor. At times, breath holding spells can occur as well.
- Children who have been involved in some sort of traumatic event often reexperience the event in the form of flashbacks or nightmares.

- Adjustment difficulties are common in children following stressful events such as death of a loved one or change of residence. Changes in mood and behavior are common symptoms.
- Unlike the adult patient, your primary evaluation should include the family as well as the child. Parents may be interviewed first so that important information and appropriate history could be obtained which would aid in the interview of the child.
- Adolescence is often a difficult period for many patients, and adolescents often consider or attempt suicide.

step can be achieved by isolating the patient from the people or events that are causing additional agitation. It is helpful to reduce noise, movement, and bright lighting, and to control environmental factors, such as heat and cold.

Specific small tasks can be delegated to family members, friends, and others who appear to be helpful, because this will mobilize the patient's resources. The presence of a loved one or a respected clergy member can do much to calm the patient.

The patient should be well informed as to what steps are being taken to manage the situation. Surprises tend to add to the chaos and cause further distress. The paramedic should offer continual reassurance of the intention to protect and not to hurt the patient.

Crisis Intervention

Crisis intervention is the immediate, active, but temporary entry into another person's or group's life situation during a period of acute stress and turmoil. People do not have to be mentally ill to benefit from crisis intervention. Because high stakes are present, such as physical or emotional deterioration as a result of stress reactions, the speed of intervention is important.

Crisis intervention has four major goals:

1. Stabilizing the situation
2. Mobilizing individual or group resources
3. Normalizing the reactions to the experience
4. Restoring the individual or group to routine functions

There are five steps in the process of achieving these goals (Box 45-3). The first step is to make psychological contact with the patient(s). The paramedic introducing himself or herself and expressing the intent to help is an example of psychological contact. Second, the dimensions of the problem must be explored by asking questions to help understand the current situation as well as relevant past history.

The third step is to examine possible solutions to the situation. The fourth step is to take concrete action. The paramedic can help the patient choose the best option for imple-

mentation. The development of this action plan gets the patient personally involved in controlling the crisis.

The fifth crisis intervention step is follow-up. It is important for the paramedic to make sure that the option chosen is working. Ultimately, the solution is likely to require transportation for definitive evaluation or release of the patient to family or friends for a less-urgent intervention.

A crisis situation is considered resolved when emotional equilibrium has been restored and the individual or group has mastered the experience and developed new coping skills. Crisis intervention prevents damage to the patient by stabilizing the situation and aims to restore patients to the highest levels of function in accordance with their capacity. This intervention is not always concluded in the prehospital setting.

Patients in crisis are part of families, organization, and communities. Therefore, it is important that crisis intervention services be provided to these key elements of a patient's environment.

Psychotic Patients

When working with psychotic patients, the paramedic must never agree with irrational, distorted thinking and must not encourage hallucination, delusion, or illusions by agreeing with the patient that these false beliefs exist. This agreement can drive the patient deeper into the psychosis. The presence of these disturbed thought patterns, especially if they are severe, indicates that the person is psychotic and requires rapid transport to a hospital for further evaluation and treatment.

BOX 45-3	**Five Steps of Crisis Intervention**

1. Establishing psychological contact
2. Exploring the dimensions of the problem
3. Examining possible solutions
4. Assisting in concrete action
5. Follow-up

Physical or chemical restraint may be necessary when a patient remains combative and threatens himself or herself or the ambulance crew (see Chapter 56). Be sure that adequate personnel are available should restraint become necessary.

Suicidal Patients

A suicidal patient should be taken seriously. Expressions of support and concern that no harm come to the patient are important. There is always a need to listen to crisis victims intently, but in suicide cases this need is heightened. The rescuer should try to build trust by moving slowly and by avoiding any attempts to hold onto the patient or use physical restraint. It is important to ask directly about suicidal thinking and planning so the patient understands that the paramedic is taking the risk seriously.

CRITICAL ISSUE

Suicidal patients may give a history "accidental" trauma or deny suicidal thoughts. If a different history is obtained from family or friends or if the suicide concern remains, the patient should be transported for further evaluation.

The paramedic must keep the suicidal patient focused on the immediate situation. If the patient's thoughts continue to wander to past troubles, he or she may become more depressed and intent on suicide. The patient's feelings can be validated by letting him or her know that having suicidal thoughts is common but acting on those thoughts is not acceptable. Many patients who are contemplating suicide have a limited range of thinking and do not see any other alternatives. The paramedic must help the patient to see that there are other possibilities for improving the situation.

Unnecessary risks should not be taken with suicidal patients. These patients can easily take helpers to their deaths, as well. All patients expressing suicidal thoughts require transport for further evaluation. A rescuer should consult with local law enforcement if a mental health "hold" is required to transport against the patient's will. Usually, the legal requirement is that a patient be a danger to himself or herself or others or be gravely disabled and unable to function independently.

Alcohol and Substance Abusers

Few factors can complicate an intervention in a behavioral situation as seriously as alcohol or substance abuse. Crises, emotional disorders, and behavioral emergencies become unpredictable in the presence of substance abuse. The potential for violence is increased, and effective management is blocked or delayed.

Intoxicated patients are prone to misinterpret the speech and actions of others, because the chemical impairment decreases their thinking ability. A misinterpretation of the rescuer's actions can lead to resisting care or to a violent outburst. It is important for the paramedic to move and talk in a slow and deliberate manner. Lowering environmental stimulus can

help the patient focus on instructions from paramedics. The rescuer should avoid making any moral judgments about the patient's lifestyle or behavior. The patient's needs should be anticipated before they become issues that disrupt the scene.

Psychological Component of Illness and Injury

Illness and injury are not only physical experiences, but they have a psychological component, as well. In fact, the psychological aspects of pain, sickness, incapacitation, and disfigurement can have a remarkably negative impact on physical illness and injury. Treatment of the whole person entails a number of important elements. The ability to communicate effectively with people is one of the most important skills, manifested by the demonstration of genuine concern, kindness, and sensitivity to the needs of others.

Sick and injured people are frightened, anxious, irritable, demanding, and emotionally needy. They need guidance, direct contact, warmth, and understanding. The challenge for the paramedic is to integrate technical skill and experience with the human elements of communication, understanding, and emotional support. Such an integration takes much practice and a considerable expenditure of energy. Adding psychological skills to technical skills humanizes both the patient and the paramedic, and both are better for the change.

Children, more than any other group of patients, have higher needs for reassurance, physical contact, reduced stimuli, alteration in wording, and orientation to place and time than adults do (see Chapter 25). Children suffer more intensely when they are in unfamiliar environments, especially when they are separated from their parents. When frightened, they may resist efforts to help.

When possible, the child should be removed from the scene and environmental stimuli should be reduced. The paramedic should speak in calm tones and use simple language. Children should be warned when a procedure is begun that the procedure may be painful. The paramedic should praise the child for being brave or cooperative. A child should never be left alone.

Being old does not always imply that a person is sick and unable to function, but many elderly patients do have medical problems and paramedics frequently come into contact with them. These patients face special problems and require special care (see Chapter 26).

The elderly are experiencing many changes. They face alterations in their physical appearances and their emotional being. They have experienced grief over the deaths of loved ones and made the adjustments required by job retirement. The elderly sometimes feel guilty over lost opportunities; many are lonely and depressed. Other elderly people suffer from anxiety and a sense of vulnerability. Elderly patients often live in fear of crime, impending death, financial problems, and the potential loss of control of physical and social capacities.

The paramedic should keep the following suggestions in mind when handling elderly patients. Family members and friends can be used to assist in communications. The patient should be touched gently; elderly patients need this direct contact. Accurate information should be provided and repeated as often as necessary. Elderly patients should not be restrained unless it is truly necessary. Family members or friends should be permitted to stay with the patient whenever possible.

Multicasualty Incidents and Disasters

Few emergency calls will be as challenging to paramedics as a multicasualty incident or a disaster. In cases such as these, every possible resource is stretched to the limit. There are several groups of people such as actual victims, community groups, disaster relief organization members, and even EMS personnel who may all be negatively affected by the incident. Disasters by nature are filled with confusion, disorganization, frustration, and a wide range of emotions.

In disasters, rescuers should remove distressed victims from the scene as soon as possible. Hysterical people should be transported early to cut down the possibility that the hysteria will spread to others. Sedation in these patients is not helpful, because it is hard to keep track of who has been medicated at a diaster and complications may arise when patients cannot be monitored effectively after being medicated.

Family members and groups that belong together should be reunited as quickly as possible. Shelter, privacy, and protection from the media should be provided for all. Frequent updates of accurate information are much more valuable to victims and those affected than are promises or false assurances.

SUMMARY

This chapter emphasizes the human elements necessary to effectively work as a paramedic and describes the various forms of emotional disorders and the appropriate management techniques for each. Paramedics are encouraged to learn behavioral patient management techniques so that they may function in the safest possible manner under field conditions.

REFERENCES

1. **American Psychiatric Association:** *Diagnostic and Statistical Manual of Mental Disorders (Third Edition - Revised) DSM-III-R,* Washington, 1987, American Psychiatric Association.

2. **Bassuk EL, Fox SS, Prendergast KJ:** *Behavioral Emergencies: a field guide for EMTs and paramedics,* Boston, 1983, Little, Brown, & Co.

3. **Guggenheim FG, Weiner MF (eds):** *Manual of Psychiatric Consultation and Emergency Care,* New York, 1984, Jason Aronson.

4. **Hafen BQ, Frandsen K:** *Psychological Emergencies and Crisis Intervention: a comprehensive guide for emergency personnel,* Englewood, 1985, Morton Publishing.

5. **Heckman JD(ed):** *Emergency Care and Transportation of the Sick and Injured,* ed 5, Park Ridge, 1992, American Academy of Orthopaedic Surgeons.

6. **Henry MC, Stapleton ER:** *EMT Prehospital Care,* Philadelphia, 1992, WB Saunders.

7. **Jones SA, Weigel A, White RD, McSwain NE, Breiter M (eds):** *Advanced Emergency Care for Paramedic Practice,* Philadelphia, 1992, JB Lippincott.

8. **Mitchell JT, Resnik HLP:** *Emergency Response to Crisis, a crisis intervention guidebook for emergency service personnel,* Ellicott City, 1981, Chevron Publishing.

9. **Salby AE, Lieb J, Trancredi LR:** *Handbook of psychiatric emergencies, second edition,* Garden City, 1981, Medical Examination Publishing.

10. **Slaikeu KA:** *Crisis Intervention: a handbook for practice and research,* Boston, 1984, Allyn & Bacon.

11. **Wolman BB:** *Dictionary of Behavioral Science,* New York, 1973, Van Nostrand Reinhold.

Section

Patient Presentations—Trauma

4B

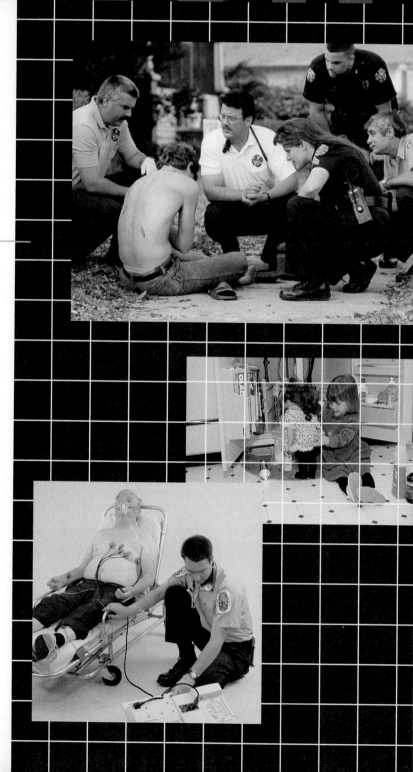

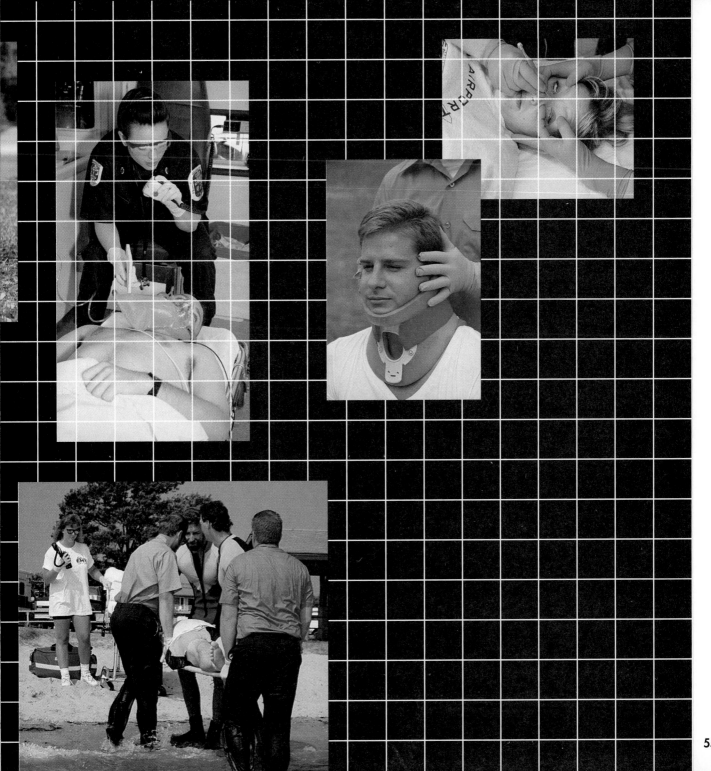

Richard Wolfe, MD, FACEP

Chapter 46
Truncal Trauma

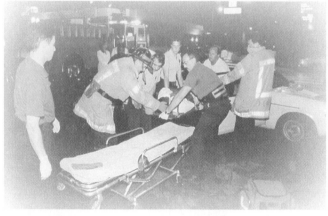

A paramedic should be able to:

OBJECTIVES

1. Describe anatomy of the chest and abdomen, including organs located in each area.

2. Describe and discuss mechanism of injury and potential organ damage for blunt and penetrating trauma.

3. Explain the significance of mechanism of injury in truncal trauma.

4. Describe the prehospital management of patients with truncal trauma, and identify the most important aspect of that management.

5. Describe the appropriate assessment of the chest and abdomen in a patient with truncal trauma.

6. Describe the correct procedure for chest decompression.

7. Describe the pathophysiology of the types of shock seen in truncal trauma and the appropriate field management of each type.

8. List five findings from recent studies regarding PASG use in the prehospital setting.

9. List the signs and symptoms, potential problems, and field management for the following:
   - a. Impaled objects
   - b. Open pneumothorax (sucking chest wound)
   - c. Flail chest
   - d. Pulmonary contusion
   - e. Evisceration
   - f. Suspected abdominal injury
   - g. Pneumothorax
   - h. Tension pneumothorax
   - i. Cardiac tamponade
   - j. Myocardial contusion

10. Define the following terms:
   - a. Mediastinum
   - b. Pleural space
   - c. Peritoneum
   - d. Deceleration injury
   - e. Pneumothorax
   - f. Flail chest
   - g. Evisceration
   - h. Hemothorax

KEY TERMS

1. **Deceleration injury**—Injuries that occur after falls from significant height or ejection from vehicles.

2. **Evisceration**—The protrusion of an internal organ through a wound or surgical incision, especially in the abdominal wall.

3. **Flail chest**—A thorax in which multiple rib fractures cause instability in part of the chest wall and paradoxical breathing, with the lung underlying the injured area contracting on inspiration and bulging on expiration.

4. **Hemothorax**—An accumulation of blood and fluid in the pleural cavity, between the parietal and visceral pleura, usually the result of trauma.

5. **Mediastinum**—A portion of the thoracic cavity in the middle of the thorax, between the sternum to the vertebral column and contains all the thoracic viscera except the lungs.

6. **Peritoneum**—An extensive serous membrane that covers the entire abdominal wall of the body and is reflected over the contained viscera.

7. **Pleural space**—The potential space between the visceral and parietal layers of the pleurae.

8. **Pneumothorax**—A collection of air or gas in the pleural space that causes the lung to collapse.

Truncal trauma, which means injuries to the organs or tissues in the chest or abdomen, is a leading cause of death for persons less than 40 years of age. Chest injuries are responsible for 25% of the 100,000 annual deaths from trauma in the United States.[7]

Anatomy

The trunk consists of two compartments, the chest and the abdomen. The chest is further separated into two parts: a central area, the mediastinum, which contains the heart, the esophagus, and the large blood vessels; and laterally, the lungs, which adhere to the chest wall because of the negative pressure in the pleural space (Fig. 46-1).

The abdomen is separated by the peritoneum into two areas: an intraperitoneal cavity, which contains the liver, spleen, and intestines; and posteriorly, the retroperitoneum, which contains the kidneys, bladder, and pancreas. The intraperitoneal cavity is spacious. Uncontrolled bleeding in this area requires prompt surgical intervention.

Determining the location of truncal injuries is important in determining hospital procedures and the need for surgery, but less critical in the prehospital setting. The diaphragm does little to prevent transmission of injury from one area to the other, so it will often be difficult to pinpoint injured organs. Fortunately, treatment does not depend on exact diagnosis. Rapid transport, intravenous access, and oxygen are needed for all truncal injuries, regardless of their location.

Mechanism of Injury

Mechanism of injury is one of the most important factors in determining the risk and type of truncal organ damage (Table 46-1). All information pertaining to the mechanism of injury should be described to the trauma team on arrival at the hospital. This information plays a critical role in determining the need for hospitalization and diagnostic procedures. Inadequate communication frequently results in poor patient care.

Blunt trauma is made up of a combination of crushing, stretching, and shearing that causes injury when forces are great enough to disrupt the strength and mobility of truncal organs. Penetrating trauma, on the other hand, injects energy along and around the path of the penetrating object, resulting in tearing and bruising of the tissue (Fig. 46-2).

Deceleration injuries occur after falls from significant height or ejection from vehicles. Large vessels such as the thoracic aorta or renal pedicle (stem), which are fixed in place at one point of their anatomy but mobile at others, will tear when the mobile portion moves following an impact.[4] Although most patients with a torn aorta die at the accident scene (Fig. 46-3), the adventitia (thin fibrous tissue surrounding the aorta) will temporarily hold the aorta together in approximately 15% of cases. With prompt surgical intervention, many of these patients can be saved.[6,16]

Occasionally, patient instability prevents a comprehensive history or a detailed picture of the mechanism of injury. In these cases, the paramedic must perform a rapid assessment and transport the patient. The life-threat survey should be performed in less than 1 minute and should provide enough information to determine the need for an endotracheal tube, the number of intravenous lines required, and, rarely, whether needle decompression of a tension pneumothorax is indicated.

Patient Assessment and Management

Truncal trauma is a true indication for rapid transport and intervention. The time saved in the field is a key factor in reaching an early diagnosis in the emergency department, reducing the interval between injury and the operating room, and decreasing overall mortality. During this first critical stage, the paramedic must record the mechanism of injury, detect life threats, and stabilize the patient for transport.

Whenever possible, field interventions should be performed during transport to minimize time on the scene. The decision to manage the airway should not be based on chest or abdominal findings, but more on the patient's overall condition: inability either to protect the airway or oxygenate adequately. Endotracheal intubation is not always a safe procedure in the setting of truncal trauma. Intubating a patient with a pneumothorax may rapidly convert a "stable" injury into a critical problem; the positive pressure delivered by bagging may push air into the pleural space. This may lead to tension pneumothorax, shock, and cardiac arrest if the pressure is not relieved by venting the chest.

Once the problem of the airway has been addressed, assessment of breathing and circulation should be performed. Breathing is assessed by looking at the chest, palpating the chest wall, and listening for breath sounds.

TABLE 46-1	Mechanism and Specific Organ Injury
Mechanism	**Organ Injury**
Blunt Trauma	
Crushed steering wheel	Rib fractures, flail chest, myocardial contusion, spleen and liver injuries
Ejection	Shearing of thoracic aorta, renal pedicle
Lap belt	Bowel perforation
Car wall intrustion	Rib fractures; spleen, liver and kidney injuries
Penetrating Trauma	
Upper chest	Hemopneumothorax, cardiac tamponade, large vessel injury
Lower chest	Hemopneumothorax, cardiac tamponade, diaphragm, intraabdominal injury
Right upper quadrant	Liver, right kidney, diaphragm, gallbladder
Left upper quadrant	Diaphragm, stomach, left kidney, spleen, pancreas

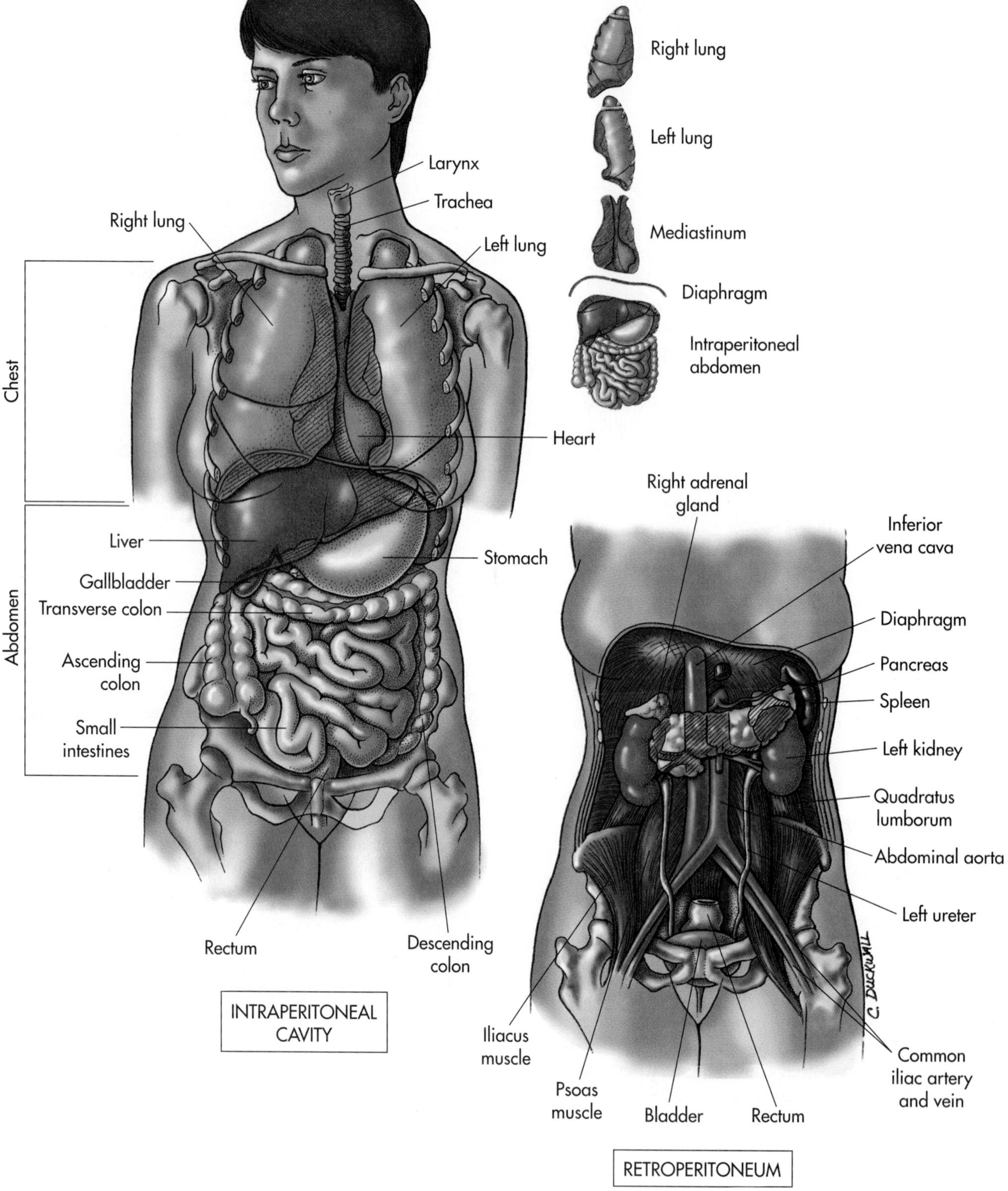

Right lung

Left lung

Mediastinum

Diaphragm

Intraperitoneal abdomen

Larynx

Trachea

Left lung

Right lung

Chest

Abdomen

Heart

Liver

Stomach

Gallbladder

Transverse colon

Ascending colon

Small intestines

Rectum

Descending colon

INTRAPERITONEAL CAVITY

Right adrenal gland

Inferior vena cava

Diaphragm

Pancreas

Spleen

Left kidney

Quadratus lumborum

Abdominal aorta

Left ureter

Common iliac artery and vein

Iliacus muscle

Psoas muscle

Bladder

Rectum

RETROPERITONEUM

C. DUCKWALL

Figure 46-1

The anatomy of the anterior and posterior cavities of the trunk.

Inspection of the Abdomen and Chest

Impaled Objects

If an impaled object remains in the patient's chest or abdomen, it is best removed in the operating room. Penetrating objects still in place can tamponade a major artery and, if removed prematurely, result in massive bleeding at the scene (Fig. 46-4). Leaving the object in place is also helpful to surgeons who must determine the potential depth of the damage. Field removal should only be performed with medical direction, when the object prevents extrication and resuscitation.

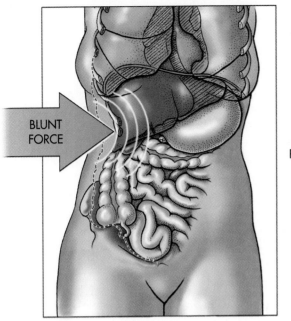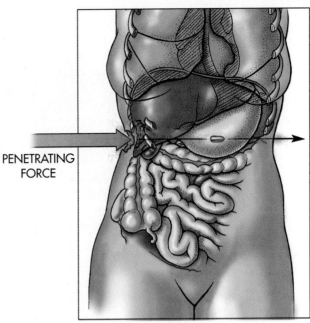

BLUNT FORCE

PENETRATING FORCE

Figure 46-2

Energy dissipation in blunt vs. penetrating trauma.

Penetrating Wounds

As soon as possible, the patient should be fully exposed and the chest and abdomen carefully inspected for wounds. When time and stability permit, the underarms, back, and flanks should also be examined. Only the most careful inspection will provide complete information. Certain injuries can be difficult to locate, such as ice pick wounds that may be the size of a pinprick. If possible, the patient should be rolled to inspect the back for injuries. The number of wounds should be recorded, especially if gunshot wounds are suspected.

If a wound is bleeding, apply direct pressure to control hemorrhage and to prevent air from entering a vein and causing an air embolus. Blood loss at the scene and in the ambulance should be estimated. Even if inaccurate, this estimate will help in determining the need for blood transfusion.

Open Pneumothorax

Wounds that violate the pleural space may appear to leak air during expiration or suck air on inspiration. These "sucking chest wounds" imply a serious underlying injury: an open pneumothorax (Fig. 46-5). Sucking chest wounds occur when the opening in the chest wall is greater than two thirds the diameter of the trachea; air then passes more easily through the chest wall than through the patient's airway. To counteract this air leak, chest wounds should be dressed with a Vaseline-type gauze taped on three sides, leaving the fourth side open. Although an open pneumothorax is not an immediate life threat, air trapping may lead to high pressure in the pleural space if all four sides of the dressing are taped. This is a life threat known as tension pneumothorax. The high pressure prevents the return of venous blood to the heart, causing shock and ultimately cardiac arrest. If a patient deteriorates after a dressing is applied over a sucking chest wound, remove the dressing immediately.

Flail Chest and Pulmonary Contusions

Observation of ventilation in blunt thoracic trauma may reveal a segment of the chest wall that paradoxically moves inward with inspiration and outward with expiration. This is **flail chest**, which occurs when one segment of the chest is broken off from the thoracic cage (Fig. 46-6). This is caused by multiple **rib fractures** or a combination of rib fractures and costal cartilage dislocations. Flail chests have traditionally been stabilized by placing sandbags against the injury or positioning the patient with the injured side down.[3] Although this is probably not harmful, there is little to suggest that external stabilization offers any benefit. The primary treatment is to ensure adequate oxygenation. Flail chest does not mandate intubation unless supplemental oxygen by itself fails to provide adequate oxygenation.

Pulmonary contusions can cause such oxygenation problems and are a common, potentially lethal complication associated with flail chest. Following a traumatic event, shearing forces can cause a disruption of the alveolar-capillary membrane and bleeding into the alveolar space (Fig. 46-7). This can also occur without rib fractures and is common following the blast effect of a gunshot wound. Pulmonary contusions progressively impair the lung's ability to exchange oxygen and carbon dioxide. The condition is similar to a severe, localized pulmonary edema. As the injury progresses, a patient with pulmonary contusions may require endotracheal intubation and mechanical ventilation to maintain minimal oxygen requirements. Although intubation is not always indicated, it should be strongly considered in the presence of shock, more than three major injuries, or cyanosis during administration of 100% oxygen. Because aspiration dramatically increases mortality in patients with pulmonary contusions, airway protection is mandatory in patients with altered mentation.

A

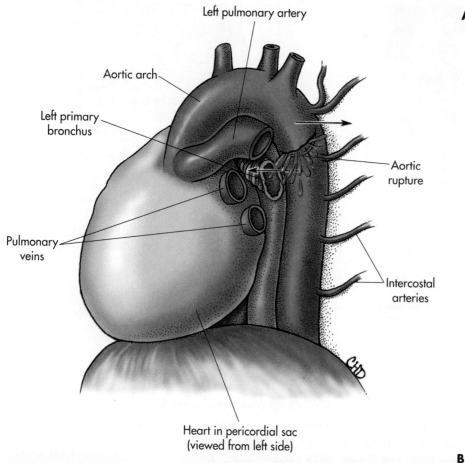

Left pulmonary artery

Aortic arch

Left primary
bronchus

Aortic
rupture

Pulmonary
veins

Intercostal
arteries

Heart in pericordial sac
(viewed from left side)

B

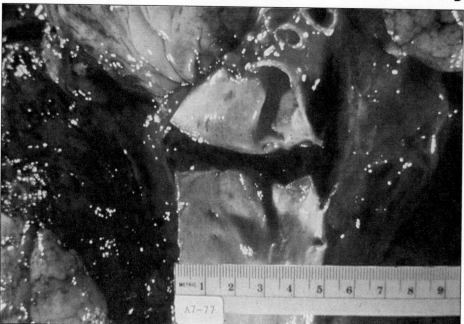

Figure 46-3

A, Aortic rupture is often seen following
deceleration injuries, The injury results
from the pulling of the structure away
from its support tissues. B, Aorta with a
tear at the junction of the arch and descending aorta. From PHTLS: Basic and
Advanced Prehospital Trauma Life Support, ed 3, 1994, Mosby Lifeline.

Evisceration

Open wounds of the abdomen may cause evisceration of
peritoneal contents such as bowel. Eviscerated abdominal contents should be covered with a moist saline gauze to prevent
further contamination and drying. Attempts should not be
made to push eviscerated organs back into the peritoneal cav-

ity; this will increase the risk of infection and complicate surgical evaluation of the injury.

A distended abdomen may be noted in patients with massive peritoneal hemorrhage, but this finding is unreliable. It is
commonly absent with serious injury, and its presence may
also be due to bowel gas, obesity, or ascites (serous fluid accumulation caused by disease).

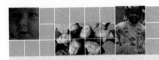

- Approximately 90% of all cases of thoracic trauma in children are associated with blunt trauma (falls, MVA, etc.). On the other hand, penetrating trauma is less common but is on the rise.
- The child's chest wall is more flexible and compliant than that of adults and thus allows transfer of energy from blunt trauma to the internal organs, often without any signs of surface injuries. Pulmonary and cardiac contusions can occur without external signs.
- The liver and spleen are the most common abdominal organs damaged in the child with thoracic or abdominal trauma. The intestines may be damaged from deceleration injuries when a lap belt is worn. Internal bleeding should be suspected in any child with blunt or penetrating thoracic trauma.
- The most difficult task to perform in a child with thoracic trauma most likely will be the assessment of the severity of the injury. Depending on their age, children cannot accurately give specifics regarding the injury and certain key signs or symptoms. The child may also be afraid of impending harm if they say that something hurts or frightened that they may be in trouble for doing something wrong.

"Guarding" of the injured site is a helpful clue in a child with suspected thoracic or abdominal trauma. Some other signs and symptoms include agitation, lethargy, tachycardia, tachypnea, diaphoresis, and signs of decreased perfusion. Instability may present rapidly (severe hemorrhage) or slowly (peritonitis). The child should be observed carefully because the initial exam may be unremarkable except for the mechanism of injury. If possible, measure the girth of the abdomen, because periodic measurements may show distention that may be caused by hemorrhage.

- The elasticity of the chest wall and the mobility of mediastinal structures in the pediatric patient results in a different clinical presentation of a tension pneumothorax. Diminished breath sounds may be heard bilaterally, and tracheal deviation and jugular venous distention may be absent.
- Traumatic asphyxia can occur from a crush injury and presents with petechiae and a bluish discoloration of the skin of the upper chest and face. This can be confused with cyanosis from other causes.

REFERENCES

1. Aoki, BY, McCloskey, K. Evaluation, stabilization, and transport of the critically ill child, ed 1. St. Louis, 1992, Mosby-Year Book, Inc.

2. Nichols, D. Et al. Golden hour. The handbook of advanced pediatric life support, ed 1., St. Louis, 1991, Mosby-Year book, Inc.

3. Silverman, BK. APLS: the pediatric emergency medicine course, ed 2. American Academy of Pediatrics and American College of Emergency Physicians.

Palpation of the Chest and Abdomen

Palpation of the chest wall is a reliable method of detecting chest injuries. A flail chest missed on inspection may be detected by feeling the paradoxical motion of the chest wall and the bony crepitus of fractured ribs. If the pleural space has been disrupted, air will leak into subcutaneous tissue of the chest and the examiner will feel air bubbles under the skin. Subcutaneous air strongly suggests a pneumothorax or, more rarely, mediastinal air from an injury to the tracheobronchial tree or the esophagus. When present in a prearrest patient, needle decompression of the chest should be considered.

When abdominal injury occurs in blunt trauma, the spleen is the most common organ injured, followed by the liver. Thus, palpation of the abdomen may reveal tenderness in the upper quadrants. Intraperitoneal hemorrhage will irritate the peritoneum, causing rebound tenderness and guarding. Either

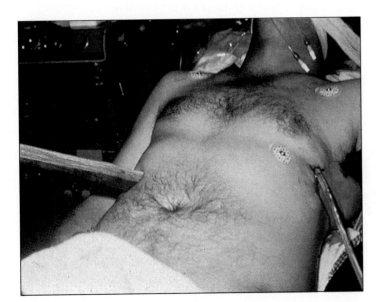

Figure 46-4

This impaled wooden spike brought clothing into the wound as it entered the body. The diaphragm was pierced and the liver, stomach, and spleen were torn. The patient recovered following appropriate EMS care and surgical intervention. From London: A Colour Atlas of Diagnosis After Recent Injury, 1990, Wolfe Medical Publications.

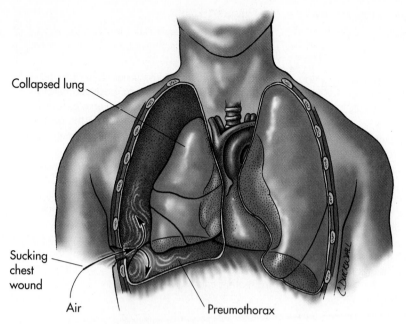

Collapsed lung

Sucking chest wound

Air

Preumothorax

Figure 46-5

An open pneumothorax, also called a "sucking chest wound," requires rapid treatment aimed at sealing the wound. If all four sides are sealed, a tension pneumothorax could develop.

abdominal tenderness or peritoneal irritation is present in 90% of patients with intra-abdominal injury, though either may be masked by alcohol or head trauma.[2]

Auscultation of the Chest and Abdomen

Unilateral Loss of Breath Sounds

A patient may develop decreased breath sounds following a traumatic event. If the patient has been intubated and left breath sounds are absent, the endotracheal tube may be lodged in the right main stem bronchus. Checking the endotracheal tube to see if it is deeper than 24 centimeters at the incisors is a reliable method of detecting bronchial tube placement.

Pneumothorax

Unilateral loss of breath sounds otherwise suggests a pneumothorax. The pleura normally allow the lungs to expand throughout the entire chest cavity and yet slide on the inner chest wall. The parietal and visceral sheaths of the pleura are held together by negative pressure, much like two panes of wet glass stuck together. If this space is torn and exposed to air by a broken rib, a bullet, or a knife, for instance, air will rush into this space and cause the lungs to "collapse" in the chest cavity (Fig. 46-8). The collapsed lung will not exchange oxygen well, but the other will remain functional. Patients with a "simple" pneumothorax usually remain stable. If air is trapped in the pleural space by a one-way valve system, high pressures can develop and cause a complete collapse of the lung and compression of the heart. Cardiac compression leads to diminished venous return, shock, and eventually death without prompt intervention (Fig. 46-9).

Intubated pneumothorax patients are at risk for a tension pneumothorax because ventilation through an endotracheal tube delivers pressure which can cause a dramatic rise in air flow to the disrupted pleural space. Patients who require air

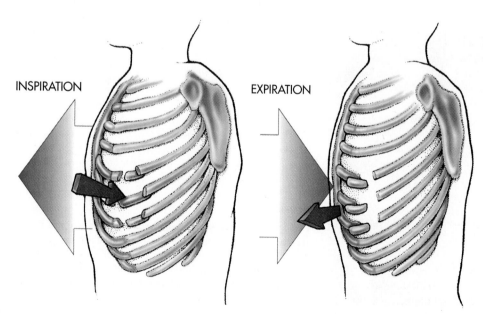

INSPIRATION

EXPIRATION

Figure 46-6

A flail chest has an unstable segment of fractured ribs or dislocated cartilage, which has lost the attachment to the rib cage. These segments will exhibit a paradoxical movement (opposite to the rest of the rib cage), during deep inspiration or exhalation.

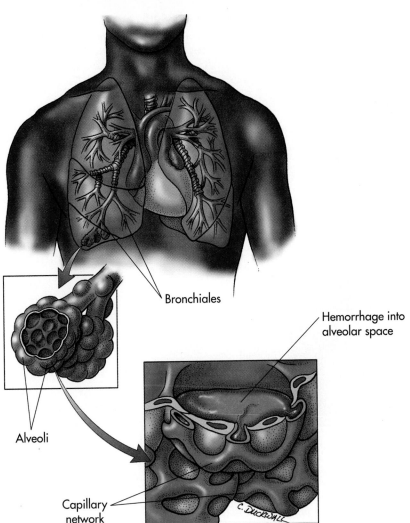

Bronchiales

Hemorrhage into
alveolar space

Alveoli

Capillary
network

C. DUCKWALL

Figure 46-7

A contused lung results from bleeding between the
alveolar-capillary membrane. Dyspnea results from
blood collecting in the airways.

transport are also at risk because the change in altitude causes an expansion of the gas trapped in the pleural space.

Tension pneumothorax is rarer and more difficult to diagnose than simple pneumothorax, which usually need not be treated in the field. A simple pneumothorax will cause decreased breath sounds, chest pain, subcutaneous air and some degree of air hunger, but the patient's vital signs will remain stable. On the other hand, a tension pneumothorax is associated with respiratory and cardiovascular collapse. The patient may present with a hyperexpanded chest and distended neck veins, although the latter may be absent if significant blood loss has also occurred. Often described as a classical sign, tracheal deviation occurs only rarely after severe hemodynamic compromise.[8]

Auscultation of the abdomen provides little information. Bowel sounds are absent in 65% to 93% of internal organ injuries but are unreliable in separating patients with and without injury.[12]

Needle Decompression

Needle decompression of the chest should be restricted to rapidly deteriorating patients. The second intercostal space, the midclavicular line, is a common site for needle decompression of the chest. However, the difficulty of correct inser-

tion through the pectoralis major and the risk of injury to the internal mammary artery suggest that the 4th or 5th intercostal space, the anterior axillary line (just posterior to the lateral edge of the pectoralis muscle), may be a better site. The 5th intercostal space is at the nipple line in men and at the margin of the breast in women.

After appropriately prepping the skin at the selected site, a large bore (14-gauge) needle is inserted through the chest wall into the pleural space. If a tension pneumothorax is present, a rush of air through the venting needle will be noted.

Needle thoracostomy is an invasive procedure that carries significant risks. If a pneumothorax is not present, opening the pleural space with a needle will complicate the patients's condition by causing a pneumothorax in 10% to 20% of cases.[11] Placing the needle too high or too anterior in the chest may injure a vessel (subclavian artery or vein) or the heart. Attempts to vent the chest below the 5th intercostal space may result in trauma to the liver or the spleen.

Cardiac Auscultation

Auscultation of the heart may on rare occasion, reveal muffled heart tones, leading one to suspect **pericardial tamponade**. This finding does not require any change in field management other than rapid transport.

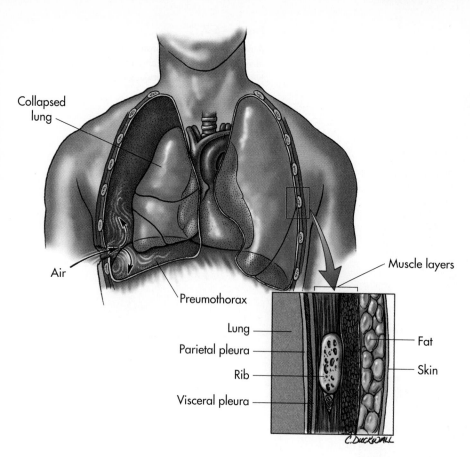

Figure 46-8

A pneumothorax results when lung tissue collapses from injury or disease.

Collapsed
lung

Air

Preumothorax

Lung

Parietal pleura

Rib

Visceral pleura

Muscle layers

Fat

Skin

C. DUCKWALL

Shock

Evaluation of circulation involves assessing vital signs, jugular veins, and skin temperature, to estimate cardiac output and blood volume.

Shock associated with truncal trauma is a complex problem. The most common cause of shock is hypovolemia, but all types of shock may be seen (Box 46-1). Clinically, the different classes of shock can be distinguished by the physical examination. One of the most helpful tests is feeling the skin of the extremities. Warm, flushed skin with shock is helpful in identifying vasogenic causes such as spinal shock. Cool skin and prominent jugular vein distention suggest cardiogenic and mechanical causes. Cool skin and flat jugular veins suggest hy-

povolemia. Regardless of the type of shock, field management should focus on establishing large bore intravenous lines and beginning volume resuscitation.

Hypovolemic Shock

Hypovolemic shock may occur secondary to bleeding in the chest (hemothorax), the peritoneum (most often involving the spleen or liver), or the retroperitoneum (after a major pelvic fracture). Massive hemothorax is defined as a blood loss greater than 1500 mL. Resuscitation with crystalloid fluid in the field, and early blood transfusion in the emergency department, are the mainstays of therapy. The definitive treatment of shock from intraperitoneal injury is surgery. Thus, short scene and transport times are the keys to improving survival in hypovolemic trauma patients. Intravenous lines should be started during transport.

Massive pelvic fractures may cause considerable bleeding. If instability is noted with pelvic compression in an unstable patient, consider placing and inflating the pneumatic anti-shock garment (PASG) to stabilize the fracture.

Cardiogenic Shock

Cardiogenic shock may be due to pump failure (cardiac tamponade or myocardial contusion) or mechanical obstruction (tension pneumothorax or air embolism). However, this difference has little relevance in the prehospital setting. Other than a rare indication for needle decompression of a suspected tension pneumothorax, field management should focus on fluid resuscitation and rapid transport.

BOX 46-1	Traumatic Causes of Shock

Hypovolemic
    Hemothorax
    Thoracic Aortic Injury
    Intraperitoneal Hemorrhage
    Retroperitoneal Hemorrhage
Cardiogenic
    Cardiac Tamponade
    Myocardial Contusion
Mechanical
    Tension Pneumothorax
    Air Embolism
Vasogenic
    Spinal Cord Injury (Cervical or Thoracic)

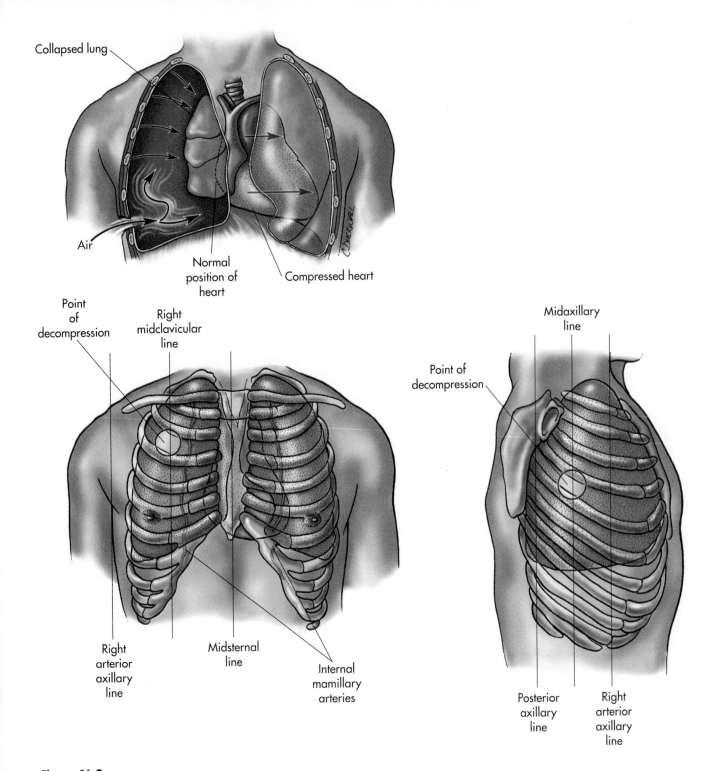

Figure 46-9

As a pneumothorax worsens and a tension pneumothorax develops, a life-threatening situation develops. Pleural decompression evacuates the build-up of air, allowing the compressed heart, uninjured lung, and mediastinum to return to their normal positions. Respirations and circulation should improve dramatically following this procedure.

Acute pericardial tamponade occurs in approximately 2% of penetrating chest trauma; it is more common with stab wounds than gunshots.[14] Tamponade after blunt trauma is extremely rare and usually due to a tear in the right atrial wall. If a myocardial rupture is contained within the pericardium, tamponade will occur (Fig. 46-10). The pericardium is minimally distensible; small amounts of blood can cause large rises in pressure, decreased venous return and shock.

by George M. Stohr, BS

In 1903, George Washington Crile introduced the predecessor to modern day PASG during his efforts to control hypotension in patients requiring surgery in a sitting position.[1] Although he was successful at maintaining blood pressure, he had to abandon his work for practical reasons, long before any studies to verify the garment's effectiveness. Although he was unable to design a suit capable of maintaining a desired volume of air, his work did inspire later researchers. The "G-Suit," developed during World War II, prevented syncopal episodes in fighter pilots exposed to extreme gravity forces. During the Vietnam War, the concept was modified further. Physicians hoped that autotransfusion would increase the survival rate among wounded soldiers during helicopter evacuations by increasing blood pressure and perfusion to the head and torso.[2]

Though the concept behind PASG was certainly a logical one, no controlled studies were conducted on the device prior to its use in Vietnam. Using Bernouilli's Equation, researchers hypothesized that a change in pressure in the lower extremities would result in autotransfusion of blood to the head and torso.[3] Using the same equation, they theorized that the applied pressure would also result in a decrease in the size of any laceration under the garment, and ultimately a reduction in the rate of bleeding from the wound. Based on such reasoning, PASGs were first used by civilians in 1973 by the Miami Fire Department. Just prior to their civilian use, one study said that the suit ". . .may be helpful in providing temporary cardiovascular support while other conventional means of rescue are begun. . ."[5]

It was not until 1984 that the first controlled study was done to compare PASG versus non–PASG groups in the prehospital setting.[6] When blood pressure, trauma score, and mortality were measured, no significant differences were found between the PASG group and those treated using only conventional methods. The study concluded that "the cost, potential disadvantages, and absence of additional benefit derived from PASG use suggest that the general use of external counterpressure garments is unwarranted in a short transport time."[6]

In the late 1980s, researchers began studying both the advantages and potential drawbacks of PASG.[7] Contrary to the original belief, changes in blood pressure were attributed to an increase in systemic vascular resistance in the lower extremities rather than an autotransfusion of blood. In fact, less than 5% of the circulating blood volume is actually displaced by the application of external pressure.[8] And while PASGs were seen to raise blood pressure,[9] but is a higher blood pressure necessarily better for a trauma patient? If the brain and heart are receiving a sufficient supply of oxygen, would raising the blood pressure too much result in an increased rate of blood loss?

Studies on the effectiveness of PASGs are contradictory and some indicate no benefit.[10] In one study, certain conclusions regarding the use of PASGs in penetrating traumatic injuries were evident: 1) PASG application did not increase the length of total prehospital time; 2) PASG application did increase the

blood pressure; 3) PASG application did not decrease the length of time in the emergency department, operating room or hospital; 4) When PASG was applied, an overall increased mortality was seen for all patients; 5) Patients with prehospital time of greater than 30 minutes and PASG application did not have a better survival rate; 6) Patients with thoracic injury had a greater chance of dying before arriving at the hospital if PASG was applied; 7) Patients with major abdominal injury did not have an overall better survival rate nor did they have a better chance of seeing a trauma surgeon.[11]

A 1991 study found that there was no statistically significant difference in survival rates between PASG and non–PASG groups, in patients presenting with shock secondary to blunt trauma.[12] All patients in the study had a prehospital time of under thirty minutes. Since such a time frame is quite common in most urban and many suburban areas, these results indicate the need for more research into the effectiveness and possible limitations of PASG.

REFERENCES

1. Gardner WJ, Dohn DF: The antigravity suit (G-suit) in surgery. *JAMA* 162(4):274–276, 1956.

2. Cutler BS, Daggett WM: Application of the G-suit to the control of hemorrhage in massive trauma. *Ann of Surg,* 173(4):511–514, 1971.

3. Soler J, Muller HA, Kennedy TJ: Clinical use of the G-suit. *J Am Coll Emerg Phys,* 5(8):609–611, 1976.

4. Kaplan BC, Civetta JM, Nagel EL, *et al*: The military antishock trouser in civilian prehospital emergency care. *J Traum,* 13(10):843–848, 1973.

5. MacKersie RC, Christensen JM, Lewis FR: The prehospital use of external counterpressure: does MAST make a difference? *J Traum,* 24(10):882–888, 1984.

6. Clark DE, Demers ML: Lower body positive pressure. *Surg Gynecol Obstet,* 168:81–97, 1989.

7. Bivins HG, Knopp R, Tiernan C, *et al*: Blood volume displacement with inflation of antishock trousers. *Ann Emerg Med,* 11:409–412, 1982.

8. McSwain NE: PASG: state of the art. *Ann Emerg Med,* 17:506–525, 1988.

9. Mattox KL, Bickell WH, Pepe PE, *et al*: Prospective randomized evaluation of antishock MAST in post-traumatic hypotension. *J Traum,* 26(9):779–786, 1986.

10. Mattox KL, Bickell W, Pepe PE, *et al*: Prospective MAST study in 9-1-1 patients. *J Traum,* 29(8):1104–1112, 1989.

11. Berendt BM: A study of MAST in injured patients presenting in shock (master's dissertation). New York Medical College, Valhalla, 1991.

12. Schneider PA, Mitchell JM, Allison EJ, Jr.: The use of military antishock trousers in trauma. *J Emerg Med,* 7:497–500, 1989.

Diagnosis of cardiac tamponade is difficult. Distended neck veins, decreased arterial pressure and muffled heart sounds (Beck's triad—the classical findings of cardiac tamponade) are present in only one third of patients.[15] However, reporting the occurrence of any hypotensive episode in the field will suggest procedures to the hospital team that may lead to the diagnosis before the patient decompensates. Atrial rupture from blunt trauma, as opposed to ventricular rupture, is a sal-

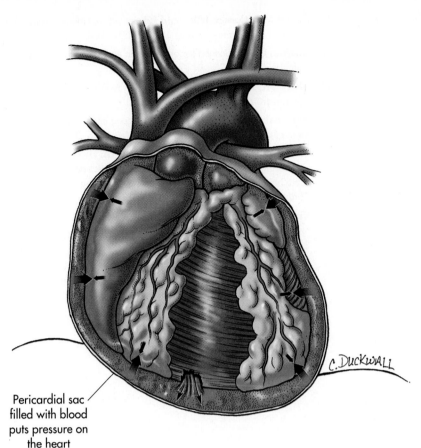

Figure 46-10
Pericardial tamponade results from a collection of blood in the pericardial sac which leads to compression of the heart muscle and ineffective pumping.

Pericardial sac filled with blood puts pressure on the heart

C. DUCKWALL

vageable injury. Rapid transport to the emergency department in any patient with blunt or penetrating trauma who arrests during the prehospital course is critical; emergency thoracotomy (chest surgery) may be life saving. On the other hand, if a trauma victim is in full cardiac arrest on initial presentation, there is little chance that thoracotomy will be successful.[5,13]

Myocardial contusion will usually present with tachycardia and electrocardiographic changes. Close attention should be paid to the cardiac monitor and dysrhythmias. Patients suspected of having a myocardial contusion should be monitored carefully.

Air embolism should be considered when a patient experiences sudden deterioration, particularly following penetrating chest trauma. This occurs when a large air bubble enters the venous circulation after an injury to a pulmonary or systemic vein. Air entering the heart through an injury to a central systemic vein will lodge in the right ventricle and prevent the heart from pumping effectively. It is difficult to distinguish air embolism from other causes of cardiogenic and mechanical shock. When air embolism is suspected, the patient should be placed on 100% oxygen and attempts should be made to trap the bubble in the right apex of the heart by having the patient lie in a Trendelenburg position on the left side.[17]

Controversies in Shock Management

The PASG has not been shown to be beneficial in controlling shock in trauma patients, and some studies have suggested that they may be detrimental, especially in patients with chest trauma.[9] Prehospital fluid resuscitation is also controversial, particularly in patients with penetrating chest injuries.[7] However, intravenous access should be obtained rapidly in the field as it is of significant benefit to subsequent care.[10]

SUMMARY

With aggressive stabilization and rapid transport, prehospital management of truncal trauma may decrease the mortality and morbidity of trauma patients. Field personnel must be knowledgeable in detecting life-threatening conditions, such as tension pneumothorax, and possess the technical skills to address reversible life threats. Prolonged scene times and failure to appreciate the severity of injury are the main pitfalls to be avoided.

REFERENCES

1. **Center for Disease Control and Prevention:** Premature mortality in the United States. *MMWR Suppl* 1986, 35:1s–11s.

2. **Colucciello SA:** Blunt abdominal trauma. *Emerg Med Clin North Am* 1993; 11(1):107–123.

3. **Corso PJ:** Chest Trauma. *Prim Care* 1978; 5:543.

4. **Dougall AM, Paul ME, Finley RJ, et al:** Chest trauma—current morbidity and mortality. *J Traum* 1977; 17:574–553.

5. **Markovchick VJ, et al:** Traumatic acute pericardial tamponade. *Ann Emerg Med* 6:562, 1977.

6. **Markovchick V, Duffens KR:** Cardiovascular trauma. In Rosen P, editor-in-chief: Emergency Medicine Concepts and Clinical Practice, St. Louis, 1992, Mosby–Year Book.

7. **Martin RR, Bickell WH, Pepe, et al:** Prospective evaluation of prehospital fluid resuscitation in hypotensive patients with penetrating truncal injury: a preliminary report. *J Traum* 1992; 33:354–362.

8. **Miller KS, Sahn SA: Chest Tubes:** Indications, technique, management and complications. *Chest* 91:258, 1987.

9. **Pepe PA, Bass RR, Mattox KL:** Clinical trials of the pneumatic antishock garments in the urban prehospital setting. *Ann Emerg Med* 1986; 15:1407–1410.

10. **Pons PT, Honigman B, Moore EE, et al:** Prehospital advanced trauma life support for critical penetrating wounds to the thorax and abdomen. *J Traum* 1985; 25:828–832.

11. **Seneff MG, Corwin RW, Gold LH, et al:** Complications associated with thoracentesis. *Chest* 1986; 90:97–100.

12. **Shaftan GW:** Indication for operation in abdominal trauma. *Am J Surg* 1960; 99:657.

13. **Sharp JR, et al:** Hemodynamics during reduced cardiac tamponade in man. *Am J Med* 29:640, 1960.

14. **Shoemaker WC:** Algorithm for early recognition and management of cardiac tamponade. *Crit Care Med* 1975; 3:39.

15. **Shoemaker WC, Carey SJ, Yao ST, et al:** Hemodynamic monitoring for physiologic evaluation, diagnosis, and therapy of acute hemopericardial tamponade from penetrating wounds. *J Traum* 1973; 13:36.

16. **Vukich DJ, Markovchick V:** Thoracic trauma. In Rosen P, editor-in-chief: Emergency Medicine Concepts and Clinical Practice, St. Louis, 1992, Mosey–Year Book.

17. **Yee ES, Verrier ED, Thomas AN:** Management of air embolism in blunt and penetrating thoracic trauma. *J Thoracic Cardiovasc Surg* 85:661, 1983.

Chapter 47

Head, Eyes, Ears, Nose, Mouth, and Throat Trauma

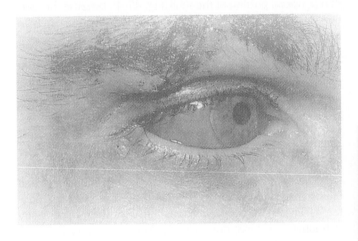

OBJECTIVES

A paramedic should be able to:

1. Describe the key anatomic structures of the head, eyes, ears, nose, and throat.

2. Describe the various mechanisms of head injury leading to unconsciousness and injuries to the head, eyes, ears, nose, and throat.

3. List signs and symptoms that may be detected on physical examination of a trauma patient with injuries to the head, eyes, ears, nose, and throat.

4. Calculate a patient's level of consciousness according to the Glasgow Coma Scale and the AVPU system.

5. Describe signs of increased intracranial pressure and cerebral herniation.

6. Describe measures that can limit or decrease intracranial pressure.

7. List three causes of altered mental status frequently found in trauma victims but not caused by trauma.

8. Describe how to manage injuries to the head, eyes, ears, nose, and throat.

KEY TERMS

1. **Arachnoid membrane**—Middle meningeal layer covering the brain; this tissue is loose, weblike, and absorbs cerebrospinal fluid.

2. **Decerebrate posturing**—Rigidity of extremities with extension at wrists and elbows.

3. **Decorticate posturing**—Rigidity of extremities with flexion at wrists and elbows.

4. **Dura mater**—Outermost and strongest meningeal layer covering the brain.

5. **Hemiparesis**—Paralysis or weakness limited to one side of the body.

6. **Herniation**—The movement, under pressure, of a tissue or part of organ outside the cavity or structure in which it is normally located.

7. **Intracerebral hematoma**—A collection of blood within the brain tissue.

ew things evoke more tension in an EMS provider than a call to the scene of an unresponsive trauma victim. Once the presence of a patent airway and reasonable respiratory effort, pulse, and blood pressure are confirmed, the paramedic is left to evaluate the patient by examination. The exact condition of the brain is unknown, and the luxury of verbal answers to questions is absent. Consequently, keen observation and inspection are required during physical assessment.

TABLE 47-1	Cerebral Divisions and Primary Functions	
Divisions	**Function**
Cerebrum	
Frontal Lobe	Emotion, motor
Parietal Lobe	Sensory, motor
Temporal Lobe	Memory
Occipital Lobe	Vision
Cerebellum	Balance, gait and coordination
Brainstem	Alertness, some automatic functions

Anatomy

A brief review of pertinent anatomy and physiology follows.

Head

The scalp has a very rich blood supply, so serious and even life-threatening hemorrhage can occur from a simple scalp laceration that is left unattended. Long, dark, or thick hair may make it difficult to appreciate the true nature of scalp injuries.

The skull consists of several bones which have joined together (Fig. 47-1). Scalp findings are described according to the bones underneath. For example, a cut on the back of the head is an occipital laceration, and a bruise on the forehead is a frontal contusion. Most of the inside surfaces of the skull are smooth. However, at the base, jagged edges lie next to the brain (Fig. 47-2). This is important because these bony projections can damage the brain in deceleration-type accidents.

The meninges lie between the skull and the brain (Fig. 47-3). The outermost layer, the dura mater, is a tough fibrous tissue that is attached directly to the inner surface of the skull. Arteries course through its outer layers. Of particular interest is the middle meningeal artery, which runs directly under the thin temporal portion of the skull (Fig. 47-4). Because this portion is thin, it is a common fracture site. That fracture can then tear the middle meningeal artery and cause an intracranial hemorrhage.

Beneath the dura mater is the arachnoid membrane, named for its spider-weblike appearance. Small bridging veins run between the dura and the arachnoid. The subdural space is the area between these two layers. Normally it is a small, potential space but it can expand greatly when bleeding occurs within it. Innermost is the pia mater, an extremely thin layer that covers the brain very closely.

The brain is divided into the cerebrum, cerebellum, and brainstem. (The structures of the brain are illustrated in Chapter 7.) These structures' locations influence their vulnerability to trauma. The cerebrum itself is further divided into two hemispheres, each with four lobes: frontal, parietal, occipital, and temporal. Table 47-1 shows some of their functions.

The cerebellum lies under the tentorium (a fold in the dura mater) in the occipital region of the skull. Its primary functions are balance and coordination. The brainstem lies anterior to this and below the cerebral hemispheres, deep within the cra-

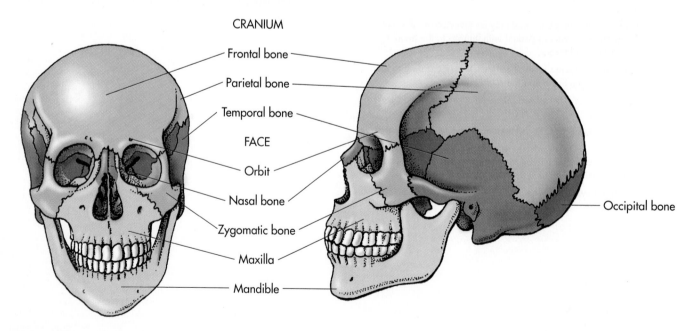

CRANIUM

Frontal bone
Parietal bone
Temporal bone
FACE
Orbit
Nasal bone
Zygomatic bone
Maxilla
Mandible

Occipital bone

Figure 47-1

Bones of the skull. *From McSwain, et al: The Basic EMT, Hanover 1996, Mosby.*

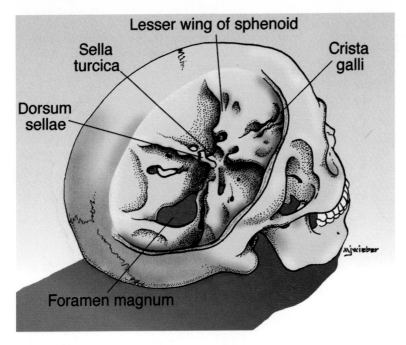

Figure 47-2

View of internal jagged edges of the skull bones. It is easy to imagine how jarring forces to the head could damage the delicate tissues of the brain and spinal cord.

nium. It consists of the pons, midbrain, and medulla. Together these three regions control alertness and regulate cardiorespiratory functions. The medulla is continuous with the spinal cord, which begins at the foramen magnum.

Eyes

The orbital bones provide excellent protection for the eyes. Immediate reflex closure of the eye lids, stimulated by rapidly approaching objects, also often spares the eyes from direct

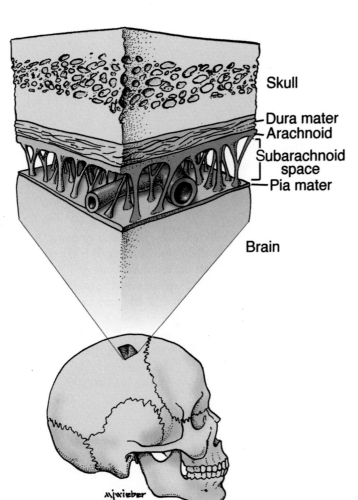

Figure 47-3

Cutaway section of the tissue layers below the skin of the head. The three meningeal layers offer protection as a shock absorber and nourishment for the brain from their blood vessels.

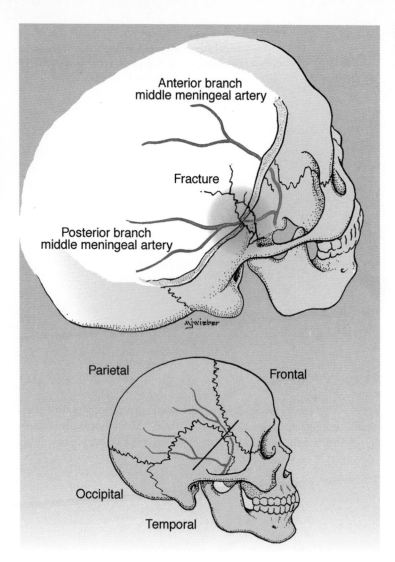

Anterior branch
middle meningeal artery

Fracture

Posterior branch
middle meningeal artery

Mjwieber

Parietal

Frontal

Occipital

Temporal

Figure 47-4

View of the meningeal artery. This is a common fracture site due to the thinness of the temporal bone. If the artery is disrupted, an intracerebral bleed occurs.

injury. The eye is a complex structure consisting of the conjunctiva, sclera, cornea, anterior chamber, iris, lens, posterior chamber, and retina.

The conjunctiva is loose connective tissue with small vessels traversing it. It overlies the white sclera, a more dense fibrous tissue that encircles the entire globe. The cornea is not covered by conjunctiva and is normally clear. This allows the paramedic to see through the anterior chamber to the iris. The state of contracture of the iris determines pupil size, influenced by a variety of cranial nerves and some drugs that control autonomic tone. The lens lies immediately behind the iris. It is a clear structure that aids in focusing.

The fluid in the anterior chamber is referred to as the aqueous humor, and that in the posterior chamber is the vitreous humor; these are also clear. Light that passes through these structures strikes the retina, the sensory end of the second cranial nerve. The images, colors, and movement in that light stimulate nerve impulses in the retina. These are conveyed to the central nervous system, especially the occipital cortex, where they are interpreted. The retina is firmly attached to the sclera. The pupils are usually equal in size and both react by constricting when a light is shined into either eye. Thus, in the normal patient, the pupils are equal, round, and reactive to light (PERRL).

Ears

The external ear is referred to as the auricle or pinna. It consists of firm cartilage without blood vessels. The external auditory canal passes through the temporal bone and ends at the tympanic membrane (ear drum), a delicate disk-shaped structure. The tympanic membrane is attached to one of three small bones, the stapes, incus, and malleus. Vibrations of the tympanic membrane by sound of different frequencies create a chain reaction of signals and stimuli. Nerves that pass through the internal auditory canal forward this data to the central nervous system for interpretation by the cerebral cortex, primarily in the temporal lobes.

Nose

The nose is formed by a combination of thin nasal bones and uniquely shaped cartilage. The nasal cavity lies within it, di-

- Closed head trauma in children is a common presenting complaint due to the greater mass of the child's head in relation to the rest of the body. It accounts for approximately 50% of all pediatric trauma.
- Children with head injury may initially present with benign signs and symptoms, however, profound lethargy, vomiting, and a decrease in the level of consciousness can occur rapidly. Often, the parent may state that the child is not acting "right" or normally.
- The modified Glasgow Coma Scale can be used to assess the infant to age 3 pediatric patient with a head injury.
- Impacted objects in the child's ears and nose are common presentation for the paramedic and can occur accidentally or intentionally. If the object can be removed without causing additional harm, gentle attempts can be made. If unable to remove the object, leave it in place, stabilize if indicated, and transport the child to the emergency department.

REFERENCES

1. Aoki BY, McCloskey, K. Evaluation, stabilization, and transport of the critically ill child, ed 1, St. Louis, 1992, Mosby–Year Book, Inc.
2. Nichols D, et al. Golden hour. The handbook of advanced pediatric life support, ed 1. St. Louis, 1991, Mosby–Year Book, Inc.
3. Silverman BK. APLS: the pediatric emergency medicine course, ed 2. American Academy of Pediatrics and American College of Emergency Physicians.

vided by a thin bone and cartilage structure called the nasal septum. The anterior septum possesses a rich vascular supply and it is often the source of **epistaxis** (nosebleeds).

The floor of the paired nasal chambers is horizontal when the head is upright. Knowledge of this anatomy is useful during nasogastric and nasotracheal intubation.

Mouth and Throat

There are normally 32 teeth in the adult, although many patients have 28 because of third molar (wisdom tooth) extraction. Dentures are also very common; removing them prior to endotracheal intubation in the unconscious patient improves access and prevents breakage and possible aspiration.

The tongue is a large, vascular muscle. Generally, it rests in the oral cavity where it is protected from trauma by the mandible and teeth. When a patient is awake, the muscle tone and the ligamentous structure at its base maintain the tongue in an anterior position that allows air to pass freely. In the unresponsive state, it becomes flaccid and may fall back into the oropharynx of the supine patient, causing complete airway obstruction. This can often be overcome by a jaw thrust or placement of a nasopharyngeal or oropharyngeal airway.

The roof of the mouth is known as the palate. The uvula hangs posteriorly from the soft palate in the midline, and the tonsils and tonsilar pillars are positioned laterally. These structures are rarely involved in blunt trauma but can be involved in penetrating injury. They are in close proximity to the neurovascular structures of the neck: carotid arteries, jugular veins, and vagal and phrenic nerves.

Head/EENT Trauma

The paramedic has the responsibility of gathering information at the scene of trauma. Descriptions of vehicular damage, the estimated height of a fall and the amount of lost blood are examples of valuable information that should be communicated verbally and in writing to the receiving physician. Paramedics also have access to additional information from witnesses regarding mechanism of injury, and the status of the patient both prior to and immediately following head trauma. Such individuals may also be the only sources of an unresponsive victim's past medical history, medications, allergies, alcohol intake, or substance abuse.

It is helpful to think of head trauma as having two components. The first is the internal component—the potential for injury inside the skull. The second is the external component, involving assessment of all the other structures of the head including the face, ears, and scalp. Careful and repeated examinations are often necessary to recognize the life threat from intracranial injury.

Assessment Considerations

Assessment of airway, breathing, and circulation takes the usual precedence in the head-injured patient. Because most head-injured patients have a mechanism of injury that indicates a possible **spinal cord injury**, cervical spine immobilization should also be done. Once the ABCs have been addressed and required corrections are underway, the degree of disability ("D"), or neurologic impairment, should be assessed. This is a dynamic assessment; paramedics should reassess it frequently on the scene and during transport. Changes, either improvement or deterioration, serve as feedback about ongoing treatments and guidelines for future interventions. Paramedics often determine the level of responsiveness by the AVPU system (See Chapter 17) and Glasgow Coma Scale (See Chapter 21).

In review, AVPU stands for Alert, Verbal, Pain, and Unresponsive. The last three refer to the patient's response to stimulus and give a gross estimate of awareness of environment.

The Glasgow Coma Scale, which is more descriptive, judges verbal, ocular, and motor responses. The best responses by the patient are totaled into a numeric score. For example, a patient who opens eyes to painful stimuli (E=2), withdraws a hand from this stimulus (M=4) and only groans (V=2) would have a score of 8. Scores range from 3 to 15; a patient with a score less than 8 is considered to be in a coma. Such patients should be intubated to increase oxygenation, decrease CO_2, and prevent aspiration.

Next, paramedics should check pupillary response to light. A normal response requires intact cranial nerves. An unreactive dilated pupil ("blown pupil") in the setting of depressed mental status is an ominous sign indicative of critically elevated intracranial pressure. Rapid transport of this patient is imperative.

The last portion of the initial field neurologic assessment is evaluating motor and sensory function. Findings such as one-sided weakness or outright paralysis can indicate significant intracranial injury, but may also be caused by spinal cord or peripheral nerve damage.

Intracranial Injuries

Perhaps the single most important observation made by paramedics is the patient's level of responsiveness and how it changes over time. A variety of traumatic mechanisms can cause impaired level of responsiveness. One example is cerebral hypoxia from airway obstruction or inadequate breathing. Another is hypoperfusion. The paramedic must ensure that oxygenated blood is arriving to the brain by providing an adequate blood pressure with fluid volume maintenance when necessary.

Bleeding and swelling in the cranial vault itself are two more common mechanisms that cause alteration of responsiveness. Both relate to the fact that there is no room for expansion. The increase in pressure can result in herniation, or in hypoperfusion when the pressure on the brain tissue is greater than the pressure pushing blood into these areas. Herniation occurs when brain tissue is pushed through openings such as the foramen magnum at the base of the skull (Fig. 47-5).

As the pressure increases, the first sign is a change in the level of responsiveness. Patients often become sleepy or lethargic, although in some cases they become agitated. As the pressure continues to increase, the patient becomes more difficult to wake and eventually becomes comatose. Physical signs vary depending on the part of the brain being compressed as the pressure inside the skull increases. Further increases in pressure lead to hemiparesis on the opposite side of the body as the hematoma or swelling, and a dilated, unresponsive pupil on the same side of the body. The dilated pupil occurs because the third cranial nerve, which normally causes pupillary constriction, is compressed and ceases to function (Fig. 47-6).

Compressed motor fibers, which cross the spinal cord and supply the opposite side of the body, cause the paralysis. Compression of the brain stem results in abnormal respiration. In addition, abnormal reflexes known as decerebrate or decorticate posturing may occur, as well as Cushing's reflex. Decerebrate posturing is usually manifested by extension of the arms and pronation of the hands, and decorticate posturing is recognized by flexion of the arms. Both are grave signs indicating serious brain injury (Fig. 47-7). Cushing's reflex is manifested by increasing blood pressure and slowing heart rate as a result of increasing intracranial pressure. It is important to remember that all of these reflexes are late signs of increased intracranial pressure caused by brain swelling or intracranial bleeding. The paramedic who waits for these findings to develop before recognizing the problem or intervening in the process has waited too long. The patient's chances lie in recognition of the early

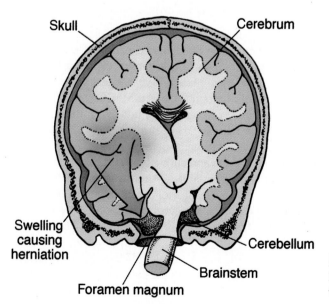

Figure 47-5

Herniation occurs when the swelling brain tissue has no place to go except through the foramen magnum, the opening found at the base of the skull.

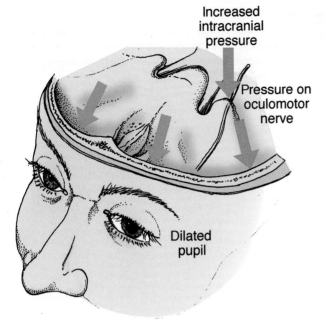

signs of increasing intracranial pressure: changing mental status or level of responsiveness.

Paramedics can begin to control or lower this pressure before the victim arrives at the hospital. Intubation and controlled hyperventilation, at no more than 20–22 breaths per minute, lower the blood carbon dioxide level, which in turn causes constriction of the cerebral arteries. This limitation of blood flow to the brain allows more intracranial space for expansion caused by swelling or bleeding. Failure to lower the CO_2 level can result in dilation of these vessels, which increases the intracranial pressure. Too much hyperventilation, however, can cause too much vasoconstriction and greatly reduce blood flow to the brain. In the case of head injury without clear signs of increased intracranial pressure, ventilation at 12–18 breaths per minute is appropriate, as prophylactic hyperventilation can reduce blood flow to the brain unnecessarily.

In isolated head injuries where ongoing blood loss is not a major concern, the paramedic must be cautious with IV fluids. These are temporary measures only, used to maintain the patient until specific injuries are identified and additional treatments performed.

Certain intracranial injuries offer typical presentations during physical assessment. Paramedics may encounter patients who are awake and talking during initial examination but later lose consciousness. Bleeding into the epidural space, or epidural hematoma formation, can result in such a history (Fig. 47-8A). The victim may have had a brief loss of responsiveness, be awake on paramedic arrival, and later become lethargic or comatose. Although this injury is relatively rare (approximately 1% of coma-producing head injuries), it must be recognized and treated early.[1] Recovery is directly related to the depth of coma and the time elapsed before surgical treatment.

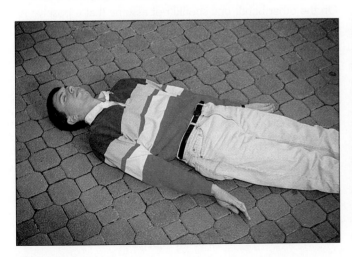

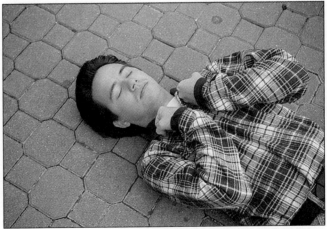

Figure 47-7
Decerebrate and decorticate posturing indicate severe brain injury.

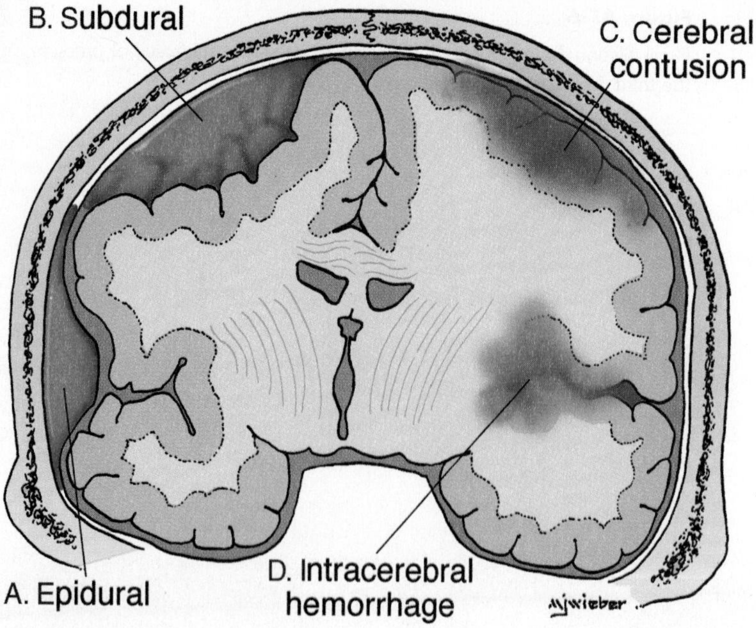

B. Subdural

C. Cerebral contusion

A. Epidural

D. Intracerebral hemorrhage

Figure 47-8

Types of brain injuries due to the presence of bruising or bleeding of brain tissues. A, epidural hematoma, B, subdural hematoma, C, cerebral contusion, and D, intracerebral hemorrhage.

It is common for a head-injured patient to bleed underneath the dura mater (30% of severe injuries). This is called a **subdural hematoma** and usually results from disrupted veins rather than arteries (Fig. 47-8B). Physical findings can be the same as in epidural hematoma. Distinguishing between epidural and subdural hematoma is far less important than recognizing the signs of an intracranial injury hematoma of any kind. If left untreated, these lesions can rapidly become fatal. Rarely, a subdural hematoma can accumulate slowly and present in a delayed fashion. Patients may complain of headaches, behavioral changes, or weakness which develops or persists over days to weeks.

Some patients have bruises inside the brain tissue, referred to as cerebral contusions (Fig. 47-8C). These can occur when the surrounding cerebrospinal fluid (CSF) fails to keep the brain from striking the inside of the skull. Typically, this occurs at the frontal lobes or temporal tips where the intracranial surface is jagged. A small bruise can occur at the site of a blow (coup) or opposite to the location of the blow (contra-coup) as the brain strikes the far side of the skull upon rebound. Deep bleeding or intracerebral hematomas (Fig. 47-8D) can occur from shear force that occurs during twisting or deceleration injuries. Both injuries can result in bleeding or swelling that causes herniation.

The paramedic usually cannot distinguish between these entities; a computerized tomography (CT scan) may be required. In fact, these injuries often occur together in severe trauma. However, the initial management is essentially the same and should be followed in all patients with significant head injury and impaired level of consciousness (Box 47-1).

The paramedic should avoid the pitfall of withholding naloxone (Narcan®) or glucose, assuming that trauma is the cause of altered mental status. **Hypoglycemia**, narcotic overdose, and alcohol abuse are common precipitating factors to trauma. They complicate field assessment and management. On the other hand, one should not assume that a positive response to one of the above agents rules out an accompanying head injury.

The paramedic should anticipate vomiting and seizures from the head-injured patient. If the patient is not intubated and vomits, he or she must be log-rolled onto the side to prevent aspiration. Seizures in head-injured patients can occur from hypoxia or from direct insult to the brain and its structures. Airway control, oxygenation, and ventilation are important preventive management interventions. Seizures may require IV medications, because persistent seizure activity can aggravate the patient's condition.

External Injuries

Once the paramedic completes the neurologic evaluation, the patient's external head should be examined. Paramedics

---

BOX 47-1	**Summary of Management of Head-Injured Patients**

- Secure and maintain an open airway (intubate if necessary)
- Stabilize patient on a spine board with cervical immobilization
- Ventilate the patient 12–18 breaths per min.
- If clear signs of increased ICP, hyperventilate no more than 20–22 breaths per min.
- Hyperventilate the patient to lower CO_2 levels
- Administer high-flow oxygen
- Treat shock with intravenous fluids
- Restrict fluid if no shock or active bleeding is noted
- Determine level of responsiveness
- Repeat and record neurologic assessment frequently

often encounter bleeding from scalp lacerations; control of active bleeding, whether arterial or venous, should be accomplished immediately by direct manual pressure. This procedure may require help, because the paramedic assessing the patient must continue the assessment. Dressings alone may fail to stop scalp bleeding; direct pressure over a 3 to 4 minute interval will be more effective. Don't assume that a 250-mL pool of blood is the only blood lost or the only cause of a patient's low blood pressure. When communicating with medical direction, try to estimate the amount of blood loss despite the fact that these estimates may not be very precise.

Scalp lacerations can result in a great deal of blood loss. When the laceration is associated with a skull fracture and the fracture is depressed, bleeding may be difficult to stop with direct pressure alone. Paramedics should also avoid further displacing the fracture with direct pressure, which can cause more injury to the underlying brain. Such injuries can be covered with sterile gauze and should be kept free from gross contamination. Impaled objects, such as knives, should be left in place for treatment at the hospital. Once there, consequences of removal, such as internal hemorrhage, can be appropriately managed. Eye, external ear, external nose, and oral lacerations can be managed in a similar way. Facial lacerations that do not involve arterial bleeding frequently clot after a few minutes of direct pressure.

Paramedics are often challenged with intraoral bleeding from tongue or cheek lacerations. If the blood amount is minimal or moderate, the awake patient can be asked to spit out the blood periodically. For persistent bleeding, direct pressure is appropriate. If the unresponsive victim has lost airway protection reflexes, suction and direct pressure may be applied after endotracheal intubation. Blood can cause severe bronchoconstriction and hypoxia when aspirated.

Bleeding from the ear canal may be the result of local trauma or may be mixed with cerebrospinal fluid leaking out of a basilar skull fracture. This condition can occur when the fracture involves the part of temporal bone that encircles the external canal. Attempts to stop such bleeding are usually futile and possibly harmful; the loss of fluid may be relieving pressure buildup in the cranial vault. Hematoma behind the ear (Battle's sign) (Fig. 47-9A) or bilateral orbital bruising (raccoon eyes) (Fig. 47-9B) can also indicate basilar skull fracture. Cerebrospinal fluid may also leak from the nose when the cribriform plate of the skull is fractured.

Blood loss from the nose, called epistaxis, can often be stopped by pinching the nose. However, if the paramedic fails to detect ongoing hemorrhage in an unresponsive victim, asphyxiation or airway obstruction may occur. Nasal trumpets can restrict bleeding in addition to providing a temporary airway. However, they do not protect against aspiration or obstruction. Consequently, endotracheal intubation is advised in unresponsive patients.

Trumpets or endotracheal tubes placed nasally are usually not recommended in severe facial trauma with unstable fractures or distorted normal anatomy, particularly midface fractures, because nasal tubes can be accidentally placed into the cranial vault with disastrous consequences. Determination of movement in the maxilla by grasping the upper teeth provides clinical evidence of a midface fracture.

After controlling hemorrhage in or near the eye, the eye itself should be examined. Assessment of pupillary response has already been mentioned; it may be repeated at this time. Although rarely the source of ongoing hemorrhage, bleeding

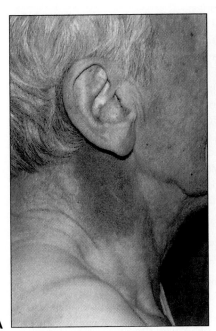

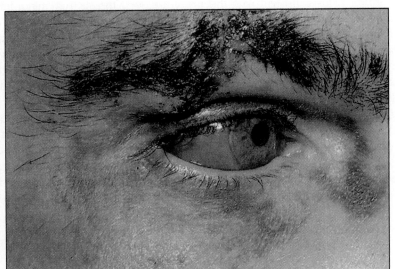

Figure 47-9

A, A hematoma seen behind one or both ears is called "Battle's sign." B, Bilateral, periorbital ecchymosis is called "raccoon eyes." Rupture of the small vessels in the conjunctiva results in a subconjunctival hemorrhage. *From Mills, et al: Color Atlas and Text of Emergencies, ed 2, London, Mosby Wolfe.*

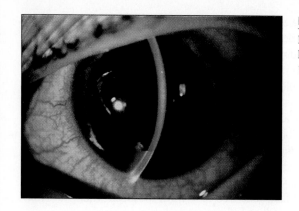

Figure 47-10

Blood seen in the anterior chamber of the eye as a result of blunt trauma is called a hyphema. *From Zitelli and Davis: Atlas of Pediatric Physical Diagnosis, ed 3, London, Mosby Wolfe.*

within the ocular tissues can be important for other reasons. A direct blow resulting in rupture of the small vessels in the conjunctiva almost always results in the subconjunctival hemorrhage rather than external bleeding. On examination of the eye, blood is noted over the white sclera (Fig. 47-9B). This injury can also occur with forces such as blunt chest or abdominal trauma, hanging-type injuries, or even simple coughing or sneezing. All of these mechanisms increase the pressure inside the chest or prevent blood flow from the head in the case of hanging, and thus cause conjunctival blood vessels to rupture. Although striking in appearance, subconjunctival hemorrhage is a minor injury that causes no serious disability.

Blunt trauma to the eye can also result in blood in the anterior chamber. This condition is called a **hyphema** (Fig. 47-10) and can cause long-term complications including **glaucoma** and impaired vision. A physical examination reveals visible blood in the anterior chamber. The most serious eye injury is a **ruptured globe**. This injury usually results from a penetrating mechanism. Signs consistent with this injury are severely impaired vision (not always present), an abnormally shaped pupil, and leakage of the internal contents. The paramedic should take care to avoid applying pressure to an eye that may be ruptured. Pressure can result in loss of intraocular contents, particularly vitreous humor, which cannot be replaced. Field treatment consists of carefully placing a hard shield over the eye to protect it from additional damage, covering the other eye to prevent parallel movement, and transporting the patient in a supine position.

Occasionally, the paramedic will encounter a patient who has sustained head trauma resulting in an avulsed tooth. If the tooth can be located and is completely intact, it should be transported in saline or milk for possible reimplantation. If transport time is greater than 30 minutes, the tooth can be placed back into the empty socket after irrigation of the tooth with saline.

Trauma to the face may produce fracture of facial bones. A physical examination will usually reveal swelling and bruising over the fracture site, tenderness, and sometimes crepitus. When the mandible is fractured, the patient will often note misalignment of upper and lower teeth, and pain when clenching the jaw. The misalignment may also be discovered visually during the physical examination. The mandible forms a complete ring with the skull and, similar to the pelvis, usually fractures in two or more places. Patients with blunt or penetrating trauma to the neck may have distorted airway anatomy, meaning that endotracheal intubation and cricothyroidotomy are likely to be difficult. However, these procedures should not be attempted unless the patient is in respiratory distress.

SUMMARY

Trauma to the head and face can produce a wide variety of injuries, ranging from a single external contusion or laceration to a life-threatening intracranial hematoma. Not all serious injuries are manifested immediately after the traumatic event. Only careful assessment and reassessment can distinguish life threats from minor injuries.

Paramedics have a great opportunity and responsibility in managing the head-injured patient. Great harm can result if a seemingly alert trauma victim is not adequately assessed, and is presumed well, and released at the scene. Emergency department care and ultimately patient outcome are enhanced when timely airway control, oxygenation, and appropriate hyperventilation are instituted early in the course of treatment of a head-injured patient, as well as appropriate immobilization, bleeding control, IV access, and precise radio communication to the receiving hospital. Finally, constant observation, reassessment, and questioning by the paramedic are crucial to detect any changes in the patient's condition.

REFERENCES

1. **American College of Surgeons Committee on Trauma:** Advanced Trauma Life Support, Chicago, 1993, American College of Surgeons.

2. **Bledsoe BE, Shade BR, Porter RS:** Paramedic Emergency Care, Englewood Cliffs, 1991, Prentice Hall.

3. **Caroline NL:** Emergency Care in the Streets, Boston, 1991, Brown and Company.

4. **Jones SA, et al (ed):** Advanced Emergency Care for Paramedic Practices, Philadelphia, 1992, JB Lippincott.

5. **Moore KL:** Clinically Oriented Anatomy, Baltimore, 1980, Williams & Wilkins.

6. **Rosen P, et al:** Emergency Medicine: Concepts and Clinical Practices, St. Louis, 1992, CV Mosby.

7. United States Department of Transportation Guidelines, Washington, 1983, United States Depatment of Transportation.

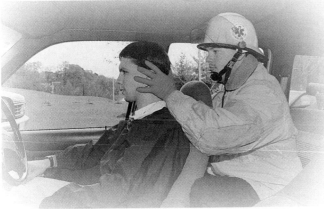

A paramedic should be able to:

OBJECTIVES

1. List the common signs, symptoms, and complications associated with fractures.

2. Describe general principles of fracture management.

3. Describe how to assess a patient for potential spinal injury.

4. Explain the appropriate use of the common types of spinal immobilization devices and extremity splints, and list the advantages and disadvantages of each.

5. Describe airway management in patients with potential cervical spine injuries.

6. Describe the situation in which it is appropriate to attempt to realign an angulated fracture before splinting, and explain the correct method for doing so.

7. Describe the procedures used to determine the nerve and vascular function of extremities.

KEY TERMS

1. **Axial traction**—Pulling force applied along the long axis of a bone or group of bones such as the spine.

2. **Compartment syndrome**—A pathologic condition caused by the progressive development of arterial compression and reduced blood supply.

3. **Crepitus**—A grating vibration or crackling sound heard on movement of the broken bone ends against each other.

4. **Dislocation**—The displacement of any part of the body from its normal position, particularly a bone from its normal articulation with a joint.

5. **Ecchymosis**—Discoloration of an area of the skin or mucous membrane caused by bleeding beneath the skin; bruising.

6. **Fracture**—A traumatic injury to a bone in which the continuity of the tissue of the bone is broken.

7. **In-line immobilization**—A manual stabilization maneuver in which the head and neck are maintained in line with the long axis of the body.

rthopedic injuries, particularly fractures, are commonly encountered by prehospital providers. All fractures have common presenting complaints and findings, regardless of location. Careful physical assessment will help identify the likelihood of a potential fracture.

Patients usually complain of pain at the injury site, often note associated swelling and bruising from bleeding at the site, and sometimes even report feeling the broken ends of the bone moving or grating against each other. Typically, patients will hold the injured body part still to minimize pain.

Recognition of a possible fracture involves finding one or more of the following physical signs:

- tenderness of the bone or injury site upon palpation
- swelling over the injury site
- ecchymosis (bruising) over the injury site
- obvious deformity
- bony crepitus
- shortening of the extremity
- abnormal rotation of the extremity
- decrease or complete loss of function because of pain

These findings are found in broken bones regardless of location, although they may be present in different combinations. For example, fracture of the nasal bones usually reveals tenderness, swelling, ecchymosis, and crepitus. Occasionally, there may be an obvious deformity. Fracture of the femur reveals tenderness, bony crepitus, leg deformity, shortening of the length of the leg, and sometimes abnormal rotation. Often swelling and ecchymosis are not noted. Fracture of the spine at any level often reveals tenderness as the only finding, although loss of function may also be noted with associated spinal cord injury.

The basic principle of management for all fractures is the immobilization of the injured site. This is true for any fracture injury. Complete immobilization includes splinting the joints above and below the injury site whenever possible. The key is to limit movement of the fracture and prevent additional complications such as nerve, spinal cord, or vascular damage.

Although most fractures are not life-threatening, several can result in significant hidden blood loss. Specifically, fractures of the pelvis and femur can lead to hypovolemic shock without obvious visual external signs of hemorrhage. Thus, whenever these fractures are suspected, the paramedic must observe the patient closely for signs of developing shock.

The Cervical Spine

Management of cervical trauma begins the moment the paramedic arrives at the scene. The question of which field interventions are appropriate for the traumatized patient is controversial; however, there is no debate that spinal immobilization and airway management are the highest priority interventions. A protected airway and adequate oxygenation should be as-

tained throughout the process.

The prevention of additional spinal injury is accomplished through careful patient handling and immobilization of any potential injuries. The use of in-line stabilization, log-rolling techniques, and backboards is essential to the protection of the patient's spinal cord.

Patients with possible cervical spine injuries must be immediately protected. Traditional teaching has recommended immobilization when the patient has "altered mental status," complains of neck pain, has muscle tenderness or spasm around the spine, or displays a neurologic deficit.[11] This is much more important in blunt trauma than in penetrating trauma, which does not cause cord injury by the mechanism of cervical instability.[1] Penetrating injury produces spinal cord damage at the time of penetration as a direct result of the penetrating object; the likelihood of penetrating trauma causing an unstable spine fracture is extremely low.

However, more recent studies have suggested that these criteria alone are only 79% predictive of identifying conscious patients with cervical fractures.[16] Another common teaching—that head, facial, and clavicular trauma should be used as predictors of cervical trauma in awake patients—has serious limitations as well. One study demonstrated that a Glasgow Coma Scale of 14 or less was associated with a greater incidence of both cervical spine and cervical cord injuries, and therefore, was a better predictor than any of the other criteria.[21] In another study of 1000 consecutive conscious trauma patients, it was found that using the findings of midline neck tenderness, evidence of intoxication, altered level of respsonsiveness, or severe painful injury elsewhere as criteria for suspecting a possible cervical spine injury, did not miss any of the 27 fractures that were ultimately discovered.[7]

Neurological Assessment

The field evaluation of neurological status in patients with potential cervical spine injury should not be extensive or time consuming. Checking for grasp or light-touch sensation is all that is necessary in the upper extremities. In the lower extremities, checking sensation and light touch, having the patient resist against pressure to flex or extend the toes, and extend and flex the knees against resistance without actual movement, identifies any gross neurological deficit that could indicate spinal cord injury (Fig. 48-1).

If the patient complains of a specific inability to move an extremity or a loss of sensation, this should be checked and recorded. Priapism (sustained penile erection) is not usually evaluated in the field, but if it is discovered during examination, it suggests a complete cord lesion. Generally speaking, if significant cervical cord involvement is suspected, motor function in the upper extremities will be compromised and the lowest intact sensation will be at or above the clavicle (Fig. 48-2).

Patients who present with altered mentation and significant injuries after blunt trauma cannot be evaluated reliably by history or physical examination for the presence of cervical spine injuries. Although several contradictory studies have been published,[6,7] it is currently recommended that any pa-

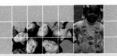

- Children's bones are more flexible than those of adults; therefore, unique fractures may occur which are rarely seen in the adult patient. Children's bones may actually bend without producing a fracture.
- Fractures that occur at or near the growth plate may appear to heal initially, yet deformities and complications may occur at a later time, caused by injury to the growth center of the bone.
- Elbow injury can occur in infants and toddlers as an acute subluxation of the radial head ("Nurse maid's elbow"). This can be witnessed every day when parents are seen "jerking" the child back toward themselves, thus causing the subluxation.
- The child's spine is made up of a larger amount of cartilage, which makes it more flexible than that of adults. Nevertheless, orthopedic spinal injuries can occur in any child with severe trauma, most commonly seen with MVAs, crushing injuries, and others.
- Cervical spine injuries in children tend to occur higher in the cervical spine.

- Atlantoaxial subluxation may occur from minor trauma in children with Down's syndrome.
    Neurologic deficits may not be apparent initially following the event; therefore, attempts should be made to prevent further movement of the potentially unstable cervical spine.
- Osteogenesis imperfecta is a hereditary disorder of the bone characterized by extremely fragile bones. Extreme gentleness should be used as even the slightest trauma or pressure can fracture the bone.

REFERENCES

1. **Aoki BY, McCloskey K:** Evaluation, stabilization, and transport of the critically ill child, ed 1, St. Louis, 1992, Mosby–Year Book.

2. **Nichols D, et al:** Golden hour. The handbook of advanced pediatric life support, ed 1, St. Louis, 1991, Mosby–Year Book.

3. **Silverman BK:** APLS: the pediatric emergency medicine course, ed 2, American Academy of Pediatrics and American College of Emergency Physicians.

tient with craniofacial trauma who is less than fully responsive deserves complete cervical immobilization.

Management of Cervical Spine Injuries

The medical literature is replete with studies that evaluate cervical spine immobilization devices.[4,6,8,9,10,13,17] The halo-vest is presently the gold standard against which all others are measured. Because it requires surgical application, it is not used in the prehospital setting[9], but recent technical advances in this area are based on simplified application of the same engineering principles.

The use of a blocking technique combined with a rigid cervical collar is the most commonly used method of cervical immobilization in the United States today (Fig. 48-3).[5] Velcro and composite materials mimic the sandbag-tape concept of the 1970s, and the results are similar.[5] One study demonstrated that blocking the head and neck without the use of a cervical collar allows 15° of flexion-extension.[15] The addition of a Philadelphia-type collar restricts flexion-extension to 7° (Fig. 48-4).

Newer devices reduce flexion-extension even further. Another study evaluated the limitations of four cervical collars, concluding that a rigid cervical collar that incorporates part of the thorax will provide better immobilization than shorter, less rigid collars[17] (Fig. 48-5).

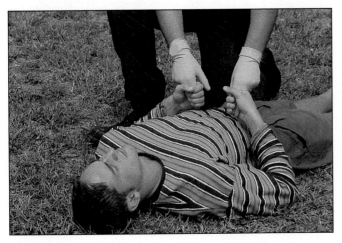

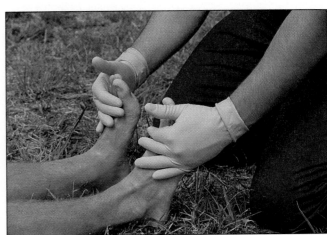

Figure 48-1

Methods of identifying gross neurological deficit include checking grasp, sensation, flexion, and extension in the extremities.

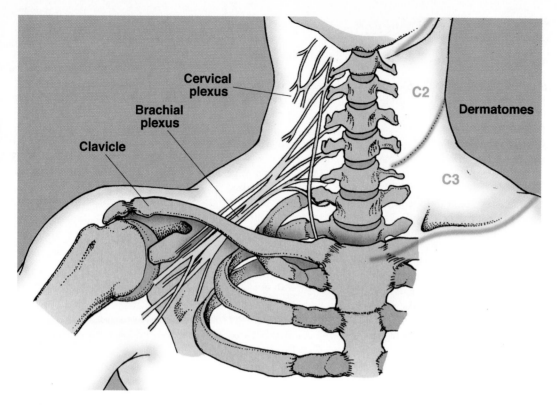

Figure 48-2

Nerve pathways in the neck and shoulder. Injury of the cervical vertebra can compromise the upper extremity in addition to the trunk and lower extremities.

Although effective in the unresponsive or cooperative patient, all of these approaches fall short of being acceptable for the combative patient. These patients require a team member to manually stabilize the head and neck to prevent self-inflicted spinal cord injury.

Airway Management with Cervical Spine Injuries

Since the advent of prehospital intubation in the 1970s, there has been an ongoing debate about what constitutes optimal

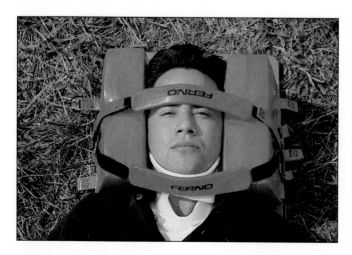

Figure 48-3

Cervical immobilization is accomplished with a combination of a rigid collar and a cervical immobilization device (CID) that "block" the head in place.

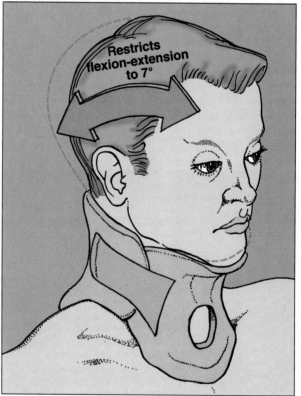

Figure 48-4

The greatest limit to flexion and extension is achieved with the use of a rigid cervical collar in addition to blocking techniques.

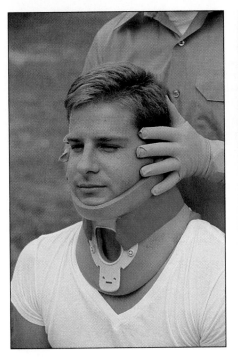
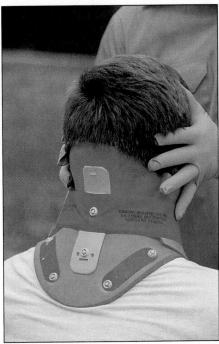
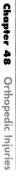

Figure 48-5

Newer version of cervical collars incorporates part of the thorax in the immobilization of the neck.

airway management in patients with potential cervical spine injuries. The introduction of nasotracheal intubation techniques in prehospital training curricula was supposed to end the controversy but may, in fact, have fueled it.

Conventional wisdom had held that endotracheal intubation in the presence of blunt head or facial trauma is dangerous because of the need to extend the head and neck. More recent, carefully controlled studies suggest that, properly performed, endotracheal intubation in these circumstances is safe and effective and can often mean the difference between life and death.[19,20] One study demonstrated that movement of the cervical spine is no more severe than with nasotracheal intubation.[22] Finally, if the decision is between intubation and bag-valve-mask ventilation, the latter may actually cause more cervical spine motion.[12]

With any of these techniques, it is important to maintain cervical spine immobilization at all times. Throughout the past 20 years, the literature has referred to axial traction as the method of choice. However, too much traction can also cause injury.[2] Thus, the more appropriate procedure is in-line immobilization (stabilization) in a neutral position without actual traction[2] (Fig. 48-6). This job is best designated to a specific team member.

Assessing Thoracic and Lumbar Spine Injuries

The vertebrae of the thoracic and lumbar spine are among the most protected bones in the human body. Consider the amount of muscle and ligamentous support surrounding the spine at these levels. This architecture provides a natural splint when injury does occur because of reflex spasm in the strong paraspinous muscles (Fig. 48-7). The complex innervation of lumbar structures helps explain the diffuse nature of pain associated with lumbar injuries.

A number of other important organs are situated in the retroperitoneum, anterior to the lumbar spine, including the kidneys, ureters, aorta, inferior vena cava, pancreas, and colon. Injuries that affect these organs may also result in referred pain that is localized to the lumbar spine.

With blunt trauma, the lumbar vertebrae may be exposed to tremendous forces. Because each intervertebral disc is a fluid system, hydraulic pressure is created when blunt trauma puts an unusual load on the spine. This increases the chances of disc injury, especially in older patients whose discs are more fragile (Fig. 48-8).

The lumbar spine is not the only structure that has to absorb these stresses. The muscles of the thoracic and abdominal cavities act as a cylinder that helps to decrease the load on the lumbar and thoracic spine. The muscles and ligaments of the spine also help to support the load.

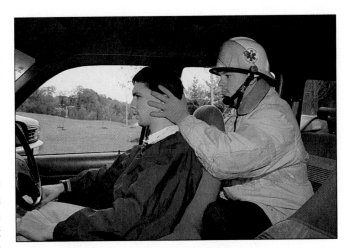

Figure 48-6

In-line immobilization in a neutral position without the application of traction is the preferred method of cervical spinal support.

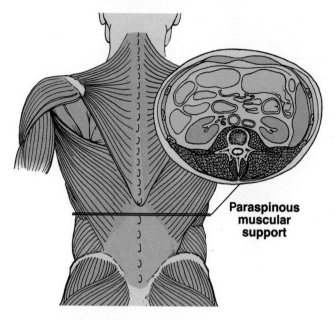

Paraspinous muscular support

Figure 48-7

Many layers of muscle help to protect the bones of the spine.

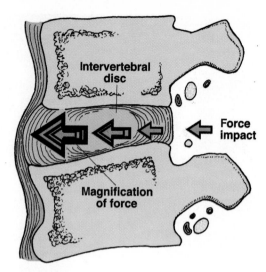

Intervertebral disc

Force impact

Magnification of force

Figure 48-8

Blunt trauma can result in a transmission of force across the vertebra and a disruption of the position of the intravertebral discs.

Vertebral compression fractures are common with falls and deceleration injuries, and are usually the result of severe flexion. The thoracic spine is most commonly involved. The force needed to compress a vertebral body is considerable, but if the patient's bones are weakened by disease, such as osteoporosis or cancer, the mechanism of injury may seem relatively insignificant.

The barriers to prehospital evaluation of thoracic and lumbar spine injuries are numerous. Because the patient has to remain stationary, the patient's back cannot be visualized and can be difficult to palpate. Immobilization must begin during the physical assessment. If the patient complains of pain in the thoracic or lumbar region, or of loss of sensation or motor function in the lower extremities, a spine injury should be presumed. If these are not present, palpation of the paravertebral muscles and of each vertebral spine can be performed by running a hand underneath the supine patient, feeling for muscle spasm or "step-off," a distinct difference in the prominence of two adjacent spinous processes (Fig. 48-9). Firm paraspinous muscles result from spasm secondary to local injury or referred pain.

If the patient is being log-rolled for some other reason, a quick examination can be done at that time. Next, sensory assessment can be accomplished in an abbreviated fashion. Skin should be evaluated by pinprick and light touch. Because the patient is being stabilized and packaged for transport at the same time, the examination should not require extremity movement. Much of the evaluation in awake patients will depend on historical data. Abnormalities will help localize an injury. Figure 48-10 is a dermatome map showing the relationship between skin surface area and spinal nerves. If the

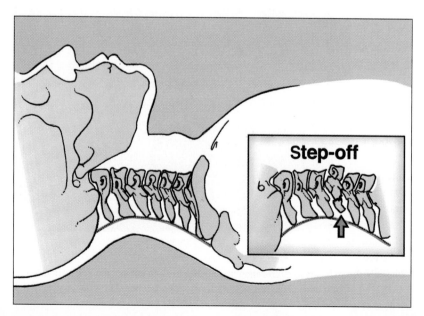

Step-off

Figure 48-9

A "step-off" is detected upon palpation of the spinal column and indicates anterior displacement of a vertebra.

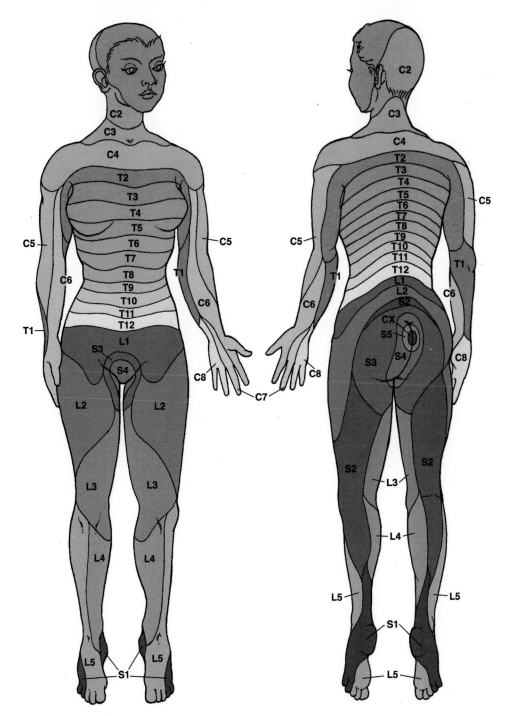

Figure 48-10

A dermatome map shows the relationship between areas of touch sensation on the skin and the spinal nerves that correspond to that area of sensation. Loss of sensation or altered sensation in that area may indicate an injury to the spinal nerve.

situation is emergent, the neurologic examination can take place during transport.

Vertebral compression fractures most commonly occur at the level of the thoracic spine. The pain associated with such fractures is localized and immediate. Tenderness over a single vertebra is the usual presenting symptom. If neurologic involvement is present from a thoracic spine injury, the sensory deficit level may begin anywhere from the clavicles (T1) down to a point just below the umbilicus (T12).

Management of Thoracic and Lumbar Spine Injuries

Loss of motor function in the lower extremities suggests complete cord injury. Every EMS system has its own protocols for managing spinal injuries. Medical direction should be notified as soon as possible in these cases to institute the established protocol.

Numerous variations of the basic backboard have been introduced over the past decade without much scientific data to support claims of superiority (Fig. 48-11). Improved x-ray transparency, incorporated cervical immobilization, lateral hip supports, special padding, and easier strapping have all been cited as claims of significant advancement by equipment manufacturers. However, the basic underlying theory remains the same. The spine board is meant to stabilize by providing a system of en bloc (in one piece) movement for transferring the patient from the ground to the rescue unit, the emergency department, and the operating room.

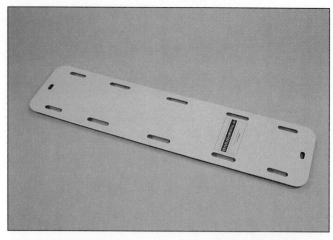

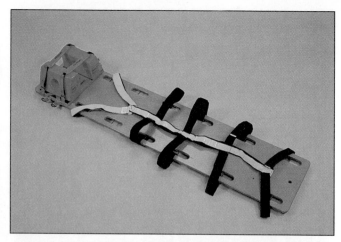

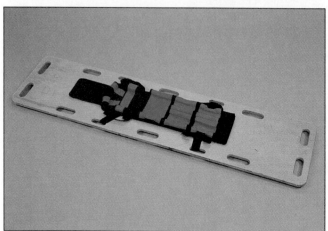

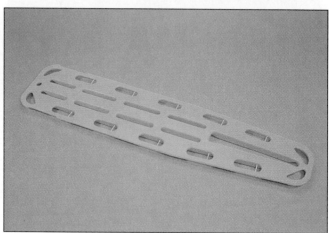

Figure 48-11

Many different styles of backboards are currently available.

One of the unsolved problems of EMS is how to get equipment back to the paramedic after a patient is delivered to the hospital. Many busy Emergency departments have had to devote space and personnel time to storing and cataloguing equipment for various EMS systems. In addition, some of the more innovative (and thus more expensive) immobilization devices have not found favor with many EMS systems because of the fear of loss within the hospital. The most logical alternative to this approach has been the development of "breakaway" backboards that can be released and removed from either side once the patient is placed on the hospital's immobilization equipment (Fig. 48-12).

Extremity Trauma

Fractures, dislocations, and sprains comprise a significant portion of EMS business. Couple those injuries with a multitrauma situation, and management priorities begin to become less clear. Certainly there is no debate against the postulate that isolated orthopedic problems are not life threatening. However, the early management can have a long-term impact on the function of the involved extremity, as well as on the psychological challenges the patient will face during rehabilita-tion. These injuries frequently occur in young, otherwise healthy individuals. The ultimate goal of the health care team, including EMS, is to return the patient to functional status. With these factors in mind, the following section will outline a

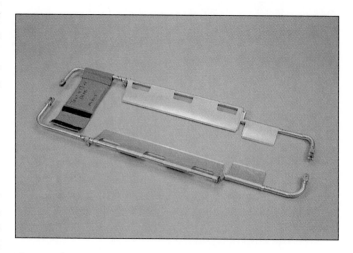

Figure 48-12

Breakaway backboards allow the EMS provider to retrieve equipment once the patient is placed on an immobilization device at the hospital, without excessive movement to the patient.

method of rapid assessment of extremity injuries and review the various issues involved in field management.

Open Fractures

If a fracture breaks the skin, it is "open" (Fig. 48-13). Often the paramedic will be left to decide whether the small cut that is near but not actually over the fracture site is caused by the fracture or is just a laceration that happens to be near the fracture. As a general rule, assume the worst and treat these as if they are open fractures.

Conventional wisdom has long dictated the golden rule, "Splint it as it lies." However, modern surgical techniques, improved broad-spectrum antibiotics, and new, aggressive approaches to rehabilitation bring that time-honored axiom into question. Case law, too, is dictating a new standard of care that rejects the concept that angulation and vascular compromise cannot be corrected in the field. Paramedics should be given "hands-on" experience under the supervision of a trained specialist in the management of angulated fractures.

Vascular Compromise

Conventional wisdom has also dictated than an open fracture with exposed bone should never be reduced. This is based on the theory that the contaminated bone end will expose deep tissues to dirt, foreign bodies, and bacteria. The surgical management of these injuries has become significantly more aggressive in the past 10 years to include extending the skin opening and surgically flushing the wound under pressure with a mixture of saline and antibiotics. These patients usually receive a preoperative dose of an antibiotic that is continued after the surgical procedure. Hospital management of open fractures is the same whether or not the bone was pulled back into the soft tissues. Thus any sign of vascular compromise from an open fracture mandates a correction attempt by EMS personnel just as with angulation. Again, the method of realignment is continuous traction along the axial length of the extremity applied distal to the fracture site (Fig. 48-14).

The absence of pulses distal to the fracture site is an important sign. If pulses are not present, an attempt to restore blood flow should be made in the field. If a fracture is angulated, the paramedic should apply manual traction to the extremity distal to the fracture site in an attempt to realign the

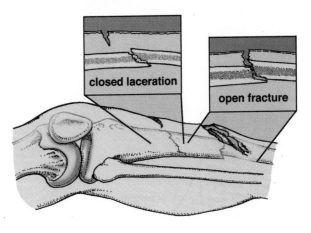

Figure 48-13

An extremity may have a fracture and laceration in close proximity without the injury being an "open fracture." A fracture and laceration together indicate an open fracture. When in doubt, treat the injury as an "open fracture," because this injury is worse than a closed fracture.

bone fragments (Fig. 48-15). In many cases, this procedure will restore blood flow to the distal extremity. The realignment must then be maintained throughout stabilization and transport. If this requires continued manual traction, a trained responder should be assigned to the task.

Monitoring Vascular Status

In the abbreviated trauma examination, the extremities should be evaluated by visualization and palpation, but actual movement of the limbs should be minimized. The following is a review of the evaluation of peripheral circulation specifically as it may be affected by extremity fractures.

The evaluation and management of life-threatening conditions always take priority. If time allows, the circulation in the extremities can also be evaluated by palpation of the pulse volume in the pairs of brachial, radial, femoral, dorsalis pedis, and posterior tibial arteries. Complaints of pain, coolness or numbness in an extremity, or signs of masses, swelling, localized pallor, erythema (reddening), or cyanosis should trigger closer examination. When a circulatory deficit is found, the cause should be sought by backtracking proximally along the artery.

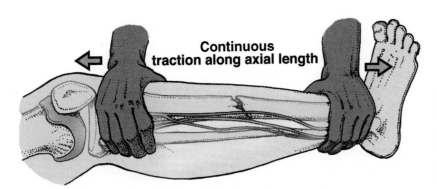

Continuous traction along axial length

Figure 48-14

Axial traction is accomplished by gently and firmly pulling the bone end apart until the extremity length approximates that of the uninjured extremity. The splint must then be applied in such a way that traction is maintained.

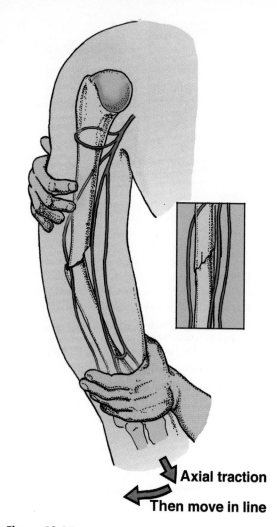

Axial traction

Then move in line

Figure 48-15

Axial traction, followed by in-line stabilization, often restores blood flow to distal parts of the extremity.

Examination of Large Arm and Leg Arteries

Systematic comparison of the pulse volumes at similar levels or symmetric arteries should be performed to assess vascular compromise. This is particularly important whenever realignment of a displaced fracture is considered. In the upper extremity, palpation of the brachial, radial, and ulnar arteries should be performed. Injuries that particularly threaten distal arterial supply in the arm include fractures and dislocations of the elbow, fractures of both bones of the forearm, and severely displaced Colle's fractures and dislocations of the wrist.

In the lower extremity, the paramedic should palpate the thighs and legs for abnormal distribution of skin temperature, comparing symmetric areas. The pulse of the posterior tibial and the dorsalis pedis arteries should be evaluated. Although it is common not to be able to palpate both arteries usually one or the other can be located. Injuries most likely to cause vascular compromise of the lower extremity include displaced fractures of the femur, anterior hip dislocations, dislocations of the knee, proximal tibia and fibula fractures, and both bone tibia-fibula fractures.

Extremity Splinting Techniques

Numerous types of splints and splinting techniques have evolved over the years for splinting fractures (Fig. 48-16). For fractures distal to the knee or the elbow, the air splint is a time-honored method. The air splint stabilizes the fracture in alignment and can be used as a pressure dressing for lacerations or open fractures. Most air splints are constructed of clear plastic material and zip up the front for each application and removal. This allows for viewing the wound and lowers the likelihood that the emergency department physician will overlook any lacerations or open fractures. Additionally, air splints can remain in place during the x-ray process. The disadvantages of air splints are that they are expensive, can compromise the circulation to the distal extremity and may require excessive manipulation to apply.

The ladder splint is widely used by EMS agencies and, like the air splint, has applications for use in both upper and lower extremities. Ladder splints are constructed of soft wire that can be bent to conform with the shape of the extremity. They are relatively strong, lightweight and impervious to blood and water. They are also low in cost and easy to store.

The disadvantages of the ladder splint are threefold. First, the splint shows up on x-rays and may cover the fractures. Second, these splints do not immobilize as well as the air splint. An agitated or unruly patient may be able to bend or re-shape these devices, which, in turn, causes the fracture to be resplinted in an undesirable position. Third, these splints must be applied by wrapping the splint to the extremity, which ultimately hides any open fractures or lacerations from view. This potentially allows the injury to be overlooked by the physicians and other hospital personnel whose attention is usually focused on the life-threatening injuries.

The box splint came into favor with many EMS agencies during the 1980s. The advantages are, for the most part, the same as the ladder splint. These devices are made of inexpensive cardboard, fold flat for easy storage, and can be left on

Arterial deficit causes skin pallor and coldness. When arterial flow is completely cut off by compression of an artery from a fracture or a compartment syndrome, the veins empty and the skin becomes chalky white. Partial but inadequate flow may produce red or cyanotic skin. Since the degree of deoxygenation varies directly with temperature, the same pooled blood may be red in cold weather and blue at higher temperatures.

Skin temperature is often a reliable indicator of blood flow in the skin vessels. In clothed patients, the skin of the head, neck, and trunk is usually warmer than that of the extremities. The fingers and toes in turn are colder than their respective hands and feet. The paramedic must try to distinguish between hypovolemic shock, vascular compromise, and simple exposure to cold. Most reliable are the differences between symmetric parts when they have been exposed to the same external temperature. When the arterial deficit is one-sided, the color of the compromised extremity may be directly compared with the other side. If both are affected equally, the paramedic must make a judgment call based on all of the data available.

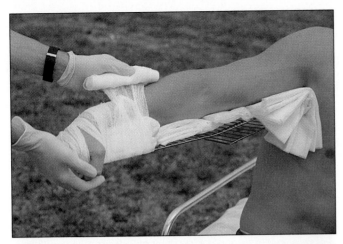

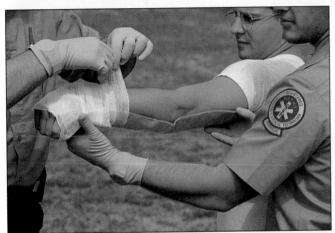

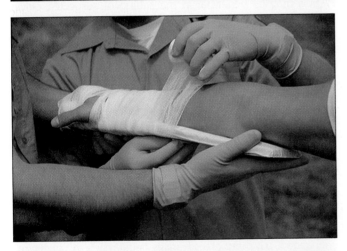

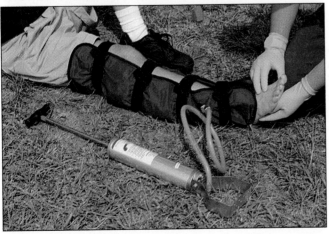

Figure 48-16

Splints from the past and present.

during x-ray procedures and even into surgery. Because they are disposable, EMS personnel do not have to worry about losing them.

The disadvantages of box splints are that they become weakened when they get wet, and they may hide serious wounds when applied to extremities with a bandage or Ace wrap. Strong patients who are intoxicated or combative are not restrained by these devices, and fractured bone ends can cause serious damage to the surrounding soft tissues if the strength of the splint is overcome.

Wooden board splints, padded for comfort, are also widely available and used in many EMS systems. They are relatively inexpensive and come in various sizes so they can be used for pediatric and adult patients, as well as upper or lower extremities.

Vacuum splints are the most recent technical advance in extremity splinting. These are pads filled with tiny plastic beads that can be molded around an extremity. A vacuum pump sucks the air out, and the outside atmospheric pressure forces the beads together so that they form a rigid mass. They retain that shape until the valve is opened to release the vacuum. These splints are versatile, reusable, and nonconstrictive. They are also expensive. Cost aside, however, these splints have many advantages over their predecessors, and can be fitted to angulated fractures; the injury is not forced to fit the splint.

The use of traction splints (Fig. 48-17) in the prehospital setting has historically been reserved for use on the lower extremities when the fracture is at or above the level of the knee. The Sager Traction Splint and the Hare Traction Splint are the most commonly used traction splints. The Hare Splint is a modification of the old Thomas device and is commonly carried on ambulances. It has adjustable extension supports for patients of different sizes, smooth operation of the ratchet traction, softer padding for patient comfort and Velcro straps

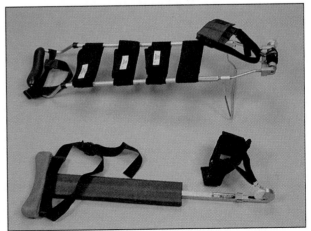

Figure 48-17

Traction splints allow traction to be maintained mechanically on the powerful muscles and heavy femur of the upper leg.

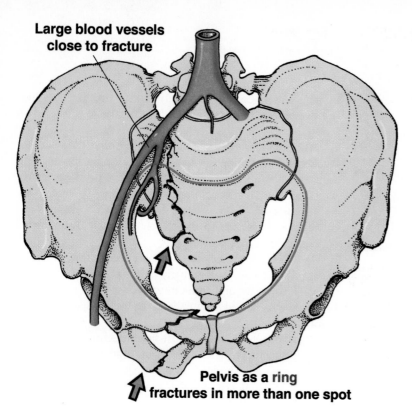

Large blood vessels close to fracture

Pelvis as a ring fractures in more than one spot

Figure 48-18
When enough force is applied to the pelvis to fracture the internal ring, expect at least two fractures to occur, as well as the possibility of severe compromise of nerves and vessels.

to wrap around the leg at four levels to provide additional stabilization.

The advantages of the Sager splint are that it can be used to immobilize both extremities if bilateral femur fractures are suspected, it has a gauge to measure the force of the traction being applied, and it has found favor with helicopter crews who often have to work in tight spaces, because there is little overhang at the end of the stretcher, unlike the Hare Splint.

All of these factors should be taken into consideration before deciding to use a certain type of splint. The final decision should be a negotiated solution with all parties in the EMS system involved.

The Pelvis

The pelvis is a somewhat unique bone in that it forms a complete ring. Therefore, when it sustains enough force to fracture it, it usually fractures in two places (Fig. 48-18). In addition, there are a large number of blood vessels which are located in close proximity to the pelvis. Fractures of the pelvis can tear these vessels and lead to life-threatening blood loss internally.

Recognition of a pelvis fracture on physical examination can be difficult. Often there are no externally visible signs of the fracture. There is usually no obvious deformity. Fracture is instead detected by compressing the pelvis both anteriorly over the symphysis pubis and laterally over the iliac crest (Fig. 48-19). Because the pelvis is usually a solid ring, it normally feels stable and has no give to it when compressed. On the other hand, when the ring is disrupted, the pelvis will feel unstable and the patient will localize pain during the compression.

There is little that can be done in the field to stabilize a pelvic fracture directly. Shock should be aggressively managed according to local protocols. Some physicians believe that PASGs may be beneficial in the setting of suspected pelvic fracture with shock; however, controlled studies are lacking in availability; therefore, many systems continue to utilize them for this indication until such time as formal research reveals a lack of benefit to do so.

SUMMARY

Fractures of the extremities and the spine are common findings in the multiple trauma patient. After attending to the ABCs, spine evaluation and immobilization are the next orders of business. New extrication collars on the market use the principles of the older neurosurgical halo-vests and provide more stability for cervical spine injuries. Backboards are fairly unchanged, but there are advances being made in patient removal that eliminate log rolling maneuvers.

Extremity fractures are third-priority items in the management scheme. Air splints and ladder splints are the standard tools of the modern EMS system, but vacuum splints may replace them if the prices become more feasible. Use of traction for femur fractures has been, for the most part, unchanged over the past 15 years.

REFERENCES

1. **Arishita GI, Vayer JS, Bellamy RF:** Cervical spine immobilization of penetrating neck wounds in a hostile environment. *J Trauma* 29(3):332–337, 1989.

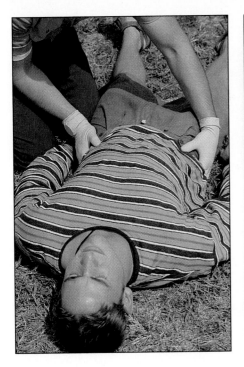 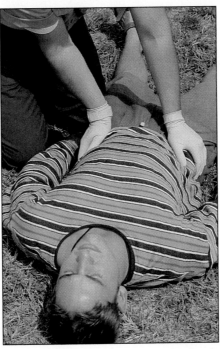

Figure 48-19

Examination of the pelvis to detect fractures involves compression anteriorly on the symphysis pubis and laterally on the iliac crests.

2. **Bivens HG, et al:** The effect of axial traction during orotracheal intubation of the trauma victim with an unstable cervical spine. *Ann Emerg Med* 17:53–57, 1988.

3. **Chandler DR, et al:** Emergency cervical spine immobilization. *Ann Emerg Med* 21(10): 1185–1188, 1992.

4. **Fisher SV, et al:** Cervical orthoses effect on cervical spine motion: Roentgenographic and goniometric method of study. *Arch Phys Med Rehab* 58:109–115, 1977,

5. **Hartman JT, et al:** Cineradiography of the braced normal cervical spine. *Clin Orthop* 109:97–102, 1975.

6. **Heary RF, et al:** Acute stabilization of the cervical spine by halo/vest application facilities evaluation and treatment of multiple trauma patients. *J Trauma* 33(3):445–451, 1992.

7. **Hoffman JR, et al:** Low-risk criteria for cervical-spine radiology in blunt trauma: a prospective study. *Ann Emerg Med* 21(12):1454–1460, 1992.

8. **Johnson, et al:** Cervical orthoses, *J Bone Joint Surg* 59A:332–339, 1977.

9. **Jones MD:** Cineradiographic studies of the collar-immobilized cervical spine. *J Neurosurg* 17:633–637, 1960.

10. **Kaufman WA, et al:** Comparison of three prefabricated cervical collars. *Orthot Prosthet* 39:21–28, 1986.

11. **Kreipke DL, et al:** Reliability of indicators for cervical spine films in trauma patients. *J Trauma* 29:1438–1439, 1989.

12. **Ligier B, et al:** The role of anesthetic induction agents and neuromuscular blockade in the endotracheal intubation of trauma victims. *Surg Gynecol Obstet* 173:477–481, 1991.

13. **McCabe JB, Nolan DJ:** Comparison of the effectiveness of different cervical immobilization collars. *Ann Emerg Med* 15:50–53, 1986.

14. **O'Malley KF, Ross SE:** The incidence of injury to the cervical spine in patients with craniocerebral injury. *J Trauma* 28:1476–1478, 1988.

15. **Podolsky S, et al:** Efficacy of cervical immobilization methods. *J Trauma* 23:461–465, 1983.

16. **Roberge RJ, Wears RC:** Evaluation of neck discomfort, neck tenderness, and neurologic deficits as indicators for radiography in blunt trauma victims. *J Emerg Med* 10:539–544, 1992.

17. **Rosen PB, et al:** Comparison of two new immobilization collars. *Ann Emerg Med* 21(10):1189–1195, 1992.

18. **Scher AT:** Unrecognized fractures and dislocations of the cervical spine. *Paraplegia* 19:25–30, 1981.

19. **Talucci R, et al:** Rapid sequence induction with oral endotracheal intubation in the multiply injured patient. *Am Surg* 54:185–187, 1988.

20. **Turner LM:** Oral endotracheal intubation in cervical spine injured patients. *J Emerg Med* 8:650–651, 1989.

21. **Williams J, et al:** Head, facial, and clavicular trauma as a predictor of cervical injury. *Ann Emerg Med* 21(6):719–722, 1992.

22. **Wright SW, et al:** Cervical spine injuries in blunt trauma patients requiring emergent endotracheal intubation. *Am J Emerg* 10:104–109, 1992.

Marilyn K. Bourn, RN, MSN, CEN, NREMT-P

Chapter 49

Burn Injuries

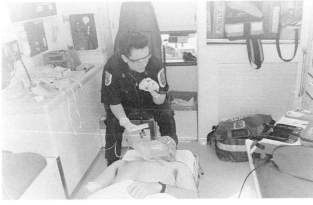

A paramedic should be able to:

1. Identify high risk groups and sources of burn injury.
2. Describe the structure and function of the skin.
3. Describe the pathophysiology and complications of burn injury in local and systemic responses.
4. Classify burn injury according to depth, extent, and severity based on established standards.
5. Identify measures that the paramedic should take to ensure personal safety and the safety of others at the scene of patients who have burn injuries.
6. Describe the assessment of the burn-injured patient.
7. Outline the prehospital management of the burn-injured patient.

1. **Adult respiratory distress syndrome (ARDS)**—a form of restrictive lung disease due to abnormal permeability of either the pulmonary or alveolar epithelium.
2. **Carbon monoxide**—a colorless, odorless gas produced by nearly all fires as a by-product of combustion.
3. **Dermis**—dense, irregular connective tissue that forms the deep layer of the skin.
4. **Epidermis**—the outer portion of the skin; formed of epithelial tissue that rests on or covers the dermis.
5. **Eschar**—dry, stiff slough or necrotic tissue; result of a full thickness burn.
6. **Rule of Nines**—guide for estimating the percentage of total body surface area burned.
7. **Subcutaneous tissue**—the adherent layer of adipose tissue, just below the dermal layer. Also known as the hypodermis.

Burns can be one of the most devastating of injuries. As well as being painful, they can be disfiguring and induce profound depression. Caring for a burned patient can often be frightening, stressful, and even nauseating to the EMS provider. This chapter will provide the information necessary to an understanding of thermal and other types of burns.

Each year, more than 20,000 adults and children die from burns, and an additional 75,000 to 100,000 individuals are hospitalized because of them. Fire is the fourth leading cause of accidental death in the United States, surpassed only by motor vehicle accidents, falls, and drownings.[22] Fires are the most common causes of fatal burns, accounting for nearly 75% of all occurrences.[27]

Children and the elderly are more likely to suffer thermal injury than any other age groups. Active and curious children are unaware of the dangers associated with fires, stoves and hot liquids. The largest number of burn victims are less than 6 years of age.[22] Burn injuries in the elderly are often a result of carelessness, senility, or infirmity. Stoves, open flames, hot liquids, and radiators cause many of these injuries.

These statistics have led to an emphasis on prevention, including stricter government regulations regarding nonflammable textiles, flammable liquids, and the use of sprinkler systems and smoke detectors. Prevention awareness is also receiving more attention. Hot water burns in the home can be reduced by lowering the setting on a water heater to approximately 120° F.[22] Education by teachers, firefighters, EMS providers, and other health care professionals provides the public with more awareness of potentially dangerous situations and can help prevent thermal injury in the future.

Types of Burns

Burns are classified as thermal, inhalation, electrical, radiation, and chemical. Thermal burns, which are the most common types of burns, are further subdivided into flame, flash, scald, and contact types. Most major injuries are the result of flame burns.

Thermal Burns

Thermal burns are caused by exposure to some form of heat, such as flames, hot liquids, or hot solid objects. Major burns are usually the result of flames. Children and adolescents often receive flame burns as a result of the misuse of matches, whereas adults may suffer major burns when flames ignite clothing. Many flame burns have associated inhalation injury. Flash burns involve brief exposure to extremely high temperatures and are often associated with explosions. Consequently, associated trauma, such as blunt trauma, fractures, and neurotrauma, may be present in addition to a major burn. Scald injuries are the result of hot liquids or molten substances. Bathtub accidents and overturned hot liquids account for the

majority of scald burns. Children are more frequently scalded than adults. Water heaters are usually set at temperatures above 60° C (140° F). At this temperature, a serious burn may occur from a 5-second exposure. Conversely, a water temperature of 48.8° C (120° F) would require at least a 5-minute exposure to cause a burn (Fig. 49-1). Intentional scaldings, often seen in child abuse, and hot drinks are common mechanisms of injury. Contact burns are the result of touching a hot solid object, such as a stove or oven. Quick reflexes usually help prevent serious injury in these cases. However, if the exposure is prolonged because of altered mentation (drugs, alcohol), poor reflexes (neurological deficit), or inability to retreat (trapped extremity), deep injury can occur.

Inhalation Burns

The National Fire Protection Association estimates that there are more than 1 million fires each year and that 73.5% of the deaths in these fires result from smoke inhalation.[19,21] Pulmonary injury may occur as a direct result of the inhalation of superheated gas, steam, smoke, or other toxic fumes. Indirectly, pulmonary injury may be the result of burns to the chest, neck, and face, aspiration of vomitus, or impaired oxygenation when fluid shifts cause hypovolemia (discussed in the section entitled Pathophysiology of Burns).

Air that is heated to 150° F or more usually causes burns to the face, oropharynx, and upper airway. Because of the effective cooling system of the respiratory tract, however, lower airway injury is much less frequent. Hot steam is an exception; it contains 4000 times the heat capacity of air.[7] Consequently, steam inhalation can easily injure the airway mucosa, major bronchioles, and alveolar beds. The extreme heat results in damage to the pulmonary tissues and can also cause airway swelling or obstruction. Within hours, this edema may be sufficient enough to produce hoarseness and early airway obstruction.

Smoke inhalation and carbon monoxide poisoning are by far the most common and well-recognized complications of fire-related accidents. Because carbon monoxide (CO) is a colorless, odorless gas and is produced by nearly all fires as a by-product of combustion, it must be assumed to be present in all fire situations.[27] CO has an affinity for hemoglobin 200 times greater than oxygen does, so the CO readily combines with the hemoglobin and displaces oxygen from the system. Cells throughout the body are deprived of oxygen and symptoms develop.

A small amount of CO exists in nearly all of us; "normal" levels are higher in those who smoke tobacco. When the levels exceed normal and reach concentrations of 20% to 30%, mild symptoms may be experienced (Table 49-1). As levels rise further, the symptoms become much more pronounced and coma or death may follow. Although the oxygen content of the blood is abnormal, clinical signs can look deceptively normal: the partial pressure of oxygen (PaO_2) will remain normal, the patient may not experience any symptoms, and pulse oximeter readings can be high. Because the carboxyhemoglobin is bright red, cyanosis may not be seen.[6,11] The absence of tachypnea can also falsely suggest an adequate oxygen supply.

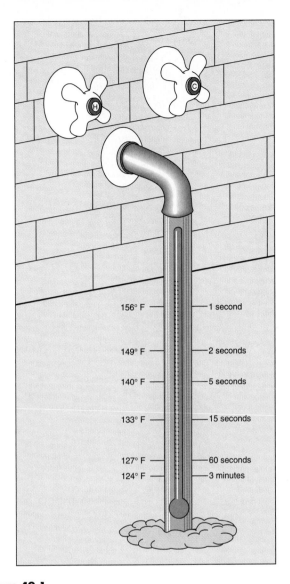

Figure 49-1

Time required to receive a third-degree burn at various temperatures.

Carbon monoxide poisoning should be assumed in all fires, especially if the patient was in an enclosed space for significant periods of time. CO poisoning is also likely if the patient experienced a loss of responsiveness for any reason during the incident (*see* Table 49-2). People most frequently affected by CO poisoning are prehospital rescuers and firefighters who fail to recognize the early warning signs of smoke inhalation such as headache, dizziness, and nausea. Anyone involved in a fire scene who experiences even the mildest symptoms should be relieved from duty, assessed, and administered 100% oxygen.

Smoke inhalation can cause exposure to other substances as well. Wood smoke alone contains more than 280 separate toxic products of combustion. Modern science, petroleum engineering, and automotive technology have developed a large number of synthetic materials that, when burned, produce a variety of toxic gases and particles.[8] For years, discussion of toxic products of combustion was limited to industrial fires only. It is important to remember that toxic gases and by-products can be produced by residential, vehicle, and other kinds of fires as well.

Chemical by-products of combustion generally fall into two major categories: those with local effects (local irritants) and those with general effects (systemic poisons).[26] Carbon monoxide and cyanide are considered systemic poisons. Cyanide, like CO, causes systemic hypoxia. Although the chemical mechanism of injury may differ for each of the systemic toxins, overall the tissue response is similar: alveolar air sacs collapse, edema develops, and sloughing and hemorrhaging occur in the respiratory tract.[12] The patient often develops **adult respiratory distress syndrome (ARDS)** and bacterial **pneumonia**. The injury may be fatal despite medical intervention.

Electrical Burns

Electrical burns may result from a variety of sources. A common misconception is that low voltage (house current, 120v)

TABLE 49-1	Symptoms of Carbon Monoxide Poisoning
Level of Carbon Monoxide (CO)	**Symptoms**
1%-5%	None
20%-30%	Headache, throbbing in the temples
30%-40%	Severe headache, weakness, dizziness, alteration in vision, nausea, vomiting, collapse
40%-50%	As above, increase in pulse and breathing rates, greater possibility of asphyxiation, collapse
50%-60%	As above, coma, intermittent convulsions, and Cheyne-Stokes respirations
60%-70%	Coma, intermittent convulsions, depressed heart action, and respiratory rate, possible death
70%-80%	Weak pulse, slowing of respirations leading to death within a few hours
80%-90%	Death within less than 1 hour

From Olsen MF: Toxic fire gases: treating the victim of inhalation injuries, *JEMS* June 24-28, 1983. Original source: Hilado CJ: *Flammability Handbook for Plastics*, ed 2, Westport, 1981, Technomic.

TABLE 49-2	Indications of Smoke Inhalation	
History		
Burned in a closed or confined space		
Loss of consciousness during the burn accident		
Signs and Symptoms		**Location of Injury**
Facial burns, singed facial hair		Upper airway
Circumoral burns		
Intraoral burns		
Dry, raspy voice or cough		
Development of hoarseness		Middle airway
Dyspnea		
Cough producing carbonaceous material		
Wheezing		Lower airway
Hemoptysis		

From Bourn MK: Fire and smoke: Managing skin and inhalation burns. *JEMS* 14(9):62-84, 1989.

is not as dangerous as high voltage (7620v) and is not potentially fatal. This is certainly not true. Significant injury may result from either low voltage or high voltage; factors such as amperage, resistance and alternating versus direct current all influence the extent of injury.[10] Electrical injuries fit the iceberg description; the majority of the danger is hidden beneath the surface. The external burns of an electrical injury may appear minor compared with the extensive internal damage (Fig. 49-2). Deep tissues such as muscle, nerves, blood vessels, and bone can be destroyed even though the skin appears normal. This is because electricity is a current, and thus flows through the body. The current will enter at a point of contact, travel along the pathway of least resistance causing direct and heat damage, and then exit at a secondary point of contact. Cardiac **dysrhythmias** are also an immediate and major concern when treating the patient with an electrical injury. Electrical energy can also ignite clothing and cause associated flame injury. Furthermore, the patient may be thrown from the power of the voltage and have associated blunt trauma or skeletal injury (*see* Chapter 43).

Electrical burns may be the result of lightning injury as well. Approximately 1000 people a year are killed as a result of direct lightning strikes; thousands more experience arc or flash injuries which are generally not fatal.[18]

Radiation Burns

Radiation burns occur as a result of exposure to ultraviolet radiation or ionizing radiation from a radioactive substance. Ultraviolet radiation (UV) rays are found in the light from the sun and are relatively harmless, although prolonged exposure may lead to thermal injury. The second form of radiant energy, known as ionizing radiation, is found in four forms: alpha, beta, gamma, and neutron radiation. Exposure to alpha and beta radiation is less dangerous than gamma. Gamma rays penetrate body tissue and damage cells, while alpha and beta particles are easily stopped at the skin.[27] Neutron radiation occurs as a result of radioactive fallout. (*see* Chapter 52 for more on this subject).

Chemical Injury

Chemical injury results from exposure to a variety of solids, liquids, powders, and gases. In addition to localized injury, many of these chemicals may also cause a serious systemic reaction. It is imperative that chemical exposure be stopped as rapidly as possible. Industrial thermal injuries often have associated chemical exposure. Early assessment of this potential is critical. The vast numbers of chemicals and the wide diversity of components and effects make specialized training in hazardous materials essential (*see* Chapter 52).

Associated Trauma

The presence of physical trauma often complicates major burns. Depending on the specific mechanism of injury (e.g., auto accident, industrial explosion, or residential fire), the pa-

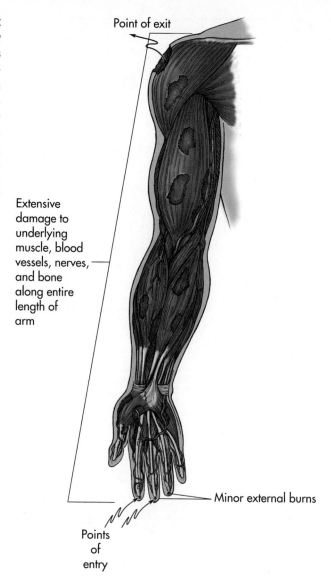

Figure 49-2

The full extent of damage due to an electrical burn may take several hours to several days to develop. Expect massive damage has occurred between the entrance and exit wound.

tient may incur fractures, lacerations, blunt trauma, and internal injury. The associated injuries may be far more serious than the thermal injury and require immediate stabilization. Management of the burn injury itself will sometimes be delayed. It is important to prioritize treatment of associated major injuries in relation to that of the burn injury. This requires careful assessment of the scene and a good understanding of the mechanism of injury, to prevent one from overlooking potentially fatal complicating trauma.

Skin Anatomy and Physiology

The skin is the largest organ of the body (16 to 20 square feet). To many, the skin's major function relates to appearance. The skin, however, does much more; it conserves body

- In children, the third most common cause of injury-related death is burns. Infants and toddlers are most frequently involved in scald injuries; older children are most commonly injured by flames.
- Burns are one of the most frequently seen forms of physical abuse in children. Deliberate burns to children most often involve liquid splash burns, hot water immersion (dunking), or burns with hot solid metal objects (branding).

   Splash burns may occur from hot water, hot coffee, or cooking oil, being thrown on the child or poured over the child. The pattern will show a large concentrated area of burn and a spattering or "run-off" pattern.

   Hot water immersion burns typically show a "stocking-glove" pattern as the feet or hands are immersed into the hot liquid. The burn often has a very clear border created by the waterline. Immersion of a child's buttocks first into the tub causes a classic dunking pattern. The burn usually injures the peritoneum, genitals, and parts of the lower extremities. The groin areas with its skin fold may be spared.

   Burns inflicted by hot objects are less common than scald burns, but often show very unusual or distinct patterns. Objects such as clothing, irons, curling irons, or electric range elements show clear and distinct patterns of injury. Cigarette burns show circular, ulcerating type patterns, often on the soles of the feet and palms of the hands. These burns may mimic infected bug bites.
- Full thickness burns occur more rapidly in children because of their thin skin.
- Children have a large relative surface area and tend to lose more body fluid and body heat than adults.

- Estimation of burn surface area is altered in the child and infant (see Figure 49-9).
- The small trachea of a child makes airway obstruction from airway edema a constant concern in the child or infant that has respiratory burns.
- Fluid resuscitation is critical in the pediatric patient, but it may be difficult. The relative lack of experience, technical difficulty, and anxiety associated with the seriously burned child may affect the paramedic's ability to gain IV access. Some medical directors believe that IV insertion may delay transport, increase the child's anxiety, and increase the risk of infection. Others believe that IVs in the field help prevent the onset of burn shock.
- The use of the intraosseous (IO) technique is controversial and must also follow local protocols. When the decision is made to initiate an IO, avoid placing it through burned tissue. The amount of fluid infused is the same as by the IV route.
- Children and infants are more susceptible to carbon monoxide poisoning.

REFERENCES

1. Aoki BY, McCloskey, K. *Evaluation, stabilization, and transport of the critically ill child,* ed 1. St. Louis, 1992, Mosby-Year Book, Inc.

2. Nichols D, et al. *Golden hour. The handbook of advanced pediatric life support,* ed 1. St. Louis, 1991, Mosby-Year Book.

3. Silverman BK. *APLS: the pediatric emergency medicine course,* ed 2, American Academy of Pediatrics and American College of Emergency Physicians.

---

fluids and acts as a barrier to bacteria and other foreign substances. In addition, the skin contains nerve endings which are sensitive to touch and temperature. When a burn injury breaks the integrity of the skin, the victim may suffer from disturbances in appearance, fluid status, infection, and temperature irregularities.

The skin is very sensitive to heat. Necrosis of the cells is dependent on the intensity of heat and the length of exposure. Local cellular damage usually does not occur at temperatures below 44° C (111° F), as confirmed by the fact that many people use hot tubs at this temperature. Temperatures between 44° C and 51° C (123° F) can cause significant cellular damage. At temperatures greater than 51° C, destruction of the skin will occur with even a brief exposure.

Layers of the Skin

The outermost portion of the skin is the epidermis. It is relatively thin (about as thick as a piece of paper) and very durable (the skin anatomy is illustrated in Chapter 7). Areas such as the soles of the feet and palms of the hand have a great deal of epidermis, and therefore more protection. The epidermis

may be burned by the radiant heat of the sun, as well as hot water or more significant heat.

Beneath the epidermis lies the dermis, which contains such structures as nerve endings, sebaceous glands, capillaries, sweat glands, and hair follicles. Slightly more heat or exposure is required to cause injury to the dermis, because this layer is covered by the epidermis. Because of the nerve endings, injury to the dermis is very painful. Blister formation and "weeping" of fluid are associated with dermal burns.

The third layer, known as the subcutaneous tissue, provides a layer of thermal insulation for muscles and bones. Areas of the body such as fingers, toes, ears, and eyelids have much less subcutaneous tissue than others and are thus more susceptible to thermal injury. Deep in the dermis, above the subcutaneous tissue, lie the epithelial buds. Their survival or destruction determines whether damaged skin will heal or regenerate.

Although not considered a skin layer, underlying muscles and bones also play an important role in burn injury and depth. In cases of prolonged exposure and in electrical injury, burn injury may actually progress into the muscles and bones. These burns indicate intense, severe heat exposure and very serious injury.

Pathophysiology of Burns

In addition to the effects on the skin, thermal injuries cause alterations in fluids, electrolytes, and circulation at both local and systemic levels. Hypovolemic and cardiogenic shock frequently accompany major thermal injury.

Shortly after injury, fluids, and electrolytes begin to shift within the burned tissue and potentially throughout the entire body (Fig. 49-3). Because of increased capillary permeability, the vascular bed leaks fluids into the interstitial spaces. This leaking may in part be related to an increase in interstitial osmotic pressure. The shift of fluids from the vascular space to the interstitial space (called "third spacing") is a beneficial compensatory mechanism; it cools and hydrates the burned tissue. However, when a large amount of fluid shifts out of the circulation, intravascular volume falls. This fluid is then lost through evaporation from the burned skin surface. Cardiac output is initially reduced because of hypovolemia; however, the release of catecholamines such as epinephrine will maintain a normal blood pressure. This fluid shift into nonburned tissue can cause numerous other problems including airway edema, pulmonary edema, cerebral edema, and compartment syndrome. Although burn shock is a slower process than other forms of hypovolemic shock, it can lead to profound hypotension, hypoxemia, and multiple organ failure. Hypovolemic shock, which occurs rapidly (within 30 minutes), is probably the result of other associated trauma. Early and aggressive airway management, oxygenation, and fluid resuscitation are imperative to help prevent profound shock and the negative effects on various organ systems.

One of the unique aspects of thermal injury is its ability to affect nearly every organ system of the body. In addition to the significant damage done to the skin, damage to the nervous, cardiovascular, renal, gastrointestinal, and respiratory systems can compound the injury, producing fatal complications.

Organ System Failure

By either direct or indirect mechanisms, the nervous system of the burned patient may be damaged or compromised. Direct head and spinal trauma may be associated with patients burned in explosions and motor vehicle collisions. The presence of alcohol or drugs has been shown to be present in a significant number of burn injuries,[1] and hypoxia, as a result of shock or inhalation injury, can compromise neurologic and respiratory function.

In an explosion or motor vehicle collision, the myocardial muscle may be damaged directly, leading to myocardial contusion, cardiac tamponade, or rupture. Patients burned during electrical accidents may also suffer direct burns to the aorta or myocardium, and hypoxia can damage the heart as well. Cellular death and increased capillary permeability lead to edema even in nonburned tissue. This capillary permeability combined with the necessary fluids for resuscitation may lead to pulmonary edema and congestive heart failure.

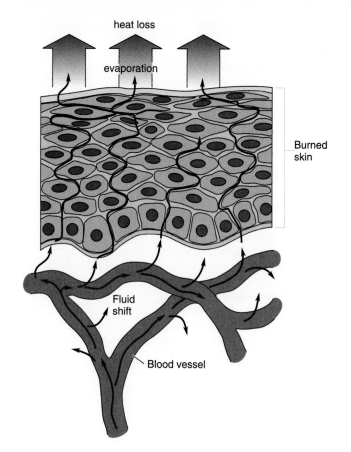

Figure 49-3

Fluid shifting occurs immediately following a significant burn injury. This event, also called "third spacing," initially has a beneficial effect by cooling and hydrating the injured tissues.

Burn Assessment

Assessment of the burn-injured patient not only includes the type of injury but also its location and extent. A general estimate of the degree and depth of burn should be made by prehospital care providers.

Burn Depth

Initially, it may be difficult to determine the depth of a burn. Burns have a variety of appearances and may also be covered with dirt or other contaminants. It is often days before depth can be determined accurately. Typically, burns are thought of as first-, second- and third-degree, from least to most severe. The terms partial thickness and full thickness are also used (*see* Fig. 49-4). First- and second-degree burns are usually considered partial-thickness burns, which can also be divided into superficial or deep categories. Third-degree burns are categorized as full-thickness burns.[13,27] Some authorities also refer to fourth-degree burns, which involve deep muscle, tissue, and bones.

Partial-thickness burns may be superficial and involve only the epidermis and upper portion of the dermis (Fig. 49-5). The skin appears reddened, pink, and glistening and may have

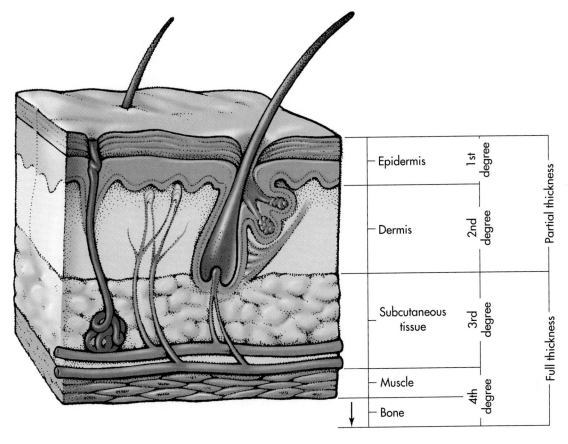

Figure 49-4

Burns are classified by degree (first to fourth degree) and thickness (partial and full), depending upon how many tissue layers are involved.

serous (clear) blisters. Superficial burns tend to be very painful and sensitive to temperature changes and exposure to air and touch. Deep partial-thickness burns damage the entire epidermis and deep into the dermis. This burn may leave the hair follicles, sweat glands, and epithelial buds intact. For this reason a partial-thickness burn can regenerate itself. Deep partial-

thickness burns may appear waxy, weep serous or bloody fluid, and have large blisters (Fig. 49-6).

Full-thickness burns involve the entire epidermis and dermis. The epithelial buds have been destroyed and no spontaneous regeneration is possible. The area may appear dry and paperlike or be covered with a charred, inelastic covering

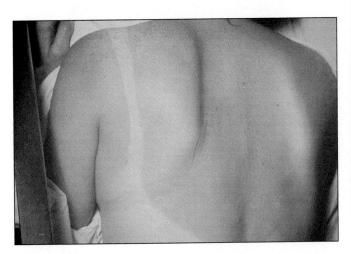

Figure 49-5

A first-degree burn is superficial and involves the epidermis and only the upper layer of the dermis. *Courtesy of C. Edward Hartford, MD*

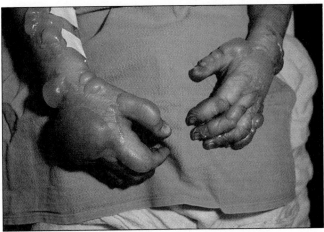

Figure 49-6

A deep partial-thickness burn (severe second degree) is waxy in appearance and has blister formations which contain serous or bloody fluids. *Courtesy of C. Edward Hartford, MD.*

called eschar (Fig. 49-7). Eschar is hard, dried tissue that cannot expand as the tissue below it swells. This inelasticity causes pressure to develop, which may impair circulation. Eschar surrounding areas such as the chest or neck may also compromise respirations. A procedure called escharotomy, which means surgical cutting of the eschar to allow for swelling beneath it, must be done to relieve pressure and restore circulation or respiratory efforts (Fig. 49-8).

Percentage of Burns

A standardized chart is used to determine the percentage of body surface burned. The "Rule of Nines" serves as a guide for estimating the total body surface area (TBSA) burned[23] (Fig. 49-9). This is the simplest and most frequently used guide. Each major portion of the adult anatomy is considered 9% or 18%, with the remaining 1% assigned to the external genitalia. Percentages differ for a small child, who is proportioned differently.

Controversy exists as to the importance of this calculation in the field. Many authorities agree that it is difficult to accurately determine the percentage and depth of the burn in the early stages. However, most EMS medical directors believe that attempting to determine the TBSA burned is important in the field assessment, treatment, and triage of patients. In particular, TBSA estimation helps calculate the amount of fluids needed for resuscitation during long transport times. It is very easy to underestimate the extent of an electrical burn. The external signs of injury may be limited to the burns at the entry and exit points, yet significant internal injury may have produced along the current pathway.

Location of Burns

The burn assessment should also include what areas of the body are burned. The hands, feet, face, and perineum are considered high-risk areas. Although the TBSA percentage may be low, injuries to these areas are more significant and more difficult to treat because of problems with mobility, cosmetics, and infection. It is also important to assess for burns that are circumferential, such as burns around the entire arm or the entire chest (Fig. 49-10). These types of burns may cause compartment syndromes because of the internal tissue edema and the limited ability of these areas to allow for expansion and relief of underlying pressure.

Classification of Burns

The American Burn Association (ABA) has identified three categories of burns: minor, moderate uncomplicated, and major. These categories are based on the depth of burn, extent of TBSA, patient age, location of injury, and any special considerations[4] (see Box 49-1). The classification of burns, although academic, assists the paramedic in understanding the level of burn severity and in making appropriate triage and destination decisions in the field.

Field Assessment

The precise order of assessment will be based on the individual patient and circumstances. There will be times when the

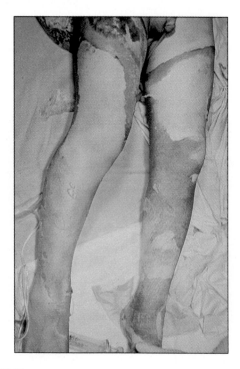

Figure 49-7

A full-thickness burn involves both layers of the skin and can go deeper into underlying tissues. This is also known as a third-degree burn. *Courtesy of C. Edward Hartford, MD.*

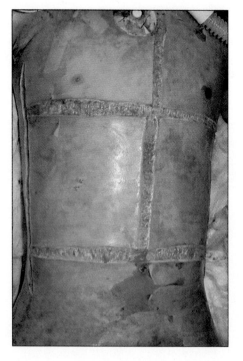

Figure 49-8

An escharotomy is performed to relieve pressure and restore circulation to underlying tissues. Eschar is very fibrous and inelastic, making respirations and movements difficult. *Courtesy of C. Edward Hartford, MD.*

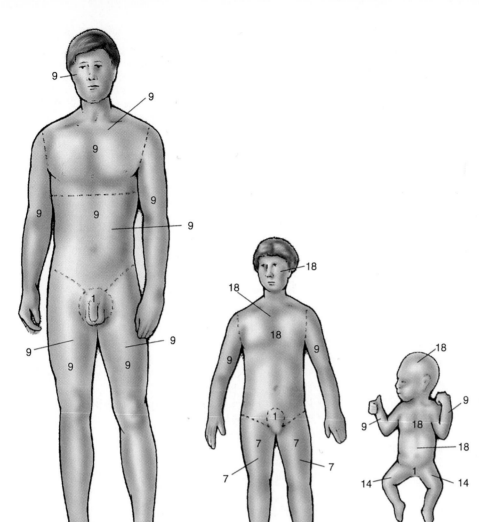

Figure 49-9
The Rule of Nines is modified depending upon the age of the patient. *From McSwain, et al: The Basic EMT: Comprehensive Prehospital Patient Care, St. Louis, 1996, Mosby Lifeline.*

Adult	
Body Part	**% TBSA**
Arm (shoulder to fingertips)	9%
Head and Neck	9%
Chest	9%
Abdomen	9%
Back (upper)	9%
Back (lower) and buttocks	9%
Leg (anterior)	9%
Leg (posterior)	9%
Genitals	1%

Child and Infant	
Body Part	**% TBSA**
Arm (shoulder to fingertips)	9%
Head and Neck	18%
Trunk (anterior)	18%
Trunk (posterior)	18%
Leg (anterior)	7%
Leg (posterior)	7%
Genitals	1%

history precedes the initial assessment, and other times when the initial assessment is immediately completed to assess and stabilize the ABCs. At the appropriate moment, depending on other priorities, a thorough, continued assessment is also important. The final element of assessment is accurate and complete documentation.

Scene Assessment

Prehospital personnel must always assess the potential danger before entering a scene. When fire is present, the first personnel on the scene help to determine the strategic positioning and use of fire units. Triage and patient care should take place

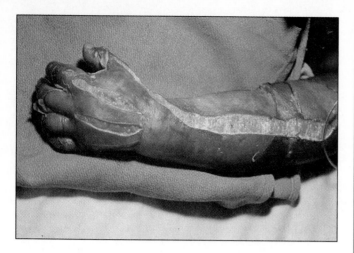

Figure 49-10

A circumferential burn is especially damaging because of compression of tissues underneath and the development of compartment syndrome. An escharotomy will relieve the pressure. *Courtesy of C. Edward Hartford, MD.*

---

close enough to the patient's location to allow rapid access, yet far enough away to be safe from explosion, water runoff, and airborne chemical contaminants (*see* Chapter 51). Field personnel who lack the proper training or equipment should not risk entering a burning building or vehicle to rescue a patient. Seemingly small residential fires can create temperatures as high as 1000° F, produce toxic products of combustion, and cause unstable building structures. Smoke inhalation and panic often lead to lost and disoriented rescuers who hurt themselves and can't help their patients. Paramedics encountering victims of electrical injury should ensure that the patient is no longer in contact with the electrical source before touching the patient and that the source does not pose a hazard to any rescue personnel.

Patient History

An understanding of the mechanism of injury (e.g., house fire) and the type of injury sustained (e.g., flame and inhalation) should begin the history. It is important to correlate the mechanism of injury with the injuries seen. Inflicted burns from matches, hot metals, and hot water are common forms of child abuse. The possibility of associated trauma must also be considered. Explosions and motor vehicle collisions frequently cause internal, neurologic, and orthopedic injuries. Patients who were trapped in an enclosed space are at high risk for inhalation injury. If possible, the field history should also include the patient's medical history. Existing medical conditions may alter the response of the patient to standardized care. Obtain any information possible regarding medications or allergies to medications. This information will be important in the hospital setting.

Physical Assessment

Physical assessment includes initial assessment, continued assessment, monitoring, and documentation. Tachycardia and tachypnea should be anticipated in every patient due to pain. Accurate breath sounds and respiratory rate should also be documented to assess for possible inhalation injury. In the patient with burns only, blood pressure should initially be normal. Burn shock is a slower process than other forms of hypovolemic shock. The patient who shows signs and symptoms of hypovolemic shock within 30 minutes may have other acute traumatic injuries causing the hypovolemia. The paramedic should consider the shock to be caused by other injuries until proven otherwise. Most importantly, level of responsiveness should be normal in the burned patient. Abnormal level of responsiveness may be the result of carbon monoxide, drugs, alcohol, neurotrauma, shock, **hypoglycemia,** or hypoxia. Each of these causes must be ruled out and treated appropriately.

Initial Assessment

The initial assessment should rapidly identify the patient's ABC status and level of responsiveness. The ABCs are observed for a few seconds to determine the general status of the patient. The level of responsiveness in the burned patient should be normal. Cervical spine immobilization should be initiated, as appropriate, during the initial assessment.

Continued Assessment

The unpleasant appearance and odor of the severely burned patient often distracts field personnel and prevents a complete continued assessment, but this examination must be completed, not only to accurately assess the burns but also to look for the associated complications. In particular, the paramedic should look for those signs and symptoms specifically associated with inhalation injury. Soot around the mouth or in the oral pharynx, singed nasal or facial hairs, respiratory distress, wheezing, and raspy voice are classic signs (Fig. 49-11).

Monitoring

Vital signs and level of responsiveness should be monitored frequently. Blood pressure may vary; hypotension is typically delayed and occurs as a result of massive fluid loss and third spacing of plasma. A cardiac monitor should be used when possible; electrical injury or hypotension may affect cardiac rate and rhythm. The patient's respiratory rate and breath sounds also require frequent assessment. The onset of respiratory distress, even if minor, may be an indication of serious respiratory complications. A decreasing level of responsiveness can indicate shock, cerebral hypoxia, edema, injury, or other impending complications.

Documentation

Careful field documentation is imperative to assure a smooth transition from the field to the hospital. The history, mechanism of injury, and initial and continued assessments should be conveyed to the hospital in verbal and written documentation. Only those facts needed to establish priorities and make triage and destination decisions should be reported by radio. When trying to prioritize information, the paramedic should include information which is used to classify the burned patient (as described above). Other pertinent information should be conveyed upon hospital arrival and in the written report.

Management of Minor Burns

Victims with minor burns will constitute the majority of prehospital providers' burn experience. These patients may require the assistance of field and emergency department personnel, but rarely need emergency resuscitation or prolonged hospital stays. The patient's fear, anxiety, pain, and apprehension will require most of the paramedic's attention. Placing the injured area in cool, clean water or covering it with a cool, moist, and clean dressing (sterile if possible) will help to alleviate the pain. Sterile saline may be used, but it is not required in the emergent phase.

The paramedic must never place ice on the burned tissue, because this may cause additional damage. Home remedies, such as butter and oil, and topical ointments should also be avoided. These remedies tend to cover the wound and hamper assessment by hospital personnel. When possible, elevating

the affected area may also help lessen pain. A calm, comforting attitude can have a significant positive effect on the anxious patient, especially the frightened child.

Transport decisions for the patient with minor burns are based on individual circumstances and local protocols. If protocol permits, many patients will be able to have family or friends transport them to the hospital. The patient, family, and friends should be instructed as to the importance of proper treatment and follow-up. If for some reason the paramedic suspects the patient will not receive follow-up care, transporting by ambulance should be considered. If the patient is not properly treated or the wound becomes severely infected, even minor burns can lead to debilitating complications.

Management of Major Burns

A major burn is a terrifying experience for both the patient and the prehospital care provider. Priority setting and rapid transport are imperative. Stopping the burning process and managing the airway are considered highest priorities. Once the burning is stopped and the airway is stabilized, field personnel can begin to replace fluids, manage concurrent injuries, and treat for pain (Box 49-2). As with any major trauma, field scene time should be short (preferably less than 10 minutes), and treatment that can wait even briefly can begin during transport.

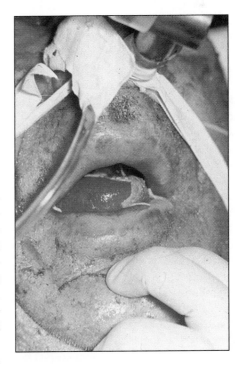

Figure 49-11

Respiratory burns are a high priority emergency. Airway compromise can occur because of swelling of the injured tissues. Courtesy of C. Edward Hartford, MD.

Priorities in Management

- Rapidly assess scene
- Establish triage priorities
- Maintain safe environment for prehospital personnel and patient
- Extinguish fire
- Stop the burning process
- Conduct initial assessment, stabilize critical findings
- Manage airway, supplemental oxygen
- Never delay transport
- Remove clothing, jewelry, boots, etc.
- Conduct continued assessment
- Apply moist dressings and maintain body temperature
- Initiate fluid resuscitation and shock management
- Initiate cardiac monitoring, frequent monitoring of vital signs
- Manage associated injuries or complications
- Administer pain medications
- Transport rapidly to proper destination

From Bourn MK: Fire and smoke: Managing skin and inhalation burns. *JEMS* 14(9):62-84, 1989.

Stopping the Burning Process

Because the severity of a burn is directly related to the length of exposure, it is essential to stop the burning process as soon as possible. Flames should immediately be extinguished by "dropping and rolling" or wrapping the patient in a blanket. Although not the best option, a multipurpose (ABC) dry chemical extinguisher may be used under dire circumstances.[9] Throwing dirt or sand on the victim should be avoided. Clothing, jewelry, shoes, and belts can retain heat and chemicals for a prolonged period and should be removed. Rings and jewelry impair circulation as burned tissue swells.[14] Remove all clothing, even if there appear to be no burns in the area. Third-degree burns can occur from heated air and yet leave 100% cotton jeans intact. If fabric is adhered to burned tissue, cut around the fabric; forceful removal of melted fabric will lead to increased tissue damage. Burns to the back are frequently missed on initial assessment, causing the patient to lie supine and retain heat in that area. It may be necessary to place the patient in a lateral position, or place moist towels underneath.

Once clothing has been removed, applying moist, clean dressings prevents further damage helps prevent fluid loss and alleviates some of the pain. The water and dressings must be clean; sterility is preferred but not necessary.

At this point, the patient will begin to lose body heat rapidly through evaporation, conduction, convection, and radiation. It is essential to prevent hypothermia. Avoid drafts, turn up the heat in the rescue unit or ambulance, and cover the patient with a dry blanket. The dressings should be damp not soaked; remoisten them intermittently. Some protocols suggest that only dry dressings be applied. However, dry dressings do not alleviate heat or pain and may stick to burned tissue, causing more pain and damage when removed. They do have an advantage; hypothermia is not as likely when dry dressings are used. Kerlix®, Kling®, 4×4s, sheets, and Chux® may be used as dressings. In addition, several companies man-

ufacture kits containing dressings and bandages designed for burn care. These may be costly and are not mandatory.

Airway and Breathing

As with all patients, management of the airway is critical. The patient may not complain of respiratory distress initially, but later rapidly develop complications. Carefully evaluate for inhalation injury; assume this injury until proven otherwise. Indications for intervention include: burns to the head, face, and neck, singed nasal hairs, presence of soot in or around the mouth, wheezing, difficulty in breathing, and decreasing level of responsiveness.

Properly position the patient and maintain an open airway. Keep suction available at all times. Provide emotional support to help prevent fear-related hyperventilation. Administer oxygen by a nonrebreather mask at a high flow, humidified if possible. Rapid and preventative endotracheal intubation may be necessary in those patients with respiratory burns. However, while the patient is still conscious it is extremely difficult to insert a tube. The experienced paramedic may be able to nasally intubate the responsive, breathing patient.

Delay in intubation may allow the trachea to close off due to edema, making intubation very difficult or impossible. In this case the patient may require chemical sedation or paralysis before intubation. If the airway has swollen shut, a surgical airway (cricothyrotomy or tracheotomy) must be performed. Even then, a patent airway is not ensured. Therefore, it is important that prehospital care providers recognize and treat the potential for airway disaster and transport immediately to the hospital when it exists. When transporting, the paramedic can provide high-flow oxygen and ventilatory support to the patient as needed. The noncritical patient with no signs of respiratory compromise will benefit from a nasal cannula at 4 to 6 liters. Any patient with signs or symptoms of respiratory involvement should have an oxygen mask at 10 to 15 liters per minute.

Fluid Resuscitation

Major burns lead to a shift of fluids from the intravascular spaces to extravascular or interstitial tissue, causing diminished blood volume.[17] Serious volume shifts and deficits must be corrected with fluid replacement. Disagreement exists as to whether this fluid replacement should begin in the field or in the emergency department. Much of the decision is based on the distance from the hospital and the expertise of the field personnel. When transport time of the burned patient is less than 60 minutes, IV volume replacement may be delayed until arrival at the receiving facility.[23] Field placement of the IV line should not delay the transport of the patient. If therapy is initiated, a large-bore (16-gauge) catheter with Ringer's lactate or normal saline should be started. If possible, the rescuer should avoid starting the line through burned tissue; however, this may not always be possible. The arm is usually the most easily accessible; the leg and external jugular should be considered as well. In major burns, a second IV can be initiated en route.

Numerous formulas exist to determine the amount of fluid needed for resuscitation of the burned patient. In the hectic prehospital phase, these formulas are usually not practical. However, knowledge of this concept will provide an understanding of the importance of vigorous fluid replacement. The modified Parkland Formula suggests that Ringer's lactate be administered, according to a detailed calculation, over the first 24 hours (*see* Fig. 49-12).[13,23,27]

Monitoring

A cardiac monitor should be applied to all patients suffering from major burns. Pad placement may require ingenuity to find nonburned areas where the pads will stick. If the patient's chest is severely burned, the paramedic should consider placing the pads on the shoulders or back. This may not be a standard lead, but the paramedic will be able to distinguish a normal rhythm from severe dysrhythmias. Electrical burns, in particular, may cause cardiac dysrhythmias. These should be treated with high-flow oxygen according to ACLS standards. The use of pulse oximetry and end tidal CO_2 monitoring may also be useful, but should never replace frequent, direct patient assessment.

Associated Injuries

Associated injuries are common. When dealing with multiple injuries, it is essential to prioritize care. Accepted protocols for backboarding, splinting, and dressing wounds should be followed. The effectiveness of PASGs is questionable in the treatment of burns, and the use of these devices may actually hold heat in against the tissues. Options should be carefully considered before applying the PASGs over burns.

Medications

Once the patient has been stabilized (which may not be completed in the field), pain medications can be administered per local protocol. Many paramedic units carry morphine sulfate (MS) for the treatment of pain. Morphine can be used via slow IV push.[15] Pain medication should never be administered by IM injection. The medication will remain in the muscle and may not be rapidly absorbed because of fluid shifts. The paramedic must remember that respiratory depression is common with the use of MS; naloxone (Narcan) should be readily available. Nitrous oxide is also used in the burn patient for pain management. Many systems require base station contact prior to the administration of pain medications. Use of other medications, such as diazepam (Valium), (Nubain), or (Stadol), is discouraged until emergency department assessment is completed, because this medication may interfere with the ability to assess mental status. Any burn patient with an altered level of responsiveness should receive dextrose 50% (D50) and naloxone (Narcan) according to protocol.

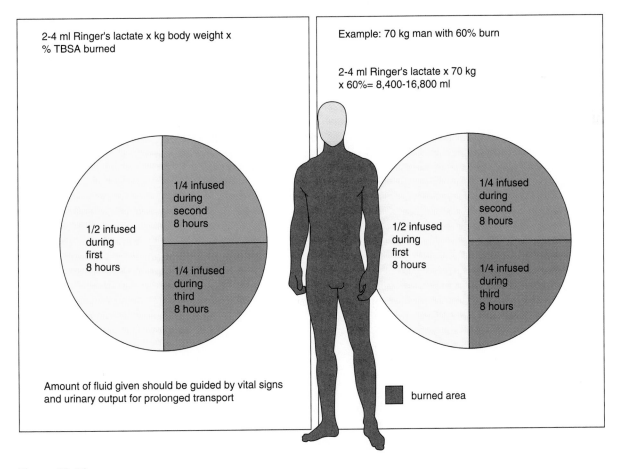

Figure 49-12

The Modified Parkland Formula is one method of fluid resuscitation for a burn patient.

SUMMARY

Burns injure and kill thousands of children and adults *every year*. Many of these injuries are a result of carelessness and accidents. The prehospital care provider can have an effect on these numbers through involvement in prevention and treatment.

Treating a patient who has suffered a major thermal burn requires a calm, organized approach. Before arrival on the scene, prehospital personnel must plan their approach to the scene and the patient. Vital elements of patient assessment will provide prehospital and base station personnel with the facts necessary to make accurate triage and transport decisions. Aggressive airway management and oxygen therapy will ensure good tissue oxygenation and help prevent potentially fatal respiratory complications. Airway management combined with fluid resuscitation and rapid transport are among the most important initial steps in treating the critical burn victim.

REFERENCES

1. **Barillo D, et al:** Is ethanol the unknown toxin in smoke inhalation injury? *Am Surg* 52:641, 1986.

2. **Baxter CR, Waeckerle JF:** Treatment of burn injury. *Ann of Emerg Med* 17(12):1305-1314, 1988.

3. **Bourn MK:** Fire and smoke: managing skin and inhalation burns. *JEMS* 14(9):62-84, 1989.

4. **Braen GR:** *Emergency management of major thermal burns*, 1977, Marion Laboratories.

5. **Braen GR:** Thermal injury. In Rosen P, et al (ed): *Emergency medicine: Concepts and clinical practice*, St. Louis, 1992, CV Mosby.

6. **Chalane M, Demling RH:** Early respiratory abnormalities from smoke inhalation. *JAMA* 251(6);771-773, 1984.

7. **Cioffi WG, Rue LW:** Diagnosis and treatment of inhalation injuries. *Crit Care Nurs North Am* 3(2):191-198, 1991.

8. **Demling RH:** *Physiologic changes in burn patients*. Scientific American, 1990.

9. **Edlich R, et al:** Prehospital treatment of the burn patient, *EMT J* 2(3):42-48, 1978.

10. **Fontanarosa PB:** Taking charge of patients with electrical injuries. *JEMS* 50-70, 1992.

11. **Heimbach DM:** Inhalation Injuries. *Ann Emerg Med* 17:12, 1988.

12. **Heimabach DM:** *Smoke inhalation: Current concepts*, Rockville, 1983, Aspen Systems.

13. **Helvig EI:** Burn Injury. In Dossey BM (ed): *Nursing*, Philadelphia, 1992, JB Lippincott.

14. **Hills S, Birmingham J:** *Burn care*. Bethany, 1981, Fleschner Publishing.

15. **Hummel R (ed):** *Clinical burn therapy: a management and prevention guide*, Boston, 1982, John Wright, PSG.

16. **Kerns DL:** Child abuse. In Mayer TA: *Emergency management of pediatric trauma*, Philadelphia, 1985, WB Saunders.

17. **Kinney MR, Packa DR:** *AACN's clinical reference for critical-care nursing*, ed 3, St. Louis, 1993, Mosby-Year Book.

18. **Kobernick M:** Electrical injuries: Pathophysiology and emergency medicine. *Ann Emerg Med* 11(11):633-637, 1982.

19. **Loke J, Mattay R:** Managing victims of smoke inhalation, *J Resp Dis* June:87-98, 1981.

20. **McGuire A:** Burn management. *Crit Care Q* 1(3), 1978.

21. **Mierley MC, Baker SP:** Fatal house fires in an urban population. *JAMA* 249:1466-1468, 1983.

22. **Munster AM:** *Severe burns*. The Johns Hopkins University Press, 1993.

23. **Nebraska Burn Institute:** *Prehospital advanced burn life support*, Lincoln, 1991.

24. **Olsen MF:** Toxic fire gases: treating the victim of inhalation injuries. *JEMS* June:24-28, 1983.

25. **Smith RJ, Keseg DP, Manley LK, et al:** Intraosseous infusions by prehospital personnel in critically ill pediatric patients. *Ann Emerg Med* 17:491-495, 1988.

26. **Thom SR:** Smoke inhalation. *Emerg Med Clin North Am* 7(2):371-387, 1989.

27. **Trofino RB:** *Nursing care of the burn-injured patient*, Philadelphia, 1991, FA Davis.

28. **Walter GP, Clark MR:** Emergency intraosseous infusions in children: a practical method of teaching prehospital personnel. *Ann Emerg Med* 16:48, 1986.

Section

Special Situations

5

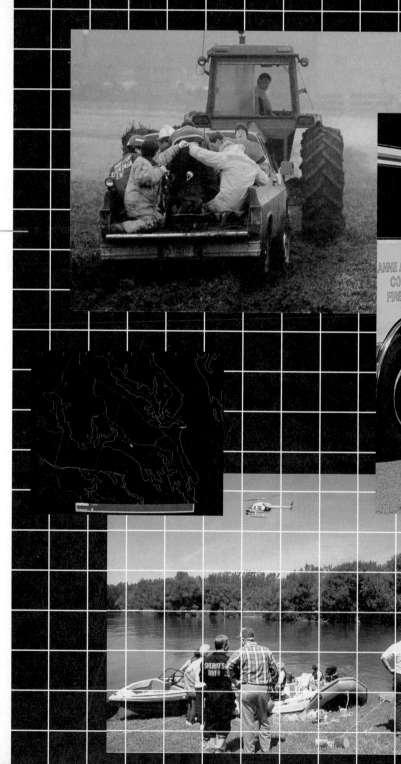

Included In This Section:

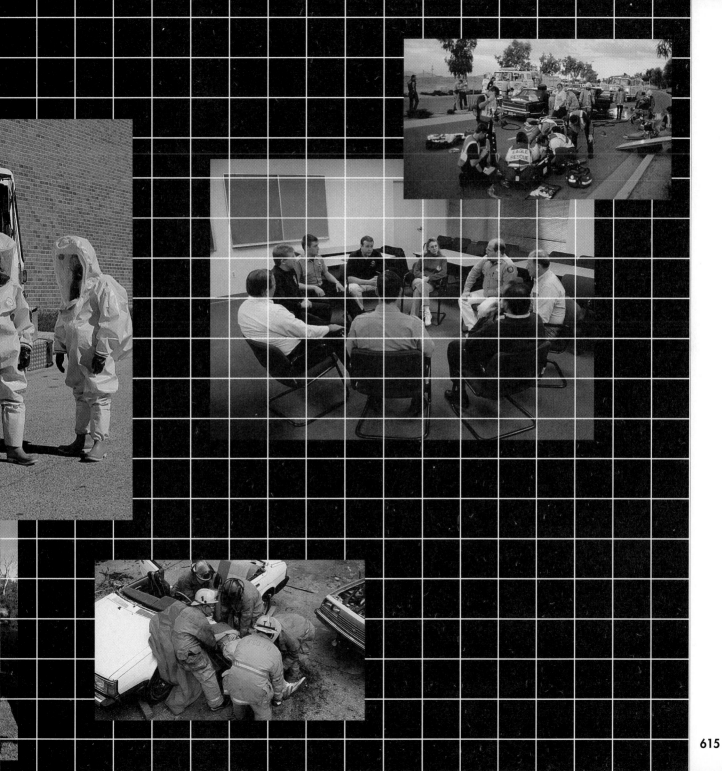

Chuck Stewart, MD, FACEP
Keith Conover, MD, FACEP
Mark Terry, BA, NREMT-P

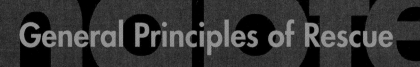

chapter 50

General Principles of Rescue

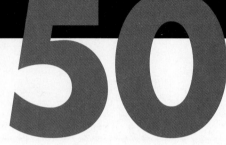

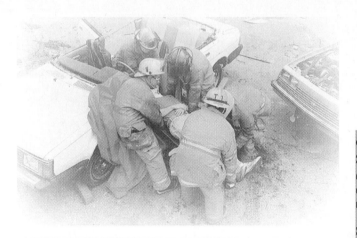

A paramedic should be able to:

OBJECTIVES

1. Discuss the significance of rescue safety.
2. Identify and discuss principles for scene evaluation and control as related to the following potential hazards:
   a. traffic
   b. environmental protection
   c. fire
   d. electrical
   e. glass and plastic hazards
   f. bumper and shock absorptions
   g. unstable vehicle hazards
3. List the three general phases of rescue operations.
4. Describe appropriate methods for extrication of patients involved in motor vehicle collisions.
5. Identify the overall goal in the prehospital setting for patients in rescue situations.
6. Describe the following special rescue environments in terms of their potential hazards and principles of patient management:
   a. wilderness
   b. gunfire zones
   c. water and ice rescue
   d. high-angle rescue
   e. farm rescue
   f. building collapse
   g. confined space

KEY TERMS

1. **Confined space rescue**—rescue in any space that is not intended for continuous occupancy, with limited or no ventilation and limited entrance/exit. Examples: water and waste removal pipes and systems, wells, caves, and silos.
2. **Disentanglement**—the systematic moving or removing portions of wreckage (e.g., motor vehicle, structural collapse, cave-ins) to make the patient readily accessible and removable.
3. **Extrication**—process of physically (by the use of force) freeing/removing a patient from entrapment.
4. **High-angle (vertical) rescue**—a specialized rescue operation.

Experience and general training allow the paramedic to handle most patient care situations, including those requiring basic rescue and removal of patients from vehicles. However, there are some rescue situations that require specialized preparation, equipment, and training. A patient might be injured on a mountainside, trapped in a trench, buried by an earthquake, found in a silo, or entangled in a wrecked vehicle. This chapter addresses general considerations for rescue situations, as well as some of the unique features of specialized rescue environments. The reader will discover an important common denominator to every rescue situation: risk to the rescuer.

The paramedic's role during rescue may vary from being completely responsible for the rescue, to being a rescue team member, to receiving a patient for care following rescue by more specialized personnel. Special rescue circumstances such as water, wilderness, farm, and high-angle rescue are reviewed in this chapter.

General Considerations

When a motor vehicle collision occurs, extrication may be required, or the victim may be located away from the road. In either situation, the rescue becomes more complex. Each rescue circumstance is unique, yet they all share common elements in terms of rescue efforts.

The paramedic should first evaluate the scene for safety and control or stabilize any hazards. A search is performed if the victim's location is unknown. The number of patients and available resources are assessed. Appropriate additional resources are requested. Rescue begins by gaining access to the patient. Initial care is provided, and patient care priorities are established. The rescue process is completed by extricating and removing the patient. Patient care is continued at the scene as resources and circumstances allow. Finally, transportation to definitive care providers is accomplished.

Search

A search is performed if a victim's location is unknown. The terms *search* and *rescue* are often used together, yet they are distinctly separate processes. Search refers to methods used to locate the patient, whereas rescue refers to gaining access to the patient, providing initial care, and extricating and removing the patient.

In most cases, the rescuers know exactly how many patients are involved and can focus their efforts on removing the patients and providing medical care for them. There are times when the patient cannot be readily located, because of geographical constraints or other limitations, such as fire and building collapse. In these cases, it is necessary to search for the patient.

Search techniques vary depending on the situation (Table 50-1); those used to locate a lost camper will differ from those used to find an entrapped person in a building collapse or fire. Generic search techniques include gathering information about the possible victim, interpreting clues in the area, and adapting a search pattern to the environment. Safety of rescuers is an important consideration as the search plan is developed. A medical area should be established within the incident command system to better facilitate communications, access, and patient care.

TABLE 50-1	**Summary of Active Search Tactics**		
	Type I	**Type II**	**Type III**
Criterion	Speed	Efficiency	Thoroughness
Objective	Quickly search high-probability areas and gain information on search area	Rapid search of large areas	Search with absolute highest probability of detection
Definition	Fast initial response of well-trained, self-sufficient, and very mobile searchers, who check areas most likely to produce clues or the subject the soonest	Relatively fast, systematic search of high-probability segments of the search area that produce high results per searcher hour of effort	Slow, highly systematic search using the most thorough techniques to provide the highest possible probability of detection
Considerations	Works best with responsive subject; offers immediate show of effort; helps define search area; clue consciousness is critical; planning is crucial for effective use; often determines where not to search	Often employed after hasty searches, especially if clues were found; best suited to responsive subjects; often effective at finding clues; between-searcher spacing depends on terrain and visibility	Marking search segment is very important; should be used only as a last resort; very destructive of clues; used when other methods of searching are unsuccessful
Techniques	Investigation (personal physical effort); check last known position for clues; follow known route; run trails and ridges; check area perimeter, confine area; check hazards and attractions	Open grid line search with wide between-searcher spacing; compass bearings or specific guides are often used to control search; often applied in a defined area to follow up a discovered clue; no overlap in area coverage; critical separation; sound sweeps	Closed grid or sweep search with small between-searcher spacing; searched areas often overlap adjacent teams for better coverage
Usual team makeup	Two or three very mobile, well-trained, self-sufficient searchers	May include three to seven skilled searchers, but usually just three	Four to seven searchers, including both trained and untrained personnel
Most effective resource	Investigators; trained hasty teams; human trackers; dogs; aircraft; any mobile trained resource	Clue-conscious search teams; human trackers and sign-cutters; dogs; aircraft; trained grid search teams	Trained grid search teams

From Auerbach, PS: Wilderness Medicine, ed 3, 1995, St. Louis, Mosby-Year Book, Inc.

Scene Evaluation and Control

The first priority is rescuer safety. The forces involved in dismantling an automobile, for instance, pose certain dangers (Fig. 50-1). Even with proper training, scenes involving hazardous materials or hazardous environments are dangerous. Without proper training and appropriate equipment for a rescue situation, the paramedic should not enter the scene. Other rescue personnel can bring the patient to a safe area for treatment by the paramedic. The paramedic serves as a medical adviser when not directly involved in rescue efforts.

As safety issues are identified at the scene, they are controlled or plans are formulated to stabilize them. For situations in which an incident command plan is established, a safety officer may be appointed to ensure rescuer and scene safety. The safety officer will stop a rescue operation if it becomes unsafe. Ideally, the safety officer has limited involvement, or none at all, in the rescue itself.

Traffic

Traffic is a major hazard in all road and freeway extrications. Paramedics should be aware of safe parking and approach techniques for various settings, such as residential streets, rural roads, and freeways. Police will assume responsibility for traffic control, but EMS personnel should remain alert to this hazard; other collisions may occur as passersby slow to view the scene.

Traffic hazard control devices include flares, warning flags, vehicle warning lights, traffic control lights, traffic cones, and safety vests. Traffic must be slowed and diverted away from the work scene. There are three general choices in traffic control: divert around the scene, detour on another road, or stop the traffic (Fig. 50-2). If there is any question about the

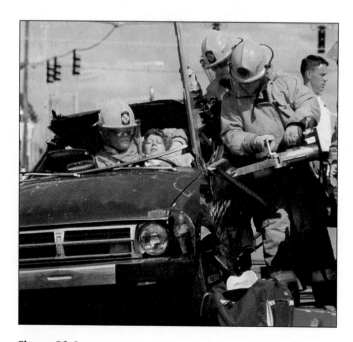

Figure 50-1

Every rescue situation poses dangers for the crew. Rescuer safety is a concern for every call. Photographed by Craig Jackson.

| BOX 50-1 | Use of Flares at Emergency Scenes |

- Flares, lights, and warning reflectors should be arranged in patterns to divert the traffic around or away from the accident scene.
- Flares should be placed to cover all possible traffic, including both directions on two-lane highways and all four directions at intersections.
- Traffic should be kept moving, if possible.
- Flares should not be set near flammable materials such as gas, brush, or dry grass.
- Flares should be lit downwind from the accident.
- Flares should be stacked so that as one burns out, it ignites the next one in a "domino" fashion.
- Flares should not be held by rescuers, because the hot liquid can cause burns.

safety of a diversion around the scene, then the entire road should be closed for the duration of the rescue and extrication. A temporary detour may be arranged by police while the road is blocked. Box 50-1 contains information on flare arrangement.

Additional traffic control is achieved by appropriate positioning of rescue vehicles; the vehicle can act as a buffer to protect rescue personnel (Fig. 50-3). For a single rescue vehicle situation, the vehicle should be parked at least 50 feet from the emergency. If there is a chemical or fuel spill, this distance may be much larger.

Environmental Protection

The rescuer should have appropriate protective gear and equipment for the rescue and weather conditions. Protective gear includes helmets, goggles, hand protection (e.g., rubber gloves), and rescue jackets or turnout gear. Potential additional equipment includes SCUBA (self-contained underwater breathing apparatus) devices, SCBA (self-contained breathing apparatus) devices, and full environmental protection suits. The type of gear required is dictated by the nature of the rescue. Specialized gear requires appropriate training.

Fire Hazards

Fire is a consideration in motor vehicle collisions and other rescue situations, and may be part of the initial incident itself. An ABC dry chemical fire extinguisher can be used to control small fires in or around motor vehicles (Fig. 50-4). The rescuer should be cautious not to spray extinguisher contents on patients. The paramedic should also wear appropriate protective gear; even when fire is not present, the danger of fire should always be considered.

Tires superheated by fire may explode, propelling pieces of tire, reinforcing wires, hubcaps, or tire rims. Fuel is an additional danger, especially considering alternative fuel vehicles that may be powered by dual-fuels, methane, propane, or electricity. Electrical fuel pumps may continue to function after the collision, spilling fuel. Catalytic converters operate at temperatures of 1000° F or higher and can ignite fuel or dry grass.

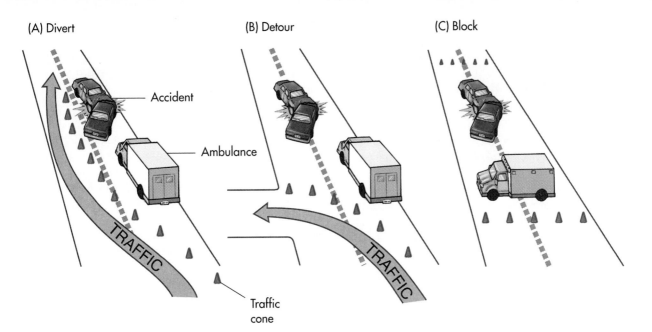

(A) Divert — Accident — Ambulance — TRAFFIC

(B) Detour — TRAFFIC — Traffic cone

(C) Block

Figure 50-2

Traffic control involves A) diverting the traffic flow, B) providing a detour, or C) blocking traffic flow completely.

Electrical Hazards

If a vehicle strikes a utility pole, electrical hazards may be present as downed wires. The danger area around a downed electrical line or charged transformer may extend for quite some distance. Wood poles are used to carry lines conducting up to 500,000 volts. These lines may have little or no insulation, and visible arcing and sparks are often not present. Computerized power switches may sense a short circuit in the line and turn power off, but the same computer may also be programmed to cycle power every few minutes.

Rescuers should look for signs that the power has been interrupted. If all of the lights are off, especially store and roadside lights, around an accident scene, an electrical hazard should be presumed to exist. All wires, utility poles and their support struts and wires, and surrounding structures, such as fences, should be considered electrically energized until an appropriately trained person (generally a power company employee) verifies otherwise. A danger zone should be established around the electrical hazard. Occupants of vehicles that are touching downed electrical lines should be advised not to get out of the vehicle and not to touch outside objects.

Glass and Plastic Hazards

Automobile windshield glass can either be laminated with plastic that holds the glass together or tempered so that it shatters into many little pieces. Older pickup trucks and vans may have side windows of plate glass. This glass will produce sharp pieces that can cause serious lacerations. Both patient and rescuer must be

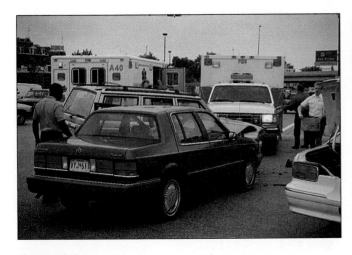

Figure 50-3

Staging the vehicle as a buffer can offer protection to the crew.

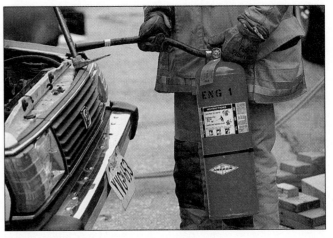

Figure 50-4

An ABC Dry Chemical extinguisher works on all types of fires and is required equipment for ambulances.

protected against these hazards. Plastic parts on a car may cause burns or break and cause lacerations. Another hazard is the toxic fumes and smoke that occur when these plastics burn.[2]

Bumper and Shock Absorber Hazards

The advent of the shock-absorbing bumper brought an additional hazard for the rescuer. The hydraulic cylinder can be pushed back and left in a "loaded" mode. If the pressure is released, the bumper is violently rammed back to its original position.

The pressure can be released by movement of the vehicle, change in temperature, pressure against the bumper, or even being struck by a rescuer's leg. If the patient or rescuer is in contact with the bumper at this point, serious injury can result. If the shock absorber is heated in a fire, it can explode, throwing parts of the bumper or shock absorber up to 150 feet. This can also happen with suspension shock absorbers.

Unstable Vehicle Hazards

Every vehicle involved in a collision should be considered unstable. The environment around the patient should be stabilized as much as possible before the rescuer approaches the patient; this may require special training. Unstable vehicles may be supported by cribbing, which is the placement of supports at strategic points under the vehicle to prevent movement, or by inflatable air bags (Fig. 50-5). Blocks are placed behind and in front of wheels. Cables or chains can also be used to secure the vehicle to a pole or to a rescue vehicle.

Bystanders

Bystanders can pose significant hazards to themselves and the overall rescue operation. Appropriate control of the environment should include control of bystanders. Some EMS systems routinely prohibit bystanders from participating in rescue efforts or patient care to decrease the potential for liability, inappropriate patient care, and conflicts. The bystander is more likely to play an active role in a rural environment. One potential role for the bystander is to assist in crowd control after they are given appropriate instructions by rescue teams. This may be especially necessary in a single rescue vehicle situation, when the need is highest for paramedics to focus on patient care. Law enforcement agencies will assume the responsibility for crowd control on arrival. Local protocol should dictate management of bystanders.

Number of Patients

The number of patients should be assessed as quickly as possible. If the patients are not visible, bystanders or other involved personnel may provide helpful information. When there are multiple patients, multiple vehicles, or large vehicles such as a bus, paramedics may need to request additional resources.

Resources

Early in a rescue scene, paramedics should evaluate available resources including vehicles, communications equipment, the number and training backgrounds of personnel, and any other specialized equipment present or needed.

Communications are important for rescue situations. Virtually every ambulance is equipped with one or more radios. Often the paramedic may have a low-power, hand-held unit for direct communication with dispatch, the base station, and the receiving hospital. Many ambulance radio systems suffer from overcrowding, a problem that may become severe in a major incident.

Ultra-high frequency (UHF) equipment exists for both the 400-megahertz (mHz) and the newer 800-mHz bands. Agencies within a city may operate on different frequencies than other agencies to limit overcrowding of channels, but communications between agencies is essential. In the event of a major incident, all parties must be able to speak in the same language on at least one frequency without codes or jargon.

The cellular phone can provide direct communication with hospitals, base station, incident command, and other rescue personnel. Transmission quality is usually high and ECGs can be transmitted over cellular phones, as well. Limitations include short battery life and areas where transmission is not possible.

Amateur radio operators can provide equipment that ranges from hand-held walkie-talkies to digital teleprinters, faxes, and portable repeaters with sophisticated antennas. The amateur radio operator often possesses radios capable of both over-the-horizon and line-of-sight communications.

If the rescue or extrication efforts occur after dark, lighting will be needed. Lighting may include flashlights, vehicle lights, generator-powered lights, and lights from other sources such as rescue vehicles. Light sources must be sufficient to illuminate both the general area and close working spaces.

Rescuers require food and water for rescue operations that last longer than 2 hours. Patients who are minimally injured also require food.[1] Although cold sandwiches or field rations refuel metabolic machinery, a hot meal and a comfortable place to eat it make the situation more tolerable for rescuers. Chilled beverages for warm climates and warm beverages for cold climates are helpful for both rescuer comfort and efficiency.

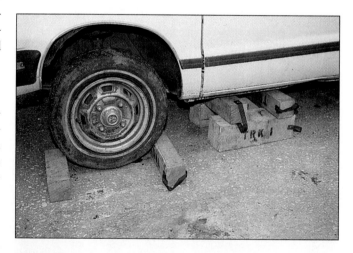

Figure 50-5

Vehicles must be stabilized to prevent further movements which could result in injury to patients or rescuers.

Rescues that last longer than 24 hours require rest and sleep planning for the rescuers, in a secured area that is both quiet and accessible.[10]

Rescue

Once the scene is assessed, hazards are controlled, and resources are determined, rescue is undertaken. The level of participation of EMS personnel in the rescue depends upon their training and experience. It is always best to assume that patients still inside a vehicle have critical injuries, so patient access should be obtained as quickly as possible. Speed of access is tempered by safety constraints. The three phases of rescue are patient access, initial patient care, and extrication and removal.

Patient Access

When a door cannot be readily opened by patient or rescuer, the quickest entrance may be through the side windows. Glass windows can be shattered by striking the glass in a lower corner or by using a spring loaded center punch. However, it is not wise to remove the patient through a side window opening. In most cases, these openings are small, and the patient may be cut by the glass fragments. It is better to remove patients through door openings, or as a second choice, front windshield or rear window openings.

Older vehicle windshields can be removed by ripping off the metal trim and cutting the rubber channel. Newer windshields are more difficult to remove and frequently require removal in pieces using an axe.

The roof may also be used to enter a vehicle. The roof frequently has the thinnest sheet metal and supports of any part of the vehicle. The roof can be cut away with cutting tools, air chisels, or other hydraulic equipment (Fig. 50-6). Removal of a section of the roof will give access to the patient while more resistant structures are cut to allow removal.

Initial Patient Care

Once access to the patient is obtained, one of the rescuers should quickly initiate and maintain in-line cervical spine stabilization and airway control. Proper airway care may be difficult to maintain during extrication if the patient is trapped in an awkward position. Positive pressure ventilation for the patient under these circumstances can also be difficult. These patients should be removed as quickly as possible for more controlled airway care.

It is often difficult to perform a direct laryngoscopy on a patient who is trapped either sitting or in some other awkward position; nasal intubation should be considered for the breathing patient requiring intubation. Use of oral or nasal airways and maintaining the patient's head in a neutral position may help to maintain the airway until intubation is possible. Suction is also useful.

Some patients will receive oxygen therapy during the extrication, unless this action is contraindicated by the conditions of the rescue, such as fire hazard. Because of the extended scene times of complicated extrications, extra oxygen supplies should be available.

Circulatory support may be necessary while the extrication is in progress. If the extrication is expected to be prolonged and the situation allows, the paramedic may initiate IV access while the patient is trapped. If the scene is cramped or IV sites are not accessible, it may be necessary to wait until the extrication is complete before IV access is attempted.

If the patient has significant compression injury to the torso that will be relieved suddenly by the extrication process, IV therapy should be started prior to releasing the torso pressure. This situation is analogous to sudden deflation of a PASG, which causes a sudden decrease in peripheral vascular resistance. The paramedic must be prepared for circulatory collapse when the torso pressure is released.

It is extremely difficult to perform cardiac resuscitation, including CPR, in a crushed vehicle. Efforts should focus on ventilation and rapid patient removal. Local protocols will dictate management of patients who are presumed dead on the scene.

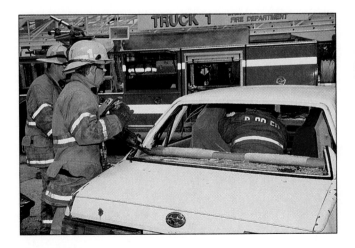
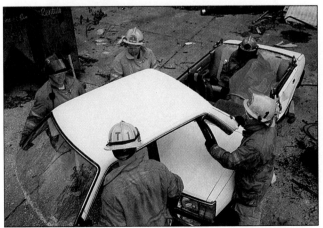

Figure 50-6
One of the easiest methods of accessing a patient is to cut the roof off of the vehicle.

The rescuer should keep the responsive patient informed of the progress of the rescue. This information includes what can be expected during the rescue such as loud noises, instructions on what the patient should do, and answers to questions. The patient should be protected during the rescue with a drape or other protective gear, and provided with heat insulation in a cold environment (Fig. 50-7).

Extrication and Removal

Extrication, or disentanglement, refers to the process of removing the wreckage from around the patient. The goal is expedient and full access so that the patient can be removed. Hydraulic tools, which are used for cutting, spreading, and pulling in rescue situations can be a big help (Fig. 50-8).

Removal of the patient is generally performed using a long spine board (Fig. 50-9). If possible, spinal immobilization should be completed before removing the patient. This may be quite complex to perform. Car seats can be moved to allow the best access to the patient. Rapid removal of patients with limited spine immobilization may be necessary for critically injured patients and those immediately threatened by fire or other scene hazards.

Patient Care

Once rescue is effected, further patient care is provided at the scene. The type and amount of care is dictated by the severity of injury or illness, the circumstances of the rescue situation,

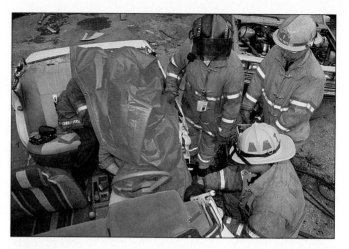

Figure 50-7

Protect the patient from further injury while performing any rescue operation.

and local protocols. For critical patients, the goal is to provide critical field interventions as quickly as possible and to transport the patient to an appropriate hospital.

Not all rescue patients are critically injured. If circumstances allow, further care can be provided, including more thorough patient assessment, stabilization of fractures, warming or cooling, and administration of IV fluids and medications.

If there are multiple patients, triage is done to determine transport priorities and hospital destinations. Chapter 51 contains further information on management of multiple-patient incidents.

Patient Transport

Ground transportation will depend on the terrain and may include the vehicles that are familiar to the EMS provider, such as ambulances, fire trucks, rescue trucks, and police cruisers. Improvised ambulances include two- and four-wheel drive trucks, vans or other trucks, or even 18-wheel semi-trailers.

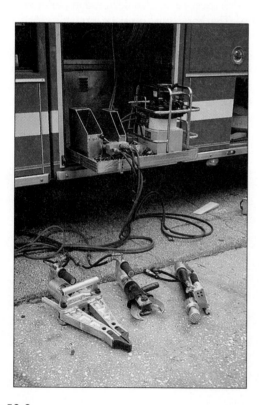

Figure 50-8

Various tools used in rescue.

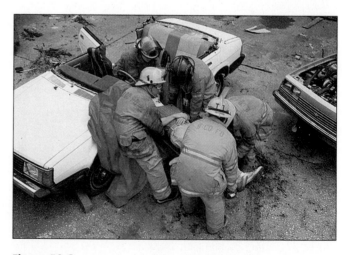

Figure 50-9

Patients are generally removed directly to a long backboard.

Ground transportation can also include long-distance stretcher carries or other methods used for wilderness terrain.

Scene response by helicopter is particularly useful for situations where there are conditions limiting access or prolonging transport time, such as difficult terrain or heavy traffic. When deciding to use helicopter transport, the paramedic should consider the time necessary for a scene response (Fig. 50-10). The helicopter's personnel may be the primary responders to the scene or serve as a secondary response for the ground-based EMS crew. In addition to risks associated with this form of transport, weather and weight limitations can be restricting factors. The helicopter agency will decide whether the crew is able to participate in a rescue. In some cases, helicopters or fixed-wing aircraft may be used to resupply the rescue. Aircraft also may be of great benefit in search efforts (see Chapter 53).

Water ambulances may be available in some areas. Water conditions and availability will dictate the choice of water craft to be used (Fig. 50-11). Combined air and water searches are employed to minimize the chance of a missing a victim.

Special Rescue Environments

Paramedics may be faced with a variety of special rescue environments, such as situations in which patients are injured in the wilderness, trapped in confined spaces, or injured by farm machinery. This section provides an introduction to some special rescue environments, with special attention to the hazards faced by the rescuer.

Wilderness Rescue

The wilderness rescue environment entails more than the ups and downs along trails. It may mandate high-angle rescue

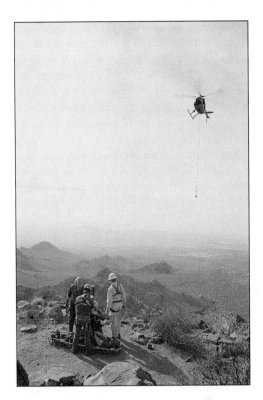

Figure 50-10

Scene response by helicopter may be necessary to access the patient. Photographed by Colin Williams.

techniques, combined with transporting patients on portable litters over long distances. There may also be sun, snow, rain, and high-altitude hazards. The paramedic should be familiar with wilderness rescue and survival techniques before attempting a wilderness rescue.

Proper stabilization of the patient for transport from wilderness environments presents unique challenges. The

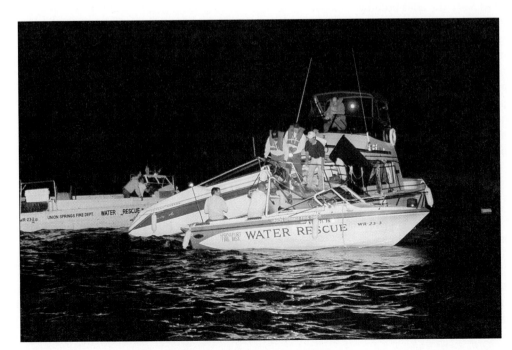

Figure 50-11

Water ambulances offer medical services to patients directly on the scene. Photographed by Craig Jackson.

transport itself is usually accomplished by directly carrying the patient out of the area. Search and rescue operations may use aeromedical services for more rapid evacuation. Spinal immobilization is a significant challenge for the paramedic charged with packaging and transporting victims from wilderness settings, and it is imperative that the patient be properly immobilized.[8] Fractures and dislocations should be properly splinted before the patient is evacuated.

Hypothermia is another concern for the paramedic managing victims in the wilderness. Both rescuer and patient must be properly protected from the environment. Additional blankets, ground cloths, sleeping bags, or even portable heaters may be valuable.

Gunfire Zones

Medical personnel may be called to the scene of gunfire in cases of civil disturbance, robbery or other criminal action, hostage-taking terrorist activity, or riot. During these disturbances, violence is usually directed at police, but fire personnel and paramedics can also be targets. As always, the rescuer safety is the highest priority. Rescue personnel should not enter the area until cleared to do so by law enforcement agencies. Under these life-threatening circumstances, removal of the patient from the threatening area may take precedence over medical assessment and stabilization, including even the ABCs. Care may also have to be provided in suboptimal areas and without adequate equipment.

Identification should be prominently visible during these operations, including uniforms or colored vests. Vehicles should also have identifying markings. Picture identification is very useful for security.

Hostage situations are managed by law enforcement agencies. Paramedics may be called to treat hostages if they become ill or injured during the crisis. The injuries that may present in these cases are diverse, including penetrating trauma from gunfire, blast injuries from explosive devices, burns from incendiary devices (such as flash grenades used by entry teams), stress-induced conditions (chest pain), chemical exposure (smoke or tear gas), or psychological trauma. Additional ambulances and personnel may be needed.

Suspects and perpetrators may be injured and require medical care. Law enforcement personnel must maintain constant physical security of these suspects. Restraints should only be removed when law enforcement officers can easily provide appropriate security. Suspects should be carefully searched for concealed weapons before restraints are removed.

Water and Ice Rescue

In many cities, specialized water rescue units are available.[14] The paramedic may be a member of the water rescue team directly involved in the rescue or may receive the patient after rescue. Appropriate training and equipment are necessary to safely provide water or ice rescue (Fig. 50-12). The water rescue team ensures both team member and patient safety. In ice rescue, danger areas and safe areas must be well defined.

Providing an airway and ventilation is of paramount concern to patient care because near drowning is primarily a problem of hypoxia. Appropriate cervical spine precautions should be observed, especially if the incident involved diving into shallow water, a high-speed power boat, moving water, or surf. Positive pressure ventilation and high-flow oxygen should be provided and endotracheal intubation accomplished as soon as possible. Victims frequently swallow large amounts of water, and vomiting is common during resuscitative efforts. Aggressive suctioning may be required. CPR performed in the water is an unproven procedure. Chest compressions should be deferred until the patient is on a stable surface.

Water temperature is a significant hazard. Hypothermia occurs rapidly in cold water; patients submerged in 35° F water for more than approximately 15 minutes have a high risk of lethal immersion hypothermia.[11] Any patient who has been in the water should be carefully evaluated for hypothermia.

Water flow hazards include currents that may entrap people or boats. They also make rescue more difficult. The entrapped victim may drown or receive serious injuries during repeated collisions with other objects in the river bed.

It is wise for the paramedic to treat rescue situations involving power boats with the same degree of caution that is used with high-speed motor vehicle collisions. Hazards include fuel spills, fires, toxic fumes, propellers, and other sharp objects.

High-Angle Rescue

High-angle rescue (also known as vertical rescue) is a technical aspect of rescue operations that requires much training, equipment, and practice (Fig. 50-13). In cities, high-angle rescue is most often a function of the fire department. In rural areas, a special high-angle rescue team can be created, similar to wilderness and water rescue teams.

The role of the paramedic in high-angle rescue teams is variable. With appropriate training, the paramedic may be an active member of the team. Because of the technical limita-

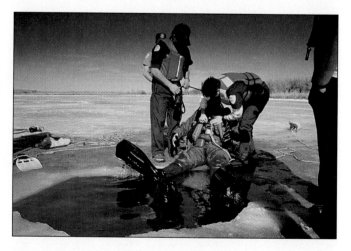

Figure 50-12

Ice rescues are especially dangerous and pose special hazards to the crew, including thin ice and dangerous environmental temperatures. Photographed by Howard Paul.

tions of providing treatment during rescue, as well as the dangers of the rescue itself, the rescue may also be performed by more specialized rescuers, who then deliver the patient to the paramedic for medical care.

Farm Rescue

Farming is a hazardous industry that produces more fatalities per capita than mining or construction.[9] The paramedic may encounter a wide variety of accidents on the farm (Fig. 50-14). The most common of these is the tractor rollover (*see* Chapter 16, for more on tractor rollovers)[7]. Farm implements can cause crushing musculoskeletal injuries.

Specialized training is required to successfully manage victims of accidents caused by heavy farm machinery. The equipment may still be running when the paramedic approaches the scene, which can present a great hazard for the paramedic. In equipment rollovers, the equipment must be stabilized with chocks and cribbing so that it does not shift and cause further injury to the victim or injure the rescuer. Other tractor-related injuries include those from power takeoff (PTO) devices such as augers, grinders, choppers, and shredders. The exposed PTO may entangle hair, clothing, or limbs. PTO injuries are more common when machine guards have been removed or when the farmer tries to step over the PTO. Skilled mechanics or other personnel familiar with the equipment may be needed to disassemble it.

Building Collapse Rescue

Numerous disasters ranging from earthquakes to terrorist explosions can leave people trapped under buildings and other structures. Building collapse rescue is complex, frequently involves large numbers of personnel and specialized equipment, and requires a substantial knowledge of building design and construction materials.

The last known location and activity of those believed to be in the structure will greatly assist in developing a plan to rescue victims. One person should be designated to interview witnesses and those who have escaped from the building or who have already been rescued.

Small organized teams should be sent to the surface of the pile to search for survivors. These teams should mark the locations that have been searched and those that may contain more victims. As many as half of the survivors of building collapse rescues have been rescued near the surface of the debris and early in the process.[10]

Rapid cardiovascular collapse may occur after a heavy weight has been removed from a victim.[5] Sudden cardiac arrest may occur from acidosis and hyperkalemia.[3] Consideration should be given to early initiation of IVs, administration of bicarbonate, and the use of PASGs for victims with crushing injuries.[12] If the victim has been entrapped for any length of time, dehydration should be corrected prior to release from the entrapment. In some cases, field amputation may have to be considered.

Careful overhead lifting of debris is vitally important to patient care. As many as one third of the victims who are subsequently rescued will be found in the spaces that are created when a building falls. Construction companies and military agencies can be called upon to provide necessary heavy construction equipment. This type of rescue may require large numbers of both rescue and medical personnel.

Most successful rescues will take place in the first 24 hours, but people have been successfully rescued after as many as 12 days of burial in earthquake debris.

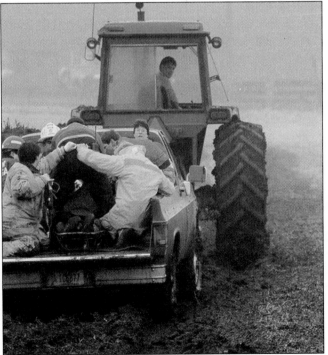

Figure 50-14

Farm machinery can crush, maul, burn, entrap, or electrocute patients. Photographed by Craig Jackson.

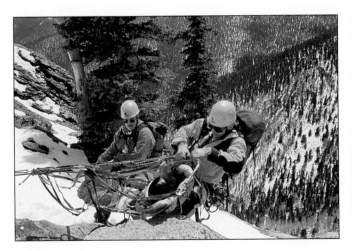

Figure 50-13

High-angle rescue teams are called upon to rescue in both urban and rural areas. Photographed by Howard Paul.

Confined Space Rescue

Confined space rescue situations include silos, storage tanks, mines, trenches, septic tanks, sewers, and any other restricted area with limited space and entrances in which a victim may become trapped. These spaces may contain less oxygen than in the normal atmosphere and often contain toxic gases. More than one victim may be involved, especially if another worker attempted to rescue a victim and then was overcome by the same toxic gases that caused the first victim to collapse.

Some situations, such as silo rescue, may require high-angle approaches. Many storage tanks or silos have a markedly reduced oxygen content. In addition, toxic gases pose a serious threat to those who work in confined spaces, as well as rescuers. Industrial workers may use full or partial protection from these substances. Silos can contain carbon monoxide, methane, nitrogen dioxide, nitric acid, and nitrogen tetroxide. Sewers and septic tanks may have methane, carbon monoxide, and sulfur dioxide. Many of these gases are heavier than air and therefore occur in a higher concentration toward the bottom of the container (Fig. 50-15). These toxic atmospheres may also be potentially explosive.

Conventional silos have a sheet metal roof or no roof, multiple doors, and a silo chute. Fermentation in conventional silos can produce toxic gases and reduce levels of oxygen. An oxygen-limiting silo is completely sealed, and because this is a closed environment, there is little oxygen and a high concentration of toxic gases.[4] Appropriate protection for the rescuer is essential, including self-contained breathing apparatus. If removal of patients cannot be done through silo doors or openings created in the wall of the silo, high-angle techniques may be employed.

Ninety percent of fatal trench accidents occur in trenches less than 20 feet in depth; most trenches are less than 12 feet deep and 6 feet wide.[6] Most trench collapses occur in good weather and the same trench often collapses twice or more. Clay soils are the most dangerous type of soil prone to trench collapse.

The reason for trench fatality is simple: compression forces. Two feet of soil on the surface of the chest or back weighs approximately 700 to 1000 pounds. This weight pressing on the thorax will cause traumatic asphyxia.[13] When unsupported trench walls collapse, tons of earth and stone can bury a worker. If emergency personnel enter the area, they may be buried by more of the same dirt as unstable walls collapse further. Shoring and excavating a trench collapse is a laborious and difficult task, but is necessary to effect a safe rescue.

Mine and cave rescue is a dangerous and physically demanding task. It should be attempted only by those with special training. Mines are even more dangerous than caves to both rescuer and victim alike. Dangers include noxious gases, cave-ins, equipment injuries, and explosion. Commercial mines often have established rescue teams with both the experience and equipment to handle these difficult situations. Since many of these rescues involve wet environments, the victim should be dried and rewarmed as soon as possible.

Other confined spaces include wells, water and waste removal pipes and systems, grain storage facilities, reaction ves-

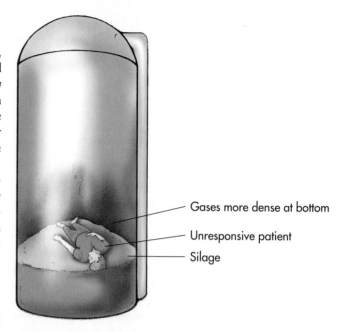

Figure 50-15

A silo can contain toxic gases, as well as an unstable platform from which the rescuers must work.

Labels on figure:
- Gases more dense at bottom
- Unresponsive patient
- Silage

sels, liquid storage tanks, tank cars, ship holds, and vaults. In many cases, the contents increase the hazards of the confined spaces.

Rescuers should gather as much information about the container, contents, and patient situation as possible. Of great importance are the oxygen content, potential noxious gases, and flammable and other dangerous products. Appropriate equipment should be gathered before entering the space, including SCBA, appropriate rescue lines for each rescuer, and protective garments if required. The rescuer should never enter an environment that poses immediate dangers to life and health without proper protective gear. Hazardous conditions should be controlled, including the disabling of electric or hydraulic lifts and machinery in the area. Steam and air operated equipment should be disconnected.

Because communications in confined spaces may be difficult, training and preplanning are especially important.

SUMMARY

The paramedic is confronted with a wide variety of rescue situations. Many of these situations can be comfortably managed without special resources. However, the paramedic's ability to recognize situations that require special training and equipment is of great importance.

The paramedic that chooses rescue as a primary or special interest should expect a considerable increase in training demands. In addition, the EMS service must define carefully what the exact paramedic roles are in special rescue operations within the agency, or as part of a multiple-agency team.

REFERENCES

1. **Beinin L:** Towards a medicine of hope: Perspectives on the Armenian earthquake tragedy. *J Wilderness Med* 1:103–114, 1990.

2. **Clark D:** Rescuer survival. *Rescue-EMS News* 16, May-June 1990.

3. **Eneas J, Schoenfeld PY, et al:** The effect of infusion of mannitol sodium bicarbonate on the clinical course of myoglobinuria. *Arch Int Med* 139:801–805, 1979.

4. **Hill DE:** Farm silo rescue and clinical care. *Rescue-EMS News* 24–27, Jan-Feb 1993.

5. **Moede JD:** Medical aspects of urban heavy rescue. *Prehosp Dis Med* 6:341–348, 1991.

6. **Naum CJ:** Rescue and EMS considerations for Trench and excavation collapse response. *Rescue-EMS News* 36–40, May-June 1993.

7. **Purshcwitz MA, Field WE:** Scope and magnitude of injuries in the agricultural workplace. *Am J Ind Med* 18:179–192, 1990.

8. **Rural Affairs Committee, National Association of Emergency Medical Services Physicians:** Clinical guidelines for delayed or prolonged transport. III Spine injury. *Prehosp Dis Med* 8:369–371, 1993.

9. **Smith RB:** Perils in the fields. *Occup Health Safety* 76–80, May 1993.

10. **Staten C:** Building-collapse rescue. *Emerg Med Serv* 56–60, July 1992.

11. **Stewart CE:** Hypothermia in Environmental Emergencies, Baltimore, 1990, Williams & Wilkins.

12. **Stewart C:** Crushing Injuries. *Emerg Med Rep* 1993.

13. **Stewart CE:** Crush injuries, compartment syndrome, and traumatic asphyxia. *Emerg Med Rep* 14:227–236, 1993.

14. **Weiss LD, McCaughan RJ, Paris PM, Kennedy RA:** The development of a water rescue unit in an urban EMS system. *Ann Emerg Med* 18:884–888, 1989.

15. **Zhi-yong S:** Medical support in the Tangshan earthquake: A review of the management of mass casualties and certain major injuries. *J Trauma* 27:1130, 1987.

John C. Johnson, MD, FACEP

Chapter 51

Multiple-Casualty Incidents and Disasters

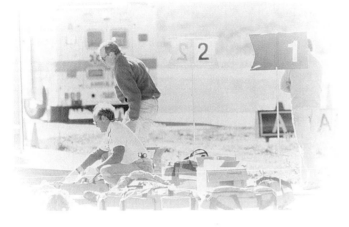

A paramedic should be able to:

OBJECTIVES

1. Define multiple-casualty incident.

2. Describe the differences in approach to patient care between single- and multiple-casualty incidents (MCIs).

3. Explain the steps of a systematic approach to an MCI.

4. Describe the actions required of the initial responder to an MCI.

5. List the roles of the first and subsequent responders to an MCI.

6. Differentiate between triage and treatment in an MCI.

7. Define and discuss examples of four patient triage categories: critical, urgent, delayed, and dead.

8. Define START and discuss how the four components are implemented.

9. Describe how transportation priorities are assigned to the victims of an MCI.

10. Describe the role of physicians and hospitals in an MCI.

11. Discuss the importance of planning for an MCI and the role of critique sessions and drills in the planning process.

12. Briefly discuss the role of critical incident stress debriefing as related to multiple-casualty incidents.

KEY TERMS

1. **Multiple-casualty incident (MCI)**—an incident, frequently called a *disaster*, in which the type of incident and the number of victims overwhelms the normal capabilities of the EMS service or system in the area. The approach to patient evaluation and care must be modified to accomplish the most good for the greatest number of victims.

2. **START plan**—an example of an MCI triage or priority assignment scheme utilizing the victims ability to understand commands, ventilate and perfuse to assign a triage priority and define minimal initial treatment intervention during the triage phase prior to the formal treatment function.

3. **Incident command system (ICS)**—an MCI management program that includes aspects of MCI control, direction, and coordination of emergency response operations and resources.

As education in EMS progresses from basic to advanced levels, prehospital personnel are taught to focus on patients' immediate problems, stabilization, treatment, and transport. They then follow these priorities as they approach each individual patient encounter. Multiple-casualty incidents, however, require a different approach.

A multiple-casualty incident (MCI) occurs when the number of victims exceeds the number of medical personnel immediately available to handle the priorities listed above. From a different perspective, an MCI exists when EMS personnel must determine which patients initially will be evaluated, stabilized, and transported and which patients will be delayed. For example, if two EMS personnel arrive on-scene and three patients require care, an MCI exists, albeit a small scale incident.

EMS personnel may not be heavily outnumbered, although the presence of a large number of victims is the most common concept of an MCI. MCI conditions are in effect whenever the imbalance exists between resources and patient needs and decisions must be made about care priorities and limitation of field intervention.

One of the most difficult MCI concepts for prehospital personnel to master, is the switch from the normal operating mode used with one or two patients. In this mode, every prehospital effort that can be executed is immediately completed. Most paramedics will face an MCI at some point in their careers. The incident may involve less than 10 patients or as many as hundreds. The principles involved will be the same, regardless of the situation encountered. The paramedic's key to handling these incidents successfully is the understanding of the principles that separate MCIs from other EMS calls.

A Systematic Approach to MCIs

First on the Scene

As a paramedic approaches a small number of patients, his or her normal tendency is to treat the patient who appears to be most in need of care and to remain with that patient through stabilization and transport.

Until the rescuer is faced with an MCI, this philosophy of attending to the most critical patient remains valid. However, as the number of patients exceeds the number of rescuers, a new philosophy takes over—the philosophy of providing the most benefit to the greatest number of patients.[1,2] If two paramedics respond to five critical patients, two victims could be saved by each paramedic concentrating on one patient. With a philosophical change, the paramedics might improve the outcome of three or four patients by intentionally limiting the care of a patient who is alive but unsalvageable, given the available resources. However, if none of the patients are critical, treatment of lesser injuries can safely be delayed while the paramedics concentrate resources and treatment on patients with immediate needs.

For an organized approach to MCI situations, paramedics must learn the sequence of the major steps to be taken (Box 51-1). The details of each scene will be different, but the general sequence remains the same.

BOX 51-1	Steps to Follow in a Multiple Casualty Incident
1. Protection	5. Triage
2. Assessment	6. Treatment
3. Communication	7. Transport
4. Command	8. Debriefing

Protection

When EMS personnel approach the scene of any accident, MCI or not, the scene should be surveyed for visible and predictable dangers, which are sometimes not obvious. Paramedics must keep an open mind and be on the lookout for potential threats (Fig. 51-1). When the dispatch call notes "shots fired," responders will naturally be cautious when approaching the scene. But what caution when approaching the isolated building, the train wreck, or the stadium collapse? How were the patients injured? Was there a toxic level of carbon monoxide, an outbreak of homicidal violence, an ingestion of bad food, or a chlorine tank leaking gas? Is diesel fuel about to explode on the train or are there electrical lines down along the track? Did the stadium simply collapse or was there a gas explosion in a concession stand? Is the collapsed structure now stable, or might it give way with minimal movement? Responding personnel should not enter such situations until they can rule out dangers to themselves and their patients. EMS personnel are of no help to victims if they become victims themselves.

Calling for the appropriate specialists is a key part of securing the scene. Gas company personnel can best handle gas-related leaks and explosions. Likewise, hazardous materials (HazMat) teams are best equipped to enter areas that are possibly toxic.[6] Unless EMS personnel have the specific equipment and expertise for the special circumstances they face, waiting for the experts is the only safe choice.

Assessment

Initially, responding personnel must focus on assessing the total situation.[4,10] Once the scene is safe for entry, EMS personnel must resist the temptation to intervene with each patient, despite potent visual stimulus and possible verbal pleas for help. Granted, if a simple maneuver can stabilize an airway or minimize bleeding, or a less-injured patient can be quickly recruited to help a fellow victim, then these choices should be done.

What should the initial responder look for?

1. *How many total victims are involved?* At this stage, the paramedic should make a quick estimate, not an exact count. Are there 10, 30, 60, or 100 patients?
2. *What is the severity of the victims and the number in each category?* Categorization of patients is explained in the Triage section of this chapter. Again, in the Assessment phase, this number is only an estimate.
3. *Will there be any special extrication needs?* Although some EMS vehicles carry hydraulic equipment for vehicle access, few have scuba gear or a crane.

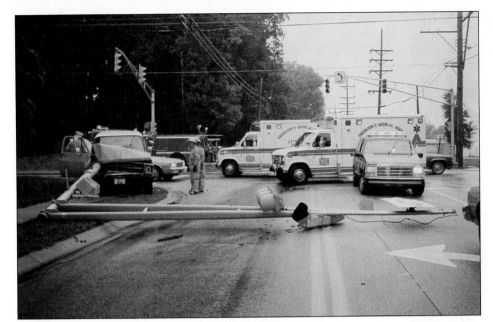

Figure 51-1
Every scene should be evaluated for potential dangers to the responding crew.

4. *Are special resources needed at the scene or the receiving hospital?* These resources may include extra burn packs, HazMat data sheets (documents that describe special treatment for a given chemical exposure), or neurosurgical or pediatric specialists required at the hospital.

Here is an assessment scenario:

A paramedic and his partner are called to a train derailment 15 miles out of town. Other EMS units are busy and the magnitude of the problem is unknown. Upon arrival, the paramedics find 20 victims trapped in a mangled train car. By quickly assessing this scene and communicating what they find, they activate a response that will benefit the greatest possible number of these critical patients. The difficult part is that both paramedics must initially pass all 20 patients without treating them.

Their initial assessment:

1. The scene is safe except for risk of fuel fire.
2. There are 20 victims total.
3. Estimated patient severities: 3 critical, 6 urgent, 7 delayed, 4 dead.
4. Rescuers will need equipment to cut steel seats off the victims, the fire department must neutralize diesel fuel spilled from engine; and a HazMat team must manage liquid leaking from the tank car (placard #1012 on side of car).

Once this initial assessment is complete, the two paramedics devote their time to coordinating the growing response, maintaining communications, initiating formal triage and treatment, and recruiting assistance from bystanders and less-injured patients in maintaining open airways, controlling blood loss, and calming the victims. The result: 4 dead, 16 survive. Without an MCI procedure, the result could have been seven survivors and the remainder lost.

From this initial information, dispatchers will coordinate the response of additional vehicles (e.g., ambulances, vans, buses, heavy equipment) and personnel. Communication with receiving facilities will alert them to prepare for the arrival of patients in the emergency department and assess the availability of resources to meet their needs (e.g., surgical suites, critical care beds, specialty physicians). If a facility determines that the number of victims will overwhelm its resources, it can arrange for direct transport from the scene to alternate sites.

Communication

Critiques often reveal communication to be the weakest link in MCI responses.[4,8] After assessment, on-scene personnel should begin to establish communication links with numerous individuals and agencies that will be involved. Good communications may do more to save patients than the actual care rendered. In fact, of the two paramedics initially arriving at an MCI, one may be diverted from patient care entirely by the need to move the ambulance to a good communications site and begin making the necessary contacts.

Traditional communication uses radio links, but increasing numbers of EMS systems are turning to cellular telephones (Fig. 51-2). Depending on the incident location, conventional telephone lines may also be available. However, none of these may work during an MCI. In one structural disaster, paramedics found that structural steel in the building blocked their portable radio signals, forcing them to leave the building to communicate. Busy phone lines and cellular cells, damaged lines and towers, and radio and cellular "dead spots" can all be problems during MCIs. Backup communication methods have to be included in MCI plans, as do procedures for situations in which the backups are not adequate.

Once it is determined what type of communication will work at an MCI scene, confirmation should occur among all involved parties that:

- an MCI situation exists
- one or more frequencies is designated as a priority frequency until the situation is stabilized
- all other traffic on the chosen frequencies is minimized

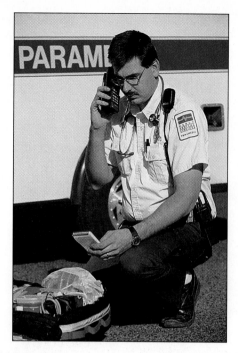

Figure 51-2

Advances in telecommunications have benefitted EMS.

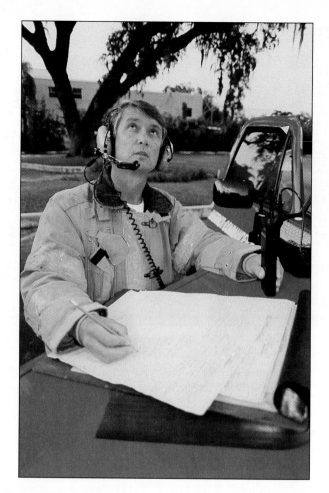

Figure 51-3

A single communications center at a disaster site will help to prevent the breakdown in communications that often occurs in disasters. *Photographed by Craig Jackson.*

- everyone who should be involved with the disaster by local protocol is monitoring these frequencies

Generally, a single location or communication center should be established at the disaster site. This center helps focus communication and minimize confusion (Fig. 51-3). In many cases, the communication center and the command center are located together. At other times, the availability of communications resources (e.g., telephone lines) or the inability to transmit radio signals from the most desirable area for command efforts will require that the communication center be separate. In this case, a communication link between the command center and the communication center is crucial. This may consist of a secondary radio or telephone system, or simply a runner system using bystanders or less-injured victims.

Command

Although initial assessment, communication, and command are covered sequentially in this chapter, all three functions actually must occur simultaneously. The first unit responding to an MCI is obligated to take charge of the scene (command), evaluate the magnitude of the situation (assessment), and convey that evaluation and summon additional resources required (communication). Should the initial responder be alone, command and communication must take precedence. When two rescuers arrive, one should begin initial assessment while the other establishes a command center and initiates communication.

Communication is the key to incident command.[8] As the initial communicators at an MCI, the first responding EMS personnel assume the command of the scene until additional assistance arrives. Establishing command and communications centers, preferably together, is the first step. Later responders can then report to the Command Center for information and assignments.

In some systems, the initial paramedic will retain command throughout the incident. In others, a senior individual or someone from another agency will take over. Even in the latter case, the initial commander may be asked to remain at the Command Center as a medical resource.

MCIs occur with no regard for the political boundaries that govern EMS, fire, and law enforcement agencies. Most MCIs will overlap public safety jurisdictions and require a coordinated effort by several public safety agencies (Fig. 51-4). As a consequence, an Incident Command structure that can effectively deal with the multijurisdictional coordination must be in place in advance. Regular drills to test the advance plan will reduce, although probably not entirely eliminate, command problems.

Initial responders will locate the Command Center in an easily recognizable area in a safe zone away from any immediate hazard (Fig. 51-5). The most senior or responsible individual from each responding agency will report to this Command Center upon arrival. Some systems use colored flags or colored lights at night to indicate key designated areas at an MCI scene (e.g., command, communications, treatment,

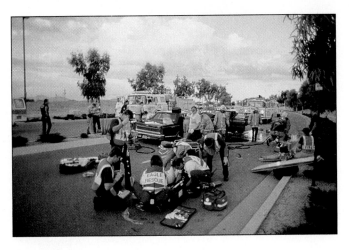

Figure 51-4

Cooperation is necessary for a smooth resolution to most MCIs. *Photographed by Colin C. Williams.*

transport, etc.) (Fig. 51-6). These agency representatives must cooperate to ensure scene safety and optimal patient care, putting aside jurisdictional and authority disputes.

Formal training in Incident Command Systems is often available through fire and law enforcement agencies. Depending on the size of the jurisdiction involved and its level of MCI preparedness, the Incident Command System can be simple or quite complex. A formal system embodies the five elements of:

1. Command—defined objectives for stabilizing and resolving the incident.
2. Operations—tactical activities necessary to accomplish the command objectives.
3. Planning—evaluation of the current status of the incident

and prediction of the future needs to resolve it. Technical specialists such as heavy equipment operators may be involved.

4. Logistics—acquisition of resources needed to resolve the incident such as transportation, personnel, fuel, supplies, equipment, and food.
5. Finance—financial accountability of the operation, including documentation of personnel involved, hours worked, and authorization for equipment purchase or rental. This element may not be used in small incidents but becomes essential in more complex and prolonged situations. Each of these areas can be further stratified depending on the complexity of the MCI (Fig. 51-7).

A detailed discussion of formal Incident Command and the necessary structure to accomplish this task is beyond the scope of this text. The Federal Emergency Management Agency (FEMA) and state emergency management agencies can provide additional information.

Medical Direction

Preestablished local protocol dictates medical direction in an MCI. In larger metropolitan systems with full-time medical directors, it is quite common for one or more physicians to be present on-scene at major MCIs and provide direction in conjunction with the Command Center operation. More often, however, medical direction is provided by part-time physicians who will be obligated, except in extreme casualty situations, to be present in the emergency department during an MCI. In this case, and to a lesser degree in the metropolitan example, preexisting protocols provide direction regarding communication, treatment, and transport or destination. When the MCI situation or patient condition does not clearly fall within existing protocols, on-line consultation should be sought from the base hospital.

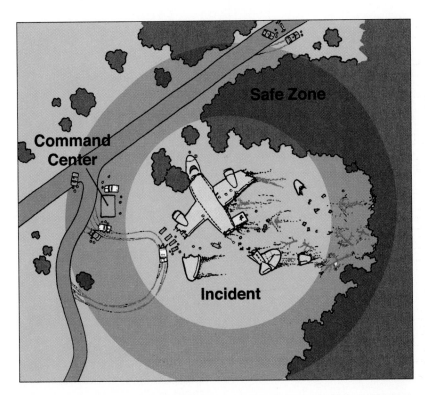

Figure 51-5

The Command Center should be established in the safe zone and be easily accessible to the incident and incoming responding agency personnel.

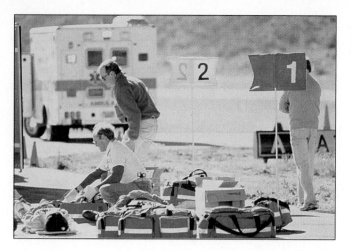

Figure 51-6

Colored flags and colored lights help to distinguish various areas, such as triage and vehicle staging, during an MCI incident. *Photographed by Howard Paul.*

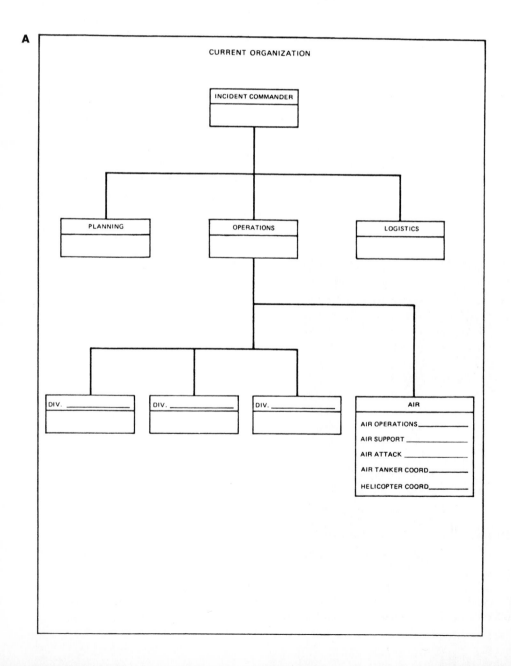

Figure 51-7

The Incident Command System can be A) simple or B) complex, depending upon the size and complexity of the incident. From Auf de Heide: Disaster Response: Principles of Preparation and Coordination, 1989, Mosby-Year Book Inc.

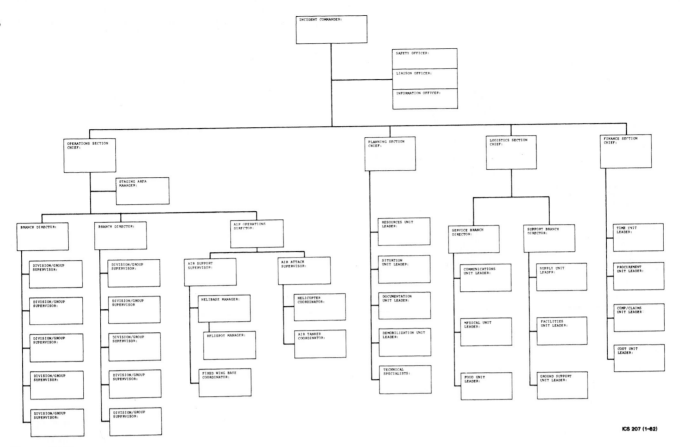

ICS 207 (1–82)

Figure 51-7

continued

In addition to MCI responsibilities, medical direction also takes into account the EMS system's needs that are unrelated to the MCI. Patients uninvolved in the MCI do not disappear. However, on-line support for non–MCI activities should be kept to a minimum. Communication channels must be available for MCI traffic.

Triage

Triage is the sorting of patients by priority based on the severity of their condition. In an MCI, the triage goal is to meet the needs of the most individuals possible by delaying treatment of selected patients.[2,8] Don't confuse assessment with triage. The assessment phase gathers preliminary data to determine the level of response necessary. Triage occurs after initial rescuers have assessed the total scene, estimated the numbers of victims and communicated the information, requested additional resources, and established a central command and communication site.

The triage team locates and evaluates all patients and establishes the priority by which patients should be treated and transported. Those individuals who are dead, or could reasonably be expected to die before sufficient secondary responders can arrive, become the lowest transport priority and must not be treated. The job of the initial responder is to salvage the most number of patients. Triage personnel provide no treatment beyond simple life-saving maneuvers.

Triage sorts patients into four categories.[2,10] Most EMS systems use commercial triage tags printed on card stock or plastic. These tags, which offer only limited area for writing, classify patients either with words or colors. They typically are

numbered sequentially to facilitate the logging of victims, which will be discussed later (Fig. 51-8). Common word and color descriptors for the four triage categories are (*see* Table 51-1):

1. CRITICAL (RED)—patients who are salvageable with timely and appropriate intervention. These patients require early transport.

    Patients who will normally be categorized as CRITICAL include those with airway problems or respiratory distress (tension pneumothorax, upper airway obstruction, flail chest, open chest wound), possible cardiac injury (tamponade, penetrating injury, severe contusion), uncontrolled hemorrhage, including internal, and altered mental or neurological status (concussion, skull fracture, spinal cord injury).

2. URGENT (YELLOW)—patients who have been initially stabilized but may deteriorate. These patients require timely transport, but only after CRITICAL patients. Patients in this category include those with major extremity or soft-tissue injuries, dislocations, burns, electrical injuries, blunt abdominal or thoracic trauma that is initially stable, and head injuries without a changing level of responsiveness.

3. DELAYED (GREEN)—patients who are salvageable, do not appear to have life-threatening injuries and will probably not be harmed by delayed treatment. Patients in this category will include those with simple fractures, lacerations, small burns, or sprains. These patients, who are often referred to as the "walking wounded" are transported after CRITICAL and DELAYED patients, and may be

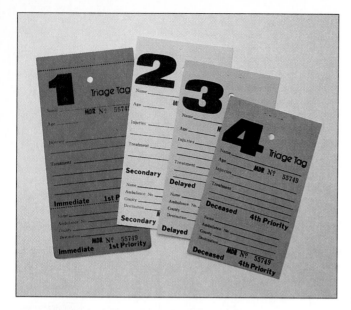

TABLE 51-1 | **Triage Priorities**

Category	Color	Examples of Patients	Transport Priority
Critical	Red	Significant airway problems Significant respiratory distress Cardiac injury Uncontrolled hemorrhage Altered mental/neuro status	1
Urgent	Yellow	Major extremity or soft-tissue injury Dislocations Major burns Electrical injuries	2
Delayed	Green	Simple fractures Lacerations Small burns Sprains	3
Dead/Dying	Gray or Black	Dead or not salvageable	Last

Figure 51-8

A triage tag is used to sort and identify the patients at a large incident.

transported by less conventional means (e.g., school bus, van, or other non–EMS vehicles).

4. DEAD or DYING (BLACK or GRAY)—patients who are either dead or are deemed to not be salvageable given the medical resources available to deal with the number of victims who appear to be salvageable and are classified as either CRITICAL or URGENT. (Patients initially categorized as DYING may later be reclassified as CRITICAL or URGENT as resources become available and reassessment takes place.) Patients in this category are the lowest transport priority.

One system of triage that has recently been developed is the Simple Triage and Rapid Transport or START Plan (Fig. 51-9).[9] The START system requires no new knowledge or skills. It follows the basic tenets of airway, breathing, and circulation (ABCs) and includes minimal treatment that can be performed briefly during triage. In most MCI situations, patients will be moved after triage to a central treatment and transportation center where they can be reassessed. The START plan relies on this secondary triage function to catch anything that the simple initial procedures miss.

START involves the sequential evaluation of the patient's ventilation, perfusion, and mental status (i.e., ABCs and mental status) as follows:

1. *Ability to walk.* If a patient can comprehend the question, "Can you walk?" and he or she is able to ambulate, they are categorized as DELAYED (walking wounded) and asked either not to move until further assistance arrives or to walk to the treatment and transportation site, where a secondary assessment will occur. If the patients cannot ambulate on their own, their respiratory rate is assessed.

2. *Breathing and rate.* The absent breathing places the patient in the DEAD/DYING category. In adult patients, a rate of less than 10 or more than 30 per minute indicates

a CRITICAL patient. This can be modified for children and extreme states; if compelling evidence argues against a critical situation, the initial triage classification is either URGENT or DELAYED. A breathing rate of 10 to 30 per minute is by itself inconclusive and the circulation is assessed next.

3. *Perfusion.* The absence of a pulse places the patient in the DEAD/DYING category. A present carotid pulse but absent radial pulse defines a CRITICAL patient. In some systems, capillary refill is used as a perfusion assessment criterion and would be significant if refill was delayed more than 2 seconds. When both a carotid and a radial pulse are present, mental status is the last assessment before assigning a triage classification.

4. *Mental status.* The patient is asked to perform two simple commands. Each system can design its own test. For example:

   1. Touch your index finger to your nose (eyes may be open).
   2. Stick your tongue out.

Other motor functions appropriate to known existing injuries or an orientation examination (i.e., person, place, time, and event) can also be used. If patients can perform both functions appropriately, he or she is classified as DELAYED. Failure of either test indicates an altered neurological state, and the patient is classified as CRITICAL.

The paramedic should note that all four steps in the START triage process are performed only if the patient passes the early steps. A positive classification at any step concludes the initial triage and allows the rescuer to move on to the next patient.

The only treatment provided during the START plan occurs during ventilation assessment, if respirations are absent, or during the perfusion assessment, if external bleeding is

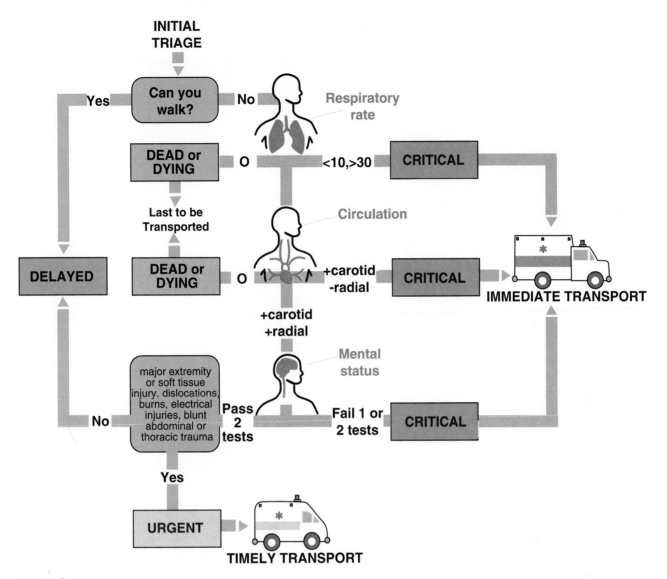

Figure 51-9

The START triage system sorts patients into critical or delayed categories. Patients are then quickly removed from the scene based upon which group they fall into.

present. The absence of respirations calls for the rescuer to reposition the airway and reassess the victim's ventilations. If they remain absent, the patient would be classified as DEAD/DYING. Major external bleeding requires simple measures to control it. However, such measures cannot tie up a rescuer. An active arterial bleed will require intervention, but slower bleeds can be ignored if further help is only a short time away and the total number of patients dictates a lowered priority.

Alternatives to delaying triage for bleeding control include having a patient apply pressure if able and recruiting the walking wounded or bystanders to help. The walking wounded and patients categorized as DELAYED can provide solace to the more severely injured patients.

In large-scale MCIs, patients are moved from their initial locations to an organized area for further evaluation. Triage personnel are often unaware of the number and severity of victims in other sectors. As the patients are brought to a central location, their priorities can be reassessed.

Reassessment and Treatment

Except for brief, life-saving interventions during triage, treatment should occur after all patients have undergone initial triage and usually after additional help arrives. Unless the patients are all initially grouped in a safe environment accessible to transport vehicles, they will next be moved to a central area for reassessment. This area may be referred to as the treatment center (Fig. 51-10). In some MCI plans, the treatment and transport centers are at the same location.

Treatment begins at this site as necessary and as time permits before transport, in triage priority order. During treatment, priorities for transport become more obvious. The paramedic develops a better feel for which patients may die despite treatment, which patients will survive with rapid transportation to a definitive facility, and which patients can wait for delayed transport. When there are a significant number of casualties, transport may occur prior to any significant treatment (see Box 51-2).

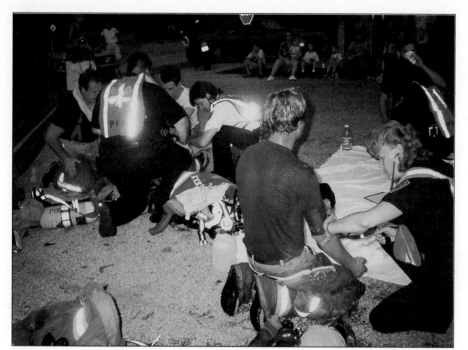

Figure 51-10

A treatment sector is established to allow for on-scene treatment and further care by physicians, nurses, and EMS personnel.

In the case of large-scale MCIs, the treatment area should be directed by one senior medical person designated as the treatment officer. This individual prioritizes treatment and resources and is responsible for securing additional resources as needed. In the case of multiple treatment centers, the treatment officers should communicate with each other to ensure that the rescue personnel and resources are properly allocated to provide the most benefit to the greatest number of patients.

Second and Subsequent Units on the Scene

As additional units and personnel arrive, they report to the Command Center for assignment unless system protocol specifies another location (e.g., treatment or transportation center) or they are otherwise instructed while en route (Box 51-3). Assignments vary depending on the number and distribution of patients and stage of the response. Assignments for responding units will depend on progress made prior to their arrival.

Transport

Once all patients with major injuries have been stabilized, they may be moved to a secondary location or Transportation Center designated by the incident commander.[4] This provides a single rendezvous point for patient pick-up, rather than requiring transport personnel to enter and roam the scene (Fig. 51-11). This final grouping of patients according to their

---

BOX 51-3   **Priorities for Secondary Responding MCI Units**

1. Complete triage.
2. Establish central treatment area and deliver equipment, when appropriate.
3. Move patients from their initial location to central treatment area, when appropriate.
4. Initiate treatment of life-threatening conditions.
5. Begin transport of CRITICAL patients.
6. Complete treatment of life-threatening conditions.
7. Initiate treatment of other injuries.
8. Complete transport of CRITICAL patients.
9. Initiate transport of URGENT patients.
10. Group DELAYED patients not involved in patient care or assisting at the scene into identifiable areas for later transport as buses or other appropriate vehicles arrive.
11. Group DEAD/DYING patients. If there are significant numbers of dead, create a temporary morgue area until later transport.
12. Complete transportation of all patients involved in MCI.
13. Survey area for noninjured individuals who either assisted as bystanders or observed the incident who may need support or subsequent care.
14. Secure the scene—gather up equipment and supplies being especially careful to seek out and properly dispose of materials which had contact with bodily fluids.

BOX 51-2   **Treatment Considerations During MCIs**

- **Treatment Provided During Assessment Phase:** NONE
- **Treatment Provided During Initial Triage Phase**: Airway opening and severe hemorrhage control.
- **Treatment Provided After Triage Phase and Prior to or During Transport**: Oxygen therapy, endotracheal intubation, cricothyrotomies, seal sucking chest wounds, flutter valves for tension pneumothorax, assisted ventilation, spinal injury immobilization, intravenous therapy, head and abdominal wound dressings, ECG monitoring, and pharmacological intervention.
- **Additional Treatment to be Considered if Time and Resources Permit**: Additional wound dressings and specific fracture splinting.

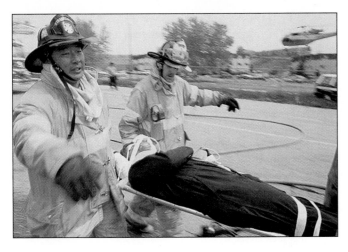

Fig. 51-11

A transportation sector will allow for coordinated interaction between transport units and patients during the incident. *Photographed by Howard Paul.*

BOX 51-4   **Transportation Priorities**

Priority 1 RED—severe respiratory or hemorrhagic problems
Priority 2 YELLOW—blunt, nonpenetrating chest and abdominal injuries, nonairway compromising facial trauma, major extremity injuries, spinal injuries, and burns
Priority 3 GREEN—soft-tissue and musculoskeletal injuries, emotional problems
Priority 4 BLACK—dead or dying victims with limited salvageability, even in a non–MCI situation

Note: The types of injuries listed are representative, but these diagnoses should not be used in determining the patient's transport priority. A START–type of approach that relies on physiologic parameters rather than presumptive diagnosis is best suited for determining transport priority in an MCI.

transport priorities provides a good summary of patient numbers and of the resources still required to resolve the incident.

Transportation depends on triage and will follow triage classifications (*see* Box 51-4). However, transport may begin before treatment, depending on the number of patients and availability of transport vehicles and personnel.

When time and resources permit, patients should be prioritized within each triage category. Within the CRITICAL category, for instance, there may be patients more in need of rapid transportation than others. In larger-scale MCIs, in which patients are moved from the site of their injury to a staging area for transportation, patients with similar triage levels can be located together, giving the designated transportation officer the ability to see and count the number of patients in each category. In some situations, ambulances may transport one critical patient with one or two urgent or delayed patients as resources permit.

The second transport priority includes patients who are not in as great a danger of dying as those classified as CRITICAL, but who do require definitive care in a short period of time. Bystanders may serve as a valuable resource in comforting these patients during what can be a long and frightening wait.

The third transport priority includes patients for whom a delay of several hours or more will not cause great harm. Patients requiring general medical screening or emotional assistance can be added at the end of this group.

The lowest transport priority includes those patients who have died either as a result of the primary accident or who were triaged as a low survival priority. In major MCIs, a morgue area is established at the scene.

In major MCI situations, one individual should be designated the transportation officer. In addition to determining transport priorities, he or she gathers information about patient capacity and specialty care capabilities at receiving hospitals. Head-injured patients may be transported to the only facility with neurosurgical coverage, for example, and chest-injured patients will go to a hospital with an open-heart surgical team.

Such facility distinctions should be worked out in advance through disaster planning. Medical directors can develop protocols to address these issues. When such protocols do not exist or the MCI circumstances do not clearly fit them, on-line medical direction can help determine destination. In some communities, the primary receiving hospital will receive the initial assessment data from responders, query other community hospitals about their availability of beds, personnel, and specialty physician coverage, and transmit destination recommendations back to the field.

The transportation officer also documents triage tag numbers, the order and time of transports, and their destinations. In very large MCIs, multiple transportation centers must communicate to ensure transport of all patients in correct priority order.

The Role of Physicians and Hospitals

As a general rule, people work most efficiently in familiar environments. Emergency physicians typically operate more efficiently in the hospital unless they have training and experience in field MCI operations, just as surgeons generally perform more decisively in the operative suite and cardiologists in the cardiac care unit. Remove any one of these individuals from their environment, and their efficiency will likely suffer. The prehospital environment, with its limited equipment and support personnel and lack of ancillary services, such as a laboratory and an x-ray, will prove foreign to most physicians unless they have had prior field experience.

However, in some communities there is a group of physicians who are experienced in prehospital care. In most communities, emergency physicians serve in this capacity because of their experience in the prehospital and hospital management of emergencies. Although EMS and disaster medical services differ in some ways, the emergency physician's background is well suited to assuming a leadership role in the planning and activity associated with MCIs.[1] Some physicians participate in the National Disaster Medical System (NDMS).[3] The NDMS program brings health care providers, including prehospital personnel and nurses, together to form disaster medical assistance teams (DMAT) capable of rapidly responding to national and international disasters.[7] These teams can also help with local MCI activities, both in the planning and response phases.

In some MCIs, extrication of some victims may not be possible. In such cases, physicians may need to respond to free the patient from the scene by surgically cutting the patient or amputating an extremity. A physician on-scene can certainly be advantageous, whether or not he or she is experienced in field care. In major MCIs with high numbers of patients, a physician who is familiar with working with prehospital personnel can help with field triage, treatment and transport decision-making, and scene coordination with other agencies. This physician may never become involved in actual patient care at the scene.

At the hospital, the physician continues the triage of incoming patients. The hospital also serves as a resource to field responders by providing supplies, support personnel, and even food in prolonged MCIs.

Other hospital personnel may be helpful at the scene when the number of injured patients overwhelms the EMS system's resources. Nurses and respiratory technicians can assist paramedics with triage and stabilization. Social service and psychological support from counselors and chaplains can help victims and families. If the scene resolution is prolonged, the hospital dietary service can provide food and beverage to workers.

Mutual Aid and Other Resources

Most emergency medical services throughout the country have evolved, either intentionally or unintentionally, into networks of emergency care. Some of these networks are formal, with extensive written agreements between services and an established command hierarchy. Others may be less structured, but still perform well when needed. All EMS services, formal or informal, must have agreements with services from adjoining geographic areas to provide response and assistance during MCIs. This may entail sending units and personnel to assist with the triage, treatment, and transport functions of MCIs, or covering routine calls while the local EMS service devotes its resources to the MCI. Fire and law enforcement services must also have similar arrangements.

As an EMS service prepares for MCIs in its area, it is important to anticipate the potential incidents that could occur and develop a list of resources needed to meet the demands of each incident type. Once this list is developed, planners can contact the sources and request their commitment to assist in time of need. Schools or regional transportation systems, for example, can provide buses to transport the walking wounded.

Anticipating MCI needs involves evaluating the local environment. If the tallest building in the community is only two

stories, high-rise rescue capabilities are not likely to be required, but a community with taller structures will have different rescue needs. Is the entire community made of wood, or are there concrete and steel structures that might require cranes to move debris after a collapse? Are chemicals or radioactive materials used, stored, or transported in the area that may require HazMat expertise? Resource lists should include names and after-hours telephone numbers for the resources that may be needed. Those lists are updated regularly and kept at hand in dispatch centers or hospitals.

Preparation Makes It Work

The MCI is unlike any other type of EMS response. It cannot be predicted, and it is difficult to simulate realistically. Planning and coordination are the best line of defense (Fig. 51-12).

Advance details include who will be in charge at the scene, with contingencies for substitution when designated people are unavailable. Plans must determine communication weaknesses in the area. What are the alternatives when the

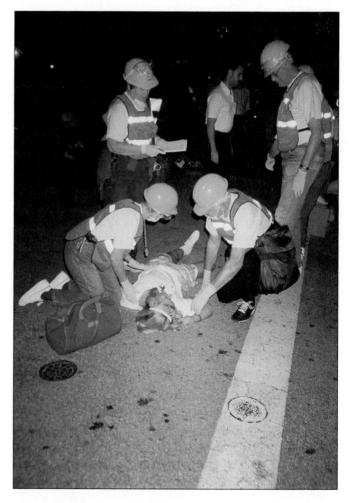

Figure 51-12

Disaster drills allow the various public safety agencies to practice ICS and work out problems with communications and intra-agency cooperation before an incident occurs. *Photographed by Craig Jackson.*

first line of communication fails? Does each EMS unit carry enough supplies? Where do paramedics quickly get additional supplies when the system is under stress? Do the rescuers require different types or quantities of supplies than are normally present in the ambulance? Does the community have the potential for disasters that require protective gear, equipment, or treatments not normally available (e.g., HazMat antidotes, radiation safety monitoring equipment and clothing)? The reader is referred to more definitive sources or to their state emergency management agency for further information on MCI planning.[2,5,8]

Although the likelihood of an MCI may be rare in a particular region, EMS continuing education programs should annually review local MCI plans and the basic principles of MCI management. The education process also requires hands-on practice in drills. A disaster or MCI drill can be as complex as total simulation of an incident scene with moulaged victims, or as simple as a table-top discussion of triaging victims who exist only on slips of paper. Although the latter is more convenient, every system should hold MCI drills at least every 2 years and preferably more frequently. The Joint Commission for the Accreditation of Health Organizations requires hospitals seeking accreditation to hold at least two disaster drills per year. Participation of the EMS system will further both agencies' training needs. Joint training ventures also pay dividends when the real event occurs, and hospital and EMS personnel are ready to function as a team.

Critique Sessions

Whether an MCI response is the real thing or a drill, it is imperative that all those involved meet and talk about the incident afterward. Recreate the scene on a flip chart or with pictures. Seek input from law enforcement, fire, EMS, hospital, and other personnel. Patients may even be willing to share their perspective. What worked, what went wrong, and what could have been better? All personnel should be honest and learn from the experience. In most cases, communications will be the weakest link, both in drills and real MCIs.

Were the right personnel, equipment, and extra resources available? Was scene control managed effectively by law enforcement? Was the fire service able to protect the rescuers from danger? Did everyone overlook the leaking chlorine gas tanker and forget to involve the HazMat team? Discussion leaders achieve the best effects by encouraging both openness and constructive attitudes. The goal of the critique session is to learn, not to place blame.

Critical Incident Stress Debriefing

To the casual observer, the victims of an MCI are obvious— those who were injured. In reality, the victims often include rescuers.[3] The tragedy experienced, the suffering, the mutilation, and the unfairness of the situation may play on the minds of responders and bystanders long after the physically injured have been transported. Resolution of emotional trauma may actu-

ally be more complex than the healing of physical wounds.

The reactions of rescuers to an MCI can vary from simple anxiety or short-lived depression to significant depression and even suicide. Rescuers may question their own actions and feel responsible for death or injuries that were clearly beyond their control.

A formal system for identifying responders with stress-related problems and for providing access to help must be immediately available when an MCI ends.[3] Attention should be given not only to the rescuers, but also to the victims and bystanders. Additional thought should be directed to the families of the victims and the rescuers. Once a Critical Incident Stress Debriefing System (CISDS) is established, it should be available to all personnel at all times, even months after the incident. Because public health and safety personnel are faced with stressful situations on a daily basis, the emotional needs of these personnel and their families should be a daily concern, not only in times of disaster.

Some EMS and public safety programs have formal stress debriefing programs or are affiliated with a nondenominational chaplaincy or counseling program designed specifically for this purpose. In the event of an MCI, the counselors involved are mobilized quickly. In the absence of a formal system, responders can at least realize that they are not alone. Supervisors and medical directors should be available to help responders talk through their feelings of stress, whenever the need arises (see Chapter 58 for a more detailed discussion of Critical Incident Stress Debriefing).

Applying MCI Principles to Smaller Incidents

What is the likelihood that the information in this chapter will ever be used? There is no way to predict the occurance of a major MCI. But even if it seems unlikely, paramedics have frequent opportunities to apply many MCI principles with only minor modification.

An efficient and systematic approach is important for each patient or group of patients that the paramedic encounters. The need for personal protection applies whether the paramedic is responding to a single-patient incident or an MCI. Failure to heed simple warning signs and exercise due caution when approaching any scene can cost both the rescuer and the patient their lives.

Once the scene has been deemed safe for entry, paramedics must identify the patients in need of care. The fact that two victims are still trapped in the front seat of a wrecked car does not mean that there is no other patient involved. Injured pedestrians or ejected passengers may not be readily apparent on initial approach. Every scene requires a full assessment.

Unless there is only one victim, the initial management of the patients and the allocation of resources must be prioritized. Should both paramedics care for one patient or should each take one? What about other possible patients? Which patient comes first or last in the treatment order? Until the patients are assessed and severities assigned to each, available personnel and other resources cannot be properly allocated. These concepts are as important in scenes involving three to five patients as they are at large-scale MCIs. Are special extrication or rescue devices required at the scene? Must the hospital be alerted to the patient's special needs? A complicated communication link will rarely be required in MCIs involving a limited number of patients, but communication between the scene and the hospital remains vital.

Command at the scene of limited MCIs should be straightforward. The ranking paramedic remains in charge until an EMS supervisor arrives, although law enforcement and fire officers may have other ideas. Traffic flow, ambulance access to a safe patient loading area, and the simple parking of response vehicles may require diplomacy to provide good patient care.

Triage has less importance as the number of patients diminishes, but it remains a key step in the overall management of any incident. The assessment phase may blend into triage when the number of victims, their location, and their severity are readily apparent. However, this blending should not occur when incident size requires a deliberate assessment effort. Triage and treatment phases will similarly combine when the number of patients is manageable. However, the paramedic must make a conscious effort to determine which patients will be transported first (CRITICAL), last (DEAD/DYING), and in between (URGENT and DELAYED), using the same criteria described earlier in this chapter.

Although all EMS personnel would like to have a perfect run, there is a lesson to be learned from every patient encounter. A few moments for an informal conversation with involved personnel, the EMS educator or coordinator, the supervisor, the medical director, or the emergency physician may help clarify objectives and the proper approach for the next incident. Paramedics cannot overlook or hide the emotional impact that an incident can have on them. Reactions to stressful situations must be discussed among friends and coworkers. Formal or informal stress debriefing sessions play just as much of a role in everyday EMS life as they do after an MCI.

SUMMARY

MCIs are unique events that, fortunately, do not occur frequently. The event requires responders to change roles from their normal routine. Paramedics must think of the multiple patients, often sacrificing less salvageable victims. Initial scene assessment and communication are higher priorities than any initial patient care. The paramedic must remember the basic tenets of PROTECTION, ASSESSMENT, COMMUNICATION, COMMAND, TRIAGE, TREATMENT, TRANSPORT, and DEBRIEFING. After the event, an honest critique should be demanded and the next major event planned for with a vision for improvement.

REFERENCES

1. **American College of Emergency Physicians:** Policy Statement: Disaster Medical Services. *Ann Emerg Med* 14:1026, Oct 1985.

2. **Auf der Heide E:** Disaster Response: Principles of Preparation and Coordination, Philadelphia, 1989, CV Mosby.

3. **Durham TW, McCammon SL, Allison EJ:** The Psychological Impact of Disaster on Rescue Personnel. *Ann Emerg Med* 14:664–668, July 1985.

4. **Hayes BE, Dahlen RD, Pratt FD, Sullivan RM:** A Prehospital Approach to Multiple-Victim Incidents. *Ann Emerg Med* 15:458–462, April 1986.

5. Incident Command System, Stillwater, 1983, Fire Protection Publications.

6. **Leonard RB, Calabro JJ, Noji EK, Leviton RH:** SARA (Superfund Amendments and Reauthorization Act), Title III: Implications for Emergency Physicians. *Ann Emerg Med* 18:1212–1216, Nov 1989.

7. **Mahoney LE, Whiteside DF, Belue HE, Moritsugu KP, Esch VH:** Disaster Medical Assistance Teams. *Ann Emerg Med* 16:354–358, March 1987.

8. **United States Department of Transportation / National Highway Traffic Safety Administration:** Mass Casualties: A Lessons Learned Approach, DOT HS 806-302, Oct 1982.

9. Triage in Mass Casualty Incidents. *Rescue-EMS* 28–30, Jan-Feb 1991.

10. **Vayer JS, TenEyck RP:** New Concepts in Triage. *Ann Emerg Med* 15:927–930, Aug 1986.

Ralph B. "Monty" Leonard, PhD, MD, FACEP

Hazardous Materials and Radiation Incidents

chapter 52

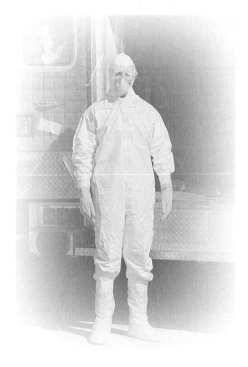

KEY TERMS

1. **Combustible**—capable of igniting and burning
2. **Corrosive**—ability to destroy tissue
3. **Flammable**—capable of being easily ignited and of burning with extreme rapidity.
4. **Hazardous materials**—any substance or material capable of posing an unreasonable risk to health, safety, and property.
5. **Placard**—square diamond-shaped signs, 10¾ inches on a side, which are official Department of Transportation labels that identify hazardous materials by means of color, symbols, and numbers.
6. **Radioactive**—having the property of emitting ionizing radiation.
7. **Toxic**—the ability to harm or poison living tissue or cells.

A paramedic should be able to:

OBJECTIVES

1. Define the term hazardous materials.
2. Describe the means of identifying hazardous materials.
3. Describe the paramedic team's role at a hazardous materials incident.
4. Given an incident's scene diagram, label and describe the three safety zones in a hazardous materials response.
5. Identify the appropriate personal protective equipment required when responding to specific hazardous materials incidents.
6. Describe the signs and symptoms of exposure to hazardous materials that require intervention.
7. Describe the emergency management of patients who have been contaminated with hazardous materials.
8. List the resources for identifying and managing hazardous material situations.
9. Outline the appropriate response to a hazardous materials emergency.
10. Describe injuries caused by exposure to hazardous materials and radiation.
11. Describe the emergency management of patients who have been exposed to radiation.

azardous materials (HazMat) are not exotic chemicals or rare substances, but rather the ordinary raw materials used daily by thousands of businesses and industries. Unfortunately, many are toxic, corrosive, flammable, or explosive, and have the potential to pose a significant threat to health and life when released into the environment during an incident. These hazardous materials are manufactured and stored by the producer, transported by truck, train, ship, barge, or aircraft, stored by the purchaser, and sold as is or used in manufacturing. At any point along this chain, a mishap may occur.

Historically, the fire service was called to manage such events. Involvement of emergency medical service (EMS) personnel in the management of hazardous materials incidents was mandated in 1986 when Congress passed the Superfund Amendments and Reauthorization Act (SARA), Title III. In 1989, the Occupational Safety and Health Administration (OSHA) required specific training for all EMS personnel who might respond to episodes involving hazardous materials.

Classes of Hazardous Materials

The Department of Transportation (DOT) regulates all aspects of transporting hazardous materials in the United States, including the design and type of container used and the means by which they are transported.

For the most dangerous materials, the shipping container and the transport vehicle must bear a placard, regardless of the quantity (Box 52-1). Hazardous materials considered to be somewhat less dangerous require placards only if more than 1000 pounds are on board (Box 52-2). However, a tractor-trailer truck may have a mixed load of hazardous materials, each in an amount of less than 1000 pounds, and thus carry far more in total without the need to display a placard.

A DOT placard immediately provides two pieces of information in most cases: one comes from the color of the placard (Table 52-1), sometimes accompanied by a specific symbol (Fig. 52-1). The color denotes the class of hazardous material, and the symbol, if present, further identifies that class. The second piece of information is a four-digit number that allows more specific identification. The number is keyed to the DOT *Emergency Response Guidebook,* which should be carried on all EMS units. This guidebook contains information on health hazards, first aid measures, and initial emergency actions at the scene. For example, #2664 (Fig. 52-2) is identified as dibromomethane and the reader is referred to Guide Number 74 (Fig. 52-3) for initial emergency actions.

Some placards also have a digit or digits at the bottom corner, which represents the United Nations hazardous materials class, but this information is not particularly useful to EMS personnel in the United States.

Unfortunately, placards may be missing, destroyed in the incident, or unreadable because of scene dangers. Hazardous materials teams should carry binoculars to observe the scene and detect placards from a safe distance.

One look at the list of hazard classes categorized by the DOT shows a bewildering array. Paramedics should know that the vast majority of hazardous materials will be toxic, corrosive, flammable, explosive, radioactive, or a combination of these. Radioactive materials are a special type of hazardous material and will be covered in a section at the end of this chapter.

Role of EMS Personnel at Hazardous Materials Incidents

EMS personnel are not expected to rescue victims from dangerous chemical environments nor are they expected to secure the scene; this manuever must be accomplished by trained teams with special equipment.

However, EMS personnel may be "first in" at an incident involving hazardous materials. Hence, paramedics must know how to evaluate the scene and gather initial information so that subsequent operations will unfold safely and effectively. On other occasions, EMS personnel will be called to a scene to stand by or to treat a contaminated patient.

BOX 52-1 — Most Dangerous Hazardous Materials

- Class A explosives
- Class B explosives
- Class A poisons
- Radioactive materials
- Water reactive flammable solids

BOX 52-2 — Less Dangerous Hazardous Materials

Blasting agents	Flammable liquids
Class B poisons	Irritating materials
Combustible liquids	Nonflammable gases
Corrosives	Nonwater reactive flammable solids
Flammable gases	Oxidizers and organic peroxides

TABLE 52-1 — Placard Color Codes for Hazardous Materials

Code	Hazard Class
White and red stripes	Flammable solid
Yellow	Oxidizer/peroxide
White	Poison
Yellow over white	Radioactive
White over black	Corrosive
White (blank)	Other regulated material
Orange	Explosive
Red	Flammable
Green	Nonflammable gas

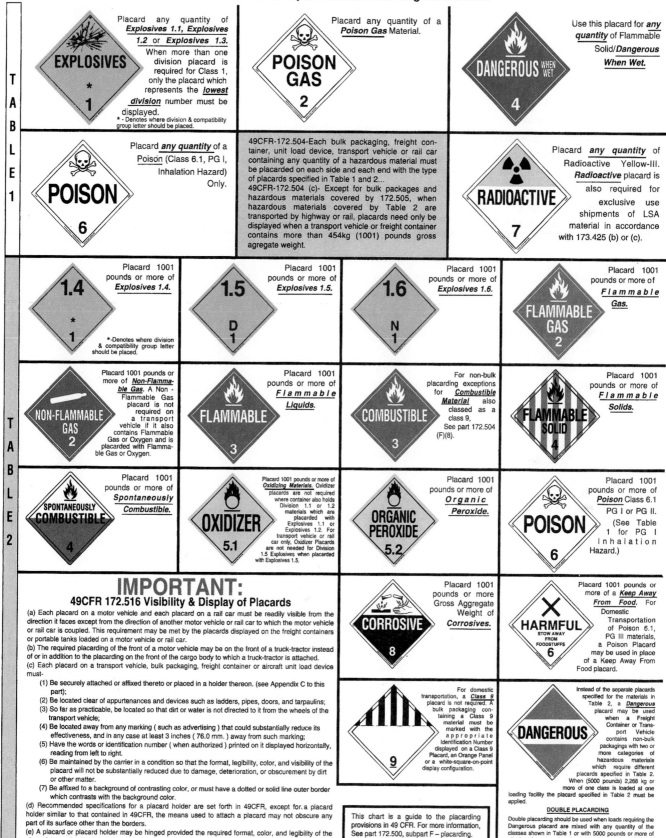

Figure 52-1

The DOT Hazardous Materials Placard contains universally recognized symbols for hazardous materials.

ID No.	Guide No.	Name of Material
2650	57	1,1-DICHLORO-1-NITRO-ETHANE
2651	53	4,4'-DIAMINODIPHENYL METHANE
2653	53	BENZYL IODIDE
2655	53	POTASSIUM FLUOROSILICATE, solid
2656	29	QUINOLINE
2657	55	SELENIUM DISULFIDE
2658	53	SELENIUM, powder
2659	53	SODIUM CHLOROACETATE
2660	55	NITROTOLUIDINES (mono)
2661	54	HEXACHLOROACETONE
2662	53	HYDROQUINONE
2664	74	DIBROMOMETHANE
2666	55	ETHYL CYANOACETATE
2667	27	BUTYLTOLUENES
2668	57	CHLOROACETONITRILE
2669	55	CHLOROCRESOLS
2670	60	CYANURIC CHLORIDE
2671	55	AMINOPYRIDINES (o-, m-, p-)
2672	60	AMMONIA SOLUTIONS with more than 10% but not more than 35% ammonia
2672	60	AMMONIUM HYDROXIDE
2673	53	2-AMINO-4-CHLOROPHENOL
2674	53	SODIUM FLUOROSILICATE
2676	18	STIBINE
2677	60	RUBIDIUM HYDROXIDE SOLUTION
2678	60	RUBIDIUM HYDROXIDE, solid
2679	60	LITHIUM HYDROXIDE SOLUTION
2680	60	LITHIUM HYDROXIDE, solid
2680	60	LITHIUM HYDROXIDE MONOHYDRATE

ID No.	Guide No.	Name of Material
2681	60	CAESIUM HYDROXIDE SOLUTION
2681	60	CESIUM HYDROXIDE SOLUTION
2682	60	CAESIUM HYDROXIDE
2682	60	CESIUM HYDROXIDE
2683	28	AMMONIUM HYDROSULFIDE SOLUTION
2683	28	AMMONIUM SULFIDE SOLUTION
2684	29	DIETHYLAMINOPROPYLAMINE
2685	29	N,N-DIETHYLETHYLENE-DIAMINE
2686	29	DIETHYLAMINOETHANOL
2687	53	DICYCLOHEXYLAMMONIUM NITRITE
2688	58	1-CHLORO-3-BROMOPROPANE
2689	55	GLYCEROL-alpha-MONO-CHLOROHYDRIN
2690	55	N-n-BUTYL IMIDAZOLE
2691	39	PHOSPHORUS PENTABROMIDE
2692	59	BORON TRIBROMIDE
2693	60	AMMONIUM BISULFITE, solid
2693	60	AMMONIUM BISULFITE SOLUTION
2693	60	BISULFITES, aqueous solution, n.o.s.
2693	60	BISULFITES, inorganic, aqueous solution, n.o.s.
2693	60	CALCIUM BISULFITE SOLUTION
2693	60	CALCIUM HYDROGEN SULFITE SOLUTION
2693	60	POTASSIUM BISULFITE SOLUTION
2693	60	SODIUM BISULFITE SOLUTION
2698	60	TETRAHYDROPHTHALIC ANHYDRIDES
2699	60	TRIFLUOROACETIC ACID
2705	60	1-PENTOL
2707	27	DIMETHYLDIOXANES

Figure 52-2

A page from the numerical index section of the DOT 1993 Emergency Response Guidebook. Chemical #2664 is highlighted. Note the reference to Guide number 74 and the listing of the chemical name. *From U.S. Department of Transportation: 1993 Emergency Response Guidebook.*

The Nature of Hazardous Materials Incidents

Many of the incidents to which paramedics are called are inherently dangerous, even in the absence of a hazardous material. Incidents involving hazardous materials have an added dimension of danger for which the paramedic requires specific training.

Many seemingly routine EMS calls actually involve hazardous materials. For example, wrecked motor vehicles carry gasoline and acid-containing batteries. However, the vast majority of these events allow EMS personnel with proper training to approach the scene and safely render aid.

Hazardous materials incident scenes are dangerous *as long as* the material is present, even if it remains within its shipping container. Hence, the paramedic must remain vigilant until the scene is cleared. Also, some hazardous materials incidents pose a threat to the surrounding population in the area.

Impact of Hazardous Materials on the Incident Scene

Usually, a person connects hazardous materials incidents with fires or explosions in chemical plants, major train derailments, or ruptured tank trucks. However, hazardous materials can be anywhere and may be present in rather small amounts. For example, the paramedic responding to a "man down" call finds a person lying on the floor of an enclosed room in which the patient was using a paint stripper containing methylene chloride. The amount may be small, but the paramedic must still recognize the chemical's presence to maintain personal safety and care properly for the patient. In fact, correct treatment and patient outcome depends on recognition of these materials and relay of this information to the treating physician. In many such instances, the victims can be treated safely by EMS personnel who are aware of the danger and take precautions to avoid contaminating themselves.

GUIDE 74 ERG 93

POTENTIAL HAZARDS

HEALTH HAZARDS
Vapors may cause dizziness or suffocation.
Exposure in an enclosed area may be very harmful.
Contact may irritate or burn skin and eyes.
Fire may produce irritating or poisonous gases.
Runoff from fire control or dilution water may cause pollution.

FIRE OR EXPLOSION
Some of these materials may burn, but none of them ignites readily.
Most vapors heavier than air.
Air/vapor mixtures **may explode** when ignited.
Container may explode in heat of fire.

EMERGENCY ACTION

Keep unnecessary people away; isolate hazard area and deny entry.
Stay upwind, out of low areas, and ventilate closed spaces before entering.
Positive pressure self-contained breathing apparatus (SCBA) and structural firefighters' protective clothing will provide limited protection.
Isolate for 1/2 mile in all directions if tank, rail car or tank truck is involved in fire.
Remove and isolate contaminated clothing at the site.
CALL Emergency Response Telephone Number on Shipping Paper <u>first</u>. If Shipping Paper <u>not available</u> or <u>no answer</u>, CALL CHEMTREC AT 1-800-424-9300.
If water pollution occurs, notify the appropriate authorities.

FIRE
Small Fires: Dry chemical or CO2.
Large Fires: Water spray, fog or regular foam.
Apply cooling water to sides of containers that are exposed to flames until well after fire is out. Stay away from ends of tanks.

SPILL OR LEAK
Shut off ignition sources; no flares, smoking or flames in hazard area.
Stop leak if you can do it without risk.
Small Liquid Spills: Take up with sand, earth or other noncombustible absorbent material.
Large Spills: Dike far ahead of liquid spill for later disposal.

FIRST AID
Move victim to fresh air and call emergency medical care; if not breathing, give artificial respiration; if breathing is difficult, give oxygen.
In case of contact with material, immediately flush eyes with running water for at least 15 minutes. Wash skin with soap and water.
Remove and isolate contaminated clothing and shoes at the site.
Use first aid treatment according to the nature of the injury.

Figure 52-3

The guides, found in the back of the DOT 1993 Emergency Response Guidebook, provide many useful pieces of information, including initial emergency actions. *From U.S. Department of Transportation: 1993 Emergency Response Guidebook.*

At the other end of the spectrum are the larger situations such as fires, explosions, and train derailments. A single EMS crew would obviously not be expected to face these incidents alone. There are also many possible situations in intermediate categories.

The following discussion will focus on small scenes that involve one or two vehicles and only a few people.

The Nature of the Event

Nature of the event refers to the degree to which hazardous materials are an active part of an emergency scene.

Paramedics commonly arrive at incidents at which the hazardous material is still intact in its shipping container. They must still be aware that the container may have sustained damage which, although it is not immediately obvious, could lead to a rupture later. This is particularly important when handling tanks that contain pressurized gases.

Scenes at which hazardous materials are already escaping from their containers are much more dangerous and complicated. These scenes require careful evaluation before approaching and in some cases cannot be approached at all.

The most obviously dangerous scene is that in which hazardous materials are burning or reacting with each other. EMS personnel should withdraw to a safe place and call for a special hazardous materials team to evaluate and deal with this type of problem.

The Scope of the Event

Most hazardous materials incidents involve small physical areas, and using routine precautions, EMS personnel often can safely approach the victims and remove them for treatment. On the other hand, the scene of a wrecked tanker truck, from which chlorine gas is escaping, may become a community disaster. Hence, the scope of the event is an important piece of information that the paramedic must evaluate upon arrival at an incident scene.

by Ralph B. "Monty" Leonard, PhD, MD, FACEP

1. *CHEMTREC.* CHEMTREC is a service sponsored by the Chemical Manufacturers Association and provides 24-hour information on emergency response to accidents involving transportation of chemicals. The service identifies industry and transportation experts who deal with hazardous materials accidents.
Emergency phone number: (800) 424-9300.
2. *National Response Center (NRC).* Federal law requires that the NRC be notified of any serious hazardous materials accident. NRC provides 24-hour assistance to emergency personnel in identifying chemical commodities.
Emergency phone number: (800) 424-8802.
3. *Agency for Toxic Substances and Disease Registry (ATSDR).* ATSDR provides 24-hour consultation to physicians and emergency response personnel on toxicological information for treating chemically contaminated patients. Their services include public health threat assessment and evacuation planning.
Emergency phone number: (404) 639-6360

4. *Nuclear Regulatory Commission (NRC).* The NRC provides emergency responders with 24-hour assistance in dealing with accidents involving radioactive materials. They also identify health physicians and other medical personnel needed to assess and treat the medical consequences of exposure to radioactive materials.
Emergency phone number: (301) 951-0550.
5. *Radiation Emergency Assistance Center/Training Site (REAC/TS).* A Department of Energy facility with a two-fold mission: 1) Teaching medical and emergency responders about radiation accidents and dealing with radioactively-contaminated patients, and 2) 24-hour consultation on any radiation accident.
Address: REAC/TS, Box 117, Oak Ridge, Tennessee 37830. Phone: (423) 576-3131; After-hours emergency phone: (423) 481-1000 (Ask for REAC/TS person on call.)

The Nature of Hazardous Materials

One aspect of a hazardous material scene, which influences the way in which the incident evolves, is the ability of the paramedic to identify the materials present. Incident scenes may involve a single, known hazardous material or multiple substances that cannot be identified. In addition to the chemical substance itself, the physical state of the substance (e.g., solid, liquid, or gas) plays an important part in the incident scene (Fig. 52-4).

Solids

Solid hazardous materials are generally comprised of a single substance. They may be an element, such as phosphorus or sulfur, or a chemical compound such, as sodium hydroxide or arsenic trioxide.

Solids are often the least dangerous form of hazardous material to deal with, because they tend to remain in the immediate vicinity when spilled. However, some have properties that increase their potential for danger at the scene.

Some solids are shipped as powders so fine that, if spilled, they are easily spread by even a light breeze. Magnesium powder burns explosively, but a solid bar of the same material is much less dangerous.

A few solids react slowly with water vapor in the air to form gaseous compounds that are flammable or toxic. For example, calcium carbide reacts with water to form acetylene, an explosively flammable gas. Elemental metals, such as sodium and lithium, react with water to form caustic lye and hydrogen gas.

Although solid materials tend to be the easiest to deal with, when an unknown solid material is out of its container, the area should be isolated to prevent the spread of materials and protect them from water, fuel, and igniting mechanisms. Victims at such scenes, if not contaminated with this material, can be removed quickly to a safe area for further evaluation and treatment.

Liquids

A liquid may be comprised of a single composition, such as benzene; a mixture of liquids such as "industrial methylated spirits," which is a mix of methyl and ethyl alcohols; or a material dissolved in a liquid, such as a solid pesticide dissolved in a hydrocarbon solvent.

All liquids and solids have what is called "vapor pressure," or the tendency for some of the material to enter the air above it. Vapor pressure of a liquid depends upon its composition and temperature. Like the liquid itself, the va-

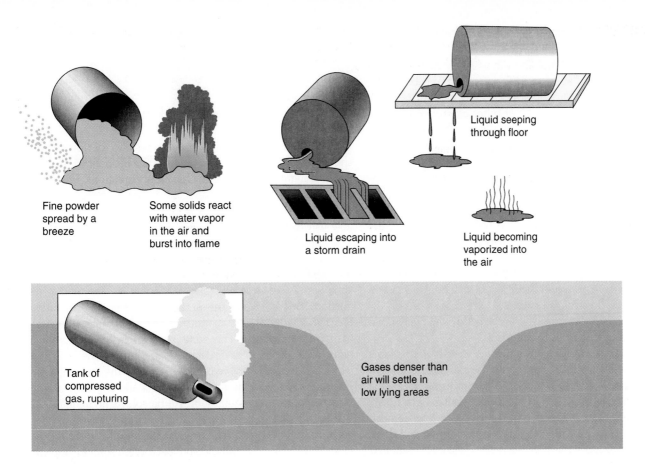

Fine powder spread by a breeze

Some solids react with water vapor in the air and burst into flame

Liquid escaping into a storm drain

Liquid seeping through floor

Liquid becoming vaporized into the air

Tank of compressed gas, rupturing

Gases denser than air will settle in low lying areas

Figure 52-4

Hazardous material can be in the form of a solid, liquid, or gaseous state, with each form representing special dangers.

por above it can be toxic, flammable or corrosive. When faced with a scene that has an unknown liquid leaking from its container, the paramedic must assume that its vapor is significantly hazardous and not enter the scene until trained personnel with proper protective equipment have evaluated the risk.

A scene that involves a liquid hazardous material leaking from its container has an added dimension of danger in that the liquid may seep through floors, escape into storm drains or otherwise spread through the physical surroundings. This danger also points to the early need to summon specially trained personnel.

Gases and Cryogenic Liquids

Many types of gases are produced and used throughout the United States. Most are shipped in compressed form in tanks of various sizes.

Any tank of compressed gas, regardless of its contents, can rupture violently if it has been damaged. Even if the tank is undamaged, both the tank and its contents must be considered a potential bomb if exposed to a temperature of 130° F or higher. The observation of flames near or on a tank of compressed gas requires quick departure from the area.

Compressed gases that are toxic, flammable, or explosive present a unique problem because the volume of gas, when released, is much greater than the size of the container. The gas spreads quickly over a large area, a process that will be hastened if a breeze is present.

When leaking gas of unknown identity is discovered at the scene of an incident, EMS personnel must withdraw to a safe area until the situation is evaluated. As they withdraw, it is helpful to register visual clues about the leaking container (e.g., size, color, identification numbers, or words or identifying symbols on the tank) for communication to the hazardous materials team.

Some gases are more dense than air, either due to their chemical composition or because they are cold, and so will settle in low-lying areas. The paramedic should therefore not walk or drive into such low-lying areas, even for a "man down," until the safety of the area can be confirmed.

Gases that liquefy when they are cooled are called *cryogenic liquids*; they are shipped under pressure in refrigerated tanks. Some cryogenic liquids, such as liquid nitrogen, are not toxic; others, such as liquid anhydrous ammonia, are highly toxic. However, because all cryogenic liquids are many degrees below zero (generally colder than -130° F), any that escape from a broken valve or pipe and contact the skin will freeze it instantly.

Evaluation of a Hazardous Materials Incident Scene

Often, the paramedic will not know in advance that hazardous materials are involved at a scene. The first clue may be a placarded vehicle. People already at the scene, such as the truck driver, chemical plant personnel, or other emergency personnel may be able to provide further information. Incidents in laboratories or factories should prompt initial questions as to whether a hazardous material could be involved.

Trucks should have shipping papers in the cab that identify the cargo. These should be retrieved if it is safe to do so. In trains, this information is in the custody of the conductor.

If the scene obviously involves a hazardous material, the paramedic must consider whether it is possible to safely approach injured victims and render aid. If it is possible to confirm that no injured people are at the scene, paramedics can withdraw to a safe area and contact a dispatcher to relay information.

The presence of victims who are already dead means that the scene is too dangerous to approach.

The situation involving hazardous materials and victims who are injured but still alive forces the paramedic to ask, "How can the victims be removed safely from the scene?" If the hazardous material is still in its intact container, it is usually possible to approach, quickly render ABC care, and remove the patient to a safe location for further assessment and treatment. If the hazardous material is already outside its container or there is smoke, fumes, or fire present, the paramedic should not approach the scene. The situation may require a hazardous materials team to rescue the victims. Familiarity with local EMS protocols is important in these situations.

The paramedic should not remain in a situation where a sudden fire or explosion could occur or a tank of compressed gas could rupture. When the scene requires the services of a hazardous materials team, the paramedic's job is to care for injured victims evacuated by the team.

Hazardous Materials Incident Scene Set-Up

Unless paramedics have a specific task to perform, they should be in a safe location away from the incident so they will not be caught up in a sudden change of conditions. Each incident scene should be cordoned off in some logical manner, usually with the help of fire and police personnel, and preferably with some type of yellow plastic warning tape or rope. The inner zone of the scene, or "hot zone," includes all areas or locations where hazardous materials either have spilled or may spill if the container is breached (Fig. 52-5). The next zone is the "warm zone," also called the "contamination reduction zone." This is the area where hazardous materials team members take patients for decontamination, assessment, and treatment. This zone is still considered a contaminated area, but to a lesser degree than the hot zone.

The "support" or "cold" zone is where the incident commander is located with a command post and any needed support personnel and equipment. All personnel and equipment that pass between zones must go through a specific "access" corridor so that commanders know what enters the areas from either direction; equipment and personnel coming out can also be checked for contamination, and be decontaminated if needed.

All personnel and equipment not immediately needed must be located in a staging area designated by the incident commander. This area should be nearby and readily accessible, but safe from any complications of the scene itself. When the sites for the command post and staging area are being

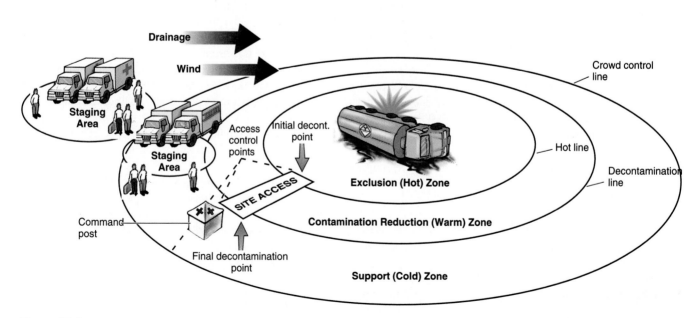

Figure 52-5

Incident zones are established to prevent the spread of contamination and to protect emergency service workers who are working on the incident.

chosen, both wind direction and drainage must be taken into account.

Scene set-up is another aspect of hazardous materials response in which knowledge of local protocols is important to optimum function at the scene.

Personal Protective Equipment

The term *personal protective equipment (PPE)* refers to both clothing and equipment used to isolate EMS personnel from the chemical, physical, and biological hazards that may be encountered at a scene of a hazardous materials incident.

OSHA standards mandate specific training requirements for personnel engaged in emergency response to hazardous materials incidents, such as firefighters, police officers, and EMS personnel. OSHA's final rule (29 CFR 1910.120) as it applies to emergency medical personnel, states: "Training shall be based on the duties and functions to be performed by each responder of any emergency response organization."

In the vast majority of cases, EMS personnel will not respond to a sufficient number of hazardous materials incidents to keep them optimally trained or to keep their PPE properly maintained. Thus, most EMS systems make arrangements with the local fire department or hazardous materials team to be ready to decontaminate patients. It should not be expected that EMS personnel deal with chemically contaminated patients if their training and equipment do not allow them to do so safely.

No single combination of protective equipment and clothing is capable of protecting against all possible hazards. The use of PPE can itself create significant worker hazards, such as heat stress, physical and psychological stress, and impaired vision, mobility, and communication. EMS personnel should not use PPE without adequate training.

Levels of Protection

The Environmental Protection Agency (EPA) has defined four levels of respiratory protection and protective clothing.

- *Level A protection* is the highest level of respiratory, skin, *eye*, and mucous membrane protection. It requires a fully encapsulating, chemically resistant suit and self-contained breathing apparatus (SCBA) (*see* Fig. 52-6).
- *Level B protection* should be selected when the highest level of respiratory protection is needed but a lesser level of skin and *eye* protection is required. It is different from Level A protection only in that it does not provide full-body protection against gases.
- *Level C protection* should be selected when the type of airborne substance is known, and air-purifying respirators of the proper type are available. This equipment includes chemically resistant clothing, a full-face mask, and a canister-equipped respirator that filters chemicals from the air. Level C protection does not contain self-contained breathing apparatus, but instead uses ambient air from which hazardous substances are filtered within the respirator.
- *Level D protection* is regular fire turn-out gear or the routine work uniform. Obviously, this protection level provides no respiratory protection and only minimal body protection.

Factors to be considered in selection of the proper protection level include the identities of the relevant hazardous materials, the rescue personnels' routes of entry into the area, the rescuers' degree of contact with the hazardous material or

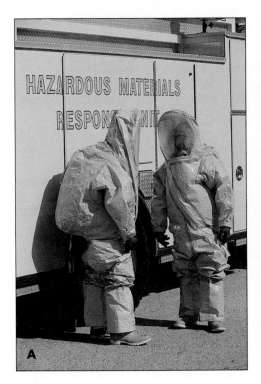
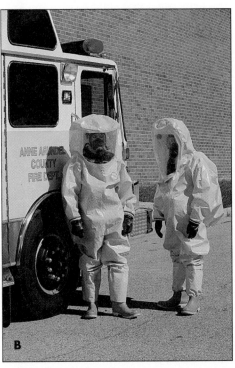

Figure 52-6

The EPA defined four levels of protective clothing and respiratory protection. A) Level A protection B) Level B protection

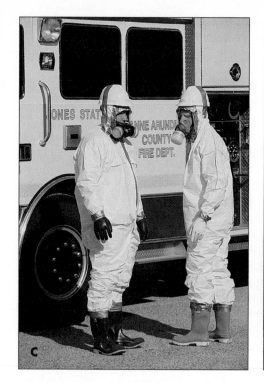

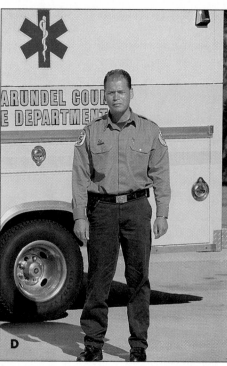

Figure 52-6 (continued)
C) Level C protection D) Level D
protection

contaminated victim, and the specific assigned task. If a rescue person is going to make an initial entry into an unknown environment or an entry into a confined space that has not been chemically characterized, it is recommended that at least Level B protection be used. The use of this protection level mandates specific training for rescue personnel.

Chemical Protective Clothing

EMS personnel who are treating a patient contaminated with a solid or liquid hazardous material should wear chemical protective clothing (CPC) in conjunction with eye, nose, and mouth protection. The person wearing the CPC shown in Figure 52-7 is wearing goggles, gloves, and a surgical-type mask. This mask prevents inhalation and ingestion of airborne droplets and particles but does not provide the level of respiratory protection that a respirator would.

CPC is designed to protect EMS personnel from hazardous materials that can affect the body by inhalation, ingestion, or direct contact. *Inhalation contamination* occurs when emergency personnel breathe in chemical fumes, vapors, or dust. Respirators are designed to protect the wearer from this form of contamination and must be fitted properly and tested frequently to ensure continued protection. Frequently, a surgical-type mask is sufficient, but selection of any specific CPC requires knowledge of the hazardous materials with which one is dealing. *Ingestion contamination* usually is the result of a health care provider inadvertently transferring hazardous materials from his hand or clothing to his mouth, such as wiping his mouth with his hand or sleeve. *Direct contact contamination* occurs when the chemical touches the skin or eye. Garments may protect the skin against direct contamination; full-face respirators protect the wearer against ingestion, inhalation, and direct contact with the eyes and face.

Many types of CPCs are available. Most are coverall-type suits with attached boots and hoods that require only the addition of gloves and face protection. No single material for either the suit or the gloves is adequate for protection from all possible chemicals, especially liquids. Therefore, if the paramedic is to use such gear, he or she should be trained in the system's protocols and equipment.

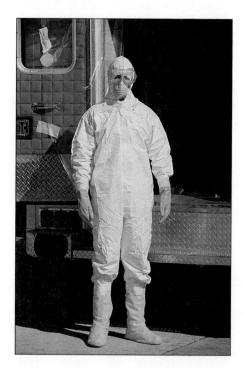

Figure 52-7

Chemical Protective Clothing offers safeguarding from splashes and inhalation or ingestion of large airborne droplets or particles. However, this equipment will not provide the same level of respiratory protection as a respirator.

Eye and Respiratory Tract Protection

If the rescuer is dealing only with solid materials, usually goggles and a simple dust mask are sufficient; exceptions would be solids that have a high vapor pressure or are chemically reactive.

For exposure to those special classes of solids, and to gaseous and liquid materials, there are many types of face protection devices with built-in respirators or cartridges to filter out harmful vapors. These devices cannot be used by untrained personnel, because each unit must be fitted to the individual wearer and a specific cartridge must be selected for the specific hazardous material present.

Patient Decontamination and Treatment

Patient Decontamination

Primary goals for EMS personnel in a hazardous materials incident include reducing the patient's exposure, removing the patient from danger, and treating the patient—all without jeopardizing his or her own health and safety. Reduction of exposure can be accomplished by moving the patient from the contaminated area and decontaminating the patient. When the patient has been removed from the immediate zone of contamination and decontaminated, the protection level for EMS personnel can be decreased to one that will better facilitate the provision of patient care. Inside the contaminated zone, the patient should not receive any treatment other than urgent basic life support.

The paramedic's initial approach to a chemically contaminated patient is two-sided: 1) the ABCs plus spine care and, 2) decontamination.

During initial patient stabilization, a gross decontamination should be carried out simultaneously. This consists of cutting away or otherwise removing contaminated clothing, including jewelry and watches, and brushing and wiping off any obvious contamination. The paramedic should be cautious to protect any open wounds on the patient from contamination. Every effort should be made by the paramedic to avoid contact with the material.

Directives for decontamination include reducing external contamination, containing the contamination that is present, and preventing the further spread of hazardous materials at the scene. In other words, the paramedics should remove what they can and contain what they cannot remove. In general, intact skin is less absorptive than injured flesh, mucous membranes, and eyes. Therefore, decontamination should begin at the patient's head and proceed downward; the paramedic should pay initial attention to contaminated eyes and open wounds. Once the patient's eyes and open wounds have been cleaned, they should be covered with waterproof dressings to prevent recontamination.

For the patient with chemically contaminated skin, adequate decontamination in the field is of the utmost importance. Copious amounts of body-temperature water with soap, if available, are usually sufficient. The use of hot water and vigorous scrubbing should be avoided because they can di-late the vessels in the skin and cause small skin abrasions, both of which increase the possibility of chemical absorption.

Three important aspects of decontamination that the paramedic must remember are: 1) avoid wash water or chemicals on the skin entering the eyes, nose, or mouth of the patient; 2) avoid vigorous cleansing of the skin, which would splash fluids on EMS personnel and about the area; and 3) avoid neglect of hidden areas of the patient's body, such as the armpits, groin, and crease of the buttocks.

EMS Personnel Decontamination

Personnel decontamination is the process of removing and neutralizing harmful materials that have contaminated personnel or equipment during the response. This decontamination is of utmost importance, because it protects all personnel by decreasing the transfer of hazardous materials from the contaminated zones into clean zones, and protects the community by preventing transportation of hazardous substances away from the site.

The easiest method of decontamination is avoiding the transferrance of material onto the body, equipment, or clothing. However, if contamination does occur, proper decontamination or disposal of outer gear is recommended.

Physical decontamination of protective clothing and equipment can be achieved by several different means; all of these include the systematic removal of contaminants by washing, usually with soap and water, and then rinsing. Occasionally, the use of solvents is necessary. Dry decontamination, or the use of disposable outer protective clothing, is the preferred method in most EMS systems.

EMS personnel leaving the "hot zone" must leave behind any contaminated or potentially contaminated tools and equipment. When entering the "warm zone," the paramedic should remove outer protective gear, which is either placed into containers or bags and secured. When approaching the contamination control line to leave the scene, rescuers should be checked by a designated safety officer to be sure that they are not accidentally carrying contaminants from the zone. Upon leaving the area, it is recommended that rescuers return to quarters, shower, and put on clean clothing.

Injuries Caused by Hazardous Materials

If the chemical contaminant is known, specific medical and toxicologic information can be gathered to aid in the assessment and treatment of the victim. Even if the identity of the chemical is not known, the paramedic can help by observing and treating symptoms as they appear. The case of a person contaminated by multiple unknown chemicals is more complex, but the same general principles of assessment and treatment apply.

Airway and Lungs

Most victims with airway or pulmonary injuries have inhaled a gaseous product (because it is rare for a patient to inhale a liquid). An immediate examination of the airway is mandatory, as are close observation and continuous re-evaluation of the patient for the delayed appearance of airway or pulmonary symptoms. Effects can be delayed for hours.

Chemical vapors that are water soluble, such as anhydrous ammonia or hydrogen chloride, can cause intense irritation of the moist upper airway, laryngeal, and tracheal tissues, leading to copious secretions, edema, and possibly airway obstruction. All of these conditions demand immediate and aggressive airway management, which may include emergent intubation.

Large and small bronchi also are susceptible to bronchospasm, and to mucosal surface damage, which can lead to obstruction from edema, secretions, or sloughed cells. Bronchospasm can be severe and life threatening and may occur in patients with or without a history of asthma. In either case, it is treated with high-flow oxygen, a bronchodilator, if indicated, and possibly intubation.

Some chemical vapors can induce a pulmonary edema, or "chemical pneumonitis," secondary to damage to alveolar cells. This condition may become evident very quickly, or be delayed for up to 48 hours. Some chemicals, such as hydrogen sulfide and carbon monoxide, do not damage the lungs themselves but enter the body through the lungs and cause systemic toxicity.

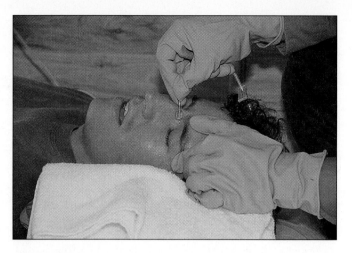

Figure 52-8

The eyes should be flushed with copious amount of water following exposure to chemicals. Be certain to lift the lid and remove contact lenses. Protect yourself from splashing runoff water.

Eyes

The eyes are very susceptible to damage by chemicals, whether in gaseous, liquid, or solid form. Unless the patient has an open injury of the globe, the paramedic should begin copious irrigation of the eyes immediately upon discovering that the organs are involved (Fig. 52-8). If present, contact lenses should be removed from the patient's eyes. The irrigation also should aim to remove all hazardous material from beneath the patient's eyelids.

Skin

The skin can be involved in chemical injuries in two ways: 1) the patient can suffer chemical skin damage called "chemical burns," or 2) the skin can be a portal of entry for chemicals that will cause systemic toxicity. Either effect may be immediate or delayed, and occasionally both will take place.

Cryogenic liquids, as previously mentioned, can cause frostbite if they contact the skin directly, but by far the most serious skin injury is a chemical skin burn. Corrosive chemicals, such as acids or alkali, can cause death of the cells and loss of skin, and be absorbed into the body. Chemical burns require fast and copious irrigation with water, a therapy that absolutely must begin in the field.

Systemic Toxicity

Although chemicals may enter the body through any part of the anatomy, the most common routes are the lungs and the skin. As a general rule, toxic gases that cause lung damage tend to produce less systemic toxicity than those that do not damage lung tissue, such as carbon monoxide and hydrogen sulfide. Chemicals that are fat soluble are most apt to be absorbed directly through the skin; organophosphate insecticides are the most common group in many communities. Chemically contaminated patients who have abraded skin or open wounds are at an even higher risk for systemic absorption.

The organophosphates, one of the most prevalent groups of hazardous chemicals, are easily absorbed by skin contact and cause a wide range of symptoms, including vomiting, diarrhea, bradycardia, and salivation. The paramedic should be alert to the development of muscle tremor and weakness in the patient, which can cause respiratory arrest as a result of paralysis of the respiratory muscles.

Many internal organs are susceptible to damage from absorbed chemicals, the damage or its degree depending upon the chemical involved. Those organs most commonly involved are the heart, central nervous system, liver, and kidneys. Liver and kidney damage may not be evident for days, weeks, or even months.

One of the many systemic effects of chemicals is irritability of the heart, which leads to cardiac dysrhythmias. Thus, every chemically contaminated patient must be placed on a cardiac monitor and closely observed for dysrhythmias and ectopic beats.

For emergency department personnel to evaluate the risk of delayed systemic reactions, the paramedic must supply them with an accurate description of what happened at the scene, what chemicals were involved (if known), to what extent the patient was contaminated, how the patient was decontaminated, and any changes in the patient's condition during treatment and transport.

Patient Transport

For all contaminated patients transported by an ambulance to the hospital, the paramedic should perform the minimal decontamination procedures of removing the patient's clothes, physically removing as much contamination as possible by brushing or wiping off solids, and washing with water.

The paramedic should exercise special care to prevent contamination of the ambulance and subsequent patients. Exposed surfaces that the contaminated patient is likely to contact should be covered with plastic sheeting (Fig. 52-9).

Fiberglass backboards and disposable plastic sheets are recommended, and EMS personnel should wear protective clothing appropriate for the conditions. Equipment that comes in contact with the contaminated patient should be segregated for decontamination or disposal.

If decontamination cannot be performed adequately, EMS personnel must at least attempt to prevent the spread of contamination. The patient's clothing shold be removed and the patient wrapped in a blanket and plastic, to maintain body heat. However, the paramedic must remember that overheating a patient accelerates skin absorption of the contaminating chemical. The paramedic also must be able to monitor the patient's ABCs, cardiac rhythm, and vital signs, especially respirations.

The chemical involved and any other data available should be collected before the patient leaves the scene. Oxygen should be administered by rebreather mask for any victim with respiratory problems; the only exception to the use of oxygen is contamination with a herbicide called paraquat. Eyes that have been exposed to hazardous materials should be irrigated with normal saline or water and such irrigation should be continued en route to the hospital.

The ambulance should park in an area away from the emergency department or continue directly to a predesignated entry point to limit exposure of hospital facilities. The patient should not be brought into the emergency department before ambulance personnel receive permission from the hospital staff, who may choose to further decontaminate the patient at or near the entry point.

Once the patient is released to the hospital, any equipment believed to be contaminated should be isolated, bagged, and labeled. Contaminated articles should be kept sealed until hazardous materials specialists provide further instructions.

If necessary, the ambulance or rescue vehicle may return to the scene to transport additional patients to the hospital. If no more chemically contaminated patients require transport, the vehicle should not be returned to normal service until it has been cleaned and inspected according to local protocol.

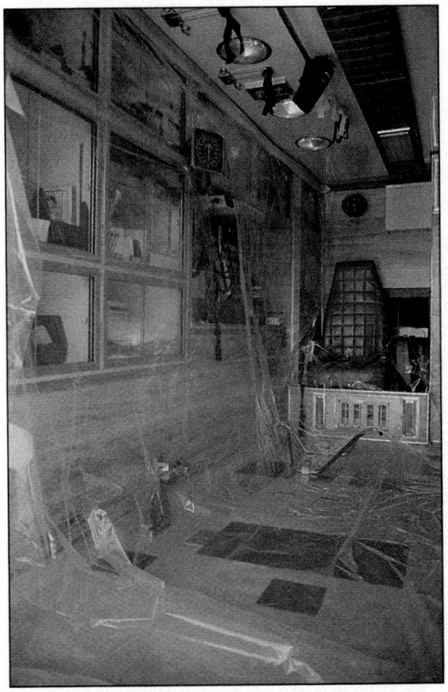

Radiation Incidents

Although radioactive materials are much feared, they actually are safer to handle than many other hazardous materials, because their presence can be determined by radiation counters.

Although many people equate radioactive materials with nuclear weapons, there is little chance that EMS personnel will be endangered by such devices. There is a slight chance that a rescuer could be involved with radioactive materials in transit to or from nuclear power reactors or when handling accidents at those sites.

The Nature of Radioactivity

The term *ionizing radiation* (generally called *radiation*) refers to electromagnetic energy or mass emitted from the material that is undergoing radioactive decay and that produces electrically charged ions in materials subjected to this radiation. Radiation can be classified as alpha, beta, or gamma. Some radioactive substances give off two of these types of radiation, but none emits all three. If the paramedic knows the exact material to be handled, a reference book will indicate the specific type of radiation involved.

Types of Radiation

Alpha particles are able to move only a few centimeters through the air. They are stopped easily by a sheet of paper or cloth, or by the skin. Thus, alpha-emitting radiation materials are not hazardous unless they are inhaled or ingested or if they contaminate open wounds.

Beta particles can pass several meters through the air and up to 5 millimeters through tissue. Thus, beta sources can be hazardous, both internally and externally, on the skin or clothes.

Gamma radiation is high-energy electromagnetic radiation similar to x-rays, but with more penetrating power. A lead shield several centimeters thick is required to stop it. Thus, gamma radiation poses the most significant medical risk.

Figure 52-9
Commercial liners or plastic sheeting offers protection from contamination to the interior of the ambulance.

The aspect of radioactive materials that separates them from all other hazardous materials is the fact that their presence and amount can be detected and measured with radiation counters. The common Geiger (or Geiger-Muller) counter detects and measures only beta and gamma radiation.

Radiation can be thought of as microscopic bullets, which harm the body by breaking up or damaging the molecules that make up living cells and the important contents of cells, such as DNA. Because radiation cannot be seen, heard, or smelled, any container, room, or area marked with a radiation sign should not be approached unless the rescuer knows that the radioactive material is safely stored within its container. Special units of measurement are used to describe the amount of radiation present.

Types of Radiation Incidents

Before EMS personnel can handle a patient involved in a radiation incident, he or she must understand the types of incidents. Each incident requires special treatment and has a different medical outcome; although of course, a patient may suffer from more than one type of radiation exposure.

Irradiation Incident

In an irradiation incident, a person has been exposed to radiation, but there is no actual radioactive material on or in the body. Because alpha particles cannot penetrate skin and beta particles can penetrate just a few millimeters, gamma radiation is the primary concern in irradiation incidents.

The patient who has suffered an irradiation incident is not radioactive. Monitoring with a Geiger counter will show only background radiation. Figure 52-10 shows a hand being held over a piece of cobalt 60, a radioactive substance that emits beta particles and gamma rays. The hand is thus irradiated by both beta and gamma radiation, but the radioactive material is not physically on the hand.

Contamination Incident

In a contamination incident, the victim may have radioactive material on the skin or clothes (external contamination), inside the body (internal contamination), or both. This type of incident requires careful decontamination while the medical needs of the patient are being attended. Figure 52-11 shows a hand that is contaminated with a radioactive material, which is giving off radiation. As long as this radioactive material is on the skin or clothes, the radiation is being absorbed by the victim's body.

Incorporation Incident

In an incorporation incident, radioactive atoms have entered the body by way of open wounds, the lungs, or the GI tract, and have become chemically incorporated into the cells of the body (Fig. 52-12). An incorporation incident poses a significant long-term health threat to the victim, primarily through the potential to cause cancer.

Basic Radiation Protection Principles

The amount of radiation injury a person sustains is related to the dose received, which in turn depends upon four factors: quantity, time, distance, and shielding.

The basic principles to follow to decrease the amount of radiation received are:

1. Spend as little time as possible in the immediate danger area (*Time*).
2. Stay as far away from the radiation source as possible (*Distance*).
3. Wear protective clothing and stay behind barriers when possible (*Shielding*).
4. Keep the amount of hazardous material in the work area contained, isolated, or limited (*Quantity*).

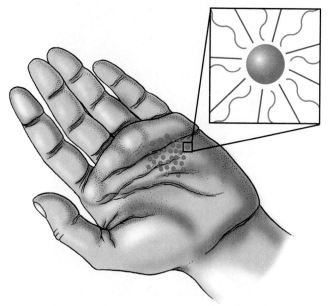

Figure 52-11

When a contamination incident occurs, the patient has radioactive particles on their clothing or skin. These patients must be decontaminated prior to handling to prevent the EMS crew's exposure.

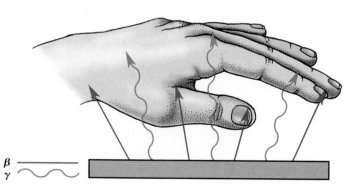

β
γ

Figure 52-10

Exposure to beta and gamma radiation results in irradiation of the skin. Beta radiation penetrates only a few millimeters, while gamma radiation can penetrate deeper.

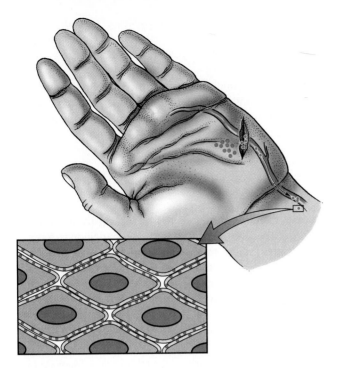

Figure 52-12

When an incorporation incident occurs, radioactive particles enter the patient's body through an open wound, the lungs, or GI tract and are taken into the various cells of the body. This results in long-term effects for the patient, often resulting in cancer.

Label	Radiation Level Associated with Intact Package
Radioactive	Almost no radiation
Radioactive Yellow-II	Low radiation levels
Radioactive Yellow-III	High radiation levels

TABLE 52-2 Requirements for Package Labels, Radioactive Materials

Scene Size-Up

Exposure to radioactive materials is most likely in university and industrial research laboratories, nuclear medicine facilities, certain industries where high-energy gamma sources are used to check industrial welds, and in transportation incidents involving shipments of radioactive materials. Emergency responders should become familiar with facilities at local industries and laboratories handling or using radioactive materials.

Motor vehicles, rail cars, and freight containers often display radioactive warning placards when transporting radioactive materials in quantity. Three different labels—white I, yellow II, and yellow III—are used to specify the radiation level at the surface of the container (Table 52-2).

Upon arrival, if the initial scene size-up reveals the presence of radioactive materials as part of the incident, the paramedic should immediately alert dispatch so that appropriate local or state radiation health teams can be alerted. As in all scenes involving hazardous materials, the paramedic must use his best judgment as to whether it is safe to enter the scene. Faced with indications that an unknown radioactive material is out of its container, the paramedic should remain outside the scene until personnel are available for proper monitoring of the area.

Care of Radiation Incident Victims

Rescuing an injured person from an area that contains loose radioactive material or a significant amount of gamma radiation is extremely rare. These situations require rescue teams with specialized knowledge, training, and equipment.

A less serious but more likely scenario for the paramedic would be handling an injured patient whose clothes and skin are contaminated. A paramedic who comes into contact with a potentially contaminated person should approach wearing eye, respiratory, mouth, and skin protection to prevent both internal and external contact, as they would for any contaminated patient.

Depending upon the substance involved, the radioactive material will emit alpha, beta, or gamma radiation. Only gamma radiation is of medical significance, as long as the paramedic does not become contaminated.

Although the paramedic does receive small amounts of gamma rays from the radioactive material on a victim's clothes or skin, the amount is only the equivalent of two or three chest x-rays. As a precaution, EMS personnel who may be pregnant should not handle possible radioactive contamination.

Emergency Medical Procedures

The emergency medical team should immediately assess airway, breathing, and circulation, and begin CPR if needed. A pocket mask or a bag-valve-mask can be used rather than mouth-to-mouth resuscitation. The victim should be moved away from areas of potential radiation exposure or contamination to lessen exposure for both the paramedic and the victim. The paramedic should never delay life-saving medical procedures to decontaminate a radiation victim.

Radiation exposure or contamination does not cause unresponsiveness or immediate visible signs of injury, unless the radioactive material is corrosive or toxic. If IV fluids are required, a routine procedure for skin preparation and fluid introduction should be used, regardless of the presence of skin contamination. However, when possible, IV fluids should be introduced through areas of uncontaminated skin. Establishing a precautionary IV line is not recommended because it may unnecessarily admit contaminants into the patient's body.

When the medical condition permits, the incident victim should be moved to the control line separating contaminated and noncontaminated areas for further care and monitoring with radiation counters. Emergency personnel need not make precise measurements of the amount of radiation present; their concern is only to detect or rule out its presence. Complete scene monitoring should be reserved for personnel with special training.

Decontamination of Incident Victims

Removing the clothing of the contaminated victim will often remove most of the contamination as well. The clothing should be sealed in plastic bags, labeled, and left at the incident scene. No other decontamination procedures are recommended, because these procedures may widen the contamination. An exception to this rule would be a victim who has corrosive material on the skin, face, or eyes.

Dry radioactive material on the skin can be brushed off into a plastic bag; small areas of wet radioactive material on the skin can be gently washed with water or normal saline and the wash water collected afterward. The paramedic must use common sense to avoid spreading contamination, and be careful not to contaminate the victim's nose, mouth, eyes, ears, or wounds, because this may lead to internal contamination. Any further on-site decontamination of the victim should be directed by specialized personnel.

Transporting Contaminated Victims

A stretcher should be covered with a sheet and placed on the contaminated side of the control line separating the contaminated and uncontaminated areas. The victim is then transferred to the covered stretcher and the sheet folded to securely "package" the victim, with the patient's arm extended through an opening in the sheet if needed for measuring vital signs or administering IV fluids or drugs. If an ambulance crew is present that has not been in the contaminated area, this crew should transport the victim to the hospital. Protective clothing worn by the paramedic should be removed at the scene and properly bagged, and the paramedic should put on clean gloves to handle the victim on the way to the emergency department. As an additional precaution, the floor of the rescue vehicle can be covered with a securely taped sheet to decrease the possibility of contamination.

Emergency Department Notification

If contamination of accident victims is suspected, emergency department personnel should be alerted as soon as possible so that a radiation emergency area can be prepared.

A more detailed report, including the extent of the patient's contamination, the body areas of greatest contamination, any evidence or suspicion of internal contamination, and the identity of the contaminating substance, can be relayed in transit.

To help control contamination at the hospital, EMS personnel should inquire about a special entrance for patients contaminated by radioactive materials. The hospital emergency response team will probably meet the ambulance outside the emergency department. The contaminated victim in stable condition should not be taken immediately into the hospital, but rather transferred to a clean hospital stretcher. This reduces the possibility that any contamination on the ambulance cot, sheet, or blankets will enter the hospital. The ambulance can return immediately to the radioactive incident site to transport additional contaminated victims, if need be. If the vehicle is no longer needed, it should be locked and kept at the hospital until it can be monitored for contamination by qualified personnel.

All EMS personnel involved in the care, treatment, and transport of potentially contaminated patients should report for radiation monitoring and follow the EMS system's protocol for such situations.

SUMMARY

Hazardous materials incidents can be among the most complex for paramedics for three reasons: 1) in addition to a physical injury, the patient may suffer from consequences of the hazardous material; 2) the hazardous material may pose a threat to the rescue personnel; and 3) some hazardous materials incidents may pose a threat to a large portion of the surrounding population. For these reasons, most EMS jurisdictions have HazMat teams with special training and equipment to handle these complex situations. Paramedics who are not part of such teams will generally find themselves involved in a HazMat scene by being "first in" at a scene or arriving to the scene to transport a victim to the hospital.

The basics of hazardous material behavior, the setup of a HazMat accident scene, and the evaluation and treatment of patients is important information for all paramedics to know. Simple observation, along with basic information, will do a great deal to protect the paramedic and render optimal care to the patients involved.

REFERENCES

1. **Borak J, Callan M, Abbott W:** Hazardous Materials Exposure: Emergency Response and Patient Care, Englewood Cliffs, 1991, Brady.

2. **Bronstein AC, Currance PL:** Emergency Care for Hazardous Materials Exposure, ed 2, Hanover, 1994, Mosby Lifeline.

3. **Carlson GP, Isman WE:** Hazardous Materials, Riverside, 1980, Macmillan Publishing.

4. **Emergency Response and Consultation Branch (E57), Division of Health Assessment and Consultation Agency for Toxic Substances and Disease Registry:** Managing Hazardous Materials Incidents: Volume I: Emergency Medical Services—A Planning Guide for the Management of Contaminated Patients, Atlanta.

5. **Meyer E:** Chemistry of Hazardous Materials, Englewood Cliffs, 1989, Prentice-Hall.

6. **Ricks RC:** Prehospital Management of Radiation Accidents, Oak Ridge, 1984, Radiation Emergency Assistance Center/Training Site.

7. **Sullivan JB, Krieger GR:** Hazardous Materials Toxicology: Clinical Principles of Environmental Health, Baltimore, 1992, Williams and Wilkins.

Nicholas Benson, MD, FACEP
Richard C. Hunt, MD, FACEP

Chapter 53

Air Medical Services

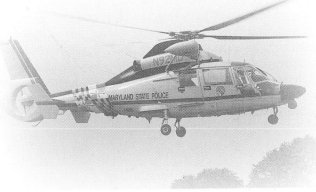

A paramedic should be able to:

Today, air medical transport is an accepted part of EMS. As the use of helicopters and airplanes for patient transportation has become commonplace over the past 20 years, the role of paramedics in air medical transport has come into focus. Indeed, there are two major roles that paramedics play in the air medical transport profession: one role is as flight paramedics, serving on the medical team in the aircraft providing patient care, and the other role is as a frequent consumer, deciding when to request air transport for a patient for whom the crew is caring. These two roles are relevant to all types of air medical services, including those sponsored by hospitals, private services, and public safety agencies.

Although physicians, nurses, pilots, communication specialists, mechanics, and other personnel play important roles in the air medical profession, paramedics have a pivotal role. The National Flight Paramedic Association recognizes this and provides educational resources for its members.[22]

Most of the air-medical focus for paramedics is on helicopters rather than airplanes. Helicopters are used primarily for emergency responses, picking up a patient at one point and delivering them to a regional receiving hospital. Airplanes are more often used for longer transports (>150 miles) and scheduled transfers involving convalescent patients. Helicopters are very useful in delivering a medical team to a scene, typically a team with a higher level of training than can be found locally. The aircraft may significantly decrease the transport time of the patient from the scene. Helicopters can fly 120 miles per hour or in a more direct line and bypass community hospitals to quickly transport the patient to a regional trauma center.

The Role of Air Medical Transport

When one or more of the following conditions exists, helicopter transport should be seriously considered: 1) lengthy extrication of a critically injured patient, especially if the aircraft can arrive at the scene before extrication is completed; 2) lengthy manual transport of the patient out of a remote area to motorized transport; or 3) extended ground transport time to get the patient to an appropriate medical facility. In each situation, the patient's clinical status should be a major guideline; it will take a certain amount of time for the helicopter to leave its base and reach the patient. The air medical service should be able to give the on-scene paramedic an estimated time of arrival. If the patient is ready for transport upon the ground EMS provider's arrival, rapid ground transport will generally be appropriate.

Frequent, inappropriate use of the aircraft increases patient care costs and exposes patients and flight teams to unnecessary risk. Most areas of the country only have one or two helicopters equipped for medical transport. Inappropriate use also increases the risk that the transport service will not be available for patients who most need it.

In 1991, nearly 140,000 patients were flown by helicopter in this country; another 24,000 traveled by fixed-wing aircraft.[18] Twenty-nine percent of the helicopter transports were from emergency scenes; the remainder were interhospital transports.

Typically, people think of scene responses only for trauma patients. But helicopters are also called for medical cardiac arrests, high-risk obstetric patients, and other medical problems where the remote location of the patient makes the helicopter a necessary resource. This is especially true in island areas.

Frequently, paramedics arrive at a scene and decide whether helicopter use is appropriate. However, ground EMS services require the paramedic to perform an initial assessment and discuss the helicopter decision with on-line medical direction. This allows the participation of a person not involved with the stress of the scene and who may be aware of other emergencies in the local area. However, it can also increase the time required to make the decision.

Air medical services are only one of numerous components in the regional EMS system. They should be used to complement the expertise and equipment that ground services provide. Air service medical directors should communicate closely and frequently with directors of ground services in their region. Joint training exercises to review protocols, equipment, and dispatch criteria are extremely useful. Practice in establishing landing zones will increase the confidence levels of both air and ground providers. The more interaction that ground and air teams have, the more smoothly they work together during emergencies.

Appropriate Use

To date, air transport has only been proven to decrease mortality when used for blunt trauma patients. Several studies, including the landmark article by Baxt and Moody in 1983, have shown that blunt trauma patients transported by air have a lower mortality rate than those transported on the ground.[1,2,6] There are fewer published studies examining the benefits of air transport for cardiac, pediatric, obstetric, and other patients, but available data does suggest that air transport contributes to decreased mortality in critical illness and other types of trauma.[3,24,20,5,16]

Paramedics and other users of air medical services can optimize use by overtriaging slightly. Overtriage is the practice of overestimating the severity of patients' illnesses or injuries, allowing the patient to receive more sophisticated or intensive care than they would otherwise. Moderate overtriage serves the patient's best interest. Undertriage, on the other hand, results in patients with significant injuries transported to facilities that are unprepared to care for them. This undertriage leads to delays in definitive care, resulting in increased patient morbidity and mortality.

One study published in 1986 reviewed a variety of potential criteria for requesting a helicopter at a trauma scene.[25] Criteria included vital signs demonstrating hemorrhagic shock, and mechanism of injury factors, such as associated fatalities and lengthy extrications. The single best triage criterion identified in this study was neurological; patients who were either unresponsive or responsive only to painful stimuli benefitted from helicopter transport to a regional trauma center.

Hospital-based helicopter providers in North Carolina have developed use-review criteria that includes guidelines for requesting a response directly to the scene of an injury.[4] These guidelines include blunt trauma, penetrating trauma, burns, objective scoring criteria, and other factors. Massachusetts and Connecticut have similar criteria[11,28] (see Box 53-1).

In 1990, the Association of Air Medical Services issued a position paper on the appropriate use of air medical transport. The paper stressed that air transport should be used when its benefits will enhance patient care in comparison with the benefits of ground transport.[15] The document also emphasizes that transport decisions should be made with several factors in mind: 1) the potential medical benefits to the patient, including the urgency of transport, the most appropriate receiving hospital, and the level of care needed in transport; 2) the safety of the transport environment; and 3) the cost of transport.

The National Association of Emergency Medical Services Physicians published a paper in 1992 with criteria for using helicopters for scene responses.[21] The paper's two cornerstones are the need to transport unstable trauma patients to recognized trauma centers as efficiently as possible, and the use of ground transport for stable trauma patients when it can be executed safely. The paper lists several specific criteria including anatomic injury, vital sign abnormalities, operational considerations, and time and distance factors (see Box 53-2). These criteria have not been prospectively studied.

Paramedics' Attitudes Toward Air Medical Services

Those paramedics who are members of air medical teams virtually always have positive attitudes about air medical transport. However, the vast majority of paramedics work in ground-based EMS systems that may call helicopters to the trauma scene. These paramedics' attitudes toward air medical services are not as clear. In some areas of the United States,

ground EMS personnel routinely call air transport to motor vehicle crashes and other trauma scenes; in other areas, helicopters are seldom or never used.[8,26]

Among 175 hospital-based helicopter programs surveyed in 1990, the percentage of flights that were scene responses ranged from 0% to 92%.[8] A nationwide survey in 1989–1990 questioned EMS personnel about their attitudes and operational procedures regarding air medical services in an attempt to understand why there is such a wide range of helicopter use for scene responses.[12] The majority of respondents were

---

BOX 53-2   National Association of EMS Physicians Guidelines for Scene Responses

A. Clinical
1. General
   a. Trauma victims need to be delivered as soon as possible to a regional trauma center.
   b. Stable patients who are accessible to ground vehicles probably are best transported by ground.
2. Specific
   a. Trauma Score <12
   b. Glasgow Coma Scale score <10
   c. Penetrating trauma to the trunk, neck, or head
   d. Spinal cord or spinal column injury, or any injury producing lateralizing signs
   e. Partial or total amputation of an extremity (excluding digits)
   f. Two or more long bone fractures or a major pelvic fracture
   g. Crushing injuries to the trunk or head
   h. Major burns
   i. Patients less than 12 or more than 55 years of age
   j. Patients with near-drowning injuries, with or without existing hypothermia
   k. Adult patients with any of the following vital sign abnormalities:
      1) systolic blood pressure <90 mmHg;
      2) respiratory rate <10 or >35 per min;
      3) heart rate <60 or >120 per min; or
      4) unresponsive to verbal stimuli.
B. Operational situations in which helicopter use should be considered:
1. Mechanism of injury:
   a. Vehicle roll-over with unbelted passengers;
   b. Vehicle striking pedestrian at >10 miles per hr;
   c. Falls from >15 feet;
   d. Motorcycle victim ejected at >20 miles per hr;
   e. Multiple victims.
2. Difficult access situations:
   a. Wilderness rescue;
   b. Ambulance exit or access impeded at the scene by road conditions, weather, or traffic;
3. Time and distance factors:
   a. Transportation time to the trauma center greater than fifteen minutes by ground ambulance;
   b. Transport time to local hospital by ground greater than transport time to trauma center by helicopter;
   c. Patient extrication time >20 minutes; or
   d. Use of local ground ambulance leaves local community without ground ambulance coverage.

From National Association of EMS Physicians Position Paper: Air medical dispatch: Guidelines for scene response. *Prehosp Dis Med* 7(1):75–76, 1992.

BOX 53-1   Sample Criteria for Helicopter Trauma Scene Transport

- Pedestrian struck by vehicle traveling >10 mph
- Automobile collision with death of another occupant in the same vehicle
- Patient fall from height of >20 feet
- Motor vehicle collision with patient thrown from vehicle traveling >20 mph
- Motor vehicle collision with patient extrication time >20 minutes
- Trauma patient unresponsive or responsive only to painful stimuli
- Champion Trauma Score ≤12
- Glasgow Coma Scale Score ≤8
- Burns of >20% of body surface area, associated with inhalation injury
- Pediatric multiple trauma, or patients >55 years old with multiple trauma
- Multiple seriously injured patients, or mass casualty incident
- Local ground EMS cannot provide advanced life support
- Patient with major trauma is more than 15 minutes to regional trauma center by ground transport

paramedics. When asked, "Who decides if a helicopter will make a scene response?", 71% answered the "squad crew chief" or "squad crew member." For 23% of the survey respondents, medical direction decided if a helicopter would make a scene response.[12]

The majority of those surveyed believed that air medical transport is safe. Eighty-five percent of respondents agreed that medical transport by helicopter could make a difference in patient outcome. This attitude is objectively supported by a 1983 study that reported a 52% reduction in blunt trauma mortality when a helicopter was used for scene responses.[1]

Only 8% of respondents felt that their EMS agency did not enjoy a good working relationship with the air medical transport service during scene responses. The perception that EMS agencies have a good working relationship with the air medical transport team during scene responses demonstrates a common goal of excellence in trauma patient care.

Generally, the survey showed a favorable inclination toward the use of air medical helicopters. Despite this favorable response, some EMS systems do not frequently request air transport. Others never request helicopter scene responses. Local or regional biases and protocols may limit or preclude helicopter use. Depending upon local availability of other advanced life support resources, this resource may have an impact on patient outcome.

The challenge for paramedics and their medical directors is to develop methods to integrate ground and air EMS services in the best interests of the patient. These methods could include educational sessions with ground paramedics on safety, patient care, and use of air services. Communication among involved administrators also facilitates appropriate employment of air transport services, as do interagency agreements and protocols. An integrated approach to patient care with defined agency and paramedic responsibilities should be the goal.

The Helicopter Environment

While the medical helicopter has been frequently called a "flying critical care unit," the air medical transport environment presents special challenges to patient care. Air medical crews are unable to hear normal breath sounds during helicopter flight, impeding assessment of breath sounds for potential tension pneumothoraces and misplaced endotracheal tubes.[13] One study also showed a substantial decrease in the ability to detect carotid pulses in both normotensive and hypotensive patients in one commonly used helicopter.[14]

Some helicopters are configured for transporting only one patient while others are capable of carrying more (Fig. 53-1). There is a wide variation in the space available for providing patient care among medical helicopters. One study measured the speed of performing emergency cardiac interventions such as application of pacemaker pads, administration of a bolus and continuous infusion of medications, defibrillation and electrical countershocks, and initiation of cardiopulmonary resuscitation. Results showed that these therapies can be performed significantly more quickly in an MBB BK-117 helicopter than in the smaller MBB BO-105 helicopter.[27]

Medical aircraft are quite different, and it is important that paramedics learn as much as possible about the limitations and capabilities of aircraft in their service area. Although the air transport environment has limitations, helicopters and fixed-wing aircraft offer two fundamental advantages in emergency and critical care transport: 1) speed and 2) the delivery of a highly trained and experienced medical team.

Effects of Altitude

The effect of altitude on gases is important both to the ground paramedic, who may be preparing a patient for transport, and the team that will provide care in flight. Boyle's Law states that gas expands as altitude increases.[7] As the aircraft ascends, the volume of air or gas in a closed space within the patient, or a piece of equipment, increases because the external pressure is decreasing (Fig. 53-2). The effects of Boyle's Law on equipment may include an increased volume of air in endotracheal tube cuffs, pneumatic antishock garments (PASGs) and glass IV bottles. Its effect on patients includes expansion of gas in the respiratory system, sinuses, and GI system.

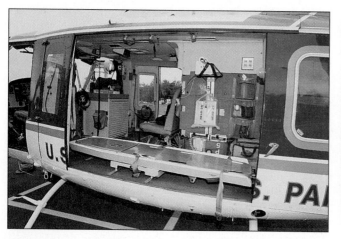

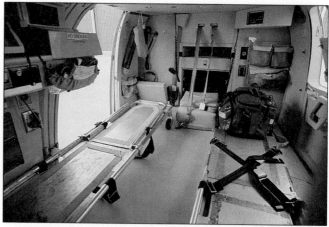

Figure 53-1

Helicopters can be set up to transport A) one or B) several patients.

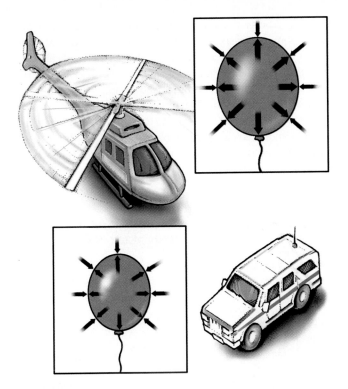

Figure 53-2

Boyle's Law describes how a given volume of air from ground level will expand as it increases in altitude, which could cause complications during flight as with a pneumothorax.

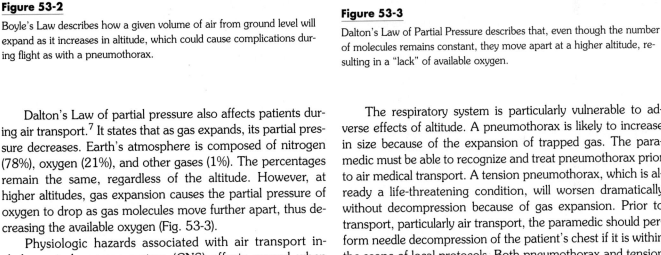

Figure 53-3

Dalton's Law of Partial Pressure describes that, even though the number of molecules remains constant, they move apart at a higher altitude, resulting in a "lack" of available oxygen.

Dalton's Law of partial pressure also affects patients during air transport.[7] It states that as gas expands, its partial pressure decreases. Earth's atmosphere is composed of nitrogen (78%), oxygen (21%), and other gases (1%). The percentages remain the same, regardless of the altitude. However, at higher altitudes, gas expansion causes the partial pressure of oxygen to drop as gas molecules move further apart, thus decreasing the available oxygen (Fig. 53-3).

Physiologic hazards associated with air transport include central nervous system (CNS) effects caused when nerve centers cannot maintain their oxygen reserves. CNS function deteriorates in hypoxic states. Cerebral hypoxia is likely at an arterial oxygen tension (PaO_2) below 50 torr, and hypoxic effects may occur even at higher PaO_2 levels if the patient is critically ill or injured, or is physically active during flight. Signs and symptoms of CNS dysfunction will be the same as any other hypoxic patient. The paramedic should keep the patient well oxygenated and observe for signs of hypoxia.

Physiologic affects of altitude on the middle ear include a "full feeling" in the ear during ascent if passive movement of gas from the nasopharynx to the middle ear is obstructed. During descent, hearing may be diminished when increased external pressure inhibits vibration of the tympanic membrane. The GI tract is affected by ascent, because gas expands in the tract. Patients with bowel problems, especially bowel obstruction, are susceptible to nausea, vomiting, and bloating. Nasogastric tubes should be left unclamped to allow for air flow during pressure changes associated with altitude.

The respiratory system is particularly vulnerable to adverse effects of altitude. A pneumothorax is likely to increase in size because of the expansion of trapped gas. The paramedic must be able to recognize and treat pneumothorax prior to air medical transport. A tension pneumothorax, which is already a life-threatening condition, will worsen dramatically without decompression because of gas expansion. Prior to transport, particularly air transport, the paramedic should perform needle decompression of the patient's chest if it is within the scope of local protocols. Both pneumothorax and tension pneumothorax are also particularly important to identify on the ground, because noise and motion can make in-flight assessment of breath sounds difficult.[13] Oxygen therapy is another altitude-sensitive care component. As the aircraft ascends, the oxygen flow must be increased to compensate for gas expansion, as explained above (Dalton's Law).

The patient and the flight team are affected by environmental factors during flight, especially air turbulence. Turbulence worsens motion sickness and can cause disorientation in flight team members. Gravitational forces also influence the body in ascent and descent, but these are minimal in helicopter transport and have no significant adverse effects.

Altitude also significantly affects medical equipment. Chest tubes should never be clamped during air transport because doing so will exacerbate a tension pneumothorax. Altitude also affects IV fluids. The use of pressure infusers on plastic IV bags will maintain the flow of fluid when gas bubbles expand and threaten to slow or stop it (Fig. 53-4). Air pressure in the PASG should be monitored, in conjunction with the

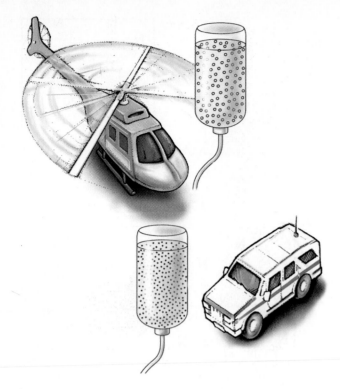

Figure 53-4

As altitude increases, the size of the air bubbles in intravenous fluids grows larger and can slow or stop the flow of the intravenous fluids.

patient's vital signs, to prevent the garment from becoming too tight or loose. If an endotracheal tube is in place, the rescue team should ensure there is always a slight air leak around the cuff so it does not become over- or underinflated.

In summary, the paramedic must understand, anticipate and minimize the effects of altitude on the patient, the medical team, and their equipment.

Dispatch

Paramedics are often familiar with the functions of ground-based emergency medical dispatch, but typically do not interact frequently with air medical communications centers. It is important to understand what makes air medical communications different from emergency medical dispatch on the ground.

Key roles of the air medical communications center are detailed in Box 53-3 and include:

1. Mission request processing
2. Mission coordination and support
3. Program documentation and monitoring[17]

An air medical communication specialist should be assigned to receive and coordinate all requests for the air medical service. The training of communication specialists should include EMT certification or equivalent knowledge or experience. In addition, knowledge of Federal Aviation Administration regulations and Federal Communications Commission requirements is important. The Commission on Accreditation of

Air Medical Services maintains the pertinent standards.[9] Communication specialists should be well versed in general safety rules, emergency procedures pertinent to air medical transport, and flight-following procedures. (Flight following is a process that allows the communication specialist to plot the position of aircraft at any time during flight [Fig. 53-5].) Familiarity with weather interpretation, navigation techniques, and aviation and medical terminology are also important, and training in the operation and troubleshooting of air medical communications center equipment is a prerequisite.

BOX 53-3	Key Roles of the Air Medical Communications Center

Mission Request Processing
- Receive calls and communicate with individuals requesting flights
- Determine medical appropriateness and provide alternative transport arrangements
- Provide price quotes and make payment arrangements for non-emergency missions
- Schedule missions in conjunction with referring and receiving institutions
- Notify physicians, medical and aviation crews, and receiving hospital department

Mission Coordination and Support
- Coordinate with hospital admissions, receiving hospital department, and physicians
- Arrange ground ambulance transportation to and from the aircraft
- Track and communicate with flights and activate remote flight-following plans
- Activate and monitor search-and-rescue operations in the event of missing aircraft or accidents
- Maintain support activities such as weather reporting, coordination of landing sites, location of scenes and destinations, and identification of fueling and alternate landing sites
- Support customer service, including callbacks to referring institution or physician upon mission completion
- Assist the family with paperwork, access to patient, and travel to receiving facility

Program Documentation and Monitoring
- Monitor launch, scene, and travel times
- Capture program use and production information
- Track patients by typing, condition, diagnosis, and length of stay
- Identify and monitor referral and receiving patterns
- Document inventory use
- Collect billing and collection information
- Support data collection for research and program analysis
- Accumulate activity statistics regarding flights, scenes, destinations, type of mission, and time of day
- Document missed flights and alternative dispensation of patients due to weather, mechanical problems, or unavailable aircraft
- Monitor aviation operations, including maintenance and downtime, fueling activity, engine and airframe hours, pilot time and activity, and aircraft use
- Record medical crew activity, such as specialty team use, scheduling, currency, frequency of training, missions completed, and procedures attempted and accomplished

From Keller, R: Air medical communications centers, The Journal of Air Medical Transport, 1992, 11(1):13–16.

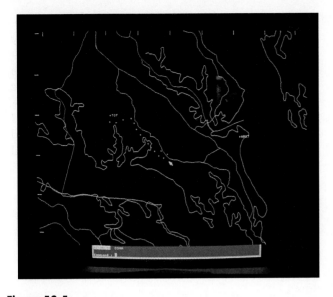

Figure 53-5

A flight following panel provides a visual orientation of the helicopter during flight for the communications center personnel.

Safety

Although the mid-1980s were a time of frequent medical helicopter crashes, considerable improvement has been made in the past few years. For example, in 1986 there were 13 crashes reported.[19] Investigations by the National Transportation Safety Board typically pointed to weather, engine failure, and obstacle strikes as the primary causes.[23] Human decision-making problems were interwoven with these mechanical factors. Recent efforts to improve both initial and recurrent pilot training, and to remove them from pressures related to the patient's medical needs have resulted in significant improvement. There are other issues, which were discussed in the Association of Air Medical Services Safety Congress in 1986 and 1992. These include the number of pilots per aircraft, flight using navigational instruments instead of visual orientation, mechanisms that systematically track the aircraft location, safety education for medical personnel, criteria-based development of landing zones for scene responses, and many other issues.

However, the most important factor for the decrease in crashes has been the dedication of the air medical professionals themselves to an overall philosophy of safety for the profession. This philosophy helped lead to the creation of the Commission on Accreditation of Air Medical Services (CAAMS).[10] The dual mission of CAAMS in developing a national voluntary accreditation process for air medical services is to emphasize the safety of the aviation transport environment and to promote the best possible patient care.

For paramedics interacting with an air medical service, specific guidelines for safe conduct around the aircraft must be kept in mind. These are especially important when handling helicopter responses to a scene, but apply in large part to interactions with aircraft in any setting. The aircraft should only be approached from the front and never from the rear, so that the paramedic can maintain full eye contact with the pilot (Fig. 53-6). There should be no running or smoking within 50 feet of the aircraft. Objects any taller than normal head height should be held close to the ground, so that the object is not struck by the helicopter rotor blades. Hats, sheets, and other loose objects should be either removed or carefully held down, because of the air turbulence created by the aircraft rotors. In general, bystanders should be kept at least 200 feet away from the aircraft, and the aircraft should never be approached when rotor blades are in motion. Usually, the flight team prefers that no one assist them with loading or unloading the patient or equipment, unless specifically directed to do so. Similarly, only members of the flight team should open or close the doors to the aircraft. Although each air medical service will have some variation in its guidelines for interacting with the aircraft, this list is widely supported (*see* Box 53-4).

When a helicopter responds to a scene request, a paramedic is often responsible for establishing a suitable landing zone (LZ). It is important for all paramedics to become familiar with the requirements of the helicopters used in their service area, because there is some variation in size and other criteria from one helicopter to another. Typically, the helicopter will require a flat, square area that is at least 100 feet square

Probably the most vital component of the communications center is its radio capabilities. The ability to communicate with an in-flight aircraft is essential to medical direction, flight following, and safety. Radio communications and paging are often used to alert flight teams of missions. The ability to provide "patching" of radio signals and telemetry from the aircraft to on-line medical direction and others is particularly useful.

Other communications center equipment may include recording devices, weather monitors, and facsimile machines. Television monitors are frequently used in air medical communications centers to monitor the helipad and parked aircraft when communications center personnel cannot see them directly. Telephones, sometimes including 800 numbers, provide the primary means for referring parties to contact the air medical program. Some air medical communications centers use computers to integrate geographic files and radio communications to provide "real time" flight following. Statistics and flight monitoring information can also be compiled in a computer system. If this system is interfaced with the rest of the hospital's computer network, it can also handle patient billing, medical records, and emergency department registration.

Air medical communications specialists should interact on a regular basis with ground-based emergency medical dispatch centers and with referring and accepting institutions. This networking is important to the successful integration of ground and air emergency medical services.

The role of communications in air medical services is nationally recognized as an important part of the system of patient care and safety during air transport. In 1989, the National Association of Air Medical Communication Specialists was created. This organization's goals include promoting an understanding of the duties and responsibilities of air medical communication specialists and meeting the educational needs of its members. The Association of Air Medical Services sponsors an Air Medical Communications Specialist Training Course.

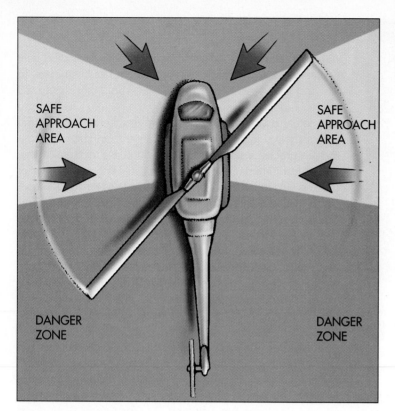

Figure 53-6

A safe approach of the helicopter allows for visualization between the pilot and the approaching personnel. The rear of the helicopter is always considered a danger zone.

SAFE
APPROACH
AREA

SAFE
APPROACH
AREA

DANGER
ZONE

DANGER
ZONE

and has no more than 8° of ground slope (Fig. 53-7). This area should be completely free of trees, shrubs, rubbish, or other loose items that may blow free in the aircraft rotor wash. Sometimes it is useful, particularly at night, to park emergency vehicles at each of the four corners of the LZ, with their emergency rotating lights on, to provide a good visual marker for the aircraft from several miles away. The region around the immediate LZ must be free of tall trees, overhead wires, light poles, and other obstructions that may present an obstacle to the flight path of the helicopter. Lights from the ground should not be shone toward the helicopter, because this can blind the pilot. Lighted flares should also not be used at an LZ, because they can create a fire hazard if blown around.

BOX 53-4	Air Medical Transport Safety Guidelines

- Bystanders should be kept at least 200 feet from the aircraft
- No running or smoking within 50 feet of the aircraft
- All hats, loose clothing, and other objects should be removed
- The aircraft should not be approached, unless instructed by the flight team
- The aircraft should be approached from the front, never from the side or rear
- No objects should be carried higher than a person's head
- Aircraft doors should not be opened or closed by any personnel other than flight crew
- Loading or unloading of the patient/equipment should be done only if instructed by flight team

From Benson, et al: Guidelines for emergency air transport developed, EPIC: North Carolina ACEP Emergency Physician Interim Communique, 2–4, Nov 1988.

When establishing an LZ for a scene response, paramedics must communicate directly with the helicopter team by radio to verify the LZ location and the estimated time of arrival. During this communication, if there are any obstacles in the potential flight path, the paramedic must identify these obstacles for the pilot. Overhead wires can be extremely difficult for the pilot to see. Failure of the ground personnel to adequately identify approximate height and location of wires for the pilot can result in tragedy. In some settings, the LZ can not be located any closer than 1 or 2 miles from the patient; this requires that the helicopter medical personnel be driven by ground ambulance from the LZ to the patient and back. Safety awareness can be enhanced by educational sessions where ground-based paramedics and air medical personnel orient each other to their respective roles and responsibilities during helicopter landing and transfer of the patient.

While part of the ground EMS team is preparing the LZ, the others must be performing the equally important job of preparing the patient. As with any other setting, this requires the standard physical assessment skills, emergency resuscitation measures, and trauma stabilization. In particular, the patient's airway should be open and secured. Although it is possible to intubate patients in most helicopters, the earlier the patient's airway is secured, the earlier optimal oxygenation and ventilation can be assured. After airway and breathing are cared for, major bleeding must be controlled by direct pressure, adding IV fluid resuscitation as needed. Immobilization of the spine and extremities should be accomplished, if appropriate. A long spine board, PASGs, femoral traction splints, and other bulky materials will usually fit in the patient care compartment of the helicopter. Depending upon the length of transport, it may be appropriate to consider placing urinary and nasogastric catheters in the patient. Patients that are com-

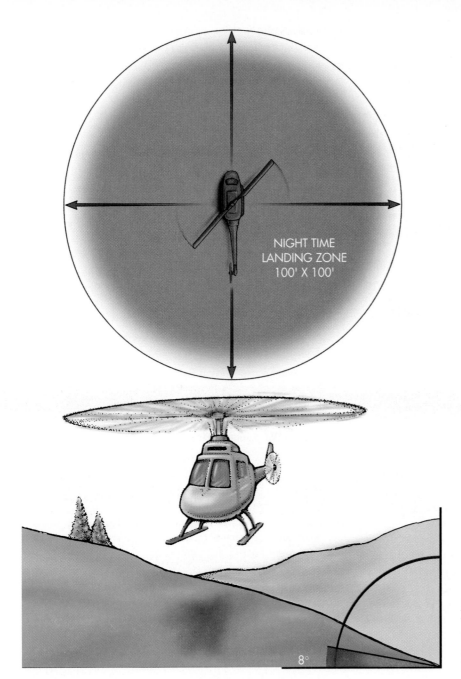

NIGHT TIME
LANDING ZONE
100' X 100'

8°

Figure 53-7

The appropriate landing zone (LZ) will be at least 100 square feet with no more than 8° of slope and free of trees, shrubs, overhead lines, and debris.

bative or restless may not be safely transportable by aircraft if they cannot be adequately sedated.

Extra care should be taken when calling a helicopter to the scene of a hazardous materials incident. The flight team should know of the material involved and the size of the affected area well before arriving. Effects of the hazardous material on the pilot or medical team may make helicopter flight unsafe. This is true whether dealing with gasoline spill from a motor vehicle collision, a hydrogen sulfide leak, or other hazardous materials. It is never appropriate to assume that the helicopter team has already been informed of the hazardous material spill. When the material is gaseous or in danger of exploding, the LZ should be located at least 1 mile upwind from the site. In an incident involving radioactive materials, the LZ should be at least ¼ mile upwind from the site.

SUMMARY

The addition of aircraft and medical and aviation personnel to the regional EMS resource pool offers clear benefits to the patients. However, these additions must be viewed as one resource in the system. Knowing the capabilities of the helicopter and the air medical team in comparison with those of the ground service is important in appropriate use of air medical services. Whether these resources are used for interhospital transfer or transport from a scene, the paramedic serves as a key consumer. The roles of flight paramedic and member of the ground team require detailed understanding of the advantages and risks inherent in air transport. The patient's safety must be a primary concern at all times.

REFERENCES

1. **Baxt WG, Moody P:** The impact of rotorcraft aeromedical emergency care service on trauma mortality. *JAMA* 249:3042–3051, 1983.

2. **Baxt WG, Moody P, Cleveland HC, et al:** Hospital-based rotorcraft aeromedical emergency care services and trauma mortality: A multicenter study. *Ann Emerg Med* 14:859–864, 1985.

3. **Bellinger RL, Califf RM, Mark DF, et al:** Helicopter transport of patients during acute myocardial infarction. *Am J Cardiol* 61:718–722, 1988.

4. **Benson NH:** Guidelines for emergency air transport developed. EPIC: North Carolina ACEP Emergency Physician Interim Communique, 2–4, Nov 1988.

5. **Black RE, Mayer T, Walker ML, et al:** Special report: Air transport of pediatric emergency cases. *N Engl J Med* 307:1465–1468, 1982.

6. **Boyd CR, Corse KM:** Outcome evaluation of trauma patients transported by a rural hospital-based helicopter EMS program. *Hosp Avia* 7:14–18, 1988.

7. **Browne-Wagner L, Bodenstedt R:** Flight Physiology, In Air Medical Crew National Standard Curriculum, Washington, 1988, United States Department of Transportation.

8. **Collett HM:** Annual transport statistics. *J Air Med Trans* 10(3):11, 1991.

9. **Commission on Accreditation of Air Medical Services:** Accreditation Standards, pp. 38–40, 46–48, 1991.

10. **Frazer E, Benson N:** Update: The Commission on Accreditation of Air Medical Services. *J Air Med Trans* 9:17–18, 1991.

11. **Gabram SGA, Jacobs LM:** The impact of emergency medical helicopters on prehospital care. *Emerg Med Clin North Am* 8(1):85–102, 1990.

12. **Hunt RC, Benson NH, Krohmer JR, et al:** Your response to air medical transport: Results of the JEMS November 1989 survey. *JEMS* 16(11):36–40, 1991.

13. **Hunt RC, Bryan DM, Brinkley VS, Whitley TW, Benson NH:** Inability to assess breath sounds during air medical transport by helicopter. *JAMA* 265:1982–1984, 1991.

14. **Hunt RC, Carroll RG, Whitley TW, Bryan D, Dufresne D:** Adverse effects of helicopter flight on the ability to palpate carotid pulses. *J Air Med Trans* 10:74, Oct 1991.

15. **Jablonowski A:** Position paper on the appropriate use of emergency air medical services. *J Air Med Trans* 9(9):29–33, 1990.

16. **Kaplan L, Walsh D, Burney RE:** Emergency aeromedical transport of patients with acute myocardial infarction. *Ann Emerg Med* 16:55–57, 1987.

17. **Keller R:** Air medical communications centers. *J Air Med Trans* 11(1):13–16, 1992.

18. **Larsen B:** Annual transport statistics. *J Air Med Trans* 11(3):27, 1992.

19. **Lillie J, Larsen B:** Safety in the 90s. *J Air Med Trans* 10:16–18, 1991.

20. **Low RB, Martin D, Brown C:** Emergency air transport of pregnant patients: The national experience. *J Emerg Med* 6:41–48, 1988.

21. **National Association of EMS Physicians Position Paper:** Air medical dispatch: Guidelines for scene response. *Prehosp Dis Med* 7(1):75–76, 1992.

22. **National Flight Paramedics Association:** The role of the flight paramedic in the prehospital environment. *Air Med J* 12(6):203–204, 1993.

23. **National Transportation Safety Board Safety Study:** Commercial Emergency Medical Service Helicopter Operations, United States Department of Transportation, Washington, NTSB/SS-88/01,1988.

24. **Oetgen WJ, Laudes RD:** Aeromedical evacuation of high-risk infants: Experience at a military medical center. *Mil Med* 143:172–173, 1978.

25. **Rhodes M, Perline R, Aronson J, et al:** Field triage for on-scene helicopter transport. *J Trauma* 26:963–969, 1986.

26. **Schwartz RJ, Jacobs LM, Juda RJ:** A comparison of ground paramedics and aeromedical treatment of severe blunt trauma patients. *Conn Med* 12:660–662, 1990.

27. **Thomas SH, Stone CK, Bryan-Berge DM, Hunt RC:** Comparison of time required for performance of ACLS interventions in the MBB BO-105 and the MBB BK-117. Accepted for presentation at the Association of Air Medical Services Annual Meeting, Oct 1993.

28. **Williams KA, Aghababian R, Shaughnessy M:** Statewide helicopter utilization review: The Massachusetts experience. *J Air Med Trans* 9(9):14–23, 1990.

Chapter 54

Rural EMS

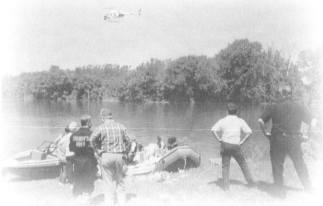

A paramedic should be able to:

OBJECTIVES

1. Describe the challenges facing rural EMS delivery systems.
2. List factors that affect communication in the rural EMS setting.
3. Explain how response times impact the delivery of rural EMS care.
4. Describe factors that can improve long response times.
5. List and describe the types of emergency situations most commonly encountered in the rural setting.
6. Describe protocol considerations that are unique to the rural setting.
7. Discuss the role of air medical transport in the rural setting.

E MS has always served as a critical but fragile link in the rural health care delivery system. With the closure and downsizing of many rural hospitals over the past 10 years, EMS has become the only health care service available in some rural communities. Personnel may be called upon to provide primary care evaluation services that would ordinarily be provided in a physician's office. As the health-care environment changes and family practice physicians become less available, the scope of practice for paramedics in these areas may change.

Defining Rural

Executive Director of the National Rural Health Association, Robert Van Hook, referred to the term **rural** as reflecting not only a state of mind, but an area with fewer resources, greater distances, smaller-scale organizations, a slower pace, and a lower intensity of services. Although there is no standardized definition of rural, approximately 25% of the Unites States population is categorized as rural by the federal government. Table 54-1 compares the distinguishing characteristics of urban, rural, and frontier areas and shows the scope of rural areas.

Rural Statistics

Department of Transportation data indicate that more than 50% of fatal traffic collisions in the United States occur in rural areas. Even though the actual accident rate is less than in urban areas, victims in rural areas are three times more likely to sustain serious or untreatable injuries.[18] Farming and mining

are two of the most hazardous occupations, and these industries tend to be located in rural communities. The older age of rural residents often results in a higher incidence of medical emergencies and a higher demand for emergency transportation services. Popular recreational pursuits, such as boating, fishing, camping, skiing, and hunting often take place in rural and frontier areas where there are limited medical resources. It is estimated that 75% of the nation is not covered by designated trauma systems, and the majority of these areas are rural.[17]

This data would seem to support the need for Advanced Life Support (ALS) services in rural communities. Unfortunately, the reality of providing ALS care in rural areas is hampered by a number of factors including a scarcity of physicians, inadequate funding levels, insufficient numbers of volunteer providers, and low call volumes that limit exposure to clinical cases.[7,12] These factors often discourage rural agencies from pursuing an ALS level of service.

Historically, funding dollars for research and development have primarily been spent for EMS projects in metropolitan areas where the majority of people reside. The results of studies conducted in urban areas, where response times are rapid and hospitals are immediately accessible, cannot be duplicated in the rural environment with the same outcomes. Among the limited number of rural EMS research and demonstration projects that have been conducted, several projects do support the feasibility and value of ALS in rural areas.[7] However, most are of limited scope, are inconclusive, or have had little impact on patient outcome.[10,15] The lack of such conclusive scientific evidence lends little support for upgrading rural prehospital care services into the realm of ALS.

Because of recent economic impacts that threaten the life of rural communities, the nation has begun to pay special attention to the value of sustaining rural services, even if it must be perpetuated through subsidies.

ALS services in rural communities can be economically feasible and effective in improving patient outcomes.[7] To operate a successful ALS program, a strong organizational infrastructure, and community commitment must exist. Needs must be demonstrated and financial resources identified to develop and sustain the service.

TABLE 54-1	Distinguishing Characteristics of Urban, Rural, and Frontier Areas		
Parameter	**Urban**	**Rural**	**Frontier**
Population	> 100/square mile	> 6 but < 100/ square mile	< 6/square mile
Driving time to hospital	< 30 minutes	30 minutes	≥ 60 minutes
Hospital size	≥ 100 beds	25 to 100 beds	< 25 beds
Technology level	High	Medium	Low/difficult access
Physician staffing	Gate keepers or specialists	Generalists	Generalists or nurse practitioners
Social structure	Individual anonymity; very dependent on others; accepts help readily from outsiders	Everyone knows everyone; interdependence; help comes from within the group	Live in isolation; self reliant; reluctant to accept outside help
EMS level of care	Paramedics rapid response times	EMT and EMT-I long response times	First aid very extended response times

Unique Characteristics of EMS Delivery

The conditions encountered in rural areas present some formidable challenges to an EMS delivery system. An understanding of these conditions is crucial for paramedics who practice in these areas and can be of considerable benefit to urban-based paramedics who interact with rural providers. Box 54-1 summarizes some of the rural EMS problems identified in a 1991 study.[14]

Communication Deficiencies

Communication in rural areas can be severely limited. Many communities do not yet have 9-1-1 or enhanced 9-1-1 (E9-1-1)

When expanding or improving rural service operations, it is always helpful to know where help can be found. The best place to start is within the rescuer's own state, speaking with those already in the business. State EMS offices have local and national resources readily available and will often provide direct assistance in expansion activities. When collecting information, the rescuer should ask each person to give names of other resources. Following are a few lesser-known resources that might also be helpful.

State Rural Health Offices

National EMS Clearing House
The Council of State Governments
Lexington, KY

National Rural Health Association
1320 19th Street, NW Suite 350
Washington, DC 20036-1610
202-232-6200

Department of Transportation
National Highway Traffic Safety Administration
Traffic Safety Programs / NTS-42
400 7th Street, SW
Washington, DC 20590
410-366-4299

National Department of Health and Human Services
Federal Office of Rural Health Policy
Division of Trauma and Emergency Medical Services
Parklawn Building, Room 11A-22
5600 Fishers Lane
Rockville, MD 20857
301-443-3401

Alpha Center
1350 Connecticut Avenue, NW Suite 1100
Washington, DC 20036
202-296-1818

Robert Wood Johnson Foundation
College Road and US Route 1
PO Box 2316
Princeton, NJ 08543-2316

WK Kellog Foundation
One Michigan Avenue East
Battle Creek, MI 49017
616-968-1611

Congress of the United States
Office of Technology Assessment
Washington, DC 20510-8025

Federal Emergency Management Association
United States Fire Administration
16825 South Seton Avenue
Emmitsburg, MD 21727
301-447-1333

telephone access for emergencies.[1] Emergency numbers frequently differ for each county or fire district, and these numbers are not posted on public telephones. Public telephones are scarce and may be some distance from the victim's location. It is not uncommon for rural residents to be without phone service in their homes. Other obstacles that hamper effective communications in rural areas include mountainous terrain, which can block signals, and outdated and inadequate equipment.

BOX 54-1	Primary Rural EMS Problems

- Inadequate public access
- Extended response times
- Lack of public education
- Shortage of volunteer personnel
- Limited training opportunities
- Absence of strong medical direction
- Inadequate funding
- Lack of a coordinated system approach

Response Times

Response times are generally longer in rural areas and probably have the greatest impact on patient outcomes. EMS incidents may go undetected for a number of hours before they are reported. Adverse road conditions (e.g., snow, ice, narrow curves, dirt) considerably lengthen response times. Some rural locations can only be reached using a combination of foot trails and water or air routes (Fig. 54-1). It is not unusual for travel time to a rural scene to exceed 20 minutes.[8]

Further delays can occur when trying to find rural locations. Residences are often not marked by street names, house numbers, or even fire numbers and can only be found by following specific landmarks.[12,18] Although local volunteers are usually familiar with many residences in the area, without a detailed mapping system, it is not unusual for the rescue team to become lost on country dirt roads.

There are several approaches that rural services find useful in improving response times. Strategic placement of response units throughout the service area makes vehicles more accessible to volunteers. Having first responders travel directly to the scene in their own vehicles to provide aid until the ambulance arrives is another approach used to improve response

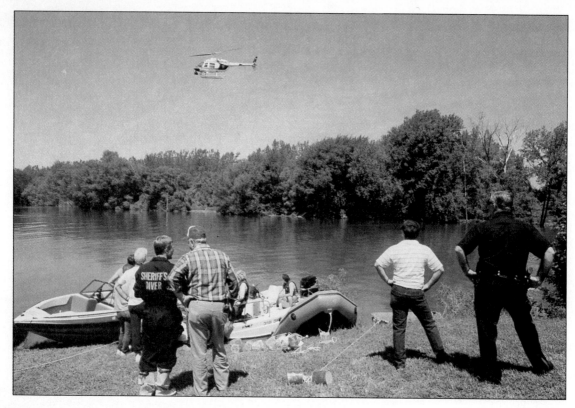

Figure 54-1

Less traditional means of patient access are necessary in some rural areas. Photographed by Craig Jackson.

times in rural areas (Fig. 54-2). Medically trained dispatchers can give initial first aid directions to callers, providing supportive treatment to the patient awaiting arrival of EMS units.

Vehicle Design

Some rural regions require nontypical ambulance response units (Fig. 54-3). Four-wheel drive and tire chains are necessities

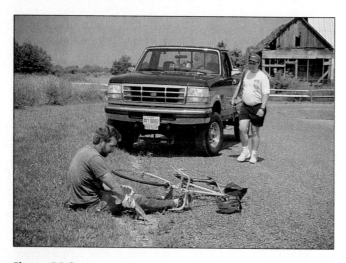

Figure 54-2

First responders often arrive to begin stabilization of the patient while awaiting the ambulance arrival.

in mountainous regions in the winter. Snowmobiles are also useful in some locations. In recreational areas, all terrain vehicles (ATVs) and helicopters are often required to reach and transport the patients to a highway or airport for further transport. Four-wheel drive pick-up trucks are useful because they can travel over off-road terrain and because they have cargo beds, which can accommodate several stretchers and providers. Sometimes, the only mode of transport is "foot power." Because of the unusual extrication requirements that are sometimes encountered in rural areas, ambulances are likely to be equipped with rescue equipment not normally found in urban units. This equipment could include items such as heavy-duty extrication equipment, mountain climbing gear, special backboards and traction apparatus, and high-angle rescue tools.

Ingenuity is one of the hallmarks of rural EMS personnel. Paramedics practicing in or interacting with rural services should be ready to adapt the principles of care learned in the classroom to the special environment and equipment found in rural areas. Thus, it is essential that rural EMS personnel be trained by individuals who understand these principles of adaptation.

Volunteer Recruitment and Retention

In most rural areas, EMS service personnel are largely or totally volunteers. It is widely believed that the number of these volunteers is decreasing.[6,9,11,12,16] As EMS has matured, the demands on volunteer time has increased. Training, recertification requirements, and long transport times have the biggest

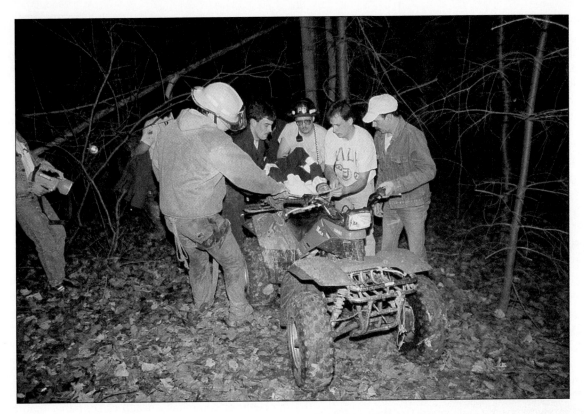

Figure 54-3

Recreational vehicles are often adapted for use by EMS services. Photographed by Craig Jackson.

impact on a volunteer's time. Job hazards, such as liability and exposure to bloodborne pathogens and hazardous materials, have also made it difficult to recruit and retain volunteers. Also, economic difficulties have displaced rural workers, resulting in a dwindling pool of potential recruits.

Community commitment is no longer sufficient to recruit and retain volunteers. Financial incentives, such as pension plans, have been extremely successful for a number of organizations.[16] Other incentives can include disability and liability insurance, pay per call, tuition reimbursement, and bonuses.

Training Demands

As requirements for EMS training and certification become more stringent, fewer volunteers are willing to make the time and financial commitments necessary to keep themselves up to date. One study reported that 30% of EMS volunteers left the field because of training demands.[1] The 1994 EMT-Basic United States Department of Transportation curriculum has tried to address this issue by making training more directly applicable to the EMTs actual duties. Increasing the availability of rural-based training programs can also ease the training burden.

As difficult as it is to train rural volunteers at the EMT-Basic level, it is harder still to support paramedics in such communities. Fortunately, the EMT-Intermediate certification has helped to bridge that gap. This level concentrates on those critical ALS skills and techniques—airway management, IV therapy, and defibrillation—that result in positive patient outcomes yet require less training than do skills at the paramedic level.[7]

In rural areas where call volumes are low, skill levels can be maintained using case discussions, simulated practice, mannequins, incident reviews, and in-service training. A New York study revealed an 88% success rate in initiating IVs when using only mannequins during training.[7] Closed circuit television and educational tapes can also augment local clinical training resources. Rural hospitals and physicians are the most obvious personnel available to assist with clinical training needs, but veterinarians and coroners are also excellent resources.

Providing Care in Rural Areas

The unique environment of rural EMS requires approaches that may differ from those in urban areas with regard to medical direction, ALS interventions, and protocols.

Medical Direction

The medical director has the responsibility to modify and adapt protocols to provide optimum levels of care. Medical direction in rural communities is best provided by a local physician, usually a family practitioner. In rural areas where there is no local physician, an urban physician, typically one affiliated with an EMS base station hospital, may serve as the physician advisor. Regardless of where the medical advisor is physically located, it is important that the individual be well versed in EMS operations and clinical therapies.

Because direct radio communication is not always available to rural EMS personnel, standing orders may be written enabling properly trained personnel to perform life-saving procedures without direct contact with a physician. This approach requires a significant commitment on the part of the medical director to ensure that responders are adequately trained and able to act independently. Regular quality assurance and run review meetings allow the physician and EMS personnel to interact directly and are an excellent continuing education tool.

Primary ALS Intervention Techniques

When initiating an ALS practice in a rural area, several factors must be considered regarding its scope. The provision of ALS services must be economically practical. Efforts are usually most effective when targeted toward treating those conditions seen most frequently, and for those in which ALS interventions can produce positive outcomes. The basics of airway, breathing, and circulation (ABCs) are still the most critical areas on which the rescuer must focus. Definitive treatment produces the most favorable patient outcomes (Box 54-2).[7]

Intravenous therapy is a skill that can be easily taught and learned using mannequins. Airway control in the arrested or unresponsive patient with a compromised airway can be treated effectively by using endotracheal intubation or other types of airway devices. Simulated practice is also useful when learning this procedure. The third procedure that can improve patient outcome is defibrillation. However, use of this procedure in rural areas has not proved as successful as its use in urban areas. The factor that determines effectiveness of defibrillation is the elapsed time between patient collapse, initiation of CPR, and arrival of the EMS unit.[5,10,15]

Special Protocol Considerations

There are several scenarios that demonstrate the need for altered protocols in rural areas. Urban-based services may require that, once initiated, CPR must be continued throughout transport until discontinued by a physician at the emergency department. This approach is difficult in a rural area where transport time to an emergency department may be 1 hour or

longer. Instead, EMS personnel may be trained and permitted to use medical criteria to determine when it is appropriate to discontinue CPR in the field. If radio communication cannot be established, the EMS provider may make an independent decision based on protocols to stop resuscitation.

Because of short transport times, urban services may require that no scene time be used to initiate an IV. In rural areas, with long transport times and rough road conditions that make it difficult to begin an IV en route, it may be more appropriate for the paramedic to take a few extra minutes to start the IV before departing the scene. Transport times also affect decisions regarding airway management techniques. A bag-valve-mask may be quite effective during short transport. However, if a 45-minute ride is part of the equation, the paramedic would be wise to take the time to secure an endotracheal tube or other advanced airway.

Transport destination protocols require modification in rural areas. In the face of limited resources, individuals who have "first-aid" level injuries may have to be treated and released at the scene because it is not feasible to transport them 30 miles to the closest hospital. In some areas, a physician's office may be the next highest level of care within many miles. Under these circumstances, it may be quite appropriate to transport a patient via ambulance to a physician's office, or to a county or community health clinic, rather than a hospital. There will also be instances when patients are released from EMS care to be transported by family. Protocols must also include these alternatives to hospital transport.

Air medical transport plays an important role in rural EMS. It offers advanced levels of care to patients and moves them quickly into tertiary centers for definitive treatment. When weather conditions preclude the use of air transport, rendezvous points can be set up with ground ALS units from metropolitan areas. Handing off the patient during transport to a higher level service not only benefits the patient, but also permits the rural unit to return to service within its community more quickly.

The key to providing good medical care when handling special protocol considerations is to adapt to the special circumstances at hand. Adequate training, written medical guidelines, and strong medical direction will enable providers to make sound medical decisions in a wide variety of circumstances.

SUMMARY

Providing quality care doesn't begin and end at the scene. An EMS system is not truly a system if the rural element of care is an isolated struggle by a few individuals to provide emergency care to local residents. With the movement toward health care reform and basic access for all, paramedicine can be a leader in expanding its influences into rural communities to help solve the problems and overcome the barriers to providing quality EMS service. The ingenuity, adaptability, and tenacity of rural EMS personnel, teamed with the resources of paramedicine can go a long way toward improving levels of care in rural areas.

BOX 54-2 **Definitive ALS Treatment Producing the Best Outcomes**

- IV therapy
- Advanced airway management
- Defibrillation

REFERENCES

1. **Center for Urban Affairs,** University at Birmingham, Emergency Medical Services in the Birmingham Region, April 1989.

2. **Campion, DM, et al:** Networking for Rural Health, Alpha Center, March 1993.

3. **Crandall LA, et al:** Recruitment and Retention of Rural Physicians: Issues for the 1990s, *J Rural Health* 6(1), Jan 1990.

4. **Doeksen GA, et al:** A Community Development Guide for Emergency Medical Services: A System Approach to Funding and Administration, Oklahoma State University, Oklahoma.

5. **Gallehr JE, Vukov LF:** Defining the Benefits of Rural Emergency Medical Technician- Defibrillation. *Ann Emerg Med* 22(1), Jan 1993.

6. **Garza MA:** Money Talks, Nobody Walks: Financial Incentives for Volunteers. *JEMS* Feb 1991.

7. **Hawks SR:** Rural ALS. *Emerg Med Serv* 20(11), Nov 1991.

8. **Johnson J, et al:** Wilderness Emergency Medical Services: The Experiences at Sequoia and King's Canyon National Parks. *Am J Emerg Med* 9(6), May 1991.

9. **National Rural Health Association and Foundation for Health Services Research, A Rural Health Services Re-** search Agenda: Summary of a Conference, December 1987, San Diego, Health Services Research 23(6), Feb 1989.

10. **Olson DW, et al: EMT-Defibrillation:** The Wisconsin Experience. *Ann Emerg Med* 18:8, Aug 1989.

11. **Ott JS:** The Wyoming Experiment: Rural EMS Issues, Needs, Problems, and Actions. *J Emerg Med* Feb 1993.

12. **Parker M, et al:** The Crisis in Rural Prehospital Emergency Care. *Emerg Med Serv* 19(5), May 1990.

13. **Reeder L:** Seeding Clouds of Change: The Drought in Rural EMS. *JEMS* 14(6), June 1989.

14. **Reich J:** Success and Failure: A Study of Rural Emergency Medical Services, Office of Rural Health Policy and National Rural Health Association, May 1990.

15. **Richless LK, et al:** Early Defibrillation Program: Problems Encountered in a Rural/Suburban EMS System, *J Emerg Med* 11, 1993.

16. **Smith, Amber:** The Changing Portrait of Today's Volunteer. *J Emerg Med* Feb 1991.

17. **Southard P, Trunkey, MD:** Rural Trauma: The Oregon Experiment. *J Emerg Nurs* 16(5), Sept–Oct 1990.

18. **United States Congress, Office of Technology Assessment, Special Report:** Rural Emergency Medical Services, GPO 4052-003-01173-5, Washington, Nov 1989.

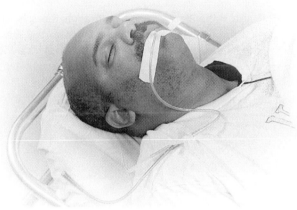

A paramedic should be able to:

1. Identify the types of patients who may have vascular access devices (VADs).

2. Describe three general categories of VADs and their appropriate uses in the prehospital setting.

3. Identify complications and emergencies that may be associated with the use of VADs.

4. Describe the steps for using VADs in the prehospital setting.

5. Identify potential emergencies experienced by hemodialysis patients and describe the proper prehospital management of those emergencies.

6. Describe the steps for using a dialysis device for vascular access in emergency situations.

7. Compare and contrast two types of tracheostomies.

8. Identify the most common complications associated with tracheostomy tubes, stomas, and mechanical ventilators, and describe the proper prehospital management of those complications.

9. Explain the purpose of enteral feedings and identify associated complications.

10. Describe the purpose of a ventricular shunt.

11. Identify the signs and symptoms of ventricular shunt occlusions, and describe the appropriate prehospital management.

12. Describe the type of patient who may require an implanted automatic cardioverter defibrillator (AICD) and discuss the prehospital management of AICD emergencies.

1. **Automatic implantable cardioverter defibrillator (AICD)**—a surgically implanted device that monitors a person's heart rate. Designed to deliver defibrillatory shocks as needed.

2. **Dialysis vascular access device**—a shunt, fistula, or graft which allows access to circulation for the purpose of renal dialysis.

3. **Enteral tube feeding**—the introduction of food or nutritive material directly into the digestive tract by nasogastric or gastric tube.

4. **Gastric tube**—a small tube inserted through the nose or mouth into the stomach, used to drain gas or gastric acid, or to provide liquid nutrition.

5. **Gastrostomy**—an artificial opening into the stomach.

6. **Hemodialysis**—a procedure in which impurities or wastes are removed from the blood, used in treating renal insufficiency and various toxic conditions.

7. **Parenteral nutrition**—provision of total caloric needs by the intravenous route.

8. **Peritoneal dialysis**—a dialysis procedure performed to correct an imbalance of fluid or of electrolytes in the blood or to remove toxins, drugs, or other waste normally excreted by the kidney.

9. **Tracheostomy**—an opening through the neck into the trachea through which an indwelling tube may be inserted.

10. **Vascular access device**—an indwelling catheter, cannula, or other instrumentation used to obtain venous or arterial access.

11. **Ventricular shunt**—a catheter inserted into the lateral ventricle which allows cerebral spinal fluid (CSF) to be drained.

he field of paramedicine is dynamic and constantly evolving. Paramedic training programs no longer teach only the basics. Patients with unusual diseases are living longer, and technical advances are sending them home from the hospital sooner. The paramedic may encounter pumps, catheters, tubes, and electrical devices not taught in the standard curriculum. This chapter is designed to acquaint the paramedic with some of the specialized treatments that were once confined to use in the hospital. Therapies such as vascular access devices, dialysis access devices, surgical airways, enteral feeding tubes, ventricular shunts, and implanted defibrillators will be discussed. These adjuncts, although relatively simple, may seem complex to the prehospital provider. Familiarity with their uses, complications, and handling will reduce the anxiety that can arise when encountering them in the field. These adjuncts may also provide a valuable and previously untapped resource for patient care.

Vascular Access Devices

Many patients with cancer and other chronic illnesses require prolonged and frequent access to venous circulation. In the past it was necessary for the patient to remain hospitalized or suffer repeated needle sticks to obtain blood at home. Today, however, medications, parenteral nutrition, and blood transfusions can be administered through a variety of vascular access devices (VADs). These tubes are inserted into the central circulation where they remain for weeks or months, allowing reliable access to circulation. Nearly 3 million VADs are implanted each year. This allows more patients to be managed at home, and as a result, paramedics encounter increasing numbers of patients with VADs. In the past, the use of VADs in the prehospital setting was strongly discouraged. In critical situations, however, VADs may provide immediate and life-saving venous access.

Although many types of VADs are currently in use, they may be classified into three general categories: central venous catheters (CVC), implanted ports, and peripheral inserted central catheters (PICC).[16] Each of these categories includes several types of catheters with a variety of uses and functions.[24] Although the specifics are complex, a working knowledge of the general types and functions of VADs is valuable for the paramedic.

Features of VADs

Catheters implanted for long-term use have many common features. Most are constructed of radiopaque silicone or, less often, polyurethane. Silicone is strong, flexible and less likely to cause clot formation than other types of materials.[24] Location of the catheter will vary based on patient characteristics, patient preference, type and duration of therapy, and self- and home-care capabilities.[8]

The venous catheter is inserted with the tip in the superior vena cava just above the right atrium, thus the descriptive name of central venous catheter. The insertion site is usually one of the major veins of the chest or upper neck, or—in the case of peripheral access—one of the large veins of the arm or leg (Fig. 55-1).[14,24] VADs are used for both bolus injections and continuous IV infusions. Examples include IV solutions, medications, total parenteral nutrition (TPN), blood, and blood products. Blood samples for laboratory studies are obtainable through most VADs.[24] The catheter may have one, two, or three lumens.

Central venous catheters (CVC) may also be referred to by the manufacturer's name (e.g., Broviac, Hickman, Groshong, Corcath). A CVC may be a single-lumen or a multiple-lumen catheter. The latter catheter is used for patients requiring complex therapy. Lumen sizes vary from 21- to 14-gauge. A small cap (referred to as an intermittent injection cap, buffalo cap, or heparin lock) covers each lumen and is filled with a heparin or saline solution to keep blood clots from blocking the catheter. These catheters are inserted through the skin and then tunneled through the subcutaneous tissue to the site in which the catheter enters the vein (Fig. 55-2). A cuff located in the subcutaneous portion of the catheter helps the catheter to imbed itself in tissue. Fibrous tissue then grows around it, stabilizing the catheter and creating a barrier against infection.[8,22,24]

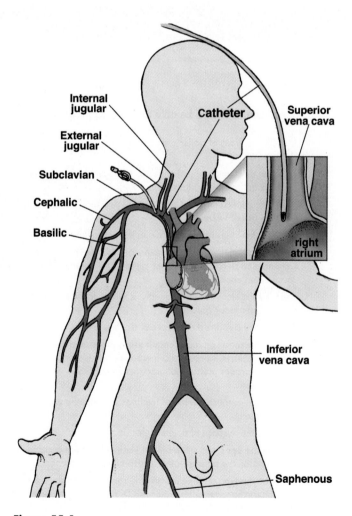

Figure 55-1

A central venous catheter shown inserted into the subclavian vein. The tip of the catheter rests in the superior vena cava.

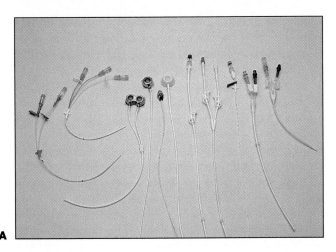

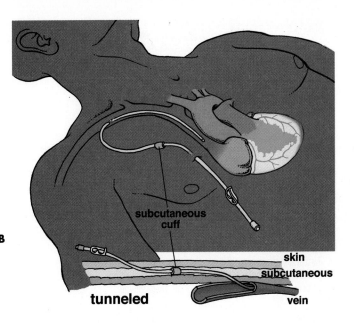

Figure 55-2

A, Central venous catheters. B, Central venous catheters are inserted into the skin and tunneled through the subcutaneous tissue and into the vein. The distal end of the catheter rests in the superior vena cava.

Unlike a CVC, there is no external infusion site in an implanted, or subcutaneous, port. This port is located at the distal end of the catheter and is implanted approximately 0.5 inch under the skin.[16,24] The port is palpated through the skin, and a needle is inserted into the self-sealing septum. Although not required, a dressing is often placed over the access site to add further protection. In routine circumstances, a special "Huber" needle is used to extend the life of the septum.[23]

PICC lines are small (23- to 16-gauge) single- or double-lumen catheters. Because of the smaller size, they are often used for neonates, very young children, or patients who require only short-term therapy.[8,14] PICC lines are less expensive than CVCs and have fewer major complications such as hemothorax, pneumothorax, and air emboli.[20] They are also called *nontunneled catheters*, because they enter the skin near the point at which they enter the vein (Fig. 55-3). PICC lines are often inserted at the antecubital space into the basilic or cephalic vein. Once inserted, the catheter may be sutured in place for stability.

VAD Complications and Emergencies

Patients with VADs may call EMS for a variety of reasons. Because many patients with VADs have chronic illnesses, they may seek help for complications of cancer, AIDS, or sickle-cell disease, for instance. Patients with VADs may be injured or have problems with unassociated illnesses. Finally, several difficulties related directly to the presence of a VAD may occur. Table 55-1 lists some of the more common possibilities.

The most common problem associated with VADs is infection of the exit site, tunnel, or port. Despite proper dressing techniques, localized redness, swelling, and drainage may develop. Patients and families are alerted to watch for any subtle signs of infection. If bacteria manage to ascend through the catheter and enter the patient's circulation, a systemic infection can also develop. The patient may present with fever, general weakness, body aches, and possibly septic shock.

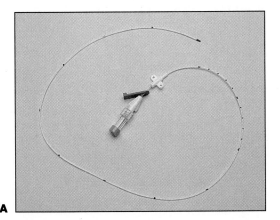

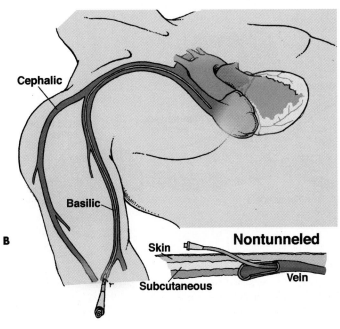

Figure 55-3

A, Peripheral Inserted Central Catheter (PICC). B, PICC lines are small and do not tunnel like CVC lines. Because of their small size, they are ideal for infants and small children.

TABLE 55-1	Complications and Emergencies Associated with VAD
Complication	**Signs/Symptoms**
Site infection	Pain Erythema Swelling Drainage
Sepsis	Elevated temperature—tachycardia Weakness Body aches Septic shock
Thrombosis (clot formation)	Sluggish fluid flow Swelling Local tenderness Ecchymosis
Torn or leaking catheter (fluid or medication) extravasation	Burning Local tenderness Fluid leakage Swelling
Air embolism	Chest pain Shortness of breath Alteration in level of responsiveness Neurological deficit

Adapted from Handelsman H: Implantation of automatic cardioverter-defibrillator: Noninducibility of ventricular tachyarrhythmia as a patient selection criterion, 10, *AHCPR Health Technology Assessment Reports*, 1990; Wickman RS: Advances in venous access devices and nursing management strategies, *Nurs Clin North Am* 25(2):345–363, 1990.

Management of local infections may begin in the prehospital setting with simple dressing changes and caution to avoid further spread of infection. Systemic sepsis or septic shock will require standard management of the ABCs. The VAD itself may be used because IV access for fluid resuscitation of the critical patient may be difficult or impossible, and aseptic technique is essential (e.g., sterile gloves, alcohol, povidone-iodine) (*see* Chapter 10). It is important for the paramedic to remember that the VAD itself may be the site of infection. If any clinical signs suggest this, the VAD should not be used for access.

VADs are usually flushed with a heparin or saline solution to prevent clotting. Despite proper care, clots may form in the catheter, disrupting the flow of solutions and medications (Fig. 55-4). Sluggish flow or inability to infuse solutions requires rapid intervention. The rescuer must never attempt to force or dislodge the clot. The catheter may require declotting with thrombolytics or may have to be replaced.

Thrombosis can develop in the vessel in which the catheter is inserted. The patient may complain of local tenderness or swelling in the arm, neck, or shoulder near the device. In addition, the patient or family may notice that the flow of solution or medication through the catheter is sluggish. Prehospital management of a thrombosis is similar to that of a deep vein thrombosis: the area should not be massaged; instead, the area or extremity must be immobilized, low-flow oxygen administered, and the patient transported to definitive care.

It is rare for the catheter or port to migrate or become displaced because VADs are secured, usually with sutures. However, physical exercise or accidental "tugging" on the external apparatus can displace the catheter. The patient may complain of bleeding, burning upon infusion, or swelling from infiltrated fluid. Upon palpation of an implanted port, the patient may have pain, swelling, and bruising in the area. In extreme cases, the tip of the catheter can migrate and puncture or become lodged in a major vessel wall or the myocardium, leading to more severe symptoms. Patients who complain of shortness of breath, chest pain, dizziness, tachycardia, or hypotension should be treated by standard emergency protocols, with an awareness that the symptoms can result either from complications related to a special device or from an unrelated and potentially life-threatening event.

Occasionally a catheter will develop a leak or tear, perhaps related to improper use. When this occurs, fluids or medications infiltrate into the surrounding tissues. The surrounding area will appear swollen and tender, and the patient may complain of burning (Fig. 55-5). The infusion should be stopped immediately; certain medications may cause significant irritation, and even necrosis of tissues, when infiltration occurs. An appropriate dressing can be applied to the area to help prevent infection and necessary measures should be used to stop bleeding.

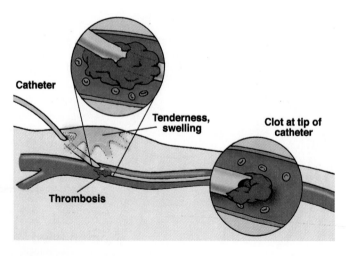

Figure 55-4

Redness, tenderness, and local tissue swelling can indicate the formation of a thrombus at the distal tip of the catheter. These patients require further evaluation in the ED.

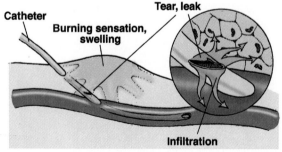

Figure 55-5

A disruption in the catheter can result in all of the signs and symptoms of infiltration seen with traditional forms of prehospital IV therapy including pain, burning, swelling, or tenderness at the site.

Either improper occlusion of the catheter port or a tear in the catheter can lead to an air embolus. Because exact prehospital diagnosis is impossible, management is by standard protocol based on a complete patient assessment. The patient should be transported in a left lateral position with the legs slightly elevated and head lowered, to prevent an air embolus from migrating to the brain and causing a stroke. Oxygen, cardiac monitor, venous access, and rapid transport are indicated in these patients.

Prehospital Use of VADs

Rapid venous access is important in many medical and traumatic emergencies. Standard methods of venous access, such as peripheral and external jugular IVs, and the intraosseous route (typically reserved for pediatric patients), should always be attempted before using a VAD. It is also important for the paramedic to remember that several medications can be administered through an endotracheal tube when IV access is not available. For the patient who requires immediate vascular access and offers no peripheral route, a VAD can provide a safe, rapid solution.[16]

The patient, family members, and other caregivers can often provide valuable information about the patient's medical condition and the use of the VAD, despite their limited knowledge of emergency situations. Because of the extremely high risk of infection and sepsis, careful aseptic technique, including sterile gloves, must be used at all times. The paramedic should identify the location of the catheter or palpate the site of the implanted port. The catheter can be clamped by folding it over, and smooth hemostats (no teeth) can be used to prevent infusion of air. When clamping, the paramedic must use care to prevent tearing the catheter. If an infusion is in progress or a pump is attached, the rescuer should ask for help from those familiar with the pump; the pump should be turned off, clamped, or the line coming from it disconnected. If the VAD has multiple lumens, the pump may be left on and a "free" lumen can be used. The paramedic should remove the small injection cap covering the hub of the lumen and attach the syringe or IV tubing directly to the catheter (Fig. 55-6).[23] The cap can also be left in place and after cleaning the cap with alcohol or povidone-iodine, a needle (20 g or smaller) can be inserted through. The paramedic should then remove the clamp or unpinch the catheter. Using a syringe, the paramedic should aspirate 3 to 5 mL of blood slowly, to avoid collapsing the catheter. This confirms placement and clears the line of heparin. If called for in local protocols, blood samples can be obtained using a syringe or vacutainer. A vacutainer should not be used for PICC lines. The paramedic must be sure to pinch or clamp the lumen when attaching and removing syringes to avoid taking air into the catheter. Using at least 10 mL of normal saline, the catheter should be flushed of blood. The paramedic can then connect the IV tubing and carefully tape it, using a loop of tubing to prevent inadvertent disconnection. The infusion site should be monitored and the patient reassessed (see sidebar).

An implanted port may be used in much the same way as a central line or PICC. The port is usually implanted in the rib area or antecubital space. Using a sterile gloved hand, the paramedic should apply pressure around the edges of the port to slightly "stretch" the skin over the injection site (Fig. 55-7). If a Huber needle is not available, as small a needle as possible (preferably a 21 g or smaller) should be used to avoid port damage and leakage at the injection site. The needle and syringe or IV tubing should be flushed first. The needle must be inserted until it touches the back of the port; this may require a great deal of pressure to puncture the skin, scar tissue, and septum.[23] The paramedic can then aspirate blood; if it does not return freely, the device should not be used. The port should again be flushed and infusion of medications or fluids begun.

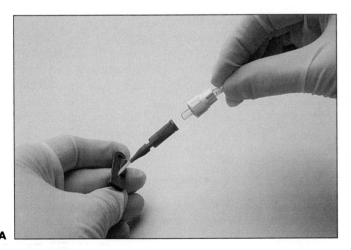
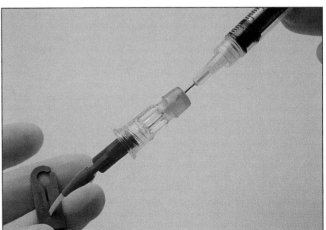

A   B

Figure 55-6

A, To use a VAD in an emergency, crimp the catheter to prevent the introduction of air into the line before removing the injections cap. B, A syringe or IV tubing can be attached directly to the hub of the catheter to inject drugs into the line. Use aseptic technique and sterile gloves throughout the procedure to prevent infection.

by Marilyn K. Bourn, RN, MSN, CEN, NREMT-P

Formal instruction in the following procedure and supervised practice are required before attempting it in the field. This procedure should only be used as a last resort. It should adhere to local protocols and be performed under supervision of medical direction.

1. Complete the primary survey on the patient and manage the ABCs.
2. Obtain pertinent medical history if possible, and any information available regarding the type of VAD.
3. Attempt peripheral, external jugular, or intraosseous access as per local protocol.
4. Identify the location and type of VAD (e.g., central venous catheter, implanted port, or peripheral inserted central catheter).
5. Use knowledgeable family members, homecare giver or others, if possible.
6. Disconnect or discontinue any pumps or medications.
7. Clamp the VAD closed to prevent air embolus by folding or using smooth hemostats.
8. If multiple lumen, identify the lumen to be used.
9. Use strict aseptic technique. Briskly wipe the injection cap with an alcohol or povidone-iodine pad.
10. Insert the needle, with syringe attached, into the cap. Aspirate slowly for a blood return. Obtain blood samples if necessary, then flush the line with solution.
11. Insert the needle, attached to a medication syringe or IV tubing, and infuse medications or fluids.
12. Secure the IV tubing.
13. Reassess the infusion site and patient condition.

THIS PROCEDURE MUST INCLUDE ANY SPECIFICS RELATED TO LOCAL MEDICAL DIRECTION.

IMPLANTED PORTS

1. Follow steps as noted above.
2. Carefully palpate the location of the implanted port.
3. Using sterile technique, prep the site with alcohol or povidone-iodine. Wipe from the center outward three times in a circular motion.
4. Using a sterile gloved hand, press the skin firmly around the edges of the port.
5. Using a syringe filled with solution, insert the needle perpendicular to the skin.
6. Aspirate for blood return and then flush the port prior to infusion.
7. Secure the IV tubing.
8. Reassess the infusion site and the patient.

Adapted from McAfee T, et al: How to safely draw blood from a vascular access device, Nursing 11:42–43, 1990; McEvoy MT: Vascular access devices, JEMS 17(5):39–50, 1992; Viall CD: Your complete guide to catheters, Nursing 2:34–41, 1990.

Dialysis Access

The kidneys are responsible for removing toxic materials from the body as well as maintaining fluid, electrolyte, and acid-base balances. When genetic, medical, or traumatic causes impair kidney function, alternatives are necessary. Dialysis uses the principles of osmosis, diffusion, and ultrafiltration to eliminate toxic materials from the body. Despite advances in therapies and transplants, nearly every patient with end-stage renal disease requires some form of dialysis.[17,18]

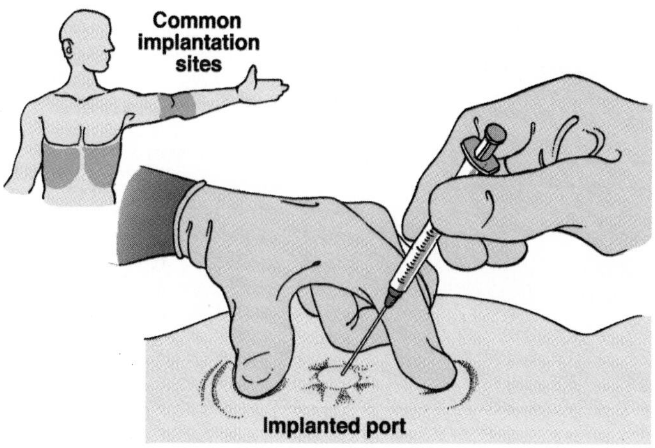

Peritoneal Dialysis

In peritoneal dialysis, sterile dialyzing fluid (dialysate) is fed through an implanted catheter into the abdominal cavity. The catheter, usually constructed of nylon or silicone rubber, is inserted in the midline abdomen (Fig. 55-8). The dialysate bathes the peritoneal membranes that cover the abdominal organs and supporting capillary beds. Blood toxins travel from the abdominal capillaries into the dialysate fluid, which is then drained back through the catheter.[22] This process lasts approximately 1 hour and is often repeated many times daily or throughout the night while the patient sleeps.[12]

Hemodialysis

Hemodialysis involves shunting the patient's blood through a dialysis machine to facilitate removal of waste and toxins (Fig. 55-9). Once the blood has been "detoxified," it is returned to the patient's circulation. Currently there are three common methods of vascular access for hemodialysis:

- arteriovenous fistula
- arteriovenous graft
- external arteriovenous shunt

Common implantation sites

Implanted port

Figure 55-7

Use Huber needles or small gauge needles to access implanted ports. Stretch the skin taut over the site, then insert the needle perpendicular to the skin.

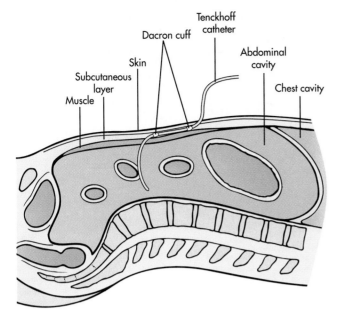

Figure 55-8

Peritoneal dialysis is performed through a catheter inserted in the midline of the abdomen. *Modified from Thelan L, Davie JK, Urden JD: Textbook of Critical Care Nursing: Diagnosis and Management, ed 2, 1994, St. Louis, Mosby-Year Book.*

Arteriovenous (AV) fistulas are created by establishing an opening in an artery and an adjacent vein. The two vessels are surgically connected (anastomosed). The high pressures associated with arterial flow creates a "bulge" or swelling of the vein (known as a pseudoaneurysm) (Fig. 55-10A); outflow of blood is accomplished by inserting a large-bore needle into this "bulge".[18]

AV grafts are the most frequently used access points for chronic renal dialysis. Synthetic materials such as Goretex®, or biological materials such as human umbilical veins, are surgically implanted in the limb to create a U-shaped tunnel. This graft is connected to the vein and artery, then secured just under the surface of the skin. The graft creates a raised area under the skin which looks like a large vessel (Fig. 55-10B).[22]

External AV shunts are seldom used today because of the advent of vascular access devices such as femoral and subclavian catheters. Similar to the AV graft, the shunt joins the vein and artery together. The tubing extends from each vessel tip outside the body and may be connected with a heparinized "T" device.[22]

Dialysis Access Device Complications and Emergencies

Problems associated with dialysis access devices are similar to those of VADs, including infection, thrombosis, obstruction, and bleeding.[17,22] As noted previously, management of these

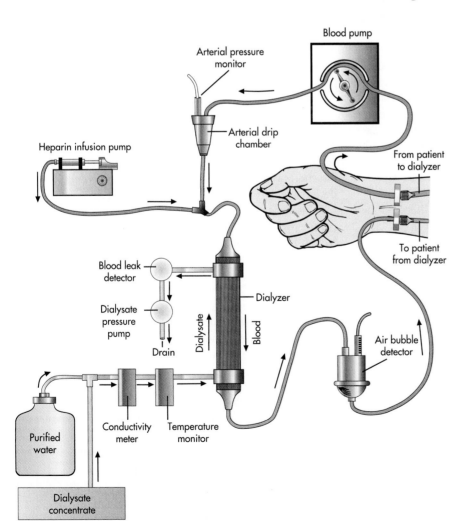

Figure 55-9

Hemodialysis is accomplished by removing blood through vascular access to a machine that cleanses the blood, restores the electrolyte balance, and returns blood to the patient. *Modified from Thelan L, Davie JK, Urden JD: Textbook of Critical Care Nursing: Diagnosis and Management, ed 2, 1994, St. Louis, Mosby-Year Book.*

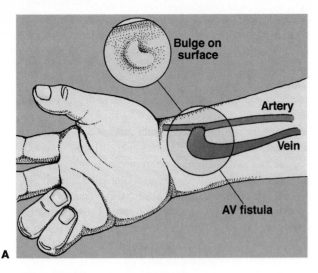

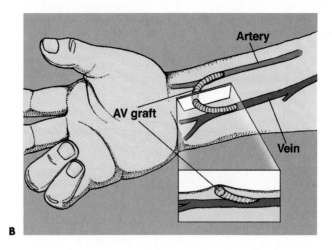

Figure 55-10

A, Arteriovenous fistulas are created when an artery and vein are surgically connected. The high pressure in the arterial side results in a noticeable bulge of the vein. B, An AV graft works along the same lines as an AV fistula, however, the vein is not connected directly to the artery and still functions as a vein by allowing venous return of blood from the extremity.

complications is based on local medical direction and established paramedic protocols, and requires careful patient assessment.

Peritoneal dialysis can also cause hypotension, **hypovolemia,** inadequate fluid drainage from the peritoneal space, pain, respiratory distress, and peritonitis.[18] Hypotension and hypovolemia are most likely a result of rapid removal of fluid from the intravascular space and should be managed according to standard prehospital protocols. IV normal saline is the crystalloid of choice for fluid resuscitation; lactated Ringer's should be avoided in dialysis patients if possible because of the higher concentration of potassium. Caution should be exercised when administering fluids to avoid inadvertently overhydrating the patient. Dialysis patients are at significant risk for developing **congestive heart failure, pulmonary edema,** and **hyperkalemia.**

Dialysate occasionally fails to drain from the peritoneal cavity because the catheter is clogged or the tip is lodged against the abdominal wall. Turning the patient from side to side or gently pressing on the abdomen may alleviate the fluid accumulation. If this does not improve the situation, it may be necessary for a physician to irrigate or replace the catheter.

Mild pain or a "pressure" sensation is often experienced with peritoneal dialysis, but severe pain is not normal. Because pain assessment and management may require a complete medical evaluation, the paramedic should care for the patient symptomatically. Do not overlook other serious causes of pain such as **gastrointestinal bleeding, myocardial infarction,** and **aortic dissection.**

As dialysate is infused, pressure rises in the peritoneal cavity. This may affect the diaphragm and cause respiratory distress. Respiratory distress is further compounded in the patient who is overhydrated. Once again, it is important that the paramedic avoid the assumption that respiratory distress is a "normal" complaint of dialysis; consider the variety of causes of respiratory distress.

Peritonitis is a serious and potentially fatal complication of peritoneal dialysis. Acute peritonitis can cause severe sepsis and a shocklike state in a relatively short period of time. Peritonitis is most often associated with organisms that have been introduced through the catheter itself. Management of the septic patient includes the ABCs, fluid management (preferably with normal saline solution), cardiac monitor, and rapid transport of the patient to definitive care.

Prehospital Use of Dialysis VADs

The decision to use a dialysis access device in the prehospital setting must be carefully assessed and discussed with medical direction prior to the insertion of any needle. A dialysis access device should be the site of last resort. Because of the very high incidence of infection associated with poor technique, the paramedic must be confident that the risks of introducing infection is outweighed by the critical condition of the patient. Thorough assessment, accurate medical history, medical direction, and local protocols must all be considered prior to initiating a "dialysis" IV line. The paramedic should first attempt to establish a peripheral, or external, jugular line. The endotracheal and intraosseous routes for medications should also be considered if appropriate.

Venipuncture of an AV shunt, graft, or fistula requires careful assessment, patience, and a confident approach. Family or home caregivers may be able to provide useful information regarding the type and placement of the device. As with VADs, these people may have limited emergency knowledge but valuable information about dialysis devices. The rescuer should note that a peritoneal dialysis catheter cannot be used for vascular access.

The area should be gently palpated to locate the fistula or graft. A "thrill" or vibration should be felt over a fistula. A synthetic shunt is located outside the skin and is easily visible. Any area that is red, tender, swollen, or draining, or shows other evidence of infection, should not be used.[17] Usually the vein is sufficiently distended, but a tourniquet can be placed proximal to the insertion site if needed.

Strict aseptic technique should be used and the area scrubbed with povidone-iodine for several minutes. Under normal "nonemergency" circumstances, a 10-minute scrub would be completed.[6,17] Alcohol should never be used to prepare the site, especially for external shunts as it will damage synthetic materials. Standard steel or teflon IV catheters may be used. Because of the large diameter of the access site, and the severity of the patient's condition, a 14- or 16-gauge needle should be used. A 16-gauge needle or smaller can be considered for use in children.[6]

The paramedic must be sure to insert the needle in the direction of venous flow (toward the head). The tip of the needle should be inserted a sufficient distance away from the connection (8 to 10 cm) to assist in blood flow and limit thrombosis formation (Fig. 55-11). The site should be stabilized as the paramedic inserts the IV needle. The skin may be approached at a slight angle (15° to 20°) to prevent penetrating the posterior lumen of the vessel. The needle must be directed and the teflon catheter advanced in the same manner as with standard IVs; the paramedic should watch for a "flashback" in the hub. Three to five mL of blood should be aspirated to confirm correct placement as well as clear the shunt of heparin. Grafts and fistulas are not heparinized.

A syringe or vacutainer can be used to obtain the necessary blood samples per local protocol; the tourniquet should be removed if one has been placed. The paramedic should attach the IV tubing and begin the infusion of normal saline or medications. IV tubing must be carefully taped and the infusion site and the patient reassessed (see sidebar). Blood pressure assessments in the shunted extremity should be avoided, because this procedure will disrupt blood flow.

Paramedics should have intensive, hands-on training prior to using either VADs or dialysis devices for access. The decision to use a dialysis access device in the prehospital setting must be made based on sound assessment and knowledge of prehospital protocols. In the critical patient when routine vascular access is not available, AV grafts, fistulas, and shunts can provide rapid and safe vascular access.

Surgical Airways and Mechanical Ventilators

A tracheostomy is a surgical opening through the third or fourth tracheal ring[3] (Fig. 55-12). The surgical opening or stoma may be temporary and sutured closed when no longer needed, or permanent, in which case a tube may be placed to keep the stoma open. Tracheostomies are performed when an endotracheal tube is contraindicated, cannot be passed, or (as is usually the case) when sustained ventilatory support is necessary.[18]

Patients may require a tracheostomy for a variety of reasons, including upper airway obstruction due to trauma, tumors, soft-tissue swelling or a foreign body,[7] and prolonged ventilatory support requiring suctioning of mucus due to profuse mucus production or inability to expectorate secretions.

Types of Tracheostomy Tubes

Modern tracheostomy tubes are constructed of polyvinyl chloride (PVC) or silastic (silicone rubber) (Fig. 55-13). These materials are flexible and comfortable and have few associated risks. Tracheostomy tubes may be of single or double construction. A single tube has a built-in tracheal cuff and an obturator or stylet is used for insertion. A double tube has a similar attached cuff but also has an inner cannula. The inner cannula is designed to be easily removed and cleaned or replaced if necessary to maintain good air exchange.[22] The cuff, similar to that found on an endotracheal tube, is inflated to prevent aspiration of upper airway secretions. Special tracheostomy tubes also exist which have a small opening in the cannula that enables the patient to whisper or talk by moving

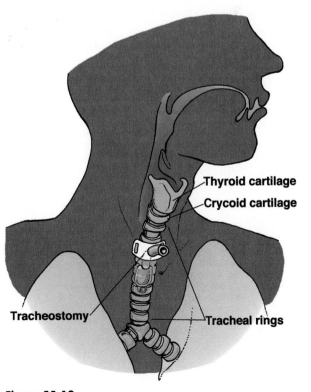

Figure 55-12

A tracheostomy tube placed through the fourth tracheal ring.

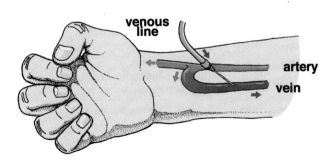

Figure 55-11

If an AV graft, fistula, or shunt is used in an emergency, be sure to angle the catheter toward the head and enter on the venous side.

by Marilyn K. Bourn, RN, MSN, CEN, NREMT-P

Formal instruction in the following procedure and supervised practice are required before attempting it in the field. This procedure should only be used as a last resort. It should adhere to local protocols and be performed under supervision of medical direction.

1. Complete the primary survey on the patient and manage the ABCs.
2. Obtain pertinent medical history if possible and any information available regarding the type of dialysis device.
3. Attempt peripheral, external jugular, or intraosseous access as per local protocol.
4. Identify the location and type of dialysis access device (graft, fistula, or shunt).
5. Assess the site for redness, tenderness, swelling, or drainage.
6. Use knowledgeable family members, home caregiver or others, if possible.
7. If additional distension of the vein is needed, apply a tourniquet.
8. Use strict aseptic technique. Briskly scrub the areas with several povidone-iodine pads. Do not use alcohol, especially with shunts.
9. Select a 14 to 16 g needle.
10. Insert the needle at a 15° to 20° angle. Watch for a flashback. Aspirate slowly to confirm blood return and remove heparin from the shunt. Obtain blood samples if necessary.
11. Attach IV tubing and secure the tubing.
12. Reassess the infusion site and patient condition.

From Gutch CF, et al: *Review of hemodialysis for nurses and dialysis personnel*, ed 4, St. Louis, 1983, CV Mosby; Nissenson AR, Fine RN, (eds): *Dialysis therapy*, Philadelphia, 1986, Hanley & Belfus.

---

air through the larynx. Once the tracheostomy tube has been inserted, it may be sutured into place or secured with soft cloth ties.

Tracheostomy Complications and Emergencies

Three common complications that EMS personnel may encounter with tracheostomy patients are obstruction, dislodgement, and infection. Some others, such as hemorrhage, subcutaneous emphysema, and mediastinal emphysema, often occur within the first 24 hours. Patients experiencing these problems are usually found in the hospital, where immediate medical and surgical intervention are available. They are less frequently seen in the field (Table 55-2). Management of tracheostomy complications and emergencies is based on good assessment and the skills necessary to maintain an open airway and adequate oxygen exchange.

Despite the placement of a definitive surgical airway, patients may experience acute respiratory distress caused by an obstruction of the tube from excessive secretions, accumulated dry secretions (encrustations), pressure on the tube from foreign bodies, or airway edema.[3] When mucus obstructs a double tube, the inner cannula should be removed and rinsed with sterile water or saline. The inner cannula can also be left in

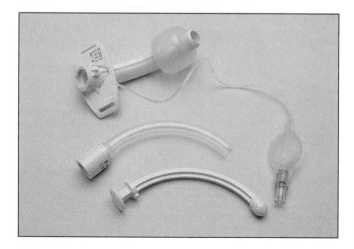

Figure 55-13

Tracheostomy tubes.

TABLE 55-2	Complications and Emergencies Associated with Tracheostomies
Complication	**Signs/Symptoms**
Respiratory distress	Shortness of breath
	Dyspnea
	Stridor
	Congestion
	Panic
Site infection	Ecchymosis
	Swelling
	Drainage
Sepsis	Elevated temperature
	Dyspnea
	Tachycardia
	Hypotension
Stenosis	Dyspnea
	Stridor
	Recurring respiratory infections
Necrosis	Infection
	Bright red bleeding
Fistula	Gastric aspiration
Subcutaneous/mediastinal emphysema	Shortness of breath
	Crepitus
	"Puffy" tissues

Adapted from Masoorli S, Angeles T: PICC lines: The latest home care challenge, *RN* 1:44–50, 1990; Phipps WJ, et al: *Medical-surgical nursing: Concepts and clinical practice*, ed 4, St. Louis, 1991, Mosby-Year Book; Thelan LA, Davie JK, Urden LK (eds): *Textbook of critical care nursing: Diagnosis and management*, St. Louis, 1991, CV Mosby.

place and cleaned of mucus with suction. Instillation of 3 to 5 mL of saline solution may help loosen mucus and allow for greater clearance during suctioning. However, this practice is controversial and depends on local protocols.

If the airway remains obstructed, it may be necessary to remove the tracheostomy tube and replace it with an endotracheal tube. This is a risky procedure that requires careful assessment and preparation, as well as medical direction. To remove the tube, the paramedic should untie the cloth tape or cut the sutures. If sterile straight or curved hemostats are available, the unclamped tip can be placed very carefully just inside the stoma next to the tube. These may be used to help keep the stoma open once the tube has been removed. The cuff can be deflated using a syringe and the tube gently removed. The paramedic should immediately insert a sterile endotracheal tube. A tube size should be chosen that will pass easily through the stoma and allow for easy suctioning and adequate ventilation. To avoid placing the endotracheal tube into the right mainstem bronchus, the rescuer should insert the tube only approximately 3 to 4 cm into the stoma. The patient can then be reoxygenated, checked for breath sounds, and reassessed shortly.

As with any invasive or surgical procedure, infection is a common complication. The stoma itself may become infected, leading to redness, swelling, exudate (pus), and temperature elevation. If the infectious organisms are introduced into the tracheal tree through suctioning, pulmonary infections, and sepsis may develop. Aseptic technique and good wound care reduce the risk of infection.

Tracheal stenosis is a narrowing of the trachea at the site of the cuff. This narrowing may develop from a week to years after the tracheostomy tube has been inserted.[3,22] Because of the reduced diameter of the trachea, the patient may complain of dyspnea, stridor, decreased exercise tolerance, and recurring respiratory infections.[22] Another complication associated with the cuff is tracheal necrosis. Tracheal necrosis may occur as early as 3 to 5 days after insertion of the tube. In some cases, the necrosis extends through the posterior wall of the trachea, causing a fistula (opening) to develop between the trachea and esophagus. This fistula allows air to escape into the stomach; oral and gastric secretions can also be aspirated into the lungs. The patient may experience dyspnea, stridor, and evidence of aspiration pneumonia. Because diagnosis of tracheal stenosis in the field is impossible, the paramedic should manage the patient according to the chief complaint, signs, and symptoms. The necrosis may also cause erosion through the anterior wall of the trachea and into the innominate artery. In this rare condition, the tube may pulsate and show bright red blood. If suction is not adequate enough to keep the tube clear, the paramedic should consider inserting a slightly smaller endotracheal tube through the tracheostomy tube, until the tip is just above the carina. If external bleeding is noted, an absorbitive dressing can be used and gentle direct pressure applied to the bleeding site. The paramedic must take caution not to occlude the airway or carotid arteries.

Although they are rare and usually immediate, complications such as subcutaneous and mediastinal emphysema may occur at any time. They are usually associated with displacement of the tube and leakage of air into surrounding tissues.

The patient may experience mild to severe respiratory distress. The area appears puffy and palpation reveals a crackling sensation or crepitus.[22] The patient will require supplemental oxygen and respiratory support. Monitor carefully; positive pressure ventilation may increase the extent of the air leak.

Mechanical Ventilators

In the past, mechanical ventilators were available only in the intensive care unit. Today however, several small and versatile ventilators are designed for home use (Fig. 55-14). Mechanical ventilators are classified according to preset parameters and the mechanism of the inspiratory phase (volume-cycled, pressure-cycled, and time-cycled).[14] These types of ventilators are typically used for home patients who are unable to maintain spontaneous respirations for any length of time. Consequently, back-up ventilator support is imperative (e.g., bag-valve-mask). The family or home caregiver may be familiar with the ventilator, but the onset of respiratory distress, or ventilator malfunctions or alarms, can cause concern. The paramedic may be called because of actual or potential loss of ventilator support. Because it is impossible to know the specific details of each ventilator, it is also impractical for the paramedic to troubleshoot the alarms or adjust settings. The patient should be treated, not the alarms. The ventilator should be disconnected from the tracheostomy tube, with the patient immediately ventilated with a bag-valve attached to the tracheostomy tube. If possible, an amount of oxygen similar to what the ventilator was providing should be administered. If the amount is unknown or the patient's status is questionable, clinical signs such as respiratory distress, skin color, and pulse oximetry measurements can be used to guide treatment.

Enteral Feedings

Adequate nutrition depends on the ability to swallow and absorb nutrients. Major gastrointestinal diseases, fistulas, trauma, burns, and side effects from radiation therapy may compromise the ability of the patient's gastrointestinal tract to digest nutrients. In some cases, total parenteral nutrition (TPN) is given through a vascular access device. For other patients who

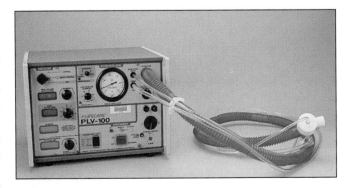

Figure 55-14

Portable ventilators are used by many advanced or critical care transport ALS units.

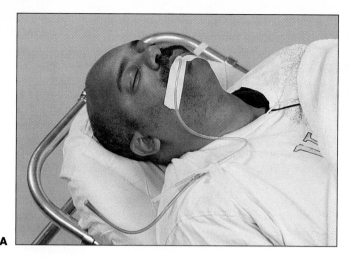 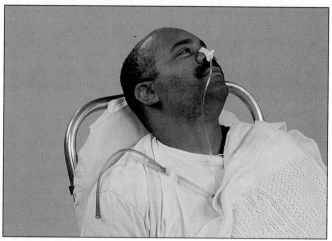

A   **B**

Figure 55-15

Gastric tubes are inserted through the A) mouth or B) nose and allow direct access to the stomach for feeding or suctioning. They are also used in emergencies for evacuation of poisons from the GI tract to "pump the stomach."

have healthy gastrointestinal systems but are unable to swallow because of difficulty swallowing (dysphagia) paralysis or unresponsiveness, enteral feedings (via the intestines) are provided.[18] There are various methods of giving enteral nutrition on a long-term basis.

Gastric Tubes

Gastric, or feeding tubes, are small polyurethane or silicone tubes that are inserted through the nose or mouth into the stomach (Fig. 55-15). Orogastric and nasogastric tubes are used to provide liquid feeding and are particularly useful in premature infants. However, patient discomfort and irritation of nasal and mucous membranes limit the long-term effectiveness of gastric feedings. When prolonged or permanent enteral nutrition is needed, a gastrostomy is performed.

Gastrostomy

Using local or general anesthesia, a surgeon makes an opening in the abdominal wall and inserts a special gastrostomy catheter through the wall into the stomach. The gastric tube extends approximately 12 to 15 inches from the skin and is sutured in place (Fig. 55-16). However, the extension of the external catheter presents problems to active patients. The protruding catheter may become tangled in clothing, is not aesthetically pleasing, and can interfere with sexual activity.[21] Consequently, the "button" device was developed, which provides a skin-level gastrostomy and eliminates the cumbersome external catheter. The button allows for attachment of a safety cap after removing the feeding tube.[10]

Enteral Feeding Complications and Emergencies

Complications associated with enteral tubes rarely require emergency medical care, but family members or others may

panic and call 9-1-1. Complications include pulmonary aspiration of formula, dehydration, nausea, diarrhea, bacterial contamination, electrolyte imbalance, and tube displacement.[1,18] If the tube has been displaced and bleeding is present, direct pressure with a sterile dressing should be applied. Transport of the patient may be necessary if careful assessment proves any of these complications to present danger.

Ventricular Shunts

Excess accumulation of cerebral spinal fluid (CSF) in the brain causes a condition known as hydrocephalus. This leads to increased intracranial pressure (ICP) and potentially serious brain damage. Drainage systems known as shunts are used to remove the excess fluid.

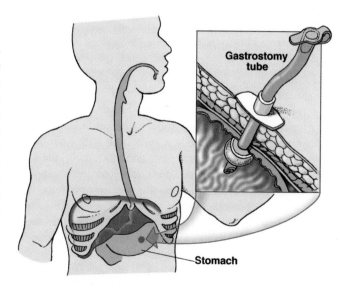

Figure 55-16

A gastrostomy tube offers long-term access to the stomach.

The shunt consists of a primary catheter, a reservoir, a one-way valve, and the terminal (drainage) catheter. The primary catheter is surgically implanted into the lateral ventricle of the brain. The reservoir collects the fluid and the one-way valve prevents the CSF from flowing back into the ventricle. The reservoir of a shunt can often be easily palpated through the skin, usually over the mastoid or parietal bone, just behind the ear. The terminal end of the catheter empties into the jugular vein or peritoneal cavity (Fig. 55-17).

Ventricular Shunt Complications and Emergencies

Despite the simple design of a ventricular shunt, complications can occur. The most common include:

- plugging of the catheter with clotted blood or other thickened fluid
- displacement of the primary or terminal end
- a break or dislodgement of one or more components
- infection[9]

With the exception of infection, these complications cause CSF to build up within the ventricle, thus increasing ICP. Early signs of increasing ICP may include headaches, nausea, vomiting, irritability, and visual disturbances. As the ICP continues to rise, the late but classical signs of increased ICP become evident: rising systolic blood pressure, abnormal respirations, and profound bradycardia. These three signs are known together as Cushing's triad.[9]

Increasing ICP is a true medical emergency and requires rapid intervention to prevent brain stem herniation. The patient's airway should be managed and high-flow oxygen administered. If possible, the paramedic should place an endotracheal tube and hyperventilate the patient. Venous access should be established, but the amount of fluid infused must be carefully limited.

Shunts that are plugged may be "pumped" in an effort to flush the system and restore function. The paramedic can locate the reservoir with gentle palpation. Using one or two fingers, the rescuer should gently compress and release the reservoir several times. This procedure should be performed in conference with medical direction and according to established protocols. Pumping the reservoir may provide only minimal or temporary relief and should not delay airway management and rapid transport to definitive care.

Automatic Implantable Cardioverter Defibrillators

Each year, more than 300,000 people die from sudden cardiac death (SCD).[8] Of those patients who receive immediate resuscitation and survive cardiac arrest, as many as 50% will experience a second cardiac arrest within 2 years. The development of the automatic implantable cardioverter defibrillator (AICD) has successfully reduced the number of deaths in high-risk patients with recurrent ventricular tachycardia or ventricular fibrillation. Since the implantation of the first AICD in 1980, more than 14,000 units have been implanted in patients in the United States.[8]

Mechanism of Action

The AICD is an electronic device used in patients who are at high risk for SCD from frequent and recurrent **ventricular tachycardia** (VT) or **ventricular fibrillation** (VF).[8] The AICD consists of a pulse generator, sensing electrodes, and two large patches. The generator is usually surgically implanted in the periumbilical area of the abdomen with the electrodes tunneled under the rib margin to the epicardium. The patches are placed on the outside of the pericardial sac or sewn to the epicardium. The generator may be seen or palpated under the surface of the skin (Fig. 55-18). The parameters are set so the device will discharge when the ventricular rate is greater than the programmed rate (e.g., >170 beats/min) for 10 to 30 seconds. The shock is usually set at 25 to 30 joules, given four times within a 2-minute period. Once sinus rhythm is restored, the device can recycle and deliver an additional four shocks within 35 seconds if VT or VF recurs.[11]

AICD Complications and Emergencies

AICDs are placed under sterile surgical conditions in the operating suite. After the generator has been implanted, the patient is monitored for several days in the intensive care unit. Consequently, problems that do develop occur most often in the in-patient setting. After discharge from the hospital, the most common problems that patients encounter are failure of

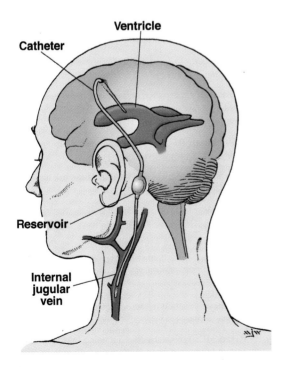

Figure 55-17

A ventricular shunt, placed into the left ventricle here, allows for drainage of excess CSF that is formed within the ventricle. The excess fluid is deposited directly into the jugular vein.

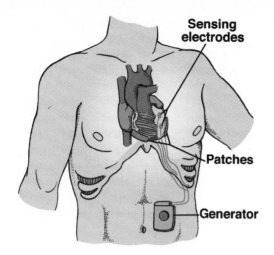

Sensing electrodes

Patches

Generator

Figure 55-18

The generator of the AICD is generally placed in the abdomen and the electrodes are attached to the heart. The generator is visible or palpable under the skin.

the AICD to fire when it should and the device discharging inappropriately.

The generator may fail to fire if it has lost stored energy or battery power. If the sensing electrodes are damaged, disconnected, or displaced, the generator will not fire. Finally, if the maximum rate is not set correctly, the generator may not discharge despite evidence of VT or VF.

Occasionally, the AICD will fire when no discharge is indicated. Unnecessary discharging of the AICD causes patient discomfort and early battery depletion.[4] However, the chance that the discharge may cause an R-on-T phenomenon and actually cause VT or VF is a much greater concern. This may happen if the leads sense a supraventricular rhythm faster than the prescribed parameter. Because these rhythms usually do not cause unresponsiveness, the patient may complain of feeling the "jolt" of the discharge. The AICD may also deliver countershocks because of certain upper-extremity movements or for no apparent reason.[4] In this case, the patient will require continuous monitoring to determine the cause of the frequent discharges.

Prehospital Management of AICD Emergencies

Prehospital management of patients with AICDs follows dysrhythmia protocols similar to those for patients without AICDs. The patient who has received an effective countershock will be in some type of perfusing rhythm and may complain of chest pain, shortness of breath, and anxiety, or be totally asymptomatic.

In addition to responding to a patient after a successful countershock, the paramedic may encounter the patient with unsuccessful countershock. The patient may be in VT, VF, bradycardia, asystole, or pulseless electrical activity. In these cases, the patient should be managed according to standard ACLS protocols. Presence of an AICD is not a contraindication for standard external countershock. Because the patient has already received one or more internal counter-

shocks, initial external shocks should be delivered at the maximum output. The external paddles should not be placed directly over the generator, because this may cause permanent damage to the device. If the first and second countershocks are unsuccessful, consider using anterior-posterior placement of the defibrillator patches or paddles.[11]

The AICD may discharge when paramedics are treating the patient. There is concern for the paramedic that contact with the patient while an internal shock is delivered may pose a hazard. Studies indicate that only approximately 2 joules of energy reach the surface of the body. Although this may cause a minor shock, there is no significant danger of physical harm. This danger can also be avoided if the paramedic wears rubber gloves, which should be standard practice anyway.

SUMMARY

Therapies such as vascular access devices, dialysis access devices, tracheostomy tubes, enteral feeding tubes, ventricular shunts, and implanted defibrillators are being used with increasing frequency. These adjuncts are relatively simple to use and are a valuable resource to prehospital care. The paramedic who understands their basic mechanisms of action, associated complications, and prehospital management will be better prepared to provide optimal patient care under critical circumstances.

REFERENCES

1. **Beare PG, Myers JL:** *Principles and practice of adult health nursing,* St. Louis, 1990, CV Mosby.

2. **Bjeletich J:** De-clotting central venous catheters with urokinase in the home by nurse clinicians. *NITA* 6:428–430, 1987.

3. **Burrell LO:** *Adult nursing in hospital and community settings,* Norwalk, 1992, Appleton & Lange.

4. **Craig SA, Hudson AD:** Emergency department management of patients with automatic implantable cardioverter-defibrillators. *Ann Emerg Med* 19(4), 1990.

5. **Goodman MS, Wickham R:** Venous access devices: An overview. *Oncol Nurs Forum* 11(5):16–23, 1984.

6. **Gutch CF, Stoner MH:** *Review of hemodialysis for nurses and dialysis personnel,* ed 4, St. Louis, 1983, CV Mosby.

7. **Handy CM:** Vascular access devices: hospital to home care. *J Interven Nurs* 12(1 suppl):S10–S18, 1989.

8. **Handelsman H:** Implantation of automatic cardioverter-defibrillator: Noninducibility of ventricular tachyarrhythmia as a patient selection criterion. 10, *AHCPR Health Technology Assessment Reports,* 1990.

9. **Hickey JV:** *The clinical practice of neurological and neurosurgical nursing,* ed 2, Philadelphia, 1986, JB Lippincott.

10. **Huth MM, O'Brien ME:** The gastrostomy feeding button. *Pediatr Nurs* 13(4), 1987.

11. **Iversen WR, Hartman JR, Foy BK, Stamato NJ:** AICDs spark hope for cardiac care. *JEMS* 14(9):37–41, 1989.

12. **Keating SB, Kelman GB:** *Home health nursing,* Philadelphia, 1988, JB Lippincott.

13. **Marcoux C, Fisher S, Wong D:** Central venous access devices in children, *Pediatr Nurs* 16(2):123–132, 1990.

14. **Masoorli S, Angeles T:** PICC lines: The latest home care challenge. *RN* 1:44–50, 1990.

15. **McAfee T, Garland LR, McNabb TS:** How to safely draw blood from a vascular access device. *Nursing* 11:42–43, 1990.

16. **McEvoy MT:** Vascular access devices. *JEMS* 17(5):39–50, 1992.

17. **Nissenson AR, Fine RN (eds):** *Dialysis therapy*, Philadelphia, 1986, Hanley & Belfus.

18. **Phipps WJ, Long BC, Woods NF, Cassmeyer VL:** *Medical-surgical nursing: Concepts and clinical practice*, ed 4, St. Louis, 1991, Mosby–Year Book.

19. **Rice R:** *Home health nursing practice: Concepts and applications,* St. Louis, 1992, Mosby–Year Book.

20. **Roundtree D:** The PIC catheter: A different approach. *Am J Nurs* 22–26, 1991.

21. **Shike M, Wallach C, Gerdes H, Herman-Zaidins M:** Skin-level gastrostomies and jejunostomies for long-term enteral feeding. *JPEN* 13(6), 1989.

22. **Thelan LA, Davie JK, Urden LD (eds):** *Textbook of critical care nursing: Diagnosis and management,* St. Louis, 1991, CV Mosby.

23. **Viall CD:** Your complete guide to catheters. *Nursing* 2:34–41, 1990.

24. **Wickham RS:** Advances in venous access devices and nursing management strategies. *Nurs Clin North Am* 25(2):345–363, 1990.

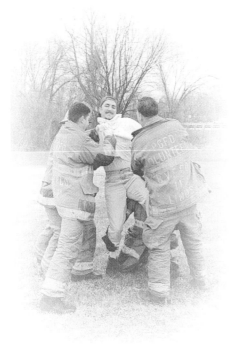

1. **Abuse**—the intentional infliction of physical or mental injury.
2. **Domestic**—regarding the home or family.
3. **Impulsive**—to act before or without thinking.
4. **Neglect**—to fail to care for or attend to properly; habitual lack of care.
5. **Sexual Assault**—an act of violence in which the victim is threatened and/or attacked and forced into unwanted sexual contact.
6. **Violence**—any verbal or physical threat or act of force against another person or group of people that places them in danger, causes harm, or produces death; any act that leaves a person feeling threatened or in jeopardy.

A paramedic should be able to:

OBJECTIVES

1. Describe the management of violent patients.
2. Describe the indications and appropriate use of restraints.
3. Explain the psychosocial factors and psychological characteristics of child, adult, and elderly abusers.
4. Describe the physical signs and management of common injuries resulting from child, adult, and elderly abuse.
5. Identify typical responses that are demonstrated by the victims of child, adult, and elderly abuse.
6. Describe and demonstrate appropriate interpersonal skills in dealing with victims or perpetrators of personal violence.
7. Describe how to care for the victim and preserve evidence in cases of sexual assault.
8. Describe the medical and legal reporting requirements of child, adult, and elderly abuse, including proper record documentation.

lssues involved in dealing with victims and suspected perpetrators of violent crimes.

- Hypoglycemia
- Hypoxia
- Ketoacidosis
- Liver failure
- Renal disease
- Severe hypertension
- Temporal lobe seizures

Recognizing Violent Behavior

When dealing with victims of violence, paramedics must be aware of potential risks so that they do not become victims themselves. If the paramedic feels unsafe in someone's presence, that person must be treated with extreme caution.[28] In fact, intuitive feelings about a potential threat can be as valid as the physical reality.[20]

With potentially violent persons, one should be concerned about impulse control, the effect of mind-altering drugs, and other medical conditions that would diminish cerebral function and control.[4] (Box 56-1)

The main perpetrators of violence today are young males. Their violent behavior is often a manifestation of feelings of anger, guilt, agitation, helplessness, and hopelessness. A threatening mannerism, a loud and forceful voice, confusion and delirium, and anxious pacing can forewarn the paramedic of violent behavior. Other clues to potential violence include drug-induced behavior, brandishing a weapon and threatening to injure or kill others with it, agitated behavior, knocking over furniture, and pounding on walls.[24]

Violent people may exhibit abnormal vital signs and excessive sweating. They may have toxic, metabolic, cardiopulmonary, or infectious disease producing their agitated and violent behavior. Such people should be restrained with a "sufficient show of force" and be immediately evaluated. Seizures, shock, hypoxia, and hypoglycemia should be considered and then appropriately treated in the field.[24]

C R I T I C A L I S S U E

Remember to consider the medical causes of altered mental status and combative behavior. Examples include hypoglycemia, hypoxia, drug ingestion, or intracranial bleeding.

Managing Violent Behavior

The situations to which a paramedic might be called involving personal violence are variable. Violence can be directed toward children, adults, and the elderly. Potentially threatening situations include those involving psychiatric patients, shooting victims, stabbing victims, armed patients, armed bystanders, and crowd tension in riot conditions (See also Chapter 45).

Frequently, paramedics are the first to arrive at a violent scene. Scene safety must be established first by police (See also Chapter 15). Paramedics are often sent to scenes of violence where the perpetrator is still present. In such cases, the potential for injury must be decreased. Never approach a dangerous person alone. Call for police protection before entering the scene. Police should quickly determine if the violent person is carrying a weapon and be on the scene so there is sufficient force to subdue the person if necessary.

When sufficient force is available, paramedics should establish their role as authority figures and maintain an attitude of active listening. The violent person should be told patiently, firmly, and with respect: "I want to help you, but you must sit down and then I'll do what I can to help you." Paramedics should be careful not to argue with violent people. Verbal conversation should immediately cease if the person becomes more threatening or if one's feelings of discomfort increase.[9]

Never let a threatening person block an exit. A means of escape should always be available to the paramedic in the event that a patient becomes violent.

Paramedics should have regular training in the management of assaultive behavior to help defend themselves. Offensive tactics learned in police training are generally not appropriate for paramedics.[28]

If it is necessary to subdue a violent person, assign one person to control each limb by grasping at clothing and large joints, such as the knees, ankles, or elbows (Fig. 56-1). The violent person should be placed on a stretcher and secured to reduce leverage and make it difficult for the person to lash out. Secure the trunk at the bony prominences (e.g. pelvis, shoulders and the extremities, proximal to the joints) (Fig. 56-2). Shoes and boots should be removed once the patient is restrained. Under no circumstances should pressure be applied to the chest, the throat, or the neck.

C R I T I C A L I S S U E

When restraining a patient, be sure adequate help is available. Utilize the assistance of local law enforcement officials if available.

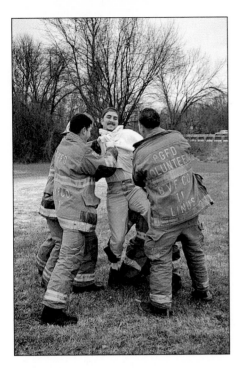

Figure 56-1

When force is necessary to subdue violent patients, use one provider to pin each limb.

Prior to applying restraints, the paramedic should ensure that one of the following conditions applies:

1. A patient has a medical or psychiatric condition that requires immediate transport and the patient is demonstrating behavior that may harm himself or others.
2. A serious medical condition exists that may threaten the patient's life by a delay in treatment or transport and there is no reasonable way to obtain consent to provide treatment or accept an informed refusal of care.
3. Paramedics are directed by appropriate authorities to transport a patient on the basis of a mental health hold or being in police custody.

Humane use of hard restraints for drug-induced violence and soft restraints for the demented or the elderly may be appropriate. Typically, gauze restraints or Velcro restraint devices are appropriate for prehospital use. Hard restraints such as handcuffs or flex-cuffs should be applied by law enforcement officials only; when utilized, a law enforcement officer should accompany the patient to the hospital so that the restraints can be removed if necessary to allow for medical care.

The goal is to restrain, not to injure. Restraining ties should be adequate but not painfully constricting when applied. A towel or sheet applied on the limbs and across the abdomen can be an additional method of restraint. Be sure to check that these restraints do not inhibit the patient's respirations. Usually, all four limbs are secured to the stretcher.

CRITICAL ISSUE

Intoxicated patients are particularly prone to aspiration, especially if they are being transported in the supine position.

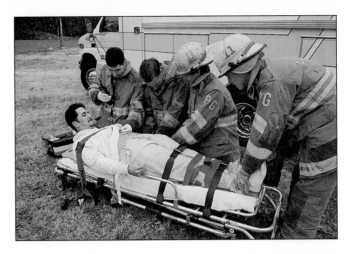

Figure 56-2

Secure patients at the bony prominence to minimize their movement.

One can also consider wrapping agitated people in a blanket. All restraint situations should be fully documented for medical-legal review. After being restrained, violent persons should be examined for trauma. Occasionally, patients can sustain **myocardial infarctions** or fractures during restraint.[21]

An alternative to physical restraint is chemical restraint of the patient with a medication such as droperidol. One study prospectively examined the use of droperidol in the prehospital setting and found significantly reduced agitation levels at 5 and 10 minutes after administration when compared to a placebo.[22] There were no significant side effect nor alteration of vital signs noted in response to the 5mg dose.

The same indications exist for chemical restraint as for physical restraint. Droperidol can be administered intravenously or intramuscularly. It should be avoided in those patients with hypotension or respiratory depression. Dystonic reactions presenting as spasm of facial and neck muscles may be noted within hours of treatment, but can be easily reversed by administering diphenhydramine.

Transport of violent patients should be performed with continuous monitoring for complications such as respiratory distress and the risk of aspiration. An EMS agency's destination policy should reflect the special needs of the violent patient in terms of facilities and personnel.

A problematic issue that can arise for paramedics when handling violent crimes is the "duty to protect" (often called "duty to warn") a potential victim. Specific threats made against another party to paramedics or other individuals must be seriously considered. If the person escapes, both police and the intended victim must be notified as soon as time permits.[32]

Child Abuse

Management of child abuse in the field requires a keen awareness of its manifestations. The Child Abuse Prevention and Treatment Act of 1974 defines child abuse as "the physical and mental injury, sexual abuse, negligent treatment, or maltreatment of a child under the age of 18 by a person who is responsible for the child's welfare."[8] Victims of child abuse may suffer injury from direct actions or through a lack of responsible care. Child abuse includes gross as well as subtle forms of physical injury, neglect, emotional trauma, and sexual exploitation.[13]

At least 1 million children are maltreated each year in the United States. At least 400,000 are sexually abused, and from 200,000 to 300,000 are psychologically abused.[7] For each child abuse case reported, there are approximately 50 others that are not detected or reported. More than 80% of all cases occur in children under 3 years of age, with more than 50% of these cases involving children less than 6 months of age.[29]

One of the most important grounds for suspecting child abuse is the child's own testimony. Child abuse must be reported when a child tells another person that he or she has been abused. Such communication is not privileged. The police, Child Protective Services, and hospital personnel should be used as a support network in these instances.

Psychosocial Contributions

While the socioeconomically disadvantaged demonstrate a greater incidence of child abuse due to an increased number of life crises and limited resources to deal with them, it occurs among the socioeconomically advantaged as well. Typically, abusive parents are poorly equipped to deal with life crises when they occur and have difficulty reaching out for help. Episodes of abuse are usually triggered by a crisis situation such as financial problems, unemployment, family arguments, eviction, personal loss, and illness.[11]

Other factors increasing the risk of abuse include the presence of drug or alcohol abuse in the family, chronically ill children, single parent family or families in which a parent is absent for a long period of time, and social and geographic mobility that produces isolation from friends, family, and social contacts.[4,11]

Psychological Characteristics

Three major factors have been identified as being the impetus for child abuse: "the right parent, the right child, and the right day."[10]

Parents who abuse their children were often victims of abuse themselves. As children, they were frequently rejected and their needs were not met. They developed no basis for trust in others. As adults, they often look upon their own child as an instrument for controlling their own needs. When a child inevitably fails to fulfill parental expectations, the parent sees this as a betrayal and becomes angry, resorting to impulsive acts of punishment.[11]

Abusive parents or caretakers typically delay or fail to seek care for their child. When exposed, abused children and abusive parents or caretakers attempt to hide injuries.

Abused children are often unwanted, the result of accidental pregnancies and illegitimate births, the opposite sex from that which the parent desired, born during a period of crisis, or the product of a former relationship. Children who are abused tend to be excessively passive, compliant, or fearful, or at the other extreme, excessively aggressive or physically violent. They are often difficult to manage because they demonstrate fussy behavior, abnormal sleep patterns, excessive crying, retardation, hyperactivity, behavioral disorders, or poor eating habits, or have handicaps and chronic diseases.[31] Children who have been abused may have also experienced poor bonding with their mother due to prematurity or lengthy separation from their mother because of illness.

Physical Signs

The instrument chosen to injure a child may depend on what is available when the parent decides to discipline or loses control. One study of children treated in a child abuse program found them to have been injured in the following manners, in decreasing order of frequency:[14]

- belt or strap
- hand open (choked, grabbed, pinched, or slapped)
- fist-propelled (thrown, dropped, pushed, pulled, or dragged)
- hit by a household object
- shot with gun or dunked in ice or hot water
- switch or stick
- paddle or board
- cord
- hot liquid
- foot
- grid of heater or stove
- cigarette
- shoe
- knife
- mouth
- shaking
- iron

All areas of the body were used as targets for the cases reported. The buttocks, back, genitals, and face were found to be the most common sites for abusive injury. The frequency of injury to the head and face, which totaled about 28%, is of special concern. Injuries to the brain, although constituting only 1% of the primary injuries, account for a disproportionate number of deaths from child abuse.[12]

Linear bruise marks, strap marks, or loop marks going around the curved body surface are almost always evidence of abuse.[2] Bruising often appears in a characteristic pattern or as an imprint of the object used. Figure 56-3 shows various types of evidence of abuse.

The location of a burn and its characteristics (i.e., shape, depth, margins, etc.) can also indicate child abuse. Burns without some evidence of withdrawal are highly suspect because a child will usually try to escape, resulting in splashes, uneven burns, or burns on the hands. Scalding a child with hot liquid is the most common burn abuse. In most cases, younger children are scalded by immersion and older children by having liquid thrown or poured on them. When an abused child is forcibly held in hot water, there are often sharply demarcated burns. If the extremities are forcibly immersed in hot water, burns resembling gloves or socks to the hands and the feet may result. "Zebra" burns are also indicative of child abuse. Such burns result when a child is held by his or her hands and legs under a running hot faucet. Another characteristic type of burn abuse is

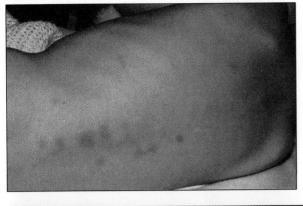

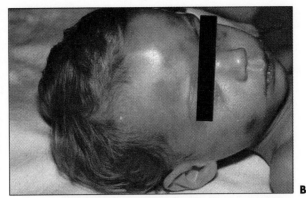

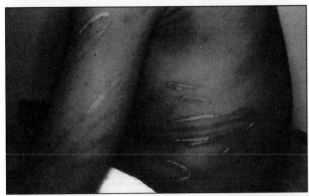

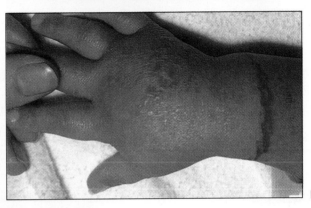

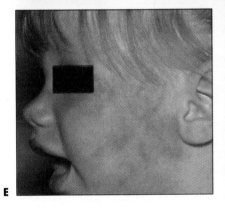

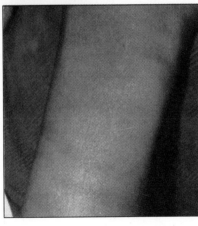

Figure 56-3

Evidence of child abuse:

A) bruising on body parts not normally bruised
B) bruising on the face
C) injuries inflicted by cords
D) injuries due to use of restraints
E) individual imprints of fingers on child's face from being slapped
F) linear contusions characteristic of child abuse

From Zitelli, Davis: Atlas of Pediatric Physical Diagnosis, ed. 2, 1992, Gower Medical Publishing.

the shape of a recognizable object evenly burned into the victim's skin. This is most commonly done with a cigarette on multiple areas, usually on the palms or soles.[25] Figure 56-4 shows various burn injuries resulting from child abuse.

Bite marks can be made on any part of the body and are usually described as doughnut- or double horseshoe-shaped. The uniqueness of the human dentation allows evidence of bite marks to be admissible in the courts of many states. Time is of the essence when recording bite marks, as they become less distinct with time. Marks should be immediately photographed by law enforcement officers and repeated daily for as long as one week.[29]

It is estimated that approximately 20% of abused children exhibit skeletal injuries.[14] The hallmark of skeletal injuries caused by abuse is multiple locations in different stages of healing, suggesting repeated assaults. Joint dislocation requires a considerable degree of force and is an uncommon accident in small children. Shaken-baby syndrome, seen frequently in in-

fants, results from holding and violently shaking the child. Hyperflexion and avulsion fractures of the thorax and lumbar vertebrae are often the result of this syndrome. "Spiral" fractures of long bones of the extremities (Fig. 56-5), which result from twisting forces, are almost always caused by abuse when they occur before a child developmentally begins to walk.[17]

CRITICAL ISSUE

The diagnosis of abuse begins with acknowledging those situations in which historical information does not match the facts evident on physical examination.

Falls from windows or fire escapes result in injuries to the proximal extremities: pelvis, thorax, and abdomen.[2] It is unusual for an infant to fall out of a bed and sustain a fracture or any permanent central nervous system injury. The force required to fracture an infant's bones (unless the impact is

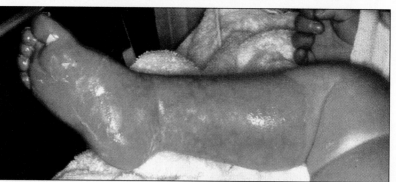

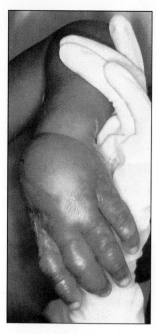

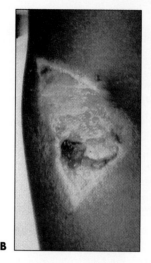

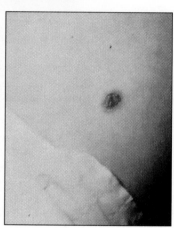

A1

A2

B

C

Figure 56-4

Burn injuries from maltreatment:
A) burns from dipping into hot liquid
B) burn from a hot iron
C) cigarette burns

From Zitelli, Davis: Atlas of Pediatric Physical Diagnosis, ed. 2, 1992, Gower Medical Publishing.

limited to a small anatomic area) must be equivalent to a fall of more than 36 inches.

Significant intracranial injury can be produced by shaking or by a blow to the head.[12] Intracranial hemorrhage associated with "shaken-baby syndrome" carries about a 15% mortality rate, and 50% of the survivors show evidence of significant neurological damage. Fractures of the skull caused by abuse tend to be multiple, bilateral, complex, and depressed.[7]

Blunt blows to the body can cause serious internal injuries to a child's liver, spleen, pancreas, kidney, and other vital organs and may occasionally produce shock and result in death. Intra-abdominal injuries rank second to neurologic injuries as the leading cause of death in abused children.[17]

Physical Neglect

In addition to recognizing physical evidence of injury to abused children, paramedics must know the signs and symptoms of physical neglect. Neglect is essentially maltreatment of a child by a parent or a caretaker. This neglect can be classified as either severe or general. Severe neglect means that the negligence has caused severe malnutrition and organ failure. This includes the intentional failure to provide adequate food, clothing, shelter, or medical care. General neglect means that the parent or caretaker has failed to provide adequate food, clothing, shelter, medical care, and supervision, but no physical injury to the child has resulted.

Physical neglect should be suspected in the following conditions:

- the child appears to be sleepy and hungry
- the child is dirty, demonstrates poor personal hygiene, or is inadequately dressed for weather conditions

- there is evidence of poor child supervision, reflected by repeated falls down stairs, repeated ingestion of harmful substances, supervision only by another child, or no supervision at all
- the home is seen as unsanitary (with garbage, animal or human excrement present)
- the home lacks heat and plumbing or has many fire hazards
- the sleeping arrangements are cold, dirty, or inadequate.[14]

Extreme neglect means that the home is unfit, justifying protective custody for the children under state child welfare laws.

Sexual Abuse

Unfortunately, child abuse also involves sexual abuse. This is often a difficult problem to uncover because it is not frequently reported by a third party. Like the physically abused child, the sexually abused child remains trapped in secrecy by shame, fear, and the threat of the abuser.[33]

There are several indicators of sexual abuse, which can be exhibited through a broad range of physical, behavioral, and social symptoms. The most important and dynamic historical clue is when the child actually reports the sexual activity to an outsider.

Paramedics should suspect sexual abuse in children who wear torn, stained, or bloody underclothing, have unexplained injuries or diseases, are pregnant, or have sexually transmitted diseases. Sexually abused children often have a detailed and age-inappropriate understanding of sexual activity, exhibit inappropriate and unusual sexual behavior with peers or toys, compulsively masturbate, show excessive curiosity about sexual matters, or are unusually seductive with classmates, teachers, or adults.

Common behavior seen in sexually abused children includes withdrawal, depression, overcompliance, fear of public showers or restrooms, extraordinary fear of males, and self-consciousness of their bodies beyond that expected for their age. Children who have been sexually abused frequently present with sexually transmitted diseases, genital discharge or infections, physical trauma to the genital areas, pain on urination or defecation, difficulty in walking or sitting due to genital or anal pain, and psychosomatic symptoms, such as stomachaches and headaches.[17]

Management

Paramedics need to immediately identify and report to police, child welfare authorities, or hospital personnel all instances of *suspected* child abuse. This is essential to protect the child victim because abusers will generally repeat the abuse. Police, paramedics, social services and court officers, and medical professionals need to coordinate the investigation and respond as a team. Any stained clothing removed from the child during the physical exam should go into a paper bag to be used as possible evidence. Plastic bags can affect the integrity of the evidence and should be avoided.

The main objective when treating an abused child is to treat the injuries. Treatment of acute injuries, such as subdural hematomas, long bone fractures, and burns, should take precedence. After the injuries have been treated, protect the child from further abuse and neglect. The paramedic's identification of child abuse is important not only because of its significant mortality and morbidity but also because of a real potential for effective remedial action and prevention.

When sexual abuse is suspected but not reported, proper authorities should be notified. When child abuse is suspected and reported, the police should then be notified.

Medical and Legal Reporting Requirements

All states require that suspected child abuse cases be reported to a child welfare agency or the District Attorney's office. This includes all cases in which there is reasonable cause to suspect child abuse and neglect, not just confirmed cases. Some states even regard the threat of abuse to be reportable. Professionals required to report abuse include child care custodians, teachers, health practitioners, and employees of child protective agencies. Paramedics should use the emergency department to coordinate the appropriate reporting requirements. Most states provide protection from liability for the reporting individual who makes a report of suspected child abuse in good faith.

Adult Abuse

Each year, 35% of the women who visit emergency departments do so for treatment of symptoms related to abuse. Unfortunately, as few as 5% of them are identified.[3] Domestic and adult violence form the second most common cause of injury to women and are the leading causes of injury among women ages 15–44, according to the U.S. Surgeon General's Office. Conservative estimates from the National Crime Survey put the annual medical costs of domestic and adult violence at 100,000 days of hospitalization, 30,000 emergency visits, and 40,000 physician visits each year.

Domestic violence often results in severe injury: 28% of the women in one study required admission to the hospital for injuries, 13% required major surgical treatment, 86% had suffered at least one previous incident of abuse, and 40% had previously required medical care for abuse.[3]

Family violence is becoming recognized as a major health and social problem worldwide. Adult abuse includes maltreatment of those who may not be able to leave or easily change their living situation. Its victims include battered women and disabled or dependent adults. Maltreatment is typically perpetrated by family members or intimate friends, but can also be done by others charged with providing care. One study suggested that physical violence occurred between family members at home more often than between any other individuals or in any other setting, except for wars and riots.[27]

Psychosocial Contributions

Families in which abuse occurs tend to be socially isolated and subjected to stress, such as low income and unwanted pregnancies. The abusive family usually holds a traditional view of marriage, wherein the man is "king of the castle." Women in abusive families may be committed to being married for life, and both men and women in abusive relationships may have witnessed their fathers abusing their mothers. There is also a high incidence of abusive adults who were abused as children. A family history of alcoholism and drug use is common for both adults and their own parents.[14]

Abuse typically occurs inside the home, usually in the kitchen, during the time of the greatest intrapersonal interactions, such as weekends and holidays. It is rarely witnessed by outsiders. Family abuse has a cyclical nature: the cycle begins with a tension-building phase marked by arguments and fights. Often, the female accepts this behavior to avoid a beating, though she fears it will occur. When the male ultimately loses control, the second phase of an acute battering episode begins, usually with a beating.

Following the battering, the male becomes remorseful, which leads to the final phase. The female, soothed by the tender, caring, and loving male, becomes hopeful that the abuse will finally cease. During this time, she experiences more nurturing, attention, and gratification than in any other part of the relationship. The cycle and her victimization are now complete, and she returns to the relationship. Ultimately, she will be abused again as the cycle is repeated. It is only during the two phases prior to reconciliation that the female may be open to outside intervention.[1, 9, 31]

Psychological Characteristics

Why does the female stay in such a relationship? Perhaps foremost is her fear of the abuser's retaliation. Additionally, the female is usually economically dependent on the abuser and has a strong desire to affirm her commitment to the relationship. She is frequently depressed and has become trained in learned helplessness.[31]

Abused women are typically young, have married early, and may have left an abusive home. They frequently have a history of psychological abuse in other dating situations. Their life experiences are usually limited, and they have few job skills and lack self-esteem. They frequently have very fragile support systems and develop multiple somatic complaints, with anxiety and depression foremost. They frequently consult mental health professionals and are diagnosed with a psychosomatic disorder. After considerable stress, there is an increased risk for mental problems, often culminating in suicide attempts that require hospitalization.[26]

The abuser is usually poorly educated. The abuser may have a criminal record of violence or spousal abuse. Some investigators have noted both antisocial personality traits and alcoholism in chronic abusers. The abuser typically suffers from a lack of self confidence, has difficulty with intimacy, and is socially isolated. He has unrealistic and traditional views of marriage, in which he overemphasizes the importance of being the primary or sole decision maker. He is frequently jealous, obsessively requires control, and interferes with other relationships that his mate may want to establish. He is likely to use alcohol and drugs as an excuse for his abusing behavior. Often irritable and explosive, the abuser exercises poor control over his aggressiveness and strikes out to avoid being hurt. He controls by using physical violence, sexual assault, or by threatening homicide or his own suicide.[11]

Physical Signs

Eighty percent of abused women report their injuries at least once to some medical personnel.[20] Battery accounts for one in every four suicide attempts in women. Fifty percent of all rapes of women 30 years of age or older are part of the battering syndrome. Using current diagnostic techniques medical personnel usually only diagnose one battered women in 25.[23]

Some of the classic injuries of abused women include black eyes and other facial injuries (typically to the midface). A fractured nose directed to the right and fractured teeth on the left side suggest that the victim was struck by the right hand. Injuries to the arms may indicate an attempt to ward off an attacker. Subdural hematomas, perforated tympanic membranes, and detached retinas have also been reported. Neck injuries, including linear strangulation marks, and injuries to the breast may be seen. Blows to the abdomen causing miscarriages have been reported in pregnant victims. Scalding burns to the chest, face, and genitals are suggestive of abuse.[23]

Abused women are frequently intentionally struck in areas hidden by clothing. Paramedics should maintain a high index of suspicion for spiral fractures of extremities caused by twisting injuries. Providers should also be aware that rape is a frequent manifestation of adult abuse and any information regarding suspected sexual assault should be shared with an emergency department nurse or physician.[26]

Management

The paramedic may initially appear imposing or threatening to a battered woman. Therefore, it is essential that she be convinced that she is safe and any disclosure is private. Supportive, nonjudgmental, nonthreatening questions are reassuring. If the abuser is present and still threatening, he should be asked to leave immediately. Treating a female patient with re-

spect, dignity, and compassion increases her feeling of well-being. In addition to encouraging disclosure, the paramedic should interact with the patient in such a way as to provide emotional support and concern. During this process, encourage face-to-face contact with a social worker, a crisis center, a shelter, or a friend. It may increase the likelihood that the patient will leave the abusive situation.

It is essential that paramedics recognize that women may return to the abusive situation several times before finally escaping it. The paramedic should avoid any personal frustration or expectation that a single encounter will change years of victimization.

Always remember to emphasize safety. The presence of weapons in the home should be brought immediately to the attention of the police. The safety of children should always be considered. If there is time, it may be helpful to explore the woman's social support system to find family or friends who can offer shelter or support.[15, 31, 32]

The paramedic may find the abused women with a variety of problems ranging from acute injuries to psychosomatic complaints. Victims often use drug overdoses and other types of suicide attempts to escape their intolerable conditions.[23]

Treatment of life-threatening injuries or illness should be the paramedic's first priority after the victim is reassured and the scene is deemed safe. Physical trauma should be evaluated, with hidden injuries sought. Historical information should be documented, particularly the mechanism of injury. An objective description of the patient's behavior must be included. Physical findings should be documented objectively and should include a diagram of the injury patterns. The assessment should include objective observations and examples of abuse even if the patient denies abuse. Women who are physically abused or raped should be brought to the emergency department for a definitive exam, psychiatric evaluation, and appropriate social services referral.

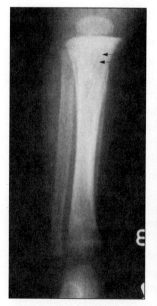
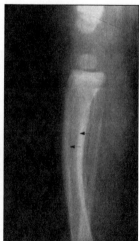

Figure 56-5

Twisting forces can cause spiral fractures. From Monteleone, Child Maltreatment, A Comprehensive Photographic Reference Identifying Potential Child Abuse, 1994, G.W. Medical Publishing Inc.

Medical and Legal Reporting Requirements

Laws vary widely from state to state in regard to the reporting of adult abuse. When they suspect adult abuse, paramedics should inform the local police force, emergency department personnel, and if appropriate, social services. If the victim refuses to be transported, every effort should be made to contact the police or social services. Carefully document all cases of alleged adult abuse for subsequent health care workers when the patient is brought to the emergency department.

Elderly Abuse

Abuse and neglect of the elderly is described by a host of terms: elder abuse, abuse of the elderly, battered elder syndrome, battered parents, geriatric abuse, and even granny battering. An elderly individual may be defined as someone of 60 years or more. They may live in a noninstitutionalized setting or nursing home, alone, with family and friends, or with a caretaker. There may be as many as 1,000,000 abused elders in the United States today.[5]

Psychosocial Contributions

To become more sensitive to elder abuse, paramedics must appreciate some of the historical indicators. Abused elders generally show a pattern of delays in seeking treatment, missed medical appointments, and have unexplained injuries or injuries inconsistent with medical findings.[16] Abused elders often have disturbed interactions with family members, companions, and caregivers, or appear fearful of their companions. There is often an absence of assistance or an attitude of indifference or anger toward the companion. Companions who deny an elder the chance to interact privately with any health care provider should also be considered suspect.[15]

Physical disability in the elderly is believed to be a risk factor for neglect. Abuse occurs more often when the elder lives with someone and is financially dependent on that individual.[16]

Psychological Characteristics

Elder victimization may be signaled by a variety of behavioral signs, including:[5]

- depression
- fear
- withdrawal
- confusion
- anxiety
- low self-esteem
- helplessness

The elder's functional status is significant, because the more dependent they are upon others for care, the more prone they are to being abused. Abuse and neglect can occur when a caregiver is overwhelmed, frustrated, or resentful of their responsibilities. However, healthy elders can also be abused. Since many elders are socially isolated, the availability of a social support system outside of the immediate residence is essential for successful intervention.

An important question to ask is whether anyone restricts the elder from maintaining social activities outside of the home. A wide variety of stresses can cause or exacerbate an abusive situation, including anyone in the home who is dependent on drugs or alcohol. When there is already a history of family violence, other external stress factors, such as loss of job, a divorce, or the death of a family member, can further increase the potential for elder abuse.[5]

When an elder reports that he or she has been a victim of abuse or neglect, the paramedic should note the following information: length of time the abuse has occurred; the number of incidences; the seriousness and consequences of abuse; and whether the abused elder has received any type of help for this problem. This information should then be passed on to the police and emergency department personnel.[5]

Physical Signs

A retrospective study of abused and neglected elderly patients found 45% with medical complaints, 25% who complained of trauma, 8% with psychological complaints, and 22% with a combination of complaints.[5]

Injuries that have been inflicted on the elderly, either maliciously or through neglect, include fractures, dislocations, lacerations, abrasions, burns in unusual locations or unusual shapes, and injuries to the head, scalp, or face. Bruises are frequently bilateral on the upper arms, indicating holding or shaking. Often, bruises are clustered on the trunk from repeated striking and are likely to be like the object that caused the injury. Bruises around the wrist or the ankles are often the result of the elder being tied down. Other more nonspecific physical findings include poor personal hygiene, signs of misuse of medication; including overmedication and undermedication, sexually transmitted diseases, and pain, itching, or bleeding in genital areas.[5]

Hair loss and bruising at the roots suggest that the victim's hair has been pulled. Welts, bruises, and burns may conform to the shape of the inflicting instrument or weapon or confining ropes. The presence of a neurologic deficit or abnormal mental status may be due to an unreported head injury. Infected wounds or those not adequately cared for are signs of neglect. Malnutrition, dehydration, or weight loss can also reflect neglect. Heat stroke or cold exposure may be due to inadequate supervision or a lack of adequate shelter.[5]

Management

Treatment of abused elders should include appropriate attention to all recent injuries, with priority directed toward the most serious ones. However, even minor injuries are important and require treatment. If sexual assault is suspected, treat the injuries first. Transport the patient to an emergency department for a thorough physical examination and definitive treatment of injuries.[16]

Proper documentation is extremely important. Observable behavior of the patient and family are also important and should be documented. Judgmental statements should be avoided. Since determination of abuse in the elderly is a legal matter, the diagnosis of abuse or neglect may be qualified as alleged or reported.

Medical and Legal Reporting Requirements

Each state has some act of legislation to provide legal protection for abused elders. The legal response varies greatly among states and includes civil injunctions, removal of the elderly from the location of the abuse, criminal prosecution, mandatory reporting, and legal protection for professionals who report suspected elder abuse.[16] When available, adult social services should be contacted.[18] Local protocols should reflect the specific reporting requirements for elder abuse enacted by the state in which the service operates.

Sexual Assault

The care of a female or male rape victim often begins in the prehospital stage. Victims should be encouraged not to wash or change their clothing, eat or drink, urinate or defecate, douche, bathe or shower, take any medication or alcohol, gargle or brush teeth, or delay in getting to the emergency department. These actions are necessary to preserve evidence.[6]

In addition, rape victims should be encouraged to notify the police as soon as possible. If the paramedics are first to arrive at the rape scene, care should be taken to not disturb any evidence at the site or on the patient.[6]

If the victim of a rape has already changed clothes, he or she should be advised to place the discarded clothes in a paper bag and bring them to the hospital. Plastic bags can affect the integrity of the evidence and should be avoided. All specimens must be correctly collected and labeled. Documentation must be made of each person who takes possession of the evidence in order to preserve the chain of custody.[16] The victim should be advised to notify the police.

SUMMARY

Cases of personal violence are underreported and underrecognized at an immense medical, social, psychological, and emotional cost. Recognizing the victim of personal violence is the first step in identification and treatment. It is extremely important that paramedics be alert to signs of physical abuse despite patient denial.

Treatment of the physical manifestations of abuse is just the initial stage of therapy. Clear documentation of an abused patient's injuries serves both the victim and the subsequent health care providers well. The paramedic is a vital member of the health care team for the victim of abuse, and should follow local protocols when reporting suspected abuse.

REFERENCES

1. Appleton W: The battered woman syndrome, *Ann Emerg Med,* 9(2): 84–91, 1980.
2. Barlow B, Neiminska M, Gandhi RP, et al: Ten years of experience with falls from a height in children, *J Pediatr Surg* 18(4): 509–511, 1983.
3. Berrios DC, Grady D: Domestic violence—risk factors and outcomes, *West J Med,* 155(2):133–135, 1991.
4. Bijur PE, Kurzon M, Overpeck MD, Scheidt, PC: Parental alcohol use, problem drinking, and children injuries, *JAMA,* 267(23): 3166–3171.
5. Bloom JS, Ansell P, Bloom MN: Detecting elder abuse: a guide for physicians, *Geriatrics,* 44(6):40–44, 1989.
6. Braen, GR: Sexual assault, in: Rosen P, Barkin RM, et al: Emergency Medicine, ed 3, pp 2003–2011, St. Louis, 1992, Mosby.
7. Carter JE, McCormick AQ: Whiplash shaking syndrome: retinal hemorrhage and computerized axial tonography of the brain, *Child Abuse Neg* 7(3):279–286, 1983.
8. Crime Prevention Center, Office of the Attorney General, Sacramento: Child Abuse Prevention Handbook, Aug 1988.
9. Dubovsky SL, Weissberg MP: Psychiatric emergencies, in: Dubovsky SL, Weissberg MP: (eds) Clinical psychiatry in primary care, ed 3, Baltimore, 1986, Williams and Wilkens.
10. Friedrich WN, Wheeler KK: The abusing parent revisited: a decade of psychological research, *J Nerv Mental Dis* 170(10):577–587, 1982.
11. Gelles RJ: Violence in the family: a review of research in the seventies, *J Marriage Fam* 42(4):873–876, 1980.
12. Hobbs CJ: Skull fracture and the diagnosis of abuse, *Arch Dis Child* 59(3):246–252, 1984.
13. Johnson CF, Showers J: Injury variables in child abuse, *Child Abuse Negl* 9(2):207–215, 1985.
14. Johnson CF: Inflicted injury versus accidental injury, in: Reese RM, Child abuse, *The Pediatr Clin North Am* 37(4):791–814, 1990.
15. Johnston SA: The mind of a molester. *Psychology Today,* Feb 1987.
16. Kapp MB, Bigot A: Elder abuse and domestic violence: In Geriatrics and the law: patient rights and professional responsibilities, New York, 1985, Springer Publishing.
17. Kempe CG, Helfer RE: Helping the battered child and his family, Philadelphia, 1971, JB Lippincott.
18. Kravitz H, Driessen G, Gomberg R, et al: Accidental falls from elevated surfaces in infants from birth to one year of age. *Pediatrics* 44(5):869–876, 1969.
19. Morrison LS: The battering syndrome: A poor record of detection in the emergency department, *The J Emerg Med,* (6):521–526, 1988.
20. Perry S: Effective management of the violent patient. *Emerg Med Reports* 4(6):31–36, 1983.
21. Rada RT: The violent patient: rapid assessment and management, *Psychosomatics,* 22(2):101–105, 1981.
22. Rosen CL, Ratliff AF, Wolfe RE, Branney SW, Roe EJ, Pons PT: The Efficacy of Intravenous Droperidol in the Prehospital Setting. *J. Emerg. Med.* 1997; 15:13–18
23. Ross DS: Adult abuse in: Rosen P, Barkin PM, et al, editors, Emergency Medicine, ed 3, Mosby, 1992, pp 2096–2109.
24. Rund DA: Evaluating and managing the violent patient, in: Rosen P, Barkin RM, et al, editors, Emergency Medicine ed 3, St. Louis, 1992, Mosby, pp. 2088–2096.
25. Showers J, Apolo J, Thomas J, et al: Fatal child abuse: a two decade review, *Pediatric Emerg Care* 1(2):66–70, 1985.
26. Straus MA, Gellas RS, Steinmet SK: Behind closed doors—violence in the American family, 1981, Garden City, Anchor Books.
27. Stuart EP, Campbell JC: Assessment of patterns of dangerousness with battered women, *Issues in Mental Health Nurs* 10:243–248, 1989.
28. Taliaferro EH: Coping with the violent patient, Emergency Medicine, pp 155–164, May 15, 1992.
29. Tercier A: Child abuse, in: Rosen P, Barkin RM, et al, Emergency Medicine, ed 3, St. Louis, 1992, Mosby, pp 2717–2734.
30. Turner JT: Violence in the medical care setting: a survival guide, 1984, Aspen Publication.
31. Walker, LE: Battered women and learned helplessness, *Victimology,* 2(3):525–529, 1977.
32. Weissberg MP: Safe strategies for recognizing and managing violent patients, *Emerg Med Reports,* 8(22):169–176, 1987.
33. Wilkins R: Women who sexually abuse children, *BMJ* 5:300(6733):115–4, 1990.

Kate Dernocoeur, EMT-P

Chapter 57

Death and Dying

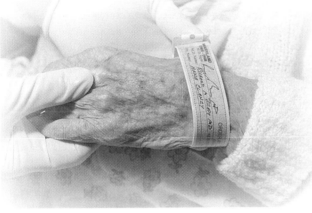

KEY TERMS

1. **Grief**—keen mental suffering or distress over affliction or loss.
2. **Hospice**—care in a facility or at home for the terminally ill that emphasizes pain control and emotional support for the patient and family, typically refraining from taking extraordinary measures to prolong life.
3. **Mourning**—the time during which a person expresses grief, often socially patterned, as in the wearing of black garments.

A paramedic should be able to:

OBJECTIVES

1. Describe factors that influence reactions to death and dying.
2. Define the terms *bereavement*, *grief*, and *mourning*.
3. Describe the three general phases of mourning.
4. Identify how critical incident stress management applies to death and dying situations.
5. Compare and contrast typical responses to a sudden versus an anticipated death situation.
6. Discuss important principles and appropriate methods to use when informing survivors about the death of a loved one.
7. Describe the paramedic's role in potential tissue or organ donation.
8. Describe the stages of death that a terminally ill patient typically experiences.
9. Explain the purpose of "hospice" and its role on behalf of terminal patients.
10. Define *DNR* and *living wills*, explaining their impact in the prehospital setting.

Paramedics witness many intensely personal events in the lives of other people. Among the most profound are those involving death and dying. There are different kinds of death, and over time the paramedic is likely to witness them all. Sometimes the paramedic actively participates in a resuscitation attempt. In other cases, death has already occurred and the paramedic must attend to the related task of informing and comforting survivors.

Rather than being an "enemy" of the paramedic, the death and the dying process can be a powerful learning opportunity, both about oneself and about other people. Every loss has an impact on the caregiver, despite the professional relationship with the patient. Everyone, including medical professionals, must heal from these losses. Unusually intense losses can have such a powerful impact that the paramedic will remember the details vividly for a lifetime. Whether or not those memories are debilitating may depend on the paramedic using the process known as critical incident stress debriefing, which is described briefly in this chapter and covered more comprehensively in Chapter 58.

Other pertinent topics related to death and dying include organ and tissue donation, "do not resuscitate" (DNR) orders, and the role of hospice.

Death and the Paramedic

Paramedics, like all people, have feelings about death and dying. However, unlike most people, paramedics witness death and dying relatively frequently, in the places where it happens in its most vivid reality. A person's attitude, perceptions, and fears about death and dying are influenced by personal background, prior experience, prejudices, and religious and cultural understanding. It is important to achieve and maintain a balanced, healthy attitude toward death, because it will ultimately affect each medical professional personally. It can help a person to think carefully about his or her feelings before entering the EMS profession, and to maintain an awareness of this matter throughout a prehospital career. The cumulative prehospital experience can be either profoundly enriching or painful, depending partly on how the paramedic chooses to approach this emotionally charged topic.

The Grief and Mourning Process

Bereavement is the state of loss. Grief is the spectrum of feelings, particularly sadness and distress, that people exhibit in response to bereavement. The feelings surrounding death and dying tend to be unusual and uncomfortable. Many people do not face these unpleasant feelings directly and lose the opportunity to learn something about life from them.

Mourning is the socially patterned expression of the bereaved person's sorrow.[3] This is the process of displaying, and ultimately working through, grief. An understanding of the mourning process and how to express grief in a healthy fashion can help a person resolve a significant loss more quickly. There are three reasons for the paramedic to understand this process: 1) the impact of multiple deaths witnessed professionally requires attention; 2) when losses are personal, medical professionals must grieve as laypersons; and 3) briefing survivors about the grief process can be an extremely valuable lesson for paramedics.

There are three general stages of mourning[5] (*see* Box 57-1). Individuals vary in the extent and length of their mourning, so paramedics must be prepared for anything. In general, the following pattern occurs:

1. Upon hearing the news that a loved one has died, people enter a 5 to 15 minute period of time known as the "psychic pain spike." Everything becomes focused on the moment of loss. This is a paralyzing surge of grief, comparable with the incapacitating pain of an acute eye injury.[5] During the psychic pain spike, survivors cannot be expected to make decisions or even converse rationally. The psychic pain spike is especially pronounced when the death is sudden and unexpected, although it may be softened somewhat during a resuscitation attempt by gradually preparing survivors for hard news.

2. For the next 4 to 8 weeks, survivors feel intense loneliness, anger, guilt, and longing for the deceased person. It is a period of nearly constant awareness of the loss. Obviously, the closer the relationship, the greater the sense of sadness and emptiness. Important issues in the relationship that remained unresolved at the time of death are likely to further intensify the distress. Gradually, a sense of revitalization—literally, the person's return toward a more regular life—occurs. The feelings continue but are less constant and intense.

3. Finally, a period of recovery begins. Absorption in the loss diminishes, and reconstruction of life begins to occur. The survivor gradually views the loss more objectively and rediscovers an interest in living. Survivors are still likely to grieve more actively, however, on important dates such as the deceased person's birthday, special holidays, and the quarterly and annual anniversaries of the death.[3]

It is entirely normal for mourning to last nearly 1 year. The mourning process is highly individual, and is essential for continuing life with a healthy emotional outlook. In some cases, it becomes a pathological problem and a person never recovers appropriately from the loss.

BOX 57-1	Stages of Mourning

Psychic Pain Spike
- Approximately 5–15 minutes of intense personal pain that begins at the moment when the news of the death of someone close has been revealed.

First 4 to 8 Weeks
- Intense loneliness, anger, guilt, and longing for the deceased. A period of nearly constant awareness of the loss.

After Approximately 8 Weeks
- Absorption in the loss diminishes, and the reconstruction of life begins to occur. It make take at least 1 year for mourning to feel complete, although the feelings of loss will never completely disappear.

Critical Incident Stress Intervention

Paramedics deal with other peoples' crises every day. Such cases can generate a normal response in the paramedic known as "uncritical incident stress." At other times, these events are emotionally overwhelming. Many critical incidents are death-related, particularly when the death involves a child or a coworker (especially suicide), occurs after a prolonged rescue attempt, involves unusual media coverage, or involves someone of similar age, background, or characteristics to the health care providers.

Critical incident stress generates a spectrum of predictable signs and symptoms. These signs usually begin within 48 hours of the event and affect the paramedic's cognitive abilities and physical and emotional health (*see* Box 57-2). Without appropriate intervention, overwhelming incidents can negatively affect the paramedic for years. In some cases in which debriefing does not occur, a single critical incident can force paramedics to leave prehospital care entirely.

There are various types of intervention for critical incident stress. Critical Incident Stress Management Teams are now widely available for education, on-site defusing, and formal debriefings. The formal debriefing process is widely recognized in EMS. The procedure is highly specific and involves a regional (not in-house) team. Debriefings executed inappropriately or facilitated by improperly trained personnel can cause further injury to already vulnerable people. However, if done correctly, they can have a rapid and extremely positive impact. (For more specific information, *see* Chapter 58.)

BOX 57-2 **Signs and Symptoms of Critical Incident Stress**

The following signs and symptoms are normal responses to an abnormal event. A person may experience any number of signs and symptoms, in any combination.

Physical
Fatigue
Insomnia or hypersomnia
Exhaustion
Change in appetite (too much or too little)
Vague health problems (e.g., headaches or digestive problems)

Behavioral
Hyperactivity or under activity
Inability to concentrate
Nightmares and/or flashbacks
Startle reactions
Memory disturbance
Desire to be isolated from others
Inability to attach importance to anything but the event

Psychological
Anxiety
Depression, especially feelings of helplessness
Fear
Guilt
Emotional numbing
Amnesia for the event
Oversensitivity
Anger, including hair-trigger irritability

Paramedics troubled by critical incident stress should seek help. Thankfully, people in emergency services are no longer expected to "tough out" the unusually difficult calls.

Sudden Deaths

Paramedics frequently respond to sudden death situations. Motor vehicle crashes, other fatal accidents, suicide, sudden infant death syndrome (SIDS), heart attacks, unexpected GI bleeding, and interpersonal violence all involve the element of surprise. Sometimes the paramedic attempts to resuscitate and sometimes does not, depending on considerations such as the number of victims involved, the length of patient "down" time, the presence of DNR orders, and physical signs of survivability.

Sudden death is particularly hard for survivors to cope with because it is unexpected. People dislike disruption and change in their lives, and the impact of sudden loss is powerful. When there are unresolved conflicts in a relationship, emotions, such as guilt and resentment, can linger for years. If the loss occurs on a symbolic occasion, such as a fatal accident involving teens the night before high school graduation, there is a heightened sense of tragedy. The paramedic is an active participant in those first moments of shock and realization endured by survivors and can provide a comforting presence.

One of the most difficult sudden deaths is that of a child, particularly that of an infant. Paramedics tend to assume that every infant has died of sudden infant death syndrome (SIDS), but SIDS is actually a diagnosis of exclusion, made after the medical examiner looks for congenital problems, abuse, underlying illness, and other causes. It is important to leave discussion of the cause of death to the medical examiner.

What to Say to Survivors

Although paramedics are well rehearsed in the medical tasks of prehospital life support, the potential for death complicates scenes of life threat. In nearly every case, highly agitated bystanders and relatives are present who add an element of unpredictability and possible safety risks to an already intense scene.

The manner in which bystanders and relatives are handled depends on whether or not the paramedics will attempt patient resuscitation. When they do, a process called "acute grief preparation" can be helpful.[2] Although hope for survival continues until the end, the paramedic can provide the family with hints that they may be facing a death situation. Every 5 or 10 minutes, someone directly involved in the resuscitation should visit briefly provide the family with a progress report. Each successive message can contain clearer clues that death could be the end result. For example, "Your wife's heart is not beating. We are pumping the heart by CPR to keep blood circulating for her." Then: "We are doing everything possible to help her, but you should understand that her condition is critical." Later: "I know this is hard for you. We'll keep you informed as we go along, but so far there's been no change. Her heart is still not beating on its own."

In this way, the family has a chance to prepare emotionally during resuscitation for the possibility an unhappy outcome. This is better than allowing them to hang on to false hopes.

Resuscitation may not be attempted for various reasons, including deaths that occur long before the patient is discovered. The paramedic faces a different sort of interpersonal task in this case. The survivors become "new" patients. The survivors must be informed of the other's death and of what to expect or do next. It is often helpful to mention that grieving can normally take up to 1 year. Many people falsely assume they will be "just fine" soon after the funeral. Knowing that this is unrealistic can be a relief. The paramedic should arrange for a neighbor, clergyperson, friend, or relative to be with survivors—especially those who are alone—before leaving.

When preparing to tell relatives that the patient has died, the paramedic should understand that the reactions are unpredictable. There are widely varying individual and cultural responses to death and dying. However, some interpersonal skills are universal. The paramedic should be positioned at eye level with the people involved. The paramedic would be wise to be positioned closest to an exit in case response to the news is violent. Ask those assembled about their relationship to the dead person; avoid making assumptions. Then, primarily addressing the closest relative, the paramedic should introduce himself or herself by name and role ("My name is Mary, and I'm a paramedic with Mountain City Ambulance") and explain what has happened. The harsh words "dead" and "died" should be introduced kindly, but clearly. These words are unmistakable, and can help reach through the intensity of the psychic pain spike. The paramedic should avoid the use of euphemisms such as *passed on*, or *gone*. Someone in denial may misinterpret such words, thinking, for example, that "gone" means going to the hospital.

When the person's psychic pain spike appears to have passed and the family is ready to receive additional information, the paramedic should reassure them that every possible action was taken to help the patient. If appropriate, it may be comforting to say that, "It appears your relative did not suffer." "Your relative felt no pain" is a statement that cannot be proven and is a poor choice of words. The local procedures for out-of-hospital death should be explained to the family. Survivors may wish to see the dead person. This is important enough to the grief process that the paramedic may even want to suggest it. If the medical examiner must assess the scene, do not allow it to be disturbed. Otherwise, straighten the room, cover the patient, and allow a private visit. Before allowing the family to enter the area, the paramedic may help to prepare them by explaining medical equipment, such as tubes and lines, that are still in place. Usually, these must be left in place for the medical examiner.

When an infant has died, parents may wish to hold the baby, wash or clean the body, or even dress or rediaper it. These are important, healthy actions which should be allowed, despite the paramedic's likely discomfort with such expressions of grief.

Giving news of a death makes many medical professionals uncomfortable. It helps to express that discomfort: "Situations like this are always difficult for me, but it's my duty to inform you . . ." It can also be helpful for the paramedic to acknowledge the pain the survivors feel: "I'm sorry this had to happen to you . . ." Offer assistance, both from a medical and an emotional point of view; some survivors develop medical crises of their own.

Organ and Tissue Donation

With the advancement of modern medicine, the opportunity for use of organs and tissues is increasing. Demand always exceeds supply, and many opportunities for transplantation are missed.

In patients who are declared brain dead but are still maintaining an adequate blood pressure, the heart, lungs, liver, pancreas, and kidneys may all be matched with needy recipients. In people who die of cardiac arrest, other tissues may be retrieved after death. These include, bone, heart valves, tendons, cartilage, veins, parts of the eye (including the cornea), and skin. These tissues are used in joint replacement, limb preservation, facial reconstruction, heart valve repair, correction of birth defects, burn dressings, plastic surgery, and research.[7] However, in certain situations, such as cancer or AIDS deaths, donation is not feasible.

The paramedic can achieve increased organ and tissue donation in two ways. First, on ambulance calls, the paramedic can check (or ask police to check) the driver's license or on donor cards for the patient's wishes regarding donation (Fig. 57-1). These findings should be reported to the receiving facility. Careful documentation of all prehospital care may also make a difference in donor eligibility. Second, the paramedic should educate the public about organ donation. When a family has talked about donation beforehand, survivors are more comfortable about making this difficult decision when faced with the stress of a sudden loss. Check to be sure that awareness of opportunities for organ donation receives priority in local emergency departments, as well.

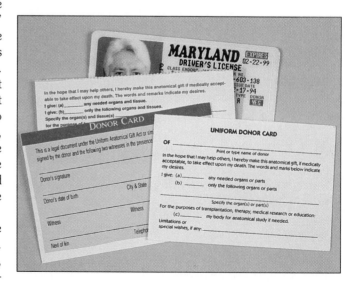

Figure 57-1

A Donor Card is a means of identifying an individual who is a voluntary organ donor. Many states place this information on the individual's driver's license.

Organ and tissue donation is an opportunity to create renewed life out of death. It can be a remarkably positive experience, and a chance to make sense out of the many tragedies the paramedic witnesses. For more information, the United Network for Organ Sharing at 1-800-243-6667 or the local or state organ procurement organization can be contacted.

Anticipated Deaths

Paramedics also respond to anticipated deaths in patients with cancer, AIDS, respiratory illness, and other chronic diseases. The paramedic often encounters these patients during transfers from one medical care setting to another. Situations of anticipated death require an attitude of patience and understanding.

Sometimes, there is a question about whether resuscitation should be attempted. Guidelines on this sensitive ethical matter should be developed by each EMS agency in accordance with local and state laws.[6] Survivors, despite having ample warning of impending death, can still respond unpredictably, so the same interpersonal communications approach discussed earlier applies here as well.

"Stages" of Death

In the late 1960s, researcher Elizabeth Kubler-Ross interviewed 200 people known to be dying. The topic was so taboo that medical staff, who thought her work was morbid and disgusting, spat at her in the hallways. Kubler-Ross discovered that dying people want to talk about what is happening and that they experience predictable stages of dying. The process in which survivors learn to cope with a loss has since been shown to follow these stages as well[4]:

- Denial
- Anger
- Bargaining
- Depression
- Acceptance

People do not always progress through these stages in order. Some people may go through a few stages or all, skip back and forth, not experience any stages, or become "stuck" in one stage. How a person dies is individual, and those in frequent contact should be prepared for anything. (If a person dies while in the "angry" stage, a survivor's last memories may be of an unreasonable, argumentative loved one which could complicate the mourning process.) It may help in recognizing the acceptance stage to know that it is not necessarily peaceful.

Families communicate about anticipated death in different ways. Some are open and speak about everything, settling unfinished logistical and emotional business, and saying goodbye. Others deny to the very end that a loss is about to occur. The paramedic must be careful not to assume anything about family dynamics, even in the relatively "planned" event of anticipated death.

Hospice and Its Role in Death and Dying

The hospice movement has taken hold in the United States since its modern beginnings in England in 1967. The goal is to provide a dignified and caring environment for dying people. There are in-patient hospices, and those serving patients who choose to die at home. Hospices provide professional medical assistance, as well as volunteer help with daily care. They also provide pre- and postbereavement counseling about the grief process and other matters. Hospices have helped to alter the perception that death is taboo and must be hidden and to reestablish it as a natural and inevitable, if sad, event.

The paramedic may occasionally encounter a hospice patient, but usually not at the moment of death. More likely, the patient will require an interfacility transfer. Such patients should be treated with the paramedic's usual compassion and gentleness.

If a family calls at the moment of death, it is often because of confusion, lack of education, or denial. The paramedic is obligated to resuscitate in the absence of clear, legally recognized DNR orders. Hospices try to preeducate families about the importance of resisting the reflexive tendency to call for help, to minimize the unnecessary emotional and financial expense of futile resuscitation. If the paramedic is unsure about what to do, the best course is still to resuscitate rather than omit any effort on behalf of the patient.

DNR Orders and Living Wills

The concept of resuscitation at all costs, regardless of patient desire or apparent futility, has declined as dialogue about death and dying has increased. Since the mid-1970s, many patients have had the option to forego CPR efforts through the use of DNR orders. This document has helped to reduce the conflict that arises when prehospital help is summoned or is already present at the time of a patient's cardiac arrest.

Many states already have policies enabling prehospital DNR orders, and numerous other states are either actively addressing the issue or planning to do so[6] (Fig. 57-2). In

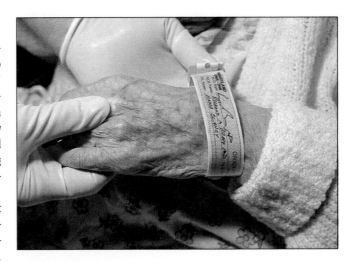

Figure 57-2

Does your state have a system for identifying individuals who have DNR orders?

addition, many local agencies have developed policies in advance of state legislation.

EMS systems vary in their determination of valid DNR orders, and whether incomplete, altered, or illegible DNR orders will be overruled by medical direction. Certain barriers to implementation of prehospital acceptance of DNR orders still exist, including questions about legal liability and administrative procedures. However, DNR orders are increasingly common in medical practice. The American College of Emergency Physicians (ACEP) has a policy statement on DNAR directives in the out-of-hospital setting.[1] Paramedics must know the status of prehospital DNR orders in their areas.

Living wills present a different legal situation. A living will is an advance directive signed by a person of sound mental capacity to avoid various medical treatments, sometimes years ahead of a life-threatening occurence. Many include the vague request that "heroic life-saving measures" be avoided. A living will is regarded as a direction to physicians; its extension to paramedics is not always clear. Legal review, separate from the general DNR topic, is needed to designate how and when paramedics can decide against resuscitation efforts solely on the basis of a living will.

Other Ethical Considerations

The paramedic must not allow his or her own perceptions, fears, and prejudices about death and dying interfere with providing appropriate emergency medical care. The paramedic does not know the patient or family rationales for the choices made about this intensely personal event. Some people fight death to the bitter end. Others seem to greet it as a relief from pain, old age, or chronic illness.

Paramedics must put aside prejudices about infectious disease risks. Bloodborne pathogens, such as AIDS and hepatitis B, and airborne ones, such as tuberculosis, have at times led to prejudicial behavior among health care professionals. The paramedic must be prepared to assist all callers equally, regardless of the nature of their diseases. A paramedic well educated in the methods of minimizing infection risk is the best way to prevent distraction in this setting (*see* Chapter 10).

SUMMARY

Death and dying can be a perplexing topic. The paramedic has a unique opportunity to recognize and appreciate the many lessons that the death process offers. Few others have the same vivid experience as paramedics who go to the homes, highways, and workplaces where people are dying. Paramedics have the chance to witness how other people handle this event. They also have a responsibility to remain compassionate and to behave appropriately at such personal moments in others' lives. The impact of prior personal experience, education about death and dying, and the paramedic's personal acceptance of death as a process all help to effectively handle this intensely personal event.

REFERENCES

1. **American College of Emergency Physicians:** DNAR Directives in the Out-of-Hospital Setting. September, 1994. *Ann Emerg Med* 17:1106–1108, 1988.

2. **Dernocoeur KB:** Street sense: Communication, Safety and Control, ed 2, Englewood Cliffs, 1990, Brady.

3. **Kastenbaum RJ:** Death, Society and Human Experience, ed 3. Columbus, 1986, Charles E. Merrill Publishing.

4. **Kubler-Ross E:** On death and dying, New York, 1969, MacMillan Publishing.

5. **Rosen P, Honigman B:** Life and Death. In Rosen P, (ed): Emergency Medicine: Concepts and Clinical Practice, ed 3, St. Louis, 1992, CV Mosby.

6. **Sachs GA, Miles SH, Levin RA:** Limiting Resuscitation: emerging policy in the emergency medical system. *Ann Intern Med* 114:151–154, 1990.

7. **Winmill D, Clawson J:** Seize the Moment: The EMS role in organ donation. *JEMS* 15:48–54, 1990.

SUGGESTED READING

Mitchell JT, Bray GP: Emergency Services Stress, Englewood Cliffs, 1989, Brady.

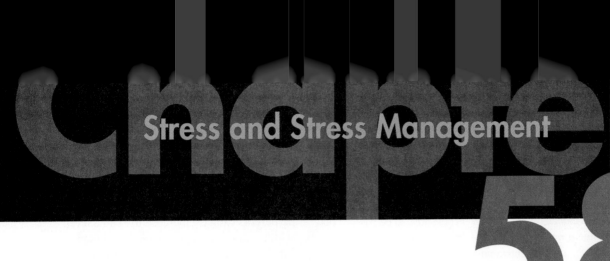

Stress and Stress Management

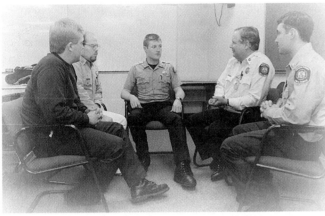

A paramedic should be able to:

OBJECTIVES

1. Define the following terms:
   a. stress response
   b. eustress
   c. critical incident

2. Describe the body's physiological response to stress.

3. Describe the three stages of the General Adaptation Syndrome (GAS) and the body's responses.

4. List the common causes and signs and symptoms of stress.

5. Discuss factors that affect an individual's response to stress.

6. Describe the three major types of stress response: acute, delayed, and cumulative.

7. Describe typical reactions of family, patients, and EMS personnel to the stress of an emergency.

8. Discuss stress related to paramedic education training and a paramedic's job.

9. Define critical incident and list examples.

10. Discuss critical incident stress management components and how they can be effective.

11. Discuss appropriate methods for coping with stress.

KEY TERMS

1. **Critical incident stress debriefings**—structured group meeting, facilitated by a CISM team, that allows for the ventilation of thoughts, reactions and feelings resulting from highly stressful events.

2. **Critical incident stress management (CISM)**—includes general stress education and prevention, on-scene management to minimize effects of stress during major incidents and techniques to help resolve stress reactions after the fact.

3. **Critical incident**—any event that overwhelms one's psychological capabilities.

4. **Distress**—negative, debilitating, or harmful stress.

5. **Eustress**—positive, action-enhancing stress.

6. **Stress**—a state of physiologic and psychological arousal.

"Stress is bad and it will hurt you. If you don't admit everything that is bothering you, whether it's a marriage or a traumatic incident, then you're never going to clear it up. There's always going to be something there telling you, 'Hey! There's this little item down here that you haven't brought up yet.' And you just have to be totally honest, dig up everything you can, and start reworking from there. If you don't, you won't survive stress. There are other people who have similar problems. They keep putting their problems on the "back burner" and one day they're going to erupt, and their mental capacity or job future will depend on how bad that emotional crash is. People have to be willing to face those things and deal with them. I'd give anything to be a paramedic in the fire department again—except my sanity—and that's what I was losing. It hurts."[18]

The paramedic quoted in the preceding interview was discussing the effects of stress, particularly critical incident stress, on his life and the lives of those around him. Little attention was given to the role of stress in the emergency service professions until the 1980s. The pioneering work of Jeffrey T. Mitchell in the area of critical incident stress heightened awareness of the vulnerability of prehospital providers to acute, delayed, and cumulative stress responses. The need for stress education, stress management techniques, and specific critical incident stress management (CISM) programs has since become widely recognized.

The Nature of the Stress Response

Stress is not necessarily a negative concept. The stress response is a natural defense mechanism that prepares the body to protect itself. Stress and stressors can produce eustress, a positive, creativity-producing stress. Eustress motivates, fuels a person's desire to excel and compete, improves performance, and provides enthusiasm and motivation. However, stressors can also be negative, resulting in distress. Distress produces frustration, poor concentration, irritability, poor performance, and other harmful, even disabling, effects. Contrary to popular belief, the nemesis of modern society is not stress but excessive stress.

Physiology of the Stress Response

Stress is a state of physiologic and psychological arousal. It is not, as some people believe, "all in the head." The stress response is a physical event, mediated by the sympathetic nervous system and certain chemicals in the body.

A *stressor* is an event or condition, whether physical, social, or psychological, that triggers a stress response. At times, EMS personnel work in hazardous or hostile environments that pose threats to personal safety. These situations can produce both physical and psychological stressors. A dispatch call for a 2-year-old child who is not breathing can initiate a stress response based on what the responder expects to find on arrival. Similarly, a dispatch call to respond to the scene of a commuter air crash is likely to trigger a stress response based on what the responder has experienced at similar calls.

The brain cortex receives input from the senses and interprets this data based on prior information and experience. In the example of the "child not breathing" call, the paramedic consciously considers the child's age, begins to formulate possible causes of respiratory failure, and develop management priorities. The responder may recall the length of time since last intubating a child or starting an IV line and previous success rates with these procedures. The stress level may increase if there has been no recent experience or there have been unsuccessful attempts.

The paramedic also has a preappraisal of the situation at a subconscious level. If the paramedic is the parent of a 2-year-old child, the situation may produce increased stress. In a small community, the possibility of the rescuer knowing the child or the parents can also increase the stress level.

All of this information is rapidly processed and interpreted, stimulating the midbrain, particularly the limbic system. This system complicates the stress with emotional interpretations such as fear, anger, and love.

The next link in the stress response chain is activation of the hypothalamus, which coordinates functions such as heart rate, blood pressure, temperature, and thirst. The hypothalamus stimulates glands such as the pituitary and nervous systems (sympathetic and parasympathetic).

Stimulation of the adrenal glands causes most of the physical signs of stress arousal. The medulla, or inner portion of the adrenal gland, responds to messages from the hypothalamus (delivered via the sympathetic nervous system) by releasing the hormones epinephrine, norepinephrine, and dopamine. These substances mediate numerous reactions, particularly cardiovascular stimulation.

Hormone secretions, rather than nerve impulses, stimulate the adrenal cortex, or outer portion of the gland, which in turn releases other substances that increase available energy by affecting metabolism. These secretions also cause sodium retention, leading to increased stroke volume, blood pressure, and blood volume (Fig. 58-1).

Once the stress response is initiated, arousal continues until physical action is completed or the secreted substances are either consumed or absorbed. Consider the dispatcher who receives a call that an EMS unit has been involved in a vehicle accident with injuries. After the call, physical signs of the stress response—elevated heart rate, blood pressure, and respiratory rate—will continue until some means of physical activity is available to consume the chemical stress mediators. The body has prepared for action without knowing what response is required.

This complex response to stress is often referred to as the "fight or flight" response. This response is protective in nature and allows for two primary options: 1) the individual can stand, meet the opposing stressor and fight; or 2) flee from it. Either action may be positive and protective. The combination of sympathetic nervous system activity and biochemical release quickly provides the necessary energy and appropriate physical response to handle acutely stressful situations.

Dr. Hans Selye, often called the father of stress research, developed the concept of the general adaptation syndrome, or GAS. The GAS includes three stages: alarm, resistance, and exhaustion. (Fig. 58-2). This syndrome occurs when normal coping mechanisms are inadequate to meet the demands of a situation. Dr. Selye noted that the body's stress response in all

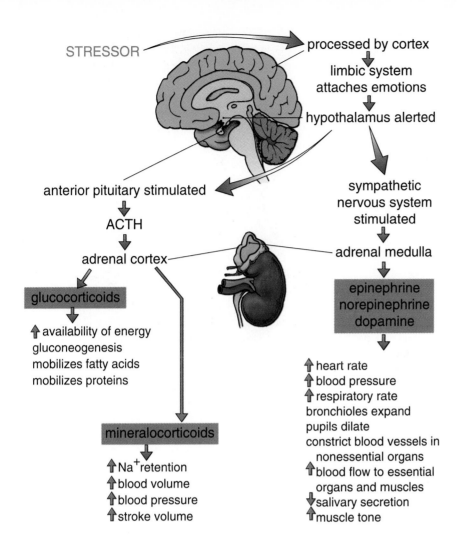

Figure 58-1

Stressors trigger the release of hormones, resulting in the chain reaction of events called the stress response.

three stages is similar whether the stressor is physical or psychological.

During the alarm stage, the body reacts to the initial stressor. There is a widespread sympathetic nervous system discharge and stimulation of the adrenal glands. Most body organs and systems are affected (Fig. 58-3).

In the resistance stage, arousal is channeled into one or more organ systems most capable of handling or suppressing the stressor. This process works effectively for the short-term stress response. However, prolonged stress responses and chronic stress can lead to stress-related illness, fatigue, and body system failure.

Prolonged stress leads to an exhaustion stage when organs and systems are energy-depleted. A recovery process follows the exhaustion stage and eventually returns the body to the prealarm level of function. The length of all GAS phases

and recovery periods varies depending on the intensity of the person's stress response.

Prolonged exposure to stress can alter the body's ability to respond, maintain the resistance phase, and recover from the exhaustion phase. Some common conditions associated with high levels of stress are identified in Box 58-1.

Causes of Stress

Stress results from a variety of sources in an individual's personal, professional, and social spheres (Fig. 58-4). Girdano and Everly identify three general categories of stress: psychosocial, bioecological, and personality.[6] Psychosocial stresses result from the way in which a person interprets and adapts to changes in relationships, the work setting, and other aspects of life. Other psychosocial factors include overload,

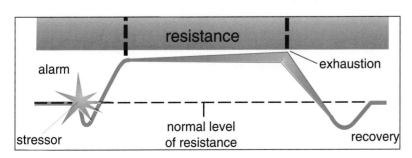

Figure 58-2

Dr. Hans Selye's General Adaptation Syndrome (GAS) has three stages and is triggered when the natural coping mechanisms are overwhelmed.

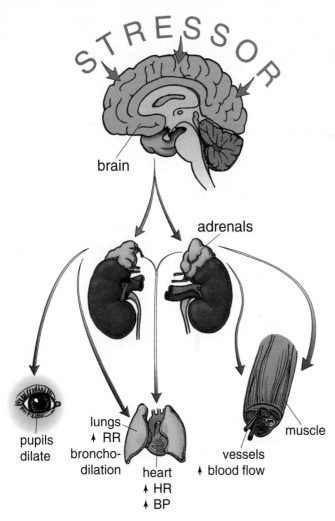

Figure 58-3

Stress triggers a sympathetic discharge that affects many organs and systems.

understimulation, and the ability to tolerate frustration. Boredom and underactivity can be as stressful to emergency responders as high-demand situations.

Bioecological stressors include biorhythms, noise levels, and thermal stresses such as heat, cold, and altitude. Nutritional factors can either contribute to or work against the stress response. Sympathomimetic substances such as caffeine mimic the stress response. Chronic stress aggravates vitamin and mineral deficiencies. Carbohydrates, proteins, and fats play important roles in the body's response to stress. A high-sodium diet causes sodium and fluid retention and can aggravate hypertension. Alcohol and other drugs taken to reduce stress and tension can interfere with healthy coping mechanisms and further compromise nutritional balance.

BOX 58-1	**Common High-Stress Conditions**
1. Asthma	**6.** Eczema
2. Backaches	**7.** Hypertension
3. Cancer	**8.** Migraine headache
4. Coronary artery disease	**9.** Peptic ulcers
5. Diabetes	**10.** Ulcerative colitis

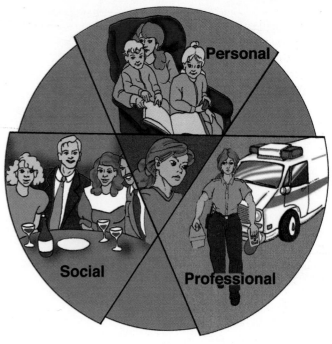

Figure 58-4

Stress can be triggered by a variety of sources.

Self-perception is a major component of personality-caused stress. Negative self-esteem can produce significant stress, while a positive self-concept enhances coping abilities. Anxiety can result from stress as well as cause it. An anxious person can repeatedly relive events and get caught in a negative feedback process. People who exhibit hostility, cynicism, time urgency, and a powerful need to be in control also suffer increased stress.

Reactions to similar stressors vary significantly among individuals. Perception of the event is a key element in determining the stress reaction. The event, individual, or situation must be viewed as harmful to produce a stress response.

Factors Affecting Stress

The magnitude of the stress response is determined by a variety of factors:

- **Intensity**—a paramedic working a cardiac arrest on his or her own father has a different degree of intensity than if the patient is a stranger.
- **Significance**—losing an anticipated promotion is less stressful than losing a job.
- **Length of time**—handling a pediatric trauma arrest for 45 minutes can have a different effect on a paramedic than would the treatment of critical patients for 12 hours at the site of a train wreck.
- **Threat to life or limb**—any situation that threatens responder safety produces tension, even if the outcome is satisfactory.
- **Threat to self-image**—failure to secure an endotracheal tube or IV line in a pediatric patient may produce a perception of failure in the rescuer, regardless of patient outcome.
- **Level of personal loss or involvement**—the responder in a small community may know the victim.

- **Responder's previous experience**—recent success in treating a patient in cardiac arrest will probably decrease the level of stress during a resuscitation attempt.
- **Suddenness or warning time**—a dispatch call for a dog bite does not prepare the responder for the sight of a 4-year-old who has bled to death from a severed carotid artery (Fig. 58-5).
- **Number of stressors present in the situation**—prolonged response time, multiple victims, inadequate manpower and equipment, extrication difficulties, hazardous conditions, and bad weather conditions will produce higher stress levels in a paramedic than a single stressor.

Types of Stress Reactions

The stress responses fall into three major categories: acute, delayed, and cumulative (Table 58-1). The acute stress response is immediate and incident specific. Signs and symptoms begin immediately or soon after the body recognizes a stressor. Acute reactions often occur in response to a particularly intense event, also called a *critical incident*.

Delayed stress reactions are also the result of a specific incident, but signs and symptoms are not immediately obvious. They may appear in the paramedic days, months, or even years later. The individual can suppress memory of an event until something, such as a smell or sound, triggers the memory's recall.

Various signs and symptoms may signal a delayed stress reaction. Intrusive images, such as the sounds, smells, or sights that occurred at the incident, may return with remarkable clarity. These are generally referred to as "flashbacks" when the individual is awake, or "nightmares" during sleep. Either form can trigger physiologic responses, such as elevated pulse and blood pressure, sweating, nausea, and others. Intrusive images are particularly distressing for emergency responders because these images seem to represent a loss of control.

Sleep disturbance is the most common physical sign of delayed stress response. Disturbances include early waking or

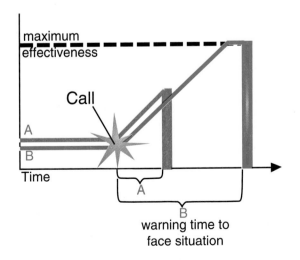

Figure 58-5

Responders react at optimal levels to stressful situations if they are given a period of time to mentally prepare for what they will encounter.

TABLE 58-1	Types of Stress Reactions		
	Acute	**Delayed**	**Cumulative**
Stressor	Intense event	Specific event	Multiple stressors
Onset of symptoms	Immediate	Days to years following event	After several events

difficulty falling or staying asleep. Other physical signs include startle reactions, hyperalertness, and emotional and physical withdrawal. The incidence of stress-related diseases also increases. Emotional signs and symptoms of delayed stress include depression, loss of emotional control, fears about the future, and feelings of isolation, grief, anger, guilt, irritability, hopelessness, helplessness, and anxiety.

Delayed stress reaction also affects cognitive abilities. A paramedic's reasoning and thought processes may be impaired. The paramedic may find that decision-making and problem-solving have become more difficult. The individual may be easily distracted and have difficulty concentrating.

The physical, emotional, and cognitive responses produce a change in the individual's behavior. Victims of delayed stress frequently withdraw from family and friends. Other signs include angry outbursts, suspiciousness, unusual silence, and excessive dark humor.

Cumulative stress reactions are the result of multiple stressors occurring over time (Fig. 58-6). The stressors typically include job-related problems and family and relationship issues. A high chronic level of stress often exists. The ability of an individual to handle stressors has an important effect on the level of cumulative stress that the individual develops. Cumulative stress may involve peers' perception of the individual, as well as a self-imposed sense of negative self-worth. Although this syndrome has been popularized as "*burnout*," *cumulative stress* is a more accurate term.

Cumulative stress is characterized by physical and emotional exhaustion and negative attitudes. This is often an insidious process that builds over time, gradually decreasing the quality of the individual's life and the ability to enjoy family, friends, job, and environment. As cumulative stress progresses, job performance declines, physical illness and work absences increase, and emotional distress grows. Personal and spiritual values may be diminished or lost. Other symptoms exemplified by the individual include feelings of disillusionment, frustration with "the system," increased use of alcohol or other drugs, apathy, withdrawal, disrespectful attitude toward patients and peers, chronic irritability and anger, and an increase in interpersonal conflict. Often a persons' denial of problems is common. Stress reactions may also include the signs and symptoms listed in Box 58-2.

Stress and the Emergency Responder

Stressors vary between professions and further within a profession, depending on roles, responsibilities, and organizational structure. In addition, each individual brings to professional life the sum of experiences and stresses from the family and social

by Rob Carter, EMT-P and Larry Newell, Ed. D., NREMT-P

PARAMEDIC WELLNESS

"Wellness" is a popular concept that encourages people to take responsibility for their health. It is an ongoing process for continous self-renewal, necessary for a healthy, fulfilling life. Wellness is based on the premise that people have control over their health behaviors.

Wellness reflects an individual's attitude and outlook toward living. Have you ever been around someone who "lives in the past," dwells on the negative aspects of his or her life, or constantly blames others for things that go wrong? This individual could benefit from adopting a wellness perspective and changing his or her behavior. A wellness perspective encourages people to focus on the present and the future, setting attainable, positive goals and measurable objectives. Wellness discourages blaming others for a particular problem.

In the 1990s, the positive impact of wellness programs has extended to schools, businesses and industry—even to the field of emergency medical services. Common wellness programs include:

• Smoking cessation
• Stress management
• Proper nutrition
• Weight control
• Cholesterol and blood pressure screening
• Physical fitness
• Safety education

WELLNESS: A NATIONAL CONCERN

The concept of wellness was conveyed in the *Healthy People 2000: National Health Promotion and Disease Prevention Objectives.*[1] This document, completed in 1990, presents a strategic plan for improving the health of the nation in this decade and into the next century. This monumental undertaking by the U.S. Department of Health and Human Services established three broad goals:

1. Increase the span of healthy life for Americans
2. Reduce health disparities among Americans
3. Achieve universal access to preventive services for all Americans

The concept of wellness was at the core of this effort. It acknowledged the important changes that occurred over the past 20 years regarding the protection and enhancement of personal health. At its cornerstone is the premise that responsible and enlightened behavior by every American is truly the key to good health.

THE COMPONENTS OF WELLNESS

Wellness has several key components:

• Physical well being
• Mental and emotional well being
• Spiritual well being

By implementing lifestyle changes in these three areas, paramedics can enhance their personal well being, and even serve as a positive role model for others.

EMS providers often find themselves in situations in which they must overcome difficulties and adverse conditions. Because of the nature of the job, they encounter a high level of job stress. Because the life of a patient may be riding on a paramedic's ability to intervene effectively, it is vital to adopt a healthy lifestyle that keeps one physically, mentally, emotionally, and spiritually able to perform at peak efficiency.

PHYSICAL WELL BEING

Physical well being includes proper nutrition, exercise, and weight control. Proper nutrition includes consuming the basic nutrients essential for a healthy body, in proper amounts, through various food groups. Proper nutrition includes reducing dietary fat, especially saturated fat. It also includes increasing complex carbohydrates and fiber-containing foods. To achieve this, adults need 5 or more daily servings of fruits and vegetables, and 6 or more daily servings of grain products.

To maintain proper nutrition, it is recommended that the average adult consume 50% of all calories from complex carbohydrates, more commonly called starches, and only 10% of the calories from simple carbohydrates, commonly called sugars. Starches are among the most important nutritional elements. They are found primarily in grains, fruits, and vegetables. Starches also contain vitamins, minerals, protein, and water. Sugars, on the other hand, offers few nutritional benefits. Sugars are commonly found in candy, pastry, and soft drinks. They are also hidden in foods such as salad dressings, ketchup, and canned fruits and vegetables.

Fats are also important to a healthy diet. Besides helping to retain body heat, providing a pleasing taste to food, and satisfying the hunger sensation, fats also serve as carriers of vitamins A, D, E, and K, which are fat-soluble. Without fat, these vitamins would pass quickly through the body. Dietary fat is comprised of three forms of fat: monounsaturated, polyunsaturated, and saturated. Saturated fat needs to be limited in a proper diet, because it is believed to promote cardiovascular disease. Saturated fat is abundant in dairy products, such as eggs, and animal products, such as meat.

Proteins are another requirement for proper nutrition. They are necessary for growth and tissue repair. Proteins are actually made up of chains of amino acids. There are two types of amino acids: essential and nonessential. There are nine essential amino acids that must be obtained from sources outside the body. Some sources, such as meat, milk, eggs, and cheese, contain all of these essential amino acids. Other sources, such as vegetables and grains, only provide some of these essential amino acids.

A proper diet is one in which a person consumes the proper amounts of simple and complex carbohydrates, fats, and proteins. By knowing the number of grams for each, one can calculate the number of calories for each and the percentage of calories that each group contributes to the total caloric intake. Follow this basic guide to a balanced diet:

• 60% Carbohydrates (10% simple and 50% complex)
• 25% Fat
• 15% Protein

Exercise also contributes to physical well being. A balanced exercise plan, like a balanced diet, helps maximize efficiency in a healthy lifestyle. A balanced exercise plan is one that improves cardiorespiratory endurance, muscle strength and endurance, and flexibility. Besides improved performance in daily activities and recreational activities, physical fitness can:

• Help improve personal appearance and self-image
• Decrease the risk of cardiovascular disease
• Decrease the risk of injury
• Prevent chronic back problems
• Maintain joint mobility

- Maintain motor skills throughout life
- Increase resistance to muscle injury and soreness

A regular exercise plan involves frequent activity, approximately 3–5 times per week. To improve cardiorespiratory endurance, the intensity of the effort should be between 60–90% of the target heart rate. The target heart rate is simple to calculate. From a maximum heart rate of 220, subtract your age. Next, multiply this number by the intensity of your effort. This provides the target heart rate that should be maintained for a period of 20–60 minutes during an activity.

Maintaining an exercise plan, along with proper nutrition, can help control weight. Eating healthy food in moderation (the average person needs 2000 calories per day, while limiting fat intake to 65 grams) and exercising regularly are the only way to control one's weight.

In addition to nutrition and exercise, maintaining physical well being also means getting adequate rest. Though this varies among individuals, an important point to remember is that the human body needs not just rest, but sound sleep. Lack of sleep affects the body and mind. If you are overly tired while at work, cognitive and psychomotor performance can be impaired. This could impair the ability to make the right decision regarding patient care and skill performance. Managing time throughout the week is important to ensure adequate sleep, especially if rotating or long shifts are inevitable.

Finally, the paramedic must take a proactive approach to the prevention of diseases such as cardiovascular disease, cancer, and infectious diseases, as well as preventing injuries through the use of proper body mechanics and safety equipment and supplies. The EMS profession has the potential to become extremely stressful. This stress can manifest itself through newly diagnosed medical conditions or injuries. Periodic risk assessments should be performed for preventive purposes. These assessments can identify the early warning signs of deteriorating physical, mental, or emotional well being.

MENTAL AND EMOTIONAL WELL BEING

Mental and emotional well being are extremely important to overall wellness. Anxiety and stress have been linked to a variety of problems that can have negative effects on a paramedic.

Stress is a physiological and psychological state of disruption, resulting from an unanticipated, disruptive, or stimulating event (also see Chapter 58). For a state of stress to occur, a person must be confronted by an event, real or imagined, that is interpreted as being disruptive, frightening, exciting, or dangerous. All of these feelings are common to the work of paramedics. The event can become the stressor, based on how a person views the event. Because people are unique, an event causing stress for one person may not cause the same stress for another. For example, a day off from work due to severe environmental conditions, such as a snowstorm, can be relaxing and enjoyable for some people, while others feel a sense of urgency to get to the office and complete work. They may feel as if they will fall behind in their work if they cannot get it accomplished at this time. The manner in which they interpret this event is causing them stress.

A positive response to a stressful event is known as "eustress" (good stress). "Distress," on the other hand, is considered bad stress, or a negative response to the environmental stimulus. Common stressors for the paramedic include:

- Employment expectations and conflicts
- Financial concerns
- Personal expectations
- Family expectations
- Time management

The ability to cope with stress is critical to one's success in the EMS field. Failure to deal effectively with stress can lead to substance misuse or abuse that could have devastating effects on the mental and emotional well being of the paramedic, as well as his or her physical well being. Because the effects of stress are cumulative, it is necessary to constantly re-evaluate stress-related behaviors. Traditional methods of coping with stressors have unfortunately included negative behaviors such as smoking, abuse of alcohol or other drugs, and overeating. They have also included short term solutions that can lead to greater long term stress, such as withdrawing from the stressor or attacking the stressor through direct confrontation.

Appropriate strategies for coping with stress include:

- Developing a structured exercise regimen
- Developing strategies for reducing everyday tension (e.g., relaxation techniques, meditation, yoga, and biofeedback)
- Making a conscious effort to slow down your life style
- Adopting a realistic perspective on stress and life. For example,
  - Do not be surprised by sudden problems
  - Anticipate problems and view yourself as a problem solver
  - Search for solutions
  - Tolerate mistakes
  - Accept the unchangeable
  - Live each day well, combining activities, contemplation, and a positive attitude
  - Remove yourself from negative influences (people or thought patterns)

SPIRITUAL WELL BEING

In addition to physical, mental, and emotional well being, spiritual wellness can contribute to a "whole" person. While this dimension can certainly include personal religious beliefs and practices, spiritual wellness is extended to include:

- Your personal relationships with other living things
- The role of spiritual direction in your life
- The nature of human behavior
- Your willingness to serve others

Cultivating one's spiritual well being requires time to be alone and with others to evaluate one's beliefs and develop inner strengths. Spending this time may help you discover how you can best "fit in" and gain the satisfaction from life that you desire. Spiritual well being can be enhanced through simple things like hiking in the woods and enjoying nature, listening to music, writing, enjoying the arts, and even pushing your body to its limits physically and emotionally.

SUMMARY

In light of the realities of the paramedic profession, providers are well-served by espousing the wellness concept in their lives. This includes taking responsibility for ensuring one's physical, mental and emotional, and spiritual well being.

REFERENCE

1. U.S. Department of Health and Human Services Public Health Service: *Healthy people 2000: national health promotion and disease preventive objectives.* 1990

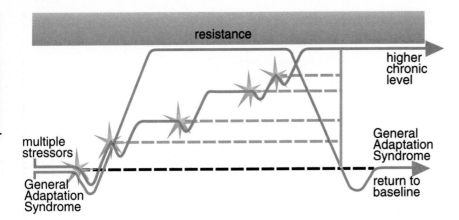

Figure 58-6

Cumulative stress results from multiple incidents occurring over time.

spheres outside of work. Some commonly reported stressors for emergency responders are identified in Box 58-3. Research on emergency responder stress and coping mechanisms for this stress are beginning to provide insight into this area.[4,16]

Paramedic Student Stress

The typical student in a paramedic training program has a foundation of field experience as an EMT-Basic and is usually familiar with the common stressors. Many students entering a paramedic program continue to maintain full- or part-time employment. The student must temporarily juggle four major compartments in the "life sphere" instead of three. The amount of time and energy devoted to the original three compartments changes. The amount of disruption this causes depends to some degree on the length of the educational program, the intensity of coursework and study, the flexibility of scheduling, and the level of need to continue working.

Additional factors that may increase student stress include:

- The length of time elapsed since the student was enrolled in a formal educational program

- The student's amount of field experience on which to build paramedic-level skills
- The adequacy of basic reading comprehension and math skills
- Current life situation, including recent marriage or divorce, birth of a baby, change in employment, or relationship conflicts
- Financial strain caused or aggravated by student status.

The paramedic student must be prudent in developing a plan to balance the time demands among the four life compartments.

- Communication with family is essential in gaining their understanding and support.
- Sound nutrition and avoidance of fast foods
- Regular exercise and time for fun and family activities, but scheduled time for coursework completion
- Avoidance of major life changes during this time, such as moving, switching jobs, starting a family, or changing relationships
- Plan ahead as much as possible

During this time, it is especially important for the paramedic student to practice the stress management suggestions in-

BOX 58-2		Common Signs and Symptoms of Stress Reactions	
Physical	**Cognitive**	**Emotional**	**Behavioral**
Fatigue	Blaming someone	Anxiety	Change in activity
Diarrhea	Poor decision making	Denial	Emotional outbursts
Difficulty breathing	Memory problems	Fear	Change in usual communica-
Thirst	Difficulty identifying familiar	Depression	tions
Grinding of teeth	objects or people	Feeling overwhelmed	Antisocial acts
Profuse sweating	Disturbed thinking	Irritability	Intensified startle reflex
Nausea	Nightmares	Feeling numb	Erratic movements
Muscle tremors	Confusion	Guilt	Excessive silence
Elevated blood pressure	Heightened or lowered alertness	Panic (rare)	Change in speech patterns
Headaches	Loss of time, place, or person	Uncertainty	Loss or increase of appetite
Weakness	orientation	Inappropriate emotional response	Nonspecific body complaints
Chills	Intrusive images	Agitation	Change in sexual function
Vomiting	Decreased attention span	Grief	Withdrawal
Chest pain	Poor concentration	Emotional shock	Suspiciousness
Rapid heart rate	Hypervigilance	Loss of emotional control	Increased alcohol consumption
Visual difficulties	Poor problem solving	Apprehension	Inability to rest
Dizziness	Increased or decreased	Intense anger	Hyperalert to environment
Fainting	awareness of surroundings	Feeling isolated	Pacing
			Excessive humor

Organizational Stressors

Lack of preparation and training
Inadequate working quarters
Outdated equipment
Inadequate equipment or supplies
Insufficient in-house recognition
Inadequate access to management
Dissatisfaction with schedules
Administrative hassles
Conflict with hospital staff

Other Job-Related Stressors

Highly charged situations with multiple demands
Life and death decisions
Boredom when there is no action
Interpersonal communications problems
Lack of public appreciation or understanding

Uncooperative or abusive patients
Feelings of isolation
Family time pressures
Dealing with the dead
Death or injury of children
Fear of own injury or death as a result of the field operations
Death of another emergency responder in the line of duty
Expanding knowledge base
Dealing with the media
Knowing the victims
Dealing with survivors
Emotional identification with the victim
Environmental stress such as extremes in weather
Waiting
Mistakes caused by stress
Feelings of intense vulnerability
Loss of control
Note: These stressors are not rank ordered.

cluded in this chapter. The ability to manage stress will affect the paramedic student's success as a student and the ability to obtain the most value from the educational experience.

Personality Factors

Various personality traits can make it more or less difficult to cope with routine and acute stressors. Individuals with certain personality traits tend to be attracted to the EMS field. Not all responders possess all of the following characteristics, but these are characteristics commonly found in emergency personnel. Typically, the individual entering EMS has a strong desire to be in control. Although this need can set up conflicts at the emergency scene, it enables the provider to manage a sometimes chaotic field environment. This need for control can also hinder the expression of thoughts and feelings.

EMS personnel tend to be action- and risk-oriented. They are easily bored waiting for the next call and have a strong need for stimulation and challenge. As the "new" becomes routine, the emergency responder looks for new ways to maintain an increased level of stimulation. Off duty, hobbies and activities frequently include some element of personal risk, challenge, and competition.

The EMS personality type is also detail-oriented; the person's desire to do a perfect job can become obsessive. A sense of idealism and a tendency to repeatedly second-guess him- or herself and others can increase stress and contribute to the damaging effects of critical incidents. Emergency workers are highly dedicated and loyal. They are more likely to be motivated by the internal satisfaction of good job performance than by external rewards.

In EMS, the ability to assist the ill and injured often provides instant gratification. The rescue personality often finds it difficult to accept a patient refusal even if it is well-founded.

Emergency responders often suppress emotions. This may be an inherent characteristic or a learned behavior that is adopted as a protective mechanism. A rescuer's failure to deal with emotions on the job can produce long-term negative effects on the individual and family.

These characteristics or personality traits are not positive or negative, good or bad. They assist the emergency responder in performing his or her job. However, many of them add to both job- and non-job-related stress. The paramedic's recognition of these characteristics in themselves and others is a key to stress management.

Critical Incident Stress

Critical incidents are extraordinary events that interfere, or have the potential to interfere, with an individual's psychological ability to cope with stress. The concept of critical incident stress is often associated with large-scale disasters or multicasualty incidents. However, most critical incidents occur on a much smaller scale, often involving a single victim. One useful definition of a disaster is any event that overwhelms the available resources. A critical incident can be defined as any event that exceeds the rescuer's ability to cope psychologically. Both definitions take into consideration not only the event, but also the resources available.

Critical incident stress can affect all levels of EMS personnel, as well as law enforcement officers, dispatchers, physicians, nurses, disaster workers, and other emergency responder groups.[3] Some critical incidents affect only one or two emergency responders; other incidents can influence the entire crew.[9] Responders vary in the type and degree of reactions they experience. The reactions identified are normal ones that occur in response to an abnormal event.

Certain events are classified as critical incidents that automatically require critical incident stress management (CISM) intervention. These include:

- Death or serious injury of an emergency worker in the line of duty
- Mass-casualty incidents resulting in serious injury or death
- Suicide of an emergency worker
- Death of a civilian as a result of emergency service or law enforcement operations.

Other incidents that can also precipitate critical incident stress reactions and require intervention include:

- Death or serious injury of a child
- Response on a call in which the victim is known to the emergency worker
- Threat to the safety of the responders, such as incidents involving a hostage or sniper, or hazardous materials
- Situations with excessive media interest or criticism
- Loss of a patient following a prolonged rescue or resuscitation effort
- Personal identification with the victim or circumstances
- Incidents in which the sights and sounds are particularly distressing.

The most common type of emergency call that initiates a request for debriefing involves a death. A recent report from an active statewide Critical Incident Stress Debriefing (CISD) Team Network reveals that 40% of requested debriefings resulted from an incident involving the death of a child or adolescent, 26% involving the death of an adult, 10% involving suicides, and 7% involving the death of emergency service personnel.[11]

Unusual circumstances can combine to transform a relatively ordinary call into a critical incident. Rescuers responding to a sudden infant death syndrome (SIDS) call may not be an unusual event, but responding on a similar call within an hour can be overwhelming. Rescuers responding to a dumpster fire may appear to be a routine call, but finding the body of a 12-year-old child burned to death in the dumpster changes the impact of the event entirely.

Characteristics of Critical Incidents

Critical incidents are usually sudden and unexpected. They disrupt a person's sense of control over, and the emotions triggered by, the situation. Critical incidents often disrupt the paramedic's beliefs and values about how the world works and may also involve feelings of emotional loss. Many emergency workers believe, at least at the subconscious level, that the incident would have resolved differently, if the job performance was better.

Assessing the Need for a Critical Incident Stress Debriefing

If a critical incident is defined by its impact, how does the responder identify the need for critical incident stress management intervention? The following are general considerations that can aid in determining the need for a formal debriefing:

- *How many individuals are affected?* If only one or two emergency responders are symptomatic, a referral may be preferable. If three or more are symptomatic, a group debriefing is indicated.
- *Does the event require debriefing?* Debriefing events that do not have significant emotional impact weakens the process.
- *What symptoms are being reported by participants in the event?* Continuing acute or delayed stress symptoms and intensification of existing symptoms are key indicators for debriefing. Group symptoms also indicate the need for debriefing. Common symptoms include fear, anxiety, confusion, sleep disturbances, acting out, unusual behavior, excessive silence, and excessive or inappropriate humor.
- *Has there been a change in the behavior of the participants in the event?*
- *Is there a regression of behavior of participants in the event?* Are crew members reverting to old (maybe destructive) forms of behavior?
- *Are group members experiencing acute or delayed stress that requires formal debriefing, or do members just need a chance to talk out their frustrations with peers and managers?*
- *Is a formal debriefing necessary, or are group members asking for general information on stress and its management?*

Importance of Critical Incident Stress Management

A CISM program is beneficial for the individual, the response team, and the organization.[14] General stress management techniques and a CISM program protect the psychological, emotional, and physical health of the individual. Managing stress levels and acute stress responses assists individuals in maintaining an optimal level of wellness, improving performance, and decreasing stress-related illness and sick time. It allows emergency workers to stay in service and remain in their careers. And, most of all, it allows providers to maintain a sense of enjoyment and accomplishment in their occupation.

CISM also contributes to the health of the group. It increases team cohesiveness and feelings of group support. Feelings of isolation are decreased, and group members learn that others share similar feelings.

Practicing the CISM concept can also improve relations between management and the workforce. Stress management programs complement health insurance, physical fitness, and employee assistance programs by showing that management is concerned about the well-being of employees.

Critical Incident Stress Management Skills

On-Scene Management

CISM includes appropriate on-scene management during large-scale events when responders will be present for prolonged periods. Some considerations for minimizing the stress effects on personnel and maximizing performance include:

- Brief rescuers before deployment about what to expect at the scene.
- Provide a 15 to 30 minute rest break, ideally every 2 hours, to help decrease injuries, fatigue, and emotional drain. Do not allow rescuers to exceed 4 hours of duty without rest.
- Allow completion of tasks before changing duty assignment.
- Locate a rest area away from the incident to decrease visual and auditory stimuli.
- Integrate relief crews with original crews to allow the "veterans" to teach the "newcomers" the task.
- Ensure that maximum exposure on scene does not exceed 12 hours.
- Provide meals and snacks that consist of complex carbohydrates and protein. Avoid foods high in sugar, fat, and sodium. Provide large amounts of water and fruit juices.
- Provide decaffeinated beverages. Caffeine exaggerates the stress response.
- Maintain normal working groups and allow them to work as teams.

CISM Team Interventions

Demobilization

Demobilization services are used during large-scale events that usually last a minimum of 8 hours and involve a large number of personnel. Crews are rotated through a demobilization center when their work at the scene is completed. Small working groups meet with a CISM team member and receive basic information on stress and immediate management techniques. Demobilization provides responders with an opportunity to discuss their feelings. Personnel are given an opportunity to rest and are offered refreshments before returning to the station or quarters, or going off duty. The entire process should last approximately 30 minutes.

Defusing

Defusings are held a short time after the incident with the units or working groups most affected by it. Defusing allows initial release of feelings, and an opportunity for the crew to share information and offer support. The session may last 30 to 45 minutes or longer, depending on the event, the impact on the personnel, and the personnel's emotional willingness to discuss feelings. The session is led by CISM team members, who provide general information on stress, hints for immediate management, and resource and referral contacts. In the process, the CISM team can determine the ability of the crew to remain in service and the need for further intervention, referral, or debriefing. A defusing may eliminate the need for a formal debriefing if the participants are able to discuss their reactions and feelings. If a defusing cannot be arranged before the end of the shift, a debriefing is scheduled within 24 to 72 hours of the event.

Debriefing

A psychological debriefing for a critical incident is a structured group meeting, facilitated by a CISM team, that allows for the ventilation of thoughts, reactions, and feelings resulting from the event (Fig. 58-7). A CISD usually includes all of the emergency responders involved in the incident, including dispatch personnel. This group process is a nonevaluative, confidential discussion among responding personnel that allows them to share and validate their responses to the incident. The debriefing process provides psychological support, a stress-education component, and suggestions on coping techniques.

Debriefings correct the common but mistaken impression that one's stress responses are unique and abnormal, accelerate recovery from stress reactions, help prevent the development of posttraumatic stress disorder, enhance group cohesiveness and support, and promote interagency cooperation. They also provide an opportunity for a mental health professional to identify any need for referral to follow-up care.

The CISD process is most effective when conducted within the recommended 24- to 72-hour time frame. If it is not possible to conduct the debriefing within this period, it should be held as soon as possible within the following week.

Referral

At times, an incident significantly affects only one person. In such cases, a CISM team can make an appropriate referral to a trained mental health professional. The group debriefing process also provides information on referral sources to personnel to be used as needed. Individuals who have experienced cumulative events or are deeply affected by a critical incident may desire additional support and counseling through a mental health professional who is familiar with the personality profile of emergency responders.

Critical Incident Stress Management Techniques

The interventions previously discussed are key elements in the CISM process. In addition, there are numerous active techniques that emergency responders can use to reduce stress and recover from acute stress responses (Box 58-4).

The ideal CISM team uses a multiagency, regional approach. Most teams provide services on a volunteer basis to fire service, law enforcement, and emergency medical personnel; flight nurses and physicians; and other emergency responders such as dispatchers, disaster response personnel, ski patrols, and search and rescue teams. CISM teams also offer spouse education programs.

A CISM team has two primary functions:

- To prepare emergency responders to manage job-related stress (education)
- To assist emergency responders following an unusually stressful event (intervention).

Stress Management Strategies

General stress management strategies are necessary on both an organizational and individual basis. Understanding the motivations, rewards and values of emergency work helps in the development of these strategies.[2]

Organizational Strategies

Three categories of organizational wellness planning have been identified. These categories include the work structure, environmental health and wellness programs, and stress reduction strategies.[17] The work structure and environmental health include the basic design and operation of the EMS organization. Proper design and implementation of the work system contribute to a positive working environment. Important elements of organizational wellness include open internal communication,

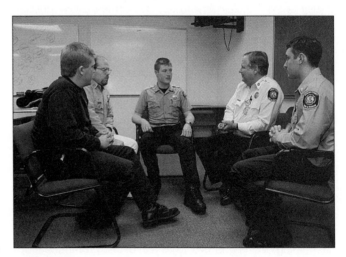

Figure 58-7

A CISM debriefing is a structured group meeting facilitated by mental health professionals and providers who are trained as peer counselors who assist in the debriefing process. Debriefings can last from one to several hours as the team members share their feelings in an environment meant to offer psychological support without criticism of the providers' performance during the event.

BOX 58-4 — Tips for Reducing Stress—and for Living with It

Many of the following ideas will help reduce daily stress if you practice them regularly. Most will be even more helpful during periods of unusually high stress, especially after critical incidents.

- *Exercise.* Develop an exercise routine that you enjoy and that includes aerobic activity. After a critical incident, exercise hard at least once in the first 24 to 48 hours, and try to alternate exercise with periods of relaxation. Walk places when it's practical, and take time to smell the flowers along the way.
- *Nutrition.* Eat regular meals and try to stick to foods that are high in carbohydrates and low in fat, sodium, and sugar. Vitamins and minerals, especially B and C vitamins, calcium, and magnesium, are particularly important. Alcohol and stimulants, including caffeine and tobacco, may add to the problem rather than easing it.
- *Plan your time.* Prepare for morning the night before, get up early, leave extra time to get where you need to go, and plan activities toward a balance of staying busy and having some quiet time. Post notes to yourself to help remember errands and commitments. Besides avoiding the extra stress of deadlines and forgotten tasks, planning maintains a sense of control over your life. Make decisions that enhance that sense of control.
- *Try to stay in a routine and optimize it to your own rhythms.* Schedule your most difficult tasks for your peak hours and less demanding items for other times.
- *Do things you enjoy and things you do well.* Plan to have some fun. Say "No" when you need time for yourself.
- *Don't disconnect.* Talking to people is therapeutic. Sharing feelings may help everyone work things out, so check on fellow responders. It's also important to spend time with people not connected with emergency work. Plan some time with family and friends. Give thought along the way to how to develop this system. Choose some "givers" along with the "takers" and let them know what you're likely to need in times of stress.
- *If you want to express thoughts or feelings that you're not ready to tell someone, try keeping a journal.* Some find it valuable even when stress is not high.
- *Think about the big picture.* Keep a sense of humor and try to control the drive for perfection. Ask yourself how much this all matters in the grand scheme of the universe.
- *Don't label yourself crazy or assume that you're all alone.* Understand that you're normal and having normal reactions. Talking to others, including those trained in critical incident stress, is very important.
- *Nurture your spirituality.* Whatever your beliefs are, your inner reserves are one of your most important resources.
- *Try not to make decisions about major life changes when stress is high.*
- *Stay open to the subject by expecting and acknowledging stress.* Maintain a regular stress management program and use peer support: discuss your stress reactions with others. Participate in critical incident stress debriefings when provided and know what other resources are available. Seek help when you need it and listen when others offer it.

Adapted from Nancy Rich, MA, Trauma Management Consultants, 1985.

---

safe work practices, adequate supplies and equipment, shared values, positive management-employee relations, pride in the quality of service, fair scheduling, and compensation policies. These areas require ongoing review and revision in a manner that shares responsibility between employees and management.

Health and wellness programs include programs that provide health insurance, employee assistance, physical fitness activities, critical incident stress management, and lifestyle counseling, such as programs to help with smoking cessation and weight loss. Fitness programs may be mandatory in some organizations such as the fire service; if such programs are not required, they should be encouraged and supported. It is well documented that physical fitness improves the ability to respond to stress.

Organizations should also create a general climate, and establish specific mechanisms, that assist the employee in future job growth and development. This includes adequate initial training, training in new skills and areas, promotional opportunities, and tuition assistance programs. Individuals who continue to learn continue to be challenged and maintain a higher level of wellness.

Individual Strategies

Just as stressors have differing effects on individuals, stress reduction techniques are also individual. And just as organizations have a responsibility to provide programs and services, the individual must be responsible for effectively using these resources.

Individual activities are varied and fall roughly into these general categories:

- Formal programs
- Fitness programs and exercise
- Diet
- Relaxation
- Recreation
- Other

Stress reduction strategies include both formal programs and individual activities. Stress management and training is important for both emergency responders and their spouses. This training should include general education about the causes and nature of the stress response and instruction in stress reduction techniques. These programs are especially effective when provided in a full-group setting. When the concept of stress is addressed as part of the organizational culture, the group begins to accept the stress response as normal. Communication training for managers and line personnel is especially beneficial and should also be offered to spouses of personnel as well. Time management courses are also useful. Many departments have established peer support programs to provide assistance to personnel as needed. Employee assistance programs provide access to confidential professional counseling on a short-term basis, and referral to further care as needed. Confidentiality is an important aspect of counseling for many individuals who may not accept that stress responses are normal.

It is important that individuals understand the difference between recreation and relaxation; each is important. Sports, for example, may be a portion of a physical fitness program that provides social interaction and is part of the individual's recreation time. However, quiet relaxation time is also needed. This time may include noncompetitive, non–ego-involved physical activity, progressive relaxation, self-hypnosis, meditation, yoga, reading, listening to music, taking long walks, or any other relaxing activity. Adequate rest on a regular basis is crucial for a person's ability to cope with stress. The EMS worker should plan frequent breaks from the job or take mini-vacations to ease stress.

Dietary considerations to relieve or reduce stress include low-to-moderate caffeine intake and weight reduction when needed.[10] Nicotine aggravates the stress response and should be avoided. Alcohol and recreational drugs, widely believed to reduce stress, actually reduce coping resources and can lead to depression.

Stress is unavoidable in both modern society and the emergency service field.

Significant-Other Stress

Many emergency responders believe that their work affects only them and not their spouses, children, or other loved ones. Those closest to emergency providers are most attuned to their moods, reactions, and pain. In addition, these individuals harbor their own fears for the health and safety of the loved one. Spouses of emergency responders often report feeling that they are somehow of secondary importance to their partners—that the job comes first. Children, especially, respond negatively to the emotional distancing that often accompanies stress.

Spouses and other family members should also receive stress management education. Communication workshops are encouraged. Too often, without ever trying to discuss the subject, an emergency responder states that the spouse "doesn't want to know about this job." A person's reasons for refusal to discuss emotional reactions are varied and include an attempt to shield or protect loved ones from the horror of the job, a need to protect confidential information, and an unwillingness to reveal himself or herself as vulnerable and less than totally in control.[5]

Men spouses of women emergency responders may find additional stress in their relationships because of the perceived role reversal and fears for their wives' safety. Ironically, many emergency responders fail to see their own family as a base for emotional support. In a society with an already high divorce rate, emergency responders must take particular care of their family relationships.[1]

Stress management training and practices are essential for spouses. Families that thrive are those that communicate openly, identify and admit to stressors, seek family solutions to family problems, play together frequently, are affectionate and loving, develop healthy coping skills, lack violence in the home, have an outside support system including friends and family, and use those resources as needed. Other resources for spouses may include a spouse support circle or group and a spouse academy to familiarize the spouse with the emergency responder role.

SUMMARY

Stress is neither good nor bad; it is an integral part of the emergency responder's daily life and career. Management techniques include a daily stress management program, lifestyle changes when needed, and intervention for acute or critical incident stress. Spouses and other family members and loved ones should be included in stress reduction programs.

Information on existing CISM teams in the United States and how to develop a team is available through the International Critical Incident Stress Foundation, 4785 Dorsey Hall Drive, Suite 102, Ellicott City, Maryland 21042. Phone: 410-730-4311.

REFERENCES

1. **Baldus R:** Marriage and the EMS Experience. *Emergency* 24(1):34–37, 1992.
2. **Becknell J:** Wants, Motivations, Values: An Informal Look at the Front-Line Provider. *JEMS* 17(6):32–37, 1992.
3. **Corneil D:** The Psychosocial Needs of Health Professionals Providing On-Scene Disaster Care. *Prehosp Dis Med* 6(4):485–487, 1991.
4. **Cydulka R:** A Follow-up Report of Occupational Stress in Urban EMT-Paramedics. *Ann Emerg Med* 18(11):1151–1155, 1989.
5. **Dunn S:** The Other Side of the Story. *Emerg Med Serv* 20(7):27–32, 1991.
6. **Girdano D, Everly G, Dusele D:** Controlling Stress and Tension: A Holistic Approach, ed 3, Englewood Cliffs, 1990, Prentice Hall.
7. **Graham N:** Done In, Fed Up, Burned Out: Too Much Attrition in EMS. *JEMS* 6(1):24–28, 1981.
8. **Graham N:** How to Avoid a Short Career. *JEMS* 6(2):25–30, 1981.
9. **Harbert K, Hunsinger M:** The Impact of Traumatic Stress Reactions on Caregivers. *J Am Acad Phys Assist* 4(5):384–394, 1991.
10. **Harrison-Davis M:** Nutrition on the Go, *Emerg Med Serv* 21(3):46–50, 1992.
11. **McHenry S:** Stress in the Pre-Hospital EMS and Disaster Setting, *Prehosp Dis Med* 6(4):483–484, 1991.
12. **Mitchell J, Bray G:** Emergency Services Stress, Englewood Cliffs, 1990, Prentice Hall.
13. **Mitchell J, Resnik H:** Emergency Response to Crisis, Bowie, 1981, Robert J. Brady.
14. **Mitchell J:** The History, Status, and Future of Critical Incident Stress Debriefings. *JEMS* 13(11):47–52, 1988.
15. **Mitchell J:** Development and Functions of a Critical Incident Stress Debriefing Team. *JEMS* 13(12):43–46, 1988.
16. **Norton R, et al:** Survey of Emergency Medical Technicians' Ability to Cope with the Deaths of Patients During Prehospital Care. *Prehosp Dis Med* 7(3):235–242, 1992.
17. **Thurnher O:** This One's For the Boss, *JEMS* 14(3):6–7, 1989.
18. **University of Maryland at Baltimore**—(Video): Critical Incident Stress, Baltimore, 1985.

Section 6

Conditions by Diagnosis

Airway Conditions

Airway Burn Airway burns are rare but serious effects of exposure to fire and the products of combustion. Along with direct heat injury, inhalation of toxic fumes can also compromise the airway. The common end point is inadequate oxygenation and ventilation.

Heat injury is usually limited to The upper airway, where it causes edema and bronchospasm. The vocal cords may also close in response to the heat exposure. Inhaled particulates cause airway irritation and can be a vehicle for delivering toxins to the lower respiratory tract. Airflow compromise from airway burns and toxic inhalations results from a combination of mucous plugging, collapsed lung tissue, laryngospasm and bronchospasm. Depending on the extent of their exposure, these patients will display minimal to major respiratory distress symptoms. Stridor, tachypnea, respiratory muscle retractions, wheezes, rales and ronchi can all be present. When present, agitation, restlessness and altered sensorium reflect hypoxia and impending respiratory failure. Because there may be a delay in symptoms for patients with minor exposures, all patients who could potentially have an airway burn or toxic inhalation should be evaluated in an emergency department. Supportive care, consisting of supplemental oxygen and elevation of the head to minimize edema, begins in the field. Patients already exhibiting signs of respiratory distress or failure should receive more aggressive airway management.

Airway Obstruction by Foreign Body The complete obstruction of an airway by a foreign body is usually a lethal condition; unfortunately, it rarely occurs in the presence of prehospital providers. An obstructed airway is an important possibility to keep in mind when confronted with an apneic patient, especially a young child or an adult who collapses while eating.

Partial airway obstruction is frequently encountered by prehospital providers. Nearly every adult patient found obtunded or unconscious with snoring, gurgling or stridorous respirations has a partial airway obstruction from the tongue, dentures, vomitus or other objects. It is not uncommon for a complete airway obstruction to start as a partial airway obstruction that is not recognized or appropriately treated.

Complete airway obstruction from a foreign body can occur anywhere from the mouth to the trachea but is most common at the narrowest point of the airway, the glottic opening at the larynx. There is no limit to the types of foreign bodies that can obstruct an airway, particularly in toddlers. Food is the most common source of obstruction but vomitus, saliva and blood can also block the airway. The object itself can occlude the airway, or irritation caused by contact with the vocal cords can trigger laryngospasm.

Patients with complete airway obstruction from a foreign body will quickly become hypoxic and, if unrelieved, will asphyxiate and suffer cardiopulmonary arrest. If the patient is still awake by the time prehospital care givers arrive, the patient will be unable to speak and will often exhibit the universal distress sign for choking. No air flow will be detected.

By far the most common cause of partial airway obstruction is the tongue; basic airway maneuvers (chin lift, jaw thrust) are designed to relieve this common obstruction. Almost any foreign object that can lead to a complete airway obstruction can also cause a partial obstruction. With a partial obstruction, the patient will initially be stimulated to cough in an attempt to dislodge the foreign body as it reaches the glottic opening. The coughing is often followed by a gasping inspiratory effort that can promote further aspiration or obstruction if the foreign body is not completely cleared from the oropharynx. Some foreign bodies will remain in place despite coughing and can easily move into a position of obstruction. The patient will be awake and usually appear agitated, restless and stridorous with coughing spells and a prolonged inspiratory time. If speech is possible, it will sound muffled.

The prehospital management of a patient with an obstructed airway is directed at relieving the obstruction. Current American Heart Association or American Red Cross guidelines for handling foreign body obstructed airway should be followed. Maneuvers to unblock the airway such as back blows or abdominal thrusts in the adult patient are performed as soon as the patient is encountered. If unconsciousness has occurred and ventilation is not possible, a finger sweep followed by back blows and abdominal thrusts should be attempted. If unsuccessful, direct laryngoscopy with Magill forceps should be performed in an effort to remove the foreign body, prior to performing needle or surgical cricothyroidotomy. Partial airway obstruction should be managed by doing nothing, beyond gently administering oxygen, as long as the patient remains conscious and breathing. A depressed level of consciousness and cessation of coughing or breathing are warnings of progression to complete airway obstruction; management should follow accordingly.

Croup/Laryngotracheobronchitis Croup, also known as laryngotracheobronchitis (LTB), is many times more common than epiglottitis. It is the most common source of stridor in children.

The cause of croup is usually a virus that causes an inflammation of the area below the glottis. The tracheal mucosa becomes swollen and inflamed, resulting in narrowing of the airway just below the cords. Because the infection affects the trachea around its entire circumference, swelling occurs inward, narrowing the airway and causing the stridorous respirations. Complete airway obstruction can occur in severe cases.

Croup typically occurs in the fall and winter months in children between six months and three years of age. Several days of upper respiratory tract infection symptoms invariably precede it. The child will appear in respiratory distress with an elevated respiratory rate, audible stridor and a "barking-seal" cough. These symptoms typically occur at night, along with tachycardia and tachypnea in most children; retractions are occasionally present. The child is usually not ill in appearance, the fever is mild and drooling is absent. Breath sounds are full, clear and equal in most patients. Progression of croup to complete airway obstruction occurs gradually, if at all. The paramedic should observe for nasal flaring, suprasternal or intercostal retractions, pallor and cyanosis as ominous indications that hypoxia is present.

Prehospital management centers around supportive care. Supplemental high-concentration, humidified oxygen is the mainstay; allowing the child to remain with a parent in a comfortable position during transport is also important. In severe cases, the patient may be lethargic or have a diminished level of consciousness, and the airway must be secured and ventilations assisted. Suctioning may be required. Only in the most severe, rare cases will intubation be necessary.

Epiglottitis Epiglottitis is the inflammation of the epiglottitis, usually from infection. It is a relatively rare condition that primarily affects children. Though uncommon, epiglottitis is life threatening if unrecognized.

In children, the most common cause of epiglottitis is *H. influenzae*. This bacteria will directly invade tissues above the glottis, causing swelling of the epiglottitis and surrounding soft tissue. The spread of bacteria into the blood stream is common. The progression of tissue swelling and inflammation is rapid, and upper airway obstruction can occur suddenly.

The classic presentation of epiglottitis is that of a child two to six years of age with a high fever, an ill appearance, drooling, severe respiratory distress, a preference for the sitting position, and depending on the degree of obstruction, may have stridor. The presentation may be more subtle, though, and epiglottitis can also occur in adults. Many children will have a recent history of upper respiratory tract infection, a low grade temperature and even a croupy cough. Older children and adults may describe only a sore throat and subtle voice changes. In both children and adults, the clinical progression of epiglottitis to complete airway obstruction can be sudden. The patient's complaints and physical findings are limited to the respiratory system; lung examination is normal, and respiratory muscle retractions are evident.

The prehospital management of epiglottitis in children and adults is primarily supportive. The patient should be allowed to sit in a position of comfort, and a child should remain with a calm parent. Humidified oxygen should be offered but not forced on the patient, particularly the young child. If respiratory failure occurs, ventilation and oxygenation can usually be maintained with a bag-valve-mask. Direct laryngoscopy should be postponed until arrival at the emergency department since the anatomy may be so distorted that successful visualization of the cords is impossible. Also, any attempt to examine the mouth or throat of a patient suspected of having epiglottitis can trigger complete airway obstruction. Intravenous access should probably not be attempted in children because it may increase agitation, with the same result.

Laryngospasm Laryngospasm is a term used to define the reflex closure of tissue in and around the glottis. It is seen most commonly after patients are extubated following a surgical procedure. Children under the age of nine seem to be the most susceptible. Laryngospasm can also be a result of any condition (infection, injury, aspiration, inhalation, allergic reaction) that irritates the laryngeal mucosa, or be provoked by unsuccessful intubation attempts.

The patient with laryngospasm will present with stridor. The complete or partial closure of the vocal cords will also be accompanied by the telltale signs of respiratory distress: tachypnea, respiratory muscle retractions, difficulty or absence of speaking, restlessness and cyanosis. Respiratory arrest can occur within minutes if the laryngospasm has completely obstructed the patient's airway. The assessment of these patients should be directed at determining the cause of the laryngospasm and the likelihood of respiratory failure.

Prehospital management begins with an attempt to overcome the laryngospasm with bag-valve-mask ventilation and supplemental oxygen. Suctioning the airway in an attempt to remove the irritant is also recommended. If laryngospasm persists, the patient should be intubated with a smaller-than-normal endotracheal tube. The use of paralytic agents such as succinylcholine is useful when available, but is controversial in the prehospital setting. Needle or surgical cricothyrotomy is the last option if intubation attempts fail.

Peritonsillar Abscess Peritonsillar or pharyngeal abscess represents an extension of a bacterial pharyngitis (sore throat) into the surrounding soft tissue of the upper airway, particularly around the tonsils, resulting in abscess formation that can partially obstruct the airway. The patient complains of sore throat, difficulty swallowing and a change in voice, and often presents drooling. The prehospital care of these patients is supportive, with supplemental oxygen and a comfortable transport position.

Tracheomalacia Tracheomalacia is an eroding of the trachea, usually caused by excessive pressure from a cuffed endotracheal tube.

Trauma to the Airway and Neck Injury to the anterior neck and upper airway, regardless of how trivial, can result in airway compromise. Neck trauma may be associated with motor vehicle accidents, falls, hanging or penetrating injury.

An injury to the neck, blunt or penetrating, can cause hematoma formation, thyroid cartilage fracture, soft tissue avulsions in the oropharynx, vocal cord paralysis and disruption of the trachea, and can precipitate airway compromise if not recognized and treated correctly. Cervical spine fracture and head or facial injuries can also lead to respiratory compromise.

The patient with a neck injury can have soft tissue disfigurement, hemorrhage, impaled foreign bodies or subcutaneous emphysema—or can seem essentially normal, depending on the mechanism of injury. Impaired speech, stridor or difficulty breathing in the absence of chest trauma may indicate impending airway collapse. Any gross deformity of the anterior neck tissues suggests airway injury and the need for aggressive airway intervention. Mild swelling or bruising, on the other hand, should serve as a reminder to monitor the patient's respiratory status regularly in anticipation of possible airway problems. This in-

cludes assessment of the adequacy of ventilation and the patient's ability to control the flow of normal secretions.

The initial prehospital management of patients with any form of neck injury is immobilization. For a patient demonstrating airway compromise, aggressive airway intervention should take place early in the patient encounter. Delays in establishing a definitive airway may lead to distortion of the upper airway anatomy, complete obstruction and the need for a surgical procedure to reopen the airway.

Behavioral Conditions

Aggressive Disorders and Aggression Many medical and psychiatric conditions can lead to aggressive behavior on the part of emergency patients. The first priority when confronting an aggressive patient must be the overall stabilization of the scene. This includes the protection of the prehospital provider, family members or bystanders, and the patient. Following scene stabilization, the patient should be assessed for possible medical conditions causing the agitation. Aggressive patients may suffer from medical conditions that include hypoxemia, hypoglycemia and head injury. Drugs and alcohol are frequently involved in situations in which patients become aggressive.

The prehospital management of the aggressive patient includes rapid and well orchestrated physical restraint. Many restraint methods have been described in the literature, but familiarity of prehospital personnel with the restraint procedure is most important. Adequate personnel must be available to safely restrain an aggressive patient. Aggressive situations may be diffused with appropriate interviewing techniques; sympathetic listening may allow patients to ventilate their frustration verbally rather than physically. Since hostile patients may change their posture rapidly, it is important for the prehospital provider to maintain an easy exit.

Alcohol Intoxication, Alcoholism Alcoholism is a chronic disease with genetic, psychological, social and environmental influences. It typically has a slow, insidious onset that may occur at any age. It is characterized by an impaired control over drinking, preoccupation with alcohol and persistent use despite adverse consequences on an individual's life. Alcoholism is also characterized by distortions in thinking, most notably denial of the problem, and is often associated with suicide attempts, homicides and fatal accidents.

Alcohol has many toxic systemic effects. The medical consequences of alcoholism include neurologic and psychiatric disorders, gastrointestinal problems (such as gastritis, ulcers and pancreatitis), blood disorders (anemia), infections (pneumonia, hepatitis), cardiovascular complications (cardiomyopathy), and metabolic disorders (hypoglycemia). The prehospital provider must assess the patient under the

influence of alcohol for possible complications, including those mentioned above. In addition, attention must be paid to the possibility of suicide or violence. Other important considerations include head injuries, especially subdural hematoma, and other serious trauma.

Prehospital management of the alcoholic patient includes a thorough assessment for complications of the disorder, possible injuries (ABCs and cervical spine control, when indicated), blood glucose testing and transportation for evaluation in an emergency department.

Anxiety Attack, Panic Disorder Anxiety disorders are the most common psychiatric disorders found in the general population. A panic attack is characterized by a sudden onset of intense anxiety associated with a fear of impending doom. The symptoms of panic attack vary according to the individual and may include palpitations or pounding of the heart, sweating, trembling, shaking, chest pain, dizziness, tingling or numbness, and a feeling of shortness of breath or choking. Panic attacks may last from a few seconds to an hour or longer.

The prehospital assessment of the patient with the signs and symptoms of panic disorder must include a thorough evaluation for possible life-threatening conditions including cardiovascular problems, respiratory emergencies and metabolic conditions. Prehospital care should focus on providing oxygen and assessing cardiovascular status. Reassurance during transport may be helpful. Sedatives are not usually given in the prehospital setting, but may be administered at the hospital after cardiovascular, respiratory and metabolic causes are ruled out.

Conversion Disorder, Hysterical Conversion An uncommon condition called hysterical conversion, or conversion disorder, occurs when physical symptoms express an acute psychological need rather than a true medical illness. The common signs and symptoms of conversion disorder may suggest neurological problems. The symptoms are usually acute in onset and may include sudden blindness, deafness, inability to smell, choking sensation, and numbness or tingling that are frequently described as involving an entire half of the body.

Although conversion disorder present physical symptoms that reflect psychological conflict, the symptoms are not under voluntary control. Surprisingly, the patient may appear emotionally indifferent in spite of the severity of the physical condition. Causal factors include a conscious or unconscious desire to avoid an unpleasant situation.

In the prehospital setting, it is very difficult to differentiate a conversion disorder from a true medical condition. It is therefore important to treat the patient as though the medical condition described is legitimate, until further evaluation can be performed to rule out organic disease.

Depression Depression is among the most common psychiatric conditions in emergency patients. It can be life threatening when it leads to suicidal impulses.

The clinical symptoms include depressed mood and loss of interest in usual activities. Anxiety may also be present. Patients often experience sleep disturbances, inability to concentrate and loss of energy and appetite. As the depression becomes more severe, patients may become psychotically depressed and have feelings of guilt, suicidal thoughts and even delusions or hallucinations. They present with a variety of physical complaints such as low energy, headache and abdominal pain.

Depressed patients can become suicidal suddenly. Vague thoughts of death can become a preoccupation, and the patient may develop a plan for suicide. Factors that increase suicide risk include advanced age, male gender, poor physical health, alcoholism, social isolation, previous suicide attempts, previous divorce or death of a spouse, and a family history of suicide.

The prehospital management of depression should include close attention to the individual and the risk of suicide. Patients who are experiencing hallucination may require restraint. Realistic reassurance is appropriate while transporting the patient to an emergency department for evaluation and psychiatric therapy.

Drug Dependence, Drug Abuse Drug or substance abuse is defined as the pathological use of a substance that includes the patient's belief that he or she cannot function without it. The definition of substance abuse requires that the use of the substance has a pathological pattern and leads to impaired social and occupational function for at least one month.

In addition to the characteristics of substance abuse, dependance also includes the patient's growing tolerance, or need for increased amounts of the substance to achieve the desired effect, and the experience of withdrawal if use is discontinued. Unsafe preparations or unsafe quantities of the substance may be used in desperate attempts to experience the expected high from the substance.

Signs and symptoms depend upon many factors such as the substance and amount used, and the method and duration of use. Prehospital management will be supportive in general. Specific antagonists may be used when available and indicated.

Manic Depressive (Bipolar) Disorder Bipolar disorder is a major psychological illness with periods of elevated, excited, hyperactive or irritable mood that may alternate with periods of depression. Mania is described as a disorder of mood that ranges from euphoria, impaired ability to concentrate and difficulty sleeping to a completely psychotic state. The elevation of mood usually lasts at least one week. Patients will frequently have inflated self-esteem and be more talkative than usual. A constant stream of conversation is typical. Ideas are scattered and poorly organized, and the patient is easily distracted. A manic episode may also involve an excess of pleasurable activities that subsequently cause problems, such as buying sprees, sexual indiscretions or unwise business investments. In the depressive phase, extreme apathy and underactivity are accompanied by feelings of profound sadness, loneliness, guilt and lowered self-esteem.

Manic depressive disorder is frequently treated with long-term medication therapy such as lithium or anti-psychotic or anti-depressant drugs. During the acute episode, patients may require sedation. Because therapy is important and suicide is a possibility, patients should be transported to an emergency department for evaluation and possible therapy.

Post Traumatic Stress Disorder Following an extraordinary or traumatic event, individuals may suffer an emotional and psychological response known as Post Traumatic Stress Disorder (PTSD). The precipitating event may be a natural disaster such as a flood or earthquake, a human or mechanical failure such as a plane crash or fire, or a personal trauma such as a sexual assault.

The symptoms of Post Traumatic Stress Disorder consist primarily of repetitive and intrusive memories of the event, or repeating dreams. An environmental stimulus may trigger the idea that the traumatic event is recurring. For example, a victim of a sexual assault may suffer recollection of the event when she hears noises in the house or someone walking behind her on the street. In addition, the victims of post traumatic stress disorder experience a type of emotional numbness. They have diminished interest in the activities of daily living, feel detached from loved ones and have a dulled mood. These victims may suffer from sleep disturbances, be hyperalert, have guilt feelings or memory impairment and trouble concentrating, and avoid the activities that stimulate memory of the traumatic event.

The Post Traumatic Stress Disorder may be acute, with an onset less than six months of the initial event. Chronic or delayed Post Traumatic Stress Disorder has an onset of symptoms at least six months after the trauma and lasts more than six months.

The long-term complications of Post Traumatic Stress Disorder can be reduced by careful attention to the victim's psychological needs in the prehospital setting. By adopting a sympathetic attitude, providing physical shelter and companionship, and being a good listener, the prehospital worker may enable the victim to begin the process of recovery. Prehospital providers themselves are at occupation risk for exposure to this condition. Disaster workers and prehospital responders are encouraged to participate in debriefing sessions, which provide a chance to work through their own psychological responses to the disaster.

Schizophrenia, Paranoid Schizophrenia Schizophrenia includes a large group of psychotic disorders characterized by severe distortion of reality, disturbances of language and communication, withdrawal from social interaction, and disorganized thought and emotional reaction. Symptoms include apathy and confusion; delusions (false beliefs) and emotional hallucinations; rambling or stylized patterns of speech, such as evasiveness, incoherence and involuntary repetition of words or phrases; withdrawn, regressive and bizarre behavior, and severe emotional instability. The condition may be mild or require prolonged hospitalization.

Paranoid schizophrenia is characterized by persistent preoccupation with illogical, absurd, and changeable delusions, usually marked by jealousy or thoughts of persecution and accompanied by related hallucinations. The symptoms include extreme anxiety, tendency to argue, exaggerated suspicion, aggressiveness, anger, hostility and violence. Although medications can help control symptoms, complete recovery is rare.

Patients with schizophrenia and other chronic psychotic conditions frequently suffer from serious medical and social problems. These patients may seek emergency medical attention for deteriorations in their condition. These include acute psychosis, agitation, severe hallucinations, increasingly bizarre behavior, withdrawal and apathy, which often occur when medications are stopped or stress increases. In addition, the patient may experience side effects from antipsychotic medications. Often these individuals will seek emergency medical therapy because of an acute medical illness or inadequate nutrition or shelter.

Individuals with the diagnosis of schizophrenia or paranoid schizophrenia who seek medical attention should be transported for further evaluation and therapy in the emergency department. Since these patients may be paranoid or hallucinating, they may become aggressive and require physical restraint. They frequently will not be competent to determine their own medical needs, so the support of family members or police may be necessary to assure safe transportation. Local protocols should be in place regarding restraint and transportation without patient consent.

Withdrawal from Alcohol; Delirium Tremens Alcohol withdrawal syndromes can be divided into early- and late-onset conditions. The most common is early-onset withdrawal syndrome, which generally begins within the first 24 hours of abstinence. Signs and symptoms of early withdrawal include tachycardia, hypertension, diaphoresis, tremor, anxiety, restlessness, irritability, poor concentration and fever associated with symptoms of agitation. This may progress to generalized tonic-clonic seizures. Patients generally will do well with outpatient therapy, and should be taken to a hospital for initial evaluation and treatment.

Delirium tremens, a rare, severe alcohol withdrawal syndrome with later onset, is a medical emergency. It generally begins within 24 to 72 hours of cessation of alcohol. The syndrome is characterized by overactivity of the sympathetic nervous system including fever, hallucinations, anxiety, agitation, confusion, change in mental status, severe motor restlessness and even combativeness. It is occasionally fatal, usually because of volume depletion, electrolyte imbalance, infection or cardiac dysrhythmias. Patients with the signs and symptoms of delirium tremens must be transported carefully for emergency department evaluation and treatment. They frequently require restraint. In addition, they should be assessed and treated as needed for hypoglycemia, dehydration, cardiac dysrhythmias and seizures. Seizures should be treated with intravenous benzodiazepines.

Withdrawal from Drugs Withdrawal from drugs such as opioids, sedative hypnotics, and cocaine is quite common. The signs and symptoms are variable but frequently include changes in blood pressure, pulse, respiratory rate and temperature. In addition, patients will frequently experience diarrhea, anxiety, nervousness and even delirium. They also have severe cravings for the addictive agent. Prehospital therapy for drug withdrawal should include routine support and comfort measures, and transport to an emergency department for evaluation.

Cardiovascular Conditions

Acute Myocardial Infarction (AMI) Myocardial infarction ("heart attack") occurs when the blood supply to a portion of the heart muscle is completely cut off. This results in infarction (death) of that area of tissue. AMI can also occur when cardiac oxygen demand of the heart is not met for an extended period of time, even though the coronary arteries are open. Many of the deaths caused by MI can be prevented by quick paramedic intervention.

AMI is most often caused by coronary artery disease and atherosclerosis. A thrombus (blood clot) is formed, usually due to disruption of the vessel wall by atherosclerotic plaque. The thrombus may enlarge and completely occlude the involved coronary artery, cutting blood flow to tissue distal to the affected site. Coronary artery spasm—caused by cocaine use, microemboli, severe hypoperfusion or severe hypoxia—can also cause AMI.

The particular location and size of the myocardium that infarcts depend on the artery involved and the exact occlusion site. The likelihood and types of complications, in turn, depend on the area of infarct. Most MIs involve the left ventricle and are the result of a lesion somewhere in the left coronary artery, which feeds the anterior, lateral and septal walls of the heart. The right coronary artery feeds the right ventricle and the inferior wall of the left ventricle. A transmural infarction refers to infarction of the entire thickness of the myocardium, which is likely to lead to complications.

The classic symptom of AMI is chest pain, but some AMI patients never experience pain. The elderly and diabetics, in particular, have these "silent MIs." Since myocardial pain is visceral, both patients and medical personnel often have difficulty identifying it as cardiac. AMI chest pain is typically severe and substernal, and may feel like crushing, heaviness or pressure on the chest. Variations include sharp pain, chest tightness and epigastric, neck, shoulder or back pain. The pain may radiate from the chest to one of these areas, or classically to the jaw or left arm. The pain usually lasts more than ten minutes and is not relieved by rest or nitroglycerin.

Accompanying signs and symptoms include sweating, dyspnea, nausea, vomiting, dizziness, weakness, anxiety, pallor, palpitations, irregular pulse, indigestion and a sense of impending doom. The patient can present with these classic symptoms or with unimpressive and non-specific symptoms such as weakness, "not feeling well," or simply breaking out in a cold sweat. Lack of patient recognition can lead to serious delays in care and increases the patient's risk of serious complications or death.

ECG findings for an AMI patient depend on what portion of the heart is affected and the point in the MI's course at which the ECG is taken. The patient's rhythm can be anything from normal sinus rhythm to a minor or major dysrhythmia; sudden death with ventricular fibrillation is sometimes the initial presentation. A 12-lead ECG may or may not reveal the classic ST-segment elevation in the prehospital setting.

Chest pain should be evaluated for its onset, duration, severity, location and any radiating patterns. Any factors which initiated the pain or change it should also be identified. Breath sounds, vital signs and cardiac monitoring are also all important. Questions about the patient's past medical history focus on:

- if the problem has occurred before and, if so, what was done for it
- current medications
- any other medical conditions
- past surgeries

The most common complications are dysrhythmias, which develop primarily because of tissue damage and changes in the cardiac electrical system triggered by hypoxia. Dysrhythmias that reduce cardiac pumping efficiency can lead to CHF and hypoperfusion.

Direct pump damage can also cause CHF, without a dysrhythmia. Fluid then backs up in to the heart, lungs and peripheral vessels. Cardiogenic shock is the most extreme and dangerous form; the myocardium is so severely damaged that systemic shock develops. Mortality is very high in cardiogenic shock.

Less common complications of MI include cardiac rupture and ventricular aneurysm. Cardiac rupture occurs three to five days post-MI, as dead muscle fibers begin to degenerate. If ventricular wall damage is extensive, a weakened area may rupture, allowing blood to fill the pericardial sac. Death usually quickly follows the development of cardiac tamponade. With ventricular aneurysm, a weakened area in the ventricular wall "balloons" out, decreasing ventricular pumping action.

Prehospital management of AMI is aimed at minimizing the oxygen demand by eliminating physical activity and decreasing anxiety and pain as much as possible. Supplemental oxygen should be administered, an IV established and any complications managed. Aspirin is given in some EMS systems to help break up the thrombus. Quick transport to an ED is important, particularly if the patient is a candidate for thrombolytic (clot dissolving) therapy. Prehospital 12-lead ECGs and thrombolytic evaluation questionnaires can aid in quick identification of patients with the potential to benefit from thrombolytics. If they are to be effective, thrombolytics must be given during the very early stages of an MI.

Angina Pectoris Angina is a form of ischemic heart disease that presents with chest pain. It represents a mismatch between available coronary blood supply and the heart muscle's demand for oxygen. If a reversible cause underlies the ischemia, such as exercise or coronary artery spasm, the pain will resolve when that cause is removed. Precipitating factors are those activities that increase the need for oxygen such as exercise, emotional upset and digestion of a large meal.

The ischemic heart muscle causes a pain or discomfort described by the patient as heavy, squeezing, constricting, pressing or tight. The patient typically perceives the pain as being substernal, with radiation to the shoulders and arms, especially on the left side. The pain may also radiate to the back, neck, epigastrium, neck or jaw. The fact that pain can also present solely in one or more of these other areas, without associated chest pain, makes recognition of angina more difficult.

Anginal pain takes about 30 seconds to reach maximal intensity and usually lasts more than one minute. If it lasts more than 10 minutes, acute myocardial infarction (AMI) must be considered.

Stable angina is recognized in individuals with known coronary artery disease (CAD), and in whom the pain appears and is relieved under similar circumstances each time it occurs. The pain description is similar each time, and the patient knows approximately how much exertion is required to trigger it (e.g., one flight of stairs). The patient also knows what it takes to bring relief, such as rest or a certain amount of sublingual nitroglycerin. Patients can experience stable angina for many years without acute problems; when the patient indicates that the pattern has changed, special concern about evaluation and follow-up treatment are called for.

Unstable angina can occur either in a patient who has known, stable angina, or in one who has no angina history at all. Unstable angina can be identified as new exertional chest pain in a previously asymptomatic individual, new pain at rest or a distinct change in a previously stable angina pattern (more frequent, less responsive to nitroglycerin or of longer duration). Unstable angina can develop when there is sudden narrowing of a coronary artery without total blockage, caused by thrombosis or arterial spasm.

Unstable angina indicates a threat of total coronary artery occlusion and AMI.

The history of the pain is the most important factor in differentiating stable angina, unstable angina and AMI. Careful attention must be paid to past history, location, character, radiation, intensity, duration, activity at time of onset and associated symptoms. Patients who experience continuing pain must be considered to have a significant coronary artery problem. Those with accompanying diaphoresis, palpitations, syncope or light-headedness are also potentially unstable.

Physical assessment in patients with true angina may reveal no abnormalities, but all chest pain patients must be evaluated for signs of hypoperfusion, cardiac dysrhythmias and signs of acute pulmonary edema and CHF.

The goal in managing angina patients is to correct, as well as possible, the mismatch between coronary blood supply and cardiac oxygen demand. This is accomplished by decreasing the patient's activity, pain and anxiety. Allowing no exertion, place the patient in a position of comfort. Give high-flow oxygen and open an IV line at a keep-open rate. Monitor cardiac rhythm and give nitroglycerin if pain persists and blood pressure allows. The paramedic should be aware that it is often not possible to distinguish between angina and acute myocardial infarction.

Cardiac Contusion This condition is the most likely injury to the heart in blunt chest trauma. The cardiac contusion may not be obvious to the patient or paramedic without ECG monitoring, so monitoring is important for any patient with blunt chest trauma.

The contusion typically occurs when the chest strikes the steering wheel during a motor vehicle collision. The heart is compressed between the sternum and the spine, bruising (or even rupturing) the myocardial wall. A less frequent mechanism of injury is a blow to the chest by a baseball. The most common result is myocardial damage similar to that caused by an MI, including dysrhythmias from electrical system disruption. These include tachycardia (by itself a more likely sign of shock), PVCs and atrial fibrillation.

Patients with cardiac contusion are likely to have chest discomfort, which may include bruised chest muscles and fractured ribs. It is also possible, however, that there will be no significant chest or cardiac complaints.

Prehospital management includes oxygen, ECG monitoring and minimizing patient activity and anxiety, much like the management of an MI. Dysrhythmia treatment also follows the MI approach.

Cardiomyopathy Cardiomyopathy is a term used to describe dilated, poorly contractile ventricles. Alcohol, pregnancy, drugs and toxins can lead to cardiomyopathy. Some cardiomyopathies are of unknown cause. The condition may present clinically as congestive heart failure.

Congenital Heart Defects Congenital heart defects are the result of malformation of a structure, or incomplete progression of a structure to its mature, functional form. This anatomic abnormality may appear benign, particularly in childhood, but cause problems later. Two examples, bicuspid aortic valve and atrial septal defects, may be asymptomatic in childhood but become clinically significant with age.

Congenital heart disease can be characterized as either cyanotic or acyanotic, depending on the oxygenation status of the patient. Some of the more common acyanotic defects include atrial and ventricular septal defects, aortic stenosis and mitral regurgitation. Tricuspid atresia, transposition of the great vessels and Tetralogy of Fallot are cyanotic defects. Tetralogy of Fallot, which consists of four anatomic abnormalities, is the most common cause of cyanotic heart disease.

In the field, the paramedic must remember that patients with congenital heart diseases have a higher risk than others of pulmonary edema (regardless of age), sudden death and cardiac dysrhythmias. A directed history and observation of the chest for surgical scars can be very helpful. Initial treatment includes oxygenating the patient and attempting to correct any dysrhythmias that occur.

Congestive Heart Failure (CHF) Congestive heart failure is an impairment of cardiac pumping function caused by myocardial infarction, ischemic heart disease or cardiomyopathy that leads to fluid congestion of the lungs and body tissues. Heart failure is a more general term that refers to an inability of the heart to pump enough blood to meet the body's metabolic needs.

Heart failure is usually categorized as left-sided or right-sided. Most kinds of heart disease initially affect the left heart, which in turn can cause right-sided failure. Right-sided failure can also be caused by disease processes that affect the lungs or the pulmonary circulation such as COPD or pulmonary hypertension (high pressures in the pulmonary artery). This type of right-sided failure is called cor pulmonale.

Left-sided failure occurs as the left ventricle fails to pump effectively and blood backs up into the pulmonary circulation. If untreated, pulmonary edema results, with its respiratory and hypoxic signs and symptoms.

As left-sided failure causes pulmonary congestion, that congestion backs up into the right side of the heart, which also weakens and fails. Signs and symptoms of right-sided heart failure are typically systemic ones that reflect congestion of the venous system. These include jugular venous distention, peripheral edema, liver engorgement and ascites.

CHF in the pediatric patient most often occurs secondary to a congenital heart defect. (See "Congenital Heart Defects" in this section.)

Field treatment begins with oxygen, which treats hypoxia and starts the process of vasodilation. It should be given through a non-rebreather mask for the highest possible percentage of oxygen. A diuretic such as Lasix may be given en route. When given intravenously, Lasix provides venous dilation as well as its diuretic effect. Nitroglycerin's arterial dilation effect helps reduce afterload. Morphine sulfate dilates peripheral vessels, also reducing myocardial work. The airway in some patients with CHF may need to be protected with endotracheal intubation.

Coronary Artery Disease Coronary artery disease (CAD), also known as atherosclerotic cardiovascular disease, is a process that narrows the coronary arteries and may eventually lead to ischemic heart disease or acute myocardial infarction (AMI). (See Angina and AMI in this section.) Its most extreme result is sudden cardiac death secondary to acute dysrhythmias resulting from myocardial ischemia.[1,2]

This ischemia is the product of reduced coronary artery blood flow and the associated reduction of oxygen and nutrient delivery to the heart muscle. The spectrum of presentations is broad. Significant restriction of coronary perfusion may cause no acute symptoms for many years, while minor disease can present with cardiac arrest.

Several factors increase the chance of developing coronary artery disease (Box 1).

Symptoms of coronary artery disease occur when cardiac oxygen demand exceeds the supply. This can happen when there is sudden narrowing of the coronary artery, caused by thrombosis or arterial spasm, that decreases blood flow. Also, when oxygen demand increases during exercise, blood flow through a previously narrowed vessel may suddenly become inadequate. Inadequate coronary blood supply can result in transient myocardial ischemia during exercise, which causes chest pain that resolves with rest or the use of a vasodilator (angina). More significant arterial obstruction can cause infarction of the heart muscle (AMI), with the further possibility of impaired cardiac pumping function. When the progression of CAD is slow and several vessels are involved, the chronic lack of nutrients and oxygen can reduce pumping function gradually, so that the individual develops congestive heart failure without ever having an MI.

Coronary artery disease must be assessed according to signs and symptoms of the conditions it causes. If there is chest pain, the patient is evaluated for angina and acute myocardial infarction. In the presence of dyspnea, the evaluation must also rule out acute pulmonary edema and congestive heart failure. The extent of CAD can be evaluated in the hospital by cardiac stress testing, angiogram and coronary artery catheterization.

In the field, any active signs or symptoms of ischemia, such as chest pain or dyspnea, are evaluated and treated according to ACLS protocols.

References:

1. Guidelines for Cardiopulmonary Resuscitation and Emergency Cardiac Care. JAMA. 1992; 268:2221.

2. **Scott JL, et al:** Ischemia heart disease. In Rosen P, Barkin RM, et al. Emergency Medicine, ed. 3, St. Louis, Mosby-Year Book, Inc.

BOX 1	Risk Factors That Can Be Modified
* Cigarette smoking	Stress
* Hypertension	* Diabetes
* Elevated cholesterol	Family history
Elevated triglycerides	Age
Sedentary life-style	Race
Obesity	Sex

*Indicates factor that by itself increases likelihood of developing CAD.

Dysrhythmias The recognition and immediate treatment of dysrhythmias are discussed in detail in Chapters 12 and 32. A more general discussion of dysrhythmias follows.

Dysrhythmias can be classified according to electrical origin, ECG characteristics and ventricular response. Treatment, particularly in the field, depends on whether there is evidence of hypoperfusion as indicated by hypotension, chest pain suggestive of cardiac ischemia, evidence of pulmonary edema, or altered level of consciousness. If the patient exhibits signs or symptoms of an unstable dysrhythmia, field treatment is by ACLS protocol. If the patient appears stable, paramedics should transport to the nearest facility with proper resources for further evaluation and treatment. The following is a list of the basic dysrhythmias:

- Sinus tachycardia is a sinus rhythm at a rate of 100-160 beats per minute (bpm). It may be brought on by hypoxia, volume depletion, fever, pulmonary embolism, drug toxicities, pain, exercise, anxiety, and so on. It is treated by treating the underlying cause.

- Sinus bradycardia is a sinus rhythm at a rate of less than 60 bpm. It may be a normal rhythm in the conditioned athlete, or the undesirable result of inferior wall myocardial infarction, drug toxicity, severe head injury or increased intracranial pressure. It is treated only if signs of hypotension or hypoxia appear. Treatment in the field can be with atropine, or an external transcutaneous pacemaker if available.

- Junctional rhythm originates in the AV node and should have a narrow, regular QRS. If patients with junctional bradycardia or tachycardia are asymptomatic, prehospital care includes frequent monitoring of vital signs, cardiac monitoring, IV access, O_2, and transport. If the patient becomes symptomatic with junctional bradycardia, atropine or external pacing may help. Digitalis toxicity can cause junctional tachycardia. Symptomatic junctional tachycardia and bradycardia can both present with hypotension, chest pain and lowered consciousness, all indicating decreased cardiac output.

- Paroxysmal supraventricular tachycardia (PSVT) can occur in the normal—as well as the diseased—patient. The rhythm begins and ends abruptly. The patient may complain of palpitations, and the rate is usually in the range of 180-220 bpm. Hemodynamic consequences depend on the rate and the patient's ability to compensate. Attempts to convert to normal sinus rhythm can be initiated in the field with vagal maneuvers, carotid massage, adenosine or cardioversion.

- Atrial flutter typically occurs in patients with underlying heart disease, and usually reverts by itself to normal sinus rhythm or atrial fibrillation. Cardioversion is indicated in the unstable patient.

- Atrial fibrillation is an irregularly irregular atrial dysrhythmia that usually signifies underlying cardiac disease. It may cause severe cardiac failure or angina, or be asymptomatic. Because of the sluggishness of blood flow through the atria, small clots can develop and migrate to cause a stroke. Cardioversion is indicated for symptomatic hypotension in association with atrial fibrillation. Otherwise, rate control with drugs should be considered. Prehospital care includes IV access, oxygenation and frequent blood pressure checks.

- First degree atrioventricular (AV) block is a conduction prolongation at the AV node that affects all impulses to the ventricles. It is often a normal variant without clinical significance.
- Second degree AV block can be divided into types I and II. Both involve conduction problems that prevent some, but not all, atrial impulses from reaching the ventricles. Type I is a conduction defect in the AV node that can be found in a variety of conditions and usually requires no treatment. Type II second degree block is never normal; it implies a conduction defect below the AV node and the HIS Bundle or the Purkinje system. Type II block may require external transcutaneous pacing in the field. Atropine may worsen the situation and should be used with caution.
- Third degree AV block, also known as complete heart block, is a complete obstruction of electrical conduction between the atria and ventricles. Treatment in the field again depends on the presence of unstable signs or symptoms. Atropine and external pacing can be used.
- Ventricular fibrillation is an unstable rhythm with no organized electrical conduction or mechanical contraction of the heart, that is fatal if not corrected. It should be treated promptly by ACLS protocol with defibrillation. It is the electrical rhythm often associated with sudden death.
- Ventricular tachycardia, a ventricular dysrhythmia that originates in the Purkinje network, is defined as three or more consecutive ectopic ventricular beats at a rate greater than 100 bpm. If the patient is hemodynamically stable, a lidocaine bolus should be given. If unstable, the patient should be treated by ACLS protocol, beginning with cardioversion.
- Asystole is the absence of electrical activity. Treatment depends on the suspected cause, and may include medications and transcutaneous pacing.
- Pulseless electrical activity (PEA) is an organized electrical rhythm without clinical evidence of cardiac contraction or cardiac output (pulse and blood pressure). Common causes are hypovolemia, hypoxia, acidosis, cardiac tamponade, pulmonary embolism and tension pneumothorax. Epinephrine and other therapies more specific to the suspected cause are the mainstays of therapy.
- Premature ventricular contractions (PVCs) can be caused by many different factors. PVCs themselves are asymptomatic, except that the patient may feel palpitations or an irregular heart beat. Their presence is less important than the clinical scenario, such as the possibility of a myocardial infarction that may cause progression to more serious ventricular dysrhythmias (ventricular tachycardia or fibrillation). Field therapy for PVCs is directed toward the underlying cause.
- Premature atrial contractions (PACs) are usually the precipitating event for other atrial dysrhythmias. Prehospital management is based on recognition of underlying the cause and treatment of more serious rhythms. No therapy is necessary for PACs themselves.
- Premature junctional contractions (PJCs) are the result

either of altered automaticity or nodal re-entry. Treatment of PJCs is the same as for PACs.

Endocarditis Endocarditis is inflammation of the endocardium (membrane line of the heart). Its causes can be non-infective, such as systemic lupus erythematosus, or infectious, such as bacteria (streptococcus and staphylococcus are the most common). Patients who use intravenous drugs are at particular risk. Patients with infective endocarditis may complain of malaise, weakness, fatigue, fever, new-onset congestive heart failure, headaches and back, muscle and joint pain. The most important complication of infective endocarditis is heart failure secondary to involvement of the valves. Prehospital management includes oxygen, limiting patient activity and immediate transport to a hospital.

Hypertension Hypertension is usually defined as a diastolic blood pressure greater than 90 mm of mercury or a systolic blood pressure above 140. Patients with hypertension have an increased incidence of stroke, cardiac events, renal disease and early death.

Sympathetic nervous system hyperactivity, salt intake, alcohol, cigarettes and the renin-angiotensin are just a few conditions that have been implicated in essential hypertension, in which there is no identified cause. Hypertension can also be the result of renal disease, endocrine disorders or an adrenal gland tumor, in which case the term secondary hypertension is used.

Signs and symptoms of mild to moderate hypertension are often absent, but can include lightheadedness, ringing in the ears and pulsating headaches. More accelerated hypertension or malignant hypertension may present with drowsiness, visual disturbances, nausea and vomiting. Patients with long-standing hypertension can present with pulmonary edema and dysrhythmias. Hypertensive crisis (usually defined as a diastolic pressure higher than 120 mm Hg) triggers a clinical situation in which rapid reduction of blood pressure is necessary to prevent serious complications. Hypertensive crisis is an emergency characterized by severe hypertension in association with neurological signs or symptoms such as severe headaches, blurred vision confusion, pulmonary edema, congestive heart failure or stroke.

In the prehospital setting, assessment for life threatening complications of hypertension is important. These include pulmonary edema, cerebral bleeding, seizures, cardiac dysrhythmias, cardiac ischemia and hypertensive encephalopathy, among others.

Prehospital management includes IV access and oxygen. If the patient is acutely hypertensive with signs or symptoms of hypertensive crisis, a nitrate or nifedipine can be given in an attempt to lower blood pressure. Lasix causes initial venous dilation that may be helpful before its later diuretic effect sets in.

Myocarditis Myocarditis is an inflammatory reaction involving the heart muscle that can result from radiation, chemicals, drugs and infections. Clinical manifestations can be non-specific, such as dyspnea or fatigue, or ECG abnormalities such as ST elevation; dysrhythmias may also be present. Heart failure and death can also occur. Prehospital treatment is aimed at managing signs and symptoms.

Pericardial Tamponade Pericardial tamponade is an accumulation of blood or fluid in the pericardial sac. It can be caused by infections, rupture of the myocardial wall or tumors of the pericardium. The result is insufficient cardiac output because the heart is being compressed by the fluid and blood return is impaired. Patients may present with distended neck veins, weak peripheral pulses, decreased heart sounds, jugular venous distention, tachycardia and pulsus paradoxus (a drop in systolic blood pressure of 10 mm mercury or more upon inspiration).

Pericardiocentesis, aspiration of the fluid in the pericardial sac, is the treatment. Otherwise, there is little to do in the field except to transport quickly and support vital functions.

Pericarditis Pericarditis is an inflammatory response that involves the membrane covering of the heart, the pericardium. It can be initiated by infections, cancer, toxin, radiation or drugs, or occur post-myocardial infarction. Clinically, pericarditis may present as right heart failure when a constriction is present. Prehospital management includes ECG monitoring and observation for pericardial tamponade.

Valvular Heart Disease, Rheumatic Heart Disease The four valves of the heart normally open fully and close completely to promote the forward flow of blood. Any one of the four valves can become narrowed (stenotic) or leaky (regurgitant) through a congenital lesion or an acquired process. Stenosis is defined as narrowing of the vascular opening. Regurgitation is the backward flow of blood that occurs as a result of incomplete valve closure. The mechanical abnormalities cause the chamber of the heart ahead of valve to increase its workload in order to maintain adequate flow through the abnormal valve. The increased workload can initially be compensated for by myocardial muscle enlargement. As the valvular disease progresses, though, the myocardium can decompensate and cause a reduction of cardiac output, decreased coronary artery perfusion and overall impairment of oxygen delivery.

Rheumatic fever is an autoinflammatory reaction precipitated by a streptococcal infection. The exact mechanism is still not known, but apparently certain proteins found in streptococcus bacteria trigger an inflammatory response in connective tissue in the heart, joints, central nervous system and skin. The inflammatory process in the heart is termed rheumatic heart disease. It can appear acutely as new mitral aortic regurgitation murmur and, in more severe cases, pericarditis and congestive heart failure.

Other possible signs are tachycardia out of proportion to the amount of fever, extra heart sounds, dysrhythmias and varying degrees of heart block.

Endocrine Conditions

Adrenal Disorders The adrenal glands are located over the kidneys. They are composed of the outer adrenal cortex and inner adrenal medulla. The adrenal medulla, part of the sympathetic nervous system, secretes epinephrine and norepinephrine. The adrenal cortex is responsible for glucocorticoid and mineralocorticoid hormone secretion. Excess adrenocortical hormone secretion will present as Cushing's syndrome. This may also occur due to prolonged use of steroid medications. Patients present with classic truncal obesity, round "moon" face and "buffalo" hump. They may show weakness, edema, and hypertension, and complain of fatigue and easy bruising.

Progressive hypofunction of the adrenal cortex is called Addison's disease. This is a rare disorder with insidious onset, characterized by easy fatigue, weakness, nausea and vomiting, weight loss, hypotension and hypoglycemia. If the adrenal glands are stressed when their reserve is exhausted from chronic hypoadrenalism, adrenal crisis can result. This may also occur if a patient is taking long-term steroids and stops suddenly. These patients appear ill, weak and confused, can be hypotensive with weak pulses, and have increased temperature and abdominal pain.

Prehospital treatment would be supportive. Definitive treatment of adrenal crisis is steroid replacement.

Diabetes Mellitus, Hyperglycemia, Hypoglycemia Diabetes mellitus is a disorder of carbohydrate (sugar) metabolism.

Glucose in the blood needs to be transported into the cell for the body to utilize it. Insulin, a hormone, secreted by the pancreas, is responsible for transport of glucose into the cell.

There are two forms of diabetes mellitus, Type I and Type II. Type I, insulin dependent diabetes mellitus (IDDM), requires insulin injections for survival as the insulin secreting beta-cells of the pancreas weaken or fail. Onset is usually during childhood, called "juvenile onset," and these patients have a tendency to become ketotic (diabetic ketoacidosis) when stressed.

Type II, non-insulin dependent diabetes mellitus (NIDDM), is due to a resistance in the body's insulin receptors to the action of insulin. Because there is generally enough insulin available to the body to prevent ketosis, these patients can usually survive without added insulin. Onset is most often during the adult years (adult onset) among obese patients. NIDDM is commonly managed with diet and oral hypoglycemic agents; most patients do not require insulin injections.

Diabetics with well controlled sugar levels can live long, functional lives. However, there are many long-term complications, especially in the poorly controlled diabetic. Complications include accelerated arteriosclerosis, kidney failure, neuropathies and blindness.

The few emergencies associated with diabetic patients can be grouped into hyperglycemic and hypoglycemic categories. Normal blood glucose levels are in the range of

80-120 mg/dl. Above that level, patients are said to be hyperglycemic, but generally are not symptomatic until the level rises to 350 mg/dl or higher.

There is a spectrum from simple hyperglycemia, through diabetic ketoacidosis (DKA) into diabetic coma (hyperglycemic, hyperosmotic coma with ketosis). As the names imply, these conditions are associated with elevated blood glucose levels that may arise from inadequate insulin dose, previously undiagnosed diabetes mellitus, or the stress of trauma, steroids or infection. Hyperglycemia has a gradual onset and is characterized by fatigue and increased thirst, appetite and urination. As glucose levels rise patients can develop DKA and experience nausea, vomiting, abdominal pain and dehydration. They may grow confused, or even comatose (diabetic coma) with the classic rapid, deep breathing of Kussmaul's respirations. The latter are the body's attempt to normalize pH and blow off CO_2 in response to ketoacidosis. The breath classically will have a fruity, acetone odor.

Hyperglycemic Hyperosmotic Non-Ketotic Coma Hyperglycemic hyperosmotic non-ketotic coma occurs in NIDDM patients, often the elderly. Precipitating events may include stroke, stress from infection or surgery, or drugs such as steroids or diuretics. Many presenting signs and symptoms are similar to those of DKA, including weakness and fatigue, thirst, frequent urination, dehydration, confusion and coma. However, in the absence of ketosis there will be no Kussmaul's respirations. Blood glucose levels are often much higher than in DKA, from 800 up to 2400 mg/dl.

There are multiple causes of hypoglycemia in the diabetic patient, the most common being excess insulin (insulin shock). Severe hypoglycemia may result from excess insulin injection, a delay in eating after insulin injections, excess physical activity or exercise, or variable absorption from injection sites. Hypoglycemia may also occur in patients taking oral hypoglycemic medications, whose effects are less predictable and longer lasting than those of injected insulin.

Presentation of hypoglycemia can be correlated to the blood glucose level. Moderate hypoglycemia (30-50 mg/dl) may present with signs and symptoms of "shock", tachycardia and diaphoretic, cold, clammy skin. This is the response of the sympathetic nervous system and may not be present if the patient is taking beta-blockers. The patient may complain of hunger, be irritable, uncooperative or confused, or have numbness of the face or hands.

Severe hypoglycemia (< 30-35 mg/dl) manifests primarily as central nervous system impairment: confusion, bizarre behavior, seizures and unresponsiveness. Occasionally the presentation includes focal neurologic signs, such as one-sided weakness or slurred speech. Checking a blood glucose level will help differentiate this from stroke and confirm the need for immediate sugar replacement.

Prehospital management of diabetic emergencies is aimed at the ABCs. Protect the airway, give supplemental oxygen—especially with seizures—and establish IV access. When starting the IV, obtain a sample tube of blood for lab evaluation of serum glucose, and immediately measure the blood glucose if prehospital method is available.

Assume dehydration if the patient is hyperglycemia, especially > 350-400 mg/dl. Volume resuscitation with normal saline or Ringer's lactate solution is indicated. Ultimately, these patients will require insulin in addition to continued volume replacement. Bicarbonate is not appropriate. The acidosis will correct with fluid and electrolyte replacement and insulin.

For the hypoglycemic adult, treat with IV Dextrose. Patients should be functioning normally in 5-10 minutes. Pediatric patients should not receive a concentration greater than D25. If IV access is unobtainable, IM glucagon is the alternative. If the patient is alert and refusing treatment or transport, give sugar and then feed a more complex carbohydrate meal. A quick boost of sugar without a prolonged carbohydrate load will end again in hypoglycemia. (See Chapter 35.)

Hypoglycemia, Alcoholic Alcohol-induced hypoglycemia is usually seen in poorly nourished chronic alcoholics. On occasion it can be seen in binge drinkers, or in children when first exposed to alcohol. Alcohol also acts as a diuretic and can cause dehydration. Management of alcoholic hypoglycemia begins with the ABCs, including IV access and volume replacement with normal saline or Ringer's lactate solution. When a patient who has consumed alcohol also has an altered level of consciousness, a blood glucose level should be checked. Hypoglycemia should be treated with dextrose. In addition, thiamine may need to be given to prevent Wernicke-Korsakoff syndrome if transport time to the emergency department is prolonged.

Thyroid Disorders, Hypothyroid, Hyperthyroid The thyroid is an endocrine gland located in the anterior neck over the thyroid cartilage. The majority of patients with profoundly abnormal thyroid gland function have a known, long standing history of hypo- or hyperthyroidism.

Hypothyroidism can be described as a progressive slowing of all bodily functions due to a deficiency in thyroid hormone. The most severe, life-threatening presentation is myxedema coma. Myxedema coma is characterized by swelling of the hands, face, feet, and periorbital tissues, as well as coma. The other extreme of this disease spectrum, hyperthyroidism, is seen with an over-active thyroid gland. Thyrotoxicosis is an increase in body functions, and thyroid storm is an exaggeration to the level of a life-threatening emergency. Thyrotoxicosis, also known as Grave's disease, may present as tachycardia or new-onset atrial fibrillation without previous cardiac disease. The eyes may appear to bulge and stare, with the lids retracted. Patients can be anxious, tremulous and sweating.

Thyrotoxicosis with fever, cardiac decompensation, CNS dysfunction and gastrointestinal symptoms is thyroid storm. The patient will be febrile, > 104°F or 40°C. The pulse pressure will widen, the heartbeat will be rapid and forceful and congestive heart failure can follow. The patient may be weak, agitated or confused, or even seem psychotic. GI symptoms of nausea, vomiting, diarrhea and abdominal pain and dehydration may also be present.

The prehospital management of thyroid emergencies is supportive care. The basic ABCs, including cardiac monitoring and IV access, are the mainstays of care during rapid transport to an emergency department.

Environmentally Related Conditions

Air Embolism Air embolism occurs when a diver breathing compressed gas at depth (as shallow as 4 feet) holds his or her breath while ascending. The air trapped in the lungs expands, rupturing alveoli and forcing air into the circulation. This may lead to impaired circulation, hypoxia, or neurologic deficits. (See Chapter 44.)

Barotrauma Barotrauma is physical injury as a result of exposure to increased environmental pressure. This increased pressure can effect the lungs, paranasal sinuses or inner ear.

Decompression Sickness (DCS) (the Bends, Caisson Disease) Also known as the "bends" or caisson disease, DCS is a painful, sometimes fatal syndrome caused by the formation of nitrogen bubbles in the tissues of divers who move too rapidly from higher-to lower-pressure environments. Nitrogen breathed in air under pressure dissolves in tissue fluids. When external pressure drops too rapidly, nitrogen comes out of solution faster than it can be circulated to the lungs for expiration. Nitrogen bubbles accumulate in the joint spaces and peripheral circulation, impairing tissue oxygenation. Disorientation, severe pain, syncope or neurologic deficits may follow. Treatment is rapid return of the patient to an environment of higher pressure, in a hyperbaric chamber, followed by gradual decompression.

Drowning, Near-Drowning and Post-Immersion Syndrome Drowning is death by submersion in a liquid. Near-drowning is a submersion accident after which the patient survives for at least 24 hours. The return of consciousness does not necessarily assure recovery. Intensive supportive therapy may be required for several days. Post-immersion syndrome, or "secondary drowning," is respiratory distress after an initial period of apparent recovery from near-drowning. This syndrome usually occurs within 12 hours of rescue but can be delayed for as long as 72 hours. Because of the possible delay in presentation of symptoms, hospital evaluation is mandatory after any submersion accident. (See Chapter 44.)

Frostbite Frostbite is the formation of ice crystals in tissue fluids after exposure to extreme cold. It is first recognized by pallor of exposed skin surfaces, particularly the nose, ears, fingers and toes. Vasoconstriction and damage to blood vessels impair local circulation and result in anoxia, edema, blisters and necrosis. Gentle warming is appropriate treatment; rubbing of the affected part should be avoided. Therapy for damaged tissue is similar to treatment of thermal burns. (See Chapter 43.)

Heat Cramps Heat cramps are any cramps or painful spasms of the arm, leg or abdominal muscles caused by depletion salt. The condition usually occurs after vigorous physical exertion in an extremely hot environment, or under other conditions that cause profuse sweating and depletion of fluids and electrolytes. The victim should be moved to a cooler place, given liquids, and kept inactive. (Also see Chapter 43.)

Heat Exhaustion Heat exhaustion, also called heat prostration, is characterized by weakness, dizziness, nausea, muscle cramps and altered level of consciousness. It is caused by depletion of body fluid and electrolytes following exposure to intense heat, and can be compounded by an inability to acclimate (adapt) to heat. Body temperature is near normal. Blood pressure may drop but usually returns to normal as the person is placed in a horizontal position. The skin is cool, clammy and pale. The patient usually recovers with rest and replacement of water and electrolytes. (See Chapter 43.)

Heat Stroke (Sun Stroke) Heat stroke, or sun stroke, is a severe and sometimes fatal condition that involves failure of the body's temperature regulating capacity caused by prolonged exposure to the sun or high temperatures. Reduction or cessation of sweating is an early symptom in classic heat stroke although sweating will be present in exertional heat stroke. Body temperature of 105°F or higher, tachycardia, hot skin, headache, confusion, unconsciousness and convulsions may be present. Treatment includes rapid cooling and fluid replacement. (Also see Chapter 43.)

High-Altitude Cerebral Edema (HACE) The most severe form of acute high-altitude illness; characterized by a progression of global cerebral signs in the presence of acute mountain sickness that are probably related to increased intracranial pressure. (See Chapter 43.)

High-Altitude Pulmonary Edema (HAPE) A noncardiac pulmonary edema thought to be related, at least in part, to increased pulmonary artery pressure that develops in response to hypoxia; results in increased pulmonary arteriolar permeability, and in leakage of fluid into extravascular locations. (See Chapter 43.)

High-Altitude Sickness Also called acute mountain sickness, high-altitude sickness occurs when an individual ascends too high (above 8,200 feet), too quickly. Environmental oxygen is less available at higher altitudes; the result is decreased oxygen saturation in the blood. As the body attempts to compensate, symptoms can range from dizziness, nausea and vomiting to pulmonary and cerebral edema. Treatment is aimed at descent to a lower altitude. (Also see Chapter 43.)

Hyperthermia Hyperthermia is a higher than normal body temperature. Causes and related factors include exposure to a hot environment, vigorous activity, medications—including anesthesia—inappropriate clothing, increased metabolic rate, illness, trauma, dehydration and inability or decreased ability to perspire. (See Chapter 43.)

Hypothermia Hypothermia is a core temperature below 95°F (35°C), usually caused by prolonged exposure to cold. Respiration is shallow and slow, and the pulse is faint and slow. The person will be pale and may appear to be dead. Patients who are very young or old, have cardiovascular problems or are under the influence of alcohol are most suscep-

tible to hypothermia. Treatment is slow rewarming. Hospitalization is necessary to evaluate and treat any metabolic abnormalities. (See Chapter 43.)

Immersion Syndrome Immersion syndrome is sudden death that occurs as a result of contact with water, usually cold water. It is probably the result of severe bradycardia or cardiac arrest with subsequent loss of consciousness. Alcohol ingestion is thought to be an important predisposing factor.

Pulmonary Over-Pressurization Syndrome Pulmonary over-pressurization syndrome, or "burst lung," occurs when a scuba diver does not exhale sufficiently during ascent. Expanding gas can reach the point where the lungs burst. Air can then leak from the lungs into the surrounding tissue and cause pneumothorax, pneumopericardium or pneumomediastinum. (See Chapter 43.)

Eye, Ear, Nose and Throat Conditions

Cataracts A cataract is an abnormal, progressive loss of transparency in the lens of the eye. A gray-white opacity can be seen in the lens. Most cataracts are caused by degenerative changes that usually begin after 50 years of age. The tendency to develop cataracts is inherited. Trauma, such as a puncture wound, may result in cataract formation; less often, exposure to poisons can cause them. If cataracts are untreated, sight is eventually lost. Vision is blurred at onset; later, bright lights glare diffusely, and distortion and double vision may develop. Uncomplicated cataracts of old age are usually treated with surgical removal of the lens and prescription of special contact lenses or glasses.

Conjunctivitis Conjunctivitis, or "pinkeye" inflammation of the conjunctiva, is caused by bacterial or viral infection, allergy or environmental factors. Red eyes, a thick discharge, sticky eyelids in the morning, and inflammation without pain are characteristic of infectious causes. Allergic conjunctivitis presents with redness, swelling, itching and clear, tear-like discharge. The cause may be found by microscopic examination or bacteriologic culture of a specimen of the discharge. Treatment at the hospital depends on the causative agent and may include antibacterial agents, antibiotics or corticosteroids. As this condition may be contagious, body substance isolation should be used, including good handwashing technique.

Corneal Abrasion or Ulcer Scratching from a contact lens or a foreign body on the corneal surface is often the cause of corneal abrasion or ulceration. Eye pain, sometimes severe, the sensation of a foreign body under the upper eye

lid, excessive tearing and sensitivity to light are typical complaints. Prehospital management includes irrigation with normal saline and patching both eyes.

Epistaxis (Nosebleed) Epistaxis can be caused by local irritation of mucous membranes, violent sneezing, fragility of the mucous membrane or the arterial walls, chronic infection, trauma, leukemia, vitamin K deficiency, other clotting disorders, or picking of the nose. Hypertension is commonly associated with hypertension but is not usually considered a cause. Epistaxis may result from rupture of tiny vessels in the anterior nasal septum; this occurs most frequently in early childhood and adolescence. In adults, it occurs more commonly in men than in women and may be severe in elderly persons. It can be accompanied by respiratory distress, apprehension, restlessness, vertigo, nausea or syncope, and may lead to hypoperfusion.

The patient with epistaxis is instructed to breathe through the mouth, sit quietly with the head tilted slightly forward to prevent blood from entering the pharynx, and avoid swallowing blood. The bleeding may be controlled by pinching the nose firmly with the fingers, occluding the blood supply to the nostrils or placing an ice compress over the nose. Pressure with both thumbs under the nostrils and above the lip may block the main artery supplying blood to the nose. Less commonly, nosebleed occurs from sites in the posterior nasopharynx. In these cases, bleeding cannot be controlled by applying pressure to the nasal septum. These are serious emergencies requiring rapid transport to a hospital.

Glaucoma Glaucoma is an elevated pressure within an eye caused by obstruction of the outflow of aqueous humor, the clear fluid circulating in the eye. Acute closed-angle, or narrow-angle, glaucoma occurs when the pupil in an eye with a narrow angle between the iris and cornea dilates markedly, causing the folded iris to block the exit of aqueous humor from the anterior chamber. Acute glaucoma is accompanied by extreme eye pain, blurred vision, a red eye and a dilated pupil. Nausea and vomiting may occur. If untreated, acute glaucoma results in complete and permanent blindness within two to five days.

Chronic or open angle glaucoma, the more common form, may produce no symptoms except for gradual loss of peripheral vision over a period of years. Sometimes headaches, blurred vision and dull pain in the eye are present. Halos around lights and central blindness are late manifestations. Chronic glaucoma can usually be controlled with eye drops such as pilocarpine.

Acute glaucoma is treated in the hospital with eye drops to constrict the pupil and draw the iris away from the cornea, and other agents to lower intraocular pressure and reduce fluid formation. Prehospital management of suspected acute glaucoma is rapid transportation to the hospital.

Globe (Eyeball) Penetration or Rupture Penetration or rupture occurs when a foreign object or external force penetrates or disrupts the integrity of the globe. Any pressure on an open globe will push out ocular contents, leading to loss of the eye. Prehospital treatment is aimed at preventing any contact with the globe by placing a metal shield or other protective eye cup over the orbital rim, and patching the other eye to prevent consensual eye movement. The patient should be made comfortable in a supine position.

Hyphema Hyphema is bleeding into the anterior chamber of the eye, in front of the iris and pupil. Although it appears alarming, hyphema is not an emergency. It does require evaluation by an ophthalmologist.

Otitis Inflammation or infection occurs both in the inner ear (otitis media) and the external ear canal (otitis externa). Otis media is common in infants and young children. Irritability, difficulty sleeping, pain, fever and loss of hearing are typical symptoms. If sufficient pressure builds up behind the tympanic membrane, severe pain will be present and rupture can occur. Otis media sometimes leads to meningitis or intracranial abscess, and chronic otitis media can result in permanent hearing loss. Management usually consists of systemic antibiotics. Otitis externa commonly occurs in swimmers and is treated with antibiotic ear drops.

Pharyngitis Pharyngitis, inflammation or infection of the pharynx, usually presents as sore throat. Some causes are herpes simplex virus, infectious mononucleosis, streptococcal infection and diphtheria. Specific treatment depends on the cause. Bacterial pharyngitis is treated by antibiotics. Symptoms may be relieved by analgesic medication, warm or cold drinks, or saline irrigation of the throat.

Retinal Artery Occlusion Retinal artery occlusion is an eye emergency triggered when a traveling blood clot occludes the blood supply to an eye. Painless vision loss is the hallmark. Immediate transportation to a hospital is necessary to preserve vision.

Retinal Detachment When the retina pulls away from the posterior wall of the eye, the patient may describe a dark curtain coming down that obstructs part of the visual field. This is an emergency that requires immediate transportation to a hospital.

Sinusitis Sinusitis is an inflammation of one or more of the paranasal sinuses. It may be a complication of an upper respiratory or dental infection or be caused by allergy, external pressure changes (air travel, scuba diving, underwater swimming) or a structural defect of the nose. Swelling of the nasal mucous membranes may obstruct the openings from the sinuses to the nose, resulting in an accumulation of sinus secretions that cause pressure, pain, headache, fever and local tenderness. Complications include spread of infection to bone, brain or meninges. Treatment includes steam inhalations, nasal decongestants, analgesics and, if infection is present, antibiotics.

Tonsillitis Tonsillitis is an infection or inflammation of a tonsil. Acute tonsillitis, frequently caused by streptococcus infection, is characterized by severe sore throat, fever, headache, malaise, difficulty swallowing, earaches and enlarged, tender lymph nodes in the neck. Acute tonsillitis may accompany scarlet fever. Treatment includes systemic antibiotics, analgesics and warm irrigations of the throat. Tonsillectomy is sometimes performed for recurrent tonsillitis or tonsillar abscess.

Fluid & Electrolyte Conditions

Calcium Level Disturbances Hypocalcemia is rarely life threatening and usually associated with renal failure, diuretics or decreased calcium absorption. Signs and symptoms may be present with severe hypocalcemia, including tetany, abdominal and muscle cramps, carpopedal spasms and seizures. Treatment of symptomatic hypocalcemia is calcium replacement with calcium chloride or calcium gluconate.

Hypercalcemia may be life threatening and is associated with multiple conditions. The signs and symptoms are nonspecific, ranging from anorexia, vomiting and abdominal pain to generalized weakness and CNS depression.

Treatment is aimed at decreasing serum calcium level with diuretics and volume administration, both of which increase urinary calcium excretion.

Dehydration Dehydration is a clinical presentation of hypovolemia. There will often be a history of poor fluid intake or excess fluid losses. These can be from the GI tract, after prolonged vomiting and diarrhea; renal losses from diuresis, or excess insensible losses such as sweating. Clinically dehydrated patients will have dry mucous membranes, thirst, poor skin tone or poor skin turgor, sunken eyes, concentrated urine and signs of circulatory compromise. Treatment is volume replacement.

Fluid Volume Disturbances, Hypervolemia, Hypovolemia Hypovolemia, or volume depletion, may produce circulatory compromise manifested with tachycardia, narrowed pulse pressure, orthostatic hypotension and shock. Treatment is volume replacement.

Hypervolemia, or excess body water (overhydration), will present as peripheral edema and circulatory overload with jugular venous distention and headache. Pulmonary edema and electrolyte disturbances are also possible. Extreme cases may present with coma and seizures. Treatment includes supportive care appropriate to presenting signs, and caution to minimize IV fluid administration.

Magnesium Level Disturbances Hypomagnesemia has a presentation similar to hypocalcemia, with jerky movements and hyperexcitability. Alcoholics and patients on diuretics are prone to hypomagnesemia. They may be tachycardiac and have ventricular dysrhythmias. Treatment is magnesium replacement, normally done in the ED.

Hypermagnesemia is usually only seen in patients with renal failure. They may be nauseous and confused, and have progressive muscle weakness and hypotension. Treatment includes IV hydration with normal saline or Ringer's lactate solution and, ultimately, dialysis.

Metabolic Acidosis, Alkalosis Inadequate tissue perfusion leads to anaerobic metabolism, lactic acid formation and metabolic acidosis. Other causes of metabolic acidosis include gastrointestinal and kidney disease, diabetic and alcoholic ketoacidosis, aspirin poisoning and other toxic ingestions. The patient with metabolic acidosis may have deep, rapid respiration, which represents an attempt to eliminate carbon dioxide and compensate for the accumulated acids in the body. The increased respiratory effort may lead to a feeling of dyspnea. Patients may also present with a decreased level of consciousness, disorientation and signs of shock such as tachycardia and hypotension. Prehospital treatment should include airway maintenance, oxygenation and—if needed—hyperventilation to compensate for any respiratory component of the acidosis. Volume expansion will increase tissue perfusion. Bicarbonate may be given if the acidosis is profound or during a prolonged cardiac arrest resuscitation.

Metabolic alkalosis is due to the loss of free hydrogen (H^+) ions, often from prolonged vomiting or renal disease.

Volume replacement with normal saline or Ringer's lactate solution is the mainstay of therapy.

Potassium Level Disturbances, Hyperkalemia, Hypokalemia Alterations in serum potassium levels are common and have a profound effect on cardiac muscle. Hypokalemia is usually due to GI losses, starvation, poor intake or diuretic use. Neuromuscular symptoms such as skeletal muscle weakness are present with mild to moderate hypokalemia. Severe depletion affects cardiac function. ECG changes seen include SVT and PVCs especially if the patient is taking digoxin, and unexplained, refractory ventricular tachycardia or ventricular fibrillation. Prehospital management is primarily supportive care, including treating dysrhythmias; definitive treatment at the hospital is potassium replacement.

ECG changes with hyperkalemia include peaked T waves, widened QRS complex and ventricular fibrillation. Prehospital management depends on the severity and the specific ECG changes. Diuretics such as furosemide will cause the patient to excrete potassium in the urine. Calcium administration counteracts the neuromuscular effects of hyperkalemia, while bicarbonate and D50 help shift potassium into the cells.

Respiratory Acidosis, Alkalosis Respiratory acidosis is produced by hypoventilation and CO_2 retention secondary to pulmonary insufficiency or CNS depression. Signs and symptoms include hypoxemia, cyanosis, irritability, headache, confusion, lethargy and coma. Treatment is aimed at maintaining adequate ventilation by assisting with bag-valve-mask, and intubating and hyperventilating if necessary.

Respiratory alkalosis is caused by acute hyperventilation. This can be precipitated by anxiety, pain, pulmonary embolism, sepsis or underlying metabolic acidosis. Patients may experience symptomatic hypocalcemia as numbness and muscle contractions leading to carpopedal spasms. Treatment is to correct the underlying problem, calm the patient and slow the breathing.

Sodium Level Disturbances, Hypernatremia, Hyponatremia Alterations in the concentration of serum sodium below the normal level is hyponatremia. Hyponatremic patients may have a history of diuretic use, vomiting and diarrhea, or kidney, heart or liver disease. The signs and symptoms are usually nonspecific and range from thirst, weakness and muscle cramps to confusion, seizures and coma.

Hypernatremia, a serum sodium level above normal, is less common and usually seen in very young or old patients. Often associated with central nervous system or renal disease, its signs and symptoms range from lethargy, confusion and restlessness to seizures and coma. These patients may appear dehydrated.

Prehospital management for both includes treating the accompanying dehydration with IV fluids, addressing any mental status changes and giving supportive care. Specific management depends on the serum sodium level.

Gastrointestinal Conditions

Appendicitis Appendicitis is inflammation of the appendix, a hollow muscular tube in the right lower abdomen at the junction of the ileum and the colon.

Almost all patients with appendicitis present with pain. The pain can begin diffusely before localizing, most commonly to the right lower quadrant. Patients also may develop loss of appetite, nausea, vomiting, low-grade fever, diarrhea, constipation, bloating and abdominal tenderness. Peritonitis and shock are also possible if the appendix ruptures.

Prehospital management includes an intravenous line, oxygen and transport to the nearest facility.

Cholecystitis, Gallbladder Disease Cholecystitis is inflammation of the gallbladder that can occur acutely or chronically. Patients usually complain of right upper abdominal pain, nausea, vomiting, fever and anorexia.

Cirrhosis Cirrhosis is the result of liver tissue destruction and the formation of scar tissue in its place. If enough damage occurs, liver failure may follow. Causes include infection, drugs and metabolic disorders. Alcohol is also a major cause.

Patients with cirrhosis may report or present with fatigue, malaise, anorexia, easy bruising, easy bleeding, jaundice, increased abdominal girth, gastrointestinal bleeding, jaundice or hepatic encephalopathy (altered mental status from inability of the damaged liver to remove toxins from the blood).

Assessment of mental status and vital signs is important, as is prompt initiation of any therapy that they indicate.

Crohn's Disease, Ulcerative Colitis These diseases are inflammatory diseases of the bowel affecting different anatomic sites within the gastrointestinal tract. Patients with these diseases present with abdominal pain, loss of appetite, diarrhea and rectal spasm. Passage of bloody stool is more common in ulcerative colitis than Crohn's disease. Prehospital care includes volume resuscitation and transport.

Diverticulitis Diverticulitis is defined as inflammation of diverticula, sac-like protrusions of the lining of the large intestine through its own muscle layer. Patients with diverticulitis typically have left lower quadrant pain, usually after a meal. Signs include low-grade fever and bloody stool. Prehospital treatment is limited to vital signs stabilization.

Esophageal Varices Esophageal varices are swollen veins at the lower end of the esophagus, caused by scarring in the liver. This disease most commonly presents with upper GI hemorrhage and can be life threatening if the bleeding is not stopped. Prehospital management includes IV fluid replacement and rapid transport to an emergency department.

Esophagitis Esophagitis is inflammation of the esophagus initiated by vomiting, infections, caustic substances, drugs, toxins or gastric reflux. The condition can lead to severe bleeding.

Evisceration Evisceration is the protrusion of an internal organ through a wound or surgical incision, especially in the abdominal wall.

Gastritis Gastritis is an inflammatory process involving the lining of the stomach. Gastritis is a common source of upper GI bleeding, and is occasionally fatal. The common agents that cause gastritis include alcohol and non-steroidal anti-inflammatory drugs.

Gastroenteritis Gastroenteritis, an inflammation of the gastrointestinal tract, consists of diarrhea, nausea, and vomiting that can be brought on by drugs and a number of infectious organisms. Prehospital care primarily involves stabilizing vital signs, which can usually be accomplished with IV fluid administration.

Gastrointestinal Bleeding Gastrointestinal (GI) bleeding is any bleeding in the GI tract. GI bleeding can be subdivided into upper gastrointestinal (UGI) bleeding and lower gastrointestinal (LGI) bleeding, depending on the site of hemorrhage. If bleeding occurs above the suspensory ligament of the duodenum, the term UGI bleed is used. Hemorrhage below this ligament is called LGI bleeding. Gastrointestinal bleeding primarily affects persons ages 50-80. UGI bleeds occur more frequently in men, and LGI bleeds are more common in women.

The causes of GI bleeding are varied. Peptic ulcer disease accounts for almost half of significant GI bleeds. Other causes of significant GI bleeding include gastritis, esophageal varices, Mallory-Weiss tear, inflammation of the esophagus and duodenum, diverticulitis, undiagnosed cancer, rectal disease and inflammatory bowel disease.

Patients with significant GI bleeding can present with a wide range of signs and symptoms. Duration and chronicity of bleeding both affect how a patient presents. In chronic bleeding, a patient may present with a history of GI bleeding but no clinical signs other than a mild tachycardia. Acute GI bleeding may present with hypotension, dizziness, tachycardia, vomiting of blood (hematemesis), bright red blood passing at the rectum (suggestive of LGI bleed), dark tarry stools (suggestive of UGI bleeding) or angina (lack of coronary blood flow).

Patients with mild or chronic GI bleeding may have few complications or symptoms. Patients with massive GI bleeding are usually in shock, and can suffer cardiac and respiratory arrest, organ damage (from decreased blood flow) or stroke.

Vital signs should be taken initially. A tilt test is appropriate if the patient is not hypotensive when supine. Large bore intravenous access is desirable at two sites if possible with Ringer's lactate or normal saline administered as vital signs indicate. The patient also needs 100% oxygen and

ECG monitoring. Medical history should focus on non-steroidal anti-inflammatory drugs and alcohol use.

Hemorrhoids Hemorrhoids are dilated venules or varicosities of the internal or external hemorrhoidal plexus in the anorectal area. These blood vessels can be a site of pain and significant bleeding.

Hepatitis Hepatitis is an inflammation of the liver. The inflammation has many possible causes including alcohol, drugs, autoimmune disorders and toxic bacterial, fungal, parasitic and viral infections.

Viral hepatitis is usually caused by the Hepatitis A, B, C or D viruses (HAV, HBV, HCV and HDV, respectively). HAV is spread by the fecal-oral route, through contaminated food or water. HBV usually spreads through contact with blood, or through sexual contact. HCV seems to be predominantly bloodborne, but fecal-oral infection has also been reported. HDV has the same transmission pattern as HBV. Liver injury in viral hepatitis apparently occurs as a result of the body's immune response to the virus, rather than a direct virus attack on the liver cells.

Patients with hepatitis present with malaise, low-grade fever, nausea, vomiting, abdominal pain, diarrhea and possible jaundice. Those with suspected hepatitis should receive medical evaluation. It is important for field personnel to observe body substance isolation procedures.

Intestinal Bowel Obstruction Bowel obstruction is a failure of the contents of the intestine to pass through the lumen of the bowel. The most common cause is mechanical blockage resulting from adhesions, impacted feces, tumor of the bowel, hernia or other conditions. Obstruction of the small bowel can cause severe pain, vomiting of fecal matter, dehydration and, eventually, a drop in blood pressure.

Obstruction of the colon causes less severe pain, abdominal distention and constipation. Since surgical repair is sometimes necessary, and fluid and electrolyte balance is often disturbed, rapid transport to the hospital is indicated, with intravenous fluid replacement en route.

Intussusception Intussusception is the prolapse of one segment of bowel into the lumen of another segment. This type of intestinal obstruction may involve segments of the small intestine, the colon, or the terminal ileum and cecum. It occurs most often in infants and young children and is characterized by abdominal pain, vomiting, and bloody mucus in the stool. Immediate transporation to a hospital is necessary for further evaluation and surgical intervention.

Mallory-Weiss Tear Mallory-Weiss tear is a tear in the lining of the lower esophageal area as a result of repeated vomiting. It can lead to severe hemorrhage.

Pancreatitis Pancreatitis is an inflammatory condition of the pancreas that can be either acute or chronic. Acute pancreatitis results from damage to the pancreas caused by alcohol, trauma, infectious disease or certain drugs. It is characterized by severe abdominal pain radiating to the back, fever, anorexia, nausea and vomiting. There may be jaundice if the common bile duct is obstructed. To prevent any stimulation of the pancreas, nothing should be administered by mouth. Intravenous fluids should be administered.

The causes of chronic pancreatitis are similar to those of the acute form. Abdominal pain, nausea and vomiting are typical. Pancreatic insulin production may be diminished, and some patients develop diabetes mellitus.

Prehospital management includes IV Ringer's lactate, since fluid and electrolyte imbalances often occur in addition to hemorrhage.

Peritonitis Peritonitis is an inflammation of the peritoneum produced by bacteria, or by irritating substances such as blood that may enter the abdominal cavity through a penetrating wound or the perforation of an organ in the GI or reproductive tract. Peritonitis is most often caused by inflammation or rupture of the appendix. In some cases, the condition is secondary to the release of pancreatic enzymes, bile or digestive juices from the upper GI tract.

Characteristic signs and symptoms of peritonitis include abdominal distention, rigidity and pain, rebound tenderness, decreased or absent bowel sounds, nausea, vomiting and tachycardia. The patient may have chills and fever, breathe rapidly and shallowly and appear anxious and often dehydrated. Electrolyte imbalance and hypovolemia are often present, and shock may follow.

Prehospital management includes intravenous infusion of normal saline or Ringer's lactate and immediate transportation to a medical facility for further management that may include surgery. Oral intake should not be allowed.

Ulcer, Gastric or Peptic A gastric or peptic ulcer is an erosion of the mucous membrane lining of the stomach that may penetrate the muscle layer and perforate the stomach wall. It is characterized by episodes of burning epigastric pain, belching and nausea, especially when the stomach is empty or after eating certain foods. Characteristically, antacid medication or milk quickly relieves the pain. Treatment includes medication to decrease the acidity of the stomach and relieve symptoms. If perforation and hemorrhage occur, shock treatment may be necessary.

Volvulus/Intestinal Malrotation Volvulus or intestinal malrotation is a twisting of the bowel on itself causing intestinal obstruction. If it is not corrected, the obstructed bowel becomes necrotic, peritonitis and rupture of the bowel occur, and death can follow. Severe gripping pain, nausea and vomiting, and a tense, distended abdomen are typical symptoms. A volvulus can occur in a newborn resulting from malrotation or nonfixation of the colon. Persistent vomiting accompanied by fecal vomiting and no stool passage occurs. Immediate transportation for surgical intervention is necessary.

Genital-Urinary Conditions

Epididymitis Epididymitis is acute or chronic inflammation of the epididymis, one of a pair of ducts that carries sperm from the testes to the vas deferens. It may result from venereal disease, urinary tract infection, prostatitis or surgical prostate removal. Symptoms include fever, chills and groin pain.

Gonorrhea Gonorrhea is a common sexually transmitted disease most often affecting the genitourinary tract and, occasionally, the pharynx, conjunctiva or rectum. Infection results from sexual contact with an infected person or by contact with secretions containing the causative bacteria. Characteristic signs include painful urination; purulent, greenish-yellow urethral or vaginal discharge; a red or edematous urethral meatus, and itching, burning or pain around the vaginal or urethral orifice. The lower abdomen may be tense and very tender. Spread of the infection is more common in women than in men, and can lead to nausea, vomiting, fever and tachycardia as peritonitis or infection of the tubes and ovaries develops. Inflammation of the tissues surrounding the liver also may occur, causing pain in the upper right abdominal quadrant of the abdomen. Severe disseminated (scattered) infection is also more common in women and can lead to pelvic inflammatory disease (PID).

Septicemia may also develop with arthritis, tender lesions on the skin of the hands and feet, and inflammation of the tendons of the wrists, knees and ankles. Gonococcal infection can involve the conjunctiva and may lead to scarring and blindness. Prehospital management is supportive. Antibiotics will be administered in the emergency department.

Kidney Stone (Renal Colic) The formation of kidney stones, and their propensity to lodge in the narrow lumens of the ureters and other parts of the urine collection system, results in the intermittent, severe flank and abdominal pain called renal colic. The pain associated with the onset of renal colic can be excruciating, often causing the patient or family to summon EMS.

Kidney stones form for a variety of reasons, often related to the body's inability to properly excrete calcium, a major component of most stones. The characteristic pain associated with kidney stones is the result of the stone moving out of the kidney and becoming lodged in the ureter's lumen. The pain increases when the wave-like contractions (peristalsis) of the ureter increase stone pressure against the wall. Most kidney stones eventually pass through the urinary system as a result of gravity, urine flow and peristalsis.

Patients with renal colic present with abrupt onset of severe, unilateral flank or abdominal pain. The onset of pain is frequently accompanied by nausea, vomiting and diaphoresis. The prehospital management of suspected renal colic should include establishing a crystalloid IV for hydration. In addition, because renal colic symptoms are similar to more life-threatening illnesses such as ruptured abdominal aortic aneurysm, it is prudent to apply a cardiac monitor and high-flow oxygen. Although pain control is one of the mainstays of emergency department management of renal stones, paramedic administration of narcotics is controversial in this setting because of the risk of "masking" more serious causes of pain.

Nephritis Nephritis is the inflammation of the kidney. This can be acute or chronic, diffuse or localized and may involve the glomerulus, tubule, or interstitial renal tissue. Acute nephritis can be caused by streptococci and occur after strep throat, scarlet fever or other strep infections. It most commonly occurs in children and young people. Chronic nephritis may follow acute nephritis or develop in individuals that have never had acute renal disease. Typically chronic nephritis is progressive, causing permanent damage to the kidneys, requiring dialysis and transplant.

Glomerulonephritis is the most common form of nephritis, and impairs the filtering process. Although acute nephritis may not exhibit signs and symptoms early, headaches, malaise, back pain, dark or smoky urine, and edema may be present. Blood pressure usually will be elevated in acute nephritis; sometimes so severely that convulsions will occur. Prehospital management is supportive with immediate transport to an ED.

Priapism The abnormal condition of prolonged or constant penile erection, often painful and seldom associated with sexual arousal, is called priapism. It may result from sickle cell anemia, or a lesion within the penis or the central nervous system. In the prehospital setting, priapism after trauma is indicative of a spinal cord injury. Spinal immobilization is important management in such cases.

Prostatitis Acute or chronic inflammation of the prostate gland is usually the result of infection. The male patient complains of burning, frequency and urgency. Treatment by a physician consists of administration of antibiotics, sitz baths, bed rest and fluids.

Renal Failure Renal failure is the reduction or complete cessation of the kidney's ability to clear certain waste products from the blood. Renal failure generally correlates with decreased or absent urine output. Renal failure can occur either acutely or chronically. Complete loss of renal function is incompatible with life. In recent decades, the advent of hemo- and peritoneal dialysis has enabled patients with renal failure to survive; dialysis filters wastes from the blood and maintains crucial fluid and electrolyte balances.

Causes of acute renal failure include interruption of adequate renal blood flow (secondary to shock or renal artery occlusion), blockage of urine flow (renal stones or blood clots) and a variety of rapidly progressive kidney diseases. Chronic renal failure is usually the result of long-standing diseases, such as uncontrolled hypertension or diabetes mellitus, which injure the kidneys.

Loss of normal renal function results in a wide range of problems. Renal failure often leads to fluid overload and electrolyte imbalances. The patients at greatest risk for these complications are those who have missed a scheduled dialysis session. Patients with systemic fluid overload will frequently present with the classic signs of pulmonary edema - shortness of breath, orthopnea and course rales on auscultation of the lungs. Electrolyte imbalances can also have life-threatening complications for the renal failure patient. Perhaps the most feared electrolyte abnormality is a high serum potassium, hyperkalemia. Hyperkalemia predisposes patients to lethal dysrhythmias and ventricular fibrillation. Renal failure patients with hyperkalemia may complain of palpitations or simply present in cardiac arrest. Those with chronic renal failure are also prone to hypertensive crisis and anemia, the latter because of reduced secretion of the hormone that stimulates bone marrow to produce red blood cells.

Finally, renal dialysis patients are subject to various complications from the dialysis itself. The two most common ones are shunt occlusion in hemodialysis, and infection of the abdominal cavity (peritonitis) in peritoneal dialysis. Hemodialysis patients with shunt occlusion will frequently state that the site suddenly lost its characteristic vibrating feeling or "thrill" to touch. Peritoneal dialysis patients who develop peritonitis often complain of abdominal pain and report dialysis fluid has become cloudy compared to its normal clear quality.

In general, the patient with renal failure should be assessed no differently than any patient, with initial attention to ABCs. Key questions include whether the patient is currently undergoing dialysis; if so, what type, and whether the patient has been compliant; and, whether the peritoneal dialysis patient has noticed any cloudiness in the dialysis fluid. Always assess the patient for signs or symptoms of the underlying disease, such as diabetes or hypertension.

Prehospital management requires careful attention to the detection of immediately life-threatening conditions such as dysrhythmias or respiratory failure from pulmonary edema. In general, all renal failure patients who are sick enough to call for EMS, with the exception of an isolated dialysis shunt occlusion, should receive oxygen, a cardiac monitor and an IV at a keep-open rate. The cardiac monitor is especially important for the detection of dysrythmias

and the characteristic large, peaked T waves typical of hyperkalemia. Patients who exhibit dysrythmias should be treated with standard anti-dysrhythmic drugs such as lidocaine. Since these dysrythmias are likely due to hyperkalemia, steps should also be taken to treat the hyperkalemia itself. The two drugs most readily available in the prehospital drug box are calcium chloride and sodium bicarbonate. Calcium chloride helps to stabilize the electrical activity of the heart in the presence of hyperkalemia. Sodium bicarbonate reduces the serum potassium level by inducing an alkalosis. The two agents are incompatible in the same IV line; flushing is required between drugs. If a renal failure patient is found in cardiac arrest, both drugs should also be administered early in the resuscitation, despite bicarbonate's late position in the normal sequence.

Two additional issues are important to the prehospital care of renal failure patients. First, dialysis shunts should not be used for routine IV access except in dire situations, such as cardiovascular collapse or cardiac arrest, as a last resort after attempts at other sites have failed. Second, the preferable transport destination for a renal failure patient is the facility where the patient's renal specialist practices. Lacking that option, the patient should be taken to a facility capable of performing hemodialysis, which is usually the definitive management of hyperkalemia and fluid overload.

Testicular Torsion Testicular torsion is the twisting of the testicle on the spermatic cord that cuts off the blood supply to the testicle, epididymis and other structures. Complete ischemia for six hours may result in gangrene of the testis. The condition presents with acute, severe, scrotal pain that may be constant and intermittent. The condition may be caused by trauma or a strenuous physical activity but most often occurs in individuals predisposed anatomically due to inadequate connective tissue. Torsion of the testes occurs most frequently in the first year of life and during puberty. Immediate transportation for surgical intervention is necessary to save the testis.

Urinary Tract Infection (UTI) Infection of one or more structures in the urinary tract, such as the urethra, bladder, ureter or kidney, is more common in women than in men and may be asymptomatic. Urinary tract infection is usually characterized by urinary frequency, burning, pain with voiding and, if the infection is severe, fever and urine with visible blood and pus. Patients with these symptoms should see a physician for further evaluation. Treatment at the hospital includes antibacterial, analgesic and urinary-antiseptic drugs.

Infectious Conditions

Acquired Immunodeficiency Syndrome (AIDS, HIV infection)
Acquired immunodeficiency syndrome (AIDS) results from infection with the human immunodeficiency virus (HIV). Modes of transmission include blood and blood products, semen, vaginal secretions and cross-placental circulation. HIV has also been detected in saliva, urine, cerebral spinal fluid, brain matter, tears and breast milk, but transmission by casual contact has not been reported.

Initial symptoms include extreme fatigue, intermittent fever, night sweats, chills, lymphadenopathy, spleen enlargement, loss of appetite and consequent weight loss, severe diarrhea, apathy and depression. As the disease progresses, there is a general failure to thrive, and a wide variety of recurring opportunistic infections, most commonly *Pneumocystic carinii* pneumonia, meningitis, encephalitis and tuberculosis. Most patients with the disorder are susceptible to malignancies, especially Kaposi's sarcoma, and non-Hodgkin's lymphoma, that both cause and result from immunodeficiency. Other manifestations of AIDS include ophthalmologic, gastrointestinal, neurological and systemic disease. Treatment consists primarily of combined chemotherapy to counteract the opportunistic disease. There is no known cure for HIV infection, though the antiviral drug zidovudine has been shown to reduce the progress of the disease and prolong the lives of patients. Patients with AIDS are at an increased risk of suicide.

Prehospital personnel should always protect themselves when dealing with any patients in which they might be exposed to blood or body fluids. Prehospital management for the AIDS patient is symptomatic and supportive.

Cellulitis Cellulitis is an acute infection of the skin and subcutaneous tissue characterized most commonly by local heat, redness, pain and swelling, and occasionally by fever, malaise, chills and headache. Abscess and tissue destruction usually follow if not treated. The infection is more likely to develop in the presence of damaged skin, poor circulation or diabetes mellitus. In addition to appropriate antibiotics, treatments includes warm soaks, elevation and avoidance of pressure to the affected areas.

Chickenpox Chickenpox is an acute, highly contagious disease caused by a herpes virus, the varicella zoster virus (VZV). It occurs primarily in young children and is characterized by crops of itching, blister-like eruptions on the skin. The disease is transmitted by direct contact with skin lesions or, more commonly, by droplets spread from the respiratory tract of infected persons, usually in the early stages of the rash. The blister fluid and the scabs are infectious until entirely dry. The incubation period averages two to three weeks, followed by slight fever, mild headache, malaise and anorexia. The lesions, which erupt in crops, appear first on the back and chest and then spread to the face, neck and limbs. In severe cases, blisters in the pharynx, larynx and trachea may cause dyspnea and difficulty swallowing. Prolonged fever, swollen lymph nodes and extreme irritability from itching are other symptoms. The symptoms last from a few days to two weeks.

One attack of the disease confers permanent immunity, although recurring episodes of herpes zoster occur, especially in elderly or debilitated people, resulting from reactivation of the virus. (Herpes zoster virus (HZV), like all herpes viruses, lies dormant in certain sensory nerve roots after primary infection.) Chickenpox in childhood is usually benign; few cases require hospitalization. It may be serious or fatal in immunocompromised people, such as those receiving chemotherapy or radiography for malignant disease, or in those who have undergone organ transplantation, have congenital defects or are receiving high doses of steroids. Common complications are secondary bacterial infections, such as abscesses, cellulitis, pneumonia and sepsis.

Chlamydia Chlamydia is a microorganism similar to gram-negative bacteria that is typically responsible for conjunctivitis and pelvic inflammatory disease. It is one of the most common sexually transmitted diseases in North America, and a frequent cause of sterility.

Gas Gangrene Gas gangrene is necrosis accompanied by gas bubbles in soft tissue after surgery or trauma. It is caused by anaerobic organisms. Symptoms include pain, swelling and tenderness of the wound area, moderate fever, tachycardia and hypotension. The skin around the wound becomes necrotic and ruptures, revealing necrotic muscle. Toxic delirium is a characteristic finding. Untreated gas gangrene is rapidly fatal. Prompt treatment, including excision of gangrenous tissue and IV administration of penicillin, can save most patients. The disease is prevented by proper wound care.

Herpes Zoster (Shingles) Herpes zoster, or shingles, is an acute infection caused by reactivation of the dormant varicella zoster virus (VZV). It mainly affects adults, and is characterized by the development of painful, blister-like skin eruptions that follow the underlying route of the cranial or spinal nerves inflamed by the virus. Distribution of the pain and eruptions is usually one-sided, although both sides of the body may be involved. The pain can be constant or intermittent, superficial or deep; it usually precedes other effects and may mimic other disorders such as appendicitis or pleurisy. Early symptoms may include GI disturbances, malaise, fever and headache.

Lyme Disease Lyme disease is an acute, recurrent inflammatory infection transmitted by a tick-borne spirochete. Knees, other large joints, and temperomandibular joints are most commonly involved, with local inflammation and swelling. Chills, fever, headache, malaise and skin eruptions often precede joint problems. Occasionally cardiac conduction abnormalities and aseptic meningitis are associated conditions. Symptoms appear in recurrent episodes, lasting usually one week, at intervals from one to several weeks, declining in severity over a 2–3 year period.

Measles, Rubella Measles, or rubeola, is an acute, highly contagious viral disease involving the respiratory tract and characterized by a spreading rash. It occurs primarily in young children who have not been immunized. Measles is transmitted by direct contact with droplets spread from the nose, throat and mouth of infected people, usually during the onset of the disease. An incubation period of seven to 14 days is followed by fever, malaise, cold symptoms, cough, conjunctivitis and loss of appetite. As pharyngitis and inflammation of the laryngeal and tracheobronchial mucosa develop, the temperature may rise. The rash first appears as irregular brownish-pink spots around the hairline, ears and neck, then spreads rapidly within 24 to 48 hours to the trunk and extremities, giving a dense red blotchy appearance. Within three to five days, the fever subsides and the lesions flatten, turn a brownish color, begin to fade and cause a fine peeling of the skin. The disease is usually benign, and mortality is extremely rare. Complications sometimes occur, the most common of which are otitis media, pneumonia, bronchiolitis, obstructive laryngitis, laryngotracheitis and occasionally, encephalitis and appendicitis.

Rubella, or German measles, is a contagious viral disease characterized by fever, symptoms of a mild upper respiratory tract infection, lymph node enlargement, joint pain and a diffuse, fine, red rash. The virus is spread by droplet infection, and the incubation time is from 12 to 23 days. The symptoms usually last on two or three days. One attack confers lifelong immunity. If a women acquires rubella in the first trimester of pregnancy, fetal anomalies may result, including heart defects, cataracts, deafness and mental retardation. The illness itself is mild and needs no special treatment.

Mononucleosis Infectious mononucleosis is an acute herpes virus infection caused by the Epstein-Barr virus. It is characterized by fever, sore throat, swollen lymph glands, bruising and enlarged spleen and liver. The disease is usually transmitted by droplet infection, but is not highly contagious. Young people are most often affected. In childhood, the disease is mild and usually unnoticed; the older the patient, the more severe the symptoms are likely to be. Treatment is primarily symptomatic. Rupture of the spleen can occur, requiring immediate surgery and blood transfusion.

Mumps Mumps is an acute viral disease characterized by a swelling of the parotid glands. Passive immunity from maternal antibodies usually prevents this disease in children under one year of age. It is most likely to affect children between five and 15 years of age, but can occur later. In adulthood, the infection may be severe. The incidence of mumps is highest during the late winter and early spring. The mumps virus lives in the saliva of the affected individual and is transmitted in droplets or by direct contact. The virus is present in the saliva from six days before, to nine days after, the onset of the parotid gland swelling. The prognosis in mumps is good, but the disease sometimes involves complications such as arthritis, pancreatitis, myocarditis, oophoritis, nephritis, meningitis and testicle in-

flammation. The common symptoms of mumps usually last for about 24 hours and include anorexia, headache, malaise and low-grade fever. These signs are commonly followed by ear ache, parotid gland swelling and higher fever.

Rabies Rabies is an acute, usually fatal viral disease of the central nervous system of animals. It is transmitted from animals to people by infected blood, tissue, or more commonly saliva.

After introduction into the human body, often by a bite of an infected animal, the virus travels along nerve pathways to the brain, and later other organs. An incubation period ranges from ten days to one year. Initial symptoms include fever, malaise, headache, paresthesia and muscle aches. After several days, severe encephalitis, delirium, agonizingly painful muscular spasms, seizures, paralysis, coma and death ensue.

Few nonfatal cases have been documented in humans; survival in those cases has been the result of intensive supportive medical care. There is no treatment once the virus has reached the tissue of the nervous system. Local treatment of wounds inflicted by rabid animals may prevent the disease. The wound is cleansed with soap, water, and a disinfectant. Great effort is made to locate, isolate and observe the animal.

Rocky Mountain Spotted Fever Rocky Mountain Spotted Fever is a serious tick-borne infectious disease occurring throughout the temperate zones of North and South America. It is caused by a rickettsii and is characterized by chills, fever, severe headache, mental confuction and rash. Untreated, the condition can lead to renal failure and shock.

Salmonella Salmonella is a genus of bacteria that includes species causing typhoid fever and some forms of gastroenteritis. It is often acquired by eating contaminated, incompletely cooked food such as poultry, eggs and hamburger.

Septic Shock/Sepsis Septic shock is the type of hypoperfusion that occurs when toxins are released from certain bacteria into the blood that cause decreased vascular resistance and increased capillary permeability. Fever, tachycardia, increased respirations and confusion or coma may occur. Septic shock is usually preceded by signs of severe infection, often of the genitourinary or GI system. Intravenous fluids (Ringer's lactate or normal saline) are given and rapid transport to the hospital for antibiotics is essential. In infants, hypoglycemia may occur with septicemia, and 25% dextrose may need to be administered.

Syphilis Syphilis, also called lues, is a sexually transmitted disease caused by a spirochete bacteria and characterized by distinct stages of effects over a period of years. Any organ system may become involved.

The first stage, primary syphilis, is marked by the appearance of small, painless red pustules on the skin or mucous membranes between 10 and 90 days after exposure. The lesion may appear anywhere on the body where contact with a lesion on an infected person has occurred, but is seen most often in the genital or anal region. It quickly erodes, forming a painless, bloodless ulcer called a chancre that exudes a fluid concentrated with spirochetes. The chancre may not be noticed by the patient, and many contacts may become infected. It heals spontaneously within 10 to

40 days, often creating the mistaken impression that the sore was not a serious event. Secondary syphilis occurs about two months later, after the spirochetes have increased in number and spread throughout the body. This stage is characterized by general malaise, anorexia, nausea, fever, headache, hair loss, bone and joint pain, and the appearance of a rash or flat white sores in the mouth and throat. The disease remains highly contagious at this stage and can be spread by kissing. The symptoms usually continue for three weeks to three months, and may be recurrent over a period of two years. The third stage, tertiary syphilis, may not develop for three to 15 years or more. It is characterized by the appearance of soft, rubbery tumors that ulcerate and heal by scarring. They may develop anywhere on the surface of the body and in the eye, liver, lungs, stomach or reproductive organs. Various tissues and structures of the body, including the central nervous system, myocardium and heart valves may be damaged or destroyed, leading to mental or physical disability and premature death. Congenital syphilis, resulting from prenatal infection, can result in the birth of a deformed or blind infant. Personal protective precautions are important while handling the patient with highly contagious syphilitic lesions because the infection may be acquired through a cut or break in the skin. The disease can be treated in its early stages with penicillin.

Tetanus Tetanus is an acute, potentially fatal infection of the central nervous system caused by a bacteria. More than 50,000 people a year die of tetanus infection worldwide. The toxin is a neurotoxin and is one of the most lethal poisons known. The tetanus bacteria infects only wounds that contain dead tissue. The bacteria is a common resident of the superficial layers of the soil and a normal inhabitant of the intestinal tracts of cows and horses; therefore barnyards and fields fertilized with manure are heavily contaminated.

The bacteria may enter the body through a puncture wound, abrasion, laceration or burn, or via the uterus into the bloodstream in a septic abortion or postpartum sepsis, or through the stump of the umbilical cord in a newborn.

The dead tissue of the area is low in oxygen, which is the environment necessary for bacteria growth.

The infection occurs in two clinical forms: one with an abrupt onset, high mortality, and a short incubation period (3 to 21 days); the other with less severe symptoms, a lower mortality, and a longer incubation period (four to five weeks). Wounds of the face, head, and neck are the ones most likely to result in fatal infection because the bacteria may travel to the brain. The disease is characterized by irritability, headache, fever, and painful spasms of the muscles resulting in lockjaw and laryngeal spasm; eventually every muscle of the body is in tonic spasm.

Prompt and thorough cleansing and debridement of the wound are essential for prophylaxis. A booster shot of tetanus toxoid is given to previously immunized individuals; tetanus immune globulin and a series of three injections of tetanus toxoid are given to those not immunized.

Treatment of people who have the infection includes maintenance of an airway, sedation, control of muscle spasm and rapid transport to the hospital.

Toxic Shock Syndrome Toxic shock syndrome is a severe, acute disease caused by infection with strains of *Staphylococcus aureus* that produce a unique toxin, enterotoxin F. It is most common in menstruating women using high-absorbency tampons, but has been seen in newborn infants, children and men. The onset of the syndrome is characterized by sudden high fever, headache, sore throat with swelling of the mucous membranes, diarrhea and nausea. Acute renal failure, abnormal liver function, confusion and hypotension usually follow, and death may occur. There does not appear to be any seasonal or geographic factor in the cause of the disease, and there is no evidence of contagion among household members or through sexual contact. Although prehospital identification is unlikely, management includes aggressive IV volume expansion, assisted ventilation and possible administration of vasopressors. Early medical intervention greatly improves survival rates and decreases both recurrence and prolonged morbidity.

Nervous System Conditions

Alzheimer's Disease; Dementia Alzheimer's disease is a specific type of dementia that involves loss of brain cells. Early symptoms are primarily related to memory loss, especially the ability to make and recall new memories. As the disease progresses, agitation, violence and impairment of abstract thinking, judgment and cognitive abilities can significantly interfere with work and social interactions. The cause of Alzheimer's disease remains unknown, and medical treatment is limited. Behavioral treatment is more valuable, particularly the use of daily routines in a familiar environment to provide a stable setting for the patient.

The demented patient is predisposed to accidents and injuries around the home. These patients also present an assessment challenge because of their inability to express pain or describe symptoms clearly. It is not uncommon, for example, to see a demented patient trying to walk on a broken hip. In advanced stages, the patient may be bedridden and totally unaware of surroundings. These patients are predisposed to typical conditions of the bedridden, such as skin breakdown, pneumonia and urinary tract infections.

Cerebral Palsy Cerebral palsy is characterized by impairment of voluntary movement. The term is applied to a number of non-progressive motor disorders resulting from CNS damage in the womb or at birth. Cerebral palsy is not a diagnosis, but a classification for children with involuntary movements or loss of coordination. A number of circumstances may be causes, including birth trauma, prenatal disorders, neonatal asphyxia and neonatal jaundice. Cerebral palsy is not always associated with mental retardation; in fact, patients often function on a mental level far above average.

Cerebrovascular Accident (CVA, Stroke): Cerebrovascular Disease, Transient Ischemic Attack (TIA) Stroke, or cerebral vascular accident (CVA), is a general term that refers to any interruption of cerebral blood flow secondary to hemorrhage or vessel disruption resulting in permanent neurologic deficit. Stroke can be fatal, and survivors are often left severely disabled.

Two general mechanisms lead to vessel occlusion: thrombosis within the vessel and embolism from another source. Plaques on the artery walls cause partial obstruction of blood flow and increase the risk of thrombus (clot) formation; this occurs with the coronary arteries in myocardial infarction.

Embolic strokes involve occlusion of a cerebral vessel by an embolus (moving object or substance) from a distant anatomic site. Atherosclerotic plaques commonly dislodge from the carotid arteries and become trapped in the narrow cerebral vessels, for example. Small emboli may be responsible for most transient ischemic attacks (TIAs). Another common origin of emboli is the heart. Atrial fibrillation is a frequent cause of embolic stroke. The fibrillating atrium encourages clot formation, and parts of the clot pass from the heart to the peripheral circulation, including cerebral vessels. IV drug users are vulnerable to the embolization of foreign materials (air, talc), as well as septic emboli from infected heart valves. Substances such as air introduced during vascular procedures and fat from large bone fractures can also cause embolic stroke.

The major types of stroke are directly related to the cerebral vessels that are occluded. A wide variety of signs and symptoms can occur. The classic stroke pattern of paralysis and loss of sensation is usually due to occlusion of the middle cerebral artery. This syndrome can also produce blindness in half of each visual field, and difficulty swallowing. Anterior cerebral artery occlusion results in lower extremity weakness.

Posterior cerebral artery stroke can also cause blindness in half of each visual field, or total blindness. Dysconjugate gaze, in which the eyes point in different directions, is commonly seen when the third cranial nerve is affected. Occlusion of the vertebral basilar artery produces cerebellar effects including vertigo, nystagmus, syncope and spasticity. This syndrome also produces a loss of pain and temperature sensation on one side.

Transient ischemic attack (TIA) is a stroke-related syndrome defined as any neurologic deficit caused by brain tissue ischemia that completely resolves within 24 hours. Although most TIAs are brief, they are an ominous sign. Many TIA patients will continue on to have a full stroke at some point, if they are not treated.

The prehospital management of the stroke patient consists of oxygen administration and, when indicated, airway management. Intravenous access should be obtained. Glucose may actually worsen brain resuscitation, except in confirmed hypoglycemia. Stroke patients should also be placed on a cardiac monitor, since dysrhythmias are a predisposing factor in stroke. A good neurologic assessment is essential; symptoms may resolve before reaching the hospital. The patient should be carefully examined for any trauma, because head injury can mimic stroke or result from a fall caused by a stroke. If a stroke victim is found late, hypothermia and dehydration can complicate the assessment. Rapid transport to a hospital is necessary as thrombolytics may be given to patients experiencing an embolic stroke.

A stroke victim may be found with a very high blood pressure, either because hypertension caused the stroke or because the high pressure is necessary to supply blood to the ischemic brain tissue. Some prehospital protocols address lowering the blood pressure in cases of extreme elevation.

Encephalopathy Encephalopathy describes an acute state of confusion with potentially reversible causes. Patients with encephalopathy have one or more of the following: inattentiveness, impaired level of consciousness, perceptual disturbances, disorganized thinking, memory impairment and disorientation to time, place or person. Causes of encephalopathy are diverse; they include infections, hypertension, drug withdrawal, ingestion of drugs, exposure to toxins, metabolic disorders (renal or liver failure, hypoglycemia), hyper- or hypothermia, trauma, vitamin deficiency, CNS disease and hypoxia, to name a few. Wernicke's encephalopathy is caused by a thiamine deficiency and is seen in association with chronic alcoholism. Treatment should focus on the ABCs while ruling out hypoglycemia and other causes listed above.

Epidural Hematoma An epidural hematoma is a collection of arterial blood between the skull and the adherent, inner membrane lining of the skull, called the dura mater. (Think of peeling a hard-boiled egg; the shell would be the skull, and the dura the thin, transparent lining stuck to the inside of the shell.) Epidural hematomas usually result from skull fractures that tear the middle meningeal artery. Classically, the condition causes a transient loss of consciousness followed by a lucid interval, with progressive loss of consciousness during the following minutes or hours. More severely injured patients will not have a lucid interval at all.

Epidural hematomas are the least common of intracranial hemorrhages. They are rare in the elderly, because dura and skull are adherent.

Prehospital management of the patient with a suspected intracranial hematoma can be challenging. Head trauma victims are often intoxicated and combative, clouding the origin of the problem. Such patients should be assumed to have a head injury until proven otherwise. The paramedic must also consider hypoxemia or hypoglycemia as possible, treatable causes.

Lowering intracranial pressure may be life saving for the patient whose brain is under pressure from bleeding or edema. Hyperventilation at a rate of no more than 20–22 breaths a minute is the most rapidly effective way to do this, and it is readily available. Signs of impending herniation, in which the brain is forced through a skull opening, include a decreased Glasgow Coma Score, a unilaterally fixed and dilated pupil, and high blood pressure with a slow pulse (Cushing's reflex).

Guillain-Barre Syndrome Guillain-Barre syndrome occurs when a preceding viral infection stimulates the immune system to produce antibodies that attack the peripheral nervous system. Afflicted patients will initially exhibit weakness or paralysis of the legs that ascends progressively to involve the arms, trunk and face. Severe cases may require endotracheal intubation with mechanical ventilation to treat respiratory failure caused by muscle paralysis. The illness is of rapid onset and short duration, with complete recovery. Patients require supportive care during the illness while the disease runs its course. Guillain-Barre syndrome is uncommon. When confronted by a patient with paralysis, attention should be focused on the ABCs, keeping in mind the more common causes of paralysis such as spinal cord problems and CVA.

Hydrocephalus Hydrocephalus, or hydrocephaly, is literally water on the brain. Decreased reabsorption of CSF results in fluid and pressure build-up in the cranium. The condition may be congenital or acquired.

Normal pressure hydrocephalus occurs in adults, and leads to dementia, urinary incontinence and gait problems. In contrast, CSF pressure is elevated in neonatal hydrocephalus because of a mechanical blockage of CSF flow.

Treatment for hydrocephalus involves the use of shunts, tubes that divert CSF from the ventricles of the brain to the abdominal cavity for reabsorption. These subcutaneous lines can be palpated in the neck. Clotting, obstruction or breakage of the shunt can cause acute illness. These problems may require urgent neurosurgical intervention.

Head Injury, Skull Fracture, Concussion In the assessment of the head-injured patient, one should determine whether or not the patient fell, height of the fall, landing surface, other mechanisms of injury, seat belt use, details of any loss of consciousness, presence of any seizure activity, and a past medical history.

As always, ABCs should be attended to, as well as spinal immobilization and vital sign assessment. Hypertension with bradycardia is an ominous sign indicating increased intracranial pressure. Neurologic exam should include pupil size, reactivity and symmetry. An enlarging pupil in conjunction with a decreased level of consciousness should be assumed to be a sign of impending herniation that requires controlled hyperventilation at no more than 20–22 breaths per minute. The presence or absence of a gag reflex is crucial to assessing the risk of aspiration. If the gag reflex is absent, the patient should be intubated to protect the airway. The general level of consciousness can be reliably assessed with the Glasgow Coma Scale. Those patients with a score of eight or less are considered to be severely head-injured, and will likely require immediate intubation, adequate ventilation (12-18 breaths per minute) and hyperventilation if clear signs of increased intracranial pressure are present.

Cerebral contusion is a bruise of the brain. There is tissue injury and small, localized hemorrhage that may be either at the site of trauma (coup injury), or directly opposite the trauma on the other side of the brain (contra-coup injury). These injuries are generally the result of a "sloshing around" of the brain within the skull, and anatomic components of the brain that are exposed to rough areas on the skull are particularly vulnerable. The localized hemorrhage and edema may lead to neurologic abnormalities which correspond to the area of the brain involved.

A linear, non-depressed skull fracture may be of little or no clinical significance. However, if the same linear fracture were to disrupt an underlying blood vessel such as the middle meningeal artery, catastrophic bleeding could occur. Skull fractures involving the middle meningeal artery are the typical injury causing an epidural hematoma.

Basilar skull fractures usually involve a portion of the temporal bone at the base of the skull, and are classically associated with bruising of the mastoid area, known as Battle's sign. Blood behind the eardrum, leakage of cerebrospinal fluid from the ear and periorbital bruising (raccoon eyes) are physical findings suggestive of basilar skull fracture. It is important to note these findings when present, because basilar skull fracture may not appear on x-ray.

Open skull fractures expose the brain and subject the nervous system to infection. Gunshot wounds are a type of open fracture that produces injury far beyond the direct path of the bullet. The extent of tissue damage is directly related to the energy of the projectile. Hemorrhage may be life threatening if significant vessels are disrupted.

Treatment of skull fractures involves C-spine stabilization, and assuring adequate ventilation. Open skull fractures should be covered with a sterile dressing. These injuries require urgent evaluation and intervention, and rapid transport. Further assessment and establishment of IV lines can be accomplished during transport.

Cerebral concussion is a diffuse injury of the brain defined as a post-traumatic neurologic deficit, usually manifested as loss of consciousness, lasting for less than 24 hours. Concussion indicates a significant head injury and symptoms sometimes forewarn of a more serious condition. A concussion is therefore a diagnosis of exclusion, after a more dangerous brain lesion has been ruled out at the hospital. Symptoms suggestive of serious head injury includes loss of consciousness, vomiting, severe headache or seizures. Post-concussion syndrome is a prolonged condition manifested by symptoms such as headache, memory problems, anxiety, insomnia or dizziness that may persist for weeks or months after a concussive head injury.

Intracranial Hemorrhage Spontaneous intracranial hemorrhage (ICH) occurs in the setting of long-standing hypertension, cerebral aneurysm or arteriovenous malformation (AVM). Chronic hypertension causes degenerative changes in the cerebral arteries, such as aneurysms and atherosclerosis, that weaken the vessel walls. Hypertensive hemorrhage occurs primarily in the elderly and is the results in ruptures of small vessels. Younger patients usually have underlying aneurysms, AVMs or tumors. A cerebral aneurysm may rupture during periods of intense physical activity or stress. Trauma to the head, particularly with skull fractures and tears of vasculature, can also cause intracranial hemorrhage. In all ages, the rapidly expanding hematoma can cause seizures, or sudden cardiovascular collapse if the cardiorespiratory centers of the medulla are compressed.

Patients with ICH are likely to present with an altered level of consciousness progressing to unresponsiveness. A primary survey assessing ABCs and vital signs should be performed, with an emphasis on blood pressure. A baseline neurologic evaluation, with attention to level of consciousness and Glasgow Coma Scale, is important to subsequent patient care. Focal neurologic deficits are extremely common with ICH and should be noted. Oxygen should be given to all patients with altered mental status; dextrose and naloxone are indicated in selected cases. Cardiac monitoring is essential during transport to a facility capable of performing CT scanning. Endotracheal intubation is needed in patients with respiratory failure, or respiratory arrest, loss of protective airway reflex (gag). Hyperventilation, at a rate of no more than 20-22 times a minute, is the quickest and most effective means of reducing elevated intracranial pressure.

Paramedics may be asked to initiate drug therapy to treat blood pressure if it is dangerously high. The drug of choice is nitroprusside, which decreases afterload and lowers systemic vascular resistance rapidly. It is easily titratable and has a short half-life. Since this drug is often not part of prehospital protocols, the paramedic may be asked to begin therapy with nitroglycerin, nifedipine or labetalol.

Meningitis and Meningococcal Meningitis Meningitis is an inflammation of the central nervous system's membrane linings—the pia mater, arachnoid membrane and dura mater. Meningitis can be caused by viruses, in which case it is referred to as viral or aseptic meningitis, or by bacteria, called bacterial meningitis. Viral meningitis usually follows a self-limited course, but bacterial meningitis can be life threatening. Infants, the elderly and immuno-compromised patients are predisposed to certain types of bacterial meningitis. Penetrating head wounds and post-surgical wounds are also particularly vulnerable to bacterial infections.

The adult with bacterial meningitis will usually have a history of recent upper respiratory infection or sore throat. Symptoms then progress to the classic findings of acute fever, headache, stiff neck and vomiting. In young children, symptoms may not be so easily detected. They include fever, irritability and confusion or coma. Any infant under two months of age with a high fever requires hospital evaluation. Ominous signs include convulsions, bulging fontanels and high-pitched, weak crying. Neck stiffness is not usually present in infants. Any suggestive case should be transported to an ED for evaluation.

Meningococcal meningitis in particular may overwhelm an individual within 1-2 hours, and antibiotics are the only definitive therapy. Prehospital providers who suspect meningitis should alert the receiving hospital so that they may be ready to administer antibiotics and perform lumbar puncture. In addition to oxygen administration, IV access should be obtained and fluid replacement given if indicated.

Patients with meningococcal sepsis, or meningococcemia, present with the usual signs of sepsis such as hypertension, fever and a decreased level of consciousness, as well a petechial or purpuric rash. (Petechiae are tiny purple or red spots that appear as a result of minute hemorrhage within the dermal layer of skin. Purpura looks similar to bruising.) Meningococcemia may present with or without meningococcal meningitis. Family members of a patient with confirmed meningococcal meningitis should be considered for prophylaxis with Rifampin. Prehospital and hospital workers exposed do not require prophylaxis unless there was significant exposure, though the event should be reported.

Migraine Headache Migraine headache exhibits symptoms caused by cerebral vasodilation, including headache, loss of appetite, nausea and vomiting. Classic migraines are preceded by visual changes, neurological deficits and photophobia caused by initial vasoconstriction. Once vasoconstriction abates and dilation follows, the headache occurs. Patients treated by EMS will often relate a history of prior migraine headaches. Patients with sudden, severe headaches should not be assumed to have a migraine even if they use the term migraine to describe it. The sudden onset of headache associated with vomiting or neurological deficits suggests intracranial hemorrhage.

Multiple Sclerosis Multiple Sclerosis (MS) is a demyelinating disease of the brain and spine. Myelin is the fatty insulation of nerve cells that aids in rapid transmission of impulses, analogous to the plastic covering of electrical wires. The nervous systems of patients with MS have widely dispersed patches of myelin loss resulting in a variety of otherwise unrelated neurologic symptoms. The disease classically runs a waxing and waning course, and over weeks, may change from severe to minor to severe again. Often, the exacerbation is triggered by infection, which should be kept in mind in any patient presenting with abrupt worsening of symptoms. Severe cases can be extremely debilitating, rendering patients unable to care for themselves.

Myasthenia Gravis Myasthenia gravis is an autoimmune disease, characterized by muscle fatigue and weakness and in severe cases, respiratory failure. The fatigue is caused by a deficiency of acetylcholine; the deficiency inhibits normal nerve impulse conduction. The onset of symptoms is usually gradual, with episodic weakness, drooping of the upper eyelid, double vision and increased fatigability of the facial muscles. The weakness may then extend to other muscles innervated by the cranial nerves, particularly the respiratory muscles. Muscular exertion aggravates the symptoms, which typically vary over the course of the day. The disease occurs in younger women more often than in older women, and in men over 60 years of age more often than in younger men. A myasthenic crisis occurs in only a few patients but may be life-threatening and may require respiratory assistance. It is important for prehospital personnel who carry paralytics to note that myasthenia patients should not be given these agents.

Organic Brain Syndrome Organic brain syndrome refers to any brain function problem that is directly related to a physical disease or disturbance. This term is most often used in reference to dementia. However, it can also refer to any delirium, or to an intoxication or withdrawal syndrome involving addictive substances. Multi-infarct dementia is a common type of organic syndrome resulting from multiple vascular insults to the brain, none of which individually causes a neurological deficit. The scar tissue and scattered loss of functioning brain matter are responsible for symptoms. This is in contrast to a stroke, which usually produces large, well defined areas of damage.

The term *dementia* describes disturbances of memory, judgment, abstract thinking and language skills. Dementia is not a normal component of aging; it always represents a pathologic change. Anxiety, depression and psychosis are behavioral findings often associated with dementia. Some causes of dementia are reversible and should be aggressively sought. These include vitamin deficiency and certain drug reactions.

Parkinsonism, Parkinson's Disease The names Parkinsonism, Parkinson's disease and Parkinson's syndrome all describe a series of related clinical findings such as absence or slowness of movement, finger rolling, resting tremor, increased muscular tone, shuffling gait, a mask-like face and rigidity and postural instability. Parkinson's disease is a slowly progressive, chronic disease caused by degeneration of a specific area of the brain stem called the substantia nigra. It is usually seen in people over 60 years of age, although it may occur in younger patients. The symptoms predispose sufferers to falls and injury. Advanced and severe cases are associated with emotional instability, dementia and autonomic disturbances, as well as difficulties with swallowing and speech. This may lead to an increased risk of aspiration pneumonia.

Secondary Parkinsonism produces similar symptoms but is caused by the use of neuroleptic drugs, which include the anti-psychotic drugs and major tranquilizers such as amitriptyline, chlorpromazine and thioridazine. (The neuroleptic drugs can also cause an acute dystonic reaction, a separate condition that presents with severe muscular stiffness, usually in the neck, and facial contortions. This reaction presents dramatically, but the symptoms are quickly abated with IV diphenhydramine.)

Reye's Syndrome Reye's syndrome is an illness that causes significant changes in mentation and liver function, primarily in children and adolescents. Fever, vomiting and altered mental status occurring after viral illnesses such as flu or chicken pox are typical of Reye's syndrome. In the late stage, respiratory arrest may occur. A higher incidence of Reye's syndrome in patients treated with aspirin has prompted its discontinuation as a fever treatment in children.

Seizures: Epilepsy; Status Epilepticus; Febrile Seizures, or convulsions are a hyperexcitation of neurons in the brain with uncontrolled electrical activity. This causes sudden, involuntary contractions of muscle groups. Different types of seizures result depending on the areas of the brain being stimulated. When the entire brain is involved, the patient experiences total-body shaking with sudden loss of consciousness. When the abnormal electrical activity is limited to a portion of the brain, the seizure activity relates to that portion only. If the area controlling motor function of the upper extremity is involved, the patient will experience shaking of that extremity without loss of consciousness. Because of these clinical differences, seizures are best divided into two broad classifications, generalized and partial (focal). There is some degree of overlap between these two classifications since episodes which begin as partial or focal seizures often progress to generalized seizures.

Generalized, or grand mal, seizures are the result of neurons throughout the entire brain firing simultaneously, producing body-wide, skeletal muscle tonic and clonic spasms, or contractions. With the sudden loss of consciousness, these patients cannot protect themselves and may sustain contusions, fractures, lacerations or abrasions. Because the sustained skeletal muscle contractions prevent normal respirations, the patient may become hypoxic. Breathing typically resumes with noisy respirations. Patients often bite the tongue, lose control of bowel or bladder function (incontinence) and are confused for up to several hours afterwards. The confusion following a seizure is called the postictal (post-seizure) period. A sensory warning, or aura, can precede each tonic-clonic seizure.

Generalized seizures may also present in a more subtle fashion, with the individual merely staring into space and appearing distracted from the environment. These petit mal, or absence, seizures usually only last several seconds, but can be life threatening if they occur while driving or operating dangerous equipment. Children are most commonly affected by petit mal seizures. Adult onset is extremely uncommon, and most children with petit mal seizures cease having attacks upon reaching adulthood.

Partial, or focal, seizures involve the stimulation of a localized area of the brain, producing a specific sensation or action depending on which part of the body the stimulated area of the brain controls. An example of a partial seizure is the psychomotor seizure, which occurs in several stages. The first stage consists of an aura, or odd feeling that a seizure is going to occur. This is followed by one or more autonomic nervous system changes, such as salivation, rapid heat rate, incontinence or apnea. Then an automatism, or involuntary motor activity, occurs. This automatism may be subtle, such as lip smacking, or more obvious with complex muscle movement. These seizures are usually of short duration but may recur frequently with associated hallucinations or memory lapses. Seizures may be caused by a variety of conditions, including electrolyte disturbance, hypoxia, hypoglycemia, head injury, high fever or epilepsy.

Causes of seizure include genetic predisposition, infection, metabolic imbalance, cancer, toxins, trauma, and fever (febrile seizures). While some patients will have only one isolated seizure in a lifetime, others are prone to recurrent seizures. Individuals suffering seizures without a known cause are said to suffer from idiopathic epilepsy.

Young children are subject to febrile seizures as a result of rapid rise in body temperature during infections. Young adults, who have a high incidence of head trauma, can suffer seizures from hypoxia and secondary scar formation in brain tissue. Older adults are susceptible to vascular disease, which may cause strokes or develop cancer that can lead to seizures.

Prehospital assessment is similar to the initial approach to any other patient. The patient's airway patency must be assessed first. The patient who is apneic and has a clenched jaw and bitten tongue, presents a special challenge. Skill in the use of airway adjuncts such as the nasal trumpet, oral airway and jaw thrust maneuver is important, but nothing must be forced into the mouth. Adequacy of breathing is assessed next. Supplemental oxygen should be provided even if breathing is adequate, since hypoxia may be causing the seizure. If possible in patients with persistent or recurring seizure activity, endotracheal intubation should be used to secure the airway and breathing.

Circulatory assessment includes inspection of the entire patient to locate any wounds that either caused the seizure or were created by it. Circulatory interventions include establishing intravenous access and obtaining blood samples for rapid glucose determination and later hospital use in determining the cause of seizures. Intravenous access also allows the administration of fluid, and medications such as dextrose, benzodiazepines, phenytoin or barbiturates that can stabilize or terminate abnormal electrical activity in the brain. Most seizures, however, are of less than five minutes duration and do not require anticonvulsant medications in the field.

The general history and physical examination are performed with attention to clinical criteria for distinguishing between seizures and other conditions that present with altered mental status, such as syncope, hypoglycemia and head trauma. Crucial historical data includes current prescription and over-the-counter medications, past history of seizures, recent head trauma, fever, drug or alcohol use, and other medical problems such as diabetes or heart disease. The epileptic may wear a medic alert bracelet or necklace. Eyewitnesses should be questioned regarding the patient's mental status, incontinence, recurrence of seizure activity, the characteristics of abnormal motor activity and actual seizure duration. The physical examination should include evaluation for head trauma, tongue biting, pupillary response, cardiac dysrhythmias and vital signs. Consideration that a seizure patient may have fallen, or been submerged in water or involved in a motor vehicle accident, calls for cervical spine immobilization and backboard placement.

Status epilepticus - persistent seizure or multiple seizures without return of consciousness - requires special attention. Prolonged hypoxia and the potential for hypoglycemia warrant emergent care to terminate the seizure activity and prevent brain injury usually be administering intravenous benzodiazepines. The seizure patient must be constantly monitored during prehospital transport for signs of subtle seizures, or return of generalized seizures. Hypoglycemia is an important and eminently treatable cause of seizures; a glucose determination should be performed in the field prior to giving 50% dextrose.

Spinal Cord Injury Spinal cord injury is one of the most devastating consequences of trauma. Automobile accidents and falls account for many of the injuries. The typical patient is male, between 18 and 25 years of age and is often intoxicated at the time of injury. Elderly patients are also at high risk, even in an apparently minor trauma, because of arthritic changes in the vertebrae.

There are four major mechanisms of injury: flexion, flexion-rotation, extension and vertical compression. The spinal cord can be damaged by both primary and secondary injuries. Primary spinal cord injury occurs at the time of impact, and involves penetrating or massive blunt trauma with disruption of the vertebral column that impinges on or transects the cord. Elderly patients can sustain primary spinal cord injury when their cervical spine is forced into extension and the spinal cord is compressed against bony spurs or ridges formed by osteoarthritis.

Secondary spinal injury occurs at any point in time following the initial injury. Spinal immobilization is performed to prevent this. Other causes of secondary injury are hypoxemia due to respiratory insufficiency, edema around the site of injury and shock—either spinal or systemic—that reduces blood flow to the injured cord.

A careful neurologic exam is helpful in diagnosing the level of the lesion in acute spinal trauma, and begins with simple observation. Look for soft tissue and bony abnormalities that may indicate level of lesion and the mechanism of injury. Abdominal breathing may indicate cervical spine trauma, since cervical nerves innervate the diaphragm. Assessment of mental status includes a Glasgow Score and determination of the areas of the body that hurt, feel numb or cannot be moved. Neurologic deficits from spinal cord injury usually progress over a period of hours, so prehospital exam results may differ from those performed in the hospital. Gross motor function can be assessed simply by asking the patient to squeeze the rescuer's hands and move the legs and feet. A quick sensory exam involves using one's hand to check response to light touch in all extremities.

Management of the patient with a spinal cord injury differs from that of a general trauma patient in only a few ways. After surveying the scene for hazards, the paramedic should immediately gain control of the patient's head and neck, then apply a rigid cervical collar (C-collar). The head and neck must stay in neutral position to prevent any secondary cord damage. The collar does not provide complete immobilization of the neck, so manual immobilization is maintained until the patient is completely secured and immobilized to a long board with C-collar and immobilization device or other lateral head support.

Spinal Disk Disease The spinal vertebrae are separated by cartilaginous disks made up of an outer annulus fibrosus and an inner nucleus pulposus. Trauma and degenerative changes can both result in protrusion or rupture of the nucleus through the annulus, at the lumbar and cervical levels. Symptoms result when the nucleus compresses a nerve root where it enters or exits the spinal canal.

In the cervical area, the most common root compression occurs in the lower vertebrae, causing problems such as the frozen shoulder syndrome. It is most common in the lumbar area to have the L5 or S1 nerve roots involved, resulting in foot drop with muscle weakness in the lower anterior leg, or calf muscles weakness and loss of the ankle tendon reflex.

Treatment is most often conservative, consisting of bed rest (supine on a firm surface). Analgesics and mild tranquilizers may be helpful to relieve pain. Surgery decompressive laminectomy may be performed when objective neurologic findings, such as sensory deficit and weakness, persist or worsen.

A similar entity, acute spinal cord compression, is caused by any structural protrusion into the spinal canal. Tumor, abscess and hematoma can cause this. Spinal cord compression and resulting neurologic deficit require immediate recognition and spinal immobilization, with emergent neurosurgical intervention on hospital arrival.

Subarachnoid Hemorrhage Subarachnoid hemorrhage is sudden bleeding into the subarachnoid space, occurring spontaneously from an aneurysm or arteriovenous malformation (AVM), or as a result of head trauma. The arachnoid membrane is the thin, transparent covering encasing the brain. Subarachnoid hemorrhage is the most common type of bleeding following acute head injury, followed in frequency by subdural hematomas.

Immediately following the vessel rupture, escaping blood mixes with CSF and irritates the meninges, increasing intracranial pressure. The increased pressure produces headache, vomiting, dizziness and alterations in respiratory and pulse rates. Typically, a subarachnoid hemorrhage presents as the patient's worst-ever headache. The patient usually does not lose consciousness immediately with the onset of headache, but initial stupor may progress to coma. Convulsions occasionally occur.

Subdural Hematoma Subdural hematomas are much more common. They occur when the veins that bridge between the skull and the brain tear, allowing blood to collect between the dura and the arachnoid membrane. A patient with an acute subdural hemorrhage presents with a deteriorating level of consciousness and requires rapid intervention to prevent further brain damage and death. Subdural hematomas may also be subacute or chronic; these are more stable and have a lower mortality.

Prehospital management of the patient with a suspected intracranial hematoma can be challenging. Head trauma victims are often intoxicated and combative, clouding the origin of the problem. Such patients should be assumed to have a head injury until proven otherwise. The paramedic must also consider hypoxemia or hypoglycemia as possible treatable causes.

Lowering intracranial pressure is often life saving for the patient whose brain is under pressure from bleeding or edema. Controlled hyperventilation at no more than 20-22 breaths per minute is the most rapidly effective way to do this. Signs of impending herniation, in which the brain is forced through a skull opening, include a decreased Glasgow Coma Score, a unilaterally fixed and dilated pupil, and high blood pressure with a slow pulse (Cushing's reflex).

Obstetrical & Gynecological Conditions

Abortion: Spontaneous, Threatened, Inevitable, Incomplete, Complete Spontaneous abortion (miscarriage) is common, though it often goes unrecognized when it occurs before a period is missed. Most spontaneous abortions are indicative of some fetal abnormality incompatible with life. Threatened abortion describes a pregnant patient who presents with vaginal bleeding. Although spotting is actually a common and normal feature of early pregnancy, vaginal bleeding indicates a high chance of miscarriage. A threatened abortion occurs early in pregnancy when the bleeding does not include products of conception or tissue and the cervical os remains closed. The occurrence of bleeding and an open cervical os is termed inevitable abortion. If products of conception (fetal tissue, placenta) are retained in the uterus or seen protruding from the os or in the vagina, the condition is called incomplete abortion. A complete abortion (miscarriage) occurs when all fetal tissue has been passed, the os is closed and the uterus contracted.

A careful history should be obtained in the pregnant patient who is bleeding. One should inquire as to the estimated number of weeks of gestation, the quantity of bleeding, any history of trauma or home abortion attempts, presence or absence of pain, and whether an ultrasound has been done to confirm normal uterine pregnancy. The presence of a fever may be important, as infection can lead to abortion or be the result of retained fetal tissue. If tissue has been passed at home, it should be saved, placed in a container and taken with the patient to the hospital. If significant bleeding has occurred, intravenous lines should be started. All bleeding, pregnant patients should be considered to have an ectopic pregnancy until diagnosis proves otherwise.

Abruptio Placenta Abruptio placenta occurs when a normally located placenta abruptly and prematurely separates from the uterine wall. The result of this abruption is blood loss into the uterine cavity. Abruption is more likely to occur in patients who smoke, have high blood pressure or have a history of trauma, multiple births or a prior episode of abruption. The blood in the uterine cavity is quite irritating and causes symptoms of painful cramping or onset of labor. Vaginal bleeding usually occurs with dark, unclotted blood. Fetal distress may be present because of the loss of maternal-fetal blood exchange. Mild cases of partial abruption can be managed conservatively with careful maternal fetal monitoring; the pregnancy may continue if there is no significant fetal distress. In cases of more severe abruption, emergency cesarean section (C-section) may be needed to save the distressed fetus. Serious complications of abruption include disseminated intravascular coagulation (DIC) and other blood clotting problems that worsen maternal bleeding.

The best way to maintain fetal well being is by preserving maternal hemodynamics. Cases of severe bleeding should be aggressively managed with oxygenation, large bore IVs and aggressive fluid replacement. Once in the hospital, fetal-maternal monitoring and ultrasound will be employed to assist in making decisions regarding emergent C-section versus more conservative care.

Braxton Hicks Contraction (Braxton Hicks Sign, False Labor)

Braxton Hicks contraction is irregular tightening of the pregnant uterus that begins in the first trimester and increases in frequency, duration and intensity as pregnancy progresses.

Dysmenorrhea, Primary and Secondary

Dysmenorrhea is pain associated with menses (menstruation). The pain is thought to result from uterine contractions and ischemia, most likely from hormones produced in the uterine lining. Primary dysmenorrhea is associated with normal cycles when there is no demonstrable lesion affecting the reproductive organs. Secondary dysmenorrhea is caused by a known problem such as endometriosis or chronic pelvic inflammatory disease. Dysmenorrhea causes crampy low abdominal pain that may be reported as a dull, constant ache. Dysmenorrhea can be extremely debilitating to women for several days during menses. Associated symptoms include headache, nausea, vomiting and constipation or diarrhea.

Eclampsia, Preeclampsia, Pregnancy-Induced Hypertension

Once grouped together under the outdated term "toxemia," the hypertensive disorders of pregnancy are now referred to by more specific names: eclampsia, preeclampsia and pregnancy-induced hypertension (PIH). PIH is diagnosed by a rise above the patient's normal systolic blood pressure of greater than 30 mmHg, a rise in diastolic blood pressure of 15 mmHg, or an absolute blood pressure above 140 over 90. Young women, especially those pregnant for the first time or with twins, are at increased risk for PIH.

PIH associated with tissue edema and protein in the urine is termed preeclampsia. If seizure activity or coma is also present, the condition is called eclampsia, which is life-threatening. The vasospams and ischemia of PIH can negatively affect the major organ systems.

Eclamptic seizures can result in maternal or fetal death.

They may be preceded by headache, visual changes or abdominal pain. Occasionally, neurologic symptoms are present without the usual edema and proteinuria. Eclampsia should be considered in any seizing, pregnant patient. The seizure can initially be managed as for any seizure victim, with airway control, oxygen and IV benzodiazepines (Valium or Ativan). Eclamptic seizures are ultimately managed with IV magnesium sulfate. Upon arrival at the hospital, blood pressure is usually controlled with IV medications, under careful maternal and fetal monitoring.

Ectopic Pregnancy

Ectopic pregnancy is defined as a pregnancy that has implanted outside of the uterus. Almost all ectopic pregnancies implant in the fallopian tubes, hence the common term "tubal pregnancy." Pregnancies may also occur in the ovaries or cervix, and more rarely on the abdominal wall or organs. Ectopic pregnancy can be caused by infections that scar and distort pelvic anatomy. Pelvic surgery, induced abortion, tubal ligation and IUD use also increase the likelihood of ectopic pregnancy. Ectopic pregnancies grow slower than normal ones and therefore may not be as readily detected by ultrasound.

The classic presentation of ectopic pregnancy is the triad of late menses with abdominal pain followed by bleeding. These symptoms differ from those previously discussed for aborted pregnancies, in which the bleeding typically proceeds the pain. Ectopic pregnancy is an event of early pregnancy, usually occurring in the fifth to eighth week. the pain of an early ectopic pregnancy may be intermittent and crampy in nature when it is associated with a minor bleed. However, in cases of rupture resulting in significant bleeding, the presentation can be acute and intense. When free blood is present in the abdomen, marked tenderness, loss of appetite, guarding and rigidity are present; the abdominal muscles are tight and the pain increases dramatically with movement, coughing, and bumps during transport. The patient with hemoperitoneum also commonly complains of shoulder pain. Life-threatening hemorrhage may be taking place in the abdomen even when vaginal bleeding is minimal.

The initial assumption that pain in pregnancy indicates ectopic pregnancy is necessitated by its high mortality rate if left untreated. Whenever there is a suspicion of ectopic pregnancy, large bore IVs should be established with normal saline or Ringer's lactate even if the patient is not yet hemodynamically compromised. Early detection and intervention greatly reduce the morbidity and mortality of ectopic pregnancy.

Endometriosis

Endometriosis is a condition in which the tissue that lines the uterine cavity is found in abnormal locations outside of the uterus. The ovaries are the most common site of endometriosis; the fallopian tubes, outer uterine surface, uterine ligaments and peritoneum can also be involved. Symptoms of endometriosis include acute pain of the ovaries, premenstrual pelvic pain, pain with sexual intercourse and dysmenorrhea. Endometriosis is often found in women seeking treatment for infertility. The most serious complication of endometriosis is bleeding, since the endometrial tissue is stimulated during the menstrual cycle.

Endometritis Endometritis is an infection or inflammation of the endometrium, usually following childbirth—especially cesarean section or abortion. Endometritis is characterized by fever and abdominal pain one to three days after delivery, and is associated with a foul-smelling, bloody discharge. The diagnosis is made when other causes of fever have been excluded. The treatment includes hospitalization with IV antibiotic therapy.

Hyperemesis Gravidarum It is not uncommon for pregnant women to experience nausea and vomiting during the latter part of the first trimester. If the vomiting is unrelenting and associated with significant weight loss, dehydration and electrolyte imbalance, it is termed hyperemesis gravidarum (literally: too much vomiting during pregnancy). Young women in their first pregnancies are particularly vulnerable.

The severely ill patient is afebrile with lethargy and dehydration. Abdominal pain may occur secondary to retching. Symptomatic relief is obtained with IV fluids and anti-emetics. If relief is not obtained, hospital admission may be required for treatment. Prehospital care givers can offer reassurance and administer IV fluids. It is important to consider other possible causes such as urinary tract infection and appendicitis.

Pelvic Inflammatory Disease Pelvic inflammatory disease (PID), an inflammatory condition of the female pelvic organs, is a common bacterial infection among women of childbearing age.

Adolescents and young women are at greatest risk for PID, especially those with a history of previous PID, frequent sexual activity with multiple partners or use of intrauterine devices (IUDs). The usual presentation of PID is lower abdominal pain and vaginal discharge. Patients usually complain of lower abdominal pain worsened by sexual intercourse. Vaginal discharge or menstrual irregularities may also be reported. The disease can also present more dramatically with fever, vomiting and an acute abdomen, requiring hospitalization and IV antibiotics.

The complications of PID include chronic and severe pelvic pain, increased risk of ectopic pregnancy, infertility, abdominal and pelvic adhesions and tubo-ovarian abscess. Because of the serious consequences of untreated disease, health care professionals have become liberal in the diagnosis and treatment of PID.

A woman of childbearing age with pelvic pain should always be considered to be pregnant until proven otherwise. In the acutely ill patient, or one in whom a serious condition such as ectopic pregnancy is suspected, lines should be started and IV fluids administered as needed.

Placenta Previa Placenta previa is the implantation of a normal placenta over or near the internal os of the cervix. Implantation can completely or partially cover the cervix. The condition is one of the common causes of bleeding in the second half of pregnancy. Factors that can inhibit normal placental implantation include multiple previous pregnancies, uterine fibroids, multiple induced abortion and multiple gestation. The patient will usually present with painless vaginal bleeding, though placental obstruction of the os may conceal blood loss until clinical signs of shock appear.

This condition can often be distinguished from abruptio placenta, in which the bleeding is painful. Internal pelvic exam is contraindicated when there is bleeding during the third trimester, as the placenta could be dislodged, causing further hemorrhage and threat to the fetus. The patient needs to be evaluated at the ED as soon as possible, with delivery by cesarean section if the hemorrhage does not stop spontaneously, or if there is fetal distress. Intravenous lines and oxygen therapy should be initiated in the prehospital setting if bleeding is significant or early shock exists.

Postpartum Hemorrhage Postpartum hemorrhage is the major cause of maternal mortality at delivery. Normal blood loss after delivery should not exceed 500 ml; greater amounts indicate significant hemorrhage that requires intervention. The site of placental separation is often the source of major bleeding, which may be caused by failure of the uterus to contract properly after delivery or by a retained piece of placenta. Other causes of significant bleeding are coagulation disorders and lacerations of the cervix, vagina or perineum.

In order to prevent postpartum hemorrhage, delivery should be accomplished in a controlled manner with minimal trauma. If the placenta is not expelled spontaneously within 30 minutes, gentle traction should be applied. With severe postpartum hemorrhage, manual uterine massage should be initiated after delivery of the placenta. IV lines should be in place prior to delivery to enable vigorous fluid resuscitation with lactated Ringer's or normal saline in the event of heavy bleeding. Oxygen therapy should accompany the fluid. When visible lacerations are the cause of significant bleeding, direct pressure or gauze packing may be indicated.

Supine Hypotension Syndrome During pregnancy, the expanding uterus considerably distorts pelvic and abdominal anatomy. Organs that are not securely attached, such as the small bowel, are displaced upward towards the diaphragm, and hollow organs such as the stomach and bladder are compressed. The usual anatomic position of the appendix between the iliac crest and umbilicus, for example, is moved superior in late pregnancy, so that appendix pain may be reported in the right upper quadrant.

The inferior vena cava, the large vein that returns blood from the body to the heart, runs along the right side of the spine. It is part of the low-pressure venous system and has thin, easily compressible walls. The considerable weight of the uterus and the added squeeze of stretched skin and muscle can completely compress the abdominal vena cava. This compression interferes with return flow to the heart, and can thereby diminish cardiac output and cause significant hypotension in the supine pregnant patient. Maternal hypotension results in decreased blood supply to the fetus, which may in turn lead to fetal distress.

Supine hypotensive syndrome can be prevented—and corrected—either by manual displacement of the abdomen to the left, away from the vena cava, or by placing the patient with the left side down. If it is necessary for the patient to be supine, pillows or padding can be utilized under the right buttocks and shoulder. If the patient is on a backboard, the entire board can be propped up on its right side.

Uterine Inversion Uterine inversion, the "turning inside-out" of the uterus, can occur spontaneously or as the result of excessive traction on the umbilical cord. The unusual condition is more likely to occur when the placenta is implanted in the rounded end of the uterus (the fundus). Because ligaments and vascular supply to the uterus are torn, severe shock usually occurs. The condition is rare, but life-threatening.

Management includes treatment for shock. Medical direction may recommend manual replacement, which is done by pushing the fundus upward through the cervical canal. If this is not done, the protruding tissues should be covered with moist sterile dressing. The patient should be transported immediately.

Uterine Rupture Uterine rupture is a life-threatening condition in which the uterine wall tears, either spontaneously or secondary to trauma. Prolonged labor or a uterine scar from a previous cesarean section, for instance, can cause spontaneous uterine rupture.

The patient with this condition will likely describe continuous abdominal pain that increases in severity. Shock will develop, although external vaginal bleeding may not be seen. The abdomen is rigid and tender, and fetal heart tones are absent.

Management includes rapid transport to a hospital where an emergency cesarean section may save the fetus. Shock treatment is important.

Vaginitis Vaginitis is defined as inflammation or infection of the vagina and external genitalia. Vaginal discharge is the most common symptom. A certain amount of vaginal discharge is normal; however, it becomes abnormal when there is an offensive odor, itching, irritation or pain, or when the amount becomes distressing to the patient. Most vaginitis is caused by bacteria, protozoa or yeast. Less common causes include viruses, foreign bodies, pinworms, fistulas, radiation and tumors of the genital tract.

Other Conditions

Allergic Reactions and Anaphylactic shock Anaphylactic shock is one of the most dramatic emergencies that paramedics encounter. The victim frequently appears near death yet prehospital personnel are often successful at reversing the deadly effects of this condition.

Anaphylactic shock is probably encountered less frequently than other types of shock. Some sources indicate that 400-800 anaphylactic deaths occur annually in the United States. The offending agents are usually either penicillin (100-500 deaths per year) or insect stings (40-100 deaths per year).

The body's immune and allergic responses are important concepts. The IMMUNE RESPONSE is a normal protective response that guards the body against dangerous foreign intruders. In this process, the protective cells of the body fight and destroy dangerous substances such as infection and antigens. The ALLERGIC RESPONSE is an oversensitive and harmful response by the body's immune system against foreign substances that may actually be harmless. The danger of these substances is overestimated and the immune system overreacts to their presence. Thus, this abnormal response can cause needless damage to body tissue while fighting these harmless substances.

The body's resistance to poisons and foreign substances is IMMUNITY. This is a natural protective state whereby the body distinguishes "self" from "non-self." Natural immunity is resistance from birth, such as the human body's resistance to the distemper virus. Immunity can also be acquired by inoculation.

An ANTIGEN is a foreign substance that causes the formation of antibodies. An ANTIBODY is a protective protein substance that is formed in the body and is caused by contact with a foreign agent (antigen). Antibodies defend the body from foreign antigen substances.

Antigens and antibodies normally work together to protect the body from disease (the immune response). The abnormal or oversensitive antigen-antibody reaction causes allergies and severe allergic shock. An ALLERGY is an abnormal and individual hypersensitivity to substances that are normally harmless.

The term *anaphylaxis* is derived from "ana," meaning without, and "phylaxis," which means protection. Anaphylaxis refers to an acute, generalized, severe allergic reaction that occurs after the body has been exposed to a foreign substance to which it is oversensitive. In most texts, this term is used when the severity of the allergic reaction causes a generalized response and shock.

An allergic reaction and anaphylactic shock cannot occur with the *first* contact with a potential antigen. The first exposure causes the antibodies to be formed, setting the stage for the antigen-antibody reaction on a subsequent exposure. This process of exposure to an allergen and the resultant production of antibodies is called SENSITIZATION. It may occur with repeated exposures to an allergen over a variable period of time or with more subtle exposures and cross-sensitivities. An example of such sensitivity would be the inhalation of horse dander, creating sensitization to horse serum, or sensitization to antibiotics by drinking milk from cows treated with antibiotics.

Common Allergens Allergens causing allergic reaction or anaphylactic shock are many and varied including drugs, insect venom, food, pollen, and other miscellaneous agents. These agents may be introduced into the body by being injected, ingested, absorbed through the skin or mucous membranes, or even inhaled.

The most common allergen causing allergic reaction or anaphylactic shock is drug-induced and is parenterally administered penicillin. Other antibodies may also be culprits as well as vaccines containing horse serum and a variety of other drugs (see box).

Hymenoptera venom is also one of the most common causes of anaphylaxis. The Hymenoptera insect order includes bees, wasps, hornets, yellow jackets, and some ants. Approximately four out of every 1,000 people are severely sensitive to these stinging insects. This order of insects has an antigen cross-sensitivity. This means an initial sting by any of the Hymenoptera insects may lead to anaphylaxis from a subsequent sting of another. Stings about the neck and head are more likely to cause a severe reaction.

Food and food additives can produce anaphylaxis but because they are ingested, the reaction occurs more slowly. Sensitive individuals may vomit the offending food before anaphylactic shock occurs. Shellfish, nuts, eggs, and legumes are common food antigens. Food additives such as tartrazine yellow (coloring agent), benzoic acid (preservative) and bisulfite (preservative) have been known to cause anaphylatic shock and death.

In some rare circumstances, highly sensitive individuals have been reported to have had anaphylactic reactions to the order of fish, walnuts, and penicillin. Cold, heat, exercise, sunlight, and human seminal fluid have also been reported to have caused anaphylactic shock.

Pathophysiology An allergic reaction is an antigen-antibody reaction; anaphylaxis is its severe form. The reaction takes place on the surface of specific types of white blood cells called mast cells and basophils, and causes the release of several chemicals. The primary chemical released is histamine, accompanied by serotonin, bradykinin, a substance called slow-reacting substance of anaphylaxis (SRS-A), and few others. These chemicals cause three primary responses in the body. They are: 1) vascular dilation, 2) increased capillary permeability, and 3) smooth muscle spasm. These chemicals travel through the body affecting specific organs and causing the patient to exhibit any of a variety of signs and symptoms. In any allergic reaction, these signs and symptoms may be mild or limited to one system (e.g., skin rash). The allergic reaction may also affect the respiratory system and cause significant or severe breathing problems due to laryngeal edema or other effects. Shock causes systemic symptoms (anaphylaxis) as the vascular system is affected.

The symptoms of shock may or may not be preceded by allergic indicators. Several body systems may be affected by the allergic response. The skin is frequently affected with urticaria (hives), itching, redness, flushing, a rash, and edema. The edema is usually noticed in the lips and eyelids. the patient may feel a warm sensation accompanied by watery eyes and an itching nose.

Airway obstruction is the primary cause of death in anaphylaxis as edema and laryngospasm can occur quickly. Stridor, choking, or tightness in the neck or throat may indicate this danger. The respiratory system may be affected by wheezing, dyspnea, bronchospasms, hemoptysis, increased mucus secreations, or pulmonary edema.

The digestive system is affected by the histamine release which may cause smooth muscle spasm, with resultant nausea, cramping, vomiting, and diarrhea. Autopsy reports on anaphylactic deaths often report hemorrhagic gastritis. The central nervous system is affected by dizziness, anxiety, and typically a decrease in the level of consciousness.

The anaphylactic shock is the result of the capillaries becoming dilated and permeable. The vascular fluid shifts into the subcutaneous and extravascular spaces and there is no longer an adequate amount of fluid in the vessels. The dilated capillaries cause a low resistance or distributive type of shock with peripheral pooling of blood, decreased venous blood returning to the heart and a fall in cardiac output. This vascular collapse and hypotension stimulate the release of adrenalin. Histamine also stimulates the adrenalin release. As the adrenalin attempts to help the body compensate for the shock the following symptoms also occur: tachycardia, pallor, dryness of the mouth, and sweating. Cardiac dysrhythmias may also be present.

A patient may experience symptoms immediately after exposure to an allergen or the anaphylactic reaction rarely may be delayed for an hour or so. In most cases, symptoms will become evident within seconds to minutes after exposure to the offending antigen. The initial signs and symptoms typically show up on the skin, but shock can occur without any skin changes. The initial signs do not indicate the severity of the reaction. However, the earlier the onset of symptoms after exposure, the more severe the reaction is likely to be. This is an important factor in evaluating the patient and the urgency of treatment.

Assessment The patient with an allergic reaction or anaphylactic shock may initially exhibit a variety of symptoms, signaling the need for EMS. If the shock occurs suddenly,

BOX 2	Common Allergens Causing Allergic Reaction or Anaphylactic Shock

Drugs	Insects
Penicillins	Hymenoptera venom
Cephalosporens	(honeybee, yellow jacket,
Tetracyclines	wasp, hornet, fire ant)
Streptomycin	Deerfly venom
Neomycin	
Bacitracin	Foods
Sulfonamides	Milk
Hydrocortisone	Egg white
Methylprednisolone	Shellfish
Allergen extracts	Beans
Vaccines	Nuts
Radiopaque contrast media	Citrus fruits
Aspirin	Bananas
Horse tetanus antitoxin	Fish
Horse rabies serum	Chocolate
	Chamomile tea
	Grains
	Sulfites

the patient may collapse and lose consciousness. Oftentimes the first symptoms that become evident are respiratory distress and/or tightness in the throat or chest. Severe itching or a feeling of warmth may also be precursors of anaphylactic shock. A simple allergic reaction without respiratory symptoms or shock can present with skin signs (urticaria, rash, itching) or other isolated symptoms.

Airway, breathing, and circulation should be immediately evaluated as laryngeal edema, pulmonary edema, and shock can develop without warning. Level of consciousness and vital signs should be evaluated frequently throughout treatment and during transportation to the hospital.

Patient history should attempt to determine when the exposure occurred, and how quickly the first symptoms became evident. Some patients may not relate their symptoms to a specific cause and some may not be conscious enough to provide a history.

Past medical history should be elicited to determine previous reactions, with particular questioning about the subsequent airway, breathing, and circulation problems. Other medical problems are of importance, especially heart disease and asthma, as patients with those conditions have a higher mortality from anaphylaxis. Known allergies and current medications are important to note. Medic-Alert tags are also helpful if available. The environment should be quickly evaluated for clues to an unknown allergen or possibly for containers indicating self-administered epinephrine was used.

Focused assessment should include a more thorough evaluation of the respiratory system and circulatory status. Dyspnea accompanied by stridor and hoarseness may indicate upper airway involvement. Wheezing is common but hemoptysis, use of accessory muscles to breathe, and tracheal tugging are findings that indicate involvement of the lower respiratory tract. Pulse rate, pulse quality and regularity, and blood pressure measurement are important to evaluate. As the capillaries become more dilated and permeable, the pulse quickens to compensate, and the blood pressure eventually falls. If the blood pressure has fallen the vascular system is not longer efficiently compensating and the patient is in late shock.

Management The patient with anaphylactic shock should be treated quickly and aggressively as follows:

1. Airway management with high flow oxygen, intubation, and ventilatory support if necessary.
2. Intravenous therapy of Ringer's lactate or normal saline wide open to maintain blood pressure about 100 mm Hg systolic.
3. Epinephrine 1:10,000 intravenously, <u>very</u> slowly or 1:1000 subcutaneously.
4. Monitor ECG.
5. Additional drug therapy as needed: Diphenhydramine
6. Rapid transport to the hospital.

The restoration of circulatory function is the primary goal of therapy in the patient is severe anaphylactic shock. If respiratory function is compromised, it also must be restored immediately.

An allergic reaction with dyspnea but without shock should also be managed with epinephrine, however subcutaneous epinephrine is appropriate. Diphenhydramine can be given IM. A patient with a simple, localized allergic reaction can usually be managed by IM diphenhydramine or it may be taken orally if the patient is not nauseated. These patients should be observed for progressive allergic symptoms.

Prevention of Anaphylaxis When appropriate, victims of anaphylactic shock should be encouraged to seek methods of prevention. Medical care is necessary to evaluate the allergen causing the reaction in order to be able to give an accurate allergic history in the future. The patient's physician can make recommendations about desensitization techniques and carrying self-injectable epinephrine. The desensitization process attempts to gradually neutralize antibodies without causing allergic reactions. the use of Medic-Alert bracelets can be helpful.

Individuals who suffer anaphylactic shock from insects should be cautious during outdoor activities. Shoes and long pants should be worn when outdoors and gloves if gardening. Cosmetics, floral perfumes, and hair spray can attract insects and should be avoided as well as flower beds, clover fields, and picnic areas.

Anemia Anemia is a reduction in the level of circulating red blood cells (RBCs). Causes include acute and chronic blood loss, disorders that destroy red blood cells, and abnormal red blood cell production.

Anemia reduces the blood's oxygen transport capacity and thus diminishes oxygen delivery to cells. In acute cases, cells begin to die, leading to ischemic events or infarction of vital organs.

Patients with an acute anemic episode may present with signs and symptoms of shock. In the earlier stages, or if onset is gradual, patients may complain of weakness, fatigue, dizziness, headache or syncopal episodes. On physical exam, tachypnea, tachycardia and orthostatic hypotension may be present. Patients with chronic anemia may also complain of weakness, and appear pale in color.

Although it can be difficult to detect anemia in the prehospital setting, all patients with suspected anemia should receive high-flow oxygen, an IV and cardiac monitoring. Vital signs should frequently be reassessed.

Arthritis; Septic Arthritis; Rheumatoid Arthritis; Osteoarthritis Arthritis is any inflammatory condition of the joints, characterized by pain and swelling. Septic arthritis is an acute form characterized by bacterial infection of a joint, usually caused by the spread of bacteria through the bloodstream from an infection elsewhere, or by contamination during trauma or surgery. The joint is stiff, painful, tender, warm and swollen. Septic arthritis is also sometimes seen as a complication of untreated or incompletely treated gonorrhea.

Rheumatoid arthritis is a chronic, destructive, sometimes deforming, collagen disease that has an autoimmune component. Rheumatoid arthritis is characterized by swelling of the joint. It usually first appears between 36 and 50 years of age, and is most common in women. The course of the disease is variable, but it usually fluctuates in intensity. Manifestations outside of the joints can include cardiac involvement and pulmonary disease.

Osteoarthritis, the most common form of arthritis, is a form in which one or many joints undergo degenerative changes. Its cause is unknown, but may include chemical, mechanical, genetic, metabolic and endocrine factors. Emotional stress often aggravates the condition, which usually begins with pain after exercise. Stiffness, tenderness to the touch, crepitus and enlargement develop, and deformity, subluxation and synovial effusion may also eventually occur. Involvement of the hip, knee or spine causes more disability than osteoarthritis of other areas. Treatment includes rest of the involved joints, heat and anti-inflammatory drugs. Surgical treatment is sometimes necessary, and may reduce pain and greatly improve the function of a joint. Hip replacement, joint debridement, fusion and decompression laminectomy are some of the surgical procedures used in treating advanced osteoarthritis.

Cancer Cancer is a devastating disease that affects millions each year. Local tumor effects and adverse reactions to chemotherapy and radiotherapy increase the severity of the disease process. Potentially life-threatening problems may arise as a direct or indirect result of the disease process. Three major cancer-related emergencies of particular concern are spinal cord compression, airway obstruction and superior vena cava syndrome.

Spinal cord compression results from tumor growth, bleeding, infections or fractures. It manifests in the form of sensory deficits, parasthesias or paralysis. Patients may require emergency surgery or radiotherapy to prevent irreversible neural damage.

Airway obstruction can also occur as a result of tumor growth, aspiration, infection or bleeding. Rapid transport with high-flow oxygen is indicated for possible surgical airway intervention, as well as correction of the underlying cause.

Superior vena cava syndrome occurs when tumor growth obstructs blood flow through the superior vena cava. As a result, blood draining from the head, face, neck and arms is compromised. Patients will have facial edema, neck vein distention and prominent upper chest veins.

The goals of prehospital management are recognition of life-threatening problems, and appropriate intervention. Patients may have legal documentation limiting or preventing transport or aggressive treatment, however. EMS services should have specific regulations available to all prehospital personnel or this matter, and responders must be familiar with the local policy.

Carpal Tunnel Syndrome Carpal tunnel syndrome is a common, painful disorder of the wrist and hand, induced by compression of the median nerve between the carpal ligament and carpal bones of the wrist, which form a tight tunnel. The syndrome is seen more often in women, especially pregnant and menopausal women. Symptoms may result from trauma, synovitis or tumor, or may develop with conditions such as rheumatoid arthritis or diabetes. Compression of the median nerve causes weakness, pain with opposition of the thumb, and burning, tingling or aching.

There may also be radiation to the forearm and the shoulder joint. Pain may be intermittent or constant, and is often most intense at night. Symptomatic treatment usually relieves mild symptoms of recent onset, but if the pain becomes disabling, corticosteroid injection or surgery is necessary.

Hemophilia Hemophilia is a group of hereditary disorders in which there is a deficiency of one of the factors necessary for coagulation of the blood. The two most common forms of the disorder are called hemophilia A and B, defined by the specific missing factor. The severity of the disorder varies with the extent of the deficiency. Nosebleed, hematoma, blood in a joint and greater-than-usual loss of blood during dental procedures are common problems in patients with hemophilia. If the deficiency is severe, life-threatening hemorrhage may occur. Treatment is aimed at replacement of the deficient factor.

Hernia; Inguinal Hernia; Hiatal Hernia; Umbilical Hernia Hernia is a protrusion of an organ through an abnormal opening in the muscle wall of the cavity that surrounds it. A hernia may be congenital, result from the failure of certain structures to close after birth, or be acquired later in life because of obesity, muscular weakness, surgery or illness.

Inguinal hernia is a hernia in which a loop of intestine enters the inguinal canal, and sometimes the scrotal sac in a male. An inguinal hernia is usually repaired surgically to prevent bowel obstruction when the herniated segment becomes strangulated or gangrenous. Most hernias are inguinal hernias.

Hiatal hernia is protrusion of the stomach into the chest through a defect in the diaphragm.

Umbilical hernia is a soft, skin-covered protrusion of intestine and omentum through a weakness in the abdominal wall around the umbilicus. It usually closes spontaneously within 1 to 2 years, although large hernias may require surgical closure.

Immunosuppression Immunosuppression (immunodepression) is an abnormal condition characterized by the immune system's decreased ability to respond to antigen invasion. This can be induced by medications (steroids, anti-rejection drugs after a transplant, cancer, chemotherapy) or occur from a genetic or acquired disease such as AIDS, diabetes, or chronic alcohol abuse. Patients who are immunosuppressed are more likely to acquire infections and less able to fight them off.

Kaposi's Sarcoma Kaposi's sarcoma is a malignancy that occurs on the skin, in the lung, and gastrointestinal tract. It has been commonly found in patients with AIDS. The skin lesions are red, purple, or dark colored and can appear anywhere in the body.

Leukemia Leukemia is a cancer of the infection-defense system of the body, characterized by abnormal numbers and forms of immature white blood cells, and by infiltration of the lymph nodes, spleen, liver and bone marrow. The origin of leukemia is not clear, but it may result from exposure to ionizing radiation, benzene or other chemicals that are toxic to bone marrow. Acute leukemia usually has a sudden onset and progresses rapidly from early signs, such as fatigue, pallor, weight loss and easy bruising, to fever, hemorrhage, extreme weakness, bone or joint pain and repeated infections. Chronic leukemia develops slowly; signs similar to those of the acute forms of the disease may not appear for years. Diagnoses of acute and chronic forms are made by blood tests and bone marrow biopsies.

Lice Lice are any of the small, wingless insect order of *Anoplura*. They are parasites that may spend their entire life cycle on a bird or mammal single host, attaching eggs to the hair shafts or feathers. They transfer to humans by direct contact. Three forms that infect humans are the head louse, the body louse, and the crab louse. Treatment is local application of a pediculicide.

Lupus/Systemic Lupus Erythematosus Lupus/systemic lupus erythematosus is a chronic inflammatory disease affecting many body systems. The pathophysiology of the disease includes blood vessel inflammation, renal involvement, and lesions of the skin and nervous system. Dysfunction of the immune system whereby the body's immune system attacks its own organs, has been suggested as the cause of the disease. The presenting symptom is often arthritis, along with a "butterfly" rash over the face, weakness, fatigue, and weight loss. Depending on the organs involved, the patient may have pericarditis, peritonities, anemia, renal failure or severe neurological abnormalities.

Lymphangitis Lymphangitis is an inflammation of one or more lymphatic vessels, usually resulting from infection of one of the extremities. It is characterized by red streaks extending from the infected area up the extremity towards the axilla or groin, and by fever, chills, headache and muscle pain. The infection may spread to the bloodstream.

Lymphoma Lymphoma is a cancer of lymph tissue usually characterized by an enlarged but painless lymph node, weakness, fever, weight loss and anemia. The spleen and liver may become involved.

Osteoporosis Osteoporosis is a disorder characterized by an abnormal decrease in bone density. It occurs most frequently in post-menopausal women, sedentary or immobilized individuals, and patients on long-term steroid therapy. The disorder may cause pain, especially in the lower back, pathologic fractures, loss of height and various deformities. The prehospital emphasis is on gentle handling of elderly patients.

Rhabdomyalsis Rhabdomyalsis is muscle necrosis caused by a variety of conditions such as heat stroke, severe burn injury, and cocaine or amphetamine overdose. The by-product of muscle necrosis is myoglobin, which can damage the kidneys.

Scabies Scabies is a contagious disease caused by the *itch* mite, and characterized by intense itching of the skin and severe abrasion from scratching. The mite, transmitted by close contact with infected humans or domestic animals, burrows into outer layers of the skin, where the female lays eggs. Two to four months after the infection, sensitization to the mites and their products begins, resulting in an itching, pimple-like rash usually on the webs of fingers, wrists and thighs. Secondary bacterial infection may occur. Scabies is treated with scabicide, applied locally at affected sites.

Sudden Infant Death Syndrome Sudden Infant Death Syndrome (SIDS) is a sudden and unexpected death in a previously health infant. By definition, the cause of death cannot be determined at autopsy. SIDS is the most common cause of death in children between 2 weeks and 1 year of age. SIDS occurs at a rate of 2 deaths per 1,000 live births each year. Ninety percent occur in the first six months of life, usually between the ages of two to four months.

Research has not yet identified the underlying cause of SIDS. Prematurity, male sex, a history of SIDS in a previous sibling and substance abuse by the mother appear to increase the risk.

Most deaths occur during sleep, and patients thus are discovered only after prolonged periods of hypoxia. Infants are most commonly found in cardiac arrest. There is no evidence of a struggle.

Resuscitative efforts should be aggressive. Though few SIDS patients survive, paramedics should assume a treatable cause of arrest in the apparent SIDS presentation. It is also important for parents to know that every effort was made for their child.

Transfusion Reactions When mismatched blood is transfused, the donor's antibodies can bind to antigens on the recipient's red blood cells (RBCs). This reaction, known as a transfusion reaction, causes clumping of RBCs in the blood (agglutination) and subsequent hemolysis (RBCs breaking apart). Transfusion reactions can only be prevented by complete and careful type matching between donor and recipient.

Paramedics will occasionally transport a patient receiving blood. These patients need careful monitoring for signs and symptoms of transfusion reaction. The severity of the reaction depends on the degree of incompatibility, the amount of blood given and the rate of administration. Onset is usually rapid either during or immediately after a transfusion. More rarely, it occurs later. Signs and symptoms include anxiety; facial flushing; pain in the neck, chest and lumbar area; tachycardia; cold, clammy skin; dyspnea; hypotension; nausea or vomiting; dizziness; hives; headaches, and fever.

When signs and symptoms of transfusion reaction appear, discontinue the transfusion immediately. Consult with a physician as soon as possible, and maintain a crystalloid infusion for drug administration. A diuretic such as mannitol, and an antihistamine such as Benadryl (diphenhydramine), may be indicated.

One of the most lethal effects of transfusion reaction is kidney shutdown, which can begin within a few minutes to a few hours and may progress to lethal renal failure.

Respiratory Conditions

Asthma, Status Asthmaticus Asthma is a respiratory problem of the lower airway that is most commonly caused by an allergic reaction to foods, pollens, mold or environmental substances such as cigarette smoke (thus "reactive airway disease"). Asthma attacks can be triggered by temperature changes, stress, physical exertion and viral respiratory infections. The pathophysiological effect of asthma is airway obstruction caused by edema, secretions, inflammation and bronchospasm. Even though school-aged children are the predominant population, asthma occurs from the one-year-old to adults.

A good medical history is important with asthma patients. The first question is the confirmation of a history of asthma. If this is the case, the patient or parent can indicate if this is the usual presentation. Determine if there is family history of asthma and if the patient has any other medical problems. If the patient is taking medication, the following information should be obtained: names of the drugs, how much is being taken, whether any has been taken for this attack, and whether there has been any relief. Medications such as standard beta-agonist bronchodilators can build up to toxic levels. It is not uncommon with severe asthma attacks, especially with inhalers, for patients to take higher than recommended doses in order to seek relief. This can result in other medical problems such as tachycardia, flushing, tachypnea and cardiac dysrhythmias.

The most typical sign seen with asthma patients is wheezing, usually heard during the expiratory phase. Remember, however, that all that wheezes is not asthma. Get a thorough history and do a complete physical exam. These patients, particularly in prolonged episodes, may become dehydrated with a build up of thick mucus. In an attempt to clear the mucus, the patient can cough hard enough to cause vomiting. Suction should be provided and the patient's anxiety and level of consciousness monitored. Tachypnea and intercostal and suprasternal retractions may also be present.

These patients should receive humidified, high-concentration oxygen. If there are signs of severe respiratory distress, ventilations can be assisted with a bag-valve. Medications that can be used, in accordance with local protocols, include albuterol, terbutaline and epinephrine. It is important to monitor these patients continually in order to be ready to respond to any change in respiratory rate or effort.

Patients with severe signs of respiratory distress whose attacks can't be terminated by medication are said to be in status asthmaticus. These patients are usually moving and have a silent chest upon auscultation. This is an ominous sign; ventilatory assistance and rapid transport will be required. Epinephrine may be ordered in this setting.

Bronchiolitis Bronchiolitis is a viral infection that affects the lower airway when the bronchi and bronchioles become obstructed. It occurs primarily in children under two years of age. Severe complications can result because of the unique pathophysiology of the small child's airway. Children with bronchiolitis may have abundant secretions. This can require placing the child in a position that allows drainage in order to keep the airway open. There may also be a need for suction.

As with other respiratory problems, it is important to get a thorough history. Determine how long the child has been ill and whether the child has been seen by a physician recently. Also learn what medications the child is taking, and if this is the first episode of these signs and symptoms.

Initially, these children can present with fever and a cough. As bronchiolitis progresses, there may be wheezing and respiratory distress. In children over 1 year of age, it may not be possible in the prehospital setting to distinguish bronchiolitis from asthma. Wheezing may be heard in both the inspiratory and expiratory phases. Nasal flaring, cyanosis and use of accessory muscles can also be seen. These patients may become too fatigued to maintain adequate respiratory effort.

As with any other respiratory problem airway maintenance and breathing are the priorities. The airway needs to be kept clear, and high-concentration, humidified oxygen should be given; use the blow-by technique if the child won't tolerate a mask. Be prepared to assist ventilations, and establish an IV at a TKO rate. Bronchodilators such as albuterol may be used according to orders or protocols. Cardiac monitoring is also indicated. Keep these children calm, in a position of comfort, and transport with a parent.

Carbon Monoxide Inhalation Carbon monoxide (CO) is a leading cause of toxic death in the United States. Because CO poisoning is often the result of faulty heating systems in older buildings, it frequently results in multiple casualty incidents (MCI's) involving an entire family or occupants of an entire building. Automobile exhaust contains CO and is a common means of suicide and suicide attempts. CO poisoning also results from smoke inhalation during a fire.

Although normal human metabolism can produce minute quantities of CO, the vast majority of CO in the body is the result of absorption of environmental CO from by-products of combustion from sources such as gasoline-powered engines and tobacco smoke. CO exerts its toxic effects on the body in several ways, the most prominent of which is displacing oxygen from hemoglobin and altering the ability of oxygen that is still bound to hemoglobin to be released to the tissues. The end-point of CO poisoning is systemic hypoxia, which depresses CNS and cardiovascular function, and—without medical intervention—eventually leads to death.

The patient with CO poisoning can exhibit a variety of symptoms, many of which are vague and nonspecific. Headache, dizziness, nausea and generalized malaise are typical symptoms of mild to moderate CO toxicity. As more CO is absorbed into the bloodstream, the patient may develop visual problems, coma, cardiac dysrhythmias and cardiopulmonary arrest. The legendary "cherry red" skin color associated with CO poisoning is, in fact, usually not seen.

The therapy of choice for CO poisoning is the administration of 100% oxygen, which works to provide maximal oxygen content in the blood and accelerate the clearance of CO from the body. All patients who present in respiratory arrest should be intubated and ventilated with 100% oxygen. If there is a local or regional center for hyperbaric medicine, direct transport to that facility should be considered for any patient with altered mentation. Because of the risk of dysrhythmias, the patient should be placed on a cardiac monitor and have an IV established. It is crucial that the paramedic takes all necessary precautions to avoid being overcome by toxic CO fumes at the scene, including using, or summoning personnel qualified to use, self-contained breathing apparatus to effect a rescue in a toxic environment. Additionally, it is important for the paramedic to recognize that pulse oximetry readings will not be accurate in the patient with carbon monoxide inhalation.

Chronic Obstructive Pulmonary Disease (COPD): Chronic Bronchitis, Emphysema COPD is an ongoing disease process most commonly occurring in male smokers over age 50, although the incidence is increasing in women who smoke. Significant lung damage results in difficulty breathing and predisposition to pulmonary infection. COPD is actually a disease continuum ranging from emphysema (type A) to chronic bronchitis (type B). More purely emphysematous patients chronically hyperventilate, maintaining adequate oxygenation ("pink puffers") despite their increased work to breathe, which causes weight loss. At the other end of the spectrum is the bronchitic patient, who frequently has some degree of cyanosis and peripheral edema ("blue bloaters") from congestive heart failure. Most patients display a mixture of these findings.

COPD is caused by destruction of lung anatomy and a reduction in lung defense mechanisms, usually from cigarette smoking leading to inflammatory tissue changes. The inflammatory reaction destroys alveolar walls, producing easily collapsible airways and a reduced number of functioning alveoli. The bronchial component also reduces airway function by secreting excess mucus into the bronchial tree. This narrows airway lumens and creates mucous plugs, both of which also predispose the patient to pulmonary infection.

These alveolar and bronchial changes result in obstruction of air flow, increased breathing effort and other ventilation changes that lower blood oxygen levels and increase carbon dioxide. The clinical result is a patient exhibiting respiratory distress and complaining of shortness of breath.

Finally, because of increased pulmonary pressures, the right ventricle of the heart needs to pump harder to move blood through the diseased lung. This eventually results in congestive heart failure (cor pulmonale).

The hallmark symptom of COPD is dyspnea on exertion. The patients know their usual baseline level of shortness of breath for a given activity, and become appropriately concerned when their breathing is worse. Similarly,

COPD patients frequently have a baseline productive cough that worsens or changes with aggravation of their disease. Prehospital personnel may find the patient seated upright, leaning on the elbows and using accessory breathing muscles and pursed lips. (Pursed lips help increase airway internal pressure to prevent airway collapse on exhalation.) Airflow obstruction may cause wheezing if the patient is able to move enough air quickly. The combination of lack of wheezing and minimal air movement is cause for concern. Crackles may be heard on lung exam, secondary to uncleared secretions, pneumonia or congestive heart failure. Cyanosis and dependent edema may be present. Patients with long-term, severe COPD are often on home oxygen therapy, beta agonist aerosols, theophylline and inhaled or oral steroids.

Complications of COPD include pneumonia, pneumothorax and congestive heart failure. Cessation of respiratory drive from high-flow oxygen therapy, though much discussed, is exceedingly rare; high-flow oxygen should never be withheld from a dyspneic patient with COPD.

Prehospital physical exam includes vital signs, skin color and general observation of the patients appearance, position, accessory respiratory muscle retractions and other signs of distress. Lung exam may reveal crackles and diminished air movement. The ankles should be examined for edema.

The prehospital history includes the patient's age, sex, number of years with COPD, current medications and when last taken, drug allergy and past medical history, and whether the patient continues to smoke cigarettes. The history of the present event should include how the dyspnea, cough and response to medications are different from the usual pattern.

Air-hungry COPD patients require high-flow oxygen (preferably humidified) by non-rebreather mask. If only mildly dyspneic, oxygen by nasal cannula will suffice. Inhaled beta agonists such as albuterol may reverse some bronchospasm and improve the dyspnea. An intravenous line for emergent medication administration should be started at a TKO rate, but must not delay transport in the severely ill patient. The patient should be in a position of comfort, with the ambulance air conditioning on high if the weather is warm and humid. Should the COPD patient decompensate to frank respiratory failure, rapid endotracheal intubation is required.

Cystic Fibrosis Cystic fibrosis is an inherited disorder of the exocrine glands that causes production of abnormally thick mucus, elevation of electrolytes in sweat, increased organic and enzymatic constituents in saliva, and overactivity of the autonomic nervous system. The glands most affected are those in the pancreas, the respiratory system and the sweat glands. Cystic fibrosis is usually recognized in infancy or early childhood, and occurs chiefly among Caucasians. Early signs are a small bowel obstruction, a chronic cough, frequent, foul-smelling stools, and persistent upper respiratory infections.

Because there is no known cure, treatment is directed at the prevention of respiratory infections, which are the most frequent cause of death. Bronchodilators are used to help liquefy the thick, tenacious mucus. Physical therapy measures, such as postural drainage and breathing exercises, can also dislodge secretions. Broad spectrum antibiotics may be used prophylactically. Life expectancy in cystic fibrosis has improved markedly over the past several decades, and with early diagnosis and treatment, most patients can be expected to reach adulthood. Prehospital management is aimed at establishing and maintaining ventilatory adequacy and oxygenation.

Diphtheria Diphtheria is an acute, contagious disease caused by the bacterium *Corynebacterium diphtheria.* It is rare in the United States, and is characterized by the production of a systemic toxin and a false membrane lining of the mucous membrane of the throat. The toxin is particularly damaging to the tissues of the heart and central nervous system, and the dense false membrane in the throat may interfere with eating, drinking and breathing. Untreated, the disease is often fatal. Immunization against diphtheria is available to all children in the United States and is usually given in conjunction with pertussis and tetanus immunization early in infancy. Prehospital treatment is supportive.

Flail Chest Flail chest is relatively common in patients with blunt chest trauma. A flail injury occurs when at least three ribs are broken in two or more places, creating one or more free-floating chest wall segments. This free segment will eventually demonstrate "paradoxical motion." When the chest expands with inspiration, the segment collapses, and the segment protrudes when the chest contracts. Breath sounds are likely to be diminished on the injured side, and frank respiratory failure is not uncommon.

The force required to cause a flail injury often results in other chest injuries such as pulmonary contusion and hemothorax, and abdominal injuries such as splenic or liver lacerations. Flail chest and associated intrathoracic injuries can result in derangements of normal oxygenation, ventilation and chest wall compliance. The patient's pain on breathing and subsequent attempts to minimize the pain by shallow breathing and splinting further contribute to hypoventilation.

Prehospital management should be directed toward maximizing oxygenation and optimizing ventilation. The patient should receive high-flow oxygen through a non-rebreather mask, and an IV once rapid transport has begun. Endotracheal intubation is indicated for the patient in obvious respiratory failure. In addition, the flail segment should be stabilized by taping a pillow or bulky trauma dressing snugly over the site. Positive pressure ventilation will help ensure an adequate ventilation volume. Overly aggressive fluid resuscitation should be avoided unless there is evidence of shock.

Hyperventilation Syndrome Hyperventilation syndrome is a common, benign entity usually occurring in teenagers and young adults. It is a physical manifestation of anxiety, recognized or unrecognized, that causes a feeling of shortness of breath. The patient responds by taking rapid breaths that lead to a respiratory alkalosis and low serum calcium, which in turn induces the characteristic tingling and muscle spasms of the extremities.

Patients with hyperventilation syndrome often present breathing rapidly and complaining of tingling sensations about the mouth, fingers and toes. The hands and feet may be awkwardly held in a tetanic position called "carpopedal" spasm. The patient may feel faint, and can occasionally pass out, with spontaneous resolution of symptoms. The primary goal in assessing a patient presumed to be hyperventilating is to exclude more dangerous causes of tachypnea such as asthma; pulmonary embolus; increased metabolism due to exercise, fever, hyperthyroidism or infections; lesions of the central nervous system is an encephalitis or meningitis; hypoxia or metabolic acidosis; hormones, and drugs.

Once more dangerous causes of tachypnea have been excluded, hyperventilation syndrome should be treated by gentle reassurance as the mainstay of therapy. Hospital transport is required mostly to rule out other potentially more serious causes and to arrange on-going medical care.

Lung Abscess Lung abscess is a complication of infection of the lung, often caused by aspiration of infected material from the mouth. Patients with signs of infection such as fever and chills, may cough up yellow-green sputum. This occurs more commonly in immune-compromised patients such as AIDS patients or alcoholics. Clinically it may be difficult to differentiate this from pneumonia until an x-ray is obtained. Treatment includes supportive therapy such as oxygen administration and intravenous fluids.

Non-cardiogenic Pulmonary Edema, Adult Respiratory Distress Syndrome (ARDS) "Permeability pulmonary edema" is a distinct form that occurs suddenly and leads to severe hypoxemia, abnormal blow flow in the lungs and damaged lung tissue. This syndrome is usually referred to as the "adult respiratory distress syndrome" (ARDS). (See Cardiovascular Conditions section for a discussion of the entirely different entity of cardiogenic pulmonary edema.) A host of non-pulmonary diseases and injuries are associated with the development of this lung syndrome (See Box 3).

In permeability edema, the alveolar-capillary wall is no longer an effective barrier to protein and fluids. These substances flow out of the capillaries into the lung air sacs (and other tissues) under force of the blood pressure.

ARDS usually develops one to three days after the initial insult. Patients complain of shortness of breath, and develop rapid, labored breathing. Blood oxygen levels fall and the patient becomes cyanotic without intervention.

Objective assessment should include vital signs and general observations of appearance. Skin exam may reveal cyanosis or diaphoresis. Lung sounds can include non-focal crackles, but their absence does not exclude the diagnosis.

Historical points of importance are the triggering event, the rapidity of disease progression and the patient's assessment of dyspnea severity. Past medical history, current medications and drug allergies should be documented.

The patient should be placed in a semi-reclining position and given 100% oxygen by non-rebreather mask. An intravenous line can be started at a TKO rate but should not delay transport to the hospital. Depending on patient condition, endotracheal intubation may be needed to maintain oxygenation.

If a transport ventilator is available, positive end-expiratory pressure (PEEP) should be used to increase oxygenation and decrease fluid influx into the air sacs. The underlying cause of the permeability change should also be treated, if possible.

Pertussis Pertussis is an acute, highly contagious respiratory disease characterized by paroxysmal coughing that ends in a loud, whooping inspiration ("whooping cough"). It occurs primarily in infants and children less than 4 years of age who have not been immunized, and can be fatal.

Transmission is by direct contact or by inhalation of infectious particles, which are usually spread by coughing, sneezing or freshly contaminated articles. The initial stages of the disease are difficult to distinguish from bronchitis or influenza. Prehospital management includes observation for airway patency and respiratory distress.

Pleurisy, Pleuritis Pleurisy, inflammation of the parietal pleura of the lungs is characterized by dyspnea and stabbing pain. It can lead to restriction of ordinary breathing because of chest wall splinting on the affected side. Common causes of pleurisy include bronchial carcinoma, lung or chest wall abscess, pneumonia, pulmonary infarction and tuberculosis. Management consists of transportation to a hospital for further evaluation and treatment.

Pneumonia Pneumonia remains a leading cause of death. Most pneumonia is caused by viruses or bacteria, but other agents such as fungi, protozoa and chemicals are seen. Pneumonia can occur in any age group and is common in immunosuppressed individuals, such as those with cancer or human immunodeficiency virus (HIV) infection.

Pneumonia is a lung infection that results when there is a failure of the pulmonary defense mechanisms (the cough reflex, mucous clearance mechanisms and the immune system). Conditions that compromise these defenses, such as diabetes, cancer, COPD, sickle cell anemia, spleen removal and cigarette smoking, place patients at increased risk for pneumonia.

The disease can present in several different ways, but the classical description is fever, chills and cough. Malaise and chest pain are frequently present, and lower lobe pneumonia can cause upper quadrant abdominal pain. Physical exam may reveal diaphoresis, tachypnea and pulmonary crackles. Use of accessory muscles, nasal flaring and grunting indicate respiratory distress; these patients can progress to respiratory failure.

Patients are usually more comfortable sitting upright. Oxygen therapy by cannula or mask may subjectively improve the patient's condition, and albuterol can be effective if wheezing is present. Only rarely will the patient progress to respiratory failure and require endotracheal intubation. Rapidity of transport to the hospital should be based on the patient's condition, as is the case in most respiratory conditions.

Pneumonitis Pneumonitis is inflammation of the lung. It may be caused by a virus or a hypersensitivity reaction to chemicals, or to organic dusts such as bacteria, bird droppings or mold. Dry cough is a common symptom. Treatment depends on the cause, but includes removal of any offending agents, oxygen administration and transport.

Pneumothorax (Spontaneous, Tension), Hemothorax A pneumothorax is the acute accumulation of air in the normally unoccupied space between the outer surface of the lung (visceral pleura) and the inner lining of the chest cavity (parietal pleura). The condition can be catastrophic, particularly when air progressively accumulates under pressure in the pleural space. This is known as a tension pneumothorax and can lead to death within minutes if not recognized and treated immediately.

As noted above, the pleural space is normally a "potential space" containing only trace amounts of fluid to allow for smooth gliding between the visceral and parietal pleura. Various types of pathologies, most commonly thoracic trauma, can result in the entry of air (pneumothorax) or blood (hemothorax) into this space. In some patients, a spontaneous pneumothorax can occur without any trauma because of a defect on the surface of the lung that permits a rupture of the visceral pleura. Most patients can tolerate a pneumothorax or hemothorax for some period of time. If a tension pneumothorax develops, in which each inhalation results in a progressive accumulation of air and pressure in the pleural space, cardiopulmonary arrest can follow quickly as the pressure compresses vital vascular structures in the chest and impairs blood return to the heart.

Most patients with pneumothorax or hemothorax complain of shortness of breath and chest pain on the affected side. In the trauma setting, the physical exam is likely to reveal signs of external trauma to the chest wall such as tenderness, deformity, contusions or penetrating wounds. Crepitus or the unmistakable "crunch" of subcutaneous

BOX 3	Partial List of Conditions That Have Been Associated with the Adult Respiratory Distress Syndrome
Shock of any etiology	Inhaled toxins
Infection	O_2 (high concentrations)
Trauma	smoke
fat emboli from long bone	corrosive chemicals (NO_2,
fractures	Cl_2, NH_3, phosgene,
lung contusion	cadmium)
head injury	Hematologic disorders
Aspiration	intravascular coagulation
gastric juice	massive blood transfusion
fresh and salt water	Metabolic disorders
drowning	pancreatitis
hydrocarbon fluids	uremia
Drug overdose	paraquat ingestion
heroin	Miscellaneous
methadone	increased intracranial
propoxyphene	pressure (including seizures)
barbiturates	eclampsia
colchicine	post-cardioversion
	radiation pneumonitis
	post-cardiopulmonary bypass

emphysema may be noticed on palpation. In the case of tension pneumothorax, the patient will appear critically ill with hypotension, jugular vein distention and respiratory distress. With a sizable accumulation of air or blood in the pleural space, the affected side will demonstrate decreased or absent breath sounds on auscultation and the trachea may deviate slightly to the unaffected side. Tracheal deviation is a late sign, which can be difficult to identify.

The prehospital care of patients with hemo- or pneumothorax is aggressive management of the ABCs. All trauma patients should be managed normally with regard to C-spine protection and minimal scene time. High-flow oxygen is mandatory and endotracheal intubation should be performed on patients in respiratory failure. (Caution: positive pressure ventilation may worsen a tension pneumothorax.) If tension pneumothorax is suspected, it will be necessary to perform a needle decompression (needle thoracostomy) on the affected side with a large-gauge IV needle.

Pulmonary Contusion Pulmonary contusion is a common, potentially lethal chest injury. It is often seen in the setting of blunt chest trauma and almost always accompanies flail chest.

Pulmonary contusion is localized bleeding and bruising within the lung tissue itself. This injury is usually the result of sufficient blunt force being applied to the chest to transfer energy through the ribs and chest wall to the lung tissue. Rapid deceleration forces can also cause the lungs to collide with the chest wall, resulting in alveolar rupture and hemorrhage. The contusion disrupts the lung's ability to oxygenate properly because of alveolar collapse and localized bleeding.

The presentation of the patient with an underlying pulmonary contusion will be similar to that of a patient with a flail chest, except that it is not possible to diagnose a pulmonary contusion in the prehospital setting. Any patient with a flail chest is likely, however, to have an associated pulmonary contusion. The patient will probably complain of shortness of breath and chest pain corresponding to the site of injury. The most common sign is an increasing respiratory rate.

Because the patient with a pulmonary contusion is likely to be the victim of significant blunt trauma, it is essential that the ABCs and cervical spine stabilization be addressed at the outset of care. Hypoxia is the most imposing complication of pulmonary contusion, so the patient should be placed on high-flow oxygen. Should respiratory failure be evident despite high-flow oxygen administration, the patient should be intubated to maximize ventilation and minimize alveolar collapse. Unless signs of shock are present, it is preferred that the patient with a pulmonary contusion not be aggressively hydrated with IV fluids, as this will complicate subsequent hospital management of the contusion.

Pulmonary Embolism Pulmonary embolism is a clot that forms in the deep venous system, usually in the thigh or pelvis, breaks off and travels to the lungs, where it lodges in the pulmonary vasculature. This leads to hypoxemia and an increase in workload on the heart. Injury to blood vessels, decreased venous blood flow and alterations in the coagulation system - as can be caused by cancer, all increase the risk of pulmonary embolism. Immobilization, especially when associated with childbirth, congestive heart failure or surgery, can also be a predisposing factor.

Because pulmonary embolism can present in a variety of ways, it should be considered in any acute, non-specific cardiopulmonary complaint. Acute onset of chest pain, dyspnea, shock and apprehension are the most common symptoms. A pulmonary embolism is difficult to distinguish from myocardial infarction and pneumonia. Physical exam may reveal tachypnea, tachycardia and pulmonary crackles. Large blockages can present with shock, or even cardiac arrest.

The patient with suspected pulmonary embolus should be transported to the hospital immediately in a semi-reclining position and on high-flow oxygen by non-rebreather mask. A large bore intravenous line with Ringer's lactate or normal saline should be started and flow rate adjusted as vital signs dictate. A decompensating patient will require endotracheal intubation. The possibility of cardiac dysrhythmias secondary to hypoxia necessitates monitoring and treatment as needed.

Rib Fractures Rib fractures are usually the result of blunt trauma to the chest. The most common location for fractures of the ribs is the lateral aspect of ribs three through eight, where there is the least muscle protection. Although typically very painful, simple rib fractures (without other injury) are rarely life threatening. Less common fractures to the first and second ribs can be associated with pulmonary or cardiac injuries, though, and lower rib fractures may accompany spleen, kidney or liver damage. Management is aimed at minimizing pain so normal respirations can continue. This can be accomplished by splinting with a sling and swathe. Supplemental oxygen should be provided during transport.

Smoke Inhalation, Toxic Inhalation, Respiratory and Pulmonary Burns The respiratory system is at particular risk for injury when a patient is exposed to a smoke- and heat-filled environment, as often occurs in a structure fire. Inhalation of toxic fumes is the most common cause of death in patients who die in fires. When the patient is exposed to a rapidly expanding fire in a confined space, there is also a high risk of direct burns to the airways.

Smoke and gases generated by combustion contain various toxic materials, including cyanide and carbon monoxide, that are absorbed through the lungs. In addition, close proximity to flame and superheated gases may result in burns to the upper, and more rarely the lower, airways. A vicious cycle then develops: oxygen use is disrupted at the cellular level by inhaled toxins, and burns impair the ability to inhale oxygen and deliver it to the alveoli by causing edema that blocks the airways. The net result can be profound hypoxia leading to cardiopulmonary collapse.

Patients with smoke inhalation or respiratory tract burns will present with shortness of breath. The hypoxic patient may also present with altered mental status. Patients with respiratory burns may have burned nasal hairs or be actively coughing up black-tinted sputum. Auscultation of the lungs can reveal a variety of findings including stridor (in upper airway burns), wheezing, rales and rhonchi.

The prehospital management of smoke inhalation and respiratory tract burns is high-flow oxygen through a non-rebreather mask and aggressive management of the airway. This includes early endotracheal intubation for patients with evidence of either respiratory failure (hypoventilation) or airway compromise from edema. These patients often also require management of thermal skin burns.

Traumatic Asphyxia Traumatic asphyxia is the result of severe blunt force applied to the upper chest, and sometimes the abdomen. Increased intrathoracic pressure forces blood from the right side of the heart into the veins of the face, neck and upper chest, giving those areas a purple-red discoloration. Petechiae and hemorrhage of the conjunctiva are also present. Although the head and neck findings in this condition may be very impressive, the associated intrathoracic and abdominal injuries are the greatest threat to life and must be aggressively identified and managed.

Tuberculosis (TB) The incidence of pulmonary tuberculosis continues to increase. TB causes lung damage and can spread to the kidney, meninges, pericardium and bones, especially the vertebrae (Potts disease).

TB is caused by an organism named *Mycobacterium tuberculosis,* which is spread from person to person by aerosolized droplets from coughing or sneezing, or by ingestion. In a healthy person, the body's defense mechanisms arrest the spread of infection. As defenses fail in a patient with a compromised immune system, the mycobacteria are reactivated, leading to the clinical manifestations of TB.

Population groups with a high prevalence of TB are alcoholics, drug addicts, the immunocompromised, immigrants, the homeless and the elderly. The patients complain of fevers, night sweats, weight loss, malaise, cough, and sputum production sometimes associated with blood streaking. The patient may appear diaphoretic, thin and wasted, and have crackles on lung exam, usually in the upper fields.

Personal protective equipment is important; an approved *M. tuberculosis* filter mask should be when TB is suspected. Oxygen may be given by nasal cannula or mask if the patient is short of breath. If the patient is not receiving supplemental oxygen, place a filter mask over the patient's mouth and nose to contain the spread of the organism. On hospital arrival, ensure that the patient is kept in respiratory isolation.

Vascular Conditions

Aneurysm: Aortic Aneurysm, Acute Aortic Dissection, Abdominal Aortic Aneurysm, Cerebral Aneurysm Aneurysm is a weakening and dilation of a vessel wall, usually an artery. A dissection occurs when the layers making up the vessel wall separate because of the weakening. Men over 60 years of age are at highest risk. The aorta is most often involved and the most dangerous clinically, and dissection is more frequent than rupture.

Atherosclerosis is the most common factor in aortic disease. Hypertension is often a predisposing factor in aneurysm formation. Dissections of the thoracic aorta usually involve the ascending aorta.

Patients with thoracic dissections will present most commonly with sudden onset of chest pain described as a "ripping" or "tearing" sensation with radiation to the back. Blood pressure in the upper extremities may be unequal and pulse deficits may be present. Patients with abdominal aortic aneurysms usually complain of abdominal, flank or back pain. A pulsatile mass may be palpable on abdominal exam. Patients may be hypertensive and anxious, or display signs and symptoms of shock if rupture has occurred. Both cases call for intravenous access, high-flow oxygen, cardiac monitoring and rapid transport. Rapid crystalloid infusion is indicated for shock.

Patients with bleeding from a cerebral aneurysm will experience neurological symptoms based on which part of the brain is affected. Symptoms and management are the same as any other bleeding in the brain (see Intracranial Hemorrhage).

Aortic Rupture, Traumatic Aortic trauma most often results from the deceleration forces produced by automobile accidents and falls from great heights. These injuries have high mortality rates and are the most common cause of sudden death from injury.

With significant deceleration forces, the ascending aorta and aortic arch shift anteriorly while the descending aorta is relatively immobile. Therefore, most ruptures of the aorta occur between the arch and the descending aorta. Initially there may be a hematoma that is contained by the outermost layer of the aorta. If the aorta has been completely transected, the patient will die within minutes.

Patients with contained rupture may only complain of chest pain. Those with full rupture of the aorta will present with signs and symptoms of shock, if they survive to EMS arrival. There may be absent breath sounds on the left side of the chest consistent with a hemothorax. Pale, cool lower extremities and absent or diminished femoral pulses are also possible signs.

Prehospital management is cervical spine immobilization, airway protection as needed, high-flow oxygen and rapid transport to the hospital, preferably a trauma center. Intravenous access should be attempted en route to the hospital. Notification to the receiving hospital is imperative if aortic injury is suspected so preparation can be made for emergency surgery.

Arterial Occlusion, Acute Acute arterial occlusion is the most common cause of arterial obstructive disease. It most often affects men between the ages of 50 and 70. Diabetes and smoking are significant predisposing factors.

Arterial occlusion results from an obstruction or narrowing of the vessel secondary to thrombus formation or embolism. Arterial emboli occur when a small piece of the thrombus breaks off and travels through the vessel. Both thrombus and embolism can obstruct or narrow the vessel and cause a sudden occlusive event.

Patients may present with pain, pallor, parasthesias, paralysis and pulselessness in the affected extremity. Prehospital management is focused on protection of the affected limb and immediate transportation to the hospital. In addition to supportive care (intravenous access, oxygen and cardiac monitor), the affected extremity should be immobilized.

Claudication Cramp-like pain in the calves caused by poor circulation to leg muscles is called claudication. The condition is commonly associated with atherosclerosis. Intermittent claudication is a form of the disorder that is manifested only at certain times, usually after an extended period of walking, and is relieved by rest.

Compartment Syndrome Compartment syndrome is caused by increased pressure in the fascial sheath that forms the confined space of a muscle compartment, usually after trauma. It leads to progressive arterial compression and reduced blood supply in an extremity. It can result in a permanent disability unless identified promptly and managed in the hospital by surgical release of the pressure.

Embolism Emboli are abnormal solid materials that travel in arteries, veins and lymphatic vessels. They may consist of clotted blood cells, fat particles, air bubbles, foreign material or bacteria. An embolus is significant when it obstructs blood flow to vital organs and causes subsequent ischemia and infarction.

Predisposing factors for thromboemboli (migrating clots) formation include atherosclerosis, atrial fibrillation, obesity, immobility, birth control pills and pregnancy. Air emboli can be formed during scuba diving accidents involving rapid ascent without exhalation, and by outside sources such as central venous cannulation and injury. Fat emboli occur secondary to traumatic events, especially femur fractures.

Patients with pulmonary emboli usually present with chest pain, and may also have dyspnea, anxiety or non-specific complaints. They may also present in cardiac arrest. Patients with cerebral embolic events present with mental status changes, parasthesias, paralysis or seizures.

Prehospital management is supportive. All embolism patients need high-flow oxygen, cardiac monitoring and an IV. In the case of suspected air embolism, the patient should be placed in a left lateral trendelenburg position.

Shock, Hypoperfusion Shock or hypoperfusion is defined as a state of inadequate tissue perfusion that will result in cell death if not corrected. Shock may be attributed to hypovolemia, cardiac failure, sepsis, anaphylaxis or neurological dysfunction.

Shock progresses through reversible to irreversible stages. The initial hypoperfusion stage is compensated by increased heart rate and constriction of peripheral vessels. This restores arterial pressure and blood flow to vital organs. As shock progresses and compensatory mechanisms

fail, perfusion to vital organs becomes insufficient (decompensation). Finally, shock becomes irreversible as cellular death begins and organ failure follows.

Clinically, the patient in the compensated stage of shock may have a normal blood pressure and only a mild increase in heart rate. As compensatory mechanisms begin to fail, blood pressure starts to fall, and heart rate and respiratory rate increase significantly. Mental status changes usually appear and skin may become cool and clammy. In the final stages of shock, blood pressure continues to fall. Heart rate and respiratory rate eventually decrease before the patient becomes comatose and dies.

The goal of prehospital care of shock is correction of the underlying cause and maximal tissue oxygenation. All patients need high-flow oxygen through a non-rebreather mask, or an endotracheal intubation if warranted. Obvious hemorrhage can be controlled by direct pressure. PASG may be used for long bone deformity or abdominal trauma. Dopamine should be considered for patients in shock secondary to cardiac failure. Rapid transport to the nearest hospital is required for all patients. Intravenous access should be attempted en route, and aggressive fluid replacement begun when needed to correct problems related to volume loss or distribution. Cardiac monitoring is important, particularly if the shock is due to cardiac failure.

Sickle Cell Disease: Anemia, Crisis Sickle cell anemia is an inherited, genetic hemolytic (breaking down of RBCs) anemia, occurring primarily in African Americans. Sickle cell crisis occurs when vessels become occluded by sickled hemoglobin, which can cause infarction of critical organs. Patients complain of severe pain in the lower extremities, chest, back or abdomen. They may also develop shortness of breath, mental status changes and shock secondary to dehydration. Prehospital management includes high-flow oxygen, intravenous fluid replacement and rapid transport to the hospital.

Thrombosis, Deep-Vein; Thrombophlebitis Acute venous disease occurs as a result of trauma, prolonged immobility from bedrest, or travel, advanced age, birth control pills, cancer, obesity, pregnancy or other states that promote clotting. It is commonest in elderly females, and the calf and thigh are most often affected.

Deep-vein thrombosis occurs when red blood cells and platelets form a thrombus that attaches to the wall of a vein and occludes blood flow. In some cases, a piece of thrombus may break off and travel to the pulmonary circulation (pulmonary embolism). Thrombophlebitis is caused by an inflammation of the venous wall where the thrombus has attached. This may occur in superficial or deep veins. However, superficial vein thrombi do not cause embolic events.

Patients with deep vein thrombosis complain of pain and swelling in the affected extremity; both are caused by partial or complete obstruction of venous blood flow. There may be redness, warmth and induration (hardness) along the affected vessel. The extremity should be immobilized and should not bear weight. Observe closely for clot movement to the lung. Signs of pulmonary embolism call for high-flow oxygen, cardiac monitoring, an intravenous line and rapid transport to the hospital.

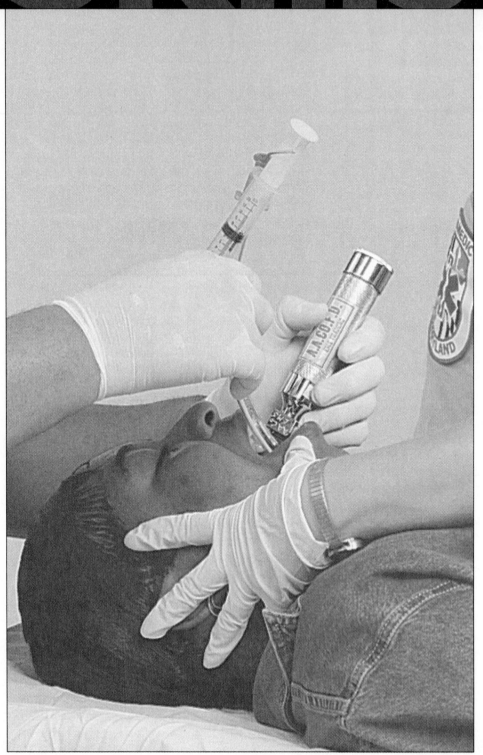

SKILL 1

Pharyngeal Tracheal Lumen Airway

Background

In the search for simple but safer airways for prehospital use, the pharyngeal tracheal lumen (PTL) airway has drawn considerable attention. Endotracheal intubation continues to be the procedure of choice for airway control, but the PTL attempts to address some of the disadvantages of older devices, the EOA and EGTA.

The PTL has two parallel tubes of unequal length. The longer tube is 31 cm in overall length; the shorter tube measures 21 cm. The longer tube has a distal cuff (for esophageal or tracheal occlusion). The short tube has a large cuff just proximal to its end (for upper airway occlusion). The long tube measures approximately 22 cm from the teeth strap (Fig. S1-1).

The airway is inserted until the teeth strap fits against the incisors. The cuffs are then inflated simultaneously by blowing into the port containing a one-way valve. The rescuer attempts ventilation through the short tube (pharyngeal lumen). The chest will rise if the long tube is in the esophagus. Ventilation is then carried out through the short tube. In this mode, it essentially acts as an EGTA. However, no facemask is necessary because the large cuff occludes the pharynx proximally.

If the long tube has entered the trachea, blowing air into the short tube will not cause the chest to rise. Ventilation is then attempted through the long tube, and tracheal placement is confirmed. The large proximal cuff is then deflated. In this mode the tube acts as an ETT.

Indications

- Deep unresponsiveness, cardiac and/or respiratory arrest
- When endotracheal intubation is not possible or available
- When BVM ventilation is not adequate or is causing excessive gastric distention

Contraindications

- Patients with an intact gag reflex
- Facial and/or esophageal trauma
- Suspected foreign body airway obstruction
- Children under 16 years of age
- Anyone less than 5 feet in height

Equipment

- PTL airway
- Water-soluble lubricant
- BVM
- Oxygen
- Stethoscope
- Gloves
- Goggles

Procedure

1. Observe body substance isolation precautions.
2. Ensure adequate oxygenation while preparing to insert the PTL.
3. Test the cuffs on the PTL. Become familiar with the various tubings in the airway. Identify the long and the short tube before insertion.
4. Lubricate the tube with water-soluble jelly.
5. Grasp the patient's tongue and jaw with the gloved left hand and pull forward (Fig. S1-2).
6. Gently insert the airway, advancing it until the teeth strap fits against the incisors.
7. Inflate both balloons simultaneously by blowing into the valve (Fig. S1-3).
8. Ventilate the patient through the short tube (Fig. S1-4). Look for the chest to rise and listen to the breath sounds.
9. *If the chest rises,* continue ventilation through the short tube. A gastric tube may be inserted through the long tube, the tip of which is in the esophagus (Fig. S1-5). Secure the teeth strap firmly with adhesive tape.
10. *If the chest does not rise,* attempt ventilation through the long tube to check to see if it has entered the trachea. The chest should rise. Continue ventilation through the long tube (Fig. S1-6). The proximal cuff may now be deflated. You have endotracheally intubated the patient successfully.

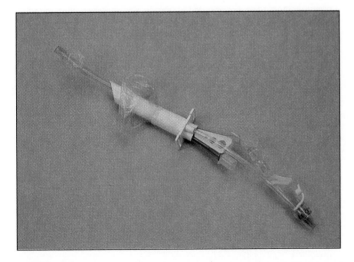

Figure S1-1

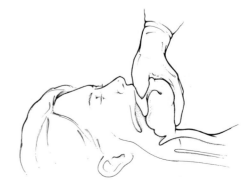

Figure S1-2

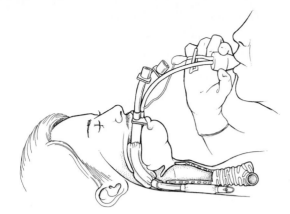

Figure S1-3

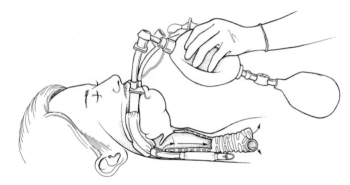

Figure S1-4

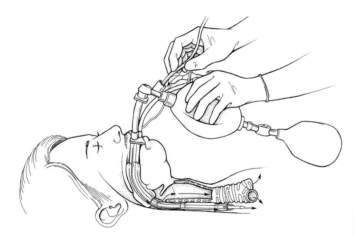

Figure S1-5

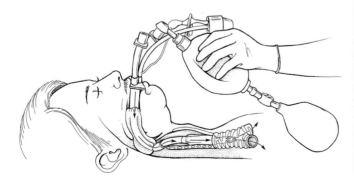

Figure S1-6

SKILL 2

Esophageal Tracheal Combitube

Background

Like the PTL, the esophageal tracheal combitube (ETC) has drawn considerable attention in the search for simple but safer airways for prehospital use. It, too, attempts to address some of the disadvantages of the EOA and the EGTA. The ETC is a twin-lumen plastic tube. One lumen resembles an EOA with a blind distal end. The other looks like an ETT (Fig. S2-1).

The ETC has two balloons: a large proximal balloon and a smaller distal balloon. The tube is inserted blindly. Ventilation can be carried out irrespective of whether the tube enters the esophagus or the trachea.

Indications

- Deep unresponsiveness, cardiac and/or respiratory arrest
- When endotracheal intubation is not possible or available
- When BVM ventilation is not adequate or is causing excessive gastric distention

Contraindications

- Patients with an intact gag reflex
- Facial and/or esophageal trauma
- Suspected foreign body airway obstruction
- Children under 16 years of age
- Anyone less than 5 feet in height

Equipment

- ETC airway
- Water-soluble lubricant
- BVM
- Stethoscope
- Gloves
- Goggles

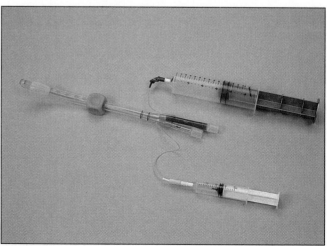

Figure S2-1

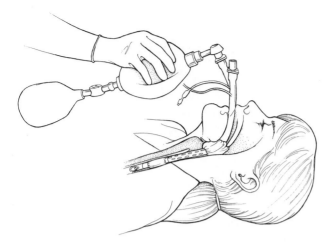

Figure S2-2

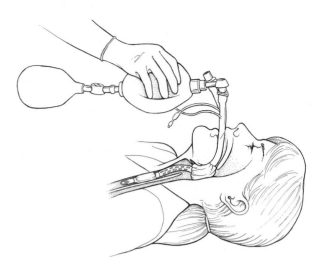

Figure S2-3

Procedure

1. Observe body substance isolation precautions.
2. Ensure adequate oxygenation while preparing to insert the ETC.
3. Test the cuffs on the ETC. Become familiar with the various tubings in the airway. Identify the long and the short tube before insertion.
4. Lubricate the tube with water-soluble jelly.
5. Grasp the patient's tongue and jaw with the gloved left hand and pull forward.
6. Gently insert the airway, advancing it until the printed ring is aligned with the teeth.
7. Inflate line 1 (blue pilot balloon) leading to the pharyngeal cuff with 100 cc of air. (The ETC is packaged with a 140 cc syringe for this purpose.)
8. Inflate line 2 (white pilot balloon) leading to the distal cuff with approximately 15 cc of air. (The ETC is packaged with a 20 cc syringe for this purpose.)
9. Ventilate the patient through the longer blue tube (Fig. S2-2). Look for the chest to rise and listen to the breath and epigastric sounds.
10. *If the chest rises and epigastric sounds are negative,* continue ventilation through the blue tube. A gastric tube may be inserted through the short tube, the tip of which is in the esophagus. The device is secured by the 100 cc pharyngeal cuff.
11. *If the chest does not rise and epigastric sounds are positive,* attempt ventilation through the shorter, clear tube, to check to see if it has entered the trachea (Fig. S2-3). The chest should rise. Continue ventilation through the shorter tube. You have endotracheally intubated the patient successfully.

SKILL 3

Nasotracheal Intubation

Background

Although the concept and technique of nasotracheal intubation were developed during World War I, the procedure was used only occasionally in the operating suite. However, emergency physicians and paramedics have sparked a renewed interest in the procedure and often utilize this technique to accomplish endotracheal intubation.

Indications

Any person who is in need of intubation and has spontaneous respirations can be intubated nasotracheally (e.g., drug overdose, head injury, COPD, congestive heart failure, pneumonia, and asthma).

Contraindications

- Apnea
- Airway obstruction caused by foreign bodies
- Severe facial injury/basilar skull fracture
- Bleeding disorders

Equipment

- ETT (7 to 8 ID for most adults)
- 10 cc syringe
- Lidocaine jelly (or water-soluble)
- Topical anesthetic spray (e.g., benzocaine)
- Laryngoscope with a No. 3 curved blade
- Magill forceps
- Tape
- Gloves
- Goggles
- BVM
- Oxygen
- Suction equipment

Procedure

1. Observe body substance isolation precautions.
2. Select an ETT (usually 7.5 mm ID in males, 7 mm ID in females). It is usually 0.5 mm smaller than the tube that would be used if orotracheal intubation were going to be performed. Check the cuff. Lubricate the tube with lubricating jelly or lidocaine jelly. Insert the distal end of the ETT into its proximal adapter to form a circle and set it

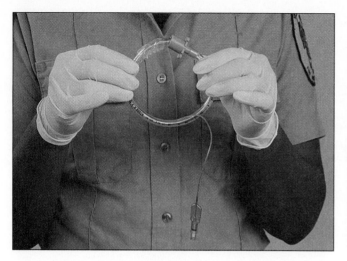

Figure S3-1

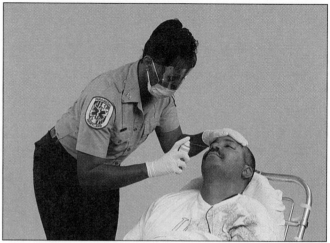

Figure S3-2

aside (Fig. S3-1). This ensures slight anterior curvature of the tube to facilitate entry into the trachea. A stylet is never used in this procedure.

3. Anesthetize the nostrils and pharynx. Benzocaine topical anesthetic spray can be used for this purpose (Fig. S3-2). Lidocaine spray (2%) can also be used. Usually, in the prehospital setting, there is no time for adequate topical anesthesia. Use a vasoconstrictor spray such as phenylephrine hydrochloride ½% or 1% to shrink the mucous membranes. Place a nasopharyngeal airway before attempting this in order to keep the nasal passage open. Have suction equipment available at all times.

4. Pick up the tube and release the circle previously formed. Taking care not to straighten the tip of the tube, insert it through the largest and unobstructed nostril. Keep the bevel of the tube toward the septum.

5. Gently insert the tube until the tip is in the nasopharynx (Fig. S3-3A). Continue to push the tube down. Listen for breath sounds and look for vapor condensation through the tube (Fig. S3-3B).

6. As the tube approaches the larynx, the sounds of breathing through the tube get louder. Gently and evenly push the tube into the larynx during inspiration.

7. The 15-mm adapter usually rests close to the nostril. On entering the trachea, the tube may stimulate the gag reflex and make the patient cough and buck. Be prepared to control the cervical spine. Watch for vomiting.

8. If the tube enters the esophagus, the breath sounds and misting of the tube will disappear. In addition, since the tube is not between the vocal cords, the patient may be able to make sounds or speak.

9. Ventilate the patient and auscultate over both lungs and the epigastrium. If the tube is found to be in the esophagus, withdraw it until the tip is in the pharynx and try again. Pushing the tube down during the patient's inspiratory efforts will greatly enhance your chances for a successful intubation.

There is no need to jab the tube unduly and forcibly through the vocal cords, "hoping to get it in quickly." Force causes

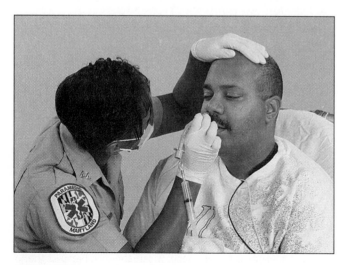

Figure S3-3A

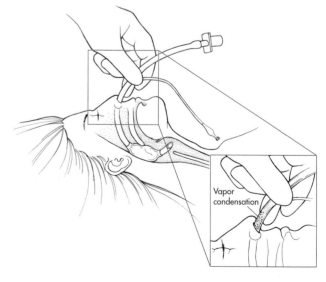

Figure S3-3B

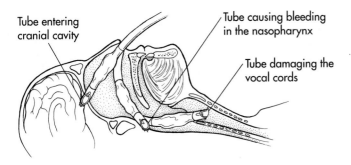

Tube entering cranial cavity

Tube causing bleeding in the nasopharynx

Tube damaging the vocal cords

Figure S3-4

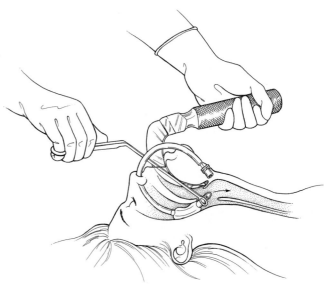

Figure S3-5

violent retching and bucking. Remember that you don't know where the tip of the tube is. You might perforate the pyriform sinus, lacerate the epiglottis, shear off the vocal cords, enter the mediastinum, or puncture major blood vessels.

Complications (Figure S3-4)

- Bleeding from the nose
- Retropharyngeal perforation, hematoma
- Nasal septal tear
- Cranial perforation in basilar skull fracture
- Infection such as meningitis, encephalitis, pharyngeal abscess, or endocarditis
- Injury to the pyriform sinus, epiglottis, vocal cords
- Subglottic stenosis
- Complications that accompany insertion of orotracheal tubes

NOTE: Most people report a 90% success rate with nasotracheal intubation. However, if two or three attempts fail, try the following:

- Withdraw the tube and try again through the other nostril. Occasionally you get a better angle from the other side.

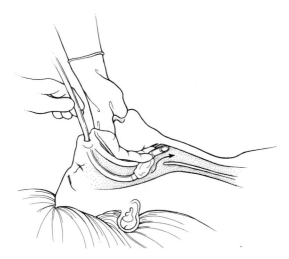

Figure S3-6

- Make sure that the cervical spine is immobilized. Insert a laryngoscope with a curved blade into the mouth. Visualize the vocal cords and the tip of the ETT in the pharynx. Sometimes the tube can be guided into the trachea under direct vision. Frequently, however, you need Magill forceps to direct the tube into the glottic opening (Fig. S3-5). Grasp the tube gently with the forceps. Do not pull the tube toward the vocal cords. Have your assistant gently push it through the nose while you guide the tip into the glottis. Remember, the teeth on Magill forceps may damage the balloon on the tube.
- Occasionally, the tube can be guided into the glottic opening by digital manipulation. You should only attempt this if the patient is comatose and therefore unable to bite your fingers. If you are on the right side of the patient, insert your right index and middle fingers into the patient's mouth. Feel the epiglottis and the tube. Gently guide the tube between your fingers under the epiglottis, as you push the proximal end toward the nostril with your other hand (Fig. S3-6).
- A ringed ETT (Endotrol) is available. A ring at the proximal end of the tube controls the tip of the tube. By pulling on the ring, the tip can be flexed anteriorly. This essentially replaces forming a circle with the tube described earlier.

SKILL 4

Orotracheal Intubation

Background

Despite recent advances in the search for superior, acceptable, and safer airway control, for over a century endotracheal intubation has remained the "gold standard" for securing and maintaining a compromised airway.

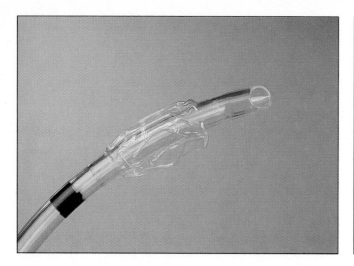

Figure S4-1

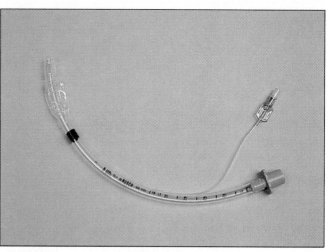

Figure S4-2

Endotracheal intubation is a skill that is mastered only after many hours of competent training and practice. If not used frequently, the skill can rapidly deteriorate. The EMS provider should be aware of this and take proper measures to maintain a high level of competence. The skill can be learned using mannequins, cadavers, or anesthetized patients in the operating room.

The ETT is a curved plastic tube with a low-pressure cuff near the distal end (Fig. S4-1). The tube is open at both ends. The proximal end is fitted with a 15-mm adapter for connection to ventilating devices. The cuff is attached to a one-way valve through a side tube that has a pilot balloon to indicate whether or not the cuff is inflated (Fig. S4-2). The tube has various markings (in centimeters) to indicate the distance from the tip. The size of the tube is expressed in terms of its internal diameter (ID).

The laryngoscope blade can be either curved (MacIntosh) or straight (Miller). The choice of which blade to use is a matter of personal preference. Since the curved blade is inserted into the vallecula and lifts the epiglottis indirectly, it is thought by some to be more "physiologic" and less traumatic. In a short, thick-necked individual, the curved blade may facilitate visualization. In children, straight blades are preferred.

Blades come in different sizes. Most adults can be intubated with a No. 3 or No. 4 blade. Infants and children, depending on their size, need No. 1 to No. 2 blades. The blade has a bulb near its distal end. It is important to check and ascertain that the bulb is tightly secured in its socket. Newer models have fiber-optic lights with the light source in the handle; hence there will not be a bulb to tighten.

The laryngoscope handle contains batteries for the light bulb in the blade. The handle has a bar at its top onto which fits the indentation of the blade (Fig. S4-3). When fitted properly and snapped into a 90-degree angle, electrical connection is made, and the bulb is turned on. When the blade is collapsed to the side of the handle, the light goes off.

The stylet is a malleable guide that can be inserted into the ETT. This allows the tube to be shaped in optimal curvature to facilitate intubation, somewhat like the letter J or a hockey stick. The stylet should be recessed ½ inch from the distal end of the tube. Once the stylet is inserted, it is advisable to bend the proximal end over the 15-mm adapter of the tube so that it will not accidentally slide down farther (Fig. S4-4). Some stylets are manufactured with a loop at the proximal end to prevent accidental slipping. Others are provided with a plastic

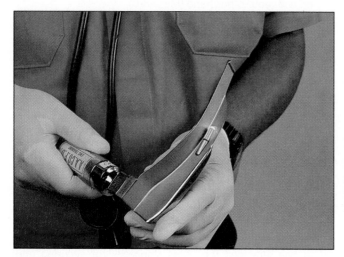

Figure S4-3

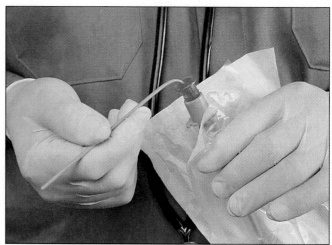

Figure S4-4

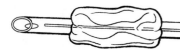

Figure S4-5

stopper to prevent them from sliding inadvertently into the tube. The stopper fits into the adapter (Fig. S4-5).

The Magill forceps have a long handle that is bent at an obtuse angle in the middle. The tips have rings with serrated inner surfaces to facilitate grasping. Occasionally these tubes are required to guide the tube into the larynx. Care should be taken not to grasp the balloon with the forceps, since the teeth on the forceps may rupture the balloon.

Indications

- Unresponsiveness, respiratory and/or cardiac arrest
- Impending airway obstruction/respiratory failure (e.g., burns to the airway, severe asthma, chronic obstructive pulmonary disease [COPD] exacerbation, severe pulmonary edema when the patient develops fatigue and may go into respiratory arrest)
- Patients without a gag reflex who need gastric lavage should be intubated first to prevent aspiration (e.g., drug overdose, bleeding in the gastrointestinal tract)
- When prolonged artificial ventilation is required

Contraindication

- When attempts at intubation could precipitate laryngospasm

Equipment (Figure S4-6)

- Laryngoscope blade
- Laryngoscope handle
- ETT
- Syringe (10 cc)
- Stylet
- Water-soluble lubricant
- Suction equipment
- Magill forceps
- Adhesive tape or ETT tube holder
- BVM
- Oxygen
- Gloves
- Goggles

Procedure

1. Observe body substance isolation precautions.
2. Continue CPR if needed and mask ventilation while preparing to intubate.
3. Set up the suction unit with a rigid tonsil-tip (Yankauer) catheter.
4. Choose the proper size ETT and blade. Women usually need a 7.0 to 8.0 mm inner diameter (ID) tube and men usually need an 8.0-8.5 mm (ID) tube.
5. Assemble the laryngoscope and check the light.
6. Check the ETT cuff for air leaks (Fig. S4-7). Open the top of the ETT package and inflate the cuff through the valve with 10 cc of air. When satisfied that there is no leak, deflate the cuff. Leave the syringe filled with air attached to the valve.
7. Insert a guide (stylet) into the ETT. Be careful not to push the stylet through the tip of the ETT. Make sure that the end of the stylet is recessed at least ½ inch from the tip. Bend the proximal end of the stylet over the ETT to prevent it from accidentally sliding farther down into the tube.

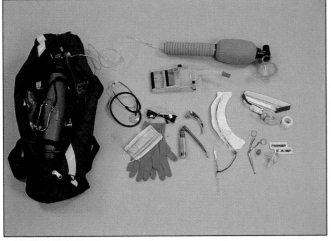

Figure S4-6

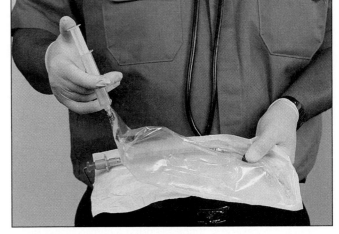

Figure S4-7

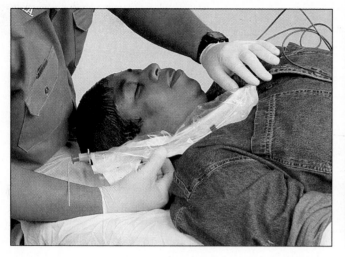

Figure S4-8

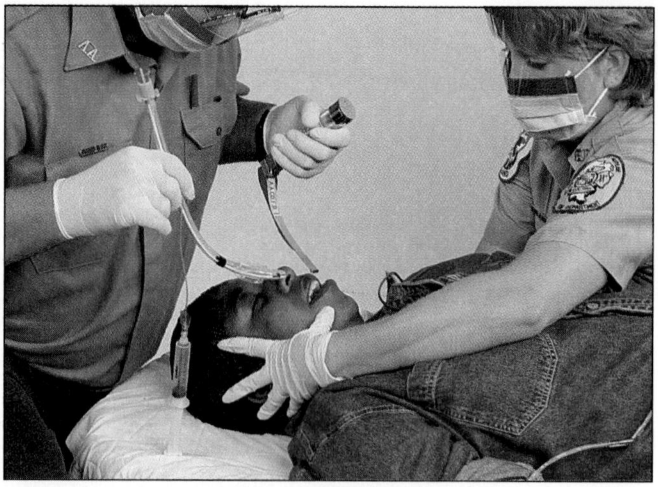

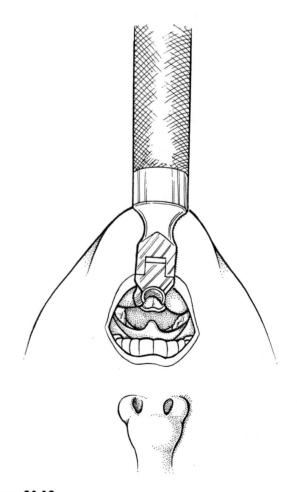

Figure S4-9

8. Estimate the length of the tube needed by placing it alongside the patient's cheek and neck to the level of the cricoid cartilage (Fig. S4-8). Remove the ETT from its package and liberally lubricate the distal 3 or 4 inches and the balloon. Lubrication may be accomplished with water-soluble lubricating jelly or, if permitted in the system, lidocaine jelly or ointment.

9. Preoxygenate the patient by bagging with 100% oxygen for one to two minutes or to a pulse oximeter reading of 100% saturation.

10. Stop ventilations and remove the facemask.

11. Use the right hand to open the mouth.

12. With the head-tilt/chin-lift maneuver, the sniffing position is achieved. This helps align the airway with the mouth. In trauma, or when cervical spine integrity is questioned, **do not** hyperextend the neck. In-line cervical immobilization should be applied by a second rescuer, who places himself or herself by the side of the patient, below the patient's shoulder level, and stabilizes the jaw, neck, and head as shown (Fig. S4-9). In this position the rescuer providing cervical spine immobilization will not hinder the intubator's line of vision.

13. While holding the laryngoscope handle in the left hand, insert the blade into the mouth on the right side of the patient, pushing the tongue toward the left. Do not touch the teeth with the blade.

14. Under direct vision, insert the blade down to the base of the tongue and visualize the epiglottis (Fig. S4-10). A common error is to push the blade down without properly visualizing the epiglottis and then to try to "fish" it out by moving the blade tip with chaotic and random motion. This not only causes trauma, but it also causes the tongue to fall around the blade, occluding landmarks. Use suction as needed. Ideally the intubating time should not be more than 30 seconds. If the intubation is difficult, stop the procedure, hyperventilate the patient with the BVM, and reattempt the procedure.

15. Once you visualize the epiglottis, the next step is to identify the vocal cords. If you are using a curved blade, direct it into the vallecula (between the tongue and the

epiglottis) and lift up on the handle and blade (Fig. S4-11A). **Do not use the patient's teeth as a fulcrum!** If you are using a straight blade, pass it below the epiglottis and lift it up (Fig. S4-11B). As you lift the epiglottis by either method, the vocal cords will come into view. Once you can see the vocal cords, try not to take your eyes off of them.

Figure S4-10

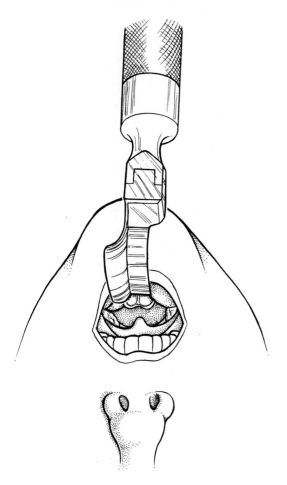

Figure S4-11A

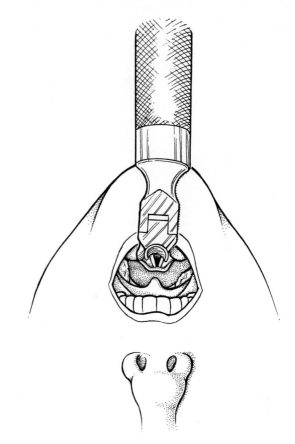

Figure S4-11B

When the trachea is positioned more anteriorly than usual, the use of Magill forceps can facilitate intubation by allowing manual guiding of the tube through the vocal cords (Fig. S4-12). Gentle cricoid pressure (Sellick's maneuver) by an assistant may help with visualization of the vocal cords (Fig. S4-13). This also helps prevent aspira-

tion of gastric contents. Do not use this maneuver when the patient is awake because it may induce regurgitation and aspiration.

16. Insert the tube into the mouth along the right cheek of the patient. Be careful that your own hand does not obstruct the view of the tube entering through the vocal cords. (Guide the tube from the side of the face.) You must be able to see the tube entering the trachea

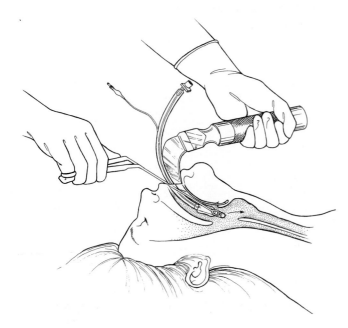

Figure S4-12

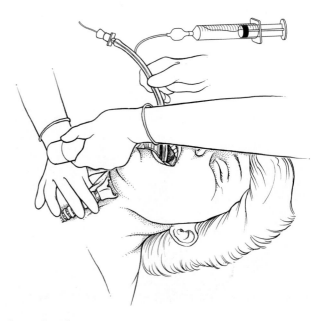

Figure S4-13

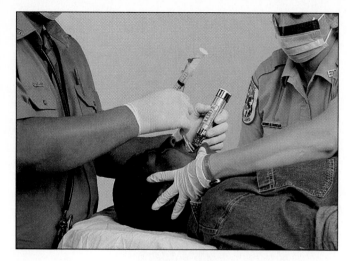

Figure S4-14

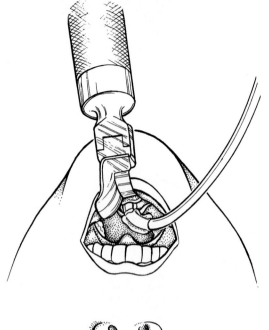

(Fig. S4-14). After you achieve some expertise, you can feel the tube pass through the vocal cords (Fig. S4-15). Be aware that the tube has been known to slip down into the esophagus at the last possible moment.

17. Insert the tube until the cuff has entered the trachea completely. Usually, the 22-cm mark for women and the 24-cm mark for men will be at the patient's incisors. The average distance from the lips to the carina is 28.5 cm in males and 25.2 cm in females.

18. Remove the laryngoscope. Secure the tube firmly with your thumb and forefinger. Remove the stylet from the tube. Inflate the cuff until the pilot balloon feels tight and there is no air leak around the balloon (about 7 to 10 cc of air). Remove the syringe.

19. Have an assistant ventilate through the tube, watching for the rising and falling of the chest. Auscultate over both lung fields and the stomach to ensure accurate placement (Fig. S4-16). CO_2 detectors, which detect carbon dioxide in expired air and indicate its presence by color change, are available for evaluating tube placement.

20. Tape the tube in place securely. This can be achieved by various means. One standard method is to use cloth

Figure S4-15

tape. Select a long piece of tape sufficient to go around the patient's head, with an extra 3 inches to spare at both ends (Fig. S4-17). The adhesive surface of another, shorter piece of tape is placed over the adhesive surface of the first tape to prevent the tape from sticking to the patient's hair. The 3-inch lengths of the first tape at both ends should have available adhesive surfaces for wrapping around the tube. These ends are split longitudinally and braided over the tube (Fig. S4-18). Commercially available tube holders may also be used and are much quicker than tape.

21. Recheck breath sounds after any manipulation.

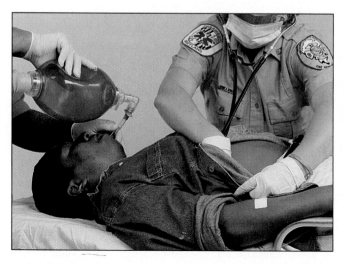

Figure S4-16

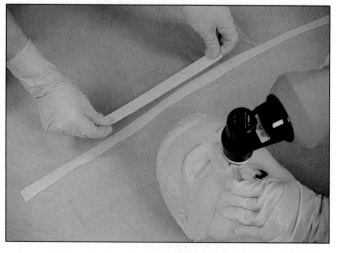

Figure S4-17

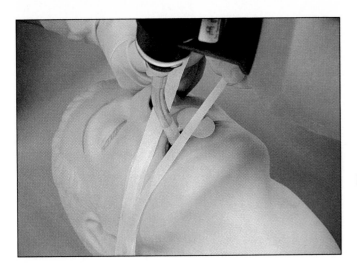

Figure S4-18

22. Check the pilot balloon periodically to ascertain proper seal and when an air leak is suspected. Also, if the patient vomits, it is prudent to check the pilot balloon to make sure that there is no danger of aspiration.

SKILL 5

Pediatric Laryngoscopy and Oral Endotracheal Intubation

Laryngoscopy is the procedure used for visualizing the upper airway using a device called a laryngoscope. The laryngoscope allows for direct access to the glottic opening by lifting the tongue and mandible. Endotracheal intubation is the process of placing an open-ended tube into the trachea to secure the airway and improve ventilation.

Background

Controlling the airway is the most crucial skill in the assessment and management of any patient. However, this is especially true for pediatrics. Unlike adults who often require total resuscitation efforts, many pediatric patients rapidly respond with aggressive ventilation and oxygenation. Each ventilation should be given gently, and just enough should be given to accomplish chest rise. High-pressured blasts of air, such as those given with a demand-valve resuscitator, are apt to cause pleural injury. A bag-valve resuscitator should be used, since chest compliance can be easily felt by the paramedic squeezing the bag.

Endotracheal intubation provides the most secure airway in the prehospital setting. The pediatric airway is anatomically different from that of the adult and thus requires special handling and equipment. Some of the anatomic differences include:

- A head that is relatively larger than the neck and torso.
- A small face with a relatively flat nasal bridge.
- A relatively large tongue in relation to the mouth.
- A larynx that is located more anterior and at the level of the cricoid cartilage.
- An airway whose smallest diameter is subglottic.
- An airway prone to more secretions, consequently necessitating careful suctioning and airway maintenance

Indications

- In any child who is unable to protect his own airway
- Ineffective BVM ventilation
- Tracheal suctioning of the neonate for meconium aspiration
- Medication route in critical patient

Contraindications

- There are no contraindications for intubation of the pediatric patient. However, special precaution should be taken with the traumatized patient. Cervical alignment must be maintained during laryngoscopy and tube placement.

Equipment

- Suction device with appropriate size catheters and bulb syringes
- Oxygen
- Pediatric BVM with reservoir bag
- Laryngoscope handle and variety of pediatric blades (sizes 0, 1, 2)
- Spare laryngoscope light bulbs
- ETTs (2.5 to 6.5 mm)
- 10-ml syringe
- Water-soluble lubricant
- 1-inch tape
- Pediatric stylet
- Gloves
- Eye protection (goggles)

Procedure

1. Observe body substance isolation precautions (gloves and eye protection).
2. Position the head in the sniffing position and hyperventilate the patient with a BVM and high-concentration oxygen. Because of the relatively large head size, some flexion of the head may naturally occur. It may be necessary to extend the head slightly so that the face looks straight up and provides an open airway (Fig. S5-1).
3. Select and check the proper equipment. (See Chapter 22.) Insert stylet into the ETT and lubricate the tube with water-soluble jelly. It may be necessary to lubricate the stylet slightly to advance it into the lumen of the tube.
4. Reposition the nontraumatized child by placing a small towel under the shoulders (Fig. S5-2). This position

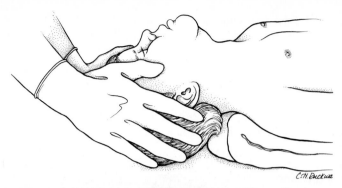

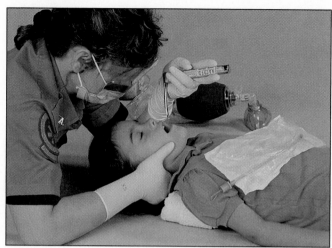

Figure S5-2

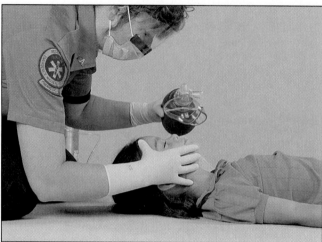

Figure S5-1

facilitates visualization of the airway because of the anatomic differences.

5. Holding the laryngoscope in the left hand, introduce the laryngoscope into the right side of the child's mouth. Sweep the tongue to the left side and simultaneously lift the chin forward. Expose the vocal cords by lifting the epiglottis with the tip of the Miller (straight) blade (Fig. S5-3). Be careful not to advance the blade too far and accidentally lacerate the vocal cords.

6. Gently insert the ETT until you see the tip of the tube advance past the glottic opening (Fig. S5-4) and the vocal cord marker on the tube is at the level of the cords. In children, the following formula will help in positioning the tube:
   Child's age/2 plus 12 = centimeter mark at the teeth

7. Remove the laryngoscope blade and stylet, while tightly holding the tube in place with the right hand.

8. If using a cuffed tube as indicated for an 8-year-old child or older, inflate the cuff until the air leak disappears. Ventilate the patient using a BVM and watch for chest rise. Confirm placement by auscultating the chest bilaterally and the epigastrium with a stethoscope (Fig. S5-5) (Adjuncts such as end-tidal carbon dioxide detectors can be used if approved by the local jurisdiction).

9. Secure the tube, by taping it to the maxilla.

10. Reassess tube placement after taping. Be aware that any substantial movement of the head may result in displacement of the tube. Reassess often.

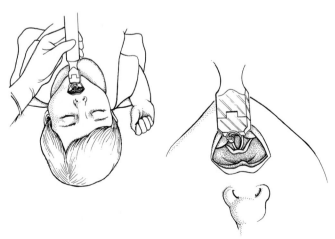

Figure S5-3

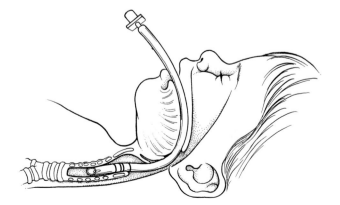

Figure S5-4

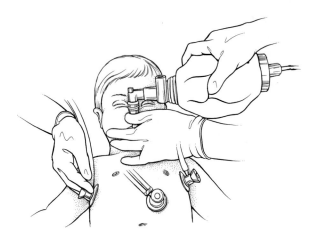

Figure S5-5

SKILL 6

Digital Endotracheal Intubation

Digital endotracheal intubation is a blind procedure that positions an ETT into the trachea without the aid of a laryngoscope. It is accomplished by placing the ETT into the pharynx of the patient with the paramedic directing the tube into the glottic opening, using the tip of the middle finger.

Background

Special situations occur that require a paramedic to use skills that are seldom performed in the prehospital setting. Digital intubation is one of those special occasions. Anatomic differences and injuries involving the airway often make traditional endotracheal intubation attempts futile.

Indications

- Inability to successfully place an ETT using a laryngoscope and blade
- Severe facial trauma that prohibits visualization of the vocal cords
- Mechanism of injury or signs indicating a possible cervical neck injury in which traditional intubation techniques may be detrimental to the patient

Contraindications

- There are essentially no contraindications to digital intubation. However, caution must be used when intubating the patient with a possible cervical injury. Neutral cervical alignment must be maintained throughout the procedure. The patient should be unresponsive before attempting the procedure.

Equipment

- Suction device
- Oxygen
- BVM with reservoir bag
- Laryngoscope and appropriate-size blades
- ETTs
- Water-soluble lubricant
- 1-inch tape
- Gloves
- Eye protection

Procedure

1. Observe body substance isolation precautions.
2. Position the head and hyperventilate the patient with a BVM and high-concentration oxygen.
3. Select and check the proper equipment. Insert the stylet into the ETT and lubricate the tube with water-soluble jelly. It may be necessary to lubricate the stylet slightly to advance it into the lumen of the tube.
4. Position yourself so that you are facing the patient and the palm of your hand rests on the patient's chin. Use a dental clamp, bite–stick, or other device to hold the patient's mouth open to protect the rescuer's fingers.
5. With the middle finger, reach into the oropharynx and feel for the epiglottis. Once located, lift the epiglottis anteriorly (Fig. S6-1).
6. Introduce the ETT into the oropharynx and supraglottic area.
7. With the middle finger still lifting the epiglottis anteriorly, identify the tip of the tube. Slide the tube between the first and second fingers (index and middle fingers) posteriorly into the glottic opening (Fig. S6-2).
8. Simultaneously advance the tube while positioning it anteriorly toward the glottic opening. Slide the tube through the cords.
9. Remove the finger and hold the tube with one hand, while applying a BVM with the other. Ventilate the patient and watch for chest rise. Confirm placement by auscultating the chest and epigastrium with a stethoscope.
10. Secure the tube using tape.
11. Reassess tube placement after taping. Reassess often.

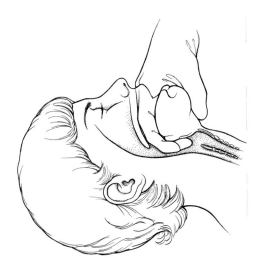

Figure S6-1

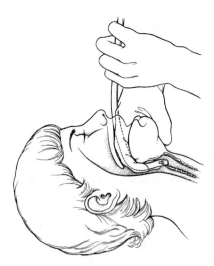

Figure S6-2

SKILL 7

Suctioning

Background

Suctioning the mouth and pharynx may be necessary to clear secretions to visualize the field before intubation.

In addition, when secretions interfere with BVM ventilation or when the patient is unable to clear secretions, aggressive suctioning may be required by the prehospital provider.

While performing direct laryngoscopy or while clearing secretions from the throat during BVM, a rigid tonsil suction device (Yankauer) should be used. Some tonsil suction catheters are equipped with a side thumb port. When the port is occluded, suction is engaged. When the port is released, air is sucked in through the side port and the suction is disengaged. In tonsil suction catheters without the side port, the suction tubing must be crimped to disengage suction.

The tonsil suction must always be used under direct vision. It should not be forced blindly into the patient's mouth because it may push an obstructing foreign body farther into the throat or cause tissue damage and bleeding.

Tracheal Suctioning

Paramedics are called on to perform deep suctioning in many situations—both medical and trauma. When the patient is unable to clear secretions because of illness, overproduction, or very tenacious secretions, airway assistance may be required. In addition, suctioning is commonly done in intubated medical and trauma patients.

Equipment

- Sterile tracheal suctioning kits are available, containing one glove (some kits contain a pair of gloves), a paper cup for sterile saline or water, a suctioning catheter with a side thumb port, a suction unit, goggles, and sterile saline or water.

Procedure

1. Observe body substance isolation precautions.
2. When opening the kit, identify the sterile glove on top. Put this on the dominant hand, taking care not to touch the outside of the glove with the other hand.
3. Grasp the catheter with the gloved hand. Keep the catheter looped around your hand.
4. With the ungloved hand pour sterile saline solution into the cup provided.
5. Connect the catheter to the suction machine, taking precaution not to touch any other part of the catheter except the proximal tip with the ungloved hand.
6. With the catheter looped around the gloved hand, you should be able to occlude and release the side port with your thumb (Fig. S7-1).
7. Feed the catheter through the patient's nose or, if intubated, the ETT (Fig. S7-2). It is suggested to use a sterile catheter with each suction attempt. If there are two gloves, you will need an assistant to give you the sterile saline; or you may pour the saline solution into the cup provided before putting on the second glove. This makes it easier to observe absolute sterile precautions.

Procedure for Tracheal Suctioning of the Nonintubated Patient

1. Place the patient in a semi-sitting position. Unconscious patients are positioned on their side.

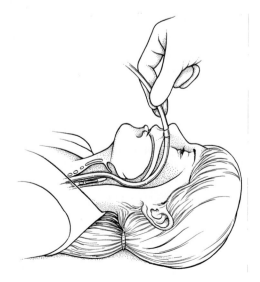

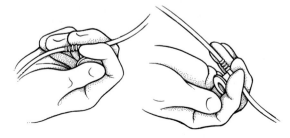

Figure S7-1

Figure S7-2

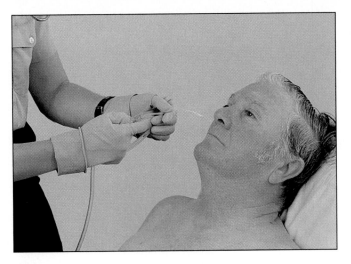

Figure S7-3

2. Supply 100% oxygen for at least 5 minutes.
3. Open the catheter kit and prepare for suctioning.
4. Insert the catheter through a nostril into the pharynx, without engaging the suction.
5. Ask the patient to assume the sniffing position and take slow, deep breaths (Fig. S7-3).
6. Advance the catheter during inspiration. Entering the larynx should induce coughing. Advance through the vocal cords.
7. Engage suction intermittently and withdraw the catheter with a rotating motion (Fig. S7-4). Count to 15 seconds or less as needed.
8. When tracheal suctioning is completed, you may use the catheter to suction around the mouth. Once you have suctioned around the mouth, do not introduce the catheter into the trachea again.
9. If you need to use tracheal suctioning again, preoxygenate the patient for 30 seconds and repeat the steps, using a new sterile catheter.
10. Dispose of contaminated materials properly.

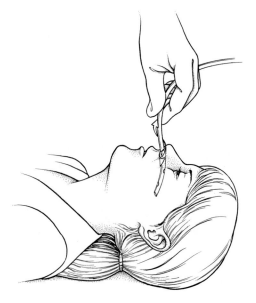

Figure S7-4

Procedure for Tracheal Suctioning of the Intubated Patient

1. Make sure the patient's cardiac rhythm is being monitored.
2. Preoxygenate with 100% oxygen.
3. Prepare for suctioning. Have an assistant disconnect the bag.
4. Introduce the catheter through the tube without touching the outside of the tube.
5. Advance the catheter as far as possible.
6. Engage intermittent suction and slowly withdraw the catheter. Do not apply suction for more than 15 seconds.
7. Monitor the patient closely. Remember to preoxygenate if you need to suction the patient again. Discontinue suctioning if you see cardiac dysrhythmias, and ventilate the patient with 100% oxygen.

SKILL 8

Nasogastric Tube Insertion

Background

Insertion of an NG tube is the placement of a specialized suction catheter through the nose, down the esophagus, and into the stomach to remove stomach contents.

Indications

NG tube insertion is indicated when evacuation of stomach contents such as air or food is required. An NG tube may also be inserted to dilute or lavage ingested poisons or to remove blood when the patient has gastrointestinal hemorrhage.

Contraindications

An NG tube should not be inserted through the nose of a patient with severe facial trauma. The patient may have a fracture of the cribriform plate, resulting in accidental placement of the tube into the cranial cavity. The tube may be inserted orally at the direction of Medical Direction. In addition, NG tubes should not be inserted in a patient with possible epiglottitis or croup.

Equipment

- NG tube
- 50-ml irrigation syringe
- Water-soluble lubricant
- Adhesive tape
- Saline for irrigation
- Emesis basin
- Gloves

Procedure

1. Assess the need for NG tube insertion.
2. Use body substance isolation precautions.
3. Assemble the needed equipment.

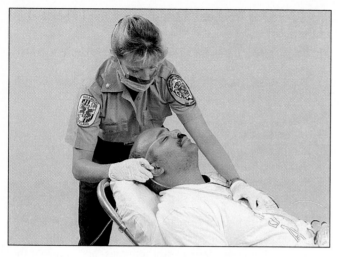

Figure S8-1

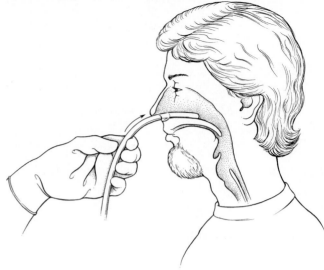

Figure S8-2

4. Explain the procedure to the patient.
5. If possible, have the patient sit up. Use a pad or towel to protect the patient's clothing.
6. Give the patient a handful of tissues because this procedure may cause tearing. An emesis basin should also be handy in case the patient vomits as a result of stimulation of the gag reflex.
7. Look at the nose for deformity or obstruction that may make it difficult to insert an NG tube. Determine the best side for insertion, usually the patient's right nostril.
8. Measure the tube from the patient's earlobe to the tip of the nose. Then measure from the earlobe to the bottom of the xiphoid process (Fig. S8-1). Total these two measurements and mark the correct length on the tube with adhesive tape.
9. Lubricate 6 to 8 inches of the tube with water-soluble gel.
10. Insert the tube in one of the nostrils and gently advance it toward the posterior nasopharynx. It is easiest if you direct the tube toward the patient's ear (Fig. S8-2).

11. When you feel the tube at the nasopharyngeal junction, rotate it 180 degrees inward toward the other nostril. Gently advance the tube until it is in the nasopharynx (Fig. S8-3).
12. As the tube enters the oropharynx, instruct the patient to swallow.
13. Pass the tube to the predetermined point. (Do not force the tube if resistance is encountered.)
14. Check the placement of the tube by two methods: aspirate gastric contents; and place a stethoscope over the epigastric region and auscultate while injecting 20 to 30 ml of air into the tube (Fig. S8-4).
15. Tape the tube in place and connect to low suction, if ordered (Fig. S8-5).
16. Document the procedure, including the following information: size of tube inserted, degree of difficulty, tube placement checked, complications such as bleeding or vomiting, and name of person performing the procedure.

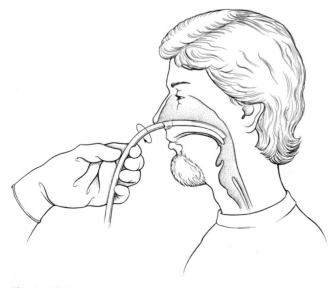

Figure S8-3

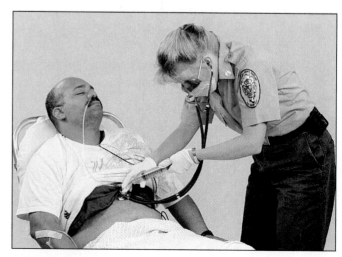

Figure S8-4

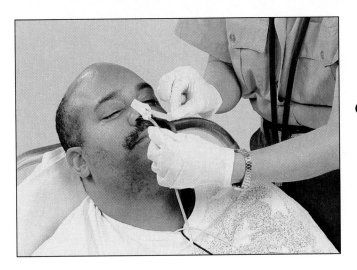

Figure S8-5

Percutaneous Transtracheal Ventilation (Needle Cricothyrotomy)

Background

In situations in which endotracheal intubation is not possible, cricothyrotomy is often the next alternative. Cricothyrotomy is a surgical procedure and requires training before it can be performed. Percutaneous transtracheal ventilation (PTV) is a viable alternative to surgical cricothyrotomy and may be more suitable in the prehospital scene.

PTV involves the insertion of a catheter through the cricothyroid membrane. The catheter is then connected to a high-pressure oxygen source, and oxygen is delivered intermittently into the trachea. The complications and difficulty that accompany performing a surgical procedure such as cricothyrotomy make PTV an attractive alternative. The procedure can be accomplished in a short time and may be used before performing cricothyrotomy.

Indications

- The only indication for cricothyrotomy is the inability to secure an airway by other procedures such as endotra-

cheal intubation (e.g., cervical spine trauma; maxillofacial trauma; and oropharyngeal obstruction caused by foreign body, masses, infections [epiglottitis], or edema resulting from allergic reactions or inhalation injury)

Contraindications

- Possibility of establishing an easier and less invasive airway rapidly
- Acute laryngeal disorders such as laryngeal fractures that cause distortion or obliteration of landmarks (e.g., children under 10 years of age, bleeding disorders, injury or obstruction below the level of the cricothyroid membrane)
- Obstruction above the level of the vocal cords, because air will not be able to escape during exhalation

Equipment

- 14-gauge or larger over-the-needle catheter, 2¼ inches long
- 10 cc syringe
- Three-way stopcock
- Two standard oxygen tubings, 4 to 5 feet each
- Y-connector
- Oxygen cylinder coupled with 50-psi step-down regulator and needle flow meter (e.g., Bourdon-type flow gauge and regulator)
- Povidone-iodine swabs
- Adhesive tape
- Suction equipment
- Gloves
- Goggles

Procedure

1. Observe body substance isolation precautions.
2. Palpate the thyroid cartilage, cricothyroid membrane, and suprasternal notch.
3. Prep the skin with two povidone-iodine swabs.
4. You may attach the syringe to the over-the-needle catheter, or you may elect to use the catheter-needle assembly by itself (Fig. S9-1). This is a personal

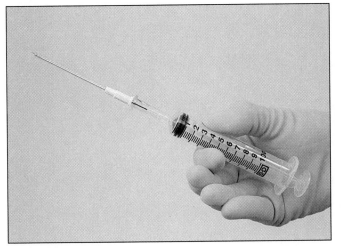

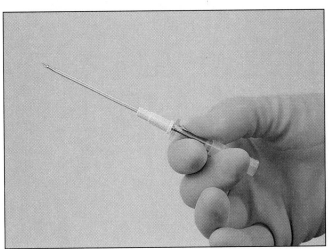

A

B

Figure S9-1

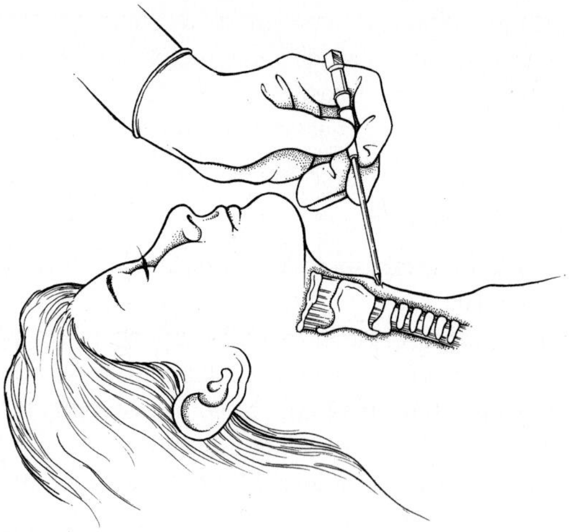

Figure S9-2

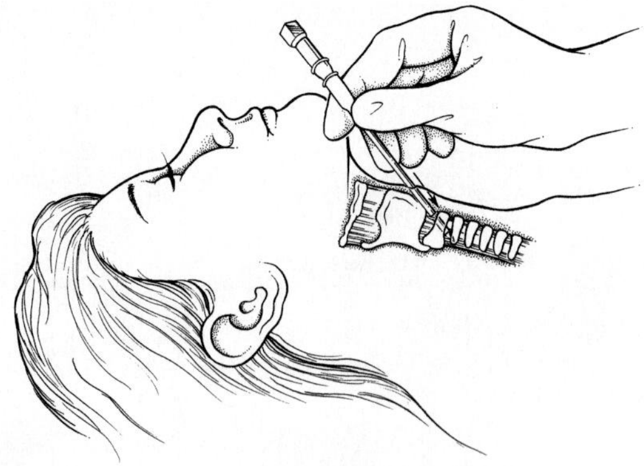

Figure S9-3

preference—some think that using a syringe makes the unit less stable. Some may argue that entry into the larynx is more readily verified with gentle suction using the syringe assembly and that this advantage somewhat outweighs the instability of the unit. Puncture the skin over the cricothyroid membrane (Fig. S9-2).

5. Advance the needle at a 45-degree angle caudally (toward the feet) (Fig. S9-3).
6. Carefully push the needle until it "pops" into the trachea (aspirating on the syringe as you advance the needle, if using a syringe).
7. Free movement of air confirms that you are in the trachea.
8. Advance the plastic catheter over the needle, holding the needle stationary, until the catheter hub comes to rest against the skin (Fig. S9-4).
9. Holding the catheter securely, remove the needle.
10. Reconfirm the position of the catheter. Securely tape the catheter to the skin.
11. Attach the three-way stopcock to the catheter hub. Connect one end of the oxygen tubing to the stopcock (Fig. S9-5).
12. Connect the other end of the oxygen tubing to the Y-connector. Attach the second oxygen tubing to the other arm of the Y-connector. This tubing is then connected to the flowmeter on the oxygen cylinder (Fig. S9-6). These connections should be made before the procedure to save time.
13. To ventilate the patient, open the regulator and set it at maximum rate (greater than 15 L/min). Occlude the third arm of the Y-connector with your thumb. Air will then flow into the lungs. When you release the occlusion on the Y-connector, air flow will be diverted outward, allowing the lungs to recoil and collapse (Fig. S9-7). By alternately occluding and releasing thumb pressure on the connector (1 second on and 4 seconds off), you can maintain adequate ventilation for approximately 30 minutes.
14. Constantly monitor the patient's breath sounds, ventilation status and color. Adequate exhalation never fully occurs with this technique. The patient may develop hypercarbia (increased CO_2) and increased air pressure in the lungs, possibly causing the alveoli to rupture.

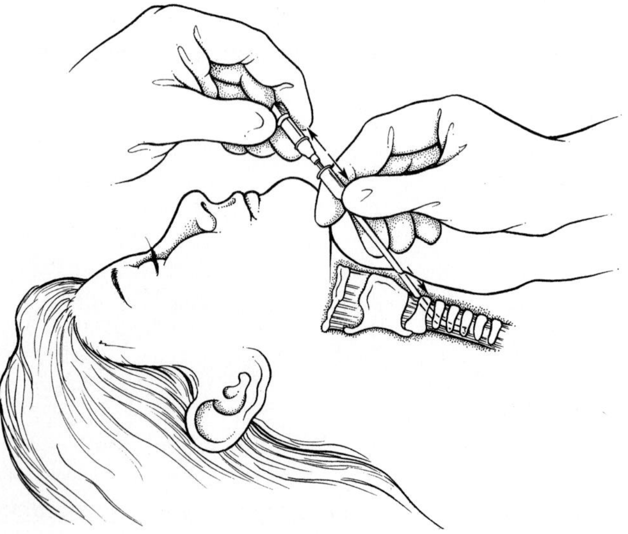

Figure S9-4

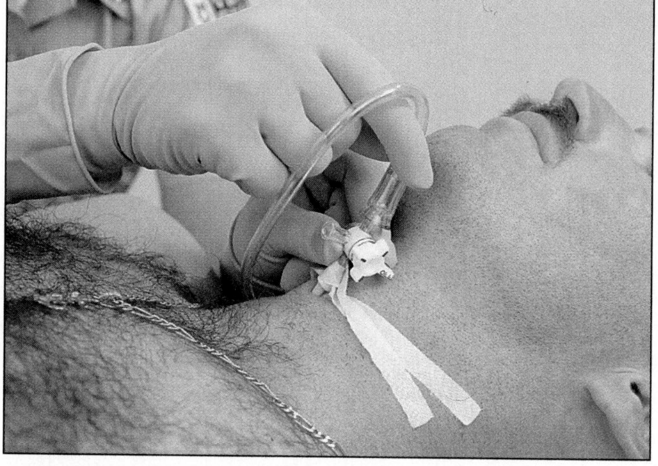

Figure S9-5

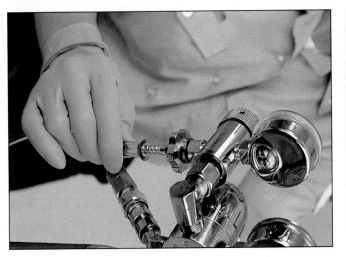

Figure S9-6

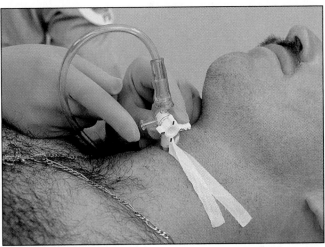

Figure S9-7

Alternative to Jet Ventilation

1. Insert large bore catheter (14G or larger) through cricothyroid membrane as described above.
2. Attach the plastic adapter from a 3.5 ETT to the hub of the catheter.
3. Fit a BVM unit to the adapter and ventilate using the bag. Allow enough time for exhalation through the small caliber catheter.

SKILL 10

Surgical Cricothyrotomy

Background

It is said that the first tracheostomy was performed by the Greek physician, Asclepiades. In the late nineteenth century, surgeons started performing cricothyrotomy because of ease of performance. The technique was not standardized. The incision was made anywhere in the anterior neck. In 1909, Dr. Chevalier Jackson, a prominent surgeon and a pioneer of his time, standardized the technique of tracheotomy. Dr. Jackson saw so many complications occur following cricothyrotomy performed by his colleagues that in 1921 he utterly condemned "high tracheotomy," as he called it.

Because of Dr. Jackson's influence in the world of medicine, cricothyrotomy became an almost extinct procedure until the 1960s. At that time, because of advances in medicine, the availability of antibiotics, and the changing pattern of disease processes, numerous investigators began "revisiting" cricothyrotomy.

Although complications can and do occur, if tracheal intubation cannot be performed, cricothyrotomy is a potential alternative.

Indications

It should be emphasized that the only indication for cricothyrotomy is the inability to secure an airway by other procedures such as endotracheal intubation (e.g., cervical spine trauma, maxillofacial trauma, oropharyngeal obstruction caused by foreign body, masses, infections [epiglottitis], edema resulting from allergic reactions, or inhalation injury).

Contraindications

- Possibility of establishing an easier and less invasive airway rapidly
- Acute laryngeal disorders such as laryngeal fractures that cause distortion or obliteration of landmarks (e.g., children under 10 years of age, bleeding disorders, injury or obstruction below the level of the cricothyroid membrane)

Equipment

- A sterile fenestrated drape (hole in the center)
- Prepared antiseptic swab sticks such as povidone-iodine
- Scalpel with a No. 11 or a No. 15 blade
- 4 × 4 gauze pads
- ETT (7.5 mm ID), or Shiley tracheostomy tube (No. 4 or No. 5), cuffed; the ETT should be shortened to about 3 inches, including the cuff and the pilot balloon; the 15-mm adapter is removed from the proximal end and fitted into the cut edge of the distal end; the proximal portion of the tube is discarded
- 10 cc syringe to inflate the cuff
- Two arterial clamps (hemostats)—8-inch and 6-inch
- Sterile gloves
- Suction equipment
- BVM
- Oxygen
- Adhesive or umbilical cord tape
- Goggles

Procedure

1. Observe body substance isolation precautions. Put on sterile gloves and goggles.
2. The patient should be in a supine position. Immobilize the neck if necessary.

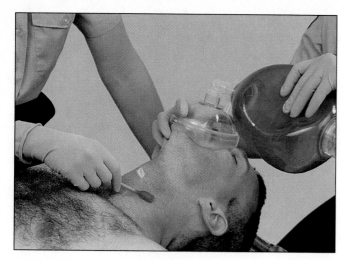

Figure S10-1

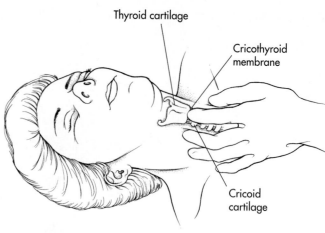

Figure S10-2

3. Open the cricothyrotomy kit.
4. Make sure that artificial ventilation is in progress by means of a BVM while preparing for the procedure.
5. Prepare povidone-iodine swab sticks.
6. Surgically prepare the entire anterior neck (Fig. S10-1).
7. Drape the area with the fenestrated sheet.
8. Palpate the thyroid notch, cricothyroid membrane, and the sternal notch; orient yourself thoroughly with the landmarks (Fig. S10-2).
9. Stabilize the thyroid cartilage with your left hand (or nondominant hand). This is the most important step. If you lose the midline, the anatomy will be distorted and you may find yourself in muscles and blood vessels on either side.
10. Make a vertical skin incision over the cricothyroid membrane. Try to cut through the skin and the subcutaneous tissue in one clean, bold stroke. Make this incision at least 2 cm long (Fig. S10-3).

11. There will be some brisk bleeding. Sponge it if necessary, but don't waste too much time trying to stop it.
12. With your index finger, feel the cricothyroid membrane. Carefully make a horizontal incision over the lower part of the membrane.
13. Insert the scalpel handle into the incision and rotate it 90 degrees to open the airway (Fig. S10-4). If the patient is breathing spontaneously, secretions, blood, and air will spray out of the opening. **Protect your face.**
14. Insert the tracheostomy tube (Fig. S10-5) into the opening. A shortened ETT (with the cuff and the pilot balloon intact) can be used in lieu of the tracheostomy tube. Remove the obturator and insert the inner tracheostomy tube.
15. Inflate the cuff and ventilate the patient.
16. Observe the chest rise and fall; auscultate the lungs and the stomach to ensure proper tube placement.
17. Secure the tube to the patient by adhesive tape or umbilical cord tape.

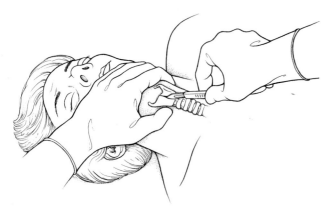

Figure S10-3

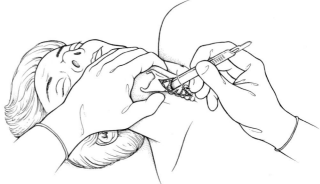

Figure S10-4

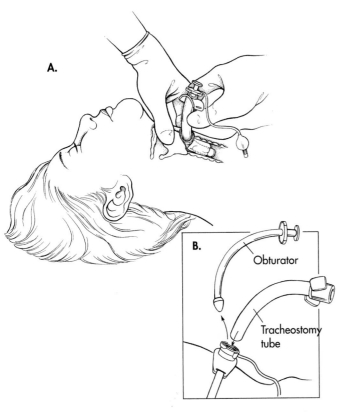

A.

B. Obturator

Tracheostomy tube

Figure S10-5

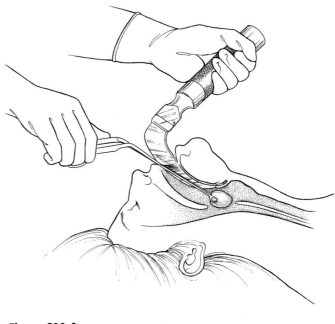

Figure S11-1

8. If unable to ventilate, there may be additional foreign bodies. Try direct laryngoscopy again. Repeat abdominal thrusts and direct laryngoscopy until the foreign body is removed. Consider needle cricothyrotomy (percutaneous transtracheal ventilation) or cricothyrotomy if all attempts fail.

SKILL 11

Direct Laryngoscopy for Foreign Body Airway Obstruction

Background

In the event of foreign body airway obstruction (FBAO), subdiaphragmatic abdominal thrusts and finger sweeps should be used to dislodge the foreign body. If these attempts fail, a paramedic may be required to perform direct laryngoscopy and Magill forceps removal of the foreign body.

Procedure

1. Observe body substance isolation precautions.
2. Have an assistant attempt BVM ventilation with 100% oxygen.
3. Proceed quickly to direct laryngoscopy.
4. Have tonsil suction and Magill forceps ready.
5. With head tilt/chin lift, bring the patient to the sniffing position and introduce the laryngoscope into the mouth with the left hand. Insert the blade on the right side of the patient's mouth and push the tongue to the left.
6. Suction if needed. Grasp the Magill forceps with your right hand. Retrieve the foreign body quickly (Fig. S11-1).
7. Immediately withdraw the laryngoscope and attempt to ventilate the patient again, holding proper head position.

SKILL 12

Lighted Stylet (Transillumination Intubation)

Background

Endotracheal intubation may be accomplished with the use of a lighted stylet. The bright light can be seen through the tissue of the neck, and this will allow the paramedic to pass an endotracheal tube through the vocal cords without having to visualize them directly. A lighted stylet consists of a malleable wire with a bright bulb at the tip (Fig. S12-1).

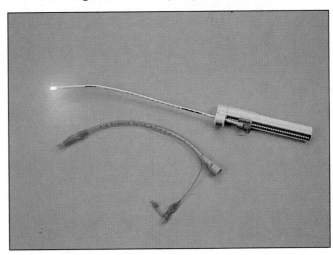

Figure S12-1

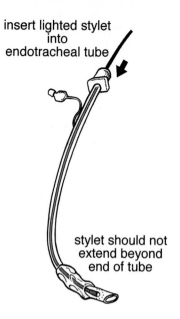

insert lighted stylet
into
endotracheal tube

stylet should not
extend beyond
end of tube

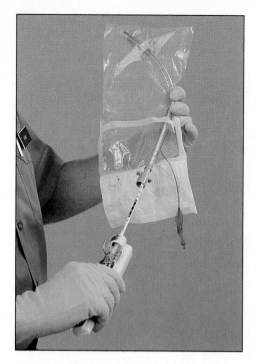

Figure S12-2

Indications

- Patients requiring endotracheal intubation

Contraindications

- Inability to completely open, or have access to, patient's mouth
- Contraindications associated with orotracheal intubation

Equipment

- Lighted stylet
- Endotracheal tube
- 10 cc syringe
- Suction unit
- Tape or tube holder
- Oropharyngeal airway
- Water soluble lubricant
- Bag-valve-mask
- Supplemental oxygen
- Personal protective equipment
- Stethoscope

Procedure

1. Observe body substance isolation precautions.
2. Assess need for orotracheal intubation.
3. Maintain airway and ventilate with BVM.
4. Select proper size endotracheal tube and prepare equipment.
5. Hyperventilate patient.
6. Insert lighted stylet through endotracheal tube (Fig. S12-2).
7. Insert endotracheal tube/stylet into mouth and advance it.
8. Look for light at the patient's larynx.
9. Advance tube approximately one-half inch and remove stylet.

Note: When endotracheal tube is in the proper place the light from the stylet should be clearly visible through the center of the patient's neck (Fig. S12-3).

10. Confirm placement and ventilate patient using BVM.
11. Inflate cuff.
12. Secure tube.

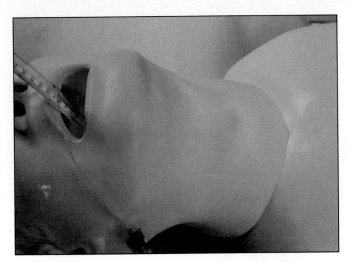

Figure S12-3

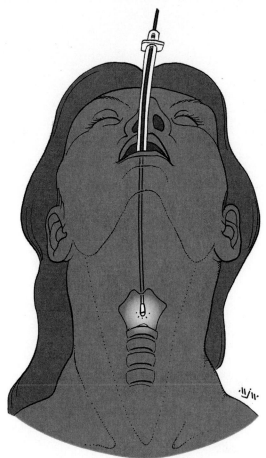

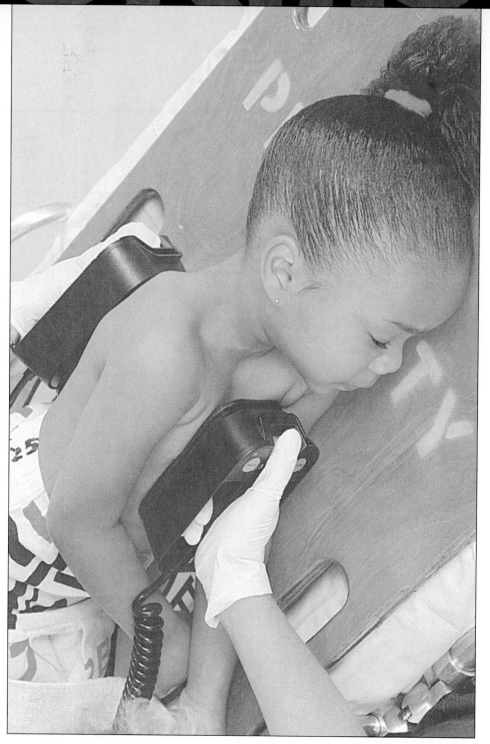

SKILL 13

ECG Monitoring and Quick Look

The electrocardiogram (ECG) is the reproduction of the electrical activity of the heart on graph paper to allow for interpretation of cardiac rhythm.

Background

Electrical monitoring of the activity and rhythm of the heart is an essential component to the appropriate assessment and intervention of patients with a wide variety of illnesses and injuries, particularly those who present with shock or suspected cardiac disease.

Indications

- ECG monitoring is indicated for any critical patient, any patient who gives a cardiac or respiratory history, or any patient who gives a medical history that does not correlate with symptomatology.

Contraindications

- None

Lead Placement and Cardiac Monitoring

Field monitoring of the ECG differs from 12-lead ECG tracing. ECG monitoring in the field generally uses only three electrodes. Generally, leads I, II, III are used. Some systems use the modified chest lead I (MCL I) and VI (MCL VI) positions. The monitoring device requires three electrodes: a positive, a negative, and a ground. Each monitoring view is simply a variation of electrode placement.

Lead II usually provides the best picture of the electrical activity of the heart because its position is quite similar to the normal electrical axis of the heart. MCL I is particularly useful when monitoring for the presence of ectopic beats.

When placing electrodes on the chest for monitoring purposes, place them high enough on the shoulders and low enough on the chest to avoid the apex of the heart. The white and black electrodes should be positioned just below the clavicle bilaterally, and the red electrode is placed at the lower edge of the left rib cage near the anterior axillary line. If the patient has a permanent implanted cardiac pacemaker, be sure to avoid placing ECG electrodes over the battery pack so that, should it become necessary to defibrillate the patient, there will be room on the chest wall for the two defibrillator paddles (sternum and apex) without moving electrodes.

Equipment

- ECG monitor (Fig. S13-1)
- Disposable electrodes
- ECG lead cables

Procedure

1. Observe body substance isolation precautions.
2. Explain the procedure and rationale to the patient.
3. Peel off the paper backing on the electrode. Check to make sure the center of the electrode is moist with conductive jelly. If the sponge is dry, discard the electrode because a poor ECG signal will result.
4. Place the electrode at the chosen sites with the adhesive side down (Fig. S13-2). Apply pressure at the center of the electrode, moving outward, to ensure a good seal.
5. Attach the monitor cables to electrodes. The electrodes will either be marked with RA, RL, LA abbreviation; or +, −, G symbols; or they will be color coded. You must know your system's markings.
6. Connect the leads to the ECG monitor.
7. Turn the monitor on and select the proper lead.

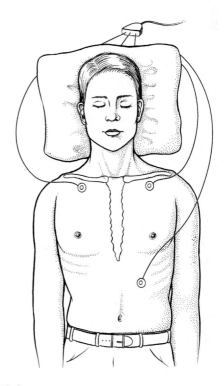

Figure S13-2

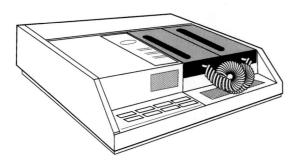

Figure S13-1

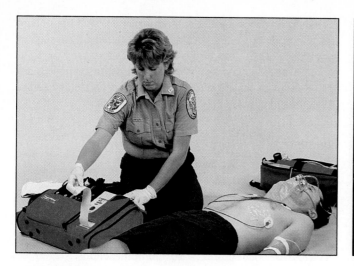

Figure S13-3

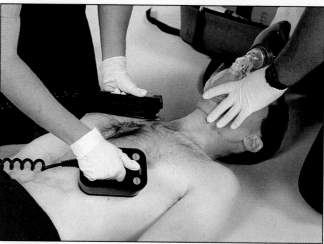

Figure S13-4

8. Observe the monitor and adjust the ECG size to the desired height. The QRS should be high enough to visualize and create a "beep" sound when the volume is increased.
9. Adjust systolic volume to desired volume.
10. Press the record button and run a tracing of the patient's rhythm. A minimum of 6 seconds is needed for each copy of the patient's chart (Fig. S13-3).
11. Label the ECG strip with the patient's name, date and time.

Use of Quick-Look Paddles

When the paramedic arrives at a scene and finds a pulseless, nonbreathing patient, he or she may use quick-look paddles to ascertain the patient's cardiac rhythm. By using the quick-look paddles, the patient can be rapidly defibrillated if ventricular fibrillation or pulseless ventricular tachycardia is found.

Procedure

1. Turn on the ECG monitor.
2. Turn the lead selector to "Paddles."
3. Apply conductive gel to paddles or use specifically designed defibrillation gel pads.
4. Place paddles firmly on the bare chest with the paddle marked STERNUM on the patient's right chest near the sternum and the paddle marked APEX on the patient's lower left chest (Fig. S13-4).
5. Adjust ECG size to the desired height.
6. Observe the scope, check pulse, and determine the patient's condition.
7. If potentially fatal ventricular dysrhythmia is noted, proceed with the defibrillation algorithm.
8. Remember, this method is for a quick-look and initial defibrillation only. It is not meant to be used for continuous patient monitoring; hence, following the initial three defibrillation attempts, the patient should be connected to the ECG monitor using traditional leads or utilize pads for both monitoring and hands-off defibrillation.

SKILL 14
Defibrillation

Definition

Defibrillation, also known as unsynchronized countershock, is the random delivery of high-intensity electrical charge to a fibrillating heart. The purpose of this charge is to depolarize the myocardium and restore the sinoatrial (SA) node as the dominant pacemaker.

Background

Ventricular fibrillation and pulseless ventricular tachycardia are potentially fatal dysrhythmias characterized by electrical and mechanical chaos. These dysrhythmias may occur in the presence of coronary artery disease, electrical shock, drowning, drug overdose, or acid/base disturbance. There is only one definitive treatment for ventricular fibrillation and pulseless ventricular tachycardia: defibrillation.

Most defibrillators are very simple to use. It is essential to become familiar with the defibrillator that is used in your department, since it may work a little differently from the one shown in this textbook.

Indications

- Ventricular fibrillation
- Ventricular tachycardia (pulseless)

Contraindications

- A patient with a pulse
- Situations in which the act of defibrillating is deemed dangerous, such as a near-drowning patient lying in water near the edge of a swimming pool

Equipment

- Monitor/defibrillator
- Monitor leads
- Defibrillator pads or conductive gel

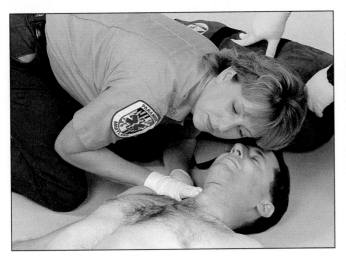

Figure S14-1

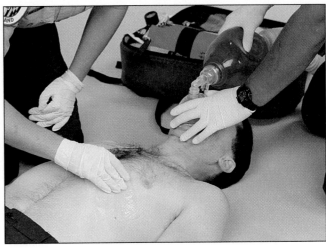

Figure S14-2

Procedure

1. Observe body substance isolation precautions.
2. Establish unresponsiveness.
3. Check to make sure patient is pulseless and not breathing (Fig. S14-1).
4. Have someone begin CPR if defibrillator is not immediately available.
5. Turn the monitor/defibrillator to the ON position (first battery) and select the "Paddle" mode in preparation for using quick-look paddles.
6. Note that "0" appears under "available energy."
7. Apply the conductive medium (Fig. S14-2). Defibrillation gel or pads may be used. The conductive material conducts electricity and at the same time reduces the risk of electrical burns. Do not use alcohol-soaked pads because they may ignite! If using conductive gel on the paddles, make sure the entire surface of the paddle is covered with jelly by rubbing them together. Take care not to rub paddles so hard that jelly oozes onto sides of the paddles

or your hands. If that happens, remove excess jelly with a cloth before proceeding.

8. Select the desired electrical charge on defibrillator paddles.
9. Press the charge button and release.
10. Place the paddles firmly on the chest, exerting 20 to 25 pounds of pressure. Place one paddle on the right of the sternum between the second and third intercostal space and the other at the fifth intercostal space, left midclavicular line, near the apex of the heart (Fig. S14-3).
11. The defibrillator is ready to fire when the charge indicator light stops flashing and glows steadily. The defibrillator will not fire unless it is fully charged to the desired energy level.
12. Call "clear" and visually survey the area to verify that no one, including yourself, is in contact with the patient (Fig. S14-4).
13. Check monitor screen one more time before defibrillating to make sure the patient is still in ventricular fibrillation.

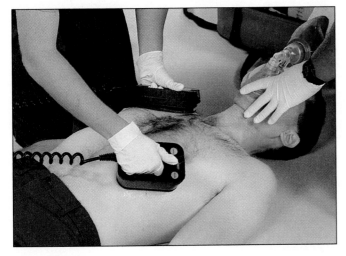

Figure S14-3

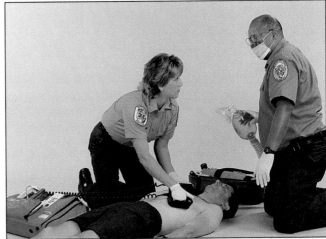

Figure S14-4

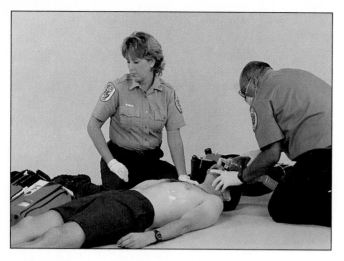

Figure S14-5

14. Depress both paddle discharge buttons simultaneously for defibrillation.
15. Check the patient's ECG strip to see if ventricular fibrillation was terminated and quickly have a co-worker check a pulse (Fig. S14-5).
16. If repeat defibrillation is indicated, depress "charge" and repeat the above steps according to the algorithms.
17. Document the procedure. Documentation should include:

    a. ECG strip of defibrillation (sometimes called "code summary" on the defibrillator).
    b. Patient's name, date, time, lead, joules delivered, and number of defibrillations.
    c. Postdefibrillation rhythm

18. If further defibrillation is unnecessary, be sure that there is no charge in the defibrillator. Most defibrillators "dump" their charge into the machine by turning the joules selection dial to another setting.
19. Once the machine is disarmed, quickly clean the paddles by wiping them with a paper towel or 4 × 4 gauze pad.

Once at the hospital, the paddles must be cleaned with soap and water. Make sure all conductive jelly is removed because any jelly that remains may corrode and pit the paddle heads, which may cause electrical arcing and skin burns in the future.

20. Contact and advise Medical Direction of the patient's status.

Procedures—Hands-Free Defibrillation

NOTE: Know your equipment. Each monitor/defibrillator with a "hands free" option will have slightly different procedures to follow. Some monitor/defibrillator units have the capability of integrating equipment from an automated external defibrillator (AED) for use with their monitor/defibrillator by using a universal cable system.

1. Observe body substance isolation precautions.
2. Establish unresponsiveness.
3. Check to make sure patient is pulseless and not breathing.
4. Have someone begin CPR.
5. Remove the electrode pads from the sealed package and attach the pads to the Hands-Free cable.
6. Attach defibrillator electrode pads to the apex-sternum or anterior-posterior placement as illustrated on the pad's package. Attach the pads firmly, pressing fingertips around the outer margin of the pad to maximize skin to electrode pad contact.
7. Attach cable for hands free mode to the monitor/defibrillator.
8. Turn the monitor/defibrillator to the ON position.
9. Select the "Paddle" mode or "lead II" mode as needed. Consult product literature for specifications.
10. Interpret the rhythm as ventricular fibrillation.
11. Make sure everyone has cleared the patient (Fig. S14-6).
12. Select the desired electrical charge (200 joules if a normal sized adult).
13. Charge the paddles.

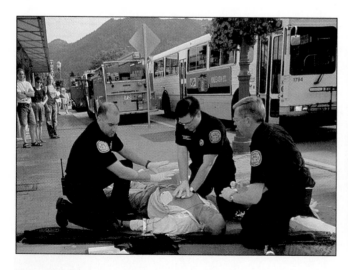

Figure S14-6
Courtesy Physio-Control Corporation, Redmond, Washington.

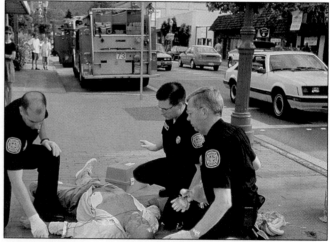

Figure S14-7
Courtesy Physio-Control Corporation, Redmond, Washington.

14. Confirm the rhythm on the monitor and run a 3-second hard copy of the strip.
15. Press the "Discharge" button(s) to deliver the energy. (The paddles should remain firmly housed in the machine throughout this process.) (Fig. S14-7)
16. Confirm the rhythm. If any rhythm other than ventricular fibrillation is present, check pulse.
17. Repeat steps 6-10 for two more cycles using 200–300 joules and 360 joules, as long as VF persists.
18. Resume CPR and continue with the ventricular fibrillation algorithm.
19. The pads remain on the patient to monitor the rhythm.

SKILL 15

Pediatric Defibrillation

Defibrillation is the process of sending an electrical current through the myocardial cells to create depolarization. This depolarization allows the heart to initiate a spontaneous organized rhythm.

Background

Pediatric defibrillation differs from the adult method in several ways. First, the pediatric paddle size is much smaller than the adult: 4.5 cm for infants up to one year or 10 kg. The adult paddle is 8 or 13 cm and is used for older children. Second, the amount of energy delivered to a child is much smaller: 2 J/kg is recommended for initial defibrillation, with repeated energy settings at 4 J/kg. (In the case of synchronized cardioversion, the procedure is the same as standard defibrillation, except that the amount of energy delivered is .5 J/kg initially and repeated at 1 J/kg. Also the synchronizer circuit must be activated by pushing the sync button. A marker will show on the monitor with each QRS complex.)

Indications

- Ventricular fibrillation
- Ventricular tachycardia (pulseless)

Contraindications

- A patient with a pulse
- Situations in which the act of defibrillating is deemed dangerous, such as a near-drowning patient lying in water near the edge of a swimming pool

Equipment

- ECG monitor/defibrillator
- Conductive interface (defibrillator gel or pads)

Procedure

1. Observe body substance isolation precautions.
2. Establish level of consciousness and evaluate ABCs.
3. Have assistants begin CPR if defibrillator is not immediately available.
4. Turn on ECG monitor/defibrillator, making sure that it is set on "Paddles."
5. Expose the patient's chest, and position the patient. Pediatric paddles should be used for the infant up to 12 months of age, with the patient in the supine position (Fig. S15-1). However, if pediatric paddles are unavailable, anterior-posterior paddle placement is necessary, with the patient rolled into the lateral recumbent position (Fig. S15-2). Adult paddles should be used after 1 year of age or in patients weighing 10 kg or more.
6. Using interface (gel or pads), perform quick-look and verify the need for electrical therapy.
7. Charge the defibrillator to the appropriate joules. The recommendation for pediatric patients is 2 J/kg initially.
8. Reconfirm that the rhythm has not changed and that the pulse is still absent. If the rhythm has changed, reassess the patient and treat accordingly.
9. Call CLEAR and visualize the area to verify that no one is in contact with the patient.
10. Apply firm pressure to the paddles and discharge the defibrillator by depressing the two discharge buttons simultaneously.
11. Following countershock, identify the rhythm on the ECG monitor. If the rhythm is unchanged, immediately recharge the defibrillator and countershock at 4 J/kg. If the rhythm changes, treat according to the appropriate American Heart Association algorithm.

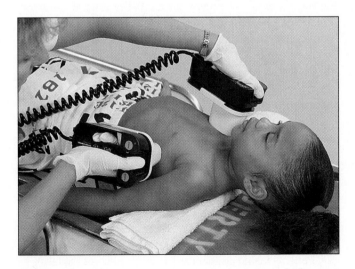

Figure S15-1

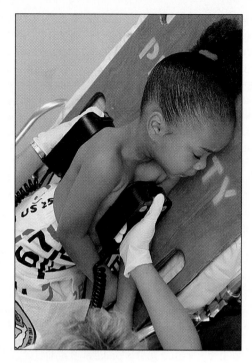

Figure S15-2

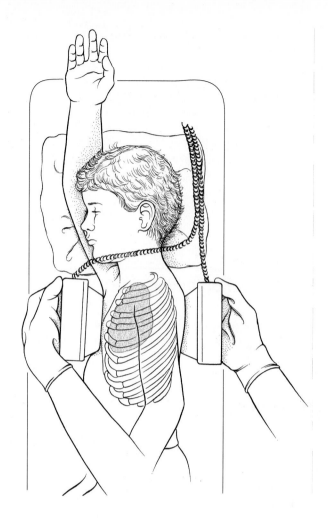

SKILL 16

Synchronized Cardioversion

Background

Cardioversion is the delivery of an electrical shock, timed to the heart's electrical activity, to avoid the relative refractory period and prevent the development of ventricular fibrillation. It is designed to interrupt an ectopic pacemaker so that the sinus node can regain control. The monitor/defibrillator senses the R-wave of the ECG and discharges at that point.

Indications

- Supraventricular and ventricular tachydysrhythmias that result in decompensation of the patient (e.g., perfusing ventricular tachycardia, rapid atrial fibrillation, 2:1 atrial flutter)

Contraindications

- Idiojunctional or idioventricular rhythms, as well as second- and third-degree block
- Patients taking certain cardiac drugs (such as digitalis), since these make the patient more disposed to serious complications such as asystole

Equipment

- BP cuff
- Stethoscope
- ECG monitor and leads
- Conductive material
- Bag-valve resuscitator
- Sedative (optional)
- Gloves

Procedure

1. Observe body substance isolation precautions.
2. Confirm the presence of the dysrhythmia and the patient's hemodynamic status (Fig. S16-1).
3. Explain the procedure to the patient.
4. Establish an IV line, if not already established.
5. Run an ECG strip to document patient's rhythm: label the patient's name, date, and time.
6. Premedicate with sedation as ordered. Be prepared to assist ventilation if necessary.
7. Turn on the defibrillator.
8. Set the defibrillator in the cardiovert mode by depressing the SYNC button. This may vary slightly on different models, so become familiar with your machine. Initial energy delivered should be 50–100 J.

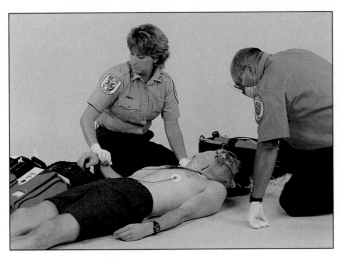

Figure S16-1

9. Examine the ECG rhythm strip again, making sure that the R-wave is at least 3 cm high. If it isn't, adjust the ECG size (gain) button until it is. The R-wave must be tall enough to trigger the cardioverter.
10. Set the control panel to the correct number of joules or watt-seconds.
11. Place defibrillation pads on the patient's chest or apply conductive gel to paddles.
12. Push the charge button. Ensure that the synchronizer is still on and is "marking" the R-wave. Marking the R-waves is recognized by a small light on each R-wave on the cardioscope.
13. Turn the recorder on to record the present rhythm and the effect of the cardioversion.
14. Position the paddles on the chest as you would for defibrillation: one paddle on the right side of the sternum below the clavicle and the other on the left side of the chest at the fifth intercostal space, midclavicular line.
15. Call CLEAR and visualize the area to verify that no one, including yourself, is in contact with the patient.

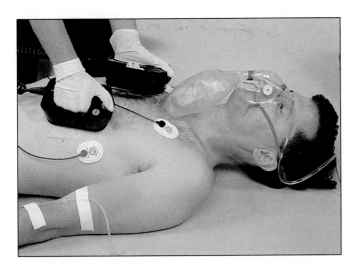

Figure S16-2

16. Simultaneously press and hold both discharge buttons until the countershock is delivered. There may be a momentary delay while the machine detects the next R-wave (Fig. S16-2).
17. Check the patient's vital signs and level of consciousness. If the patient deteriorates into ventricular fibrillation or pulseless ventricular tachycardia, prepare for immediate defibrillation.
18. Document the entire procedure and rhythm strip.
19. If repeat cardioversion is required, repeat steps 7 through 17. If it is not necessary to repeat the procedure, turn off the power. Clean paddles with soap and water to prevent corrosion.

SKILL 17

Noninvasive Pacing

Background

Noninvasive pacing is the application of an external pacemaker for the emergency treatment of symptomatic bradycardia, heart block, or asystole until transvenous pacing can be initiated.

Indications

- Symptomatic bradycardia or heart block that causes decompensation of the patient (e.g., second- or third-degree block with associated hypotension, confusion, or chest pain)

Equipment

- ECG monitor
- ECG monitor leads
- BP cuff
- Stethoscope
- Pacemaker electrodes

Procedure

Not all noninvasive pacemakers are exactly alike. If your pacemaker differs from the one illustrated, consult the operator's manual supplied by the manufacturer for specifics.

1. Observe body substance isolation precautions.
2. Confirm the presence of the dysrhythmia and the patient's hemodynamic status.
3. Receive orders from Medical Direction if needed.
4. Explain the procedure to the patient.
5. Establish an IV if not already established.
6. Run an ECG strip to document the patient's rhythm. Label the strip with the patient's name, date, and time.
7. Adjust the ECG size so the machine can sense the intrinsic QRS activity. The machine will then inhibit the pacing stimulus for the cycle.
8. Apply pacing electrodes in one of the following positions:

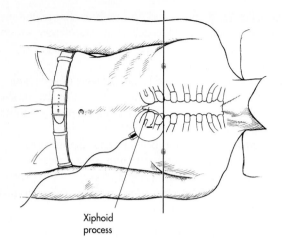

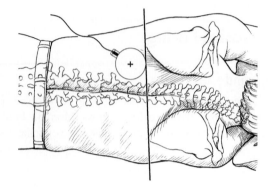

Figure S17-1

Anterior-posterior: This is the preferred placement (Fig. S17-1). Place the negative electrode on left anterior chest, halfway between the xiphoid process and left nipple. The upper edge of the electrode should be below the nipple line. Place the positive electrode on the left posterior chest beneath the scapula and lateral to the spine. The placement of the electrodes affects current threshold.

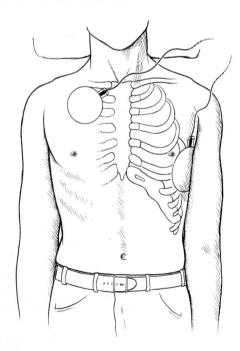

Figure S17-2

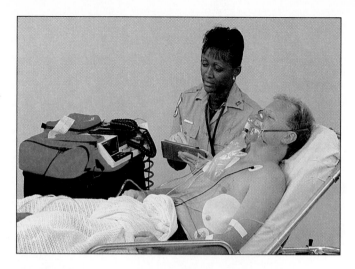

Figure S17-3

Anterior-anterior: This position should be used only if the anterior-posterior position cannot be used (Fig. S17-2). Place the negative electrode on the left chest, midaxillary over the fourth intercostal space. Place the positive electrode on the anterior right chest, subclavicular area.

8. Turn on the power.
9. Connect the pacing cable to the PACE connector.
10. Push the pacer button.
11. Select the desired pacing rate.
12. Observe the cardioscope for a "sense" marker on each QRS complex. If a "sense" marker is not present, readjust ECG size. If this fails, select another lead and readjust the size.
13. When the unit is sensing properly, activate the pacer by pushing START/STOP button. Pacer spikes should be seen with each pacer stimulus.
14. Increase the current slowly while observing the cardioscope for evidence of electrical pacing capture.
15. Assess for perfusion. Palpate the patient's pulse or check blood pressure.
16. Record ECG and document patient's rhythm, vital signs, and tolerance of pacing (Fig. S17-3).
17. Report results to Medical Direction.

SKILL 18

Automated External Defibrillation

Background

Ventricular fibrillation is a common cause of sudden death. Electrical defibrillation is the treatment of choice to correct this dysrhythmia. To be effective, defibrillation should be delivered as soon as possible.

An automated external defibrillator (AED) provides electrical defibrillation by EMS providers and first responders with a minimum of training. The device is designed to be rapidly attached to the arrested patient; it senses and interprets the

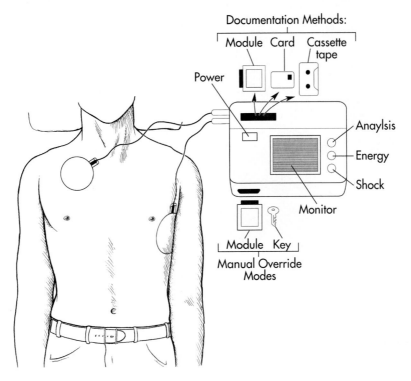

Figure S18-1

patient's ECG, and advises if an electrical shock is needed, which the rescuer must initiate. The automatic AED (as opposed to semi-automatic) is capable of delivering shocks without rescuer intervention.

AEDs are classified as either automatic or semi-automatic. An automatic AED interprets and delivers the necessary electrical shocks without further intervention from the rescuer. With the semi-automatic, the rescuer is advised when a shock is appropriate and directed to manually discharge the AED.

Indications

- Patients in cardiopulmonary arrest

Contraindications

- Patients not in cardiopulmonary arrest
- Pediatric patients weighing less than 90 pounds
- Wet, rainy atmosphere; patients lying in a puddle
- Patients on conductive surface

Equipment

- Automated external defibrillator with cable and self-adhesive defibrillation pads (Fig. S18-1).
- Personal protective equipment

Procedure

1. Observe body substance isolation precautions.
2. Assess cardiopulmonary arrest.
3. Assure that manual CPR is in progress.
4. Expose patient's chest and wipe dry if necessary.
5. Connect pads to AED cables.
6. Place pads on chest. One pad on right upper chest next to sternum and top edge below the clavicle. Place second pad on left side below and to the left of the nipple. Check that pads and cables are secure.

7. Turn on AED.
8. Follow voice commands announced from AED.
9. Stop CPR and clear all personnel from immediate area of patient.
10. If using semi-automatic defibrillator, depress shock button if voice command announces "shock advised."
11. Check breathing and pulse as directed by the AED.
12. If pulse present, continue to support patient and prepare for transport.
13. If no pulse, resume CPR.
14. Monitor AED function and be prepared to stop CPR in 60 seconds while rhythm is analyzed (Fig. S18-2). Follow voice commands if additional shocks are indicated.
15. After termination of call, remove documentation device and process as per local protocol.
16. Replace AED defibrillation pads and battery if necessary.

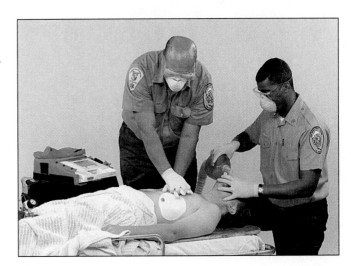

Figure S18-2

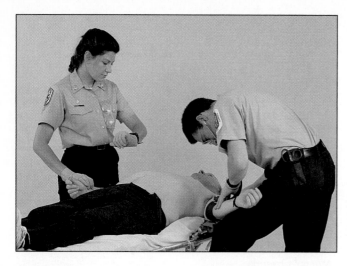

Figure S19-1

SKILL 19

Tilt-test (Orthostatic Vital Signs)

Background

The tilt-test, also known as orthostatic vital signs, is used to assess the patient for signs of compensated shock which may not be otherwise apparent. A significant change in vital signs usually indicates a hypovolemic state, and can be considered a positive tilt-test.

Indications

- Suspected dehydration
- Suspected hypovolemia
- Dizziness, fainting of unknown origin
- Abdominal pain of unknown origin

Contraindications

- Patients with suspected spinal injuries
- Patients with obvious signs of hypovolemia or dehydration (tachycardia or hypotension)

Equipment

- Appropriate size blood pressure cuff
- Stethoscope
- Watch/stopwatch
- Personal protective equipment

Procedure

1. Observe body substance isolation precautions.
2. Assess need for tilt-test.
3. Obtain patient's pulse and blood pressure while supine (Fig. S19-1).
4. Sit patient up with feet dangling. Wait 60 seconds (Fig. S19-2).
5. Obtain pulse and blood pressure with patient seated (Fig. S19-3).
6. If pulse has increased by 10 to 20 BPM, AND systolic blood pressure decreased by 10 to 20 mm Hg, the tilt-test is considered positive.
7. A positive tilt-test indicates need for fluid administration.

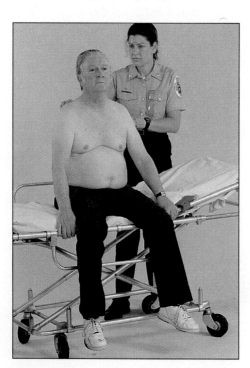

Figure S19-2

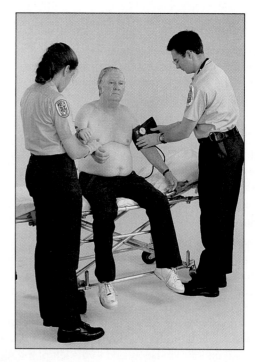

Figure S19-3

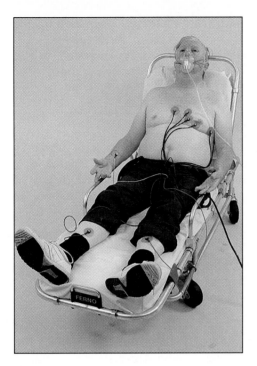

Figure S20-1a

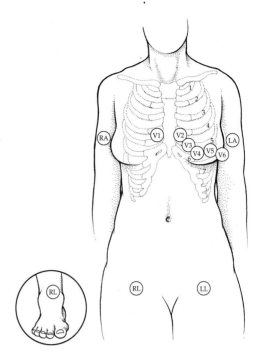

Figure S20-1b

12-Lead ECG

Background

Traditionally, the paramedic was limited to only three views of the heart in the field using leads I, II, and III. Now, with advanced in treatment of ischemic heart disease, it is desirable to diagnose myocardial infarction early in the treatment phase to initiate definitive care either in the field or immediately upon arrival at the hospital. To facilitate this rapid assessment, portable 12-lead ECG units interpret the rhythm and provide a means of transmitting the complete 12-lead ECG to the receiving hospital. With the use of a 12-lead ECG unit, thrombolytic therapy can be instituted much earlier.

Indications

- Suspected cardiac patient

Contraindications

- None

Equipment

- Portable monitor/defibrillator capable of computerized 12-lead ECG analysis
- Patient leads and electrodes for monitor
- Cellular phone and interface (system dependent)
- Personal protective equipment

Procedure

1. Observe body substance isolation precautions.
2. Assess patient and monitor cardiac status.
3. Administer oxygen.
4. Prepare ECG monitor and connect patient cable with electrodes.
5. Explain procedure to patient.
6. Expose chest and prep as necessary.
7. If patient is not in need of immediate intervention, apply standard 12-lead electrodes as in Figure S20-1. If in extremis, proceed as per protocol.
8. Instruct patient to remain still.
9. Start computerized analysis.
10. When analysis is complete, continue to monitor patient in lead II.
11. Obtain printout and review for errors.
12. Transmit 12-lead ECG data as per local protocol (cellular fax or voice) (Fig. S20-2).

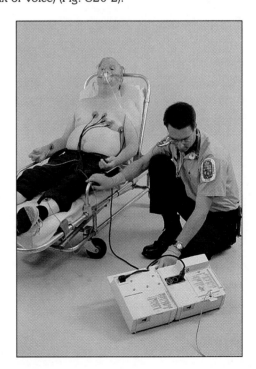

Figure S20-2

13. Monitor patient while continuing with treatment protocol.
14. After termination of call, remove recording device or download data as per local protocol.
15. Replace electrodes and battery as needed.

SKILL 21

Vagal Maneuvers

Vagal maneuvers stimulate the vagus nerve (cranial nerve X), causing a slowing of the sinus node and a decrease in conduction through the AV junction. Vagal stimulation can be used in supraventricular tachycardias as an effective method of slowing or even converting these dysrhythmias to a more stable rhythm.

Background

Two forms of vagal maneuver are used most commonly in the field: Valsalva's maneuver and carotid sinus massage. Both of these methods can be potentially lethal and should be performed with Medical Direction.

Valsalva's Maneuver

The vagus nerve is stimulated by having the patient hold his or her breath and bear down as if having a bowel movement. This is the most convenient maneuver. Although this appears to be a simple procedure, severe bradydysrhythmias or asystole may occur. The patient and the ECG must be monitored closely before, during, and after the procedure. The patient should be oxygenated and an IV line should be established before the procedure. Have the patient stop immediately when the rhythm slows. Be prepared to resuscitate the patient if necessary. If the Valsalva maneuver fails to convert the patient, be prepared to proceed to carotid sinus massage as directed by Medical Direction.

Carotid Sinus Massage

Carotid sinus massage is a noninvasive method of stimulating the vagus nerve and is often effective in slowing tachydysrhythmias.

   The vagus nerve is the tenth cranial nerve and is responsible for carrying parasympathetic nerve fibers to the heart and other organs. As the vagus nerve exits the brain, it passes through the neck in close proximity to the carotid artery. You can stimulate the vagus nerve manually by applying firm, steady pressure on the carotid artery near the angle of the jaw, causing the heart rate to decrease.

Indications

Vagal maneuvers are indicated in the treatment of symptomatic supraventricular tachycardia.

Contraindications

Carotid sinus massage should not be performed on patients who are > 65 years of age, who have known carotid artery disease, or who have a history of a cerebrovascular accident. It should be standard practice to always palpate both carotid arteries separately to check for equal pulses and to auscultate for bruits in elderly individuals before performing carotid sinus massage.

Complications

Bradydysrhythmias or asystole may occur following vagal maneuvers caused by increased vagal tone. A disruption of carotid plaque may result in a cerebral embolus, causing a cerebrovascular accident.

Equipment

- ECG monitor
- Oxygen
- ACLS equipment

Procedure

1. Observe body substance isolation precautions.
2. After evaluating the patient, receive orders from Medical Direction.
3. Place the patient on oxygen. Ensure that an IV is established and that the patient is placed on the ECG monitor.
4. Prepare all ACLS equipment.
5. Place the patient in a supine position with head hyperextended. Check the equality of the carotid pulses by gently palpating both arteries separately (Fig. S21-1). If the pulse is absent or weak on one side, do not perform the procedure and report to Medical Direction.
6. Auscultate for bruits, or vascular turbulence, by listening with the bell of the stethoscope over each carotid artery. If bruits are present, do not proceed (Fig. S21-2).
7. On the right side of the neck, locate the carotid artery.
8. Turn the patient's head slightly to the left.
9. Use the flat side of two fingers and press firmly against the carotid artery toward the cervical vertebrae. You should be able to feel the pulse below your fingertips.
10. Massage the carotid sinus by using a circular motion firmly for 5-10 seconds (Fig. S21-3).

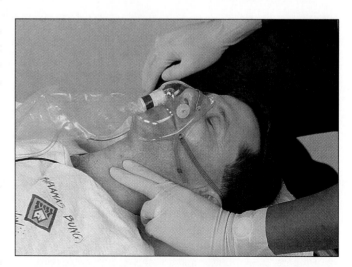

Figure S21-1

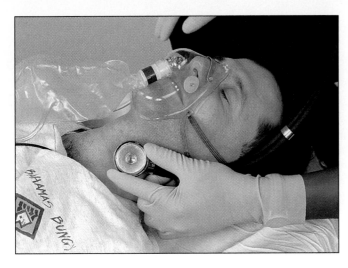

Figure S21-2

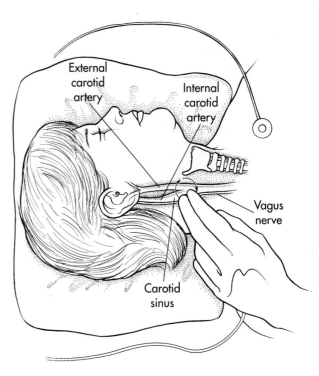

Figure S21-3

11. Keep the monitor strip running to record the procedure and *keep your eye on the monitor at all times.* The massage can be repeated 2–3 times.
12. Discontinue after 3 massages, when the heart rate starts to slow, or when the patient experiences dizziness or a change in level of consciousness.

13. If the procedure is unsuccessful on the right carotid, wait 2 to 3 minutes and repeat the procedure on the left side.
14. Report the results of the procedure to Medical Direction.
15. Document the procedure, including a copy of the ECG strip.

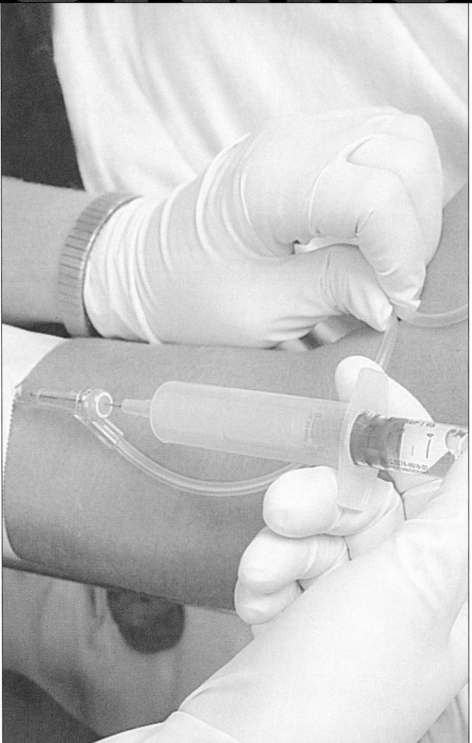

Skills
Drug Administration

Peripheral Intravenous Cannulation

Intravenous cannulation is the process of placing a catheter (metal or plastic) into a peripheral vein for the administration of fluids or drugs.

Background

Peripheral intravenous cannulation provides access to the circulation for rapid administration of fluids and drugs. Commonly, peripheral intravenous cannulation is used for fluid administration in shock and as a lifeline for various medical conditions such as cardiac disease, hypoglycemia, and seizures. Intravenous cannulation in the field is most commonly performed with a plastic catheter inserted over a hollow needle. Other types of cannulas are hollow needles and plastic catheters inserted through a hollow needle.

Indication

Intravenous cannulation is indicated for the administration of drugs or fluids in any serious or critically ill or potentially critically ill patient.

Contraindications

Although there are no true absolute contraindications, peripheral intravenous cannulation should not significantly delay scene times. Intravenous cannulation in serious trauma patients should be started while en route to the hospital when possible.

Equipment

- Intravenous fluid ordered (e.g., lactated Ringer's, normal saline, or dextrose 5% in water)
- Intravenous infusion set—use microdrip tubing for lifelines used for drug administration, and macrodrip tubing for rapid fluid administration
- Intravenous catheter (cannula)—preferably 18 gauge for lifelines and 12 to 16 gauge for fluid administration
- Povidone-iodine or alcohol preps
- Sterile dressing (e.g., 4 × 4 gauze pad)
- Adhesive tape strips, 3 to 4 inches in length
- 10 cc syringe, vacutainer tubes for blood samples
- Tourniquet (commercial or blood pressure cuff)
- Armboard
- Gloves

Procedure

1. Explain to the patient the need for intravenous cannulation and describe what will be done.
2. Observe body substance isolation precautions (glove minimally).
3. Assemble the necessary equipment.
4. Place a commercial tourniquet or inflate a blood pressure cuff just above the elbow and place the arm in a dependent position (Fig. S22-1). If using a blood pressure cuff, inflate until 20 mm Hg below the systolic pressure.
5. Select a prominent vein by feel more than sight. Choose the most distal prominent vein on the hand, forearm, or antecubital space that is straight, on a flat surface, and not rolling. If possible, avoid veins over joints, using the antecubital veins as a last resort.
6. A vein may be distended for easier cannulation by gently tapping on it with the fingers.
7. Prep the venipuncture site with povidone-iodine or alcohol prep, using a firm circular motion from the vein outward.
8. With traction on the skin below the venipuncture site, stabilize the vein.
9. Tell the patient there will be a quick, painful stick.
10. With the bevel of the needle upward, puncture the skin using a 30- to 45-degree angle. Enter the vein directly from above or from the side (Fig. S22-2).
11. When the vein is entered, you should feel a "pop" and see blood return through the catheter.
12. Carefully lower the catheter and advance the needle and catheter approximately 2 mm to stabilize the needle in the vein.
13. Slide the catheter off of the needle into the vein and then remove the needle (Fig. S22-3). Dispose of the needle into a puncture-proof (sharps) container. Do not attempt to recap the needle.
14. Consider drawing a blood sample using a syringe or luer-adapter and vacutainer.
15. Release the tourniquet and then attach the infusion tubing to the hub of the catheter (Fig. S22-4).
16. Open the flow regulator on the IV tubing. The fluid should run freely.
17. Cover the venipuncture site with povidone-iodine ointment.

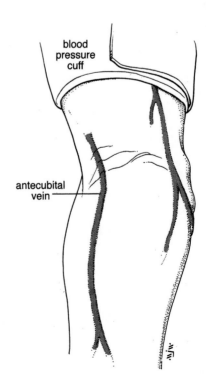

blood
pressure
cuff

antecubital
vein

Figure S22-1

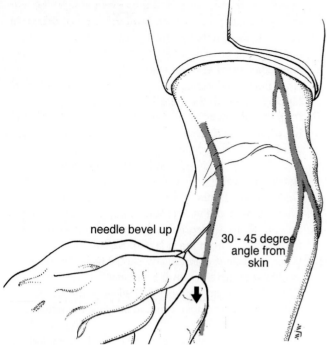

needle bevel up

30 - 45 degree angle from skin

Figure S22-2

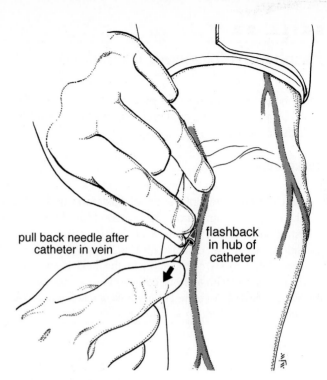

pull back needle after catheter in vein

flashback in hub of catheter

Figure S22-3

18. Tape the catheter to the skin, using any acceptable technique.

19. Make a loop with the infusion tubing and tape the loop to the arm. This will allow a little extra tubing in case the IV bag is accidentally pulled away from the patient.

20. If the vein is near or over a joint, immobilize it with an armboard to prevent dislodgement of the catheter and positional fluid flow through the tubing.

SKILL 23

External Jugular Vein Cannulation

The external jugular vein is a large vessel in the neck that may be used by paramedics for intravenous cannulation. This vein is considered to be a peripheral IV site.

Background

The external jugular vein runs from behind the angle of the jaw downward across the sternocleidomastoid muscle to pierce the fascia above the middle third of the clavicle. It joins the subclavian vein just behind the clavicle (Fig. S23-1). If EMS systems allow the procedure, external jugular vein cannulation can be used for any patient that presents with a definite need for peripheral intravenous cannulation

The external jugular vein should not be considered for a precautionary IV. The external jugular vein may be used for pediatric patients; however, the vein is difficult to visualize in infants and small children.

Indication

External jugular vein cannulation is indicated in a patient who requires peripheral intravenous cannulation in whom an extremity vein cannot be catheterized.

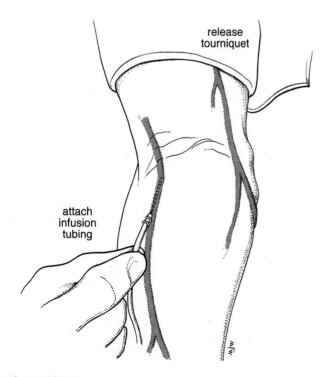

release tourniquet

attach infusion tubing

Figure S22-4

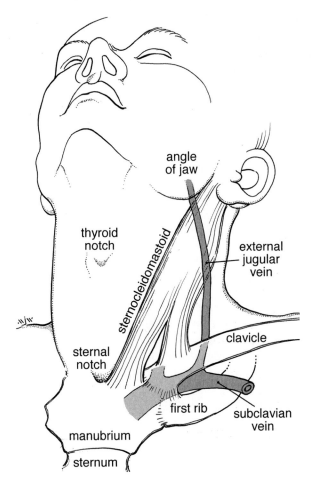

Figure S23-1

Contraindications

- Inability to visualize the vein
- Obscured landmarks caused by local trauma, hematoma, or subcutaneous emphysema
- Cervical collar

Equipment

- Intravenous fluid ordered (e.g., lactated Ringer's, normal saline, or dextrose 5% in water)
- Intravenous infusion set: use microdrip tubing for lifelines used for drug administration, and macrodrip tubing for rapid fluid administration
- IV extension tubing
- IV catheter (cannula)—preferably 18 gauge for lifelines and 12 to 16 gauge for fluid administration
- Povidone-iodine or alcohol prep
- Sterile dressing (e.g., 4 × 4 gauze pad)
- Adhesive tape strips, 3 to 4 inches in length
- 10 cc syringe, vacutainers for blood samples
- Latex gloves

Procedure

1. Explain procedure to patient.
2. Use body substance isolation precautions.
3. Position the patient supine with feet elevated (when possible).
4. Turn the head in the direction away from the side to be cannulated.
5. Prep the skin with povidone-iodine.
6. Apply traction on the vein just above the clavicle.
7. Attach a 10 cc syringe to an IV catheter. Align the catheter and point the tip of the catheter toward the feet.
8. Tell the patient there will be a quick, painful stick.
9. With the bevel of the needle upward, puncture the skin using a 30-degree angle. The needle tip should enter midway between the angle of the jaw and the clavicle, and should be aimed toward the shoulder on the same side as the vein (Fig. S23-2). Apply suction to the syringe. As the vein is entered, note a flashback of blood.
10. Carefully lower the catheter and advance the needle and catheter approximately 2 mm to stabilize the needle in the vein.
11. Slide the catheter off of the needle into the vein and then remove the needle. Dispose of needle and syringe into a puncture-proof container. Don't attempt to recap the needle.
12. Consider drawing a blood sample using a syringe or luer-adapter and vacutainer.
13. Attach the infusion tubing to the hub of the catheter.
14. Open the flow regulator on the IV tubing. The fluid should run freely.
15. Cover the site with povidone-iodine ointment.
16. Tape the catheter to the skin using any acceptable technique.
17. Make a loop with the infusion tubing and tape the loop to the neck so there will be extra tubing in case the IV bag is accidentally pulled away from the patient. Never use circumferential taping because of vascular compromise that can result in a decreased cerebral circulation.

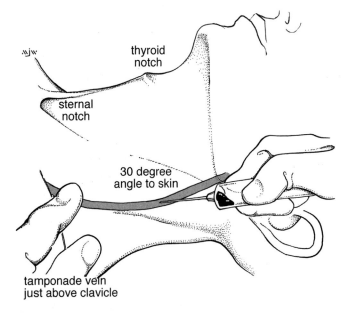

Figure S23-2

SKILL 24

Pediatric Peripheral Vein Access

- Armboard
- Latex gloves
- Eye protection

Background

Peripheral access in the neonate or pediatric patient can be very challenging, even for an experienced paramedic. The small size of the vessel, along with a child who is often uncooperative, can make this procedure very difficult. It is important to select a catheter that is not too large for the vein. Generally, the large veins of the arm, leg, or scalp are selected, using a 20-, 22- or 24-gauge over-the-needle catheter. The external jugular vein is very difficult to access because of the short neck on a child and is often not attempted.

Indications

- Any medical condition, such as cardiopulmonary arrest, accidental overdose, or sepsis, that suggests an IV or possible medication administration
- Any traumatic condition such as head injury, multiple fractures, or shock that suggests the need or potential need for volume resuscitation

Contraindications

- There are no contraindications to initiating an IV in the pediatric patient who is in need of vascular access.

Equipment

- Intravenous fluid ordered (e.g., lactated Ringer's, normal saline, or dextrose 5% in water)
- Intravenous infusion set—use microdrip tubing for life-lines used for drug administration, and macrodrip tubing for rapid fluid administration
- IV catheter (cannula): 20-, 22-, 24-guage over-the-needle
- Povidone-iodine or alcohol prep
- Sterile dressing (e.g., 4 × 4 gauze pad)
- Adhesive tape strips, hypoallergenic, ½″ to 1″ wide
- 10 cc syringe, vacutainers for blood samples
- Tourniquet (commercial or blood pressure cuff)

Procedure for an Extremity Venipuncture

1. Observe body substance isolation precautions.
2. Assemble the necessary equipment. Set up intravenous solution, flush tubing, and tear tape.
3. Immobilize the extremity, if necessary.
4. Place a venous tourniquet proximal to the proposed site. A rubber band can be used if the extremity is very small (Fig. S24-1).
5. Locate a suitable vein that will accept a catheter. Cleanse the site, using an alcohol or povidone-iodine prep.
6. Perform venipuncture, using correct, aseptic technique. Watch for blood return. Because of the small catheter lumen and lower venous pressure, the flashback may not be as apparent as it is in adults.
7. Slowly advance the catheter and remove the needle.
8. Release the tourniquet and attach intravenous solution.
9. Slowly introduce fluid into the vein. If patent, adjust flow rate.
10. Secure the catheter, using an acceptable taping method. With an active child, extra tape or roller-gauze dressing is advisable.
11. Routinely reconfirm IV patency and drip rate (Fig. S24-2).

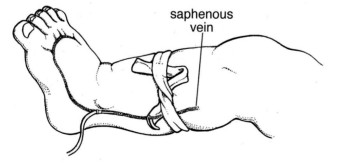

saphenous vein

Figure S24-1

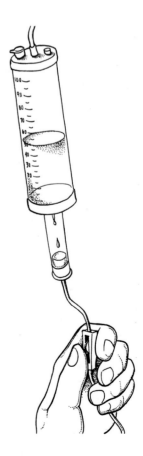

Figure S24-2

Intraosseous Infusion

Intraosseous (I/O) infusion is defined as a puncture into the medullary cavity of a bone that provides the care provider with a rapid access route for fluids and medications.

Background

The technique of I/O puncture and infusion was first described in the medical literature in 1922. It was used for several decades, but with the development of better intravenous catheters, the procedure lost its popularity until the late 1970s. Even with improved catheters, it was often still difficult to achieve vascular access. Thus there was a reemergence of the procedure, and its acceptance has grown in the prehospital setting.

Generally, I/O infusion is reserved for the pediatric patient up to 6 years of age.

Introduction of a needle into the medullary cavity is relatively rapid and simple, compared to peripheral IV insertion. The procedure only requires the addition of one instrument: a needle with a stylet. There are currently several commercially manufactured I/O or bone marrow biopsy needles available. The needle is usually large bore (12 to 16 gauge), with a shorter shaft than the standard intravenous catheter.

Three sites are suggested for the puncture. The most commonly used site is the proximal tibia, since the tibial plateau has a broad, flat surface. The distal tibia and distal femur can also be accessed.

It should be noted that the I/O site is for temporary use only. Once the child's condition has stabilized, another form of intravenous therapy should be initiated. Prolonged use of I/O infusion has proven to lead to infection more often than traditional IVs.

Indications

- Cardiac arrest
- Multisystem trauma with associated shock and/or severe hypovolemia

- Severe dehydration associated with vascular collapse and/or loss of consciousness
- Any child who is unresponsive and in need of immediate drug or fluid resuscitation (burns, status asthmaticus, status epilepticus, sepsis)

Contraindications

- Fracture above the insertion site
- Prior infection at the insertion site
- Site used for previous insertion

Equipment

- Intravenous solution
- IV tubing (microdrip or Buretrol-type)
- Commercial I/O or bone marrow biopsy needle (can substitute large-bore spinal needle)
- Povidone-iodine swabs
- Antibiotic ointment
- 1-inch tape
- Several rolls of 2- or 3-inch Kling
- 10-ml syringe
- Injectable sterile saline
- Gloves
- Eye protection (goggles)

Procedure

1. Observe body substance isolation precautions.
2. Assemble and prepare necessary equipment to be used.
3. Identify the landmark for insertion, preferably the anteromedial aspect of the proximal tibia, approximately 1 to 3 cm below the tibial tuberosity (Fig. S25-1).
4. Cleanse the puncture site.
5. Using a twisting motion, introduce the needle using a 90-degree inferior puncture, away from the joint and epiphyseal plate (Fig. S25-2). Note the decrease in resistance as the needle enters the marrow. Stabilize the needle once it has been inserted.

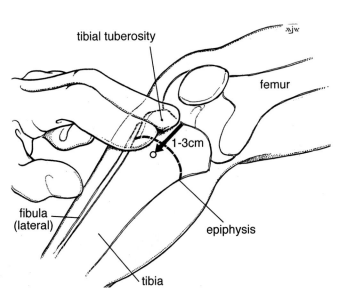

tibial tuberosity

femur

1-3cm

fibula (lateral)

epiphysis

tibia

Figure S25-1

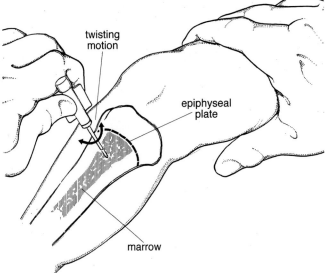

twisting motion

epiphyseal plate

marrow

Figure S25-2

6. Remove the stylet.
7. Attach a 10-ml syringe and aspirate bone marrow to verify the location of the needle. Remove the syringe.
8. Attach another 10-ml syringe filled with sterile saline. Inject 5 to 10 ml of saline to clear the lumen of the needle.
9. Attach the IV and adjust the flow rate.
10. Place antibiotic ointment around the site and secure with tape.
11. Following the administration of a medication, 10 ml of saline should be administered to expedite absorption into the circulatory system.

SKILL 26

Umbilical Vein Catheterization

Umbilical vein catheterization (UVC) is the process of gaining intravenous access by placing a specialized catheter or tubing into the umbilical vein of the neonatal umbilicus.

Background

UVC is making its way into the field setting. This procedure allows a paramedic to administer fluids or medications when percutaneous cannulation into a small vein is technically impossible.

The umbilical vein catheter is not without serious risks. Local and systemic infection, thrombus formation, and possible emboli are all potential side effects. In addition, too aggressive or poor placement by the paramedic may result in the tip of the catheter entering the portal system of the liver.

Indication

- Neonatal patient, less than one week of age, in need of IV access, but does not have accessible peripheral veins.

Contraindications

- There are no significant contraindications, especially when used in a life-threatening illness or injury.

Equipment

- Sterile scalpel
- Umbilical tape
- Two sterile, delicately curved 5-inch hemostats
- Sterile gauze pads (4 × 4)
- No. 3.5, or 5, Fr. umbilical catheter
- Luer-Lok disposable stopcock
- Sterile scissors
- Povidone-iodine swabs
- Intravenous solution
- Microdrip or Buretrol-type solution set
- Heparin (concentration of 10 U/1 ml of fluid)
- Gloves
- Eye protection (goggles)
- Sterile drapes

Procedure

1. Observe body substance isolation precautions.
2. Prepare the above equipment.
3. Restrain the infant, if necessary.
4. Clean and drape the area. The umbilicus should be cleansed, using povidone-iodine solution.
5. Place a loose tie of umbilical tape around the base of the umbilicus.
6. Locate the two umbilical arteries and one umbilical vein (Fig. S26-1). The vein has a thin wall and larger lumen compared to the thick walls and smaller lumen of the umbilical arteries. Trim the cord approximately 1 cm to provide a fresh opening.
7. Using a sterile hemostat, insert the tip of the hemostat into the lumen of the vein. Gently open the hemostat to dilate the vessel (Fig. S26-2).

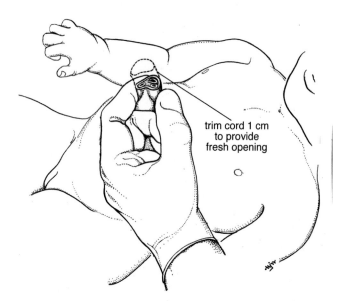

trim cord 1 cm
to provide
fresh opening

Figure S26-1

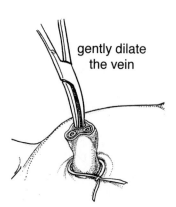

gently dilate
the vein

Figure S26-2

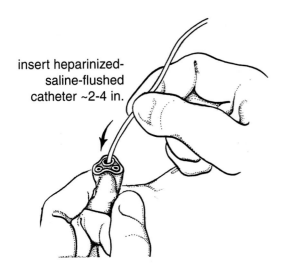

insert heparinized-saline-flushed catheter ~2-4 in.

Figure S26-3

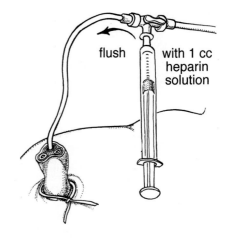

flush   with 1 cc heparin solution

Figure S26-4

8. Introduce and advance a heparinized-saline flushed umbilical catheter approximately 2 to 4 inches (Fig. S26-3). This will place the catheter into the inferior vena cava of the infant. You should note blood return after inserting the catheter. Do not force the catheter because severe hemorrhage or liver injury may occur.
9. Hook up the catheter to a three-way stopcock. Flush the catheter with 1 ml of heparin solution (Fig. S26-4).
10. Secure the catheter, using the piece of umbilical tape, by tying the tape around the umbilicus (Fig. S26-5).
11. After securing the catheter, hook the IV tubing to the stopcock to allow for the administration of fluids and/or medications.
12. Monitor the umbilicus for bleeding. A dressing is usually not used in this situation so that the umbilicus can be viewed.

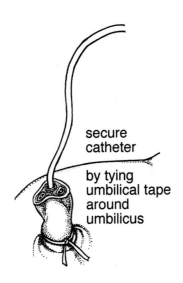

secure catheter

by tying umbilical tape around umbilicus

Figure S26-5

SKILL 27
Endotracheal Drug Administration

Endotracheal bolus is a procedure that allows the delivery of a medication directly to the tracheobronchial tree and lung tissue, via an ETT.

Background
Administration of medication via an ETT is generally reserved for use during cardiac arrest or when intravenous access is not available. The number of drugs that may be given via an ETT is limited. Paramedics most often administer three drugs during cardiopulmonary arrest: atropine, epinephrine, and lidocaine. Another medication can be given when necessary via ETT: naloxone (Narcan). The exact dose of drug administered via this route is still under investigation, but for now the ET dose of a drug should be at least equal to the intravenous dose and should be delivered in a volume of 5 to 10 ml.

Indications
Endotracheal bolus drug administration is indicated for certain drugs during cardiopulmonary arrest or when intravenous access is not available.

Contraindications
There are no specific contraindications to administering drugs via an ETT. However, the paramedic must remember the four medications listed above that can be given via ETT without detriment to the patient.

Equipment
- Prefilled syringe and needle or 18- or 19-gauge needle with syringe
- Sterile saline or water for dilution
- Sharps container

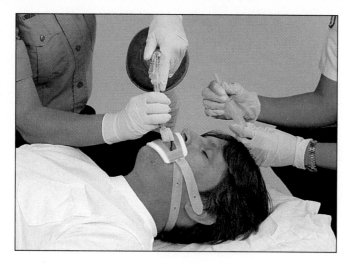

Figure S27-1

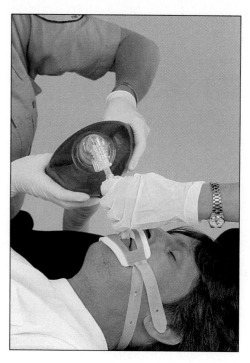

Figure S27-3

Procedure

The following procedure outlines the method used for administering a medication that comes in a prefilled syringe (it is taken for granted that this patient is already intubated).

1. Observe body substance isolation precautions (gloves).
2. Confirm the drug order, amount to be given, and route.
3. Check the medication name, expiration, coloration, and clarity.
4. Assemble the syringe.
5. Calculate the desired volume of drug. If the entire syringe is not going to be given, the paramedic can either carefully inject the appropriate amount of drug or squirt out the excess amount.

6. Hyperventilate the patient.
7. Disconnect the ETT from the bag-valve device (Fig. S27-1).
8. Stop chest compressions if CPR is being performed.
9. Place the needle into the lumen of the ETT and forcefully inject the solution (Fig. S27-2).
10. Reconnect the bag-valve device (Fig. S27-3) and hyperventilate the patient for 10 seconds to facilitate drug delivery farther into the tracheobronchial tree.
11. Resume appropriate ventilation and reinitiate chest compressions.
12. Verify the placement of the ETT. It is not uncommon for the tube to be displaced from the trachea and accidently repositioned in the esophagus during this procedure.
13. Monitor the patient for medication effect.

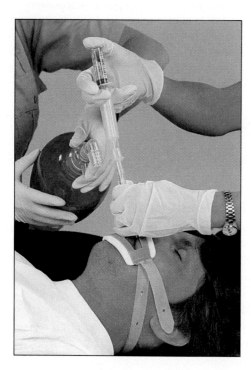

Figure S27-2

SKILL 28

Intravenous Bolus Drug Administration

Intravenous bolus, or "IV push," is a method of administering drugs directly into the vein. This method of administration allows for a rapid onset of medications, especially in critical situations.

Background

As the most rapid method of drug administration available to paramedics, intravenous bolus is most commonly used for life-threatening emergencies and cardiopulmonary arrest. These emergencies include, but are not limited to:

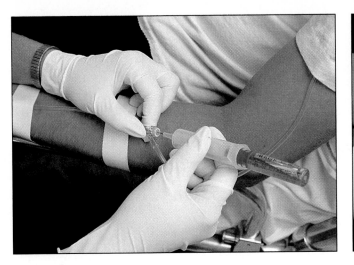

Figure S28-1

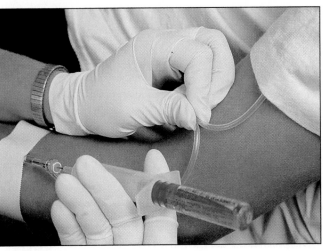

Figure S28-2

- Ventricular dysrhythmias
- Supraventricular tachycardia
- Symptomatic bradycardia
- Hypoglycemia
- Metabolic acidosis
- Seizures
- Acute pulmonary edema
- Cardiopulmonary arrest
- Narcotic overdose
- Pain control

Because of the emergent nature of these conditions, many of these drugs come in commonly used dosages in pre-filled syringes for convenience and ease of administration.

Indications

Intravenous bolus drug administration is indicated for the rapid delivery of drugs.

Contraindications

Intravenous bolus drug administration may be ineffective at sites in close proximity to dialysis shunts or traumatized areas.

Equipment

- Appropriate size syringe and needle for amount of medication to be delivered (or medication in prefilled syringe)
- Appropriate medication
- Alcohol preps
- Gloves
- Sharps container

Procedure

This procedure assumes that an IV has previously been established and that a prefilled syringe is being used.

1. Observe body substance isolation precautions (gloves).
2. Confirm the drug order, amount to be given, and route.

3. Explain the procedure to the patient and reconfirm that the patient is not allergic to the medication.
4. Check the medication name, expiration, coloration, and clarity.
5. Assemble the appropriate equipment.
6. Reconfirm that the IV is patent and running by observing fluid freely flowing.
7. Calculate the desired volume of drug. If the entire syringe is not going to be given, the paramedic can either carefully inject the appropriate amount of drug or squirt out the excess amount.
8. Eject any air from the syringe.
9. Cleanse the rubber injection port with an alcohol prep.
10. Insert the needle into the rubber injection port (Fig. S28-1).
11. Pinch off the IV tubing just above the injection port (Fig. S28-2).
12. Inject the desired amount of medication into the injection port. Speed of administration is based on the individual drug (Fig. S28-3).

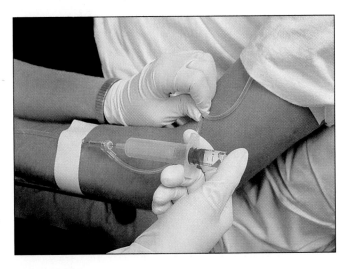

Figure S28-3

13. Release or unpinch the IV tubing.
14. Flush the IV tubing. Run enough fluid in (no greater than 20 cc) to ensure delivery of drug through the tubing into the circulation.
15. Readjust the IV flow to the previous rate.
16. Properly dispose of the syringe and medication container.
17. Monitor the patient for medication effect.

SKILL 29

Intravenous Drip Infusion (IV Piggyback)

Intravenous drip infusion or IV piggyback (IVPB) provides a route for continuous administration of a medication. This is accomplished by connecting an IV infusion containing a medication to a preexisting IV site.

Background

Intravenous drip infusion is a method of continuous medication administration. It offers the advantage of being easily titrated to increase or decrease the rate of flow or to discontinue the infusion, depending on the patient's response. The correct computation of the amount of medication to be added to the intravenous solution and the rate at which it should be delivered are most important.

Indications

Intravenous drip infusion is indicated for drugs that require continuous infusion and/or titration of dose.

Contraindications

None

Equipment

- Intravenous solution to which the medication will be added, usually 5% dextrose.
- Mini-drip (micro) IV tubing
- 19-gauge needle
- Alcohol preps
- Gloves
- Syringe and needle
- 1-inch tape
- Medication label

Procedure

This procedure assumes that an IV has already been established.

1. Observe body substance isolation precautions (gloves).
2. Confirm the drug order, amount to be given, and route.
3. Explain the procedure to the patient and reconfirm that the patient is not allergic to the medication.
4. Check the medication name, expiration, coloration, and clarity.
5. Assemble the equipment and attach the needle to the syringe if not preattached.
6. Calculate and draw up the desired volume of drug into the syringe.
7. Check the intravenous fluid for proper fluid, expiration date, and clarity.
8. Cleanse the injection port on the IV bag with an alcohol prep.
9. Insert the needle into the injection port on the IV bag or bottle and inject the volume of the drug ordered (Fig. S29-1).
10. Mix the drug in the intravenous solution by gently shaking the bag.
11. Using a medication label, identify the bag with the time, amount injected, concentration of medication in the fluid, and preparer's initials.
12. Attach the administration set and purge the line of air. This will provide you with a line filled with medication. A microdrip set should be used with prehospital IVPBs (Fig. S29-2).

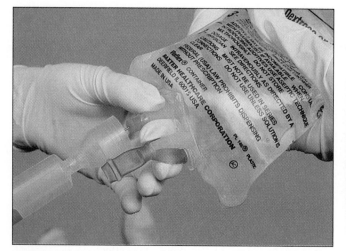

Figure S29-1

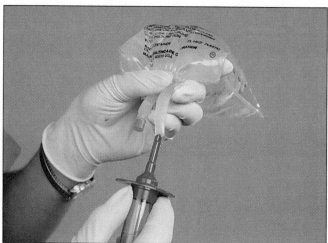

Figure S29-2

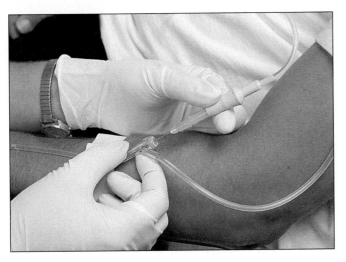

Figure S29-3

13. Attach a sterile needle to the administration set. Clean the injection port nearest to the patient and attach the IVPB to this site (Fig. S29-3).
14. Set the primary IV rate to TKO.
15. Calculate the rate of administration to achieve the desired dose and adjust the flow rate accordingly.
16. Secure the IVPB with tape to prevent accidental dislodgement of the needle.
17. Monitor the patient for medication effect.

SKILL 30

Intramuscular Injection

Intramuscular (IM) injection is a method of administering drugs directly into muscle, where they are subsequently absorbed into the general circulation.

Background

The administration of intramuscular drugs in the field is relatively uncommon. Prehospital drugs that may be administered intramuscularly include, but are not limited to, diazepam, meperidine, morphine, and glucagon. This method is particularly useful when other administration routes fail. Compared with intravenous injection, absorption via the intramuscular route is slower and requires adequate perfusion. For example, the intramuscular route may be ineffective when the patient is hypotensive.

Indications

Intramuscular injection is indicated for the administration of specific drugs in the prehospital setting when slow absorption is acceptable, or when other administration routes are unsuccessful.

Contraindications

Intramuscular injections may be contraindicated in patients with coagulopathies (a defect in the clotting mechanism of the body) or those who take anticoagulants.

Equipment

- 21-gauge needle
- Syringe
- Povidone-iodine or alcohol preps
- Gloves
- Sharps container

Procedure

1. Observe body substance isolation precautions (gloves).
2. Confirm the drug order, amount to be given, and route.
3. Explain the procedure to patient and reconfirm that the patient is not allergic to the medication.
4. Check the medication name, expiration, coloration, and clarity.
5. Assemble equipment and attach the needle to the syringe if not preattached.
6. Calculate and draw up the desired volume of drug into the syringe.
7. Eject any air from the syringe.
8. Identify an appropriate injection site. The deltoid muscle of the shoulder and upper arm and the upper outside quadrant of the gluteus muscle are commonly used sites (Fig. S30-1). The preferred injection site for children is the vastas lateralis muscle (Fig. S30-2). It is midway between the knee and the greater trochanter, just lateral to the midline. The rectus femoris muscle can also be used in children.
9. Cleanse the injection site with alcohol or povidone-iodine.
10. Stretch or "flatten" the skin overlying the site with your fingers.
11. Advise the patient to expect a painful stick.
12. Insert the needle at a 90-degree angle (Fig. S30-3).
13. Pull back, or aspirate, on the syringe. If a blood vessel has been entered, blood will return in the syringe. If this happens, withdraw the needle, apply direct pressure with a sterile gauze pad, and prepare to restick the patient with a new needle.
14. Inject the drug into the muscle slowly.
15. Withdraw the needle and apply pressure to the site with a sterile gauze pad or iodine/alcohol prep.
16. Properly dispose of the syringe and medication container.
17. Monitor the patient for medication effect.

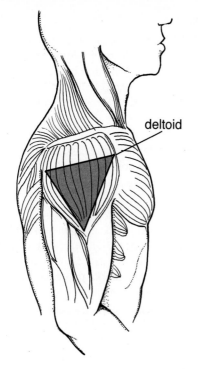

deltoid

Figure S30-1a

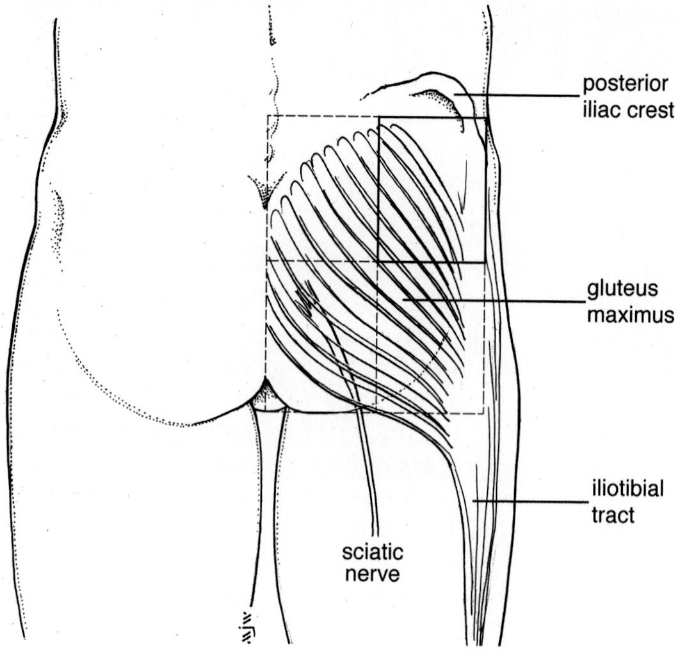

posterior
iliac crest

gluteus
maximus

iliotibial
tract

sciatic
nerve

Figure S30-1b

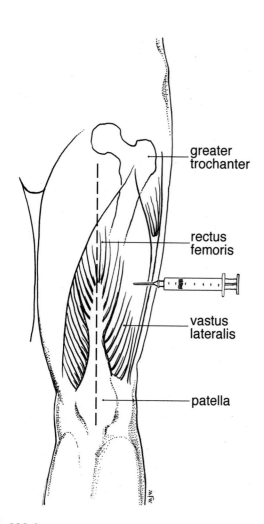

greater
trochanter

rectus
femoris

vastus
lateralis

patella

Figure S30-2

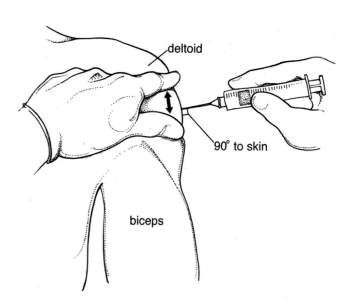

deltoid

90° to skin

biceps

Figure S30-3

SKILL 31

Subcutaneous Injection

Subcutaneous (SQ) injection is a method of administering drugs directly into subcutaneous or fatty tissue where they are absorbed into the general circulation.

Background

Subcutaneous injection is one of the simpler forms of drug administration that indeed may be lifesaving in cases of severe asthma or allergic reactions in which epinephrine 1:1000 is required. Some EMS systems carry glucagon for insulin shock, which may be administered subcutaneously when other routes are not easily available. It is important to ensure that the subcutaneous injection is an administration of drug into the subcutaneous tissue rather than into the more superficial dermis or deeper muscle, connective tissue or blood vessels. Medication injected subcutaneously is typically absorbed more slowly than the intravenous or intramuscular routes, but faster than the oral route.

Indications

Subcutaneous injection is indicated for administration of a limited number of drugs in specific clinical settings, commonly asthma and allergic/anaphylactic reactions.

Contraindications

There are no contraindications to subcutaneous injection, except for medications not delivered by that route.

Equipment

- 25-gauge, ½-inch needle
- Tuberculin 1-cc syringe
- Povidone-iodine or alcohol preps
- Gloves
- 2 × 2-inch sterile gauze pads
- Sharps container

Procedure

1. Observe body substance isolation precautions (gloves).
2. Confirm the drug order, amount to be given, and route.
3. Explain the procedure to the patient and reconfirm that the patient is not allergic to the medication.
4. Check the medication name, expiration, coloration, and clarity.
5. Assemble the equipment and attach the needle to the syringe if not preattached.
6. Calculate and draw up the desired volume of drug into the syringe.
7. Eject any air from the syringe.
8. Identify an injection site—the area below the deltoid muscle of the shoulder is commonly used but other subcutaneous sites are also available (Fig. S31-1).
9. Clean the injection site with alcohol or povidone-iodine.
10. Apply tension to (or tent) the skin to pull it away from underlying muscle.
11. Advise the patient to expect a stick.
12. Insert the needle at a 45-degree angle into the subcutaneous tissue (Fig. S31-2).
13. Pull back, or aspirate, on the syringe. If a blood vessel has been entered, blood will return in the syringe. In the event that this occurs, remove the needle and begin again, using a different site. Apply pressure over the site with a sterile gauze pad. If performed correctly, air bubbles may appear in the syringe.
14. Inject the drug into the subcutaneous tissue slowly.
15. Withdraw the needle and apply pressure to the site with a sterile gauze pad.
16. Properly dispose of the syringe and medication container.
17. Monitor the patient for medication effect.

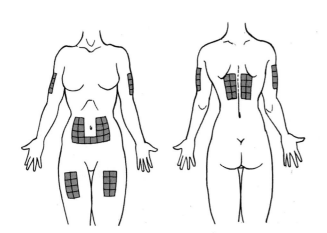

Figure S31-1

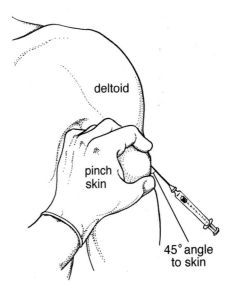

deltoid

pinch skin

45° angle to skin

Figure S31-2

SKILL 32

Nebulized Inhalation

Nebulized inhalation of drugs is a method of delivering medications via the tracheobronchial tree, using a device known as a nebulizer. This process mixes high-flow oxygen and a medication, which results in a vapor that the patient can inhale.

Background

Paramedics frequently see patients with hand-held nebulizers. Many EMS systems have incorporated nebulized drug administration into their treatment regimens for asthma and chronic obstructive pulmonary disease (COPD). Inhaled bronchodilators, such as albuterol (Proventil) and metaproterenol (Alupent), are commonly used in hand-held and side-stream nebulizers. Most prehospital medications are given via side-stream devices, which mix oxygen with the medication. Some attachments also allow a nebulized mist to be forced into a patient, using a bag-valve-mask when the patient is unable to adequately ventilate himself.

Indications

Nebulized inhalation is indicated for patients with asthma or COPD, who are in need of rapid bronchodilation.

Contraindications

The procedure of nebulized inhalation is not contraindicated for any patient. Specific contraindications are reserved to the medication (bronchodilator) to be inhaled by the patient.

Equipment

- Side-stream nebulizer, which is driven with oxygen
- Medication to be administered
- 0.3 cc of normal saline for dilution of the bronchodilator

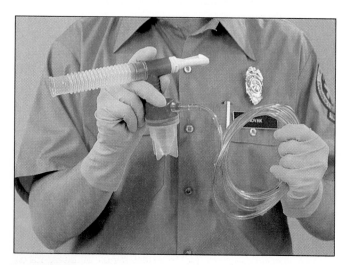

Figure S32-1

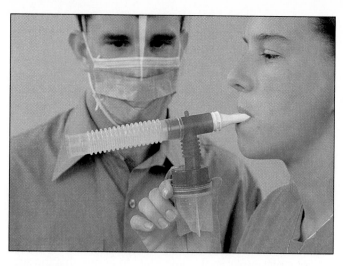

Figure S32-2

Procedure

1. Observe body substance isolation precautions (gloves are a minimum; mask and goggles are recommended since patients often experience coughing during treatments).
2. Explain the procedure to the patient.
3. Take the patient's vital signs and connect the patient to a cardiac monitor.
4. Assemble the nebulizer device. Place the bronchodilator and saline solution in the reservoir well of the side-stream nebulizer (Fig. S32-1).
5. Connect the device and administer oxygen at 6 to 12 L/minute (according to the specific device) to start nebulizer treatment.
6. Have patient inhale normally through mouthpiece of nebulizer. The aerosol inhalation should start at the end of one tidal breath just as the patient initiates the next breath. The inhalation should continue until the patient fully expands his or her lungs (Fig. S32-2).
7. Have the patient take a deep breath every 3 to 5 inhalations.
8. The treatment should last until the solution is depleted.
9. Place the patient back onto supplemental oxygen following medication administration.
10. Monitor the patient, ECG, and vital signs for medication effect. Treatment should be discontinued if tachycardia greater than 120 beats per minute, ventricular ectopy, or paradoxic bronchospasm is noted.

SKILL 33

Self-Administered Nitrous Oxide

A 50:50 nitrous and oxygen mixture allows the patient to regulate his pain control by self-administering this gas, commonly known as "laughing gas."

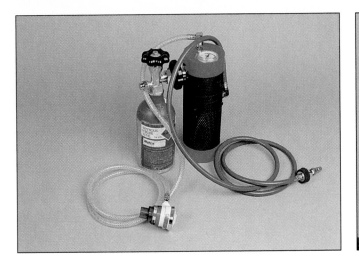

Figure S33-1

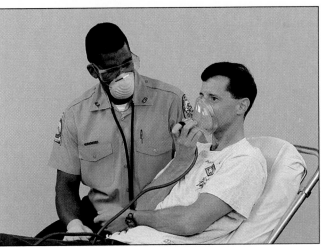

Figure S33-2

Background

Inhalation of a preset 50:50 mixture of oxygen and nitrous oxide through self-administration is an important method of pain management in the prehospital setting. It can exert analgesic effects equivalent to 10 to 20 mg of intravenous morphine, without the side effects. Approximately 10% of patients are "nonresponders" to the gas. When effective, maximum analgesia is obtained within 5 minutes of inhalation. Although the inhalation of nitrous oxide produces a rapid effect on the central nervous system and depresses cortical function, there are no direct effects on the respiratory system. Cough and gag reflexes are not altered. Its extremely short half-life makes it a valuable prehospital medication.

Indications

- Musculoskeletal trauma
- Myocardial infarction
- Thermal burns
- Childbirth

Contraindications

- Altered mental status
- Alcohol intoxication
- Head injury
- Abdominal or chest trauma
- Shock
- Pneumothorax
- Pulmonary disease (COPD or asthma)
- Inability to comprehend or respond to verbal commands
- Inability to self-administer
- Abdominal distention suggestive of bowel obstruction

Equipment

- Nitrous oxide–oxygen blender with facemask (Fig. S33-1)

Procedure

1. Use body substance isolation precautions.
2. Invert the nitrous tank several times to create vaporization.
3. Open the pressure valves on the oxygen and nitrous oxide tanks.
4. Make sure the pressure gauges are reading in the green bands, indicating proper pressure, and record the pressure.
5. Instruct the patient on the use of the device and what effects to anticipate.
6. Place the patient in a sitting position. Instruct and assist the patient in creating a tight facemask seal.
7. Encourage the patient to inhale and exhale normally (Fig. S33-2). If the patient feels uncomfortable for any reason during the procedure, he or she should simply remove the mask and breathe normally.
8. No one should apply the facemask to the patient except the patient himself.
9. Monitor the patient for changes in level of consciousness and other vital signs.

SKILL 34

Epinephrine Auto-Injectors

Background

Many patients who have experienced a severe allergic reaction now carry epinephrine in auto-injectors. The auto-injector will deliver a dose of 0.3 mg of epinephrine for adults or 0.15 mg for children intramuscularly.

Indications

Severe allergic reaction due to insect stings or bites, foods, drugs, or other allergens.

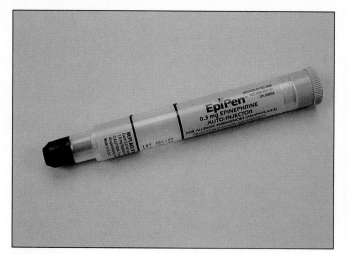

Figure S34-1

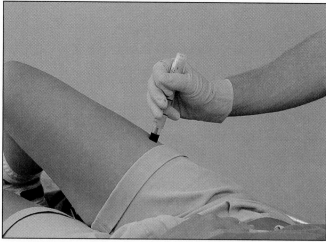

Figure S34-2

Contraindications

None in the emergency setting.

Equipment

- Epinephrine auto-injector (Fig. S34-1)
- Personal protective equipment

Procedure

1. Observe body substance isolation precautions.
2. Assess need for epinephrine administration. Check expiration date on auto-injector.

3. Remove safety cap from auto-injector.
4. Place auto-injector onto outer thigh.
5. Press hard until you hear the injector function (Fig. S34-2).
6. Hold the auto-injector in place for several seconds.
7. Gently massage the injection area for 10–15 seconds.
8. Monitor the patient for change; reassess, vital signs.

NOTE: The auto-injector may be used through clothing if necessary. Observe patient after injection. If condition does not improve, the paramedic should consider additional doses of epinephrine SQ or IV according to local protocol and Medical Direction.

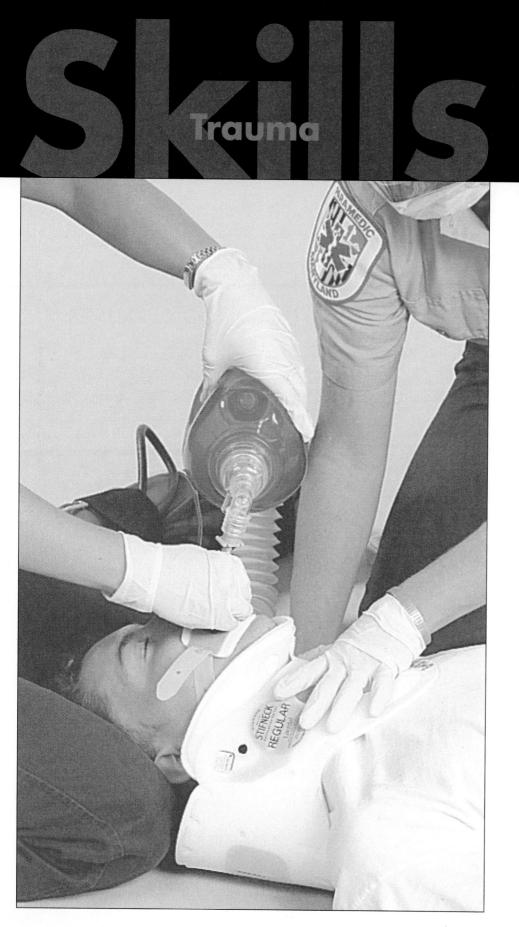

Skills

Trauma

SKILL 35

Pneumatic Antishock Garment Application

The pneumatic antishock garment (PASG) surrounds the lower extremities and abdomen and is used to control bleeding, increase perfusion to vital organs, and splint the pelvis and/or lower extremities.

Background

The PASG has many names, but most commonly is called the pneumatic antishock garment, or medical or military antishock trousers (MAST). It is most commonly used to treat hypotension following trauma. The device increases peripheral vascular resistance, but only autotransfuses cephalad approximately 250 ml of blood from the lower extremities and the abdomen in the adult.

Indications

- Stabilization of pelvic or lower extremity fractures
- Compression of external bleeding
- Intraabdominal bleeding, ruptured aortic abdominal aneurysm
- Other causes of shock for which MAST may be helpful: spinal shock, overdose, septic shock, anaphylaxis
- Hypovolemic shock

Contraindications

Absolute:
- Pulmonary edema
- Congestive heart failure

Relative:
- Abdominal injuries with protruding abdominal contents
- Cardiogenic shock

- Impaled objects to the leg or abdomen
- Lumbar spine instability—use lower extremity compartments only
- Penetrating thoracic injuries
- Pregnancy—use lower extremity compartments only during third trimester
- Isolated head trauma
- Use legs only with pediatric patients

When a patient's respiratory condition becomes markedly worse after inflation, consider diaphragmatic rupture or tension pneumothorax. Deflation under Medical Direction should be considered.

Equipment

Two major types of PASG devices are available. One type has pressure gauges for monitoring the suit pressure, whereas the other type has pop-off valves that limit pressures to approximately 106 mm Hg.

Procedure: Methods of Application and Inflation

1. There are three methods to apply the PASG. The logroll method is most commonly used when a spinal injury is suspected and at least three team members are available to properly logroll the patient. The garment should be fan-folded, or layered, and placed next to the patient. The cervical area and head are protected by one member, while a minimum of two others support the body and roll the patient onto the rescuer's knees (Fig. S35-1). The garment is then slid into place, under the patient and just inferior to the twelfth rib. The patient is then rolled as a unit onto the garment, and the velcro is secured (Fig. S35-2). Careful alignment of the velcro straps will prevent the straps from popping loose during inflation.

   The second method is the diaper method, which consists of simply placing the garment flat, in the open position, at the feet of the supine patient (Fig S35-3).

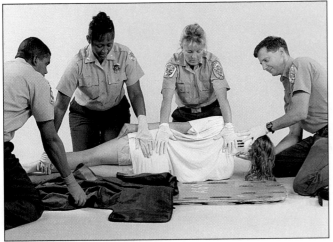

Figure S35-1

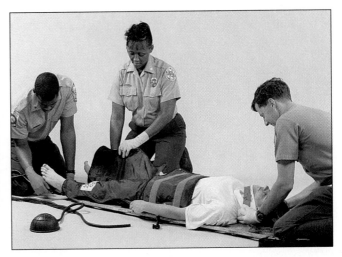

Figure S35-2

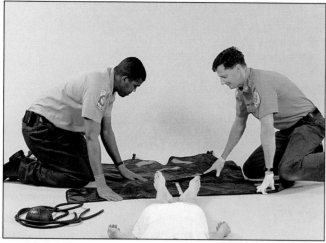

Figure S35-3

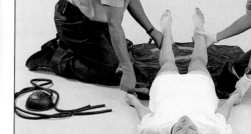

Figure S35-4

Two team members simultaneously lift the legs, slide the garment up under the patient, and lower the legs onto the garment. The hips are then lifted, and the garment slid up just inferior to the twelfth rib (Fig. S35-4). The garment is wrapped around the patient, and the velcro secured.

The third method is the <u>trouser</u> method. To begin, open the trousers and attach the velcro in the wide-open position, creating a very large pair of pants. One team member can place an arm up each leg of the garment, or more easily, two rescuers can place one arm each (one right arm, one left arm) up the respective leg of the garment (Fig. S35-5). Next, place a hand over the patient's foot, lift the legs, and slide the garment off onto the patient's extremities. Lower the legs and move up to the pelvis. Lift the pelvis slightly and slide the abdominal section up under the torso, just inferior to the twelfth rib and secure as previously described (Fig. S35-6).

2. Consideration should be given to placing the patient on a backboard, both for immobilization as well as for ease of moving the patient.
3. Once the garment is secured, attach the tubing–foot pump apparatus to the trousers.
4. Open all stopcock valves so that all three compartments can be inflated simultaneously. (Some areas will require that the leg compartments be inflated first, then the abdominal section.)
5. Inflate the garment, using the foot pump, until the velcro crackles, air exhausts through the "pop-off" valves, and/or the patient's blood pressure exceeds a systolic pressure of 100 mm Hg (Fig. S35-7).
6. Close all stopcocks. (The foot pump should remain attached and stay with the patient until the garment is removed.)
7. Monitor the patient for hemodynamic and respiratory changes, as well as air leakage from the garment.

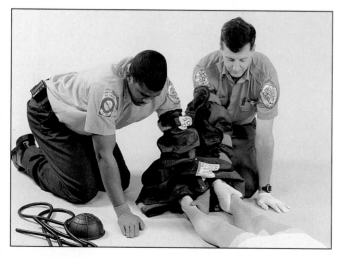

Figure S35-5

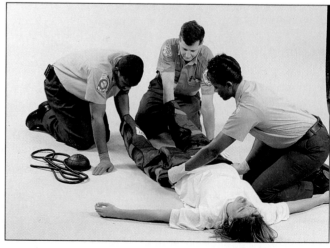

Figure S35-6

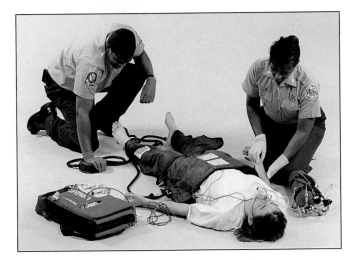

Figure S35-7

Procedure: Deflation and Removal

Deflation of the PASG is generally reserved for the controlled environment of the emergency department. Occasionally though, deflation in the field must be considered when a patient develops respiratory distress following inflation of the garment. If time permits, you should consult Medical Direction for advice. However, if distress is severe and the patient is decompensating, take immediate action. Deflate the abdominal section of the garment and monitor the patient closely. This deflation procedure is usually guided by local or state protocol.

1. Evaluate the patient's vital signs and verify the patient's stability.
2. Ensure that IV lines are accessible, that the patient has received proper fluid replacement, and that support teams such as a surgical crew are available.
3. Check the garment to ensure that the foot pump is still attached (in case the need arises to rapidly reinflate) and that all stopcocks are in the closed position.
4. Remove the abdominal hose and open the stopcock for approximately 2 seconds, releasing about one third of the pressure in the abdominal section. Close the stopcock.
5. Reevaluate vital signs and, if no significant change occurs, continue the procedure until deflated. A rule-of-thumb is that a rise in heart rate of 5 beats per minute or a drop in blood pressure of 5 mm Hg represents a significant change. If an increase in heart rate or drop in systolic pressure occurs, cease the deflation procedure and open the IV lines. An infusion of 250 ml of lactated Ringer's or normal saline serves as a fluid challenge.
6. Repeat steps 4 and 5 with each leg until the garment is fully deflated. It may take up to 30 minutes to properly remove the PASG.

Thoracic Decompression

Thoracic decompression is placement of a needle through the chest wall of a patient whose lung has collapsed as a result of a one-way valve air leak.

Background

Recognition of tension pneumothorax is facilitated by understanding that it results from a one-way valve air leak from the lung and/or through the chest wall. Air enters one side of the thoracic cavity without any means of escape, thus producing total collapse of the lung on the affected side and pressure against the mediastinum and lung on the uninvolved side. The rise in intrapleural pressure decreases venous return to the heart and decreases cardiac output. Ventilation and perfusion are rapidly compromised. This is a life-threatening condition that will result in death if not recognized and treated rapidly. It occurs most commonly in the clinical settings of chest trauma and in manually or mechanically ventilated patients with chronic lung disease.

The initial signs of tension pneumothorax may be subtle, such as restlessness. However, these patients have an extremely rapid downhill course over a period of just a few minutes.

The clinical signs of tension pneumothorax are:

- restlessness and agitation
- increased airway resistance on ventilating patient
- neck vein distention
- respiratory distress—severe dyspnea, tachypnea, air hunger in the conscious patient
- unilateral absence of breath sounds on affected side
- hyperresonance to percussion on affected side
- hypotension
- cyanosis
- tracheal deviation toward unaffected side
- respiratory arrest

A high index of suspicion and repeated assessment in patients with clinical profiles at risk for tension pneumothorax are extremely important. Although tension pneumothorax is not an everyday experience for a paramedic, its prompt recognition and treatment are dramatically lifesaving.

Indications

Thoracic decompression is indicated in patients with clinical signs and symptoms consistent with tension pneumothorax.

Contraindications

There are no contraindications for performing a needle decompression for patients meeting the above criteria; however, Medical Direction may be required in your locale before executing this skill.

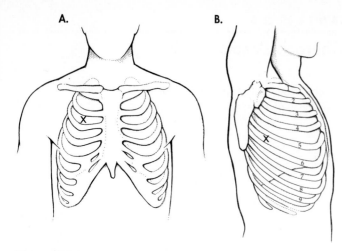

Figure S36-1

Equipment

- Large-bore over-the-needle catheter (14-gauge or larger)
- 10 cc syringe
- Povidone-iodine preps
- Finger cut from a sterile glove for flutter valve (alternatively, a Heimlich flutter valve may be used)

- Sterile dressing
- Sterile gloves
- McSwain Dart is used in some systems

Procedure

1. Observe body substance isolation precautions (gloves and eye protection).
2. Locate the landmark for decompression on the affected side (Fig. S36-1) and cleanse the chest povidone-iodine solution.
3. Attach a 10 cc syringe to a 14-gauge (or larger) over-the-needle catheter. Puncture the skin perpendicularly just superior to the third rib (second intercostal space) in the midclavicular line (approximately in line with the nipple) until the thoracic cavity is entered (Fig. S36-2). The fifth intercostal space in the mid-axillary line is an alternate site.
4. On entering the thoracic cavity with a tension pneumothorax, you should feel a pop, and then, depending on the level of ambient noise, you may hear a "hiss" as air is decompressed. Alternately, you may see the plunger of the syringe push outward.
5. Advance the catheter and remove the needle (Fig. S36-3).
6. A Heimlich valve or the finger cut from a surgical glove may be used to create a one-way valve allowing air to

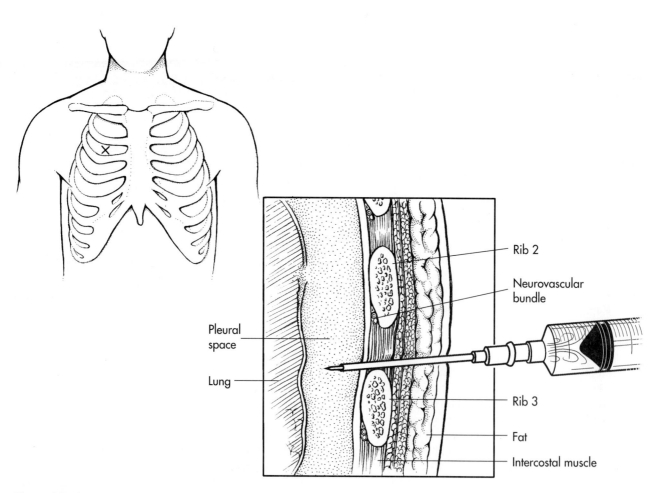

Pleural space

Lung

Rib 2

Neurovascular bundle

Rib 3

Fat

Intercostal muscle

Figure S36-2

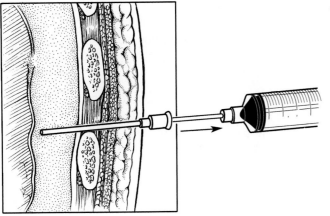

Figure S36-3

escape, but not enter, the chest. Place a finger from a surgical glove over the catheter hub. Cut a small hole in the end of the finger to make a one-way or flutter valve. Secure the glove finger to the catheter, using tape or a rubber band. The flutter valve collapses during inspiration and opens during expiration (Fig. S36-4). In some EMS systems a Heimlich valve is used in place of the surgical glove finger.

7. Secure the catheter to the chest wall with a dressing and tape (Fig. S36-5).

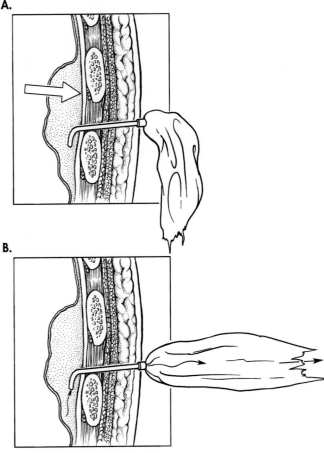

Figure S36-4

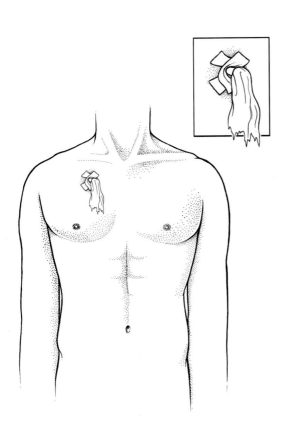

Figure S36-5

SKILL 37

Intubation with Cervical Spine Stabilization

Background

Trauma patients routinely have cervical spine stabilization applied. When these patients need intubation, the paramedic must use special care to limit movement of the cervical spine during laryngoscopy.

Indications

- Patients with spinal immobilization applied requiring orotracheal intubation

Contraindications

- Inability to completely open, or have access to, a patient's mouth
- Contraindications associated with non-traumatic orotracheal intubation

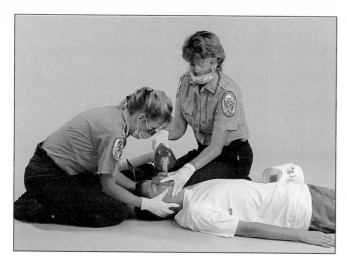

Figure S37-1

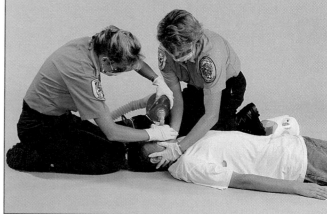

Figure S37-2

Equipment

- Laryngoscope handle and blade
- Endotracheal tube
- 10 cc syringe
- Stylet
- Suction unit
- Tape or tube holder
- Oropharyngeal airway
- Water-soluble lubricant
- Bag-valve-mask
- Supplemental oxygen
- Personal protective equipment

Procedure

1. Observe body substance isolation precautions.
2. Assess need for orotracheal intubation.
3. Paramedic #1 maintains manual in-line stabilization of cervical spine from behind patient.

4. Maintain airway and ventilate with BVM (Fig. S37-1).
5. Select proper size endotracheal tube and prepare equipment.
6. Paramedic #2 takes control of spine from the front of patient while kneeling at patient's side.
7. Paramedic #1 hyperventilates patient (Fig. S37-2).
8. Paramedic #1 performs laryngoscopy without manipulating cervical spine (Fig. S37-3).
9. Additional personnel apply cricoid pressure if needed and not contraindicated by patient condition.
10. Endotracheal tube is placed, placement confirmed, and secured.
11. Paramedic #1 continues to ventilate patient using BVM (Fig. S37-4).
12. Cervical stabilization is transferred from Paramedic #2 to Paramedic #1 during a pause in ventilations.
13. Paramedic #2 applies cervical collar (Fig. S37-5).

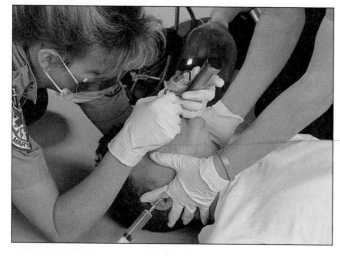

Figure S37-3

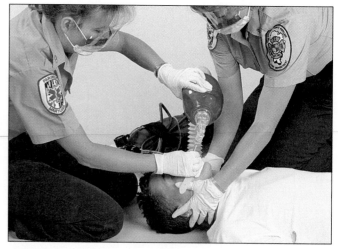

Figure S37-4

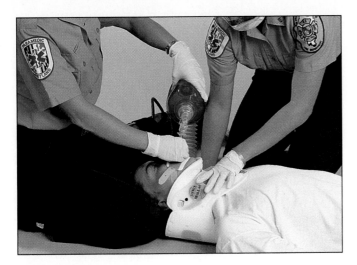

Figure S37-5

Mark A. Kirk, MD and S. Rutherfoord Rose, PharmD

Appendix A

Patient Medications by Generic Name

This appendix lists many medications that are commonly taken by patients. Knowing certain medications are being taken by patients helps in assessment and determining appropriate interventions. Knowing the category of a drug is also helpful in evaluating the patient and in guiding the course of treatment.

The generic name of each drug is alphabetized and is followed by one or more trade names and then the category of the drug.

Appendix A	Patient Medications by Generic Name				
Generic Name	Trade Name	Category	Generic Name	Trade Name	Category
acebutolol	Sectral	Beta-blocker	bitolterol	Tornalate inhaler	Bronchodilator
acetazolamide	Diamox	Diuretic, Anti-Glaucoma	bromocriptine	Parlodel	Antiparkinsonian
acetohexamide	Dymelor	Antidiabetics	bumetanide	Bumex	Diuretic
acyclovir	Zovirax	Antiviral (herpes simplex)	bupropion	Wellbutrin	Antidepressant
albuterol	Ventolin, Proventil	Bronchodilator	buspirone	Buspar	Antianxiety
allopurinol	Zyloprim	Gout agent	butalbital	Fiorinal	analgesic
alprazolam	Xanax	Tranquilizer	captopril	Capoten	Antihypertensive
amantadine	Symmetrel	Antiparkinsonian	carbamazepine	Tegretol	Anticonvulsant
amiloride	Midamor	Diuretic	carbidopa-levodopa	Sinemet	Antiparkinsonian
amiodarone	Cordarone	Antidysrhythmic	carisoprodol	Soma	Skeletal muscle relaxant
amitriptyline	Elavil, Endep	Antidepressant	carteolol	Cartrol	Beta-blocker
amlodipine	Norvasc	Calcium channel blocker	cefaclor	Ceclor	Antibacterial
amoxapine	Ascendin	Antidepressant	cefadroxil	Duricef	Antibacterial
amoxicillin	Amoxil, Polymox	Antibacterial	cefuroxime	Ceftin	Antibacterial
ampicillin	Amcill, Omnipen	Antibacterial	cephalexin	Keflex	Antibacterial
astemizole	Hismanal	Antihistamine	chloral hydrate	Noctec	Sedative/Hypnotic
atenolol	Tenormin	Beta-blocker	chlorazepate	Tranxene	Tranquilizer
azatadine	Optimine	Antihistamine	chlordiazepoxide	Librium	Tranquilizer
AZT (zidovudine)	Retrovir	Antiviral	chloroquine	Aralen	Antimalarial
baclofen	Lioresal	Skeletal muscle relaxant	chlorothiazide	Diuril	Diuretic
beclomethasone	Beclovent	Steroid/Antiinflammatory	clorpheniramine	Chlor-Trimeton	Antihistamine
benazepril	Lotensin	Antihypertensive	chlorpromazine	Thorazine	Antipsychotic
benztropin	Cogentin	Antiparkinsonian	chlorpropamide	Diabinese	Antidiabetic
bepridil	Vascor	Calcium channel blocker	chlorthalidone	Hygroton	Diuretic
betamethasone	Celestone	Steroid/Antiinflammatory	chlorzoxazone	Parafon Forte DSC	Skeletal muscle relaxant
betaxolol	Kerlone	Beta-blocker	cholestyramine	Questran, Cholybar	Lipid-lowering
bethanechol	Urecholine	Cholinergic	cimetidine	Tagamet	Antiulcer
biperiden	Akineton	Antiparkinsonian	ciprofloxacin	Cipro	Antibacterial
bisacodyl	Dulcolax	Laxative	clemastine	Tavist	Antihistamine
bisoprolol	Zebeta	Beta-blocker	clofibrate	Atromid-S	Lipid-lowering

Continued

Generic Name	Trade Name	Category	Generic Name	Trade Name	Category
clomiphene	Clomid	Ovulatory stimulant	furosemide	Lasix	Diuretic
clomipramine	Anafranil	Antidepressant	gemfibrozil	Lopid	Lipid-lowering
clonazepam	Klonopin	Anticonvulsant	glipizide	Glucotrol	Hypoglycemic
clonidine	Catapres	Antihypertensive	glutethimide	Doriden	Sedative/Hypnotic
clozapine	Clozaril	Antipsychotic	glyburide	Diabeta,Micronase	Hypoglycemic
codeine	none	Narcotic analgesic	griseofulvin	Fulvicin, Grisactin	Antifungal
colchicine	none	Gout agent	guanabenz	Wytensin	Antihypertensive
colestipol	Colestid	Lipid-lowering	guanadrel	Hylorel	Antihypertensive
cromolyn	Intal	Antiallergic	guanethidine	Ismelin	Antihypertensive
cyclobenzaprine	Flexeril	Skeletal muscle relaxant	guanfacine	Tenex	Antihypertensive
cyproheptadine	Periactin	Antihistamine	halazepam	Paxipam	Tranquilizer
desipramine	Norpramin, Pertofrane	Antidepressant	haloperidol	Haldol	Antipsychotic
dexamethasone	Decadron,Hexadrol	Steriod/Antiinflammatory	HCTZ with triamterene	Dyazide, Maxide	Diuretic
dextroamphetamine	Dexedrine	CNS stimulant, appetite suppressant	hydralazine	Apresoline	Antihypertensive
			hydrochlorothiazide (HCTZ)	Hydrodiuril	Diuretic
dextromethorphan	Delsym, others	Anticough	hydrocodone with acetaminophen	Lortab, Vicodin	Narcotic analgesic
diazepam	Valium	Tranquilizer			
diclofenac	Voltaren	Antiinflammatory/analgesic	hydrocortisone	Hydrocortisone	Steroid/Antiinflammatory
dicloxacillin	Dynapen	Antibacterial	hydromorphone	Dilaudid	Narcotic analgesic
didanosine (ddI)	Videx	Antiviral	hydroxyzine	Atarax, Vistaril	Antihistamine, anti-emetic
diethylpropion	Tenuate	Appetite suppressant	ibuprofen	Motrin, Rufen	Antiinflammatory/analgesic
diflunisal	Dolobid	Antiinflammatory/analgesic	imipramine	Tofranil	Antidepressant
digoxin	Lanoxin	Antidysrhythmic	indapamide	Lozol	Diuretic
diltiazem	Cardizem	Calcium channel blocker	indomethacin	Indocin	Antiinflammatory/analgesic
dimenhydrinate	Dramamine	Anti-emetic	insulin	Humulin, Iletin	Antidiabetic
diphenhydramine	Benadryl	Antihistamine	ipratropium	Atrovent inhaler	Bronchodilator
diphenoxylate with atropine	Lomotil	Antidiarrheal/Antispasmodic	isoniazid (INH)	same as generic	Antituberculin
			isosorbide dinitrate	Isordil, Sorbitrate	Antianginal
dipyridamole	Persantine	Vasodilator/Anti-platelet	isosorbide mononitrate	ISMO, Imdur	Antianginal
disopyramide	Norpace	Antidysrhythmic	isotretinoin	Accutane	Antiacne
docusate calcium	Surfak	Laxative	isradipine	DynaCirc	Calcium channel blocker
docusate sodium	Colace	Laxative	ketoconazole	Nizoral	Antifungal
doxazosin	Cardura	Antihypertensive	ketoprofen	Orudis	Antiinflammatory/analgesic
doxepin	Adapin, Sinequan	Antidepressant	ketorolac	Toradol	Antiinflammatory/analgesic
doxycycline	Vibramycin	Antibacterial	labetalol	Trandate, Normodyne	Beta-blocker
doxylamine	Unisom	Antihistamine/Hypnotic	levodopa	Larodopa	Antiparkinsonian
enalapril	Vasotec	Antihypertensive	levothyroxine	Synthroid, Levothroid	Thyroid hormone
encainide	Enkaid	Antidysrhythmic	lindane	Kwell	Antiparasite
ergotamine	Ergostat	Antimigraine	lisinopril	Prinivil, Zestril	Antihypertensive
erythrityl	Cardilate	Anti-anginal	lithium	Lithobid, Eskalith	Antidepressant
erythromycin	E-mycin, EES, Ilosone, EryTab	Antibacterial	loperamide	Imodium	Antidiarrheal
			lorazepam	Ativan	Tranquilizer
estrogen	Premarin	Hormone	lovastatin	Mevacor	Lipid-lowering
ethacrynic acid	Edecrin	Diuretic	loxapine	Loxitane	Antipsychotic
ethambutol	Myambutol	Antituberculin	maprotiline	Ludiomil	Antidepressant
ethchlorvynol	Placidyl	Sedative/Hypnotic	meclizine	Antivert	Antihistamine, anti-emetic
ethosuximide	Zarontin	Anticonvulsant	meclofenamate	Meclomen	Antiinflammatory/analgesic
etodolac	Lodine	Antiinflammatory/analgesic	mefenamic acid	Ponstel	Antiinflammatory/analgesic
famotidine	Pepcid	Antiulcer	meperidine	Demerol	Narcotic analgesic
felodipine	Plendil	Calcium channel blocker	mephenytoin	Mesantoin	Anticonvulsant
fenoprofen	Nalfon	Antiinflammatory/analgesic	meprobamate	Equanil, Miltown	Sedative/Hypnotic
flecainide	Tambocor	Antidysrhythmic	mesoridazine	Serentil	Antipsychotic
fluoxetine	Prozac	Antidepressant	metaproterenol	Metaprel, Alupent	Bronchodilator
fluphenazine	Prolixin	Antipsychotic	methadone	Dolophine	Narcotic analgesic
flurazepam	Dalmane	Hypnotic	methamphetamine	Desoxyn	CNS Stimulant/appetite suppressant
folic acid	Apo-Folic, Folvite	Vitamin			
fosinopril	Monopril	Antihypertensive	methocarbamol	Robaxin	Skeletal muscle relaxant

Generic Name	Trade Name	Category
methyldopa	Aldomet	Antihypertensive
methylphenidate	Ritalin	CNS Stimulant
methysergide	Sansert	Antimigraine
metoclopramide	Reglan	Anti-emetic
metolazone	Diulo, Zaroxolyn	Diuretic
metoprolol	Lopressor	Beta-blocker
metronidazole	Flagyl	Antibacterial
mexilitine	Mexitil	Antidysrhythmic
minoxidil	Loniten	Antihypertensive
misoprostol	Cytotec	Prostaglandin
morphine	MS Contin, Roxanol	Narcotic analgesic
nadolol	Corgard	Beta-blocker
naltrexone	Trexan	Narcotic antagonist
naproxen	Naprosyn, Anaprox	Antiinflammatory/analgesic
niacin	Nicobid	Lipid-lowering
nicardipine	Cardene	Calcium channel blocker
nifedipine	Adalat, Procardia	Calcium channel blocker
nimodipine	Nimotop	Calcium channel blocker
nitroglycerin	Nitrostat, Nitro-Bid	Antianginal
nizatidine	Axid	Anti-ulcer
norfloxacin	Noroxin	Antibacterial
nortriptyline	Pamelor, Aventyl	Antidepressant
omeprazole	Prilosec	Anti-ulcer
orphenadrine	Norflex	Skeletal muscle relaxant
oxazepam	Serax	Tranquilizer
oxycodone with acetaminophen	Tylox, Percocet	Narcotic analgesic
paroxetine	Paxil	Antidepressant
penbutolol	Levatol	Beta-blocker
penicillin	Pen Vee K, Veetids	Antibacterial
pentaerythritol	Peritrate	Anti-anginal
pentamidine	NebuPent	Antibiotic
pentazocine with naloxone	Talwin Nx	Narcotic analgesic
pentoxyphylline	Trental	Hemorheologic agent
pergolide	Permax	Antiparkinsonian
perphenazine	Trilafon	Antipsychotic
phenazopyridine	Pyridium	Urinary analgesic
phenobarbital	none	Anticonvulsant
phenylbutazone	Butazolidin	Antiinflammatory/analgesic
phenytoin	Dilantin	Anticonvulsant
pimozide	Orap	Antipsychotic
pindolol	Visken	Beta-blocker
piroxicam	Feldene	Antiinflammatory/analgesic
potassium	K-Phos, K-Lor, Slow K	Electrolyte replacement
pravastatin	Pravachol	Lipid-lowering
prazepam	Centrax	Tranquilizer
prazosin	Minipress	Antihypertensive
prednisone	same	Steroid/Antiinflammatory
primidone	Mysoline	Anticonvulsant
probenecid	Benemid	Gout agent
probucol	Lorelco	Lipid-lowering
procainamide	Pronestyl, Procan SR	Antidysrhythmic
prochlorperazine	Compazine	Anti-nausea
procyclidine	Kemadrin	Antiparkinson
promethazine	Phenergan	Antihistamine
propafenone	Rythmol	Antidysrhythmic
propantheline	Pro-Banthine	Antispasmodic
propoxyphene	Darvon	Narcotic analgesic
propranolol	Inderal	Beta-blocker
propylthiouracil (PTU)	none	Antithyroid agent
protriptyline	Vivactil	Antidepressant
pseudoephedrine	Sudafed	Decongestant
pyrazinamide	None	Antituberculin
quazepam	Doral	Hypnotic
quinapril	Accupril	Antihypertensive
quinidine	Quinidex, Quinaglute	Antidysrhythmic
ramipril	Altace	Antihypertensive
ranitidine	Zantac	Anti-ulcer
reserpine	Serpasil	Antihypertensive
rifampin	Rifadin	Antituberculin, Antimeningitis
scopolamine	Transderm-Scop	Anti-emetic
secobarbital	Seconal	Hypnotic (Barbiturate)
selegiline	Eldepryl	Antiparkinsonian
sertraline	Zoloft	Antidepressant
simethicone	Mylicon	Antiflatulant
spironolactone	Aldactone	Diuretic
sucralfate	Carafate	Anti-ulcer
sulfasalazine	Azulfidine	Antibacterial
sulindac	Clinoril	Antiinflammatory/analgesic
temazepam	Restoril	Hypnotic
terazosin	Hytrin	Antihypertensive
terbutaline	Brethine, Bricanyl	Bronchodilator
terfenadine	Seldane	Antihistamine
tetracycline	Sumycin, Robitet, Achromycin V	Antibacterial
theophylline	Aminophylline, TheoDur, Slo-bid	Bronchodilator
thioridazine	Mellaril	Antipsychotic
thiothixene	Navane	Antipsychotic
timolol	Blocadren	Beta-blocker
TMP-SMX	Septra, Bactrim	Antibiotic
tocainide	Tonocard	Antidysrhythmic
tolazamide	Tolinase	Hypoglycemic
tolbutamide	Orinase	Hypoglycemic
tolmetin	Tolectin	Antiinflammatory/analgesic
trazodone	Desyrel	Antidepressant
triamterene	Dyrenium	Diuretic
triazolam	Halcion	Hypnotic
trifluoperazine	Stelazine	Antipsychotic
trihexyphenidyl	Artane	Antiparkinsonian
trimethobenzamide	Tigan	Anti-emetic
tripelennamine	PBZ	Antihistamine
valproic acid	Depakote, Depakene	Anticonvulsant
verapamil	Calan, Isoptin	Antidysrhythmic
warfarin	Coumadin	Anticoagulant
zalcitabine (ddC)	Hivid	Antiviral
zidovudine (AZT)	Retrovir	Antiviral
zolpidem	Ambien	Sedative/Hypnotic

Glossary

Abandonment — termination of patient care without consent, and which results in harm to the patient.

ABC dry chemical fire extinguisher — a class of fire extinguishers which may be used for Type A (wood), Type B (chemical), or Type C (electrical) fires.

Abdominal aortic aneurysm — a weakening and dilation of the abdominal portion of the descending aorta.

Abduction — movement of an extremity away from the body.

Abruptio placenta — the premature and usually painful separation, partially or completely, of the placenta from the uterine wall. *See Conditions by Diagnosis section.*

Abscess — a cavity containing pus and surrounded by inflamed tissue.

Accessory respiratory muscles — muscles which assist with respiration during labored breathing, e.g., neck, back and abdominal muscles.

Acclimatization — the physical adjustment to a different climate or to changes in altitude or temperature.

Acetylcholine — a neurotransmitter substance widely distributed in body tissues, with the primary function of mediating the synaptic activity of the nervous system.

Acetone — ketone metabolite normally found in the urine in trace amounts; blood and urine concentration increase in diabetic ketoacidosis and starvation.

Acid — substance that releases hydrogen ions when dissolved in water and reacts with bases to form salts; sour-tasting substance.

Acidosis — a condition in which the blood is abnormally acidic, i.e., the arterial pH is below 7.35; an abnormal increase in hydrogen ion concentration in the body resulting from an accumulation of an acid or loss of a base.

Active transport — the movement of materials, e.g., molecules or ions, across the membrane of a cell by means of energy consuming chemical reactions.

Acute abdomen — an abnormal condition characterized by the acute onset of severe pain within the abdominal cavity.

Acute aortic dissection — sudden tear in the inner lining of the aorta that allows blood to enter the space between the inner and outer layers. *See Conditions by Diagnosis section.*

Acute glaucoma — rapid increase of pressure within the eye. *See Conditions by Diagnosis section.*

Adduction — movement of an extremity toward the body.

Adipose tissue — a specialized connective tissue that stores lipids. Also known as fat tissue.

Adrenal glands — two glands located superior to each kidney which release catecholamines; they are responsible for many of the physical arousal mechanisms in the stress response.

Adrenergic — of or pertaining to sympathetic nerve fibers of the autonomic nervous system that respond to epinephrine and other catecholamines.

Adrenocorticotropic hormone (ACTH) — a hormone secreted by the pituitary gland, which stimulates the adrenal cortex.

Adult Respiratory Distress Syndrome (ARDS) — a form of restrictive lung disease characterized by respiratory insufficiency and hypoxemia, and which results from abnormal permeability of either the pulmonary or alveolar epithelium. *See Conditions by Diagnosis section.*

Adulterate — the debasement of purity or dilution of any substance, process, or activity by the addition of extraneous material (adulterant).

Advance directive — a legal document, such as a "Living Will," in which a patient has signed a statement expressing his or her wishes to receive, or not to receive, specific medical procedures in the event of being unable to express his or her wishes at a later date.

Advanced cardiac life support (ACLS) — clinical care, or guidelines for care, of severe, life-threatening cardiovascular and respiratory disorders.

Advanced life support — provision of care rendered by paramedics or allied health professionals that includes advanced airway management, defibrillation, intravenous therapy, and medication administration.

Adventitia — the outermost layer of an artery, organ, or other structure, composed of connective tissue with elastic and collagenous fibers.

Adverse effect — unintended, undesirable or harmful effect; especially pertaining to adverse drug reactions.

Aerobic metabolism — biochemical reactions that involve oxygen.

Aeromedical communication specialist — person trained to coordinate air medical service flights by radio and other modes of communication.

Affective disorders — a class of disorders characterized by feelings, emotions, moods and dispositions.

Afferent (sensory) neuron — nerve fibers that transmit impulses from the periphery toward the central nervous system.

Afterload — the load, or resistance, against which the left ventricle must eject blood during systole.

Air embolism — an air bubble in a blood vessel.

Air medical service — a service designed to provide medical care during air transport of patients directly from the scene of an emergency or from hospitals; an air medical service is a component of a regional emergency medical service system.

Airway obstruction — a blockage of the airway, which may result from the presence of a foreign body, such as food or vomitus, or as a result of an anatomical disorder such as tongue displacement or tissue swelling.

Aldosterone — a corticosteroid produced by the adrenal cortex to regulate sodium and potassium balance in the blood.

Alkali — compound with the chemical characteristics of a base; pH greater than 7 in water solution.

Alkalosis — an abnormally high concentration of alkali or bases in the blood; an arterial pH greater than 7.45.

Allergic reaction — a hypersensitive response to an allergen to which an organism has previously been exposed and to which the organism has developed antibodies. *See Conditions by Diagnosis section.*

Alpha adrenergic receptors — sympathetic binding complexes that, when stimulated, cause vessels to constrict by increasing peripheral vascular resistance and cause pupillary dilation.

Alternating current — electrical current in which the wave form fluctuates between positive and negative.

Alveolus — a small cavity; the terminal ending of a secretory gland. Alveoli of the lungs are microscopic dilations of terminal bronchioles.

Alzheimer's Disease — a disease marked by progressive loss of mental capacity (e.g., impaired memory, thinking, and behavior) resulting from degeneration of the brain cells. *See Conditions by Diagnosis section.*

Amniotic fluid — the fluid contained in the gestational sac which surrounds the fetus.

Amperage — the measurement of electrical current expressed in amperes, or in units of ohms (resistance) and volts (force).

Amphetamine — a group of central nervous system stimulants often prescribed for depression or obesity. This class of drugs are often abused because of their ability to produce feelings of euphoria.

Anaerobic metabolism — biochemical reactions that occur in the absence of oxygen.

Anaphylactic shock — shock due to a severe, rapid onset of an allergic reaction that results in widespread vasodilation and tissue permeability. *See Conditions by Diagnosis section.*

Anaphylaxis — acute, severe immune response resulting in a life-threatening emergency reaction. *See Conditions by Diagnosis section.*

Anastomosis — a connection between two vessels, which may be natural, surgical or pathologic.

Anatomical position — a position of the body in which the person stands erect, facing directly forward, feet pointing forward, arms hanging down at the side with palms facing forward. This is the standard position of reference to describe sites or motion of various parts of the body.

Anatomy — the study, classification, and description of structures and organs of the body.

Anemia — disease in which the oxygen transporting capacity of the blood is diminished; may be due to loss of whole blood, inadequate development or destruction of erythrocytes, or an inadequate amount of hemoglobin. *See Conditions by Diagnosis section.*

Aneurysm — a localized dilation of the wall of a blood vessel, usually caused by atherosclerosis and hypertension, or, less frequently, by trauma, infection, or a congenital weakness in the vessel wall. *See Conditions by Diagnosis section.*

Angina — chest pain due to myocardial ischemia; stable pattern angina occurs with exertion and is relieved by rest or vasodilators such as nitroglycerin. *See Conditions by Diagnosis section.*

Angioedema — an acute, painless, dermal, subcutaneous or submucosal swelling of short duration involving the face, neck, lips, larynx, hands, feet, genitalia or viscera.

Angiotensin — a substance released by angiotensinogen and acted upon by a converting enzyme in the lung to become a powerful vasoconstrictor.

Angiotensin I — inactive precursor to angiotensin II.

Angiotensin II — active form of angiotensin; a vasopressor.

Angiotensin-converting enzyme (ACE) inhibitor — an agent which blocks the effects of angiotensin converting enzyme thus producing decreases in systemic peripheral vascular resistance; these agents are useful in treating hypertension.

Angiotensinogen — plasma globulin protein formed in the liver which is converted to angiotensin by the action of renin.

Anions — negatively charged ions that are attracted to the positive electrode (anode) in electrolysis.

Antagonist — a drug or substance which blocks or counteracts the actions of another drug or substance.

Anterior — the front, or ventral surface.

Antibody — a protein produced by the body to provide immunity or fight infection against a specific antigen, pathogen or other foreign substance. Antibodies can be measured in the blood, and the presence of antibodies indicates previous exposure to a disease. *See also* "seroconversion."

Anticholinergic — of or pertaining to the blocking of acetylcholine receptors which results in the inhibition of parasympathetic nerve impulse transmission.

Anticoagulants — substances that prevent or slow the clotting of blood.

Antidiuretic hormone (ADH) — a hormone that decreases the production of urine by increasing the reabsorption of water in the renal tubules. It is released in response to a decrease in blood volume, an increase in the concentration of sodium or other osmotic substances in the blood, and also to pain, stress or the action of certain drugs.

Antidote — a drug that antagonizes the action of a poison.

Antigen — a substance or pathogen that the body recognizes as foreign, causing activation of the immune system.

Antispasmodic — a drug or other agent that prevents smooth muscle spasms, as in the uterus, digestive system, or urinary tract.

Antivenin — a suspension of venom-neutralizing antibodies prepared from the serum of immunized horses; confers passive immunity and is given as a part of emergency first aid for various snake and insect bites. Also called antivenom.

Aortic aneurysm — a structural defect in the lining, or linings of the aorta. *See Conditions by Diagnosis section.*

Aortic stenosis — a cardiac anomaly characterized by a narrowing or stricture of the aortic valve secondary to congenital malformation or of fusion of the cusps, as may result from rheumatic fever.

Aortic valve — valve between the left ventricle and the aorta.

APGAR score — a post-partum numeric score based on infant heart rate, respiratory effort, muscle tone, color and response to stimuli.

Aphasia — a neurologic condition in which language function is defective or absent.

Apnea — absence of breathing; respiratory arrest.

Appendicitis — an infection of the vermiform appendix. *See Conditions by Diagnosis section.*

Appendicular skeleton — the bones of the upper and lower extremities of the body.

Appendix (vermiform appendix) — a wormlike blunt process extending from the cecum.

Arachnoid membrane — middle meningeal layer covering the brain; vascular, loose and weblike, it absorbs cerebrospinal fluid.

Arterial insufficiency — physiologic condition in which an artery or arteries do not function to normal capacity to supply sufficient blood the body.

Artery — a vessel that carries blood away from the heart.

Arthritis — a disease of inflammation and destruction of joints which is accompanied by pain and leads to loss of function in affected joints. *See Conditions by Diagnosis section.*

Artificial pacemaker — electronic device used to stimulate the heart beat when the electrical conduction system of the heart malfunctions.

Aseptic — sterile; a condition free from microorganisms.

Aspiration — the inhalation or entry of substances such as food or fluid into the trachea and lungs.

Asterixis — hand flapping tremor; often seen with hepatic encephalopathy.

Asthma — respiratory disorder characterized by recurring episodes of paroxysmal dyspnea, wheezing on expiration due to constriction of the bronchi, coughing, and viscous mucoid bronchial secretions. *See Conditions by Diagnosis section.*

Asymmetry — the lack of similarity or equality between opposite side anatomical structures of the body.

Asymptomatic — without symptoms.

Asystole — an absence of electrical and mechanical activity in the heart. *See Conditions by Diagnosis section.*

Ataxic gait — a staggering gait in which the person walks with a wide base and has difficulty turning. The feet are thrown outward and the person comes down first on the heel and then on the toes. The condition is caused by a lesion in the cerebellum or cerebellar pathways.

Atherosclerosis — thickening, hardening and loss of elasticity of arterial walls; atherosclerotic heart disease (ASHD). *See Conditions by Diagnosis section.*

Atria — the two upper chambers of the heart.

Atrioventricular node — junction in the heart where atrial conduction pathways converge to pass electrical impulse transmission to the bundle-of-His.

Atypical — a condition or object that is not of a usual or standard type.

Autoimmune — pathologic condition where the body develops antibodies in response to the body's own tissues or protein.

Automatic implanted cardiac defibrillator (AICD) — a surgically implanted device that monitors a person's heart rate and which is designed to deliver defibrillatory shocks as needed.

Automaticity — a property of specialized excitable tissue that allows self-activation through spontaneous development of an action potential, as in the pacemaker cells of the heart.

Autonomic — Self regulating, or automatic functioning.

Autonomic nervous system — the involuntary nervous system consisting of the sympathetic and parasympathetic nervous systems.

Axial skeleton — the bones of the head, neck and torso.

Axial traction — tension applied along the long-axis of a bone or group of bones such as the spine.

Axon — the main central process of a neuron that normally conducts action potentials away from the neuron cell body.

Barbiturate — a derivative of barbituric acid that acts as a sedative or sleeping pill.

Barometric pressure — the pressure exerted by the weight of the atmosphere.

Baroreceptor — one of the pressure-sensitive nerve endings in the walls of the atria of the heart, the vena cava, the aortic arch, and the carotid sinus. Baroreceptors stimulate central reflex mechanisms that allow physiologic adjustment and adaptation to changes in blood pressure via vasodilation or vasoconstriction.

Barotrauma — physical injury sustained as a result of exposure to excessive environmental pressure changes, e.g., blast injury or underwater pressure injury. *See Conditions by Diagnosis section.*

Barrel chest — increased anterior-posterior to lateral chest proportion; large, over distended chest cavity, usually associated with chronic obstructive lung disease.

Base — Alkaline; bitter tasting substance which releases hydroxyl ions (OH^-) when dissolved in water; reacts with acids to form salts.

Base hospital — hospital designated as a medical direction facility which has trained emergency physicians available at all times to provide direct, on-line medical direction to paramedics.

Basic life support (BLS) — care provided by prehospital providers that includes first aid, cardiopulmonary resuscitation and other non-invasive care; BLS includes automated emergency defibrillation and airway adjuncts.

Battery — unlawful touching or contact with a person.

Battle's sign — a contusion behind the ear over the mastoid process. It is a sign of a basilar skull fracture.

Behavioral emergency — any behavioral disorder that poses a threat to the health, safety, or life of the individual involved or to people around that person.

Benzodiazepine — one of a group of psychotropic agents, including the tranquilizers chlordiazepoxide, diazepam, oxazepam, lorazepam, and the hypnotics flurazepam and nitrazepam; often prescribed in the treatment of anxiety, and sometimes insomnia.

Beta-blocker — an agent that antagonizes the actions of the adrenergic receptors of the sympathetic nervous system; administration of *Beta*-blockers result in a decreased heart rate and dilation of the bronchioles and vessels of the cardiovascular system.

Beta adrenergic receptor — one of several types of sympathetic system binding sites, that when stimulated, causes increases in heart rate, force of cardiac contractions, and relaxation of bronchial smooth muscle.

Bile — a yellow-green fluid secreted by the liver and stored in the gallbladder; it is released in the duodenum in response to the ingestion of fats via the common bile duct; it emulsifies the fats for further digestion.

Biliary colic — a type of smooth muscle or visceral pain specifically associated with the passing of stones through the bile ducts.

Biorhythms — the rhythmic cycles of process and functions in the body.

Bipolar — having two poles or branches at extreme ends; usually applied to a disorder in which a person swings from depression to manic states. *See Conditions by Diagnosis section.*

Bleb — an accumulation of fluid under the skin.

Blood — the circulating fluid of the vascular system consisting of erythrocytes, leukocytes, platelets, albumin and globulin proteins, electrolytes, and gases.

Blood-brain barrier — a specialized membrane that blocks the passage of many drugs and toxins into the central nervous system.

Blunt trauma — a closed injury produced by kinetic compression forces.

Body substance isolation (BSI) — the practice of avoiding exposure to all the body fluids of others on the basis that they are potentially infectious.

Bone — specialized hard, connective tissue; consists of living cells in a mineralized matrix.

Bowel obstruction — a failure of the contents of the intestines to pass through the lumen of the bowel.

Boyle's Law — a gas law affecting physiology during aeromedical transport: at a constant temperature, the volume of a gas varies proportionately to changes in the temperature of the gas.

Bradycardia — heart rate slower than 60 beats per minute.

Brain — the portion of the central nervous system contained within the cranium. It consists of the cerebrum, cerebellum, pons, medulla, and midbrain. Specialized cells in its mass of convoluted, soft, gray or white tissue coordinate and regulate the functions of the body.

Breech presentation — the abnormal position of the fetus in the uterus with the buttocks or a limb directed toward the cervical os.

Bronchi — the larger airway passages in the lungs.

Bronchiole — a small branch of a bronchus.

Bronchitis — an acute or chronic inflammation of the mucous membranes of the tracheobronchial tree. *See Conditions by Diagnosis section.*

Bronchospasm — an abnormal contraction of the smooth muscle of the bronchi, resulting in an acute narrowing and obstruction of the respiratory airway.

Bullae — a thin-walled blister of the skin or mucous membranes greater than 1 cm in diameter containing clear, serous fluid.

Bundle-of-His — conduction pathway from the atrio-ventricular junction to the bundle branches and Purkinje fibers.

Bundle branches — divisions of the bundle-of-His which subdivide into right and left bundle branches

Burden of proof — the legal requirement that one establish facts in a legal proceeding.

Calcium channel blocker — a drug which blocks the uptake of calcium into cells, resulting in smooth muscle relaxation. These agents are useful in treating hypertension and angina pectoris.

Capacitance vessels — the blood vessels that hold the major portion of the intravascular blood volume.

Capillary — The segment of the cardiovascular system that connects arterioles to venules, and where oxygen, carbon dioxide, and metabolic substances diffuse into and out of tissues.

Carbohydrate — any of a group of organic compounds, the most important being the saccharides, starch, cellulose, and gum. They are classified according to molecular structure as mono-, di-, tri-, poly-, and heterosaccharides. Carbohydrates constitute the main source of energy for all body functions, particularly brain functions, and are necessary for the metabolism of other nutrients.

Carboxyhemoglobin — hemoglobin combined with carbon monoxide, which occupies the sites on the hemoglobin molecule that normally bind with oxygen resulting in inability of hemoglobin to carry oxygen.

Cardiac cycle — periodic cardiac electrophysiologic depolarization and repolarization, and myocardial contraction and relaxation (systole and diastole), in which the atria, ventricles, cardiac valves function to produce arterial pressures.

Cardiac glycoside — one of a group of compounds such as digitalis which are natural plant products and contain a carbohydrate (sugar) molecule in their structure.

Cardiac muscle — the striated heart muscle which contains intercalated disks at the junctions of fibers.

Cardiac output — the volume of blood expelled by the ventricles of the heart, equal to the amount of blood ejected at each beat (the stroke output) multiplied by the heart rate per minute; number of beats in the period of time used in the computation.

Cardiac sphincter — a ring of muscle fibers at the juncture of the esophagus and stomach which prevent gastric juices from refluxing into the esophagus.

Cardiogenic shock — inadequate tissue perfusion and hypoxemia due to inadequate cardiac pumping.

Cardiopulmonary resuscitation (CPR) — emergency procedures for basic life support consisting of initial assessment and call for help, manual opening of the airway, artificial respiration and manual external cardiac massage.

Cardioversion — delivery of a synchronous countershock to convert a pathologic cardiac rhythm.

Cardiovert — delivery of energy to correct a potentially lethal dysrhythmia.

Carotid sinus — dilation of the arterial wall at the bifurcation of the common carotid artery.

Carpopedal spasm — involuntary contraction of the hand, thumbs, feet or toes that sometimes accompanies tetany.

Carrier — a person who harbors a pathogen, but who has no current symptoms of a disease. Carriers can transmit communicable diseases while remaining symptom-free.

Cartilage — firm, smooth, nonvascular connective tissue.

Cataract — an abnormal, progressive condition of the lens of the eye, characterized by loss of transparency. *See Conditions by Diagnosis section.*

Catecholamines — any one of a group of sympathomimetic compounds composed of a catechol molecule and the aliphatic portion of an amine; agents that stimulate adrenergic, or sympathetic responses.

Cations — positively charged ions.

Cauda equina — the distal end of the spinal cord at the first lumbar vertebra; the lumbar, sacral, and coccygeal nerve roots of the spinal cord that pass through the spinal canal of sacrum and coccyx prior to reaching their intervertebral foramina.

Cavitation — the formation of cavities within the body, such as those formed in the lung by tuberculosis.

Cell — the fundamental unit of all living tissue.

Central nervous system — the brain and spinal cord.

Cerebellum — the second largest part of the brain, which controls coordination and fine motor movements.

Cerebral contusion — bruised brain tissue.

Cerebral herniation — an abnormal protrusion of the brain through a covering membrane or through an opening in the skull.

Cerebrospinal fluid — fluid that fills the subarachnoid space in the brain and spinal cord and in the cerebral ventricles.

Cerebrovascular accident (CVA) — an abnormal condition of the blood vessels of the brain characterized by occlusion by an embolus, thrombus, or cerebrovascular hemorrhage, resulting in ischemia of the brain tissues normally perfused by the damaged vessels. *See Conditions by Diagnosis section.*

Certification — a process for the evaluation of an institution or agency, and also for recognition of meeting performance or material standards.

Cervical os — the cervical outlet or opening.

Chemical pneumonitis — inflammation of the lung caused by foreign substances rather than viruses or bacteria.

Chemically contaminated patient — a patient with dangerous or potentially dangerous chemicals on the clothing and/or skin.

Chemoreceptor — a sensory nerve cell activated by chemical stimuli.

Cheyne-Stokes respiration — an abnormal pattern of respiration, characterized by alternating periods of apnea and deep, rapid breathing.

Cholecystitis — acute or chronic inflammation of the gallbladder.

Cholinergic — the effects produced by the parasympathetic nervous system, or drugs which stimulate or antagonize the parasympathetic nervous system.

Chronic bronchitis — obstructive airway disease of the trachea and bronchi. *See Conditions by Diagnosis section.*

Chronic obstructive pulmonary disease (COPD) — one or more of the respiratory illnesses which result in permanently narrowed airways, most commonly emphysema or chronic bronchitis, or a combination of the two. *See Conditions by Diagnosis section.*

Cilia — small, hairlike processes on the outer surfaces of some cells, aiding metabolism by producing motion, eddies, or current in a fluid.

Circulatory system — the dynamic cardiovascular network consisting of the heart, arteries, veins, capillaries and blood.

Cirrhosis — chronic liver disease usually caused by chronic alcoholism or chronic hepatitis; signs include jaundice, hepatomegaly and hepatojugular reflux. *See Conditions by Diagnosis section.*

Claudication — pain, usually in the calf, which occurs with exertion or walking, and may cause temporary lameness or limping. Usually due to arterial insufficiency. *See Conditions by Diagnosis section.*

Coagulopathies — pathologic conditions affecting the coagulation of blood.

Cocaine — a white crystalline powder used as a local anesthetic, and which has been used illegally as a nervous system stimulant.

Cold zone — the area around a hazardous materials incident that is free of hazardous materials which are dangerous to emergency personnel. The area in which the command post is located, along with essential supplies, equipment, and personnel; sometimes called the "support zone."

Collagen — fibrous structural protein that form skin, tendons, bone, hair and other connective tissues.

Colle's fracture — a distinctive fracture of the distal radius at the epiphysis in which the fractured tip is displaced posteriorly.

Colloid — protein molecules or aggregates of protein in solution.

Combustible — capable of igniting and burning.

Command center — a clearly marked safe area at the site of a mass casualty incident in which the senior representatives of responding agencies locate to manage the incident.

Common law — the body of principles, rules of action, and customs of society expressed in legal decisions by judges (also called precedents).

Communicable disease (contagious disease) — an infectious disease that can be spread from person to person.

Communication — the transmission and reception of information, resulting in common understanding.

Communication center — a defined area of a mass casualty incident in which all radio communication is coordinated. The Communication Center will generally be located within or near the Command Center.

Compartment syndrome — a pathologic condition caused by the progressive development of arterial compression and reduced blood supply. *See Conditions by Diagnosis section.*

Compassion — a feeling of sympathy and sorrow for those struck by misfortune, accompanied by a strong desire to alleviate the suffering.

Compensatory mechanism — physiologic increase in one or more functions to supplement or substitute for a decreased or an inefficient vital function.

Compound — a chemical substance composed of different types of atoms which are linked by chemical bonds (e.g. hydrogen sulfide (H_2S), methane (CH_3) sulfuric acid (H_2SO_4).

Compression — the act of pressing, squeezing, or otherwise applying pressure to an organ, tissue, or body area.

Computer-aided dispatch (CAD) — a dispatch communication system in which electronic (computerized) data is used to assist dispatchers in selecting and directing EMS resources.

Concurrent medical direction — the direct, on-line, physician direction of prehospital care providers via radio, telephone or another medium.

Concussion — transient loss of consciousness after head trauma. *See Conditions by Diagnosis section.*

Conduction — 1. A process in which heat is transferred from one substance to another because of a difference in temperature; a process in which energy is transmitted through a conductor. 2. The process by which a nerve impulse is transmitted.

Confidentiality — refers to a person's right to privacy and the requirement of healthcare providers to keep patient information protected from those who do not have a right to know it.

Confined space rescue — rescue in any space that is not intended for continuous occupancy, with limited or no ventilation and limited entrance/exit. Examples: water and waste removal pipes and systems, wells, caves, and silos.

Congenital — a condition or disease that exists from birth.

Congestive heart failure (CHF) — fluid accumulation in the lungs and extremities as the result of inefficient pumping of blood from the heart. *See Conditions by Diagnosis section.*

Conjunctivitis — inflammation of the mucous membrane covering the anterior surface of the eyeball and lining of the eyelids; caused by bacterial or viral infection, allergy, or environmental factors. *See Conditions by Diagnosis section.*

Connective tissue — tissue that supports and binds other tissues and anatomical structures.

Consensual — stimulation of one side of the body produces a reflex that also causes the other side to react (e.g., both pupils react to light when only one eye is exposed to light).

Continuous quality improvement — a management approach to customer service and organizational performance in which there is a process of constant monitoring, evaluation, decisions and actions.

Contractility — the force of ventricular contraction.

Constitutional law — The fundamental law of the United States, individual states and organizations; establishes the powers and principles which regulate the government and institutions.

Contamination — chemical or radioactive material on a person's skin and/or clothing (external contamination) or in the lungs and/or gastrointestinal tract (internal contamination).

Contraindication — a disease process or specific situation in which a drug is absolutely not to be given.

Convection — the transfer of heat through a gas or liquid by the circulation of heated particles.

Conversion disorder — a disorder in which a repressed intrapsychic conflicts are transferred into over physical symptoms that have no physiological basis. *See Conditions by Diagnosis section.*

Core temperature — the temperature of deep structures of the body, such as the liver, as compared with temperatures of peripheral tissues.

Corneal abrasion — scrape of the convex, transparent, anterior part of the eye. *See Conditions by Diagnosis section.*

Coronary artery disease — any one of the abnormal conditions that may affect the arteries of the heart and produce various pathologic effects, especially the reduced flow of oxygen and nutrients to the myocardium. *See Conditions by Diagnosis section.*

Corpus callosum — an arched mass of white matter in the depths of the longitudinal fissure; made up of the transverse fibers connecting the cerebral hemispheres.

Corrosive — a chemical which destroys tissues or substances which it contacts.

Cortex — the portion of the brain which forms abstract imagery and processes thoughts on an intellectual plane.

Cranial nerve — one of 12 pairs of nerves that originate from a nucleus within the brain, and which exit the cranium via openings in the skull other than as part of the spinal cord.

Cranium — the bones and cavity of the skull.

Crepitus — a grating vibration or crackling sound heard on movement of fractured bone ends; the grating sensation of subcutaneous air bubbles which is felt with palpation.

Cribbing — supports placed at strategic points under a vehicle during a rescue to prevent movement.

Cribriform plate — the bone at the anterior base of skull, and which is one of the potential site of cerebrospinal fluid leak after basilar skull fracture.

Crisis — a sudden change in the clinical condition of a patient, usually indicating an improvement; a dramatic or circumstantial upheaval in a person's life.

Crisis intervention — a set of helpful techniques designed to achieve rapid intervention in a crisis with the goals of stabilizing the situation, mobilizing the resources to resolve the crisis and restoring the person to function as quickly as possible.

Criteria-based dispatch (CBD) — a system for dispatching emergency response units based upon established guidelines.

Critical incident — any event that overwhelms one's psychological coping abilities.

Critical incident stress debriefing (CISD) — a structured process designed to mitigate the emotional distress caused by an extremely disturbing event. The process allows for the free expression of thoughts, reactions and feelings resulting from the highly stressful event.

Critical incident stress management (CISM) — agency programs, policies and procedures that address education, prevention, incident management and post-incident management of extremely disturbing incidents, and which are designed to minimize the acute and residual effects of stress during major incidents.

Critical incident stress response — behavioral, emotional, and cognitive signs and symptoms that occur in normal people in response to abnormal events; often mitigated through a debriefing process designed to accelerate normal recovery.

Croup — an acute viral infection of the upper and lower respiratory tract that occurs primarily in infants and young children 6 months to 3 years of age. *See Conditions by Diagnosis section.*

Cryogenic — relating to very low temperatures.

Crystalloid — solution formed by a solute which is in crystal form when dry.

Cushing's reflex — a reflex caused by ischemia of the brain that increases systemic blood pressure to perfuse the brain.

Cyanosis — blue coloration of the skin due to high levels of deoxygenated hemoglobin; usually found in nailbeds or around the lips.

Dalton's law — a gas law affecting physiology during air medical transport; as altitude increases, barometric pressure decreases and gas expansion causes a depletion in oxygen.

Deceleration injury — injury that occurs from a sudden stop in a high speed impact, as in a fall from significant height, or a high speed motor vehicular collision.

Decerebrate posturing — rigid position, or reflexive response to painful stimuli in a patient with severe brain injury; the upper extremities extend and internally rotate with flexion of the wrists, and lower extremities extend and internally rotate with plantar flexion.

Decompression sickness — a painful and sometimes fatal syndrome caused by the formation of nitrogen bubbles in the tissue of divers, caisson workers, and aviators who move too rapidly from environments of higher to those of lower atmospheric pressures. *See Conditions by Diagnosis section.*

Decontamination — the act of removing hazardous material from skin and/or clothes, as well as from medical and rescue equipment.

Decorticate posturing — reflexive posturing of the extremities in response to painful stimuli which occurs in patients with disruption of the corticospinal tracts; bilateral flexion at the shoulders, pronation and flexion of the elbows and wrists; extension and internal rotation of the lower extremities, with plantar flexion.

Deep fascia — the most extensive of three kinds of fascia comprising an intricate series of connective sheets and bands that hold the muscles and other structures in place throughout the body, wrapping the muscles in gray, feltlike membranes.

Defibrillation — attempted termination of ventricular fibrillation by delivering a direct current electric shock to the patient's precordium.

Delegated practice — legal means by which a paraprofessional may provide patient care under the supervision and license of a physician.

Delirium — an acute mental status change that is sudden in onset and is often reversible.

Delirium tremens (DTs) — an acute and potentially fatal reaction which occurs in patients with chronic alcoholism; caused by sudden complete abstinence from alcohol consumption after a long period of heavy consumption. *See Conditions by Diagnosis section.*

Delivery — the actual passing of the products of conception, including the placenta.

Delusion — a belief or sense of reality that is firmly held despite being completely false, or unfounded.

Demand pacing (synchronous) — electrical stimulus to the myocardium which is delivered when the hear rate falls below a determined rate, or when chemical sensors trigger a stimulus in response to pH or indicators.

Dementia — a general and gradual loss of mental function, including memory loss, poor judgment, personality changes, and loss of abstract reasoning capabilities.

Demographics — statistical data on the human population.

Dendrite — the branching processes of a neuron that receives stimuli and conducts potentials toward the cell body.

Dependence — the total psychophysical state of addiction to drugs or alcohol where one must receive increasing amounts of a substance to prevent the onset symptoms.

Depolarization — electrophysiologic action in a cell or tissue in which cellular membranes open to allow the flow of ions in the direction of the concentration gradient.

Dermatome — the area of skin supplied with sensory fibers from a single spinal nerve.

Dermis — dense, irregular connective tissue that forms the deep layer of the skin.

Dialysis vascular access device — a shunt, fistula or graft which allows access to circulation for the purpose of renal dialysis.

Diaphragm — the dome-shaped musculofibrous partition that separates the thoracic and abdominal cavities.

Diastole — relaxation phase of the cardiac cycle; period when the ventricles are filling.

Diffusion — the random, passive distribution of particles in a mixture or solution; substances move in the direction of the concentration gradient. When all parts of the solution have equal concentrations, the solute is dissolved, and the solution is homogenous.

Digestive system — the organ system of the body which prepares food and liquids for absorption; consists of the mouth and tongue, esophagus, stomach, small and large intestines, and the rectum; also includes glands which produce digestive enzymes (e.g., pancreas, gall bladder).

Dignity — bearing, conduct or speech indicative of self-respect or appreciation of the formality or gravity of an occasion or situation.

Direct current — electrical current which is constant in wave form and does not fluctuate between positive and negative; opposite of alternating current.

Direct medical direction — *See* On-line medical direction.

Direct transmission — spread of a communicable disease from person to person. *See also* Indirect transmission.

Disentanglement — the systematic moving or removing of portions of a wreckage (e.g., motor vehicle, structural collapse, cave-ins); done to access patients and prepare for extrication.

Dislocation — the displacement of any part of the body from its normal position, particularly a bone from its normal articulation with a joint.

Disorientation — a state of mental confusion characterized by inadequate or incorrect perceptions of identity, time, place, or events.

Disseminated intravascular coagulopathy — a grave coagulopathy resulting from the overstimulation of clotting and anticlotting processes in response to disease or injury, such as septicemia, acute hypotension, poisonous snake bites, neoplasms, obstetric emergencies, severe trauma, extensive surgery, and hemorrhage. The primary disorder initiates generalized intravascular clotting, which in turn overstimulates fibrinolytic mechanisms; as a result the initial hyper coagulability is succeeded by a deficiency in clotting factors with hypocoagulability and hemorrhaging.

Distal — away from or being farthest from the point of origin or midline.

Distress — negative, debilitating or harmful stress.

Distribution — the process of moving a drug through the body and delivering it to various tissues.

Distributive shock — compromised circulation and oxygenation resulting from loss of vascular tone leading to dilation of blood vessels and decreased perfusion. Causes include sepsis, anaphylaxis, drugs, toxins and spinal cord injury.

Diuretic — a drug that promotes the formation and excretion of urine.

"Do not resuscitate" orders (DNR) — documented physicians' orders not to initiate advanced cardiac life support in the event of a cardiac arrest.

Dopamine — a catecholamine secreted by the adrenal medulla; also, a drug administered for hypotension.

Dose — the total amount of a drug, toxic substance, or radiation, which a person has received.

Dose-response — the relationship between the amount of a substance received, and the effects.

Drug absorption — the process of a drug moving into the blood from oral, sublingual, transdermal, subcutaneous, intramuscular or endotracheal administration.

Drug agonist — drugs that stimulate (switch-on) a receptor.

Drug antagonist — a substance that binds to a receptor and prevents an effect of another drug.

Drug metabolism — the process of detoxification and conversion of chemicals and drugs so that they are more easily eliminated by the kidney.

Dual-fuels — alternate-fuel vehicles operating on two distinctly different types of fuels. The two most common are compressed natural gas and propane or butane.

Duodenum — the first subdivision, or segment, of the small intestine.

Dura mater — outermost, coarsest and strongest meningeal layer covering the central nervous system.

Dysphagia — inability to swallow or difficulty in swallowing.

Dyspnea — an unpleasant or uncomfortable sensation of labored or obstructed breathing, or an inappropriate awareness of breathing that is accompanied by obvious signs of difficulty in breathing.

Dysrhythmia — any disturbance or abnormality in a rhythmic pattern; irregularities in the electrical rhythm of the heart, in brain waves or in cadence of speech.

Dystonic reaction — muscle stiffness or prolonged contractions that may cause twisting or distorted movements or positions.

Ecchymosis — discoloration of an area of the skin or mucous membrane caused by bleeding beneath the skin; bruising.

Eclampsia — the occurrence of a seizure in the presence of preeclampsia. *See Conditions by Diagnosis section.*

Ectopic pregnancy — an abnormal pregnancy in which the conceptus implants outside the uterine cavity. *See Conditions by Diagnosis section.*

Eczema — a chronic skin irritation and inflammation.

Effacement — the elongating and thinning of the cervix in preparation for delivery.

Efferent (motor) neuron — nerve that transmits signals from the central nervous system to the muscles; motor nerve.

Effusion — the leaking or escape of fluids or gases from a vessel or compartment.

Electrocardiogram (ECG) — graphic display of the electrical activity of the heart generated by the depolarization and repolarization of the atria and ventricles.

Electrodes — the wires and patches that connect the patient to the ECG monitor machine or monitor and sense the flow of electrical current within the heart.

Electrolyte — a compound or substance, which when dissolved in water, ionizes and conducts electricity.

Element — atoms having the same atomic number. Examples: hydrogen, oxygen, iron, sulfur, and arsenic.

Embolus — a foreign object, tumor, gas or liquid, which is in the circulatory system; when the embolus lodges in a vessel, it results in an obstruction. *See Conditions by Diagnosis section.*

Emergency medical dispatcher — 1. a program for educating dispatchers in the appropriate use of emergency medical dispatching; including prearrival instructions, radio terminology and triage. 2. a person trained in asking the caller standard questions, prioritizing the call and providing prearrival instructions.

Emergency medical services (EMS) system — the deployment of personnel, facilities, and equipment for coordinated delivery of emergency medical services.

Encephalitis — inflammation of the brain, usually caused by an arbovirus infection transmitted by the bite of an infected mosquito, may also result from lead or other poisoning or from hemorrhage. *See Conditions by Diagnosis section.*

Encrustation — accumulation of dried pus, blood or serum.

Endocarditis — inflammation of the lining membrane of the heart. *See Conditions by Diagnosis section.*

Endocrine system — network of ductless glands that secrete hormones directly into the bloodstream;

Endometritis — an infection of the inner lining of the uterus. *See Conditions by Diagnosis section.*

Endometrium — the inner lining of the uterus.

Endorphin — any one of the neuropeptides composed of many amino acids, elaborated by the pituitary gland and acting on the central and the peripheral nervous systems to reduce pain.

Enhanced-911 (E-911) — a fully integrated, computerized 911-access telephone system; caller and dispatch information is automatically displayed and relayed from a database.

Enkephalin — one of the two endogenous pain-relieving pentapeptides.

Enteral — within or by way of the intestines.

Enteral tube feeding — the introduction of food or nutritive material directly into the digestive tract by nasogastric or gastric tube.

Enteric — pertaining to the intestinal tract.

Enterotoxin — poison absorbed through the intestines, or digestive tract.

Envenomation — a poisoning caused by a bite or a sting.

Epidural hematoma — a collection of blood between the inside of the skull and the dura mater, usually caused by broken arteries. *See Conditions by Diagnosis section.*

Epidermis — the outer portion of skin; formed of epithelial tissue that rests on or covers the dermis.

Epiglottitis — inflammation of the epiglottis, hypopharynx and trachea. *See Conditions by Diagnosis section.*

Epilepsy — nonspecific term for idiopathic seizure disorder; indicates only a propensity to having seizures. *See Conditions by Diagnosis section.*

Epinephrine — a sympathetic hormone, also called adrenalin, that primarily affects the cardiovascular system.

Epistaxis — nosebleed. *See Conditions by Diagnosis section.*

Epithelial buds — the layer of cells that generates the epidermis of the skin.

Epithelial tissue — the cellular covering of internal and external surfaces of the body, including the lining of vessels and other small cavities.

Erect — upright, vertical, straight.

Erythrocyte — red blood cell.

Eschar — dry, stiff slough or necrotic tissue; result of a full-thickness burn.

Escharotomy — removal of the eschar formed on the skin; incision through the eschar to restore circulation to underlying tissues that have been compressed as a result of swelling underneath circumferential burns.

Esophageal spasm — painful muscular contraction of the esophagus which results in dysphagia.

Esophagus — the muscular canal extending from the pharynx to the stomach.

Ether — a nonhalogenated, volatile liquid used as a general anesthetic.

Ethics — a system of moral principles or standards governing conduct; professions have a code of ethics.

Etiologic agent — a category of hazardous materials that contains living microorganisms capable of causing human disease.

Eustress — positive, performance enhancing stress.

Evidence — anything that has a bearing on or establishes an issue in a legal proceeding.

Evisceration — the protrusion of an internal organ through a wound or surgical incision, especially in the abdominal wall.

Excretion — the process of eliminating substances by body organs or tissues, as part of a natural metabolic activity.

Exocrine gland — any of the multicellular glands that open onto the skin surface through ducts in the epithelium, as the sweat glands and the sebaceous glands.

Expiration — exhalation of a breath.

Explosive — an unstable compound that breaks down with the sudden release of large amounts of energy; in psychology, an unstable, extremely violent personality.

Exposure — contact with blood, body fluids, tissues or airborne droplets through direct or indirect means.

Expressed consent — stated voluntary agreement to be treated after being informed of the risks of treatment.

Extension — movement at a joint to increase the angle between two bones, to straighten at a joint.

Extracellular fluid — the portion of the body fluid comprising the interstitial fluid and blood plasma.

Extravasation — leakage of fluids from vessels into surrounding tissues.

Extrication — process of physically (by the use of force) freeing/removing a patient from entrapment.

Exudate — accumulation of fluid, or the production of pus or serum.

Facilitated diffusion — movement of a particle through a membrane with the help of another substance, e.g., insulin helping glucose cross muscle cell membranes.

False imprisonment — detention of a person, without consent or lawful justification, so as to substantially interfere with the person's liberty.

Fascia — the loose areolar connective tissue found beneath the skin or dense connective tissue that encloses and separates muscle.

Fat — 1. substance composed of lipids or fatty acids and occurring in various forms or consistencies ranging from oil to tallow. 2. a type of body tissue composed of cells containing stored fat (depot fat). Stored fat is usually identified as white fat, which is found in large cellular vesicles, or brown fat, which consists of lipid droplets.

Febrile seizure — a seizure associated with a rapid rise in core body temperature. *See Conditions by Diagnosis section.*

Fenestration — an opening usually covered by a membrane or an artificial opening.

Fetus — a general term for an unborn infant.

Fibrillation — the chaotic, uncoordinated firing of cardiac muscle cells; though it generates electrical activity, it cannot cause organized contraction of the chamber involved, and cardiac output decreases.

Fight or flight response — the stress response, mediated by epinephrine and related hormones, which prepares the body to fight off a threat, or to flee.

Fixed-wing — aircraft in which the lifting force is generated by the aircraft's speed, and in which the wings do not move in relationship to the craft.

Flaccid — weak, soft, flabby; lacking normal muscle tone.

Flail chest — multiple rib fractures which result in paradoxical chest wall movement during breathing; hypoxia results from reduced tidal volume. *See Conditions by Diagnosis section.*

Flammable — capable of being easily ignited and of burning with extreme rapidity.

Flexion — movement at a joint to decrease the angle between two bones, to bend at a joint.

Foramen magnum — hole at base of skull where the spinal cord exits the cranium.

Fracture — a traumatic injury to a bone or solid organ in which the continuity of the tissue is broken.

Frontal — pertaining to the ventral, or anterior, surface.

Frostbite — injury to the skin caused by prolonged exposure to cold. The liquid content of the skin freezes and ruptures the cell membranes; may be superficial (frostnip) or deep. *See Conditions by Diagnosis section.*

Fundus — the bottom or rounded end of a hollow organ, such as the fundus of the uterus.

Gangrene — necrosis of tissue; typically due to ischemia, bacterial infection, and putrefaction. *See Conditions by Diagnosis section.*

Gastric lavage — flushing of the stomach, intestines or peritoneum with sterile water or a saline solution.

Gastric tube — a small tube inserted through the nose or mouth into the stomach, used to drain gas, gastric acid, or toxins, or to provide liquid nutrition.

Gastrointestinal bleeding — any bleeding from the GI tract.

Gastrostomy — an artificial opening into the stomach.

General adaptation syndrome (GAS) — the biological stress syndrome consisting of alarm, resistance and exhaustion phases.

Generic name — the unique name given to a drug which generally is adopted as the official name.

Germinal — beginning, early stage of development.

Gestation — in animals that deliver via live birth, the period from conception to birth.

Gland — organs that produce substances which affect other organs and processes; functions include lubrication, hormone production, and development of blood cells and blood components.

Glasgow Coma Scale — numerical scale developed to predict mortality in patients with head injury; commonly used as a quick and objective central nervous system assessment.

Glaucoma — localized pain, redness, visual loss, cloudy cornea and pupillary abnormalities involving one eye.

Glucagon — a hormone secreted by *alpha* cells in the isles of Langerhans; increases the concentration of glucose in the blood.

Glucocorticoids — stress hormones, secreted by the adrenal cortex, which increase the availability of energy.

Glucose — six carbon sugar used by the body for metabolic energy.

Glycogen — a polysaccharide that is the major carbohydrate stored in animal cells. It is formed from glucose and is stored chiefly in the liver, and to a lesser extent, in muscle cells.

Golden hour — principle developed by R. Adams Cowley that major trauma patients must be transported to surgery within one hour of the time of injury for a trauma system to be effective and to provide for the best chances for survival.

Good Samaritan — a person who renders first aid in an emergency situation even though he or she does not have a duty to act; from the Biblical parable.

Gravidity — the total number of pregnancies a woman has had, including abortions and miscarriages.

Grief — keen mental suffering or distress over affliction or loss.

Gross negligence — 1. a type of negligent conduct that is beyond simple negligence, usually related to intentional conduct, and sometimes to willful and wanton negligence in which an act or failure to act creates a substantial degree of risk of harm to another. 2. the failure to act or to perform to a standard which is acceptable by professional standards; does not include common errors of omission or commission.

Guillain-Barre Syndrome — an acute, more or less symmetrical paralysis of unknown cause, with loss of reflexes, and variable sensory involvement. *See Conditions by Diagnosis section.*

Hair follicle — an invagination of the epidermis into the dermis that contains the root of the hair and receives the ducts of sebaceous and apocrine glands.

Half-life — the time required for the body to metabolize or otherwise eliminate half of a drug or toxin dose; time period for one-half of an amount of radioactivity to decay.

Hallucination — a perception which is not caused by an external stimulus; hallucinations may occur in any of the senses.

Hazardous materials — any substance or material capable of posing an unreasonable risk to health, safety, and property.

HazMat — hazardous materials, often referring to the team of individuals who deal with hazardous materials incidents.

Health care professional — a person with specialized education and training who works in the health care field.

Heart — the cone-shaped muscle in the chest about the size of a clenched fist that pumps blood throughout the body.

Heart block — an interference with the conduction of electric impulses in the heart from the atria to the ventricles; an A-V block.

Heat cramps — the first and mildest form of heat exposure; muscle cramping caused by excessive loss of body fluids and salts.

Heat exhaustion — a form of heat exposure that occurs when the body's circulation system fails to maintain its normal function due to excessive loss of body fluids and salts; patients present with shock-like symptoms. *See Conditions by Diagnosis section.*

Heat stroke — a severe, potentially fatal condition that results from failure of the body's temperature-regulating capacity; primarily caused by prolonged exposure to the sun or to high temperatures. *See Conditions by Diagnosis section.*

Heimlich maneuver — manual compression of the abdomen to clear an obstructed airway; a technique developed by Henry Heimlich, also called the *abdominal thrust maneuver.*

Hemarthrosis — blood in a joint.

Hematemesis — vomiting of blood.

Hematopoiesis — the normal formation and development of blood cells.

Hematuria — a dark-colored urine due to the presence of hemoglobin.

Hemiparesis — paralysis or weakness limited to one side of the body.

Hemodialysis — a procedure in which impurities or wastes are removed from blood utilizing an osmotic gradient to promote filtration; used in treating renal insufficiency and various types of toxicity.

Hemoglobin — a protein-iron molecular complex in the red blood cells that transports oxygen from the lungs to the cells, and carbon dioxide from the cells to the lungs.

Hemolysis — the breakdown of red blood cells and the release of hemoglobin.

Hemolytic anemia — a disorder characterized by the premature destruction of red blood cells.

Hemophilia — a group of hereditary bleeding disorders in which one of the factors necessary for blood coagulation is deficient. *See Conditions by Diagnosis section.*

Hemoptysis — coughing up blood from the respiratory tract.

Hemostasis — the termination of bleeding by mechanical or chemical means or by the complex coagulation process of the body, consisting of vasoconstriction, platelet aggregation, and thrombin or fibrin synthesis.

Hemothorax — an accumulation of blood between the parietal and visceral pleura, usually the result of trauma.

Herniation — the protrusion, typically under pressure, of tissue or part of an organ, outside the cavity or structure in which it is normally located.

High-altitude cerebral edema (HACE) — the most severe form of acute high-altitude illness; characterized by a progression of global cerebral signs in the presence of acute mountain sickness that are probably related to increased intracranial pressure.

High-altitude pulmonary edema (HAPE) — a noncardiac pulmonary edema thought to be related, at least in part, to increased pulmonary artery pressure that develops in response to hypoxia; results in increased pulmonary arteriolar permeability, and in leakage of fluid into extravascular locations.

High-angle rescue — a vertical access, treatment, packaging and extrication operation.

Histamine — an amine released by mast cells and basophils that promotes inflammation.

Homeostasis — a state of dynamic physiologic equilibrium in the body.

Hormone — a complex biochemical substance which is produced in one part of the body, and which stimulates or regulates physiologic activity in another part of the body.

Hospice — holistic care for the terminally ill that emphasizes pain control and emotional support for the patient and family; hospice care may be provided in specialized facilities, long term care or acute care facilities, or the home. Extraordinary measures to prolong life are generally not provided.

Host — a person or animal which another organism, usually parasitic, harbors.

Hot zone — the area around a hazardous materials incident in which the material is known to be or suspected to be out of its container. Also includes the area in which one would be in danger if there were a sudden fire, explosion, or release of gas.

Huffing — a type of forced expiration with an open glottis to replace coughing when pain limits normal coughing; street slang term for inhalation of chemicals to obtain an altered level of consciousness, commonly termed a "high."

Hydrocarbon — any one of the organic compounds, the molecules of which are composed of hydrogen and carbon, many of which are derived from petroleum.

Hydrocephalus — increased accumulation of cerebral spinal fluid within the ventricles of the brain. *See Conditions by Diagnosis section.*

Hyperbaric oxygen chamber — an airtight chamber containing an oxygen atmosphere under high pressure.

Hypercapnia — greater than normal amounts of carbon dioxide in the blood.

Hyperdynamic — greater than normal physiologic activity (e.g., tachycardia and hypertension with increased cardiac output).

Hyperextension (of a joint) — a position of maximum extension; extension beyond comfort or stability.

Hyperglycemia — increase of blood sugar, as in diabetes. *See Conditions by Diagnosis section.*

Hypernatremia — a greater than normal concentration of sodium in the blood, caused by excessive loss of water and electrolytes resulting from polyuria, diarrhea, excessive sweating or inadequate water intake. *See Conditions by Diagnosis section.*

Hyperosmolarity — increased concentration of particles in the blood, such as glucose, electrolytes and protein; causes a fluid shift out of cells.

Hyperosmotic — solution with a greater solute concentration.

Hypersensitivity reactions — responses to drugs, therapeutic and untoward, which far exceed responses anticipated for the doses administered.

Hypertensive encephalopathy — signs and symptoms associated with glomerulonephritis; includes headache, convulsions, and coma. *See Conditions by Diagnosis section.*

Hyperthermia — significantly elevated core body temperature. *See Conditions by Diagnosis section.*

Hypertonic — having a greater concentration of solute (particles) than another solution; hypertonic saline solution contains more salt than is found in intracellular and extracellular fluid.

Hyperventilation — induced or spontaneous increase in respiratory rate that leads to a decrease in blood carbon dioxide content.

Hyphema — blood in the anterior chamber of the eye. *See Conditions by Diagnosis section.*

Hypogastric region — lower middle region of the abdomen located below the umbilicus and above the pubic bone.

Hypoglycemia — a condition in which the glucose in the blood is abnormally low. *See Conditions by Diagnosis section.*

Hyponatremia — a lower than normal concentration of sodium in the blood. *See Conditions by Diagnosis section.*

Hypoperfusion — inadequate circulation; insufficient delivery of oxygen and nutrients necessary for normal tissue and cellular function.

Hypotension — an abnormally low blood pressure.

Hypothalamus — portion of the diencephalon of the brain that activates, controls, and integrates the peripheral autonomic nervous system, endocrine processes and many somatic functions, such as body temperature, sleep and appetite.

Hypothermia — an abnormally low core body temperature. *See Conditions by Diagnosis section.*

Hypotonic — a lower concentration of solute (particles) than another solution, hence exerting less osmotic pressure than that solution, as a hypotonic saline solution that contains less salt than is found in intracellular and extracellular fluid. Cells expand in a hypotonic solution.

Hypovolemia — an abnormally low circulating blood volume. *See Conditions by Diagnosis section.*

Hypovolemic shock — the most common cause of compromised circulation in trauma and non-trauma patients; caused by decreased circulating blood volume. *See Conditions by Diagnosis section.*

Hypoxia — inadequate delivery of oxygen to the tissues of the body.

Hypoxic drive — Respiratory stimulus triggered by a very low PaO_2, e.g., <60 mm. Hg.

Hysterical reaction — a mental disorder characterized primarily by dissociation, repression, emotional instability and suggestibility.

Idiosyncratic reaction — unusual, unpredictable and unexplained response to the administration of a drug.

Ileum — the distal portion of the small intestine.

Ileus — a bowel obstruction; may be due to mechanical obstruction or inactive bowel.

Illusion — a distortion in a person's mind of things that exist in reality.

Immersion syndrome — tissue damage caused by prolonged exposure to water. *See Conditions by Diagnosis section.*

Immune system — internal defense against infectious pathogens and other foreign bodies; composed of white blood cells, the lymphatic system, antibodies, and other organ functions (e.g., genito-urinary elimination).

Immunoglobulin — any of five structurally and antigenically distinct antibodies present in the serum and external secretions of the body, including IgA, IgD, IgE, IgG, and IgM.

Implied consent — the assumed consent of an unconscious patient or other person who is unable to participate in decision-making in an emergency medical condition (e.g., a minor, or mentally incompetent patient).

Incident commander — the individual with decision-making authority in a major event in which multiple units or agencies respond; the Incident Commander is ideally predetermined by protocol defined in a system plan.

Incident command system (ICS) — a mass casualty incident (MCI) management program that includes aspects of MCI control, direction, and coordination of emergency response operations and resources.

Incompetency — legally declared to be unable to make decisions for oneself; determined by court order.

Incorporation accident — the uptake of radioactive atoms into the cells or interstitial fluid of the body.

Incubation period — the time interval between exposure to a disease and the development of symptoms.

Indication — the specific reasons or conditions for which a medication should be administered or treatment performed.

Indirect medical direction — see Off-line medical direction.

Indirect transmission — spread of a communicable disease by contact with a contaminated object such as an improperly cleaned laryngoscope blade. See also "Direct transmission."

Infection — the growth of an organism in a suitable host, with or without detectable signs of illness.

Infectious disease — any disease caused by a pathogen.

Inferior — toward the feet; below a point of reference in the anatomical position.

Infiltration — fluid leak into surrounding space (e.g., intravenous fluid leak into interstitial space).

Informed consent — agreement to medical treatment that is based on sufficient information for a reasonable person to make a decision; includes the risks of treatment.

Inhalant — medication administered by vapor or gas breathed into the lungs.

Inhibitions — the unconscious restraint of a behavioral process, usually resulting from the social or cultural forces of the environment; the condition inducing such restraint.

In-line immobilization — a manual stabilization maneuver in which the head and neck are maintained along the long axis of the body.

Innervation — the distribution or supply of nerve fibers or nerve impulses to the body.

Inspiration — inhalation of air into the lungs.

Insulin — a pancreatic hormone secreted by the *beta* cells of the pancreas which regulates blood levels and metabolism of blood sugar.

Integumentary system — skin, hair and nails; the outer covering of the body.

Intercostal — the space and tissues between the ribs.

Interhospital transport — medical transport from a referring hospital to a receiving hospital.

Interneuron — see "Motor neuron."

Interpersonal space — the physical distance maintained between two or more communicating persons; distances and degrees of comfort vary between cultures, and also depend on the interpersonal relationships involved.

Interstitial fluid — an extracellular fluid that fills the spaces between cells and provides a liquid environment for cells. Formed by filtration through the blood capillaries, it is drained away as lymph.

Interstitial space — the space between body cells that exists outside the vascular compartment.

Intracellular fluid — fluid within cell membranes.

Intracerebral hematoma — bleeding into the cerebrum.

Intracranial hemorrhage — bleeding inside the skull. *See Conditions by Diagnosis section.*

Intracranial lesion — a structural abnormality of the tissues inside the cranial vault.

Intracranial pressure — pressure within the cranium.

Intraosseous — pertaining to the medullary canal of bone; an alternate route for I.V. access in pediatric patients under the age of six.

Intravascular space — the space within the vascular compartment, i.e., the volume within the blood vessels.

Involuntary consent — consent established, usually by a court or statute, to authorize treatment of a person, such as a prisoner or person determined by a court to be lacking decision-making capacity.

Ionizing radiation — high energy *alpha* or *beta* particles, or electromagnetic radiation (*gamma* rays), that ionize molecules which they pass through.

Irradiation incident — the exposure of a person to ionizing radiation.

Ischemia — insufficient perfusion of oxygenated blood to a body organ or part, often marked by pain and organ dysfunction, as in ischemic heart disease.

Isotonic — having the same number of solute or particles as another solution, hence exerting the same amount of osmotic pressure as that solution.

IUD — Intrauterine Device; a contraceptive device inserted in the uterus.

Jejunum — the second portion of the small intestines extending from the duodenum to the ileum.

Jugular venous distention (JVD) — prominent or engorged neck veins; a sign of central venous back pressure in patient's whose heads are elevated.

Junction — an interface or meeting place for tissues or structures.

Kaposi's sarcoma — a cancer often associated with AIDS that appears as brownish or purple skin lesions. *See Conditions by Diagnosis section.*

Ketoacidosis — acidosis due to an excess of ketone bodies. *See Conditions by Diagnosis section.*

Ketone bodies — a group of compounds including acetone that are produced during the metabolism of fatty acids.

Ketosis — an abnormal accumulation of the ketones in the blood.

Kidney — the organ that cleanses the body of the waste products through glomerular filtration and urination.

Kinematics — the study of motion energy.

Korsakoff's psychosis — a form of amnesia seen in chronic alcoholics, characterized by a loss of short term memory and an inability to learn new skills.

Kussmaul respirations — deep, gasping respirations associated with severe diabetic acidosis and coma.

Labor — the coordinated sequence of involuntary uterine contractions producing effacement and dilation of the cervix, and leading to delivery.

Landing zone (LZ) — a space prepared specifically for landing helicopters; typically, this term applies only to scene responses, not to interhospital transport.

Large intestine — the portion of the digestive tract comprising the cecum, appendix, ascending, transverse, and descending colons, and rectum.

Laryngoscope — instrument used to lift the tongue and visualize the vocal cords.

Larynx — the voice box organ (glottis, epiglottis, thyroid cartilage, and cords), located inferior to the hypopharynx.

Lateral — toward the side, away from the midline.

Lateral recumbent — lying on one side; a position used for unconscious patients where there is no suspected risk of spinal injury; minimizes risk for aspiration.

Lead — a combination of three or more electrodes that make up a single channel of the ECG.

Lesion — a generic term for an abnormality of the tissues of the skin.

Leukocyte — white blood cell; there are many types of leukocytes, which are primarily involved in fighting infections.

Level of consciousness — a degree of cognitive function involving arousal mechanisms of the reticular formation of the brain.

Licensure — the process of documenting authority to engage in an activity, profession or occupation that would otherwise be illegal.

Ligament — a white band of fibrous tissue which connects bones.

Limbic system — the area of the brain that processes feelings and emotions.

Litigation — a lawsuit or legal action.

Liver — the largest and one of the most complex internal organs of the body; produces bile; secretes glucose, protein, vitamins, fats, and other compounds; processes hemoglobin to scavenge iron content; converts alkaloid toxins for harmless elimination.

Living will — a document which expresses the medical interventions a patient desires to have implemented or withheld in the event of becoming medical incompetent to express those choices at a later time. Living wills only become active after the patient is medically determined to be terminally ill, and unable to verbally express medical decision choices.

Log-rolling — a maneuver used to turn a reclining patient while maintaining spinal alignment.

Lumen — the opening, or diameter of a tubular structure (e.g., an artery, vein, airway, intestine, or catheter).

Lung — bilateral thoracic respiratory organs; airways transport gases, and pulmonary arteries and veins transport blood, to and from the lungs where exchange of oxygen and carbon dioxide are exchanged.

Lymphadenopathy — disease of the lymph nodes and vessels.

Lymphatic system — network of vessels, ducts, nodes, valves and organs that are involved in protecting and maintaining the internal fluid environment of the body; returns filtered interstitial fluid to vascular circulation, and is also involved in the production of certain blood cells and antibodies.

Lymphocyte — a type of white blood cell formed in lymphatic tissue.

Lymphoma — a neoplasm of lymph tissue that is usually malignant. Characteristically, the appearance of a painless, enlarged lymph node or nodes in the neck is followed by weakness, fever, weight loss and anemia. *See Conditions by Diagnosis section.*

Macrophage — cell in the immune system which consumes other cells.

Malpractice — professional misconduct or violation of the standard of care which causes injury to another.

Marijuana — a psychoactive herb derived from the flowering tops of hemp plants.

Mass — matter; physical substance.

Mast cell — cells of connective tissue that release histamines, heparin, and other substances in response to injury and infection.

Mechanism of injury — the physical manner and forces in which an injury occurred; a criterion for assessment in which the potential for the severity of trauma is estimated by analyzing the physical forces which caused the injury.

Medial — toward the midline.

Median plane — a vertical plane that divides the body into equal right and left halves.

Mediastinal emphysema or pneumomediastinum — pathological accumulation of air in the mediastinum.

Mediastinum — a portion of the thoracic cavity in the middle of the thorax, between the sternum to the vertebral column and contains all the thoracic viscera except the lungs.

Medical audit — a component of quality assurance; a systematized method of monitoring and evaluating patient care.

Medical direction — physician-directed supervision of prehospital care.

Medical practice act — state law which grants authority to provide patient care and determines the scope of practice for healthcare providers.

Melena — abnormal, black, tarry stool containing blood.

Membrane — a thin layer of tissue that covers a surface, lines a cavity, or divides a space.

Meninges — three layers of fibrous tissue that cover the brain. See Arachnoid membrane, Dura mater, and Pia mater.

Meningitis — any inflammation of the membranes covering the brain and spinal cord. *See Conditions by Diagnosis section.*

Menstruation — the periodic sloughing of the uterine lining, which is composed of blood, tissue, and cells.

Mental status — the degree of competence shown by a person in intellectual, emotional, psychologic, and personality functioning as measured by psychologic testing with reference to a statistical norm.

Metabolic acidosis — disease in which the arterial bicarbonate ion concentration is abnormally low, e.g., <22 meq/L. *See Conditions by Diagnosis section.*

Metabolism — the aggregate of all biochemical reactions that take place in living organisms, resulting in growth, generation of energy, elimination of wastes, and other bodily functions.

Methaqualones — a group of sedative-hypnotics.

Microorganism — life form such as a bacterium, virus, fungus or parasite which is too small to be seen without magnification.

Midaxillary line — a line extending from the axilla to the iliac crest.

Midbrain — the area of the brain that integrates messages from the cortex and lower brain.

Midclavicular line — an imaginary line that extends from the midpoint of the clavicle down the anterior chest wall.

Midline — an imaginary line denoted by the median plane dividing the body into equal right and left halves.

Midsagittal plane — see median plane.

Migraine headache — a severe, often debilitating throbbing headache; may be unilateral or bilateral. *See Conditions by Diagnosis section.*

Mineral — naturally occurring metal, nonmetal, radical, or phosphate. Minerals play many vital roles in regulating body functions.

Mineralocorticoids — stress hormones, secreted by the adrenal cortex, that cause retention of sodium and water.

Mitral valve — bicuspid valve between the left atrium and the left ventricle of the heart.

Monoamine oxidase inhibitor (MAOI) — any of a chemically heterogeneous group of drugs used primarily in the treatment of depression.

Morbidity — degree or severity of illness or disability.

Morgue — a temporary storage area for dead patients.

Mortality — death rate, as in the mortality associated with a certain disease.

Motor (efferent) neuron — a neuron that innervates skeletal, smooth, or cardiac muscle fibers. Also known as an interneuron.

Mourning — the expression of grief over the death of a loved one, often socially patterned, as in a period of wearing of black garments or refraining from social activities.

Multigravida — having been pregnant more than once.

Multipara — a woman who has had two or more deliveries.

Multiple casualty incident (MCI) — an incident, sometimes called a disaster, where the incident and number of victims overwhelms the capabilities of the EMS service or system. The approach to patient evaluation and care are modified due to the overwhelming needs of the particular event.

Muscle tissue — contractile tissue that provides kinetic energy for the body.

Muscular system — the complex dynamic network of muscles, nerves, bones and tendons that function to maintain body posture and provide motion.

Myocardial infarction — necrosis of a portion of heart muscle caused by obstruction in a coronary artery from either atherosclerosis or an embolus. Also called heart attack. *See Conditions by Diagnosis section.*

Myoglobin — a ferrous globin complex consisting of one heme molecule containing one iron molecule attached to a single globin chain; responsible for the red color of muscle and for its ability to store oxygen.

Narcotics — a class of drugs derived from opium that depress the central nervous system. Legally used to relieve pain; illicitly used to produce an intense state of relaxation.

Necrosis (necrotic) — death of a cell or group of cells as the result of disease or injury.

Near-drowning — survival from submersion in water for a duration that usually causes drowning or disease. *See Conditions by Diagnosis section.*

Negligence — a failure to act as a reasonably prudent person would, and which directly results in harm to another.

Negligence per se — legal determination, as in a tort ruling, that a violation of a regulation or statute has occurred, and which has directly caused harm to another person in a manner in which no prudent person would have acted.

Nephritis — renal inflammation or infection. *See Conditions by Diagnosis section.*

Nephron — the functional unit of the kidney.

Nervous system — network of conductive tissues which transmit impulses to and from the brain, and processes thoughts, impulses and reflexes.

Nervous tissue — collection of interconnected conductile cells which transmit electrical impulses.

Neuralgia — pain originating from a nerve or nerves.

Neurogenic shock — a type of distributive shock that results when sympathetic control of the vascular system is lost.

Neuroglial cell — supportive cells of the nervous system (e.g., protective membrane cells).

Neuron — the functional unit of the nervous system, consisting of the nerve cell body, the dendrites, and the axon.

Neuropathy — disease of the nervous system.

Neurotransmitter — any one of numerous chemicals that modify or result in the transmission of nerve impulses between synapses.

Neutrophil — a small, phagocytic white blood cell with a lobed nucleus and small granules in the cytoplasm; stains readily with neutral dyes.

Nitroglycerin — a potent smooth muscle relaxant and vasodilator; often prescribed for the relief of heart symptoms.

Norepinephrine — a sympathetic hormone secreted by the adrenal medulla, catecholamine vasopressor.

Nystagmus — rhythmic involuntary oscillations of the eyes; occurs in various orientations: lateral, circular, vertical or combinations.

Obstinate — inflexible persistence or an unyielding attitude; stubborn.

Occlusion — blocked, closed or bound, e.g., an artery is blocked by an occlusion caused by a thrombus.

Off-line medical direction — also called indirect medical direction. Refers to the medical oversight of EMS patient care, which occurs before and after the care of the individual patient.

On-line medical direction — also called direct medical direction; involves direct data and voice communication between a field unit and a physician during patient care.

Oophoritis — inflammation of an ovary.

Opiate — a narcotic drug that contains opium, derivatives of opium, or any of several semisynthetic or synthetic drugs with opiumlike activity.

Opioid — pertaining to natural and synthetic chemicals that have opium-like effects although they are not derived from opium.

Opportunistic infection — an infection occurring in an immune-suppressed patient that a functioning immune system would resist.

Organ — a structure composed of two or more types of tissue, which jointly perform certain functions.

Organophosphates — a family of toxic compounds widely used as pesticides.

Orthopnea — dyspnea which occurs in the supine position.

Orthostatic hypotension — a drop in blood pressure occurring when a person sits or stands rapidly from a reclining posture.

Orthostatic vital signs — pulse rate and blood pressure changes which occur when a patient is moved from a supine to an elevated position

Os — an opening, passage.

Osmolarity — the osmotic pressure gradient expressed in osmoles or milliosmoles per kilograms of the solution.

Osmosis — the movement of fluid across a semipermeable membrane in the direction against the concentration gradient of solutes; fluid movement and pressures are created by the partial pressures of dissolved gases in the fluid.

Osteocyte — a bone cell; a mature osteoblast that has become embedded in the bone matrix.

Osteoporosis — a disorder characterized by abnormal rarefaction of bone, occurring most frequently in post-menopausal women, in sedentary or immobilized individuals, and in patients on long-term steroid therapy. *See Conditions by Diagnosis section.*

Otitis — inflammation or infection of the ear. *See Conditions by Diagnosis section.*

Ovary — one of the pair of female gonads found on each side of the lower abdomen beside the uterus.

Ovulation — release of an ovum or secondary oocyte from the vesicular follicle.

P-wave — the ECG wave representing atrial depolarization.

Pacemaker — the cell that initiates a cardiac impulse; it is usually the sinus node but can be any cell of the atrium, AV node or ventricle; a pacemaker can also be an artificial electronic device implanted in the heart to stimulate the formation of an electrical conduction.

Palpitation — a sensation of fluttering or slipped beats caused by a dysrhythmia.

Pancreas — a nodular transverse gland on the posterior abdominal wall in the epigastric and hypochondriac regions which secretes digestive enzymes, insulin, and glucagon.

Pancreatitis — inflammation of the pancreas, most often caused by alcoholism or gall bladder disease. *See Conditions by Diagnosis section.*

Panic attack — periods of intense fear or discomfort; they are unexpected and not associated with any immediate threat or uncomfortable situation. *See Conditions by Diagnosis section.*

Paranoia — a personality disorder whereby the person views others with suspicion, believing them to be untrustworthy and devious. This term can also be applied to the psychotic patient (schizophrenia) who has hallucinations, delusions of persecution, sense of grandeur, and misinterprets real or minor incidents.

Parasympathetic nervous system — the division of autonomic nervous system that controls vegetative functions and relaxes the body.

Parens patriae — doctrine of law by which the government supervises or protects the welfare of children or other incompetent persons.

Parenteral nutrition — provision of caloric needs by the intravenous route. TPN is "total parenteral nutrition."

Paresthesia — sensation of numbness or tingling.

Parietal — of or pertaining to the outer wall lining of a cavity or organ.

Parietal peritoneum — the portion of the largest serous membrane in the body that lines the abdominal wall.

Parity — the total number of live deliveries a patient has experienced.

Paroxysmal — sudden, unprovoked occurrence.

Partial pressure — the pressure exerted by one gas in a gaseous or liquid solution containing several dissolved gases.

Pathogen — a microorganism capable of causing disease.

Pathological grief — grief that overwhelms and debilitates, or causes physical complaints or disorders.

Pathophysiology — the study of the biological and biochemical processes of diseases.

Patient care report — the document completed by EMS personnel to record all pertinent patient information; often called a run report, or run sheet.

Pedicle — a narrow stalk, stem, or tube of tissue attached to a tumor, skin flap, or organ.

Pelvic inflammatory disease — any inflammatory condition of the female pelvic organs, especially one caused by bacterial infection.

Penetrating trauma — an injury or wound in which the integrity of the skin is broken and underlying organs or tissues are affected.

Peptic — pertaining to the digestive system or digestive processes and juices.

Peptic ulcer — defect in the mucous membrane lining of the esophagus, stomach or small intestine. *See Conditions by Diagnosis section.*

Perfusion — the circulation of blood to the tissues.

Pericardial tamponade — disease in which fluid effusion fills the pericardial sac and mechanically interferes with ventricular refilling. *See Conditions by Diagnosis section.*

Pericardiocentesis — procedure for withdrawing blood or fluid from the pericardial sac.

Pericarditis — inflammation of the membrane surrounding the heart (pericardium). *See Conditions by Diagnosis section.*

Pericardium — protective sac surrounding the heart.

Periosteum — tough connective tissue covering the bone.

Peripheral nervous system (PNS) — subdivision of the nervous system outside the protective cover of the central nervous system.

Peripheral vascular resistance — resistance created by constriction of arterioles.

Peritoneal dialysis — the continuous sequential lavage and gavage of fluid in the peritoneum over periods of several hours for the purpose of removing waste.

Peritoneum — an extensive serous membrane that covers the entire abdominal wall of the body and is reflected over the contained viscera.

Peritonitis — inflammation of the membranous lining of the abdominal cavity and viscera. *See Conditions by Diagnosis section.*

Peritonsillar abscess — an infection of tissue between the tonsil and pharynx. *See Conditions by Diagnosis section.*

Permeability — degree to which fluid or dissolved material passes through a membrane or barrier.

Personal protective equipment — equipment worn by emergency responders to prevent contamination, exposure to infectious or dangerous materials, or injury.

Petechiae — tiny purple or red spots that appear on the skin as a result of minute hemorrhages within the dermal or submucosal layers. They range from pinpoint to pinhead size and are flush with the surface.

pH — a measure of the acidity or alkalinity of a solution; the hydrogen ion concentration expressed as the negative *base 10* logarithm of the moles of hydrogen ions per liter.

Pharynx — a tubular structure anterior to the cervical vertebrae, about 13 cm long in the adult, that extends from the base of the skull to the esophagus; the joint passageway for the respiratory and digestive tracts; actively changes shape in forming sounds.

Phencyclidine — a piperidine derivative administered parenterally to achieve neuroleptic anesthesia. Slang term is angel dust, when used as an illegal psychoactive substance of abuse.

Phenothiazine — a yellow to green crystalline compound that is a source of dyes and is used in veterinary medicine to treat infestations of threadworms and roundworms. It is too toxic for humans, but derivatives or phenothiazine are used in tranquilizers and antihistamine medications. *See also phenothiazine derivatives.*

Phenothiazine derivatives — any of a group of drugs that have a three ring structure in which two benzene rings are linked by a nitrogen and a sulfur. They represent the largest group of antipsychotic compounds in clinical medicine.

Phlebitis (thrombophlebitis) — inflammation of a vein, often accompanied by formation of a clot. *See Conditions by Diagnosis section.*

Phlebotomy — surgical opening (needle insertion) into a vein to draw blood.

Phobia — a persistent irrational fear of some stimulus or of humiliation or embarrassment. Exposure to the stimulus almost always provokes an immediate anxiety response.

Photophobia — ocular pain or unpleasant sensation upon exposure to light.

Physiology — the study of the processes and function of the human body.

Pia mater — thin and delicate innermost meningeal layer covering the brain.

Placard — square, diamond-shaped signs, 10-3/4 inches on a side, which are official Department of Transportation labels that identify hazardous materials by means of color, symbols, and numbers.

Placenta — the vascular structure in the uterus that connects to the maternal circulation and exchange nutrients and wastes for the fetus.

Placenta previa — the location of the placenta over the cervical outlet or os. *See Conditions by Diagnosis section.*

Plasma — fluid components of lymph and blood in which the leukocytes, erythrocytes, and platelets are suspended.

Platelet — smallest cells of blood; active in coagulation, contain granules in the central part and clear protoplasm peripherally, but have no definite nucleus.

Pleural space — the potential space between the visceral and parietal pleurae.

Pleuritis — inflammation of the lining of the lung tissue. *See Conditions by Diagnosis section.*

Plexus — intersecting network of nerves, blood vessels or lymphatic vessels.

Pneumonia — an acute inflammation, infection or infiltration of the lungs. *See Conditions by Diagnosis section.*

Pneumothorax — air or gas in the pleural space; collapse of a lung, or lungs. *See Conditions by Diagnosis section.*

Poisoning — the act of administering a toxic substance; the condition or physical state produced by ingestion, injection, inhalation or exposure to a poison.

Polydipsia — excessive thirst.

Polyphagia — excessive hunger.

Polyuria — excessive urination.

Positive pressure ventilation — the active delivery of air into the airway and lungs via a pressure ventilation device, e.g. autovent or bag-valve-mask and reservoir.

Post partum — the time period after delivery.

Posterior — behind, pertaining to the back of a structure; the dorsal surface.

Postictal — altered mental and physical state immediately following a convulsion.

Post-traumatic stress disorder (PTSD) — the physical and psychological effects produced from exposure to a severely disturbing event (e.g., a brutal murder of a child). See Critical Incident. *See Conditions by Diagnosis section.*

Postural hypotension — abnormally low blood pressure occurring when an individual assumes the standing position.

Potentiation — the enhancement or stimulation of the effects of one drug by the administration of another.

Precautions — information regarding the handling of a drug that will avoid adverse drug effects.

Preeclampsia — the presence of hypertension, proteinuria and edema associated with pregnancy, generally occurring in the later half of pregnancy. *See Conditions by Diagnosis section.*

Prejudice — any preconceived opinion or feeling, either favorable or unfavorable.

Preload — the stretch of myocardial fiber at end diastole. The ventricular end diastolic pressure and volume reflect this parameter.

Premature delivery — the birth of an infant before the 37th week of gestation.

Premature labor — regular uterine contractions with dilation of the cervix after the 20th week and before the 37th week of gestation.

Presence — the ability to project a sense of ease, poise or self-assurance; especially the quality or manner of a person's bearing before an audience.

Priapism — an abnormal and painful condition of prolonged or constant penile erection; often a sign of spinal cord injury.

Probable cause — level of proof required to detain a person in an emergency when the person appears to be a danger to himself or others.

Prolapse of the umbilical cord — the pinning or entrapment of the umbilical cord by the fetal head as it enters the birth canal.

Pronation — positioning the body face downward.

Prone — face down position.

Prospective medical direction — proactive physician involvement in EMS administration to assure quality patient.

Prostaglandins — one of several potent unsaturated fatty acid hormones that act in exceedingly low concentrations on local target organs.

Protein — structural molecular complexes of living organisms composed of linearly linked amino acids; the fundamental structural molecules of all tissue.

Protocol — a written procedure for clinical treatment.

Protoplasm — the internal substance of cells, composed of myriad molecules of water, minerals, and organic compounds, and excluding the nucleus.

Proximal — closer to the heart; nearer to the point of reference.

Proximate cause — an injury which has occurred as the result of an act or the neglect to act.

Proxy — appointment of a person to represent another person in matters, such as medical treatment decisions.

Psychic pain — intense, incapacitating anguish with no organic cause which occurs immediately after notification of a affliction or loss.

Psychosis — mental disorder in which senses and reasoning are not based on reality, and in which physical evidence does not alter the misperceptions.

Psychotic — person who suffers from a psychosis.

Pulmonary embolism — the blockage of a pulmonary artery by foreign matter such as fat, air, tumor tissue, or a thrombus that usually arises from a peripheral vein. *See Conditions by Diagnosis section.*

Pulmonary-over-pressurization syndrome — hyperbaric trauma to the respiratory system. *See Conditions by Diagnosis section.*

Pulse oximetry — non-invasive measurement of arterial oxygen saturation utilizing infrared absorption frequencies.

Pulseless electrical activity (PEA) — organized electrical activity observed on a cardiac monitor (other than VT or VF) which produces no palpable pulse. *See Conditions by Diagnosis section.*

Pulseless ventricular tachycardia — regular, rapid, wide-complex cardiac contractions which do not produce a palpable pulse. *See Conditions by Diagnosis section.*

Purkinje fibers — endocardial electrophysiologic conduction pathways through the ventricles.

Purpura — any of several bleeding disorders characterized by hemorrhage into the tissues, producing ecchymoses or petechiae.

Pyloric sphincter — a thickened, muscular ring in the stomach, separating the pylorus from the duodenum.

Pyrogens — any agent or substance that tends to cause a rise in body temperature, such as some bacterial toxins.

Q-wave — a negative deflection from the baseline that precedes the R wave; it may not be present at all times.

QRS complex — ventricular depolarization wave.

QRS interval — the width of the QRS from the start of the Q wave to the end of the S wave; if one or more portions are not present, then it is measured from the beginning deviation above or below the isoelectric line to the end of whatever waves are present.

Quality assurance (QA) — a systematic evaluation method used to assure quality care and provide information to caregivers about how to improve it.

Quality improvement — See Continuous Quality Improvement (CQI).

R-R interval — section of the ECG between the onset of one QRS complex and the onset of an adjacent QRS complex or the distance between two adjacent R waves.

R-wave — the first positive deflection of the QRS complex. The QRS complex is sometimes referred to as the "R wave."

R-wave (R prime wave) — the second positive deflection of the QRS complex; it is only seen occasionally.

Rabies — an acute, usually viral disease of the central nervous system of animals; transmitted from animals to people by infected blood, tissue, or most commonly, saliva. *See Conditions by Diagnosis section.*

Raccoon eyes — bilateral periorbital bruises; an indication of basilar skull fracture following trauma.

Radiation — 1. The emission of energy, rays, or waves. 2. The use of a radioactive substance in the diagnosis or treatment of disease. 3. transmission of pain from a point of origin toward another anatomical location; energy transmission via electromagnetic or nuclear force.

Radioactive — a substance which emits ionizing radiation.

Radioactive decay — the degradation of atomic nuclei which results in the emission of *alpha*, *beta*, or *gamma* radiation.

Rapport — psychological connection, especially harmonious or sympathetic.

Receptor — the basic site of drug interaction, composed of a protein that has a specific shape.

Reciprocity — the process by which an agency grants automatic licensure or certification to an individual with comparable licensure or certification from another agency or association.

Recompression — hyperbaric procedure to reverse the physiologic effects of decompression sickness.

Rectum — the segment of the large intestine, continuous with the descending sigmoid colon, just proximal to the anal canal.

Re-entry — a defect in the cardiac conduction pathway in which a charge, through contact, depolarizes a previous segment causing a premature complex or tachycardia to result.

Referred pain — pain felt at a site different from that of an injured or diseased organ or part of the body.

Registration — data base record of professional qualifications.

Renin — a proteolytic enzyme, produced by and stored in the juxtaglomerular apparatus that surrounds each arteriole as it enters a glomerulus. The enzyme affects the blood pressure by catalyzing the change of angiotensinogen to angiotensin, a strong presser.

Repolarization — recharging of cardiac cells after they have been depolarized. This phase allows the cell to accept and transfer the next electrical impulse.

Reproductive system — the organ systems involved in conception (in males and females), and gestation, labor and delivery, and mammalian feeding (in females).

Rescue breathing — the process of oxygenating and ventilating a patient who is in respiratory arrest.

Resin — an amphorous, nonvolatile substance secreted from plants.

Resistance — opposition to the flow of electrical current.

Respiration — the molecular exchange of oxygen and carbon dioxide within the body.

Respirators — a mask worn over the nose and mouth with a special filter which removes a designated dust, vapor, or chemical.

Respiratory arrest — prolonged period of apnea with no spontaneous return to breathing.

Respiratory failure — inability of the lungs either to adequately provide oxygen to the body or to eliminate carbon dioxide.

Retinal artery occlusion — decreased blood supply to the retina caused by a clot or embolus in the retinal artery. *See Conditions by Diagnosis section.*

Retrospective medical direction — the review of patient care after the fact to assure that care is appropriate and to find areas for improvement.

Revised trauma score — numerical scale used for assessment of trauma patients and prediction of mortality which incorporates the Glasgow Coma Scale and vital signs.

Reye's Syndrome — a combination of acute encephalopathy and fatty infiltration of the internal organs that may follow acute viral infections. *See Conditions by Diagnosis section.*

Rhabdomyolysis — an acute, sometimes fatal disease characterized by destruction of skeletal muscle. *See Conditions by Diagnosis section.*

Rotor-wing aircraft — helicopters; aircraft powered by vertically mounted propellers.

Rural — geographical area with sparse population and resources.

S wave — a negative origin deflection that returns to the baseline that follows the R wave; it may not be present in all cases.

ST segment — the segment between the end of the QRS complex and the beginning of the T wave.

Safe zone — an area in a hazardous materials incident (HazMat) or mass casualty incident (MCI) which is designated to be safe from environmental dangers.

Schizophrenia — large group of mental, behavioral disorders involving distortion of reality and disorganization fragmentation of thought processes. *See Conditions by Diagnosis section.*

Scope of practice — specified medical practices that may be performed by a licensed or certified health care provider, usually established in statute or regulations.

Sebaceous (oil) gland — a gland of the skin, usually associated with a hair follicle that produces sebum.

Seizure — a hyperexcitation of neurons in the brain; presentation may vary from partial (localized), subtle signs, e.g., minor transient aphasia, to a sudden, violent involuntary series of muscular contractions which are paroxysmal and episodic, as after a head injury. *See Conditions by Diagnosis section.*

Sellick maneuver — pressure placed on the cricoid cartilage using the thumb and fingers; prevents passive aspiration and gastric insufflation during positive pressure ventilation.

Semi-Fowler's position — placement of the patient in an inclined position, with the upper half of the body raised by elevating the head of the bed.

Sensory (afferent) neuron — nerve that conducts impulses from the body to the central nervous system.

Sepsis — infection, contamination. *See Conditions by Diagnosis section.*

Septic shock — type of hypoperfusion that occurs when toxins are released from certain bacteria into the blood that cause decreased vascular resistance and increased capillary permeability. *See Conditions by Diagnosis section.*

Septicemia — infection in which pathogens are present in the blood.

Serial — in numerical order.

Seroconversion — the development of blood antibodies to a disease following an exposure in a person who has not previously tested positive for antibodies.

Sexual assault — an act of violence in which the victim is threatened and/or attacked and forced into unwanted sexual contact.

Shear — an applied force or pressure exerted against the surface and layers of the skin as tissues slide in opposite but parallel planes.

Shock — a state of inadequate tissue perfusion that will result in cell death if not corrected. *See Conditions by Diagnosis section.*

Side effect — common, undesired effect that occurs with routine, therapeutic doses of a drug.

Simple triage and rapid transportation plan (S.T.A.R.T. Plan) — an example of a mass casualty triage or priority assignment scheme utilizing the victims ability to understand commands, ventilate and perfuse; to assign a triage priority and define minimal initial treatment intervention during the triage phase prior to treatment.

Simplex — method of radio transmission in which both transmission and reception occur on the same frequency. Simultaneous transmission cannot occur without blocking a message.

Sinoatrial node (SA node) — primary cardiac pacer in the right atrium; the SA node initiates conductive impulses automatically and rhythmically at a rate between 60 and 100 times per minute, or faster, during exercise or excitement etc.

Sinus node — the primary pacemaker of the heart, located in the high right atrium, below the opening for the superior vena cava.

Sinusitis — inflammation of the sinuses.

Skeletal system — the structure of bones which provide posture to the body.

Slough (sloughing) — necrotic tissue in the process of separating from viable portions of the body; to shed or cast off.

Small intestine — the longest portion of the digestive tract; divided into the duodenum, jejunum, and ileum.

Smooth muscle — contractile tissue composed of elongated, spindle-shaped cells not under voluntary control, (e.g., muscle of the intestines, stomach, and other visceral organs). Also known as visceral muscle and nonstriated muscle.

Somatic — the body.

Sphincter — a circular band of muscle fibers that constricts a passage or closes a natural opening in the body.

Spinal cord — nerve complex in the vertebral canal which extends from the foramen magnum at the base of the skull to the upper lumbar region.

Spinal nerve — one of 31 pairs of nerves formed by the joining of the dorsal and ventral routes that arise from the spinal cord.

Spotting — blood stained vaginal discharge which appears between menstrual periods, during pregnancy, and at the onset of labor.

Standard of care — minimum performance criteria.

Stare decisis — a principle of law in which a legal decision acts as a precedent to be followed when deciding future disputes.

Status asthmaticus — bronchspastic disease in which the patient is refractory to treatment with bronchodilators. See Conditions by Diagnosis section.

Status epilepticus — continuous seizure activity, or repeated seizures without regaining consciousness. See Conditions by Diagnosis section.

Statute of limitations — the period in which a person may initiate legal action, typically two years after knowledge of the possible cause for action is known.

Sternocleidomastoid — the muscle of the neck which extends from the mastoid to the clavicle and sternum.

Stimulus — anything that excites or incites activity or function.

Stomach — the organ of digestion between the esophagus and the small intestine located in the right upper quadrant of the abdomen.

Stress — a stimulus which causes physiologic and psychological arousal.

Striated muscle — muscle tissue that appears microscopically to consist of striped myofibrils. Also called skeletal muscle or voluntary muscle.

Stridor — a shrill, harsh sound, especially the respiratory sound heard during inspiration in laryngeal obstruction.

Stroke volume — amount of blood pumped from a ventricle.

Subarachnoid hemorrhage — an acute often spontaneous bleed in the brain, usually caused by cerebral artery aneurysm or an arteriovenous malformation. See Conditions by Diagnosis section.

Subarachnoid space — potential area between subarachnoid layer and pia mater.

Subconjunctival hemorrhage — bleeding under the white portion of the eye.

Subcutaneous emphysema — pathological accumulation of air in the subcutaneous or interstitial tissues; often associated with pneumothorax or pneumomediastinum.

Subcutaneous tissue — the third layer of the skin.

Subdural hematoma — a bleed inside the dural membrane. See Conditions by Diagnosis section.

Subjective — reported by the patient but impossible to verify by testing. e.g., pain.

Subluxation — partial dislocation or separation of a joint resulting in a darkening of an x-ray.

Sudden infant death syndrome (SIDS) — the unexpected sudden death of an apparently healthy infant that occurs during sleep and with no evidence of disease or disorder. See Conditions by Diagnosis section.

Superficial fascia — pertaining to the outer layer of skin or covering.

Superior — situated above or higher than a point of reference in the anatomical position.

Supination — position on the back, face up; rotating the hand so that the palm faces upward.

Support zone — See Cold Zone.

Supraventricular — impulse origin from above the ventricle; the term is used to describe an impulse or rhythm that begins in the sinus node, the atrium or the AV node.

Surfactant — lipoprotein fluid in the alveoli that reduces the surface tension of pulmonary fluids and contributes to the elasticity of pulmonary tissue.

Surfactant washout — loss of surfactant on the alveolar membrane leading to loss of pulmonary compliance, alveolar function and atelectasis.

Surrogate decision maker — See Proxy.

Sympathetic nervous system — division of the autonomic system that energizes the body in response to an alarming or arousing stimulus.

Sympathetic response — the defensive or arousal response of the body in which catecholamines are released and sudden stores of energy are released.

Sympatholytic — an agent which opposes or blocks the effects of the sympathetic (adrenergic) system.

Sympathomimetic — an agent which mimics the function of sympathetic substances such as epinephrine and norepinephrine.

Synapse — functional contact of nerve cells, muscle cells, glandular cells, or sensory receptors; location of chemical transmission of action potentials from one cell to another.

Synchronized cardioversion — delivery of an electrical pulsation that is timed so it does not fall during the relative refractory period.

Synergism — the combined effect of two medications, which is greater than the sum of their individual effects.

Synovitis — inflammation of the synovial membrane in a joint.

System — interconnected functions and organs in which a stimulus or action in one area affects all other areas. Physiologic systems, such as the cardiovascular or reproductive systems, are made up of structures specifically capable of compensating processes that are essential for homeostasis.

T wave — the wave representing repolarization of the ventricle.

Tachycardia — rapid heart rate; pulse rate > 100 beats per minute.

Tachydysrhythmia — heart rate greater than 100 beats per minute.

Tachypnea (tachypneic) — rapid respiration.

Target organ — the tissue or organ ultimately affected by a drug.

Technician — a person with the knowledge, certification and skill required to carry out specific technical procedures.

Tendon — a band or cord of dense connective tissue that connects muscle to bone or other structures; characterized by strength and inelasticity.

Tension headache — headache commonly caused by tension or traction on anatomical structures. Tension can cause spasm in scalp and neck muscles.

Tenting — evidence of poor skin turgor; describes the "tent" of skin left when skin does not resume normal contour after being pinched up.

Tentorium — a horizontal, folded portion of the dura mater that separates the cerebrum from the cerebellum.

Tetany — spasms, convulsions or twitching of muscles; often related to serum calcium imbalances and metabolism.

Therapeutic action — the desired beneficial effect of a drug.

Therapeutic window — the margin between the level at which a drug in the body acts therapeutically, and the level at which it becomes toxic.

Thermoregulation — the control of heat production and heat loss, specifically the maintenance of body temperature through physiologic mechanisms, activated by the hypothalamus.

Thiamine — a water-soluble, crystalline compound of the B-complex vitamin group, essential for normal metabolism. Thiamine combines with pyruvic acid to form a coenzyme necessary for the breakdown of carbohydrates into glucose.

Thoracotomy — surgical opening in the chest wall.

Thought disorder — any mental disturbance in which the thinking process is seriously disturbed. Hallucinations, paranoid thinking and illusions are examples.

Thrombosis — a clot within a blood vessel.

Thrombus — a clot consisting of platelets, fibrin, clotting factors and other components of blood. *See Conditions by Diagnosis section.*

Tidal volume — the amount of air inhaled or exhaled in one respiratory cycle.

Tilt test — cardiovascular vital sign changes which occur when the pulse and blood pressure are compared between the supine and sitting or standing positions. The tilt test is positive for possible hypovolemia when the pulse rate increases by 10–20/minute and the systolic blood pressure drops by 10–20 mm Hg.

Tissue — similar cells which perform a particular function.

Tolerance — the tendency of some drugs to lose the intensity of their effect after repeated doses are administered.

Tonic-clonic — seizure contractions characterized by intermittent sustained and transient spasms. *See Conditions by Diagnosis section (Seizure Disorders).*

Tonicity — the concentration, or size, of particles in solution compared to another. For instance, a hypertonic saline solution has a tonicity greater than that of blood.

Torr — the pressure of one millimeter of mercury (mm Hg).

Toxic — the ability to harm or poison living tissue or cells.

Toxic delirium — altered level of consciousness with hallucinations as a result of the poisonous effect of a drug.

Toxic effect — harmful effect from poisoning, overdose or chronic misuse of a medication.

Trachea — cylindrical airway tube in the neck composed of cartilage and ciliated mucus membrane.

Tracheal deviation — slight tracheal angling to the right or left side felt at the sternal notch in the direction away from the side of a tension pneumothorax.

Tracheal tugging — an effect of an aortic aneurysm in which the trachea is tugged downward with each heart contraction.

Tracheostomy — an opening through the neck into the trachea through which an indwelling tube may be inserted.

Trade name (brand name) — registered trademark name created by a manufacturer to identify a specific drug.

Transcutaneous pacing (TCP) — rhythmic external electrical cardiac stimulus applied across the chest via precordial electrodes.

Transient personality disorder — usually the least serious of the three main categories of mental disorders (psychoses, anxiety states and transient personality disorders). Usually associated with crisis events. In most cases when the events are resolved, the person returns to a normal level of behavior.

Transportation center — a site selected within or near a mass casualty incident (MCI) which is used to deploy ambulances.

Transportation officer — individual responsible for recording assigned triage tag numbers, time of transport, and assigned designation. Transportation officers assure that all *critical* patients are transported first, *urgent* second, *delayed* third, and finally the *dead* or *dying* last.

Transverse plane — plane that divides the body into equal upper and lower halves.

Trauma — an injury; physical trauma is caused by transfer of energy from some external source to the human body; emotional trauma is caused by a disturbing event.

Trauma center — medical center officially designated by government or EMS system to receive and provide advanced care for major trauma patients; tertiary receiving facility for major trauma patients.

Treatment center — a safe site selected within or near a mass casualty incident (MCI) where patients are initially moved for treatment. The treatment and transportation centers may be located in the same place. *See transportation center.* Large MCIs may have more than one treatment and transportation center.

Treatment officer — individual in mass casualty incidents (MCI) who is responsible for triage and directing patient care activities; also responsible for the acquisition of additional resources.

Trendelenburg position — supine position with the legs elevated; the "shock" position (head, neck and back level; legs elevated) has been commonly called the Trendelenburg position.

Triage — the sorting of patients by priority.

Trimester — pregnancy is divided into three equal intervals, each approximately three months in length, referred to as first, second and third trimesters.

Tubal ligation — one of several sterilization procedures in which both fallopian tubes are blocked to prevent conception from occurring.

U wave — although the origin is uncertain, it is thought to represent repolarization of the Purkinje fibers.

Ulcer/ulceration — defined necrotic skin lesion resembling a crater.

Ultrafiltration — filtration of a colloidal substance in which dispersed particles, but not the liquid, are held back.

Umbilical cord — the cord containing the blood vessels that connect the fetus and the placenta, transporting nutrients and wastes.

Unilateral — one sided; occurring on the right or left side only.

Unipolar — having only one pole; a description of the movement of a person from a normal state to a manic state and back to a normal state, or from a normal state to a depressive state and back to normal.

Universal precautions — infection control practices in health care which are observed with every patient and procedure, and which prevent exposure to blood-borne pathogens. Universal precautions were initially developed in 1987 by the Centers for Disease Control in the United States, and in 1989 by the Bureau of Communicable Disease Epidemiology in Canada. The guidelines for universal precautions include specific recommendations for use of gloves, masks and protective eyewear when contact with blood or body secretions containing blood is anticipated.

Urea — Ammonium (nitrogen and hydrogen) waste product.

Ureter — one of the pair of tubes that carry urine from the kidney to the bladder.

Urethra — a small tubular duct that drains urine from the bladder. In men, it also serves as a passageway for semen during ejaculation.

Urinary bladder — the muscular, membranous sac in the pelvis that stores urine for discharge through the urethra.

Urinary system — the organs of the body which filter, store, and then eliminate urine; includes the kidneys, ureters, bladder and urethra.

Urine — waste fluid produced by the urinary system; includes water, urea, sodium chloride and potassium chloride, phosphates, uric acid, organic salts, and the pigment urobilin.

Urticaria — a pruritic skin eruption characterized by transient wheals of varying shapes and sizes with well-defined erythematous margins and pale centers. Also called hives.

Uterine rupture — the tearing or traumatic opening of the uterus, usually the result of uterine contractions or trauma. *See Conditions by Diagnosis section.*

Uterus — the pear-shaped muscular organ that houses the fetus in pregnancy, also often called the womb.

Valvular stenosis — a hardening and narrowing of any of the valves of the heart.

Vapor pressure — gas pressure of a solid or liquid.

Varicosity — swollen, torturous vein.

Vascular — pertaining to, or provided with, blood vessels.

Vascular access device — a device or instrumental used to obtain venous or arterial access (e.g., catheter, cannula, or Intraosseus needle).

Vasoconstriction — vascular constriction, or increase in vaso tone, which narrows of the lumen of blood vessels. Also called vasopression.

Vasodilation — an increase in the diameter of a blood vessel caused by inhibition of its constrictor nerves or stimulation of dilator nerves.

Vasomotor — refers to the blood vessels that regulate the lumen of the arteries and veins.

Vasovagal response — increased parasympathetic tone which results in slowing the heart rate and possible syncope. The stimulus may be grunting or bearing down on the gut (Valsalva maneuver), a suppressed sneeze, or other maneuvers such as carotid sinus massage or ice packs applied to the face.

Vein — a vessel which carries blood toward the heart.

Velocity — the rate of movement in a particular direction.

Venom — a toxic fluid substance secreted by some snakes, arthropods, and other animals and transmitted by their stings or bites.

Ventilation — the movement of gases into and out of the lungs; clearing of CO_2 via exhalation.

Ventricles — larger and inferior pumping chambers of the heart; small cavities in the brain that produce, store and circulate cerebral spinal fluid.

Ventricular fibrillation — a pulseless cardiac dysrhythmia marked by rapid, disorganized depolarizations of the ventricular myocardium. *See Conditions by Diagnosis section.*

Ventricular shunt — a catheter inserted into the lateral ventricle which allows cerebral spinal fluid (CSF) to be drained.

Vertex presentation — the normal position of the fetus in the uterus, with the head directed downward.

Vertigo — a sensation of faintness or an inability to maintain normal balance in a standing or seated position.

Vesicle — a small bladder or blister, such as a small, thin-walled, raised skin lesion containing clear fluid.

Villi — tiny projections, barely visible to the naked eye, clustered over the entire mucous surface of the small intestine. The villi absorb fluids and nutrients.

Violence — any verbal or physical threat or act of force against another person or group of people that places them in danger, causes harm, or produces death; any act that leaves a person feeling threatened or in jeopardy.

Virulence — the relative strength of a pathogen.

Visceral — internal organs; internal tissues.

Visceral pleura — the inner layer of the pleura that lines the lungs.

Vitamin — organic compound which the body requires in small quantities; most vitamins are not produced by the body and must be obtained from outside sources.

Walking wounded — individuals injured in a mass casualty incident (MCI) who are ambulatory, and who can, to some degree, assist themselves and others. They are generally a low priority for treatment and transportation.

Warm zone (yellow) — the area around a hazardous materials incident in which there is a lessened danger of coming into contact with the hazardous materials, but precautions are still required. Decontamination is done in the "warm zone."

Wernicke's syndrome — an inflammatory, hemorrhagic, degenerative condition of the brain, characterized by lesions in several parts of the brain, including the hypothalamus, mammillary bodies, and other tissues.

The White Paper — a landmark study, "Accidental Death and Disability: The Neglected Disease in Modern Society," by the National Academy of Sciences and National Research Council. This document identified key issues and problems facing the U.S. in providing emergency care, and proposed recommendations for comprehensive and organized EMS development.

Window phase of testing — the time between exposure to a disease and the development of measurable levels of antibody. During the window phase, a person may have a disease and be capable of spreading it, and yet test negative.